GW00862580

The Arterial Anatomy of Skin Flaps

Detailed knowledge of the vascular anatomy of the arterial circulation in the skin and subcutaneous tissue is of practical importance to the reconstructive surgeon who must form and transplant pedunculated flaps, the viability of which depend upon this vascularity.

Herbert Conway 1953

Qu'ils n'oublient jamais que sans anatomie il n'y a point de médecine; et que toutes les sciences médicales sont greffes sur l'anatomie comme sur un sujet; que plus ses racines sont profondes, plus ses branches sont vigoureuses et chargeront de fleurs et de fruits.

J. Cruveilhier 1791–1874
Professeur à la Faculté de Médecine de Paris

The Arterial Anatomy of Skin Flaps

George C. Cormack MA MB ChB FRCS(Ed)
Consultant Plastic Surgeon,
Addenbrooke's Hospital, Cambridge.
Associate Lecturer, University of Cambridge

formerly
Department of Anatomy,
University of Cambridge.
Fellow of Queens' College, Cambridge

B. George H. Lamberty MA MB BChir FRCS
Consultant Plastic Surgeon,
Addenbrooke's Hospital, Cambridge.
Associate Lecturer, University of Cambridge

SECOND EDITION

CHURCHILL LIVINGSTONE
EDINBURGH LONDON MADRID MELBOURNE NEW YORK AND TOKYO 1994

CHURCHILL LIVINGSTONE

Medical Division of Longman Group Limited

Distributed in the United States of America by Churchill Livingstone Inc., 650 Avenue of the Americas, New York, N.Y. 10011, and by associated companies, branches and representatives throughout the world.

First edition 1986
Second edition 1994
Reprinted 1995

ISBN 0 443 045674

British Library Cataloguing in Publication Data
A catalogue record for this book is available from the British Library.

Library of Congress Cataloging in Publication Data
A catalog record for this book is available from the Library of Congress.

For Churchill Livingstone

Commissioning Editors Miranda Bromage, Sheila Khullar
Senior Project Controller Mark Sanderson
Sales Promotion Executive Marion Pollock

Printed in Hong Kong
NPC/02

Contents

Preface to the Second Edition

The aim of this Second Edition remains as it was for the First Edition, namely to provide a basic text for the trainee in plastic and reconstructive surgery. Revision has increased the amount of text and the number of illustrations with the regrettable result that the book is likely to be priced higher than most trainees will wish to pay. There seems no solution to this problem.

In this second edition the central core of anatomy contained in Chapter 6 remains essentially unaltered with only a few additions where recent anatomical studies have added to our knowledge of vessel variability. There have been no changes or advances in International Nomina Anatomica in the interval and therefore many vessels still lack an official name and some vessels have acquired extra unofficial ones as surgeons report clinical experiences with flaps that they invent new terminology for. In some areas the situation is ludicrous with, for example, the layer of fascia lying beneath the extension of the galea in the temporoparietal area having 13 different names in 5 separate languages – with a new name introduced in 1991 this brings the total to 14.

All the other chapters have undergone updating with most of the changes being in Chapter 7. This reflects the fact that many new flaps have been described since the first edition was prepared and more information has accrued concerning established ones. 91 new illustrations have been added to this chapter alone. The original intention of restricting the number of references on each flap in this chapter to six has had to be modified but the aim of presenting only selected helpful papers rather than a list of almost everything published has been retained.

The understanding of flap physiology has not advanced as much in the last 8 years as one would wish. Advances in the concept of free radical mediated damage have undoubtedly occurred and some of this information has been incorporated in Chapter 2. Endothelins may be the next breakthough but their role in the context of flaps is not yet defined and therefore they are only briefly mentioned. Further progress in understanding flap physiology is still needed.

Increased sophistication in flap design has led to more compound flaps incorporating bone being used. A new chapter reflects this progress over the last decade. Chapter 8 describes the basic anatomy of the blood supply to bone and periosteum and lists the majority of bone containing flaps.

The debate over flap nomenclature and classification has been reviewed in a new chapter at the end of the book. Whether this is helpful or simply adds to the confusion only the reader can judge. Some people find classifications helpful while others do not. The purpose of presenting these choices is to give each individual reader an opportunity to choose a scheme which suits his or her particular requirements, as an aid to understanding cutaneous vascular anatomy and as a basis on which to develop new flap variations. What Chapter 9 does not attempt is to present a consensus view on flap terminology since the prospects for unanimous agreement in a speciality with so many individualists is non-existent. This, of course, is part of the fun of it all – nothing is written in 'tablets of stone' and we can confidently expect many more developments over the next decade in this continuously evolving field.

Cambridge
1994

G.C.C.

Preface to the First Edition

In the past 20 years there have been dramatic advances in reconstructive surgery largely attributable to a better understanding of cutaneous vascular anatomy. This renaissance of anatomy may be considered to have started with the discovery of axial pattern skin flaps in the early 1960s and to have proceeded to the development of muscle and musculocutaneous flaps in the 1970s. These new flaps coincided with developments and advances in microsurgical techniques so that free tissue transfer was rapidly established for skin flaps, muscle flaps, musculocutaneous flaps, bone and various combinations of these. The wish to exploit the enormous versatility and reliability of these new flaps to some extent blinkered the search for a new flap concept and it was not until the 1980s that another milestone was reached with the development of the fasciocutaneous flap. This brings us up to a point where for the first time we are in a position to be able to integrate the three separate anatomical discoveries into a comprehensive account of the principles underlying the blood supply of skin. An historical overview of this process of development forms the short first chapter of this book.

Chapter 2 includes information on the structure and function of the microcirculation and summarises some of the published information on the pharmacological manipulation of flaps and on the effects of the delay procedure. These aspects are integral to the vascular basis of flaps and may serve to remind the reader that in striving for technical mastery of the relatively well documented anatomy of skin flaps, one must not lose sight of the fact that our understanding of the various phenomena of flap physiology is still rudimentary and inadequate.

The direct cutaneous, musculocutaneous and fasciocutaneous systems are each explained in turn in Chapters 3, 4 and 5 which together form the second section of this book. The manner in which these systems interact in the supply of different skin areas of the body is then covered region by region in Chapter 6 which forms the third section. The cutaneous vascular territories described in this section are essentially anatomical ones.

In the final chapter the potential territories of individual vessels are described with text, line drawings and illustrative injection studies. These are the dynamic and potential territories which are of surgical importance and have been demonstrated clinically. This section presumes a thorough knowledge of the anatomical principles elaborated earlier in the book and on this basis it aims to give a brief and concise guide to those flaps that may be based on specific vessels. It is not an exhaustive study of each and every flap but rather a pointer to some of the important anatomical features. It also draws together information from the authors' own studies and multiple published works about the constancy and position of each vessel, and relates their surface markings to fixed anatomical features such as bony points. It is *not* intended as a surgical operative manual and therefore clinical photographs taken during and after surgery have been expressly excluded although they might have enhanced the text here and there. Instead, this last section should provide a rapid reference source for the original material and clinical data, which has been restricted to six references for each flap. It is hoped that, by presenting the history, principles and details in this way, a fuller knowledge and understanding of the blood supply to skin will be obtained by the reader, whether anatomist or surgeon, and provide him with a sound basis of anatomy from which to pursue his craft and the development of improved designs of flaps.

The fundamentals of cutaneous vascular anatomy are of importance to both professional anatomists and those in postgraduate surgical training. For those who are not in surgical training the brief Appendix I defines some of the technical surgical terminology.

Cambridge
1986

G.C.C.
B.G.H.L.

Acknowledgements

First Edition

We are grateful to Philip Wilson, Medical Illustrator, for the line drawings without which this book would not have been possible. All the illustrations are unsigned but they are nearly all his work. John Bashford of the Anatomy Department, University of Cambridge, exposed and processed all our radiographs in trying circumstances using obsolete and temperamental equipment and we are very appreciative of his expertise and willingness to help. John also prepared the montages of prints for Figures 6.17 and 6.25. We have produced all the other photographic work but should like to thank Tim Crane and Roger Liles for generously giving technical advice, and Bert Williams for the use of his darkroom. We are indebted to the following for typing parts of the manuscript: Caroline Hunt, Karen Cullum, Susan Curry, Sarah Page, Janet Wrightson and Pamela Morley. Finally we wish to thank Churchill Livingstone for their kind co-operation throughout the production of this book.

Cambridge 1986 — G.C.C. B.G.H.L.

Second Edition

The second edition contains a further 131 new illustrations. We are greateful to Colin Hollidge, illustrator, for producing Figures 2.1, 7.3 and 9.5, and to Roger Liles and his team in the Anatomy Department who carried out the photographic work for Figures 2.15, 7.61, 7.137, 7.140 and 7.186. The deficiencies in the remainder are entirely my responsibility.

The mark-up for the Malaysian typesetters has been carried out by a freelance copy editor, Susan Beasley, in Edinburgh. Her work has been quite superb and her eye for detail a great asset. She has maintained the basic style given to the first edition by Erik Bigland, the in-house designer who succeeded in giving the first edition the clean, up-to-date look for a manual. For this reason the unjustified format, criticised by some reviewers of the first edition, has been retained and the 'manual look' further enhanced by the introduction of colour bars to highlight the start of each chapter. Erik Bigland's major contribution was not acknowledged in the first edition and I would like to take this opportunity to correct that omission while also thanking all the other unseen members of the production team at Churchill Livingstone.

Cambridge 1994 — G.C.C.

Introduction

1

1

The development of regional and free flaps has been, and continues to be, the most exciting and essential of the advances in plastic surgery. This chapter gives a brief account of the historical development of the flap concept, introduces the terminology used in this book, and puts the present stage of development into perspective.

TERMINOLOGY

Historically the word *flap* originated from the 16th century Dutch word 'flappe' – this being anything that hung broad and loose, fastened only by one side. *Graft* derives from 'gryft' which in the same period was used in horticulture to describe a shoot inserted into a slit of another stock so as to allow the sap of one to circulate with the other. However, commensurate with the historical process of diversification of reconstructive techniques there has been a proliferation of flap neologisms. At the present time the term 'a flap' has come to mean, through common usage, anything from the basic pedicled flap to a complex microvascular free composite tissue transfer. Since O'Brien first referred to a one-stage flap transfer as a 'free flap' at the British Hand Society Meeting in May 1973, many published articles have used the term *free flap* in a way which renders it synonymous with microvascular graft. We will adopt the convention that if a specific type of flap is intended then this will be indicated e.g. pedicled flap, island flap, random flap, axial flap etc. For anatomists and other readers unfamiliar with fundamental techniques in plastic surgery, these and other terms are defined in Appendix I. A free flap will generally be referred to as such although the alternative of a microvascular graft (strictly speaking a more accurate term) may be used.

The term *flap* without further qualification, is a general term encompassing both pedicled flaps which are attached to the body at their base, at least during the initial stage of transfer, and microvascular grafts which involve complete separation and then reattachment at a distant site.

HISTORICAL DEVELOPMENT

The history of the development of flaps can be conveniently divided into four phases (represented diagrammatically in Fig. 1.1):

1. An early period culminating in the extensive use of pedicled skin flaps in the First and Second World Wars.
2. A period during the 1950s and 1960s during which what we now recognise as regional axial pattern flaps were developed mainly in the area of the head and neck. Some flaps included muscle.
3. A third period, mainly in the 1970s, during which the distinctions between axial and random skin flaps were elaborated and the principles extended to all other areas of the body. Muscle and musculocutaneous flaps were developed and a concomitant expansion of free tissue transfer occurred.
4. In the 1980s it was realised that many vessels to skin passed round, rather than through, muscles and this led to identification of the fasciocutaneous system of perforators. Flaps based on these vessels were developed throughout the 1980s and all flap types were refined and became more sophisticated, e.g. by incorporating bone.

The early period

A résumé of the early period could start almost anywhere: with the Susruta Samhita c. 700 BC; with the work of the Sicillian Antonio Branca c. 1430; with the Calabrian Vianeo family c. 1549; with Tagliacozzi's rhinoplasty of 1597; or with the effect of the so-called Indian rhinoplasty on the plastic operations of 19th century European surgeons such as Carpue, von Graefe and Dieffenbach.

Because of the central role played by nasal reconstruction in the evolution of skin flaps it is worth recounting the story of the Samhita rhinoplasty – particularly so as the misconception has arisen that this was a pedicled forehead flap. The following translation from this ancient Indian medical treatise shows that the procedure involved a full thickness skin graft from the cheek (Jolly, 1901).

'If one has lost his nose, the surgeon should cut a leaf of equal size from a tree, place it on the cheek and cut out from the same an equal-sized piece of skin and flesh, suture the cheek with needle and thread, scarify the existing piece of nose, put on quickly but carefully the cut up skin on it. Join it properly with a large bandage and stitch the (new) nose firmly. Then he should put in carefully two reeds in order to ease the breathing and when it is elevated thereby, he should moisten it with oil and sprinkle it with red sandal and other blood-sucking powders. White cotton should then be placed on it and it should often be sprinkled with sesame oil. The operated person should then be given ghee and later a purgative.'

In India the use of a pedicled forehead flap for rhinoplasty probably dates from a later period. The operation was performed in Kangra by the Kanghiara family from about AD 1440 onwards and near Poona by a family belonging to the class of potters. Hakim Dina Nath Kanghiara, the last surviving descendant of the Kanghiara family, who secretly carried out this operation until recently, claimed that his family had been practising the art since 1000 BC.

Tagliacozzi's rhinoplasty is also well known among plastic surgeons. His procedure, perhaps learnt from his professor Aranzio, used a distally based upper arm flap for nasal reconstruction and was later modified for cheiloplasty (see Fig. 2.9). His method was successful and he was really the first surgeon to write on the subject from his own experience. The publication of this work in Venice in 1597 two years before his death, and subsequently in three further editions (1597, 1598, 1831) ensured his lasting fame. The statement has often been made that following his death the method was not used and was eventually forgotten until revived in the 19th century. Gnudi & Webster (1950) in an extremely scholarly review of the life and times of Gaspare Tagliacozzi concluded that after his death there were isolated examples of serious interest in Tagliacozzi's work all over Europe including a complete reprint of his work in the Bibliotheca Chirurgica (Geneva 1721), but

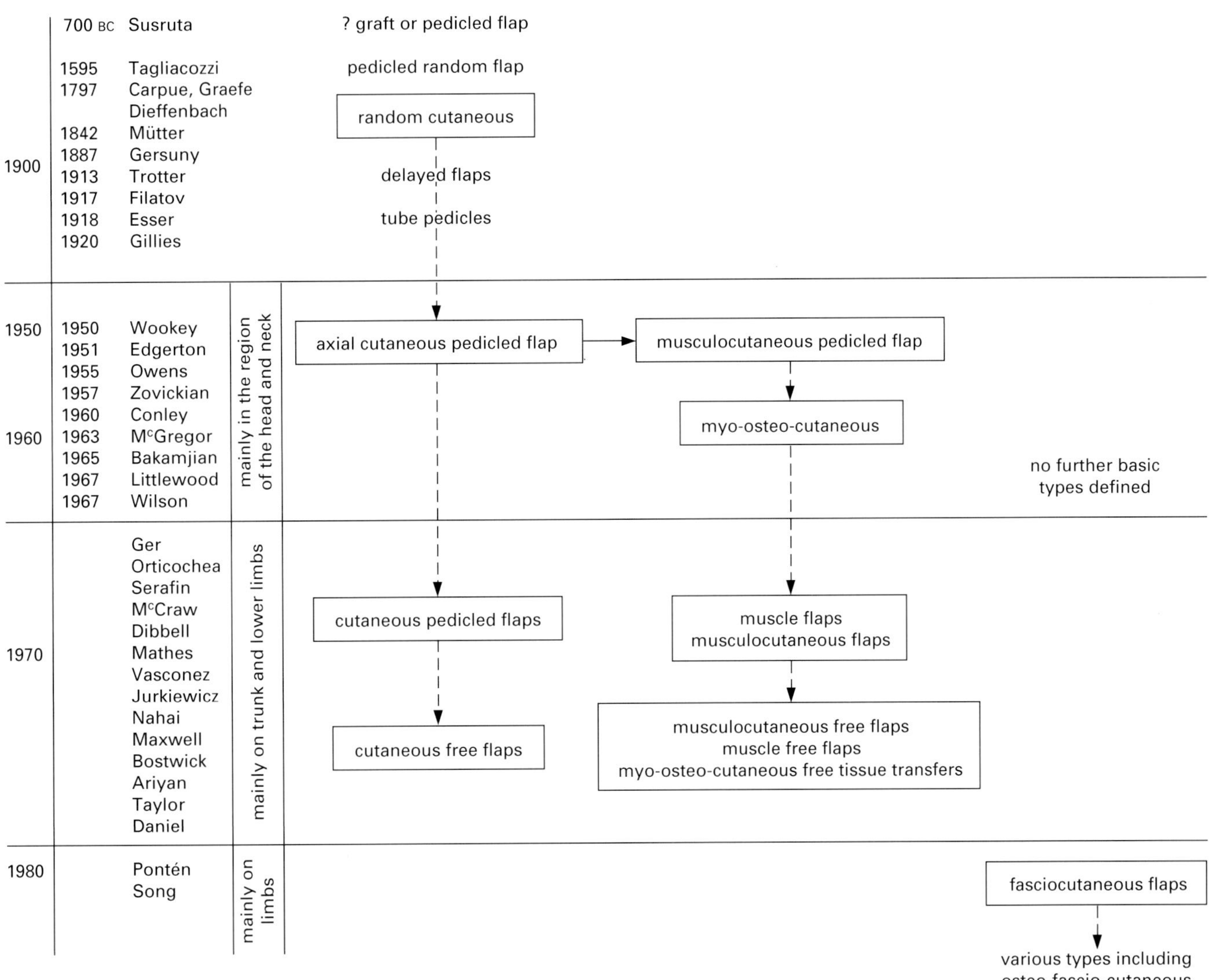

Fig. 1.1 The historical development of the present concept of flaps.

these were largely lost sight of among the jokes, satire and mass of misinformation that developed about the method.

Indeed the 17th and 18th centuries were a period of decline and neglect of plastic surgery and it was only at the beginning of the 19th century that a true revival of interest in rhinoplasty took place. In India the custom of cutting off the nose for vengeance or as a punishment for crimes was widespread and had led to a flourishing practice in corrective surgery using a forehead flap. It has frequently been stated that the event which initiated the revival of plastic surgery in Europe was the publication in the Gentleman's Magazine of 1794 of a letter accompanied by an engraving, describing such a rhinoplastic operation on a bullock-driver named Cowasjee who had been punished by having his nose cut off. (The B.L. letter, 1794.)

It is doubtful whether so much can be ascribed to so slight a communication but it is probably the case that among English surgeons, Carpue at least learnt of this procedure. After practising on cadavers he successfully employed the forehead flap method in 1814 and 1815 on two army officers. A description of these cases was published in 1816 and stimulated surgeons in Germany, France and Italy to follow his example. Carpue's publication is a landmark in the development of flap surgery, both as a record of his own surgical achievement and as a classic in the history of plastic surgery. In Germany a further stimulus arose when in 1818 von Graefe reported three cases illustrative of the Italian, the Indian, and what he termed the 'German' method in his book 'Rhinoplastic'. This was a comprehensive survey of the three methods both historically and clinically, although the pretentiously named German method was no more than a shortened version of the Italian technique. In Europe, Delpech (1821), Labat (1834), Dieffenbach (1845), Blasius (1848) and Volkmann (1874) also made contributions to flap surgery and in the United States Mütter (1843) was a pioneer in applying flap surgery to the correction of extensive burn scars of the neck.

By and large these were all isolated events but in the late 19th and early part of this century the scope of plastic surgery widened rapidly. It was here that the principles of flap surgery were conceived, laying down the bedrock of modern plastic surgery. It would be tedious to give a comprehensive list of all those who published papers in this field but worthy of note are the early flaps of Gersuny (1887), Morax (1908) and Snydacker (1906).

At this time the majority of flaps had in common that the unepithelialised undersurface of the bridge was left raw resulting in the free exudation of blood and serum and the ready invasion of bacteria. The next milestone was to recognise the value of closing the parallel skin edges of these open pedicle flaps by suturing them together to form tubes. In 1916 and 1917 three surgeons independently practised such advances; they were V.P. Filatov, ophthalmologist at the Novorossiisk Eye Clinic, Odessa; Dr Hugo Ganzer of the Charlottenburg Hochschule Hospital, Berlin; and Major Harold Delf (later Sir Harold) Gillies of the Queen's Hospital, Sidcup, England. Filatov's original article was published in Russian in 1917, followed over the next ten years by three further articles in Russian, three in German and one in French which undoubtedly helped to disseminate the method in Europe. Ganzer described his tube pedicles, including one of an upper arm flap for repair of a palatal defect, at a meeting in Berlin in 1917 and in two articles in the same year. Gillies' first tube pedicle was in fact a bipedicled flap taken from the anterior chest and used to reconstruct the face of a badly burned sailor in 1917. This first case was, with other examples of the technique, presented in New Orleans and New York in 1919 and published in 1920. In his work with the war wounded at Sidcup, Gillies directed teams of surgeons who had come from both the Dominions and America to study his techniques. Later these men returned to their respective countries and not only used the tubed pedicle procedure, but published papers in which Gillies was credited with having devised the method (e.g. Smith, 1920; Arbuckle, 1920). Thus, although conceiving and performing the tube pedicle procedure after Filatov, Gillies has been regarded in the English speaking work as being chiefly responsible for its wide dissemination.

Interestingly enough, apparently quite independently of Gillies although working at the same surgical centre, Captain J. L. Aymard performed a tubed flap transfer from shoulder to nose in late 1917. Aymard published an account of his operation in December 1917 and later tried to claim priority but the facts are that Gillies' operation preceded Aymard's by two weeks. Of the many flaps raised during this early period, large and small, tubed and untubed, all had one thing in common – they were random pattern flaps and an increase in the length-to-breadth ratio of these flaps could be achieved only by the delay phenomenon.

Despite this, the random tube pedicle flap was exploited with a vigour and a resoluteness imbued by the stature and reputation of Sir Harold Gillies. Of course it must be remembered that in Britain there were very few plastic surgeons, indeed at the outbreak of the Second World War there were only four recognised plastic surgeons in England – Gillies, McIndoe, Kilner and Mowlem all working within the London area. Later during the War, two further centres were set up in Scotland near Glasgow (Tough) and Edinburgh

(Wallace). These surgeons, with their trainees and assistants, developed specialised units and established the speciality of plastic surgery on a national basis (Cope, 1953).

To some extent the search for a new flap concept was delayed and the concept of axiality was passed over. This is remarkable when one considers that the classical delay procedure consisting of double parallel incisions with undermining, effectively axialised the flow in a flap. The breakthrough of the post-War period was the recognition of this concept of axiality in a flap, in many cases allied with the application of regional flaps around the head and neck, the need for which had arisen as a result of the more radical ablative surgery that had become possible in this region as a result of other medical advances.

The second period

The second major period of discovery came in the 1950s and 1960s with a surge of reports by, for example, Bakamjian, Conley, DesPrez, Edgerton, Littlewood, McGregor, Owens, Shaw, Wilson, Wookey and Zovickian, describing the ingenious creation of a variety of flaps from the scalp, forehead, neck, chest, supraclavicular area and upper back. This inventiveness was again inspired by the nature of the clinical problems confronting the surgeons of the time, whilst anatomists, unaware of these problems, did little to further the knowledge of the blood supply to skin. But in this respect we shall say something more later. Many of the principles governing the flap surgery of this period were elaborated with much empiricism in the region of the head and neck. Many of these advances in understanding were formalised when McGregor & Morgan defined the distinction between axial and random pattern flaps. New donor sites based on the principle of axiality were now exploited outside the area of the head and neck in such places as the groin, dorsum of foot, thigh and abdomen.

The third period

Almost concurrently, technological advances were producing better operating microscopes, smaller needles and finer sutures so that it became feasible to consider the transfer of many of these same units of tissue as free flaps. Indeed, Krizek and others reported experimental free tissue transfers in 1965 some three years after Kleinert & Kasdan had performed the first successful replantation of an incompletely severed thumb (Kleinert & Kasdan, 1965), and in the same year as Komatsu & Tamai replanted a completely severed thumb (Komatsu & Tamai, 1968). Cobbett (1969) carried out the first great toe to thumb transfer in 1967. Improvements in microvascular anastomotic techniques were developed by Buncke et al (1965, 1966) and Cobbett (1967) and helped to improve the reliability of both replantation and free flap surgery. And so it was that free tissue transfer became a major feature of this third phase of flap development with McLean & Buncke (1972) and Antia & Buch (1971) carrying out the first human free flap transfers to be reported in the English literature in 1971. Harii et al (1974) completed a free flap in 1972 to be followed by Hayhurst in 1973 and Taylor and Daniel working with O'Brien in 1973. Acland (1973) and others helped to solve some of the problems of thrombus formation in microvascular surgery.

Unbeknown to the Western world, throughout this period, Chinese surgeons had been independently developing an extensive experience in microsurgery following the first successful hand replantation in Shanghai in 1963. The Chinese had carried out second toe transfer as early as 1966 and a free groin flap in 1973 but this only became known to the English speaking world much later (Chen et al, 1982). The amalgamation of the Western experimental background in microsurgery with the considerable Chinese clinical experience gave a significant boost to the worldwide development of microsurgery (Zhong & Kong, 1989).

Another milestone was the move away from the old concept of flaps as consisting of skin only. This was a consequence of the second major feature of this period, namely the discovery of muscle and musculocutaneous flaps. The first description of a muscle flap is attributed to Ger (1968) but it was from Atlanta, Georgia that the growth spurt came. It is to names such as Jurkiewicz, McCraw, Dibbel, Furlow, Vasconez, Mathes, Nahai, Bostwick, Maxwell, Daniel, Ariyan, Orticochea and Serafin that we are indebted for the rapid delineation of muscle and musculocutaneous flaps used both as local and as free flaps. These discoveries highlighted the importance of knowing about each and every vessel supplying the skin. Thus a major feature of this third period of development was a renaissance of anatomy – the knowledge of the blood supply to units of skin and muscle, no longer just in the region of the head and neck but to the whole integument.

The fourth period

Both the direct cutaneous and the musculocutaneous concepts were taken up so widely and with such speed and enthusiasm that little consideration was given to the possibility of the existence of a third system of vessels contributing to the blood supply of skin. To some extent it is the development of the fasciocutaneous concept that marks the fourth phase. It is indeed remarkable that the existence of a third system of blood supply to the skin, consisting of perforators passing along the fascial septa between certain muscles and spreading out at the level of the deep fascia, should have been neglected until now. The role of the fascia and the vessels in it were not scientifically analysed prior to 1980 despite the fact that both Esser in 1918 and Gillies in 1920 had suggested that it might be advantageous to include the deep fascia in what we now regard as random pattern skin flaps. Instead, delayed flaps and tube pedicles continued to consist of skin and fat alone and an opportunity to discover the existence of a fascial plexus fed by septal perforators was missed. Even during the second period of flap development the concept of axiality in a flap was still confined to specific axial cutaneous vessels and the concept of axiality in anastomosing small vessels at the level of the deep fascia was missed. Perhaps this is not surprising since fasciocutaneous flaps depend on less immediately obvious anatomy and the concept is one of potential skin vascular territories not readily demonstrable by in vivo injection techniques rather than the more readily definable anatomical territories of the axial cutaneous flaps.

So it was that in the 1980s it was the turn of the fasciocutaneous system. Although not as dramatic an advance as the discovery of the musculocutaneous flaps, the elucidation of the details of the fasciocutaneous system resulted in the development of some extremely useful and versatile flaps. Many of these have been combined with bone and the development of such compound flaps, and of free microvascular bone transfers, has been a continuing process through into the 1990s.

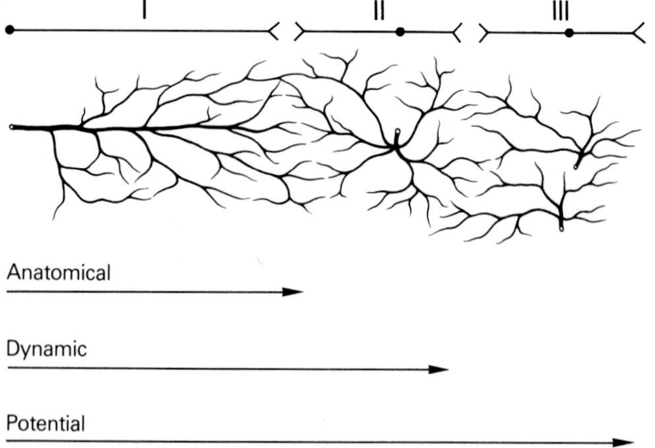

Fig. 1.2 A simplified concept of the anatomy underlying the different sizes of anatomical, dynamic and potential territories (see text for explanation).

CONCEPTS OF TERRITORIES

It would be appropriate at this stage to introduce some explanation of the various current concepts of cutaneous vascular territories and to define the terms used in this book. Figure 1.2 is a schematic diagram illustrating the differences between anatomical, dynamic and potential territories.

Anatomical territories

The anatomical territory of a vessel is one based on observation of structure, and is delineated by the extent to which the branches of that vessel ramify before anastomosing with adjacent vessels. Anatomical territories were essentially what the German anatomist Carl Manchot purported to show when in 1889 he published his now famous work 'Die Hautarterien des Menschlichen Körpers' in which he described the results of his dissections of the human integument. His account was based on dissection studies of whole cadavers and resulted in a demonstration of the cutaneous territories of the major named arteries of the body, although his original intention had been to compare the cutaneous arterial and nerve supplies and investigate the interrelationships that might exist between arterial distribution and the somitic arrangement. His conclusions, as summarised in the final illustration of his book and reproduced in Figure 1.3, are a mixture of veracity (e.g. the anterior chest) and inaccuracy (e.g. the groin).

Just as Tagliacozzi's work was not entirely forgotten until its relatively recent 'rediscovery', so Manchot's work was known to a few surgeons who used his diagrams as the basis for designing their flaps. In 1931 Joseph reproduced Manchot's chest diagram in his book 'Nasenplastick und Sonstige Gesichtsplastik', to justify the unusual length of a transverse chest flap which he had designed for reconstructing post-burn neck scars. Also in the 1930s Webster had relied on Manchot's work and published his diagram of the anterior trunk arteries to explain the basis of the thoracoabdominal tube pedicle with which his name is associated (Webster, 1937). Milton had recognised the importance of Manchot's book when he wrote, 'Those who have not seen the segmental vessels in man during paramedian incisions or radial mastectomies might dismiss the monograph of Manchot (1889) for lack of clear experimental details and evidence but it is a remarkable coincidence that his description of the largest vessel of the ventral chain (second intercostal) is the one included in the versatile deltopectoral flap.' Milton arranged for an English translation of Manchot's book to be done

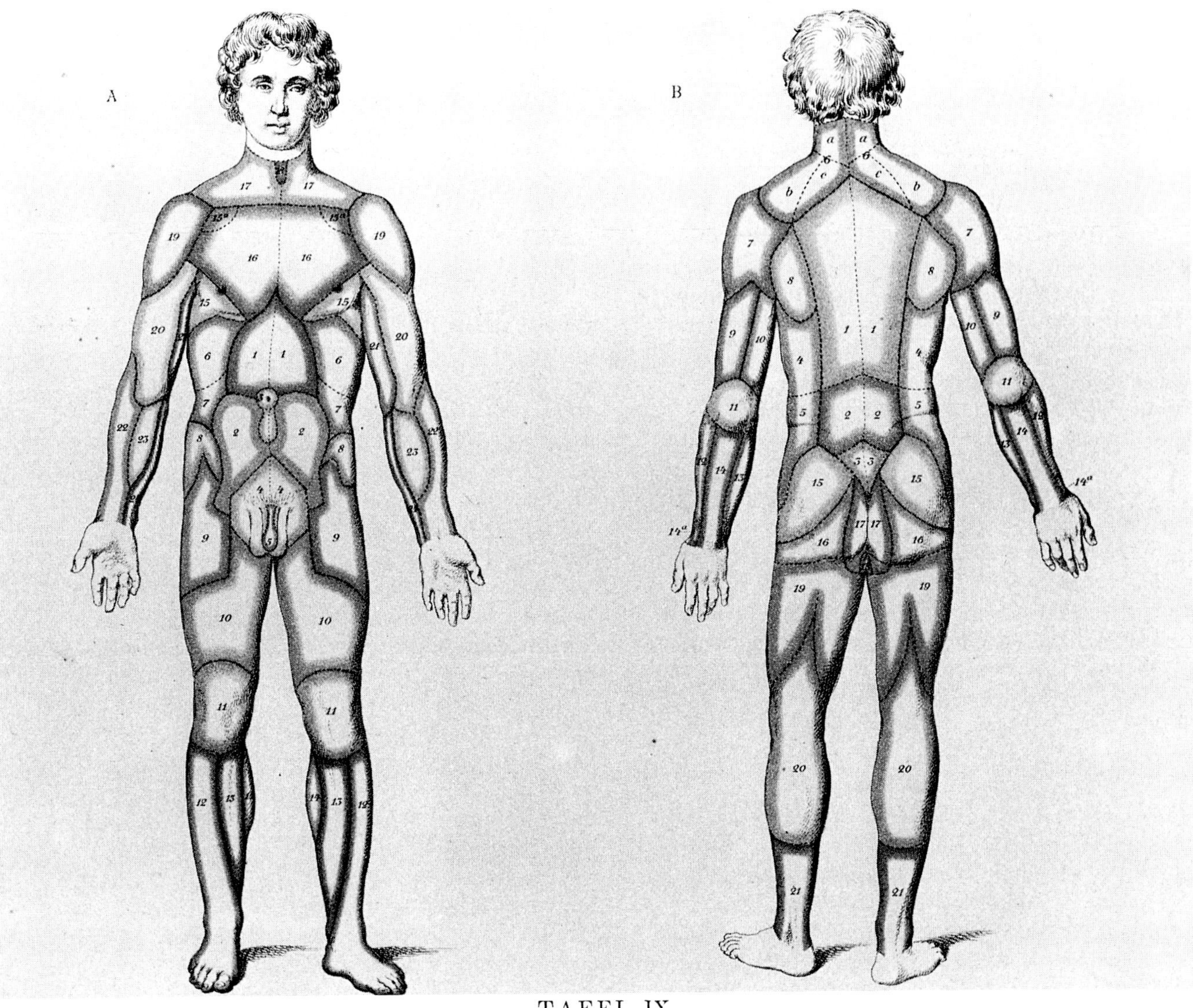

TAFEL IX.

Uebersichtsschema der Hautarteriengebiete.

Figur A.

1 Hautgebiet der A. epigastrica superficialis superior.
2 Hautgebiet der A. epigastrica superficialis inferior.
3 Hautgebiet der Aa. epigastrica superior und inferior.
4 Hautgebiet der Aa. pudendae externae.
5 Hautgebiet der Aa. dorsales penis.
6 Hautgebiet der Rr. perforantes aus den Aa. intercostales.
7 Hautgebiet der Rr. perforantes aus den Aa. lumbales.
8 Hautgebiet der A. circumflexa ilium superficialis.
9 Hautgebiet der A. profunda femoris (Aa. circumfl. femor.).
10 Hautgebiet der A. femoralis.
11 Hautgebiet des Rete superficiale genu.
12 Hautgebiet der A. tibialis antica.
13 Hautgebiet der A. tibialis postica.
14 Hautgebiet der A. poplitea (Aa. surales).
15 Hautgebiet der Aa. thoracicae.
15*a* Hautgebiet der A. thoracico-acromialis.
16 Hautgebiet der Rr. perforantes der A. mammaria interna.
17 Hautgebiet des Truncus thyreocervicalis.
18 Hautgebiet der A. thyreoidea superior.
19 Hautgebiet der A. deltoidea subcutanea anterior.
20 Hautgebiet der A. brachialis.
21 Hautgebiet der A. collateralis ulnaris superior.
22 Hautgebiet der A. radialis.
23 Hautgebiet der A. mediana.
24 Hautgebiet der A. ulnaris.

Figur B.

1 Hautgebiet der Rr. dorsales aus den Aa. intercostales.
2 Hautgebiet der Rr. dorsales aus den Aa. lumbales.
3 Hautgebiet der Rr. dorsales aus den Aa. sacrales.
4 Hautgebiet der Rr. perforantes posteriores der Aa. intercostales.
5 Hautgebiet der Rr. perforantes posteriores d. Aa. lumbales.
6 Hautgebiet des Truncus thyreocervicalis.
a der A. cervicalis superficialis.
b der A. transversa scapulae.
c der A. transversa colli.
7 Hautgebiet der A. deltoidea subcutanea posterior.
8 Hautgebiet der A. circumflexa scapulae superficialis.
9 Hautgebiet der A. collateralis radialis inferior.
10 Hautgebiet der A. collateralis ulnaris superior.
11 Hautgebiet des Rete cubitale.
12 Hautgebiet der A. radialis.
13 Hautgebiet der A. ulnaris.
14 Hautgebiet der A. interossea externa und interna.
15 Hautgebiet der A. glutaea.
16 Hautgebiet der A. ischiadica.
17 Hautgebiet der A. pudenda interna.
18 Hautgebiet der A. obturatoria.
19 Hautgebiet der Rr. perforantes der A. profunda femoris.
20 Hautgebiet der A. poplitea.
21 Hautgebiet der A. tibialis antica und postica.

Fig. 1.3 Plate IX from Carl Manchot's book, Die Hautarterien des Menschlichen Körpers (1889).

and took this with him to America when collaborating with Myers and Cherry in the early studies of the delay phenomenon. In America several plastic surgeons at the forefront of the advances in flap design saw this work and must have been influenced by it. This translation was not published, and neither it nor its copies have resurfaced. However, a separately commissioned translation has recently been published (Morain & Ristic, 1983) with an historical assessment of Manchot's work in the light of contemporary medical and world history.

Recently many descriptions of new flaps have made reference to Manchot and his work has come to be regarded as authoritative. One wonders, however, how many other anatomists have produced work on the vascular system which temporarily rests forgotten awaiting re-evaluation. The studies of Dubreuil-Chambardel (1925), Belou (1934) and Salmon (1936) have all been notable but neglected in the English speaking world. Certainly a most significant contribution to the understanding of the blood supply of skin was made by the French surgeon and anatomist Michel Salmon. His work advanced that of Manchot by the extensive use of radiography which enabled demonstration of much smaller vessels than Manchot had been able to show. Salmon dissected 15 adult cadavers and took 150 radiographs of the integument of three whole cadavers, of four isolated upper and lower limbs and of six heads after intra-arterial injection of a radio-opaque liquid mass. He thereby established the presence of intra-muscular anastomoses and elucidated the detailed supply to the skin. His work on muscles and skin was widely acclaimed at the time and won the Prix Monthyon 1935 and Prix Marc Sée 1935 from L'Institut et L'Académie de Médicine. He was aware that surgeons at that time were raising skin flaps and although his works were essentially morphological he occasionally made observations in the text on what he considered to be suitable sites for the elevation of 'grafts of the Italian kind'. We have previously drawn attention of his work in the plastic surgery literature (Lamberty & Cormack, 1982).

Certain anatomical territories have also been studied in vivo (Nakajima et al, 1981). The arteries under investigation were identified by selective angiography using the Seldinger technique and 10 ng of prostaglandin E_1 dissolved in saline were injected through the same catheter over a period of 10 seconds. The flushed area that resulted from the peripheral vasodilator effect of PGE_1 was regarded as the vascular skin territory of the artery under study. These areas corresponded well with the pattern of fluorescence after injection of fluorescein, and it was also observed that the areas delineated did not overlap with adjacent territories. Although observed in an in vivo situation these territories are approximately the same as the anatomical ones based on the physical extent of the vessels in the cadaver and reflect the fact that a pressure equilibrium exists in the vessels of neighbouring territories along the boundary line between anatomical territories.

Dynamic territories

The concept of an equilibrium point or 'watershed' was elaborated by McGregor & Morgan (1973) in their paper on 'Axial and Random Pattern Flaps' in which it was shown that if one of a pair of abutting cutaneous vessels was occluded then the other vessel would 'extend' its territory into the area of decreased intravascular pressure. Using fluorescein injection techniques this was beautifully demonstrated at the internal thoracic/thoraco-acromial interface on the anterior chest and also across the midline of the chest – a line across which virtually no flow takes place in the 'intact' resting patient. These studies clearly indicated how, for example, the territory of internal thoracic artery perforators could extend over the clavipectoral fascia to the deltopectoral groove if surgical intervention removed the contribution to this areas by the thoraco-acromial axis. This is effectively what happens when a deltopectoral flap is raised and explains why such a flap can be raised to this extent without a prior delay procedure. In this book the use of the term 'dynamic territory' implies that some interference has taken place, generally surgical (such as flap elevation or undermining), in the adjoining areas with resultant alterations in intravascular pressures and changes in the dynamic equilibria, leading to readjustments of flow and changes in the size of the areas perfused.

Dynamic territories are therefore fundamentally different from anatomical ones. It will be found that Chapter 6 is largely devoted to anatomical territories and Chapter 7 to dynamic and potential territories. Dynamic territories have largely been studied in the clinical setting on patients but corroborative studies of the principles involved have been carried out in pigs (Milton, 1969) and rabbits (Smith, 1973). The authors believe that anatomical cadaver injection studies also have something to offer in this field although others have disputed this. If a single specific cutaneous artery is injected with dye or a radio-opaque substance in a fresh cadaver, then the situation approaches that of a dynamic territory because the absence of any intravascular pressure in vessels of surrounding territories results in a shift in the boundary of the injected territory. In this situation the margins of the area indicated by the dye are likely to approach the limits of a flap raised clinically without a prior delay procedure. Clearly this is not coincidental but an expression of the underlying anatomy, its consistency, and the fact that dye will only penetrate into areas whose vessels are in physical continuity with those of the primary (injected) vessel.

The earliest so-called axial pattern flaps based on direct cutaneous arteries and their accompanying venae comitantes showed this correlation between clinical behaviour and underlying anatomy – for example the deltopectoral flap based on perforators from the internal thoracic artery, the hypogastric flap based on the superficial inferior epigastric artery, and the groin flap based on the superficial circumflex iliac artery.

From these observed patterns of extension of axial pattern flaps, has arisen the concept of a dynamic territory or flap as being made up of vascular units. The main artery supplying a flap has been termed the 'prop' artery (Wilson, 1967) and its territory termed an angiotome. An axial pattern flap consists mainly of the prop artery and its territory but may be extended in length by the addition of one or more other territories (see also p. 76). The exact factors influencing whether or not such extension into adjoining territories is possible remain unknown. Clearly anatomical vascular connections or anastomoses must be present but the size of the local vessels, the pressure in the feeding arteries, how readily reversal of flow can take place in the vessels of the adjoining territories, and the presence of venous return pathways are all likely to be important factors.

Potential territories

It has been mentioned that in the deltopectoral flap the anatomical territories of the second and third perforating branches of the internal thoracic artery may be extended into a dynamic territory which includes the thoraco-acromial area. If, on the skin overlying the deltoid muscle, a prior delay procedure is carried out by peripheral incision, undermining and ligation of perforators in such a way that the base of the delayed flap remains linked onto the end of the 'true' deltopectoral flap, then the deltopectoral flap can be extended even further. From this arises the idea of a third type of territory, namely, the potential territory. These potential territories cannot be demonstrated by either in vivo injection techniques or by cadaver studies since a potential territory incorporates a 'random' element of the flap which has undergone fundamental changes during the period between delay of the flap and its elevation. The exact nature of these changes is unknown. It is certainly the case that they are multifactorial and various hypotheses are discussed in Chapter 2. Among these events there is an element of changing the predominating axiality of the vessels in the delayed area – sometimes referred to as training the flap. As yet, no clear explanation is possible to account for why some flaps, e.g. the forehead, may be extended over four separate territories (superficial temporal – supraorbital/supratrochlear – supraorbital/supratrochlear – superficial temporal) and others over only one or two.

An aspect of anatomy that has received little attention, but which the authors feel may be important in this context, is related to the level, or depth, beneath the surface at which the anastomoses are thought to exist. As will be shown in detail in Chapters 3, 4 and 5 it is clear that the three systems of vessels supplying skin contribute to a variable extent to the arterial plexi that exist at different levels beneath the surface. Musculocutaneous perforators contribute very little to the plexus at the level of the deep fascia but pass directly through it to then fan out in the subcutaneous tissues at approximately the same level as the direct cutaneous vessels. This may be part of the reason why the potential territory of the forehead flap is so unusual in extending over four separate anatomical territories; the arteries supplying these territories are all direct cutaneous vessels anastomosing at the same level. The deltopectoral and hypogastric flaps involve direct cutaneous vessels anastomosing with musculocutaneous perforators on much the same level and extend over three anatomical territories. Fasciocutaneous flaps can be extended over multiple small anatomical territories since all the fasciocutaneous perforators anastomose at the same level. By contrast, flaps relying on anastomoses between direct cutaneous and fasciocutaneous vessels at different levels may not be capable of elevation across so many anatomical territories.

These and other aspects of the inter-relationship between adjacent territories and between vessels of the three different systems are covered more fully in Chapters 3–6.

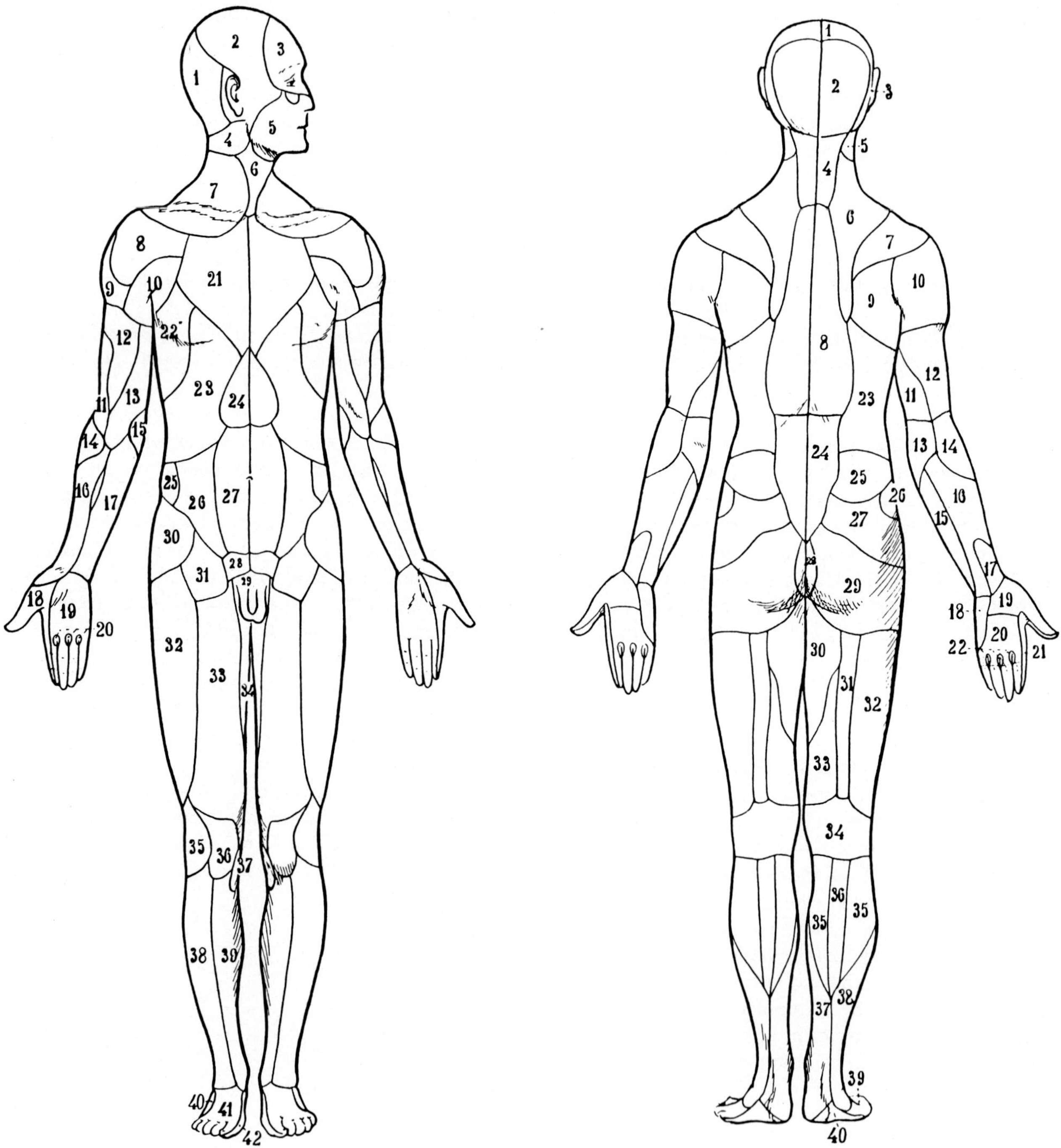

Fig. 1.4 Reproduction of Plate 70 from Michel Salmon's book, 'Artères de la peau' (1936). (Reproduced with the permission of the publishers.)

Fig. 1.5 Reproduction of Plate 71 from Salmon's book.

ADDENDUM

At the time of writing this book we were not aware of Salmon's maps of cutaneous territories as reproduced in Figures 1.4 and 1.5, and hence no reference is made at any stage in our text to Salmon's territories. This situation arose because the volume of 'Les Artères de la Peau' in our possession since 1981 appears to have been an early and incomplete edition. In this earlier version the descriptive text finishes on page 156 and is followed by 11 pages of conclusions and the list of contents. We became aware that our edition was 'incomplete' when Figure 1.4 was reproduced in the British Journal of Plastic Surgery in 1985. The illustrations come from a later edition (which features a preface by Raymond Gregoire) and in which the descriptive text is extended up to page 185 by an additional section on the external genitalia and perineum. There then follows a greatly enlarged Etude Critique which includes nine line drawings of anatomical territories (including the two reproduced here), and 18 excellent radiographic plates covering the whole integument. Both volumes are otherwise indistinguishable, are both dated 1936, and give no indication that there might be more than one edition. We regret that this oversight has meant that in our text we have not given full justice to Salmon's delineations of anatomical territories but we have subsequently taken the opportunity to include these plates and this addendum.

Salmon's book 'Artères de la Peau' is now more widely accessible since being translated into English by Michael Tempest and published in 1988. The radiographs and diagrams have been reproduced together with a foreword by G.I. Taylor.

Fig. 1.4 Schéma récapitulatif des territoires artériels cutanés du plan ventral.

1. Artère occipitale. — 2. A. temporale superficielle. — 3. A. ophtalmique. — 4. A. sterno-cleido-mastoïdienne. 5. A. faciale. — 6. A. thyroïdiennes. — 7. A. cervicale transverse et sus-scapulaire. — 8. A. delto-pectorale. — 9. A. circonflexes. — 10. A. petites thoraciques. — 11. A. humérale profonde. — 12. A. humérale (branches musculaires). — 13. A. humérale (branches directes). — 14. A. des épicondyliens. — 15. A. des épitrochléens. — 16. A. radiale. — 17. A. cubitale. — 18. Arcade palmaire profonde. — 19. — Arcade palmaire superficielle. — 20. A. interosseuse antérieure. — 21. A. mammaire interne. — 22. A. mammaire externe et scapulaire inférieure. — 23. A. intercostale. — 24. A. épigastrique superficielle supérieure. — 25. A. lombaires. — 26. A. épigastrique superficielle inférieure. — 27. A. épigastrique profonde. — 28. A. honteuse externe supérieure. — 29. A. honteuse externe inférieure. — 30. A. circonflexe iliaque superficielle. — 31. A. fémorale primitive. — 32. Grande A. du vaste externe. — 33. A. fémorale superficielle. — 34. A. des adducteurs. — 35. A. articulaires externes. — 36. A. articulaires internes. — 37. A. grande anastomotique. — 38. A. tibiale antérieure. — 39. A. tibiale postérieure. 40. A. péronière. — 41. A. pédieuse. — 42. A, plantaire interne.

Fig. 1.5 Schéma récapitulatif des territoires artériels cutanés du plan dorsal.

1. Artère temporale superficielle. — 2. A. occipitale. — 3. A. auriculaire postérieure. — 4. A. cervicale profonde. — 5. A. sterno-cleido-mastoïdiennes. — 6. A. scapulaire postérieure. — 7. A. sus-scapulaire. — 8. A. intercostale, branche dorso-spinale. — 9. A. scapulaire inférieure. — 10. A. circonflexe postérieure. — 11. A. humérale (collatérales internes). — 12. A. humérale profonde. — 13. — A. récurrente cubitale postérieure. — 14. A. récurrente radiale. — 15. A. cubitale. — 16. A. interosseuse postérieure. — 17. A. interosseuse antérieure. — 18. A. cubito-dorsale. — 19. A. dorsale du carpe. — 20. A. Interosseuses postérieures. — 21. Arcade palmaire profonde. — 22. A. digitales. — 23. A. Intercostales (rameaux perforants). — 24. A. lombaires (rameaux dorso-spinaux). — 25. A. lombaires (rameaux perforants). — 26. A. circonflexe iliaque superficielle. — 27. A. fessière. — 28. A. honteuse interne. — 29. A. ischiatique. — 30. A. des adducteurs, — 31. A. du petit sciatique. — 32 et 33. A. perforantes. — 34. A. poplitée, — 35, A. jumelles, — 36. A. petite saphène. — 37. A. tibiale postérieure. — 38. A. péronière, — 39, A. pédieuse. — 40. A. plantaire externe.

References

Acland R 1973 Thrombus formation in microvascular surgery: an experimental study of the effects of surgical trauma. Surgery 73: 766–771

Antia N H, Buch V I 1971 Transfer of an abdominal dermo-fat graft by direct anastomosis of blood vessels. British Journal of Plastic Surgery 24: 15–19

Arbuckle M F 1920 Plastic surgery of the face. Its recent development and its relation to civilian practice. Journal of the American Medical Association 75: 102–104

Aymard J L 1917 Nasal reconstruction; with a note on nature's plastic surgery. Lancet 2: 888–891

Bakamjian V Y 1965 A two stage method of pharyngo-oesophageal reconstruction with a primary pectoral skin flap. Plastic and Reconstructive Surgery 36: 173–184

Belou P 1934 Revision Anatomica del Sistema Arterial. Tomo 1, Technica. Tomo 2 + 3, Atlas Estereoscopico. Facultad de Ciencias Medicas de Buenos Aires.

Blasius E 1848 Beitrage zur praktischen Chirurgie. Forstner, Berlin

B L 1794 Letter to the editor of Gentleman's Magazine 64: 891

Buncke H J Jr, Schulz W P 1965 Experimental digital amputation and replantation. Plastic and Reconstructive Surgery 36: 62–70

Buncke H J, Buncke C M, Schulz W P 1966 Immediate Nicoladoni procedure in the Rhesus monkey, or hallux-to-hand transplantation, utilizing microminiature anastomosis. British Journal of Plastic Surgery 26: 194–201

Carpue J C 1816 An account of two successful operations for restoring a lost nose from the integuments of the forehead. Longman, London

Chen Z W, Yang D Y, Chang D S 1982 Microsurgery. Springer-Verlag, New York

Cobbett J R 1967 Small vessel anastomosis: A comparison of suture techniques. British Journal of Plastic Surgery 20: 16–20

Cobbett J R 1969 Free digital transfer: Report of a case of transfer of a great toe to replace an amputated thumb. Journal of Bone and Joint Surgery 51B: 677–679

Conley J. 1960 The use of regional flaps in head and neck surgery. Annals of Otolaryngology, Rhinology and Laryngology 69: 1223–1234

Cope V Z 1953 (ed) History of the Second World War. UK Medical Series – Surgery. John Wright and Sons, Bristol

Delpech J M 1828 Chirurgie clinique de Montpellier. Tome II. Paris

Dieffenbach J F 1845 Die operative Chirurgie. Vol 1. Brockhaus, Leipzig

DesPrez J D, Kiehn C L 1959 Methods of reconstruction following resection of anterior oral cavity and mandible for malignancy. Plastic and Reconstructive Surgery 24: 238–249

Dubreuil-Chambardel L 1925 Traité des variations du système artériel. Masson, Paris

Edgerton M T Jr 1951 Replacement of lining to oral cavity following surgery. Cancer 4: 110–119

Esser J F S 1918 Schwerer Verschluss einer Brustwand perforation. Berliner klinisch Wochenschrift 55: 1197

Filatov V P 1917 Plastika na kruglom stebl. Vestnick Oftalmologii 34: 149–158. (Translated by Labunka, Gnudi and Webster, 1959 Plastic procedure using a round pedicle. The Surgical Clinics of North America 39: 277–287)

Ganzer H 1917 Die Bildung von langgestielten Stranglappen bei Gesichtsplastik. Berliner klinische Wochenschrift 54: 1096

Ger R 1968 The surgical management of pretibial skin loss. Surgery 63: 757–763

Gersuny R 1887 Kleinere mittheilungen plastischer Ersatz der Wangenschleimhaut. Zeitblatt für Chirurgie 14: 706–707

Gillies H D 1920a The tubed pedicle in plastic surgery. New York Medical Journal 3: 1–12

Gillies H D 1920b Plastic surgery of facial burns. Surgery, Gynaecology and Obstetrics 30: 121–134

Gnudi M T, Webster J P 1950 The life and times of Gaspare Tagliacozzi. Herbert Reichner, New York

Harii K, Ohmori K, Ohmori S 1974 Hair transplantation with free scalp flaps. Plastic and Reconstructive Surgery 53: 410–413

Jolly J 1901 Grundriss der indo-arischen Philologie und Alterstumskunde. 10 Medicin. (Translated into English by Kashikar C G, Poona, 1951)

Joseph J 1931 Nasenplastik und sonstige Gesichtsplastik, 2nd edn. Kabitzsch, Leipzig

Kleinert H E, Kasdan M L 1965 Anastomosis of digital vessels. The Journal of the Kentucky Medical Association 63: 106–108

Komatsu S, Tamai S 1968 Successful replantation of a completely cut off thumb. Plastic and Reconstructive Surgery 42: 374–377

Krizek T J, Tasaburo T, DesPrez J D, Kiehn C L 1965 Experimental transplantation of composite grafts by microsurgical vascular anastomoses. Plastic and Reconstructive Surgery 36: 538–546

Labat L 1834 De la rhinoplastie. Art de restaurer ou refaire complétement le nez. Ducessois, Paris

Lamberty B G H, Cormack G C 1982 The forearm angiotomes. British Journal of Plastic Surgery 35: 420–429

Leuz C A 1977 The Leuz index of plastic surgery. 1921 AD–1946 AD. Williams & Wilkins, Baltimore

Littlewood M 1967 Compound skin and sternomastoid flaps for repair in extensive carcinoma of the head and neck. British Journal of Plastic Surgery 20: 403–419

Manchot C 1889 Die Hautarterien des Menschlichen Körpers. FCW Vogel, Leipzig

McDowell F 1977a The Honolulu index of plastic surgery. 1971 AD–1976 AD. Williams & Wilkins, Baltimore

McDowell F 1977b The source book of plastic surgery. Williams and Wilkins, Baltimore

McGregor I A 1963 The temporal flap in intraoral cancer: its use in repairing the post-excisional defect. British Journal of Plastic Surgery 16: 318–335

McGregor I A, Morgan G 1973 Axial and random pattern flaps. British Journal of Plastic Surgery 26: 202–213

McIndoe A H 1951a British contributions to plastic surgery. Medical Press 225: 457–459

McIndoe A H 1951b Fifty years of plastic surgery in Great Britain – Part II. Modern Plastic Surgery. Medical Press 226: 131–134

McLean D H, Buncke H J 1972 Autotransplant of omentum to a large scalp defect, with microsurgical revascularization. Plastic and Reconstructive Surgery 49: 268–273

Milton S H 1969 The tubed pedicle flap. British Journal of Plastic Surgery 22: 53–59

Milton S H 1970 Pedicled skin flaps: The fallacy of the length:width ratio. British Journal of Plastic Surgery 57: 502–508

Morain W D, Ristic J 1983 Manchot: The cutaneous arteries of the human body. Springer-Verlag, New York

Morax V 1908 L'autoplastie palpébrale ou faciale à l'aide de lambeau pédiculés empruntés à la region cervicale (procédé de Snydacker) et de l'autoplastie en deux temps avec utilisation du pédicule. Annales Oculist 89: 14–30

Mütter T D 1843 Cases of deformity from burns relieved by operation. American Journal of Medical Sciences 4: 66–80

Nakajima H, Maruyama Y, Koda E 1981 The definition of vascular skin territories with prostaglandin E_1 – the anterior chest, abdomen and thigh-inguinal region. British Journal of Plastic Surgery 34: 258–263

O'Brien B McC, MacLeod A M, Hayhurst J W, Morrison W A 1973 Successful transfer of a large island flap from the groin to the foot by microvascular anastomoses. Plastic and Reconstructive Surgery 52: 271–278

Owens N 1955 A compound neck pedicle designed for repair of massive facial defects. Formation, development and application. Plastic and Reconstructive Surgery 15: 369–389

Patterson T J S 1977 The Zeis index and history of plastic surgery 900 BC–1863 AD. Williams and Wilkins, Baltimore

Patterson T J S 1978 The Patterson index of plastic surgery 1864 AD–1920 AD. Williams and Wilkins, Baltimore

Salmon M 1936 Artères de la peau. Masson, Paris

Salmon M 1988 Arteries of the skin. Edited by Taylor G I and Tempest M. Churchill Livingstone, Edinburgh

Shaw D T, Payne R L 1946 One stage tubed abdominal flaps. Surgery, Gynaecology and Obstetrics 83: 205–209

Smith F 1920 Plastic surgery. Its interest to the laryngologist. Journal of the American Medical Association 75: 1554–1559

Smith P J 1973 The vascular basis of axial patterned flaps. British Journal of Plastic Surgery 26: 150–157

Snydacker E F 1907 Lidplastik mit gestieltem Lappen vom Halse. Klinisches Monatsblatt für Augenheilkunde 45: 71–76
Sun L, Shu J L 1982 Clinical and experimental microsurgery in China: an historical note. Journal of Microsurgery 3: 180–183
Susruta. Samhita (date uncertain, probably originated in approximately 600 BC but not committed to Sanskrit until 200 AD). Translated into English by Bhishagratna K K 1916 3 volumes. Bose, Calcutta
Tagliacozzi G 1597 De curtorum chirurgia per institionem. Meitti, Venice
Taylor G I, Corlett R, Boyd J B 1983 The extended deep inferior epigastric flap. Plastic and Reconstructive Surgery 72: 751–764
Volkmann R 1874 Die frontale rhinoplastik. Verhandlung der Deutschen Gesellschaft für Chirurgie 3: 20
Von Graefe C F 1818 Rhinoplastik; oder, Die Künst den Verlust der Nase organisch zu ersetzen. Berlin
Webster J P 1937 Thoraco-epigastric tube pedicles. Surgical Clinics of North America 17: 145–184
Wilson J S P 1967 The application of the two-centimetre pedicle flap in plastic surgery. British Journal of Plastic Surgery 20: 278–296
Zhong S-Z, Kong J-M 1989 Microsurgical anatomy in China. Surgical and Radiologic Anatomy 11: 115–122
Zovickian A 1957 Pharyngeal fistulas: Repair and prevention using mastoid-occiput based shoulder flap. Plastic and Reconstructive Surgery 19: 355–372

The microcirculation

2

The different layers of the integument
Blood supply to the different layers

The structural organisation of the microcirculation
The microcirculatory components
Cutaneous vascular patterns
The lymphatic system

The functional organisation of the microcirculation
Control of blood flow
Control of transcapillary fluid exchange

The ischaemic flap
Definitions
Theories of the mechanism underlying the delay phenomenon
Treatment of the failing flap

2 THE DIFFERENT LAYERS OF THE INTEGUMENT

Definitions vary but the integument may be regarded as composed of skin, subcutaneous fat and deep fascia.

The skin is supplied from two vascular plexi, the dermis from a subdermal plexus which in turn feeds the subpapillary plexus lying beneath the epidermis. These are described more fully under 'Cutaneous vascular patterns' on page 25. Veins have a similar arrangement except that they have an additional plexus in the dermis.

The subcutaneous tissues consist of the fatty layer or panniculus adiposus containing vestiges of the panniculus carnosus. This adipose tissue has its own vascular system and in this respect is different from the perivascular fat grouped around vessels which do not relate specifically to the fat cells but to their associated tissue or organ (e.g. mesenteric fat). The adipose tissue is made up of delicate lobules separated by fibrous septa which are histologically connected both to the dermis and to the deep fascia. This was well described by Spalteholz (1893) whose method of clarification of the soft tissue resulted in the fat becoming transparent and allowed the fascial septa to be visualised in three dimensions. Passing through this connective tissue network are the cutaneous nerves and vessels. Each lobule consists of hundreds, even thousands, of fat cells, and is vascularised through a single pedicle entering the centre of the lobule and is drained to a vein on the periphery (see Fig. 2.1). The capillaries are therefore located within each lobule, rather than in the connective tissue septa around them. The surrounding septa confer on these very delicate fat lobules a surprising mechanical resistance, and it is this system of supporting tissue that is in proportion to the expected mechanical stresses, the heel pad area being the most extremely developed example of this.

The blood vessels which feed the subdermal network arise in the tissues beneath the deep fascia and ascend through the subcutaneous fat in either a vertical or a horizontal-linear fashion (Fig. 2.2). In areas with thin subcutaneous fat layers the lobules are vascularised largely by descending branches from the wide-meshed subdermal plexus while in thicker fat layers the deeper lobules are supplied by branches coming directly from the ascending arteries. In these areas of thick fat the subcutaneous adipose tissue receives blood from two directions, the superficial layer from above and the deep layer from below, with a connective tissue septum frequently lying between the two and containing a further vessel plexus at this level (Pearl & Johnson, 1983). The

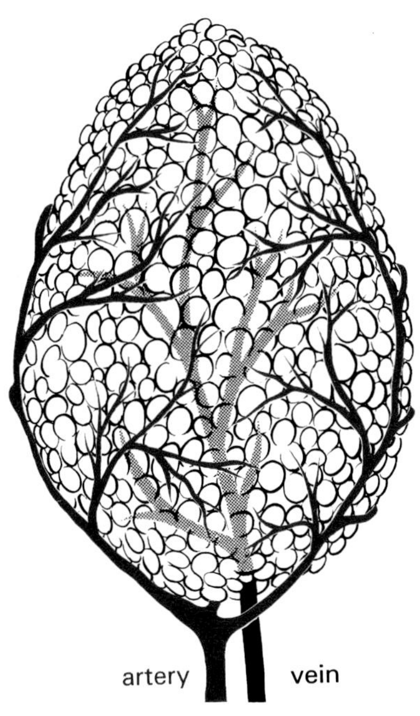

Fig. 2.1 Diagrammatic representation of the blood supply to a fatty lobule.

existence of two such relatively autonomous layers is relevant to the raising of adipo-fascial flaps in which the deeper layer of fat is moved with the deep fascia, while the skin and superficial fat nourished through the subdermal plexus remains at the donor site. The ascending branches from the deeper structures may have either a largely vertical course through the subcutis to the skin in which case the area of skin supplied is small, or alternatively they may run more obliquely, first on the superficial surface of the deep fascia and then through the subcutaneous tissues, giving off branches to the subdermal plexus as they go and supplying a longer strip of skin. The predominating direction of these vessels may be termed their 'axiality' and on the limbs this is generally found to be directed longitudinally. A clue to understanding why this is so provided by the fact that arterial branches often accompany cutaneous nerves. Frequently these vessels are reinforced at intervals along the nerve by branches of other ascending vessels, thereby forming what might be termed a 'relay' artery alongside a

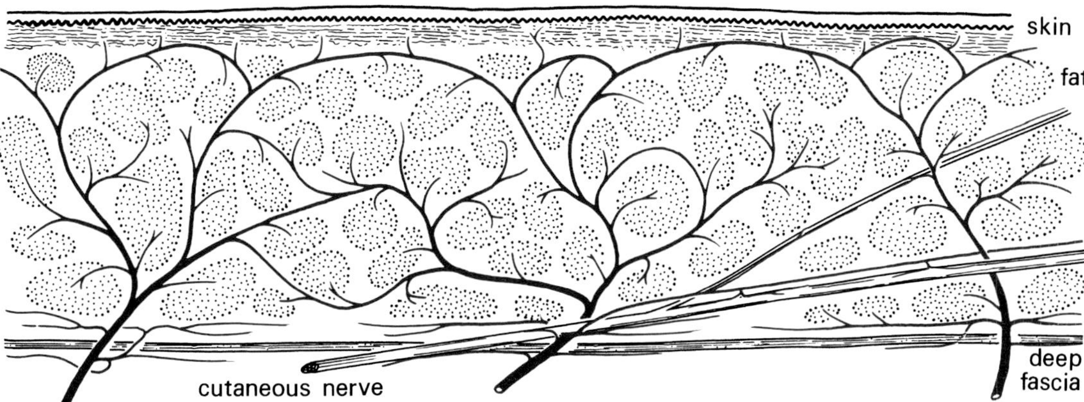

Fig. 2.2 Diagrammatic representation of the subcutaneous vascular network.

Table 2.1 Blood supply of the integument

Plexus	Fed by arteries described as	Anatomically subdivided as
subpapillary plexus subdermal plexus subcutaneous plexus superficial fascial plexus deep fascial plexus	ascending vessels or conductor arteries or perforators	direct cutaneous arteries musculocutaneous perforators fasciocutaneous perforators

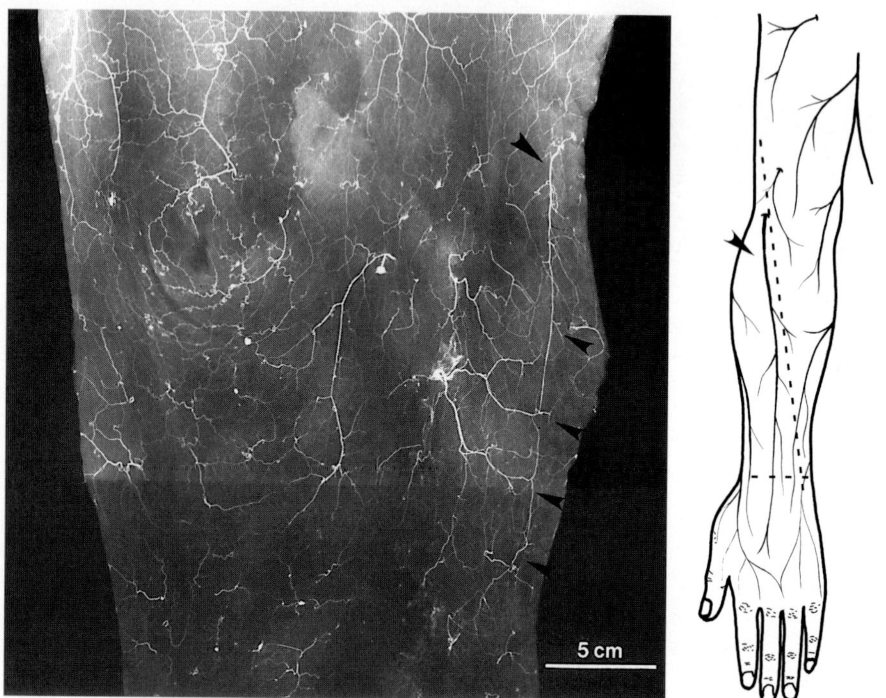

Fig. 2.3 Longitudinal 'relay artery' alongside the posterior cutaneous nerve of the forearm. The dotted line on the diagram of the forearm indicates the position of the incisions made for elevation of the skin specimen shown in the radiograph.

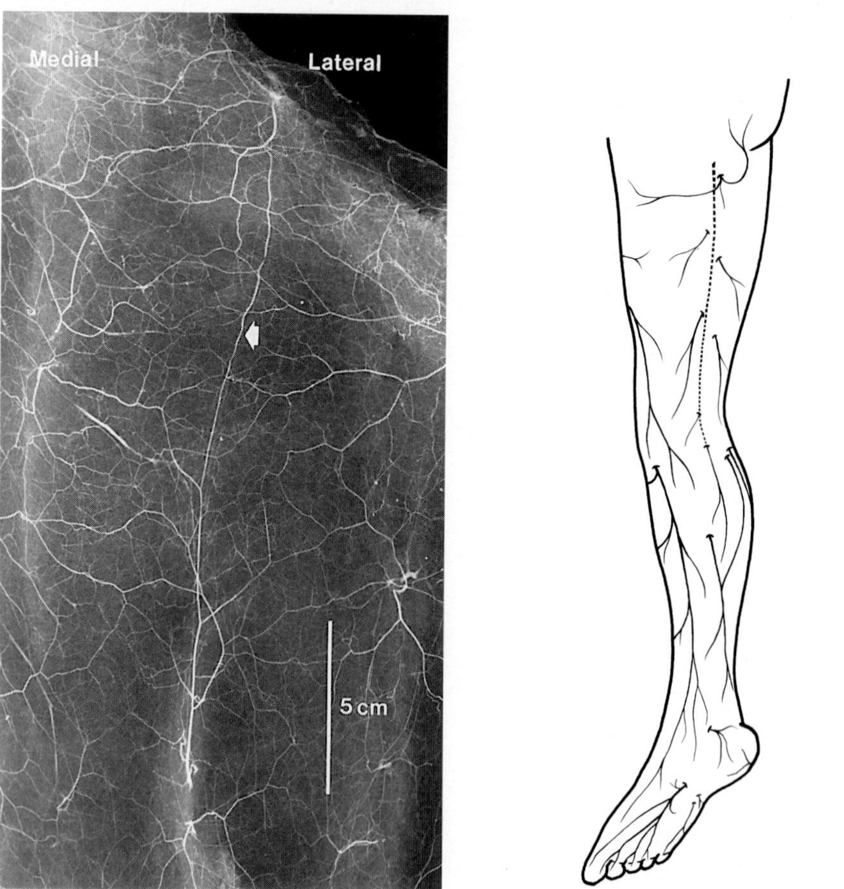

Fig. 2.4 Longitudinal artery along the posterior cutaneous nerve of the thigh reinforced at intervals by perforators from the profunda femoris.

nerve. These vessels are not 100% constant but Figures 2.3 and 2.4 show good examples from the forearm and thigh. The patterns of blood supply to cutaneous nerves have been classified by Briedenbach & Terzis (1983) in order to clarify which might be appropriate for use as free vascularised nerve grafts (Fig. 2.5).

The deep fascia is of two distinctly different types. On the trunk it consists of a well-developed epimyseal surface covering on the muscles. This is elastic in the sense that it is capable of permitting expansion of the abdominal viscera and increase in the diameter of the chest and is therefore very different from the deep fascia on the limbs which is altogether a more rigid structure. The deep fascia on the limbs is continuous with the intercompartmental fascial septa. It not only encloses the muscle groups but also acts in places as a point of origin for muscle fibres and near the joints it forms part of the retinacular system restraining the tendons and preventing bowstringing. It is not surprising that the vascularisation of the so-called deep fascia is therefore different on the trunk compared with the limbs. On the trunk the vascularisation is tied in to the anatomy of the underlying flat muscles and there are no specific fascial plexi with the exception of the area over the scapula. On the limbs the deep fascia is vascularised from vessels passing up along the fascial septa between muscles as described in Chapter 5. These vessels contribute to the formation of two vascular plexi. One is on the undersurface of the fascia and the other on the superficial surface. The deep plexus is made up of tiny branches of the ascending vessels before they perforate the fascia. The superficial plexus is more extensive and made of larger vessels, again originating from the ascending perforators but only after they have pierced the fascia. These two layers are effectively separate except for the ascending vessels themselves and some tiny capillaries which connect them through the fascia (Lang, 1962). Other terms which may be used when referring to these ascending vessels up to the point at which they pierce the deep fascia are 'conductors' and 'perforators'. The sources of origin of these vessels are identified in Chapter 6 and a fuller discussion concerning the various alternative designations for these vessels is available in Chapter 9.

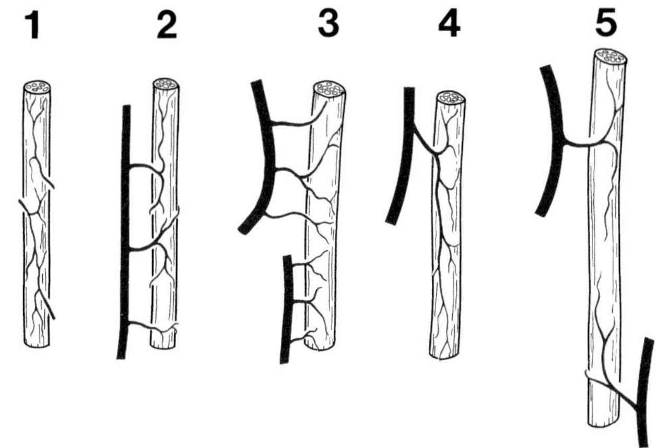

Fig. 2.5 Classification of the vascular anatomy of nerves (after Briedenbach & Terzis, 1983).
Type I nerves have no demonstrable dominant blood supply. They receive small branches along their whole length from multiple different ascending vessels which arise from multiple different musculocutaneous and fasciocutaneous perforators.
Type II nerves have one dominant blood supply which runs for the majority of the nerve length. The mesoneurium directly connects the vascular structures with the nerve. There are small branches running from the vessels through the mesoneurium to the nerve.
Type III nerves have a series of major vessels running along their whole length. When one arteriovenous complex turns away from the nerve another joins it.
Type IV is a nerve with one dominant supply which runs with the nerve for less than the majority of its length. Therefore the nerve is supplied by one dominant artery for a segment (like a Type II nerve) and the remaining segment of the nerve has no dominant system (like a Type I).
Type V has multiple major vessels supplying it (like Type III) interspersed with segments without a dominant vascular supply (like a Type I).

2 STRUCTURAL ORGANISATION OF THE MICROCIRCULATION

THE MICROCIRCULATORY COMPONENTS

The microcirculation is here used in the sense of that part of the vascular tree in which the exchange of gases, nutrients and metabolic waste products occurs. The microcirculatory bed begins with arterioles with a diameter of less than 300 μ and proceeds through terminal arterioles, precapillary sphincters, capillaries, postcapillary venules and collecting venules to muscular venules with a diameter of up to 300 μ.

Many textbook descriptions of the cutaneous microcirculation are based on the original work of Hibbs et al (1958) and on Rhodin's classification (1967, 1968). Rhodin studied the microcirculation in the fascia overlying the thigh muscles in the rabbit and provided ultrastructural criteria for subdividing the vascular tree into the vessels listed above. Recent work by Braverman & Yen (1977, 1981; Yen & Braverman, 1976) has highlighted the structural differences between rabbit and human blood vessels and has greatly clarified our understanding of the human dermal microcirculation. Despite these important differences, Rhodin's system remains a useful basis for describing the microcirculation. The concepts of location in the microcirculatory bed, size of vessels and cellular composition of the vascular wall are generally applicable principles which form the basis of the following account.

Arterioles

The arterioles supplying the skin are derived from three sources; the direct cutaneous system of vessels, the musculocutaneous perforators, and the fasciocutaneous system (described in Chapter 3, 4 and 5 respectively). These arterioles lie in the subcutaneous tissues and gradually decrease in luminal diameter to about 30 μ as they give off branches which form a network in the deep part of the dermis and on its undersurface. The wall of a deep dermal arteriole consists of endothelium, smooth muscle cells and connective tissue. The endothelial cells are squamous but may appear cuboidal in collapsed or contracted arterioles and contain microfilaments and micropinocytotic vesicles. The filaments tend to run along the abluminal border of the cells and extracellular filaments may form a connection between the intracellular bundles of two adjacent endothelial cells. In the subendothelial layer and in between the smooth muscle cells are collagen fibrils grouped in bundles of 50–100 fibrils and orientated parallel to the long axis of the vessel. In the larger arterioles a thin internal elastic lamina is present but has disappeared by the time the vessel has narrowed to 30 μ. This elastic layer is not present in the form of a continuous band but is made up of individual fibres of different lengths which branch and join one another at various points to produce an irregular network. The smooth muscle cells of the arteriolar wall lie in four or five layers and are thin, spindle-shaped cells with the polar ends divided into many long processes. The cells are arranged circularly or spirally around the long axis of most arterioles and each cell is invested by a thin basal lamina except where there is direct cell-to-cell contact at myo–myo junctions. Outside the smooth muscle cells is a thin layer of loose connective tissue composed of veil cells, collagenous and elastic fibrils, occasional macrophages, mast cells and non-myelinated nerve fibres. As the arteriole approaches the precapillary area, this connective tissue is reduced to veil cells and a loosely woven network of collagenous fibrils.

The veil cells were first described by Rhodin and are flat fibroblast-like cells which surround vessels in the dermis, but information about them is meagre. Unlike the pericytes which are an integral component of the vascular wall and are surrounded by the mural basement membrane material, the veil cells are totally external to the wall. The veil cell demarcates the vessel from the surrounding dermis and can be considered to be an adventitial cell. The veil cells are infrequently seen around the microcirculatory vessels in the subcutaneous fat, and it is not known whether they are present around the microcirculatory vessels in other organs.

Terminal arterioles

The terminal arterioles are branches off the arterioles and were so named by Rhodin because they terminate in a capillary network and have no vascular communication, such as an anastomosis or arcuate structure, with any other arterial or venous vessel. These vessels range in size from about 30–10 μ. In the papillary layer of the dermis they vary from 17–26 μ in outside diameter. (No allowance has here been made for any possible shrinkage of fixed material.) The endothelial cells are surrounded by $1–1\frac{1}{2}$ layers of smooth muscle cells. The vascular wall is composed of basement membrane material which has a relatively homogeneous appearance and completely surrounds and encompasses the elastin and smooth muscle cells. As the diameter of the arteriole diminishes from 26 to 15 μ, the elastin assumes a more peripheral position in the basement membrane material of the vascular wall. At the 15 μ level, the elastin disappears from the vascular wall and initially forms an incomplete sheath between the basement membrane and the surrounding veil cells. Smooth muscle cells, which are identified by their numerous dense bodies and myofilaments, are not found below the 15 μ level. Their place is taken by pericytes which have less well developed dense bodies and many fewer filaments, and have the appearance of poorly developed smooth muscle cells.

Precapillary sphincter

The precapillary sphincter has been variously defined. Originally it was placed at the origin of a capillary channel leaving a 'preferential channel'. (The concept of the preferential channel proposed by Zweifach (1961) in some of the early descriptions of the microcirculatory bed has not been given much support by subsequent investigators, but the term appears occasionally in current literature. Wiedeman (1981) has pointed out that the vessel called the metarteriole is perhaps its counterpart in current usage). *Anatomically* it is the area containing the final smooth muscle cell of the arterial distribution. Over this segment the luminal diameter decreases from about 30 to 10 μ. The endothelium of this area is similar to that of larger arterioles and rests on a thin basal lamina except where myo-endothelial junctions occur. The smooth muscle cells are small and few in number; they are surrounded by connective tissue containing some non-myelinated nerve fibres. *Functionally* it is the last part of the terminal arteriole that controls blood flow into the capillary network which lies distal to it. Uncertainty persists, however, concerning the contribution of the precapillary sphincter to total peripheral resistance, and the extent to which its contraction is dependent on neural or local mechanisms.

Capillaries

After the terminal arteriole has narrowed and the external elastic sheath has disappeared, one encounters a vessel with an outside diameter of 10–12 μ and a luminal diameter between 3 and 7 μ. Until relatively recently it was thought that all capillaries had the same structure but it is now recognised that the arrangement of the three structural elements of a capillary, namely the endothelium, the basal lamina and the occasional pericytes, varies between organs and even between the arterial and venous ends of capillaries within an organ.

All capillaries can be classified into one of essentially four types on the basis of their endothelial morphology. These types are (1) continuous thick endothelium, (2) continuous thin endothelium, (3) fenestrated thin endothelium, and (4) discontinuous endothelium. The arterial capillaries of the dermis are of the continuous thin endothelial type with the endothelial cells having an average thickness of about 0.1 μ and containing microfilaments and micropinocytic vesicles. Endothelial cells form tight junctions with pericytes through breaks in the basement membrane and veil cells closely surround these vessels with a thin cytoplasmic rim. Fenestrations occasionally occur in arterial capillaries but they are unusual and may be related to increased epidermal cell proliferation. As the arterial capillary is traced, the basement membrane begins to develop lamellae within its previously homogeneous framework. This is the transition zone, and leads into the venous capillary in which the entire vascular wall is multilaminated. As many as 100 lamellae have been counted in some vessels. The outside diameters of the vessels remain at 10–12 μ with a 4–6 μ luminal diameter. Pericytes and veil cells remain the important cellular elements in the vascular wall and in the immediately surrounding dermis, respectively. The veil cell is probably responsible for the synthesis and maintenance of the peripheral portion of the vascular wall in these vessels and is stimulated to produce excessive basement membrane-like material in response to ultraviolet light, factors associated with diabetes mellitus, and possibly to factors associated with the early phases of chronological ageing. With progressive ageing there is a decrease in the number and synthetic activity of veil cells which correlates with the appearance of abnormally thin-walled vessels (Braverman & Fonferko, 1982). The venous capillaries of the dermis are of the fenestrated thin endothelium type. The fenestrations are closed by a thin single-layered membrane derived from a fusion of the basal and luminal plasma membranes. The endothelium averages 800 Å in thickness and the fenestrations are round with a diameter of about 600 Å.

Postcapillary venules

Postcapillary venules have a luminal diameter which ranges between 8 μ and 30 μ and a length which can vary from as short as 50 μ to as long as 500 μ. In the papillary dermis most of the postcapillary venules measure 18–23 μ in external diameter and 10–15 μ in luminal diameter. The wall consists of endothelium, basal lamina, pericytes and fibroblasts. Pericytes are more numerous than in the venous capillary but they do not form a continuously overlapping layer. The basement membrane of the vascular wall is multilaminated. Collagen fibres may be present between the lamellae or may form a thin sheath in the outer layer of the vascular wall. Functionally, the postcapillary venule is the site of diffusion of metabolites and fluids from the interstitial tissues into the blood. However, the postcapillary venule is more sensitive and vulnerable than the true capillaries, and it is this segment which is affected by allergic reactions, inflammation and extremes of temperature. Reactivity involves an increase in outward diffusion (oedema) and, exceptionally, an extravasation of blood cells. How this is brought about is uncertain although endothelial cells and pericytes must be involved. In normal circumstances the pericyte probably functions as a stabiliser of the endothelial tube and may have some contractile properties although there is no evidence that it has any function as a postcapillary sphincter.

Collecting venules

Collecting venules follow on from the postcapillary venules and progressively increase in diameter to about 50 μ. Although the endothelium and basal lamina hardly change, the pericytes increase in number forming a complete layer around the proximal part of the collecting venule and several layers around the distal part. Among the pericytes lie primitive smooth muscle cells and fibroblasts surround the complete assembly. The functions of this segment are not clear, but may involve control of luminal diameter through smooth muscle action. In terms of reactivity, this segment is far less sensitive than the postcapillary venule.

Muscular venules

These have a wall containing fully differentiated smooth muscle cells and a luminal diameter between 50 and 300 μ. The endothelium is thicker than in the collecting venules. Around vessels in the dermis the muscle layers are usually two or three cell layers thick. The surrounding fibroblasts form, together with large bundles of collagenous fibres, the beginning of what might be termed an adventitia.

It must not be supposed from the descriptions given above that the structure and pattern of blood vessels is fixed. Changes in morphology occur gradually along the vascular tree and changes in diameter and in ultrastructure can occur within minutes of irritation.

Arteriovenous anastomoses

Arteriovenous shunts or anastomoses (AVAs) are normally occurring vessels which connect the arterial and venous sides of the circulation proximal to the terminal capillary network, and from which no significant exchange takes place between the contained blood and the surrounding tissue fluids. AVAs have been found in almost all tissues which have been examined for them. They vary in diameter between 50 and 150 μ but in the skin are fairly constantly about 50 μ in diameter. They have a well-developed connective tissue sheath which appears to be an extension of the adventitia of the arterial segment and contain pericytes (also known as epithelioid cells, myo-epithelioid cells, or glomus cells in this location) in the vascular wall.

The simplest form of AVA is the direct type in which there is no sharp demarcation between the arterial and venous segments. The musculature of the thick-walled arterial limb is often complex with circular, oblique and longitudinal fibres. The venous portion of this type of anastomosis usually has no distinguishing histological characteristics.

The more common form of AVA is the indirect type of anastomosis characterised by the presence of an intermediate segment between the arterial and venous limbs. Here the wall is made up of smooth muscle fibres and modified muscle cells, and the adventitia is thick. Anastomoses of this type may be relatively short with few of the modified muscle cells present, or they may form complex coils and have walls composed entirely of these specialised cells. This increasing complexity and tortuosity, sometimes with a double lumen, gives rise to the fully differentiated 'glomus'.

The glomus is notable for its large proportion of modified muscle cells which are large, clear, polygonal, have little chromatin in the nucleus and resemble epithelial cells. The glomus has a rich nerve plexus, and many of the fibres are cholinergic. The concept that a glomus evolves from a simple to a complex form is derived from histological studies by several authors; for example, detailed examination of fœtal and adults fingers has suggested that some anastomoses remain simple shunts while others progressively increase in complexity to the glomus organ (Hale & Burch, 1960).

Furthermore, involution has been noted of even the most complex types with age or disuse. Note that no values have been given for the number of AVAs in human skin. Values varying between 100 and 500 AVAs per cm^2 of surface have been quoted for the fingers but seem to be unrealible. For example, counts done by different techniques on rabbit ears vary from 5 to 140 per cm^2. A possible source of error in evaluating the presence of an AVA by histological techniques is the fact that, shortly after death, AVAs are in a state of extreme contraction and may be overlooked. Only from 14 to 20 hours after death do the AVAs relax, allowing study of the normal vascular anatomy. If tissue is fixed soon after death, the channels will remain closed.

In addition to AVAs, there are other specialised vascular structures which may permit local regulation of blood flow, and since these have been confused at times with AVAs they deserve comment. In the walls of some arteries and veins there are structures which project into the vessel lumen, having the appearance of a 'cushion'. These intramural pads when found in arteries are located at the origin of a branch and can apparently act as a sphincter in the vessel. Vessels with these pads have been called 'cushioned' or 'blocked' arteries or veins. Another variation on regulator structures is the 'central A–V channel' of 'preferential capillary channel' described by Zweifach and co-workers as a feature of certain capillary beds (but not human skin). These channels extend directly from an arteriole to a venule and may serve as a short-circuiting system entirely within the capillary bed. Since these central channels are within the capillary network, they are not true AVAs.

Flow through AVAs. These anastomoses are richly supplied with nerves and are capable of contraction or dilatation in response to nerve impulses and chemical stimuli, often in a manner quantitatively different from the response of neighbouring arteries or arterioles. Since the anastomoses lie proximal to the capillary network they are able to partition the circulation into or away from the functional capillary bed.

An understanding of the magnitude of this partition can be gained by applying Poiseuille's equation (1846) (as modified by Hagenbach, 1860):

$$F = \frac{\Delta P \cdot \pi \cdot r^4}{8 \cdot \zeta \cdot L}$$

in which

F = flow
P = pressure difference between the ends of the tube
r = radius of the tube
ζ = coefficient of viscosity
L = length of the system

Although this formula was designed for a system of small, rigid tubes through which a Newtonian fluid was flowing, it has been able to express, with reasonable accuracy, the flow of blood in living vessels.

If factors such as viscosity and pressure remain constant, the flow within vessels of equal length would be proportional to the fourth power of the radius of each vessel. Under these conditions, an AVA whose radius is twice that of a capillary would carry 16 times as much blood, per unit of length. An AVA 5 times larger than a capillary (i.e. 50 μ in diameter) would have a flow rate about 600 times greater than the capillary, per unit length.

On the same basis, the speed of blood flow would be related to the fourth power of the radius of the vessel. Based upon normal capillary pressures, 1 ml of blood requires about 6 hours to flow through a capillary 10 μ in diameter. An AVA with a diameter of 50 μ would pass the same amount of blood in minutes.

Actually, several factors in the Poiseuille equation do not remain constant when vessels as different as an AVA and a capillary are compared. Plasma skimming, and the pressure difference across the ends of the AVA have not been allowed for and therefore the assumption that flow volume and rates of these two vessels are proportional to the fourth power of their radii is not accurate.

Nevertheless, it is clear that these shunts can divert enormous amounts of blood to or away from the capillary bed although even when AVAs are open there may be some flow through the capillary network, depending on the arterioles nearby – if they are dilated there will be some blood flow through capillaries. Since their partitioning effect can be so great it is necessary to understand the ways in which flow through them is controlled.

Control of AVAs. Original observations of the AVAs in the living rabbit ear stressed the rhythmic contractions of AVAs occurring 2–12 times per minute which appear to occur independently of neighbouring arterioles and anastomoses. Modifying this general activity are neural, humoral and thermal influences. Rhythmic contractions are replaced by continuous constriction when the local sympathetic nerve fibres are stimulated, while injury or destruction of the nerve fibres leads to continuous dilatation of AVAs. In the rabbit ear this lasts for 10–14 days and is then progressively replaced by a degree of tone which maintains the lumen at a narrower diameter. This is thought to be attributable to denervation hypersensitivity to low levels of circulating hormones with a vasoconstrictor effect such as noradrenaline. By contrast, acetylcholine and histamine cause vasodilatation. Other influencing factors are hypoxia, pH, trauma and intravascular pressure. A fall in the oxygen tension of the blood closes AVAs, as does a rise in pH. Trauma dilates AVAs and a fall in intravascular pressure to levels below the 'critical closing pressure' leads to sudden closure of the shunts.

To a large extent these responses of the AVAs are quantitatively different from those of arteries, a fact which allows fine regulation of the terminal circulation.

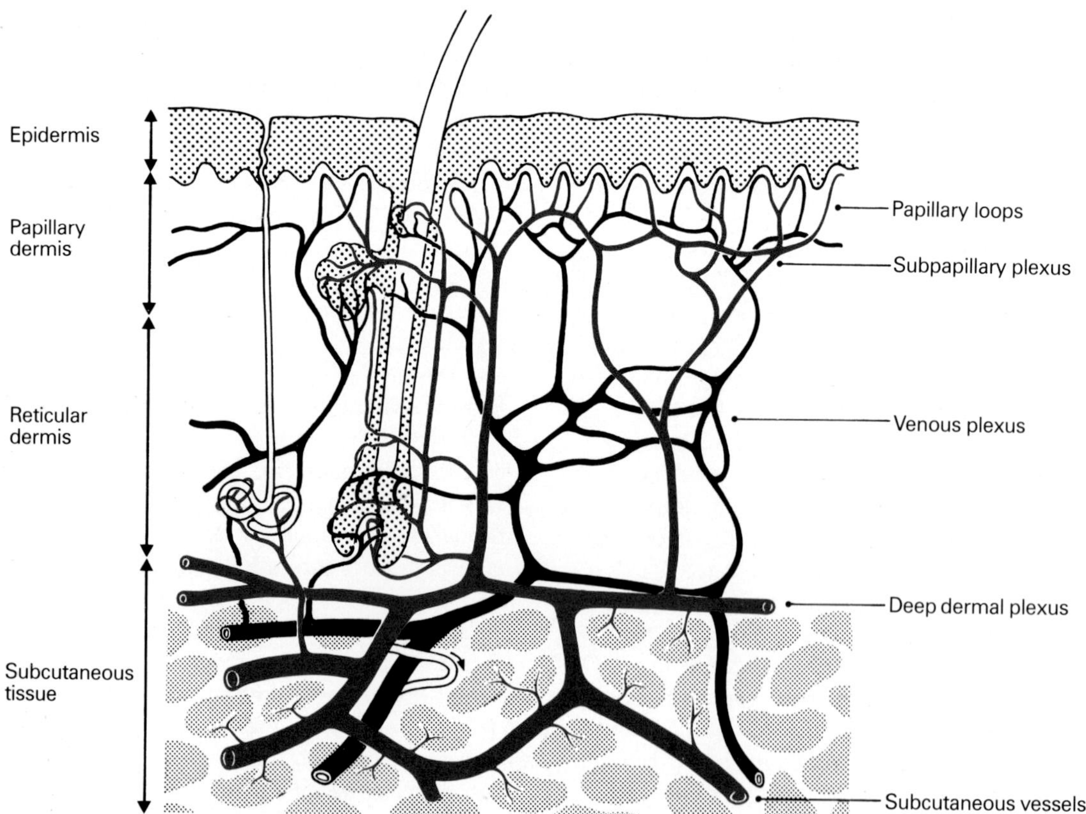

Fig. 2.6 A schematic representation of the cutaneous vascular bed.

CUTANEOUS VASCULAR PATTERNS

There is a vast literature on the subject of cutaneous vascular patterns in health and disease based on direct in vivo visualisation of vessels in implanted chambers and on large numbers of studies using the three principal post-mortem techniques of intravascular Indian ink injection, microradiography of injected barium sulphate, and alkaline phosphatase staining of capillary and arteriolar endothelium. Certain aspects of the anatomy of the dermal circulation revealed by these studies appear to be worth attention because of their possible relevance to circulation in flaps, but first the general pattern of organisation of the separate elements of the microcirculation will be presented.

The arterioles supplying the skin are derived from three sources; the direct cutaneous system of vessels, the musculocutaneous perforators and the fasciocutaneous system. These arterioles lie in the subcutaneous tissues and give off branches which form a network in the deep part of the dermis and on its undersurface (Fig. 2.6). The dermis is uneven where its outer surface contacts with the epidermis and is thrown up into dermal papillae which project into the concavities between the ridges on the deep surface of the epidermis. This sculptured portion of the dermis is termed the papillary layer, and the deeper main portion of the dermis is the reticular layer, which in certain sites may contain remnants of the panniculus carnosus (e.g. muscle fibres beneath areola, platysma, dartos and corrugator cutis ani). Whilst these two layers differ in terms of density of connective tissue, orientation of collagen fibres, content of cells and so on, it is also the case that they cannot generally be clearly separated. Similarly the undersurface of the reticular dermis blends into the subcutaneous tissues without a sharp boundary and therefore the overall thickness of the dermis cannot be measured exactly but it is approximately 1–2 mm overall, less on the eyelids (≤0.6 mm) and more on the soles and palms (≥2.5 mm). On the ventral surface of the trunk and limbs it is generally thinner than on the dorsal surface and it is thinner in females than in males.

The network of vessels which lies in and on the undersurface of this dermis (the 'deep plexus') gives off branches which supply the subcutaneous stratum with its fat cells, sweat glands and the deeper portions of the hair follicles. From the other side of this network vessels enter the dermis and form the denser *subpapillary network* at the junction of the papillary and reticular layers. (The subpapillary plexus is synonymous with the term 'horizontal network' or superficial plexus used by other authors.) This gives off small branches which form loops and plexi in the dermal papillae. Other synonyms for the *papillary loops* include 'subepidermal plexus', 'papillary plexus' and 'capillary loops'. The veins which collect the blood from the capillary loops form the first network of very thin veins immediately beneath the papillae and are part of the superficial plexus. It is this network of vessels which makes a substantial contribution to the colour of the skin. Then follow a number of flat networks of gradually enlarging veins at the junction between papillary and reticular layers of the dermis (the middle plexus) and also at the boundary between the dermis and the subcutaneous tissues where the venous network is once again on the same level as the arterial. The sebaceous and sweat glands have a dense network of capillaries surrounding their basement membranes from which veins enter this plexus. Each hair follicle similarly has an extensive capillary net around it and a knot of vessels within the dermal papilla of the hair bulb. (Note that the term dermal papilla is used both to described the dermal component of the hair bulb and also the dermal ridge containing the capillary loops supplying the epidermis.) From the deep network pass the large, independent, subcutaneous veins, and also the venae comitantes of the cutaneous arteries. Whilst the principle of arcading of vessels is not unique to skin and is in fact quite common on the venous side in other circulations, the arrangement of the arcades in layers is particular to the skin and can be related to general functions (Table 2.2). The way in which the arterioles subdivide, their mainly vertical orientation and the way in which they then link with the more horizontal subpapillary plexus from which further vertical capillary loops arise, has earned the cutaneous microcirculation the descriptive label of candelabra-shaped.

These plexi vary in importance and prominence in different areas of the body. The papillary loops are perpendicular to the surface of the skin except for those in the nailfold which are parallel to the surface and easily observable by direct microscopy. This has enabled extensive investigation of capillary flow and other parameters such as magnitude and time to onset of post-occlusive reactive hyperaemia by non-invasive means in health and disease (Tooke, 1984; Östergren & Fagrell, 1984; Bollinger et al, 1974).

Table 2.2 The layered arrangement of the vascular arcades

Location	Components	Principal functions
superficial plexus	arterial and venous	nutrition and heat exchange
middle plexus	mainly venous	heat exchange and defence (e.g. emigration of leucocytes)
deep plexus	arterial and venous	provides a bypass of the superficial plexus for heat conservation

The papillary loops have been studied in vivo for many years by a classical anatomical technique (Lewis, 1927) which consists of dehydrating the surface of a small patch of skin with alcohol, or blistering the cornified layers, applying a drop of bland oil and a glass coverslip, illuminating the skin with a concentrated beam of light, and examining it with a binocular microscope. Nowadays, the repeated application of Sellotape provides a quick and easy method for removing the cornified layers and by this technique it is possible to see not only the papillary loops but sometimes also the subpapillary plexus. By this, as well as the histological and injection methods referred to earlier, the much greater density of the subpapillary plexus and superficial papillary loops in the palms, the soles, and the tips of the fingers and toes has been established.

The papillary loops in other portions of the skin differ according to the development of the system of rete in the particular area such that where the epidermis is thin, and the rete ridges poorly developed, there are few papillary loops and a poor subpapillary plexus; this is the pattern found in the skin of the thigh and calf, on the nose, the forehead and temporal region, where the dermal–epidermal junction is nearly flat (Moretti et al, 1959). In the axilla and on the breast the loops may be short, while in the skin from the scapular region, sacral region and in the nail bed the loops may be attenuated and even have cross-shunts. It is the development of the rete ridges which correlates with the richness of the vascular supply and not the thickness of the epidermis. For example, in the forehead the epidermis is 45–65 μ thick and there are an average of 157 papillary loops per mm^2, while on the nose the epidermis is 75 μ thick and it has an average of 100 underlying papillary loops per mm^2.

Ageing. These observations must be qualified by the statement that dramatic changes may take place in the same region during the ageing process; this is particularly evident in the scalp. In the child and in the young man, the epidermal ridges of the scalp are pronounced and long papillary loops run through each of the dermal papillae. With advancing age, the dermal–epidermal junction flattens and the papillary loops are shorter and less abundant. In the bald scalp the epidermis is nearly flat along its base, with only a few low-lying arched capillaries beneath it (Ellis, 1958). A similar tendency towards reduction with age in the number of papillary loops present in the dermis has been noted in other areas such as the lower leg (Ryan & Kurban, 1970). In older skin there is also a tendency for the calibre of the vessels to increase, with aneurysmal dilatation of the loops.

Changes have also been demonstrated in the veil cells with ageing (Braverman & Fonferko, 1982). With increasing age there is a decrease in the number and synthetic activity of veil cells which correlates with the appearance of abnormally thin-walled vessels.

Changes in the vascular patterns

It might be asked whether these networks hold any importance for the surgeon. Information regarding the cutaneous microcirculatory vascular patterns may be relevant to the raising of skin flaps in various ways. The limit of viability in a skin flap which does not include an axial vessel or a plexus of fascial vessels with an axial component is determined mainly by the flow into it and along its length at the level of the deep dermal and subcutaneous plexi. Thus the much greater density of vessels in the reticular dermis of the face compared with any other region – a difference which may be up to five-fold when face and sole are compared – correlates with the greater reliability of flaps on the face and the greater length to breadth ratios of flaps that are possible here. In contrast, the much greater density of the subpapillary plexus and the superficial papillary loops in the palm and the sole compared with the face, would not be expected to correlate with greater viability of flaps on the palm and sole, since blood at these superficial levels is essentially flowing perpendicular to the skin surface with no capacity for flowing longitudinally parallel to the surface. This predominance of flow towards the surface accords with the more important role these areas have in heat regulation. Of course, all these vessels are involved in the first responses of the skin in wound healing; they undergo observable changes in various skin diseases including cutaneous malignancies and during ageing; the vessels are affected by radiation and burns; they appear to form new vessels during skin expansion with the inflatable Radovan-type tissue expander; and the vascular patterns are greatly altered in congenital haemangiomas, portwine stains, telangiectasia, spider naevi and other cutaneous vascular malformations.

In the portwine stain in particular there are specific anatomical changes in the vascular patterns, with the basic abnormalities being increases in the numbers of vessels and ectasia (dilated vessels) (Barsky et al, 1980). On vertical sections perpendicular to the surface, the number of vessels sharply decreases with depth beneath the surface and the majority of vessels are found in the dermis immediately beneath the epidermis. Ectasia, as measured by mean vessel area in histological sections perpendicular to the surface, reaches a maximum 0.2–0.4 mm beneath the epidermal/dermal junction (epidermal base averaged into a straight line); i.e.

portwine stains in respect of vessel numbers are superficial lesions, but in respect to vessel ectasia involve the vessels throughout the skin thickness. The conclusion is that the portwine stain is not a haphazard arrangement of vessels, but one with a characteristic architecture. Furthermore, the colour of the portwine stain is consistently related to the degree of vessel ectasia and the percentage of vessels containing erythrocytes (% fullness), i.e. the dark purple lesions have maximum % fullness. The lesion histologically evolves in an orderly and characteristic way with mean vessel area, vascular area, and % fullness all increasing with age which is consistent with clinical observations that the portwine stain darkens with advancing age, and that prominent ectasia is characteristic of the adult portwine stain. The 'orderliness' of such vascular patterns is significant in view of the trend towards laser treatment of these lesions. If the stain is related to only one plexus then treatment with laser radiation could markedly improve the condition, but if all plexuses are involved then destruction of one plexus may still result in at least the partial return of the condition after vascular regrowth. How these lesions develop is uncertain although histological studies suggest that aneurysmal dilatation and ectasia of an initially normal cutaneous vascular plexus occurs.

New vessel formation in skin is invariably an extension of preformed vessels and primary generation of vascular endothelium unassociated with previously formed vessels does not occur in the dermis. This raises the general question of what are the influences which bring about changes in vascular anatomy and new vessel formation? With the increasing interest developing in techniques of tissue expansion an added impetus has been given to the search for the mechanisms underlying these events. A number of studies on experimental animals have investigated the effects on epidermal proliferation and thickness of either uniaxial stretching using spring-loaded devices (Squier, 1980) or general stretching using the subcutaneous inflatable Radovan-type tissue expander (Austad et al, 1982) and some workers have carried out ultrastructural studies of the effects of tension on human skin (Brown, 1973) but the extent of knowledge about the effects of tension on the vascularity of skin are still very meagre.

Barnhill et al (1983) used a spring-loaded apparatus to apply uniaxial tension to forearm skin in 10 normal human subjects. Simultaneously, the effects of stretching on the upper dermal vasculature were observed stereomicroscopically. Progressive collapse was observed to take place in the vertical papillary loops and horizontal subpapillary plexus with increasing tension. Force and strains were recorded at the points of disappearance of virtually all vessels visualised. An average force of 11.9N, accompanied by a mean strain of 10.3%, resulted in occlusion of all vessels. This correlates with the obvious deleterious effects of tension on the survival of clinical skin flaps. Interestingly in this study, although almost all subjects were relatively young, there appeared to be a trend towards greater force being needed for vascular occlusion with advancing age. In contrast to these acute studies, experimental work on pigs (Cherry et al, 1983) and clinical experience in patients, indicate that skin expanded progressively over a period of about 5 weeks undergoes an increase in vascularity. This improved vascularity has been demonstrated experimentally by microangiography and has been suggested by an increased survival length in random flaps raised in expanded skin compared to unexpanded control skin. In patients, the appearance of the skin on removing an expander is often one of increased vascularity and the detailed changes in the dermal vascular patterns responsible for these appearances are under investigation.

The question of what the stimuli are which bring about increased vascularity is clearly an important one in this context. In general terms, new vessel formation is dependent on migration of endothelium and on mitosis of endothelial cells. Migration of endothelium probably accounts for much of the new vessel formation in the upper dermis. Perhaps the stretching 'opens' spaces in the tissues and enables vessels to extend by intercalation and formation of new sprouts. (Intercalation is the term used to describe elongation of capillary loops not by sprouting or mitosis, but by the migration of endothelial cells to new sites at a more distal location in the vessel wall.) This concept is supported by experiments which, from the way in which vessels tend to sprout into and extend along clefts in surrounding fibrin networks or connective tissue, suggest that vessels do tend to grow preferentially into areas of decreased resistance. A role for venous pressure or outflow obstruction in maintaining and encouraging capillary growth has also been postulated. Any tension or expansion technique will interfere with lymphatic drainage and perhaps there is a common pathway here in which exudation into the tissues with consequent changes in tissue proteins and tissue compliance becomes an important factor.

Mitosis also seems to be encouraged by stretching the cells, presumably through the intermediary of a chemical stimulus. There is considerable evidence for the existence of chemically mediated negative feedback control mechanisms for many mitotically active tissues and the activity of such epidermal chalones is presently receiving much attention in skin.

The immediate environment of the endothelial cell

2

obviously also plays a part in controlling mitotic activity and the relationship between the morphology of the papillary loops and the state (atrophy) of the epidermis already referred to, shows that the epidermis can influence its own blood supply. Ryan (1973) has repeatedly suggested that, in respect of papillary vessels, the epidermis produces vasoformative factors. Expanding the epidermis increases the metabolic activity of this layer and thereby may stimulate the endothelial cells but ischaemia and inflammation secondary to wounding and repair have also been suggested as stimuli. Ryan & Barnhill (1983) have listed some of the factors, both chemical and physical, which might be expected to influence the growth of new blood vessels and these are listed in Tables 2.3 & 2.4 which have been adapted from their published work.

From these few examples it can be seen that a knowledge of the normal cutaneous microvascular architecture is necessary in analysing some of the changes in cutaneous vascular patterns which the surgeon will encounter in clinical practice. The precise aetiology of these changes in the majority of cases remains unknown but constitutes an important field of investigation from which positive findings can be expected to yield clinically important applications in the future.

Table 2.3 Physical influences on growth of new blood vessels (Adapted with permission from Ryan & Barnhill, 1983)

1. *Mechanical tension*
   A. effects on cell shape and propensity for growth brought about by:
      (i) haemodynamic influences, e.g. vasodilatation
      (ii) axial stretching by outside forces
   B. effects on orientation of fibre and vascular networks, thereby providing orientated pathways for migration
2. *Substrata for endothelial migration*
   A. provided by structural elements such as fibrin, collagen and basement membrane
   B. effects on cellular adhesion and propensity for cellular migration and proliferation, e.g. fibronectin
3. *Nature of perivascular environment and its effects on facilitation or inhibition of vessel growth*
   A. cellular contact, e.g. by pericytes
   B. nature of basement membrane
   C. nature of interstitial tissue
4. *Temperature*
   A. effect on level of metabolic demands
   B. effect on compliance of tissue
   C. effect on blood viscosity

Table 2.4 Chemical influences on growth of new blood vessels (Adapted with permission from Ryan & Barnhill, 1983)

1. *Metabolic products*
2. *Inflammatory products*
   A. Cellular products:
      from neutrophils — proteases — free radicals — prostaglandins
      from lymphocytes — lymphokines
      from macrophages — proteases — prostaglandins — mitogens — 'monokines'
      from mast cells — histamine — heparin — prostaglandins — enzymes
      from platelets — histamine — serotonin — prostaglandins — ADP
   B. Products from tissue injury and circulation:
      — proteases — free radicals — prostaglandins — complement — coagulation
3. *Factors affecting cellular adhesion and/or migration*
   — fibronectin — laminin — proteases
4. *Tissue 'angiogenic' factors*
   from epidermis but also from certain other tissues
5. *Other growth factors*
   — fibroblast growth factor
   — epidermal growth factor

THE LYMPHATIC SYSTEM

Information regarding the anatomy and physiology of lymphatics in normal human skin is surprisingly incomplete, largely because of the difficulty of demonstrating these structures. On the basis of their structure, lymphatics may be broadly divided into three principal groups; lymphatic capillaries or initial lymphatics, collecting lymphatics and main lymph trunks.

Lymphatic capillaries

These begin blindly with glove-finger-like endings and form a closed endothelial tubular system in the sub-papillary dermis (Rusznyak et al, 1967). No definite statements can be made regarding the size of lymphatic capillaries because of their extraordinary distensibility and the fact that on routine histological sections they tend to be collapsed into cruciform of star-shapes. Another characteristic of lymphatic capillaries (and other lymphatics) is the shape of their endothelial cells which differ from those of blood capillaries in being larger and irregularly shaped with peculiar dentate-patterned edges when seen 'en face'. These irregular cell margins are demonstrable by silver impregnation techniques which show up the intercellular cement substance which is continuous with the ground substance of the connective tissue surrounding lymph capillaries. Another feature particular to lymphatics is the presence of collagen fibres which are attached to the endothelial cells and project outwards from them into the surrounding connective tissue. This is thought to be a feature of functional importance responsible for ensuring that when the tissue pressure rises, the lymphatics, instead of being compressed, become distended. Stretching of the connective tissue fibres pulls the endothelial cells apart so that openings of the order of 100 nm and occasionally much longer, permit tissue fluid or blood cells to pass unimpeded into the lymphatics. These lymphatic capillaries lie mainly in the dermis – some probably lie in the dermal papillae – and show varying degrees of development. Most developed are those in the skin of the finger, the palm, the sole and the scrotum where numerous papillae are present. Most of the dermal lymphatic capillaries, however, lie in two lymph plexi, a superficial and a deeper. The superficial plexus consists of small, thin vessels and is found in the papillary dermis near the subpapillary arterial network. The deeper plexus is composed of thicker lymphatics of varying calibres, and lies in the deep reticular part of the dermis near the subcutis.

Collecting lymphatics

Arising from the deeper dermal plexus of lymph capillaries are lymph collectors which possess valves. Except for the smallest ones these lymphatics possess, like other vessels, a wall consisting of three layers – intima, media and adventitia (Boggon & Palfrey, 1973). The endothelial cells of the intima are separated from the tunica media by a thin subendothelium mainly composed of collagen fibres with a few elastic fibres. The media is formed by smooth muscle cells, separated only by small numbers of collagen fibres. Elastic fibres are relatively frequent in the adventitia; blood vessels and nerves are confined to the adventitia.

Lymph trunks

The large lymph trunks have a greater number of well developed smooth muscle fibres forming walls which resemble not so much those of veins as those of arteries. However, where lymph vessels as distinct from capillaries are concerned, it is neither the appearance of muscle fibres nor the three layers of the muscle wall (of which the smallest lymph vessels are still devoid) nor their greater calibre which characterises them, but the appearance of valves. These vessels are anastomotically connected to the subcutaneous connective tissue lymphatics where lymph capillaries are sparse, and in turn lead into major lymph trunks. These, like large blood vessels, possess their own nutrient vessels and are surrounded by a capillary network and may be accompanied by an artery and a vein. The superficial lymph vessels tend not to cross fascial planes and show a tendency to run close alongside blood vessels in the loose tissues of the perivascular spaces.

The superficial lymphatics of the skin and subcutaneous tissues are separated from the deep lymphatics by the deep fascia, particularly where it is dense and strong as in the lower limb. Peripheral anastomoses between the superficial and deep sets of vessels are practically insignificant, and on the limbs the two unite only proximally where the main collecting trunks of the superficial set pass through gaps in the deep fascia to enter the underlying tissues, e.g. the cribriform fascia in the femoral triangle. The recognition of this fact formed the basis for the Thompson operation for lymphoedema introduced in 1963 in which excision of a long strip of the deep fascia is combined with infolding of a de-epithelialised dermal strip through the fascial defect into the muscles. It was originally thought that this would promote the formation of anastomoses between the obstructed superficial lymphatics and the deep lymphatics or even result in the lymphatics in the de-epithelialised skin flap linking up with blood vessels in the intramuscular spaces so making lymphovenous shunts, both processes thereby providing alternative routes for lymph drainage of the skin. Kinmonth (1982), however, has been unable to demonstrate either of these processes by postoperative lymphography and favours the massaging effect of the muscles on the buried flap during exercise as being the principal mechanism producing the beneficial effect from the Thompson procedure, aided by the general increase in tissue tension and the elimination of stagnant pools of tissue fluid in relatively avascular subcutaneous tissues.

Valves are the most important and obviously characteristic feature of the mammalian lymphatic system and it is obviously due to the valves that lymph flow is unidirectional and centripetal. In 1885 Sappey succeeded in demonstrating the presence in cadavers of 60–80 valves in an average lymph vessel running along the length of the upper limb and as many as 80–100 in vessels along the lower limb, i.e. about 1 every centimetre, although the distance between adjacent valves is obviously much less in the smaller lymphatics. Of themselves the valves do not produce flow but only determine its direction unless the vessels are so dilated that the valves become incompetent when retrograde flow may occur. In the interstitial tissues every pulsation of arterial walls or movement due to muscular activity or breathing, as well as vibration and massage exerted by external forces tend to stretch, bend or twist the fibrous connective tissue network and squeeze fluid from between its strands. Some of this escapes into the lymphatics through the junctions between endothelial cells which tend to open under the tension of the fibrils. Thereafter, direct compression of lymphatics from the contraction of surrounding muscles, massage by the tissue, and transmitted pulsations from adjacent blood vessels all tend to produce lymph flow. The importance of the pressure changes is further demonstrated by the fact that in the absence of solid tissue movement the hydrostatic pressure in the tissues is insufficient in itself to maintain movement of tissue fluid into and along lymphatics. In a moving limb this flow has been estimated at 0.003ml/min per 100 g of tissue (Jacobsson & Kjellmer, 1964) originating mainly from muscle and the average values for intra-lymphatic vessel pressures range between –0.7 mm of mercury (Allen, 1938) and –2 mm of mercury (Blocker et al, 1959).

The extent of the intralymphatic pressure changes which must inevitably take place in an elevated flap have not been measured, although measurements have been made in limbs suffering from lymphatic obstruction (Kinmonth, 1982). In the context of both lymphatically obstructed limbs and skin flaps, the question of whether or not lymphatic to venous communications develop becomes a significant consideration. The general view is that they normally exist at a peripheral level in certain animals but in man only in some lymph nodes. Communications between lymph vessels and veins have been sought in cadavers (Threefoot et al, 1963) and patients (Edwards & Kinmonth, 1969) with the result that they were demonstrable in humans only if some pathological condition had previously imposed some form of obstruction or stress on the lymphatic system, otherwise (i.e. in the normal individual) they were not demonstrable.

Lymphaticovenous communications may develop pathologically in the periphery but those that have been demonstrated were more common at or above the level of the kidneys and probably represented enlargements of pathways normally present but non-functional (and non-demonstrable) except under the stress of chronically increased volume or pressure within the lymphatics. Lymphovenous communications have not been definitively demonstrated to develop in flaps in which the major part of the lymphatic drainage has been interrupted although their development has been suggested by animal experiments. Lymphatico-venous communications may, however, be created surgically either by end-to-side anastomosis of lymphatics to veins or between sectioned lymph nodes and veins (Clodius, 1977; O'Brien et al, 1978).

The ability of lymphatics in skin flaps to link up with lymphatics of surrounding tissues is another important consideration, and has been exploited clinically since 1935 when Gillies introduced the concept of the lymphatic wick. Gillies elevated a flap on the upper limb and inset it into the lateral side of the thigh and abdomen in order to bypass a lymphatic block at the junction of the lower limb and the trunk, and thereby promote lymph drainage from the leg to the axilla. This functioned successfully over a 15-year follow-up (Gillies & Fraser, 1950). On the contralateral side, instead of an arm flap, an abdominal tube pedicle was raised and transferred but the procedure was unsuccessful. Two interesting features of these flaps, probably directly related to their success and failure, were the effect of scar tissue on the formation of lympho-lymphatic anastomoses (clearly much more scar tissue was formed with the delayed abdominal tube pedicle), and the axiality of the lymphatics in the flaps relative to the lymphatics in the recipient areas. Both considerations raise questions that are relevant to the development of lympho-lymphatic anastomoses between any flap and its surroundings. Although not investigated in man, some experimental work with a rabbit ear preparation has been carried out by Oden in an attempt to determine the influence of these factors (Oden, 1960, 1961). Using a circular rabbit skin autograft inset into a circular defect in the rabbit ear, Oden showed with microlymphangiography that link-ups did occur, but at 84 days after transplantation only coarse irregular lymphatics, constricted by surgical scar tissue, were present between the recipient site and the autograft. To investigate the importance of the axiality of the lymphatics Oden returned the circular full-thickness skin grafts to their beds, either with or without rotation. If not rotated, lympho-lymphatic anastomoses occurred and lymph was carried through the graft by a large lymph collector. If, however, the graft was rotated out of the general lymph flow axis of the rabbit ear by only 30°, then several lymph collectors did form lympho-lymphatic communications, but the lymph from the ear did not traverse the graft and instead returned towards the base of the ear by a system of dilated collaterals around the margins of the graft. The alignment of lymphatics in free flaps transferred into an area of lymphatic block is therefore significant and may be added to the factors postulated by Smith & Conway (1962) as essential for successful lymph-bearing flaps: (1) the inclusion of major lymphatics in adequate number; (2) provision of intimate contact between the functioning lymphatics distal to the site of obstruction and those of the pedicle; and (3) minimal scar at the site of junction of lymphatics between the pedicle and the diseased areas.

2 FUNCTIONAL ORGANISATION OF THE MICROCIRCULATION

Just as the traditional idea of anatomy as a body of knowledge obtained by dissection of the cadaver has been superseded by a modern discipline incorporating knowledge gained from a variety of histological, cytological, chemical and dynamic studies, so it is that an understanding of the anatomical vascular basis of skin flaps similarly extends beyond the narrow confines of structure to a wider understanding of the principles of function of the microcirculation. In this section an attempt is made to review some of these more physiological aspects of the blood supply to skin although it must be recognised that not only is this a superficial overview but that there are many facts which still remain to be elucidated. Until more is understood about the physiology of what is happening to blood flow and cellular metabolism in pedicled and free flaps, it is likely that the response of the clinician to problems such as that of a failing flap will be based largely on empiricism. Even now, after many years of research, the physiological basis of the delay phenomenon remains enigmatic and the risk exists that the technical abilities of surgeons to accomplish increasingly complex tissue manipulations will outstrip their understanding of what effects these manoeuvres are having at a cellular level.

Although the functional aspects particular to the dermal, as compared to any other, part of the microcirculation include thermoregulatory, blood 'storage' and specific defence mechanisms (Table 2.5), this section is concerned solely with the dynamic role of the microcirculation as it encompasses two elements: (1) control of blood flow, and (2) transcapillary fluid exchange. The exchange of CO_2 and O_2 takes place passively by virtue of the solubility and diffusibility of these gases in tissue components, including the vascular wall and are not considered here. Many of the

Table 2.5 Distinctive functional features of the dermal microcirculation

Thermoregulation
— dissipation of heat via blood stream
— response to ambient temperature
— cold reaction (heat conservation)
Reservoir function
— exercise, shock, emotions
Defence mechanisms
— leakage of complement, immunoglobulins, contact factors
— leucocyte emigration
— hypersensitivity

governing factors in these two dynamic processes are poorly understood. We shall first give an account of the principal mechanisms controlling blood flow in the cutaneous microcirculation and then examine various factors which are likely to significantly affect the flow in skin flaps.

CONTROL OF BLOOD FLOW

It is clear that the cutaneous blood flow must fulfil both the metabolic needs of the skin and the thermoregulatory requirements of the body, but the principal determinant of blood flow in the normal 'resting' state is the requirement for thermal homeostasis. Plethysmographic measurements on whole fingers provide an approximate quantitative measurement of the cutaneous blood flow since fingers have no muscle and only a small amount of blood flowing to bone and tendon. Such measurements have shown that the minimum value for fingers, obtained under conditions of intense vasoconstriction due to exposure to cold, is of the order of 0.5–1.0 ml/min per 100 ml tissue (Burton, 1939). The mean flow is much higher than this – values of 20 to 30 times the minimum as a rule* – while the maximum flow rates in vasodilation are over 100 times the minimum value. The conclusions drawn from this data derived from finger measurements are by no means applicable to the skin of other areas of the body, where it is known that important structural differences exist in the vascular bed of the skin. Nevertheless, from these and other measurements such as those on the O_2 consumption of viable pieces of skin, it can be estimated that 0.8 ml of blood/min per 100 ml of tissue would be perfectly adequate to supply the oxygen requirements of skin. Yet the average skin blood flow is around 20 ml/min per 100 g (with considerable regional differences) in the 'resting' state of thermal equilibrium (i.e. when naked and exposed to an environmental temperature of 25–30°C) and the maximum possible values are several times greater than this.

It is therefore clear that the skin is normally relatively 'overperfused' with blood, although not equally so in all areas since in a thermally comfortable subject nearly one-half of skin blood flow is distributed to the hands, feet and head. These are the regions with the highest densities of AVAs – as has already been described – and the greatest potential range of variation in blood flow. In the normal state these and indeed all A – V shunts and precapillary sphincters in the cutaneous circulation possess a considerable degree of basal tone which maintains these vessels in a state of partial constriction. Even after sympathectomy skin blood flow remains far below the maximum possible levels indicating that the smooth muscle activity is maintained even in the absence of nervous control. Although blood-borne excitatory and inhibitory humoral agents might be involved in this basal tone it is accepted that some activity results from intrinsic membrane instability of single-unit or 'pacemaker' cells in the vessel walls. This basic tone may then be facilitated or overridden by neural, hormonal, thermal and local factors (Fig. 2.7).

*The values found, when expressed per 100 ml of tissue, depend upon whether just the finger tip, giving the highest values, or two terminal phalanges are included.

Myogenic theory

According to the Myogenic theory associated with the name of Bayliss (1902), the smooth muscle cells in the vessel wall are partially constricted in response to distension, even under conditions when there is no innervation or exposure to blood-borne vasoactive agents. Since the vasculature would normally be in a state of partial constriction, a decrease in distending pressure would result in relaxation and a lowering of vascular resistance, whilst an increase in transmural pressure would increase resistance. In both cases the myogenic responsiveness of the precapillary vessels would tend to keep blood flow constant through the capillary bed. The mechanism of the myogenic response has not yet been fully established but it has often been suggested that wall tension might be the controlling parameter. According to this hypothesis, vascular smooth muscle is composed of two series-coupled functional units; a contractile element and a passively distensible sensory element. The sensory element is stimulated by an increase in wall tension, which in turn causes an increase in the activity of the contractile element.

The myogenic responsiveness of the vascular smooth muscle may be important not only in controlling flow through the capillaries, but also in controlling the amount of fluid filtered out of the capillaries. An increase in transmural pressure would increase filtration out of the capillaries, resulting in the formation of oedema, but the myogenic responsiveness of the precapillary vessels would tend to reduce hydrostatic pressure in the capillaries and therefore attenuate oedema formation.

Myogenic control does play a role in regulating skin blood flow and is thought to be the explanation for the eventual return of the cutaneous vascular resistance towards control levels following sympathectomy. Similarly, it is thought to be the mechanism underlying the reflex hyperaemia following transient occlusion of blood flow to the skin. It is unlikely that accumulation of vasodilator metabolites would be an important mechanism of control in such a situation since the metabolic rate of skin is very low. For the same reason it is felt that myogenic control is the principal mechanism responsible for cutaneous autoregulation (defined as the maintenance of a constant blood flow in the face of changes in perfusion pressure although the term is also used to describe the continuous local adjustment of blood flow in proportion to the need of the tissue for nutrients). The autoregulatory capability of the cutaneous vasculature is much more limited than that of other organs such as skeletal muscle, myocardium and brain, and autoregulation does not occur in skin when perfusion pressure is lower than 100 mmHg.

Endothelium-mediated vasoconstriction

Although the myogenic theory has been around for many years it is only recently that a more pharmacological explanation for vasoconstrictor tone has been developed based on the idea that the endothelium can mediate vasoconstriction via the production of contracting factors. These factors appear to be released in response to various chemical and physical stimuli such as noradrenaline, thrombin, high extracellular potassium, hypoxia and stretch. In response to stretch, endothelial Ca^{++} channels have been described and these may operate as mechanotransducers (Lansman et al, 1987). Thus, the role of endothelial cells in generation of vasoconstrictor tone may be twofold, sensory and effector, and this may occur independently of any additional vasoconstrictor action brought about by extraneous vasoactive substances (see p. 43).

Venivasomotor reflex

A further local reflex, additional to the myogenic one, has more recently been accepted to account for the observation that when the limbs are lowered, blood flow through the skin and subcutaneous tissues of the hands and feet is reduced and for the similar reductions that result when venous pressure is increased. The mechanism is much more than just retrograde filling of the capillary bed limiting inflow, and involves an increase in tone in arteriolar resistance vessels. A local nervous reflex mechanism has been proposed to account for this (Henriksen, 1976a, b). It has been noted to persist for up to four days following sympathectomy but disappears after this time, and has been found to be impaired in various conditions including diabetes mellitus. The exact nature of this venivasomotor reflex

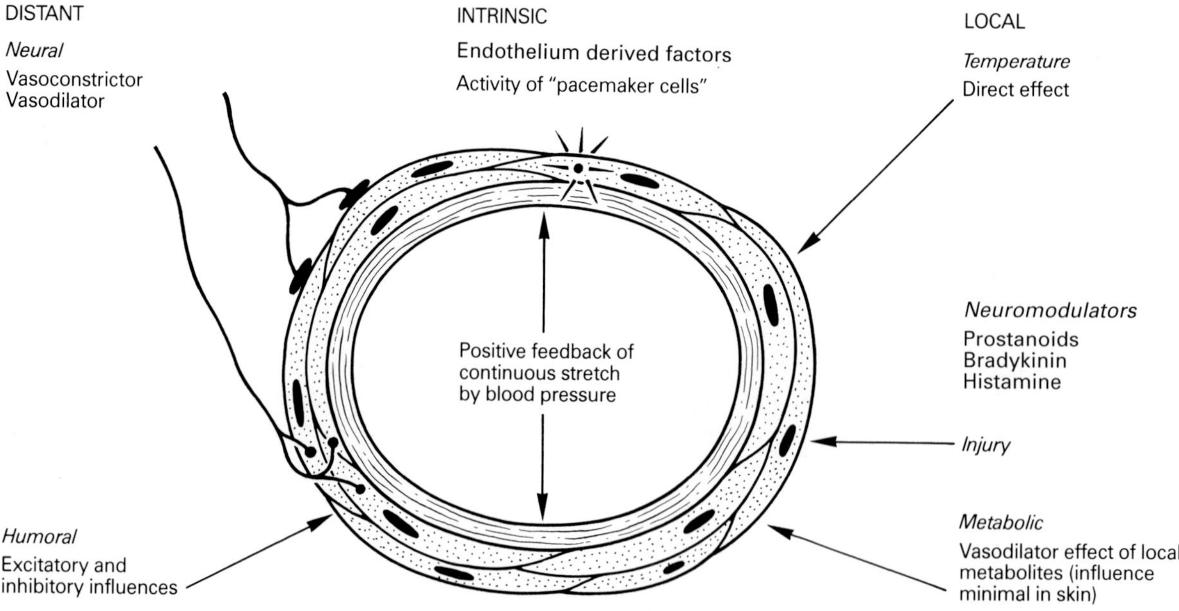

Fig. 2.7 Influences on basal vascular tone. Myogenic 'pacemaker' activity is reinforced by the continuous stretch offered by the blood pressure and via cell-to-cell excitation spread constitutes the basal vascular tone. Extrinsic excitatory and inhibitory factors modulate and sometimes dominate the local control systems.

remains obscure and its role in the congested skin flap is open to speculation.

Neural control

The earliest idea that cutaneous vessel diameters were influenced by nerves arose out of observation of the emotional blushing response. Its suddenness and vividness suggested specific vasodilator fibres but even now the blushing response is not satisfactorily explained and it is not entirely impossible to rule out an effect of kallidin-bradykinin, released from sweat glands which are suddenly activated by corticohypothalamic excitation via cholinergic sympathetic nerves. Conversely, emotional stress of the type provoking the so-called 'defence reaction' may produce the opposite of blushing, with adrenergic cutaneous vasoconstriction, often in association with perspiration ('cold sweat'). Much more important than these temporary neural reactions affecting the cutaneous microcirculation are the cardiovascular homeostatic reflexes initiated from atrial (volume) receptors and carotid sinus (pressure) receptors which provide overall remote control. Acting through medullary 'centres' these provide steady control of the vascular bed through sympathetic vasoconstrictor fibres which affect the level of basal tone resulting from myogenic activity. The cutaneous circulatory effects of exercise and severe deep pain which bring about reflex changes in blood pressure and heart rate are also mediated through this system. Finally, the thermoregulatory hypothalamic neurones provide graded and selective adjustments of the sympathetic constrictor discharge to the skin vessels. At the level of the cutaneous vessels the effects are brought about by alpha (vasoconstrictor) and beta (vasodilator) adrenergic receptors and although their relative distribution in man is not absolutely certain it appears that the majority of adrenergic receptors are of the alpha type (Brownlee, 1966).

The ways in which noradrenaline and other constrictor hormones cause contraction of blood vessels are reasonably clear in outline, through only a few of the details have been established with certainty. The initial event following binding of noradrenaline to the alpha-receptors appears to be a chemical one. The succeeding stages of activation require calcium (Ca) to be present either in the extracellular fluid or in the cells, and lead to smooth muscle contraction largely by increasing the concentration of free Ca in the cytoplasm. These events are summarised in Figure 2.8.

The gross electrical changes produced by vasodilators are in general the reverse of those produced by vasoconstrictors. Beta-adrenergic stimulation produces relaxation of arteries partly by hyperpolarising them and partly by other means. How this is brought about is unclear but the effect of hyperpolarisation must be the reverse of the entry of Ca which follows the depolarisation induced by the action of vasoconstrictor agents or by other means. Responses of vessels to beta-adrenergic stimulation are often inconveniently small, and most studies on dilator mechanisms have used artificial agents rather than natural hormones. The initial actions of vasodilators on the smooth muscle cell seem to involve a chemical event in the membrane involving sulphydryl groups (SH). In the case of beta-adrenergic stimulation and of responses to diazoxide, hydralazine, nitroprusside and the physiological vasodilator adenosine, these initial events probably lead to production of cAMP and/or cGMP. Such increases have been attributed to activation of the enzymes which produced them (adenylyl cyclase and guanylyl cyclase), rather than to inhibition of phosphodiesterases which destroy them. Evidence that cAMP and cGMP relax smooth muscle cells is in short supply but the concept is supported by the fact that papaverine and other inhibitors of phosphodiesterase, greatly increase the concentration of both cAMP and cGMP in smooth muscles, and cause powerful relaxation. Papaverine is in fact one of the most powerful of all relaxant agents in large arteries.

The non-electrical component of the relaxation produced by vasodilator agents may in theory involve increased expulsion of Ca, either indirectly by accelerating pumping of Ca from the cell and so lowering intracellular Ca, or directly by stimulating an ATP-driven Ca pump. Either process could also account for the hyperpolarisation often produced by dilator agents. In practice there is no clear evidence that vasodilator agents do reduce either intracellular Na or Ca and it is therefore doubtful if movements of Ca across the cell membrane play much part in responses to

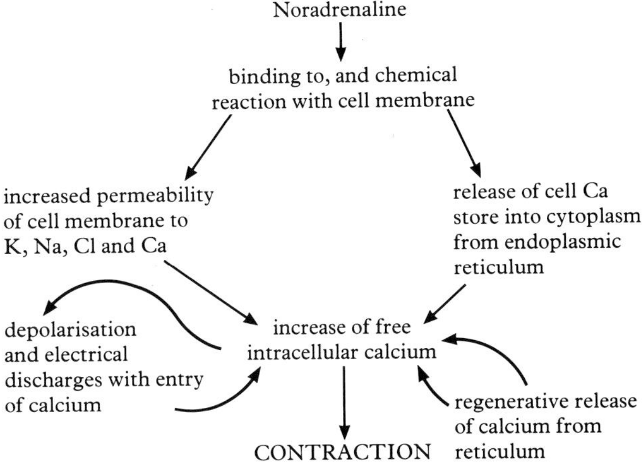

Fig. 2.8 Events leading to the contractile response to noradrenaline.

vasodilator drugs. Even if Ca is not moving across cell membranes it is still possible that vasodilator agents could lower cytoplasmic Ca by causing its increased uptake by endoplasmic reticulum, a mechanism that would be mediated by the increases in cAMP and cGMP. In any case there are indications that part of the mechanical dilator response is brought about by means independent of a fall in free cytoplasmic Ca. For example, activation of a phosphorylase (present in cells) could dephosphorylate the P light chain of smooth muscle myosin, and lead to relaxation at a given level of Ca. These considerations are relevant to the use of Ca-channel blocking drugs as vasodilators when applied topically to vessel anastomoses in free flap surgery.

General effects of temperature

The general conclusion to be drawn from quantitative data is that from the point of view of its own metabolic needs, the skin is tremendously 'overperfused' with blood, and that the purpose of this 'extra' flow lies in thermoregulation. The total skin blood flow in man exposed to cold may be reduced by sympathetic vasoconstriction to 20 ml/min or even less, so that almost the full heat-insulating power of the skin and fat is realised. Conversely, during maximal heat stress the skin blood flow may be some 3 l/min, thereby transferring heat to the overlying epithelium and also delivering the raw materials for sweat secretion (which may reach 1–2 l/hour). From the epithelium heat is conducted to the surface from where it is lost by radiative, conductive and evaporative pathways. This thermoregulatory function of the cutaneous circulation was first stated in 1882 by Leon Fredericq.

The control mechanisms governing thermoregulatory cutaneous blood flow are mainly neural and chemical in nature. In general it is the thermoregulatory hypothalamic centres which dominate except that different areas of skin respond differently and some hardly at all (Ström, 1960). The neuronal pathways act upon two separate elements of the cutaneous vascular bed – the sympathetic vasoconstrictor fibres dominate the 'specialised' A–V anastomoses which are mainly confined to skin areas in the face, hands and feet, while general vasoconstrictor discharge produces basal tone in the 'regular' cutaneous vessels, which are present everywhere. Reduction of flow in these latter cutaneous vessels is induced by vasoconstrictor discharge, whereas 'active' dilation beyond the basal level is secondary mainly, if not only, to the release of bradykinin which occurs when sweat glands are excited. In any discussion of precapillary behaviour or the phenomena associated with vessel tone and reactivity, problems of communication arise because of the various terms which have been used to described the state of a vessel. Suggested definitions for some of the terms used to describe changes in vascular tone and spasm are summarised in Figure 2.9.

With a gradual increase in heat load, first the A–V anastomoses of the ears and hands dilate due to inhibition of discharge of the vasoconstrictor fibres which supply them aided by the fact that the anastomoses are more sensitive to neurogenic discharge than are the 'ordinary' skin vessels. Then the anastomoses of the feet dilate, and gradually the vasoconstrictor fibres to the more proximal skin areas begin to reduce their discharge. If the increase in flow due to reduction of vasoconstrictor discharge is insufficient to restore heat balance, then the sweat glands become active. Again, this shows a geographical pattern, sweating usually starting on the forehead. Next, the vasodilation becomes greatly intensified in skin areas that lack A–V shunts and whose basal vascular tone is high in resting conditions. This increased dilation is induced by kinin formation and serves the dual purpose

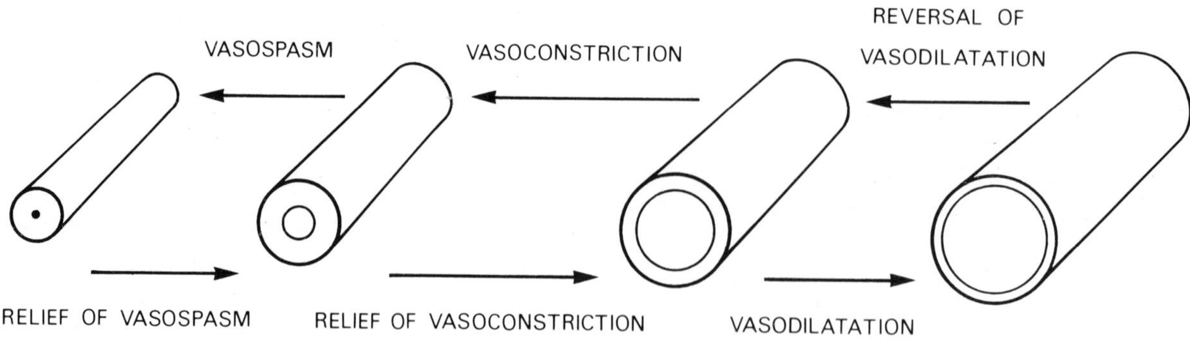

Fig. 2.9 Suggested definitions of terms to be used when describing work on vascular spasm. (Reproduced with permission from Roberts, 1984.)

of delivering enough blood flow to the sweat glands to provide the fluid they secrete and of providing a sufficient delivery of heat to the skin to warm it, thereby rendering the evaporative loss of heat more efficient in terms of heat elimination. By contrast in cool air (22°C) individuals initially lose heat from the periphery, but later maintain heat balance by an increase of metabolism due to shivering. The reverse order of shut-down is seen.

Using these mechanisms, a normal individual can regulate body temperature very adequately between about 15 and 40°C. However, patients may be subject to a variety of endogenous and external influences which affect their ability to respond. An environment that is both hot and damp interferes with the efficiency of the heat loss mechanisms and indeed patients have died in burns units from hyperthermia because much of their body surface was wrapped in gamgee and cotton wool dressings. Disorders of the nervous system may also seriously interfere with thermoregulatory capability. Guttman et al (1958) reported experiments on four patients with complete transections of the spinal cord above the level of the thoracolumbar sympathetic outflow who had all been bed-patients for many months since their injury at the air temperatures prevailing in the non-air-conditioned wards in Britain in 1958. When put into an air temperature of 36–37°C the rectal temperatures of these naked patients with cervical lesions rose to 38.5°C in $1\frac{1}{2}$ hours when distress and panting were present. At an air temperature of 18–20°C their rectal temperatures fell to 35.5°C in $1\frac{1}{2}$–2 hours. Normal subjects by comparison have no difficulty in thermoregulating over this range. The effects of the ambient temperature can also be important on the hypovolaemic patient. After severe blood loss, patients in normal thermoequilibrium show marked reflex vasoconstriction of their skin vessels. The exposure of such a patient to a heat load is dangerous because 'thermally' enforced cutaneous vasodilatation tends to overcome this reflex vasoconstriction.

Local direct effects of temperature

The neuronal reflexes described above are under the control of thermoregulatory hypothalamic centres and are the dominant influence regulating blood flow through the skin of the body as a whole. Nevertheless it is also the case that local direct effects, particularly of temperature, are important. This is especially relevant to plastic surgery where, for example, the heating effect of theatre lights on an operative site, or the cooling effect on a flap of being elevated in an operating theatre maintained at a temperature of 19–24°C, may well be significant. Even a slight increase in local skin temperature can produce a substantial increase in skin blood flow which is independent of any change in nutrient flow due to increased metabolism, while a drop in temperature has the opposite effect. These local changes in flow are brought about by changes in the calibre of resistance vessels and by changes in blood viscosity. The change in viscosity is small in relation to the changes in flow generally observed, and is of minor significance in producing them, but in low flow conditions when compensatory vasodilatation reaches a maximum, then blood viscosity may become a determinant of tissue perfusion (Schmid-Schönbein, 1981).

Much work has been done on the effects of local skin cooling. Classical experiments on the immersed finger have shown that cooling to less than 15°C produces vasoconstriction, but cooling greater than this with the temperature maintained below 12°C for several minutes, results in vasodilatation which may increase blood flow to greatly above resting levels (Hertzman, 1953).

With *moderate cooling* (down to 12–15°C) the vasoconstriction is partly the result of reflexes initiated by skin temperature receptors which result in noradrenaline release from sympathetic nerve endings on cutaneous vessels, but in addition there is a direct action of cold on vascular smooth muscle. The direct effects of low temperatures are illustrated by the vasoconstrictor response to cold seen in patients with Raynaud's disease, even after the sympathetic nerves have been cut. Since this was first pointed out by Lewis in 1927, many investigators have repeated the observation that normal blood vessels can produce a constrictor response to moderate cold even after denervation. Although the constriction usually lasts only for a few minutes in large arteries (Smith, 1952), in resistance vessels the effect often lasts for as long as the temperature remains low. The mechanism of these direct constrictor effects of moderate cold is not fully established, but arterial smooth muscle is depolarised by cooling (Keatinge, 1964). The depolarisation is likely to be due to halting of the Na pump, with immediate cessation of the electrogenic effect of the pump and a slower secondary depolarisation due to gain of Na and loss of K by the cells. It presumably causes contraction in turn by allowing entry of Ca and perhaps by releasing endoplasmic Ca. In innervated blood vessels another factor in the vasoconstrictor action of cold is prolongation of the action of noradrenaline released by vasomotor nerves, since removal of the noradrenaline from the tissue is delayed at low temperature. This fact was first suggested by experiments on cutaneous veins of dogs in which it was shown that cooling did not cause constriction, but if the vein was constricted by electrical stimulation or the application of noradrenaline then cooling below 37°C augmented the constriction and warming depressed it (Vanhoutte & Shepherd, 1970).

With more *severe cooling* to below 12°C for 2–10 minutes the response is different. Instead of vasoconstriction, the phenomenon of 'cold vasodilatation' appears, in which there are periods of intense vasoconstriction alternating with periods of vasodilatation. This was first described by Lewis in 1930. He showed that the dilatation was very localised, taking place in his experiments in the finger cooled but not in an adjacent finger which remained at a temperature above 12°C. The reaction usually started about 5 minutes after the finger was cooled, and was then intermittent, being interrupted every few minutes by waves of vasodilatation.

Cold vasodilatation occurs to different degrees in different skin areas, even with a given degree of surface cooling. The characteristic dramatic pattern of cold vasodilatation occurs in the extremities, the fingers, toes and ears, and although equivalent reactions do not occur in more proximal areas there is evidence that some degree of cold vasodilatation may take place (Clarke et al, 1958). This distribution reflects that of the arteriovenous anastomoses which are usually the first vessels to open at the beginning of cold vasodilatation. Cold vasodilatation has been demonstrated in chronically denervated fingers (Greenfield et al, 1951) and it has been concluded that the response is not dependent on nerves, although it is much larger when the nerves are functioning. Instead, it is thought to result from direct cold-induced paralysis of the peripheral blood vessels, by interfering with the early stages of noradrenaline interaction with the cell membrane. Other incompletely tested possibilities remain; for example, it may be that the coldness results in a higher blood viscosity which slows the flow through papillary loops. This could cause a higher pressure at the arterio-venous anastomoses and open these structures. The increased flow through the AVAs could then warm the capillary blood by conduction and start a new cycle. The reason why the vessels do not dilate immediately they are cooled below 12°C is because low temperature also has a direct effect on the actinomyosin in arteries, slowing its rate of relaxation following an active contraction.

Effects of temperature on experimental skin flaps

Clearly many of these findings are relevant to pedicled and/or free flaps, particularly in the range of moderate cooling which may occur clinically. Several workers have reported on the fall in blood flow which takes place on raising flaps (Fujino, 1969; Tsuchida et al, 1978, 1981). To minimise any additional fall in perfusion which might compromise the viability of the flap it is necessary to counteract cooling of the flap and of the patient. The effect of moderate cooling on the skin blood flow in the experimental dog saphenous flap model has been investigated and the flow found to vary directly with local temperature (Awwad et al, 1983). The temperature-dependent rate of change of flow in the saphenous flaps (termed the Thermal Sensitivity Index (TSI)) was 0.0341°C^{-1} which can be interpreted as meaning that the blood flow changed at a rate of 3.4% per degree Centigrade. Below 22°C and above 38°C the rate of change became greater.

Furthermore, both free flaps and island flaps (which had an intact nerve supply) behaved in the same way, reinforcing the concept that the direct action of cold on vascular smooth muscle may be more important than the nervous reflex. It was also shown that during the period of elevation of the flap (averaging 42.5 ± 5.3 SD minutes) there was considerable heat loss from it as shown by a fall in its temperature and this was accompanied by a decrease in blood flow. This fall in perfusion could be as high as 27% depending on the flap's TSI and the actual temperature drop. It therefore seems logical to suggest that deliberate measures should be taken to keep a flap warm, i.e. at its normal temperature. This conflicts with older studies which led to the claim that hypothermia was beneficial because it reduced flap metabolism (Kiehn & DesPrez, 1960). As pointed out by McGregor (1980): 'cooling of the flap is felt by some physicians to be of value, but the fact that it has not caught on suggests that this is doubtful'.

Local injury

Injury to a part of the arterial wall can completely override basal vascular tone and cause spasm. This has been known since John Hunter's day and there is no doubt that arterial injuries frequently seal off without intervention by going into spasm, whereas damaged veins cease to haemorrhage largely by the formation of clots.

Vasoconstrictor nerves would appear to be an obvious means whereby such arterial smooth muscle contraction might be produced, but in practice it has been found that injury can cause arteries to contract even after their sympathetic nerve supply has been blocked by local anaesthetics or tetrodotoxin (Graham & Keatinge, 1975), or has been removed locally by stripping the adventitia off the vessel (Kinmonth et al, 1965). The latter procedure of adventitial stripping, even if done without injury to the underlying muscle, can cause some contraction but it is small in degree. By contrast direct injury of the muscle coat (e.g. by needle puncture) can produce large persistent ring contractions. In sheep carotids these contractions are very localised and unaffected by tetrodotoxin (Graham & Keatinge, 1975). Furthermore, they occur even in the absence of bleeding and are therefore not attributable to vasoconstrictor agents in blood. The conclusion is that these ring contractions represent a direct response of the smooth muscle to injury. The reduction in circumference produced by a needle prick to the smooth muscle is much greater than that which can be accounted for by shortening of only those cells which are directly damaged by the needle. This suggests that there must be some spread of depolarisation from one smooth muscle cell to another round the artery wall. However, there is little evidence of longitudinal spread along the axis of the vessel because the contraction remains localised to a ring rather than a band. By contrast, the presence of a K channel blocking agent such as procaine 5 mmol/l, produces widespread contractions, although this is offset to some extent by a direct relaxant action which procaine produces by non-electrical means. Lignocaine, unlike procaine, does not produce any important facilitation of the arteries' electrical activity. It is therefore not liable to cause widespread contractions, and is in this respect a better local anaesthetic for procedures involving manipulation of arteries.

When injury to an artery involves more than just a pin-prick, and there is an extensive crushing or tearing injury of the wall, then spasm of the artery tends to be intense, widespread and prolonged. It has been shown experimentally that the passage of a high velocity bullet through nearby issues, can stretch a vessel wall without rupturing it, and cause several centimetres of the vessel to go into spasm (Amato et al, 1970). These intense contractions are probably induced by the injury to the smooth muscle cells causing their cell membranes to become leaky, and to admit extracellular Ca which enters the cell to cause constriction.

A third mechanism for producing contractions of blood vessels depends on the action of substances released by blood which have leaked out from a damaged vessel (Fig. 2.10). These vasoconstrictor agents are released from aggregating platelets, and probably from other constituents of the blood, as it clots. The spread of such extravasated blood along a vessel, particularly if it is tracking along the adventitia, can cause contraction of undamaged parts of the artery. The nature of the vasoconstrictors has not been fully defined and there are substantial species differences, but the majority are amines which are released by platelets. In man, serotonin (5 hydroxytryptamine) is the principal one of these, and noradrenaline and adrenaline are also present.

Apart from amines there are other vasoconstrictor agents which can be released by platelets when they aggregate to form thrombi. Thromboxane A_2 (TXA_2) is one of these substances and has been isolated from human platelets incubated with arachidonic acid or prostaglandin G_2 (PGG_2) (Fig. 2.11). TXA_2 is technically not a prostaglandin though it is structurally closely related to them and is a powerful vasoconstrictor with a half-life of only 30 seconds at 37°C. It is produced from prostaglandin endoperoxides (PGG_2 or PGH_2) by an enzyme, described as thromboxane synthetase, which has been isolated from human and other platelets (Needleman et al, 1976). Whether thromboxane A_2 is more or less important than serotonin in producing vasoconstriction during natural clotting in unknown but a role for it in determining the blood flow in flaps has been postulated (see p. 58). Thromboxane has also been implicated (together with prostaglandin $F_2\alpha$) in the progressive dermal ischaemia which follows electrical injury. Therapy to block the production of thromboxane has proved successful in providing tissue salvage in experimental burn injury in rats.

Other lipoxygenase-derived products from arachidonic acid at the cellular level are the leukotrienes which have an important role in inflammation of the skin. Leukotrienes are produced by neutrophils and are essential for the chemotaxis and emigration of leucocytes from the capillaries, and produce increases in vascular permeability but they have less effect in the regulation of blood flow.

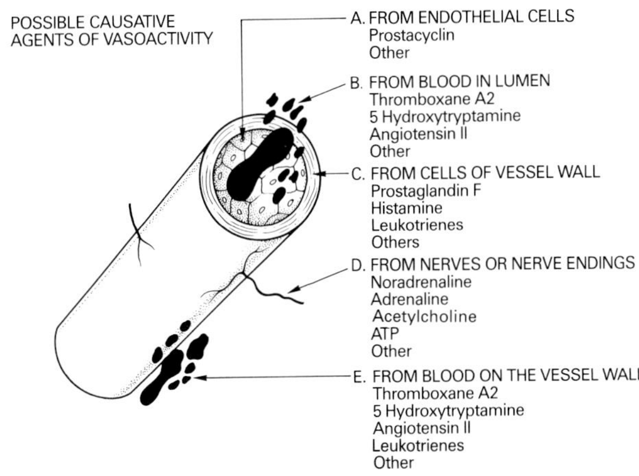

Fig. 2.10 Possible causative agents of vasoactivity. (After Roberts, 1985.)

2

Viscosity

It has been known for a long time that blood does not behave as a simple fluid. In vitro, blood exhibits anomalous viscosity, that is, its viscosity changes with velocity of flow, which changes the shear rate. At a high velocity (high shear rates), blood is less viscous than at a low velocity (low shear rates). Although several factors contribute to the anomalous viscosity of blood it is clear that the suspended erythrocytes are the main factor, while the plasma alone behaves largely like a Newtonian fluid. The parabolic flow profile in large vessels is well known and is attributed to the fact that as shear rates increase the red cells come to lie with their long axes parallel to the direction of flow but in that part of the steam where the flow rate is highest and the intermolecular differences in shear rate are least. This is sometimes called axial streaming and is associated with a progressive decrease in viscosity as the shear rate rises. Conversely, at low shear rates there is no streaming, but many collisions between cells and rouleaux formation tends to occur.

In vivo, with a normal haematocrit and sufficiently high flow rates, blood behaves largely as a Newtonian fluid with almost constant viscosity, showing a linear pressure–flow relationship. Anomalous viscosity is largely irrelevant in large vessels, and in the microcirculation where the flow rate may be greatly decreased it also appears to be a factor of minimal importance because the cells usually pass along the capillaries in single file and the blood behaves rheologically almost like plasma. The precise explanation for this is uncertain but certain surface characteristics of the vascular endothelium may be important (Copley, 1960). Anomalous viscosity becomes important, however, if blood composition is altered simultaneously with low flow rates and when the overall flow rate is grossly reduced, as in shock. Then the anomalous properties of blood raise its viscosity in the wide postcapillary bed above that of the blood passing through the precapillary vessels because the linear flow rate is always less in small veins than in small arteries owing to the dimensional difference in the size of the total cross-sectional area. For this reason the postcapillary resistance may increase relative to that of the precapillary compartment, even though the effect of such a compartmental increase of viscosity on total flow resistance is small. Nevertheless, such a 'rheologically determined' reduction in the pre/post capillary resistance ratio is serious, because it tends to raise the capillary pressure and thereby tends to cause additional fluid loss from the capillaries. The increased tendency of the cells to aggregate and sludge, particularly if sepsis and trauma coexist, further exacerbates this situation. Furthermore, cell aggregation blocks some capillaries, which reduces the total surface area available for gaseous exchange and increases tissue hypoxia. The resulting acidosis reduces cell deformability, and if the ischaemia persists, the endothelium of the blood vessels may be damaged with aggregation and adhesion of blood cells and other elements which will further obstruct blood flow. Clearly a 'vicious circle' situation may develop which in a skin flap may result in necrosis and death of the flap (Fig. 2.12).

Although it has been generally assumed that it is only a low flow situation which can lead to viscosity becoming the principal determinant of tissue perfusion, it is important to look at the other factors which, in such a situation, can affect viscosity. Analysis of regional viscosity values and viscosity changes is a

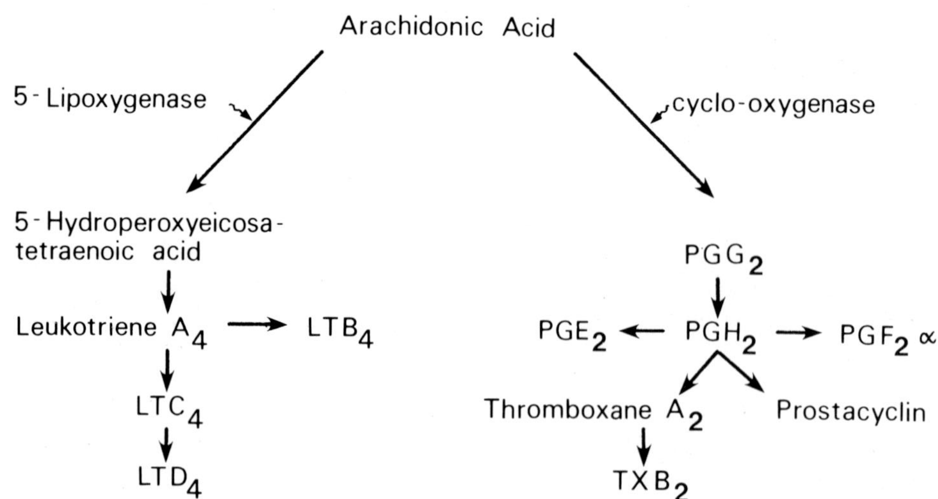

Fig. 2.11 Cyclo-oxygenase and lipoxygenase pathways.

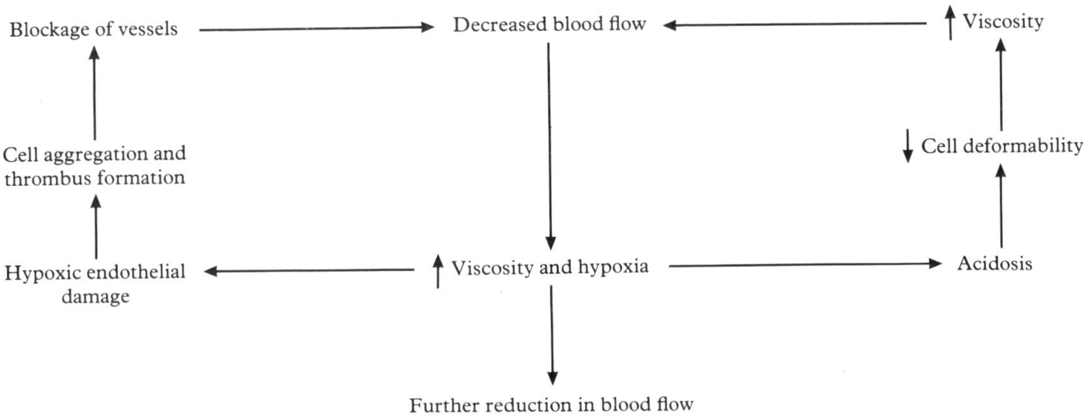

Fig. 2.12 The 'vicious circle' situation in which changes in viscosity may further compromise the circulation in low flow rate situations.

complicated problem but excellent reviews are available and should be consulted for details (Lowe & Forbes, 1981; Whitmore, 1968). Here we will adopt a pragmatic approach and consider some of the factors which affect viscosity in small vessels and which may be susceptible to therapeutic manipulation in the clinical situation of a failing flap. Much of the data is based on animal experiments and has not yet been transferred to the clinical situation, but possible areas for consideration are temperature, haematocrit, deformability of the cell wall, the tendency for rouleaux formation and the plasma viscosity.

Cold increases plasma and blood viscosity. Although an extreme example, it has been shown that in fingers cooled in ice water, regional viscosity may be increased three fold or perhaps even more. In addition, cooling may reduce the suspension stability of cells, producing a reversible aggregation which further increases blood viscosity. All these effects, together with cold-induced vasoconstriction, are responsible for the skin damage occurring under conditions of low temperature. Experiments have shown that significant falls of temperature and blood flow occur during elevation of the dog saphenous skin flap and it has been suggested that deliberate measure should be taken to prevent flap cooling (Awwad et al, 1983).

Haematocrit has a considerable influence on viscosity because even at the normal haematocrit of 40–45% there is only a limited space available in streamline flow if the cells are not to be deformed and the cell wall is to be maintained. When the haematocrit exceeds 40–45%, the viscosity measured in vitro increases out of proportion to the increase in the cell fraction. When flows are measured in tubes of a diameter similar to those of the 'resistance' section of the vascular bed, as for example in a tube of 200 μ diameter, the effect on the viscosity of halving the haematocrit from 40 to 20% is appreciable, but the oxygen carrying capacity of the blood is reduced more than the gain in oxygen supply that results from the increased flow at the lower viscosity. Conversely, at a haematocrit of 60% the increase in viscosity is great and negates any increased oxygen carrying capacity.

With smaller tubes of the dimensions encountered in small pre- and post-capillary vessels, the same haematocrit changes produce far smaller changes in viscosity. With tubes of capillary diameter, reducing the haematocrit has an insignificant effect on viscosity (Fig. 2.13). This is surprising but it has been shown that the red cells are very deformable and can be squeezed through pores of 3–4 microns with very little extra force (Prothero & Burton, 1962); therefore whether few or many erythrocytes transverse a capillary per second has little effect on the regional viscosity, which in the capillaries approaches that of plasma. Nevertheless,

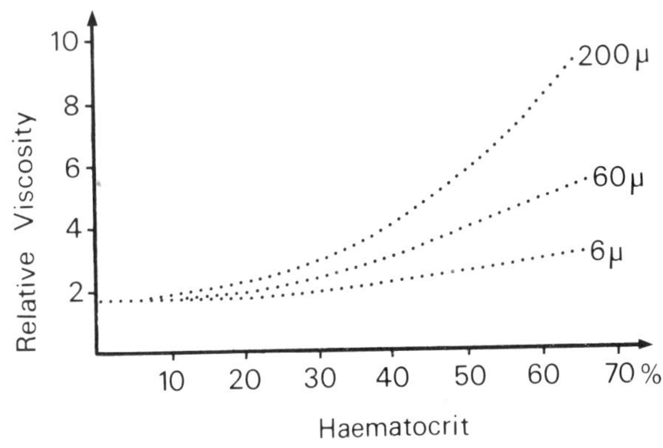

Fig. 2.13 Approximate relationship between viscosity and haematocrit when blood is passed at high rates through tubes of three different diameters (200 μ, 60 μ and 6 μ). Haematocrit changes clearly have little effect on viscosity of blood in small tubes of the approximate dimensions found in the capillary bed. (After Haynes, 1961.)

experimental studies in rabbits and dogs (Earle et al, 1974) have shown increases in the survival length of random pattern flaps in animals whose haematocrits had been lowered. (Of course, bleeding an animal to induce anaemia is also going to produce changes in blood volume, cardiac output and circulation times, blood gas tensions, and blood coagulability – to mention only a few of the most obvious changes and the effects of these on the flaps are not necessarily accounted for.) In a similar study in rats in which the serum protein concentration was also lowered, a significant increase was seen in the surviving length of random pattern flaps (Ruberg & Falcone, 1978). Intuitively it seems undesirable to decrease the oxygen carrying capacity of the blood to a failing flap if an improvement in flow can be obtained by a reduction in serum proteins alone and a number of studies have addressed this possibility.

Plasma fibrinogen. A reduction of the plasma fibrinogen level might be expected to have two effects. Firstly, it would reduce the fibrinogen component of plasma viscosity, and secondly it would greatly reduce fibrinogen-mediated red cell aggregation. The first mechanism could be effective at all flow rates, whilst the second could be expected to have marked effects only at low shear rates, as for example might be expected under conditions of greatly impaired flow as might exist in failing skin flaps.

General protein depletion is one method of producing hypofibrinogenaemia and has been used in rats to increase the survival length of random pattern skin flaps (Ruberg & Falcone, 1978). A more specific and controlled effect may be obtained by the use of defibrinating agents. One of these substances is ancrod (Arvin) which is currently being used to treat peripheral arterial insufficiency and deep venous thrombosis. It is a proteolytic enzyme, purified from the venom of the Malayan pit viper, which produces a controlled defibrination, probably by producing microclots which are quickly removed by the normal fibrinolytic system. When administered intravenously or subcutaneously it has been shown to reduce plasma and blood viscosity and it has been possible to demonstrate an increase in skin blood flow in the legs of patients with peripheral arterial disease after treatment with ancrod (Lowe et al, 1979).

The effect of ancrod therapy on the blood flow in the dog saphenous artery flap has been studied (Awwad et al, 1983). Temperature of the flap and haematocrit were held constant and the flow in the flap was measured before and after intravenous ancrod infusion at a dose of 1 unit /kg body-weight in 10 ml of normal saline administered over 1 hour. The initial blood flow (mean ± SD) was 4.36 ± 1.09 ml/min. After ancrod infusion, the mean blood flow rose to 5.44 ± 1.35 ml/min. This was statistically significant ($p < 0.02$) and the increase in mean flow was 25%. The initial level of plasma fibrinogen was 2.5 ± 0.24g/l. This dropped to zero after the ancrod infusion in all the experiments, and it is interesting to note that there did not appear to be any excessive bleeding. Although this does not directly demonstrate an improvement in survival of failing skin flaps it seems possible that ancrod could be beneficial in such a situation.

Other agents. Postoperative treatment of rat skin flaps with pentoxifyllin which is believed to increase red cell deformability and inhibit platelet aggregation (Takayanagi & Ogawa, 1980) and rabbit flaps with heparin (Sawhney, 1980) has increased flap survival. The use of dextran has not improved experimental flap viability (Myers & Cherry, 1967) but it is used in microvascular surgery. Hyaluronidase, because of possible effects in augmenting interstitial diffusion, has been tried in myocardial ischaemia (Kloner et al, 1978) and may be efficacious in peripheral vascular disease (Elder, 1980). This led to its study on dorsal rat flaps where it appeared to produce a minor degree of increased flap survival if administration was started 6 days preoperatively (Hurvitz, 1983).

Rouleaux formation. Although the aggregation and adhesion of blood cells in the microcirculation has been described as one of the consequences of reduced blood flow, visualisation of the vessels in mature skin tubes by direct microscopy using an implanted titanium chamber has shown that rouleaux can break up with the restoration of normal flow if the flow reduction has been of short duration (Brånemark, 1968). Healthy volunteers aged between 20 and 25 had skin tubes fashioned on the inner aspect of the upper arm and microcirculatory studies were conducted 2–3 months after installation of the chamber. It was seen that, under normal flow conditions, erythrocytes, granulocytes and platelets did not show any tendency to adhere to each other or to the endothelium. The red cells were very plastic, granulocytes moderately plastic and deformable, and platelets behaved like rigid discs. When flow velocities in the microcirculation were reduced to 0.2–0.1 mm per second (normal 0.5–0.8 mm/s) erythrocytes formed characteristic rouleauxs which could be short (4 or 5 cells) or long (20–30 cells). In blocked venular segments, rouleaux consisting of 5 to 10 erythrocytes were often seen moving slowly in the centre of the vessel with granulocytes and separate erythrocytes moving in the spaces between the red cells. If the skin tube was compressed for 2 hours in order to produce stasis, the rouleaux did not show any tendency to adhere to the endothelium or the endothelial plasma layer. When flow returned, the rouleaux formations immediately broke up again, and the red cells exhibited normal deformability and did not appear to adhere to each other.

This appears to indicate that after complete controlled stasis for up to 3 hours in human skin, flow can be re-established such that structurally and functionally normal erythrocytes are regained. The endothelium does not show any significant swelling under these circumstances, and there is no apparent tendency for cells to stick to it when flow is regained. Observations on animal tissues such as skeletal muscles and peripheral nerves have shown similar patterns; in fact it has been possible to regain as much as 70% of microvascular function after complete and controlled circulatory standstill for 12 hours in a peripheral nerve vessel. This contrasts to the situation in which, in addition to reduced flow rates, the tissues are damaged, as by burns, and blood cells adhere to the vessel walls singly and in clusters.

Endothelium-derived factors

Since 1985 there has been an increasing interest in the role of the endothelium in the regulation of vascular tone. Action on endothelial cell receptors by a number of vasoactive substances stimulates the production of endothelium-derived relaxing and constricting factors as well as prostaglandins. Although the nature of the endothelium-dependent contracting factor (EDCF) is still unclear, and furthermore appears to be different in blood vessels of different anatomical origins, at least three different classes of endothelial vasoconstrictor substances have been recognised: (1) metabolites of arachidonic acid, (2) polypeptide factors isolatable from cultured endothelial cells, and (3) a still unidentified diffusible factor released from anoxic/hypoxic endothelial cells. A peptide, named endothelin, has been isolated from pig aortic endothelial cells and has been shown to be a potent constrictor in the rabbit skin microvasculature (Brain et al, 1988) and in isolated human resistance vessels. Endothelium-derived relaxing factors (EDRF) have also been investigated and have been identified as including nitric oxide, substance P and other substances which, by their release, contribute to flow induced vasodilation. Once again there is considerable variation between species and vascular beds and the details of this system remain to be elucidated in humans. Interestingly the snake venom vasoconstrictor peptides, the sarafotoxins, have a high degree of sequence homology with endothelin and binding studies suggest they share common sites and mechanisms of action. Further discoveries in this area may be of great significance.

CONTROL OF TRANSCAPILLARY FLUID EXCHANGE

The second dynamic role of the microcirculation lies in transcapillary fluid exchange. Whilst the nature of the blood flow in acute and delayed flaps has been the subject of much experimental work, the problem of postoperative oedema in flaps has conversely received little attention. The presence of oedema must interfere with the diffusion of nutrients to the cells of a flap and may affect the circulation through it. It therefore seems appropriate to review some of the principles of transcapillary fluid exchange. The subject is also important in the context of increasing interest in lymphovenous anastomotic surgery and micro-lymphatic bypass operations for selected cases of chronic limb oedema.

In 1896 E. H. Starling showed that, contrary to many previous concepts, most of the fluid filtered from the capillaries into the tissues was not returned to the circulation by the lymphatics. Instead, a significant proportion of the filtered fluid was absorbed directly back into the capillary blood. In 1926 E. M. Landis confirmed and extended this concept which is now known as the Starling–Landis model of transcapillary exchange.

In the model there are four driving pressures for the movement of fluid between capillary blood and the surrounding interstitium. These are: hydrostatic pressure of the capillary blood, which tends to push fluid out of the capillary; oncotic pressure generated by the plasma proteins, which attracts fluid from the interstitium into the capillary; hydrostatic pressure in the tissue fluids, which pushes fluid into the capillary; and oncotic pressure developed by plasma proteins and other macromolecules or 'colloids' in the interstitium, which attracts fluid from the capillaries into the interstitium. It is variations among these pressures which determine the direction and magnitude of fluid exchanges across the permeable capillary wall.

Capillary hydrostatic pressure. This is the pressure that remains after the blood has passed through the large feeding arteries and experienced pressure drops, primarily in the muscular arterial portions of the microvasculature. Due to vasomotion, this is highly variable in a vessel over time but can be determined by the amount of external pressure necessary to occlude the capillaries, or the amount of pressure necessary to make saline start to flow through a micropipette which has been inserted so that its tip is directed towards the arteriolar end of the capillary (Landis, 1930). Typical values in human nail bed capillaries reported by Landis were 32 mmHg at the arteriolar end and 15 mmHg at the venous end. The pulse pressure is approximately 5 mmHg at the arteriolar end and zero at the venous end. Transit time from the arteriolar to the venous end of an average-sized capillary is 1–2 seconds.

Plasma oncotic pressure. Starling's original postulate was that the presence of protein in the plasma accounted for the reabsorption of tissue fluid into capillary blood. By in vitro measurements he found the oncotic pressure developed by the proteins to be approximately equal to the available estimates of capillary hydrostatic pressure. Recent studies have shown that the permeability of the capillary to protein and fluid varies among different organs and tissues, and at different sites along the capillary; for example, the venous end of the capillary, in addition to having a larger surface area than the arterial end, contains a few large pores and possibly pinocytotic vesicles which allow protein to leak continuously through to the interstitium.

Tissue oncotic pressure. Clearly the concentration of the tissue proteins is affected by the amount of transudation of fluid into the tissues. With a greater rate of fluid filtration into the tissues, the tissue protein concentration and, therefore, tissue oncotic pressure should decrease if the rate of protein leakage by the capillaries and removal by the lymphatics remains relatively fixed. This decrease shifts the transcapillary pressures in the direction of reabsorption of fluid into the capillary thus providing an oncotic 'buffering' mechanism for controlling fluid exchange at the level of the capillary. In fact, this buffering is observed clinically in that a substantial decrease in plasma protein concentration is required to induce significant tissue fluid accumulation and oedema formation.

Tissue hydrostatic pressure. This pressure component is the counterpart of the hydrostatic pressure in the capillary blood but acts in the opposite direction so that an increase in tissue hydrostatic pressure enhances reabsorption of fluid by the capillary. The magnitude of tissue hydrostatic pressures has not been definitely established. Measurements in artificially induced fluid spaces in tissue, yield sub-atmospheric pressures, while those involving puncture techniques generally yield positive pressures. Differences between these results may be due to oncotic effects.

More recent measurements suggest that the Landis–Starling filtration reabsorption hypothesis may need modification. The original concept that filtration of fluid from the arterial end of the capillaries was balanced by reabsorption of fluid back into the plasma at the venous end depended heavily on Landis's figures for capillary hydrostatic pressure which neatly straddled the colloid osmotic pressure. More recent nail fold capillary loop measurements by Levick & Michel (1978) have shown differences in pressure between the arterial and venous limbs of the capillary loops (15 cm H_2O) which are smaller than those reported by Landis (27 cm H_2O) while the absolute pressures are higher. In these experiments the capillary pressure at the venous end of the capillary loop in the warm hand was never less than the plasma colloid osmotic pressure and therefore fluid must flow out along the entire capillary , although the capillary filtration coefficient must be assumed to be high, and the volume of fluid filtered very low, since oedema was never apparent in these studies. These different values may be attributable to the fact that Landis' measurements were made on patients in cold hospital wards rather than in the centrally heated laboratories of Michel & Levick, a difference further magnified by the fact that Landis' measurements were made at a time when an industrial dispute had further reduced heating levels.

In addition to the four basic elements of the Starling–Landis model there are many other interacting variables. Wiederhielm (1968) has produced a mathematical simulation of the variables involved in transcapillary fluid exchange with 21 simultaneously interacting equations which were solved using a computer and values from the literature for the various parameters. Simulation of phenomena, such as the effects of reducing plasma protein concentration, increasing venous pressure, and accumulating protein in the interstitium, not only predicted many clinical features, such as degree of oedema formation, but also served to focus attention on specific areas where understanding of governing factors is lacking. One such question concerned the role of the interstitium.

For convenience of thinking, the interstitium may be considered as being made up of three components; (1) a solvent, consisting of an aqueous solution of low molecular weight substances which move essentially with the water; (2) a solute of impeded mobility, consisting mainly of serum albumin but including other macromolecules and assemblies of large molecular weight; and (3) a network of crosslinked components such as collagen, with elastin, structural glycoproteins and linkage proteins, and various network immobilised components. In the dermis the interstitium contains collagen and elastic fibres and a ground substance made up of proteoglycans and interstitial fluid. The three major proteoglycans in human dermis are hyaluronic acid, dermatan sulphate and chondroitin sulphate, and it is their water-retaining properties that maintain and determine the hydroelastic properties of skin. Any increase in the amount of interstitial fluid alters these properties and also results in an increased distance for diffusion between blood and tissue cells. Supposing oedema doubles the volume of a piece of skin in which the interstitial space normally accounts for 15% of the total tissue volume, then if all the extra fluid is contained within the interstitial space, this must have increased its volume eightfold. The increase in the mean diffusion distance is then at least twofold, which is clearly disadvantageous for cell nutrition.

In normal circumstances this does not occur because the lymphatics carry away the excess tissue fluid. The initial lymphatics function mainly as conduits but Casley-Smith (1977) has proposed a second mode of functioning that takes into consideration the finding that mean lymph protein concentrations are generally higher than those in the connective tissues. This second mechanism may be described as a force-pump powered by the colloid osmotic pressure of the concentrated lymph and depends on pressure changes brought about by tissue movement and compression. It is envisaged that the emptying phase of the initial lymphatic cycle occurs when the tissues become compressed. In addition the 'open' junctions become 'closed' as a result of the very pliable inner leaflets of the open junctions being forced close up against the outer endothelial cells and surrounding tissues, and to this will be added the effects of the 'telescoping' of the lymphatics during tissue compression. The endothelial cell junctions are therefore likely to be impenetrable to macromolecules, particles and cells but still quite permeable to water and small molecules. So these will be forced out of the lymphatics into the tissues, leaving the macromolecules to become concentrated to levels greater than those in the tissues. This colloid osmotic pressure differential then causes filling of the initial lymphatics during the next relaxation phase.

Oedema and flaps

It is clinically apparent that oedema can be a significant problem in flaps, perhaps contributing to circulatory embarrassment. To establish the fundamentals of the problem one might ask two questions: what is the degree of oedema formation in free flaps compared to pedicled flaps; and what pharmacological agents affect oedema formation in experimental flaps? Although work has been done on the latter subject, the key question of how these various agents bring about a reduction in oedema has not been answered. This remains difficult while we do not fully understand all the factors governing oedema formation.

One way of looking at oedema formation in flaps is to try to measure interstitial fluid pressure (IFP). Despite the fact that the pressure is minimal and the techniques difficult, several methods have been used for estimating subcutaneous IFP, including an open needle inserted into the tissues, implanted perforated capsules and a subcutaneous cotton wick. Despite arguments regarding the relative merits of the different methods and the variability of their results it is now generally agreed that IFP is negative in subcutaneous tissues. A correlation between IFP and the survival of skin flaps remains to be established although attempts have been made to measure pressures in pedicled flaps under changing conditions of circulation (Sundell & Patterson, 1963). These workers used a fluid filled hypodermic needle connected to a pressure measuring device and recorded the pressure required to force small amount of fluid into the tissues. This does not in fact measure IFP but the breaking point at which the tissues are forced apart by the injected fluid – the 'interstitial resistance'. A combination of the open needle and wick methods, termed the 'wick in needle' technique has been developed to overcome the problems of the open needle method and to avoid the trauma of the wick method. Jones et al (1983) have experimented with the wick in needle technique as a means of measuring intradermal IFP in the rat epigastric flap in the hope that this might prove to be a useful method for monitoring skin flaps. The technique is difficult and not really suitable for continuous monitoring because of problems with blockages but has produced some interesting results. Simply raising an epigastric flap and resuturing it in position did not significantly affect dermal IFP values. Ligation of the inferior epigastric artery supplying the flap produced, as might be expected, increases in negativity of intradermal IFP, but when the inferior epigastric vein was similarly treated, increased negativity of lesser degree was again observed, contrary to expectations. These results have not been satisfactorily explained and highlight our lack of understanding of the physiological changes taking place during elevation of flaps.

More direct methods of assessing oedema in flaps by measuring changes in thickness or volume have also been tried on experimental flaps. Aarts (1980) has studied the relative degree of oedema formation in differently treated island flaps in the rabbit ear model. In one group of animals, 3 × 5 cm island flaps were created by the division of all tissues except for the main artery and vein (the central ear vessels) and the adventitia was stripped from the vessels to ensure complete severance of all lymphatics which might have drained the flap. A standard neurovascular island flap was created on the opposite ear as a control. In a second group of animals 3 × 5 cm standard neurovascular island flaps were raised bilaterally one day after regional intra-arterial block with guanethidine had been carried out on one side. Flap oedema was measured accurately with a micrometer over the most swollen area and expressed as a difference in thickness between the flap and the surrounding ear tissue. It was found that in the first group of animals all three showed, as might be expected, a greater degree of oedema formation on the side where all the lymphatics had been divided. In the second group of animals, oedema was absent on the side pretreated with guanethidine. Groups of animals with pedicled flaps were also benefitted by regional intravascular sympathetic (RIS) blockade and it has been suggested that the mechanism may be one of improving capillary flow through relaxation of precapillary and postcapillary 'sphincters'. This could cause a decrease in capillary blood pressure and an increase in capillary oxygen tension resulting in reduced oedema formation. What has not been definitely established is a correlation between degree of oedema in flaps and their survival, but RIS blockade in the experimental pedicled flaps appeared to both reduce oedema formation and also to improve flap survival, which is promising for clinical practice.

Anderson & Zarem (1977) have studied the changes which take place in the lymphatics of the rabbit ear following a partial amputation at the base in which only the central artery and two veins were preserved. Serial lymphangiograms showed changes from 1 hour after division of the lymphatics, consisting of saccular dilatations at intervals along the lymph vessels. During the following 6–8 hours these dilatations extended along the lymphatic vessels enlarging them from an initial diameter of about 150 μm up to 400 μm. After 24 hours the ears were very oedematous but there were no further changes in the lymphatics. About two weeks later, distension of the lymphatics and clinical oedema began to subside. If the procedure was then repeated at 3 weeks after the first partial amputation, then the sequence of events was different – oedema was minimal or absent and the lymphatics showed no significant alterations in size. Similarly, if the rabbits were treated with intramuscular hexamethonium for 5 days before surgery, then the oedema and lymphatic dilatation failed to occur. Both observations could be explained by postulating the activation of lymphatico-venous communications, although their physical existence has not been demonstrated. Nevertheless, Threefoot's statement (1970) that 'the opening of lymphaticovenous communications in response to stress signifies a beneficial compensatory function' may be relevant to flap surgery.

THE ISCHAEMIC FLAP

The clinical problem of flap failure is so well known that there is no need to document its incidence here. It is well recognised that both inadequate arterial inflow to a flap and poor venous outflow may each be responsible for inadequate perfusion and consequent death of the flap. Both of these grossly obvious routes leading to flap death may be due to one or more of a constellation of factors which include such causes as poor flap design, thrombosis of the vascular pedicle, pressure on the pedicle, kinking of the flap, haematoma formation, hypovolaemia and hypotension, hyperviscosity, low haematocrit, hypothermia and infection. Correction of these adverse factors, if brought about soon enough, might be expected to improve the chances of survival of a compromised flap. However, these adverse factors are superimposed upon various physiological changes that occur whenever any skin flap, musculocutaneous flap or any other kind of flap is raised. Such inevitable physiological changes are the direct result of surgical interference with not only the blood supply but also the nerve supply and the lymphatic drainage of the flap, and these changes provide an additional, but not alternative, target for therapeutic intervention. The problem is that these physiological events are but poorly understood in respect of their nature, their timing of onset and progression, their influence and their importance to flap survival. In an effort to unravel some of these mysteries this section approaches the subject of these physiological events from the standpoint of a discussion of the delay phenomenon since the changes we are considering are inevitable and exist in a flap whether we call it simple flap elevation or delay. The following pages therefore attempt to gather together some of the experimental data on flap survival and the delay phenomenon and marshall this evidence under the titles of the various theories which have been put forward at various times to explain the delay phenomenon.

First, however, it is necessary to define some terms.

Distal ischaemia is a condition that occurs in a pedicled flap that has been acutely raised with a larger size than can be supported by its supplying vessel(s). The ischaemia is generally greatest at the point furthest removed from the vascular pedicle, hence *distal* ischaemia. Distal ischaemia if severe enough can be expected to proceed to necrosis.

Delay phenomenon. If a pedicled flap with inherent distal ischaemia is raised in two (or more) stages separated by a period of about two weeks, then a greater length will survive than if the flap had been completely elevated at the first operation. The optimum time interval varies between different species, (Myers & Cherry, 1971).

The term 'delayed transfer' was introduced by Blair in 1921 to describe these preliminary stages and this has since been contracted to 'delay'. The delay procedure has been in use in one form or another for several hundred years but even now our understanding of it is incomplete. In the 16th century Tagliacozzi delayed his upper arm flaps by making parallel incisions through the skin and subcutaneous tissues over the biceps muscle using a metal clamp with slits in it specially designed for the purpose. The strip of skin was separated from the underlying muscle, except at its proximal and distal attachments, and was prevented from reattaching to its bed by the insertion of a strip of lint soaked in melted butter between the skin strip and the muscle (Fig. 2.14). His intention was to 'train' the flap until 'firm and robust, not flaccid and feeble' and 'so strong as to endure the violence of the operation well enough'.

Global ischaemia. This describes the insult sustained by a free flap (= microvascular graft) after complete interruption of its vascular supply. This occurs either *intentionally* at the time of transfer, in which case the interruption is to arterial and venous supplies; or occurs *accidentally* in the postoperative period as a result of mechanical problems associated with the pedicle such as torsion, kinking, compression, thrombosis of anastomosis etc. in which case either arterial or venous or both vessels may be affected. Delay procedures are generally not applicable with the aim of ameliorating the effects of global ischaemia, but interest in global ischaemia and ways of reducing the metabolism in the flap are increasing.

No-reflow phenomenon. If a skin flap is kept ischaemic for long enough then it will not be possible to re-establish inflow at the end of this time as tissue death and microvascular sludging will be too far advanced. Milton's experiments suggested that a minimum of 21 hours were necessary for these changes to occur (Milton, 1972). Clearly the same considerations can be applied to traumatically separated parts and amputations. Some of the early literature on this subject used the term in a rather loose way to refer to the injury sustained by organs subjected to prolonged ischaemia and included the condition in which inflow was successfully re-established yet the tissues still died. This should not be included under the heading of no-reflow because quite clearly the circumstances do not fit with the pathophysiological events implied by the term 'no-reflow'.

Ischaemic reperfusion injury (IRI) or ischaemia induced reperfusion injury. This condition describes the cell death that follows a period of ischaemia despite the resumption of inflow and nutritive capillary blood flow at the end of the ischaemic period. Indeed the processes leading to cell death are intimately bound up with the reperfusion. Milton showed that in experimental flaps subjected to 18 hours of ischaemia, reperfusion was possible but the flap subsequently died, whereas with 15 hours of ischaemia reperfusion was associated with flap survival. There is now less concentration in the literature on no-reflow since this appears to be irreversible, and more concentration on IRI which may be modifiable by chemical agents.

It should be noted that in the context of flaps the word 'ischaemia' is rarely used in the sense of its dictionary definition of 'an absence or lack of blood'. The term is rather used to describe the condition where blood is present in the vessels but there is a lack of nutritive capillary blood flow.

THEORIES OF THE MECHANISM UNDERLYING THE DELAY PHENOMENON

Early theories

The pioneers of plastic surgery in the early part of this century all described the improvement in perfusion of the pedicled flap which was associated with the delay procedure; 'blood supply of an increased character is induced down the pedicle to the flap extremity' (Gillies, 1920); 'delicate vessels develop into spurting arteries' (Ganzer, 1943).

Milton, using thc pig, investigated the effectiveness of four different methods of delaying a flap (Fig. 2.16). He found that the creation of a bipedicled flap by making two incisions and undermining the skin between the incisions in the Tagliacottian manner, was the best form of delay (Milton, 1965).

By 1950, delay procedures were in widespread use although there was little experimental evidence to either support their value or elucidate their mechanism of action. Many thought that the basic implication of the delay was that surviving length would be doubled because the classic bipedicled flap delay appeared to join together two single pedicled flaps.

Braithwaite (1951a) suggested that in a delayed flap the number of vessels was not increased but that many of the veins of the subdermal plexus were of a larger diameter than normal. He thought that this might improve flow and thereby diminish the risks of cyanosis and thrombosis and lead to increased viability. He later suggested that the relative ischaemia produced by the delay procedure caused a release of histamine which led to the change in vascularity (Braithwaite, 1951b). Stark & DeHaan (1959) cast doubt on this by showing that histamine by iontophoresis produced an increase in the

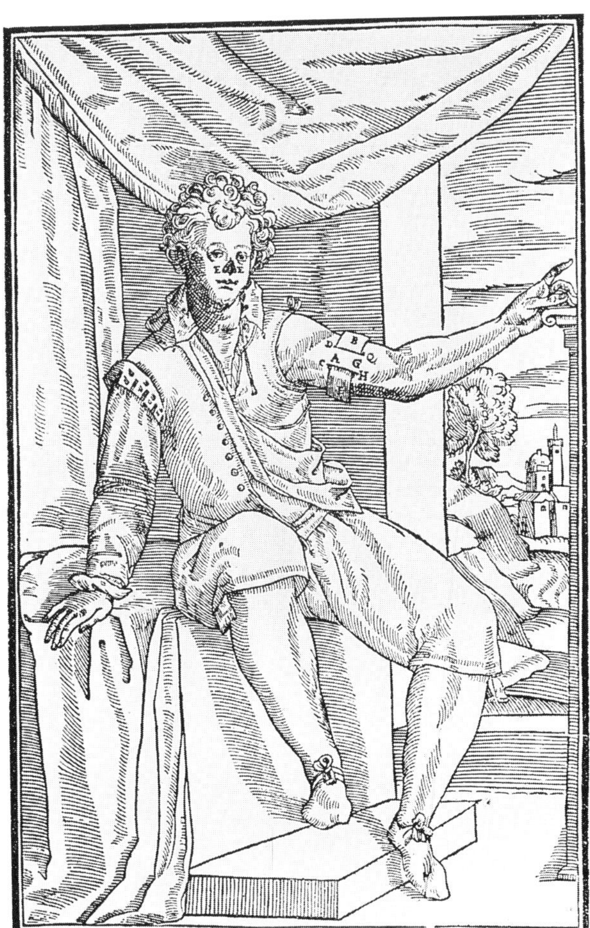

a

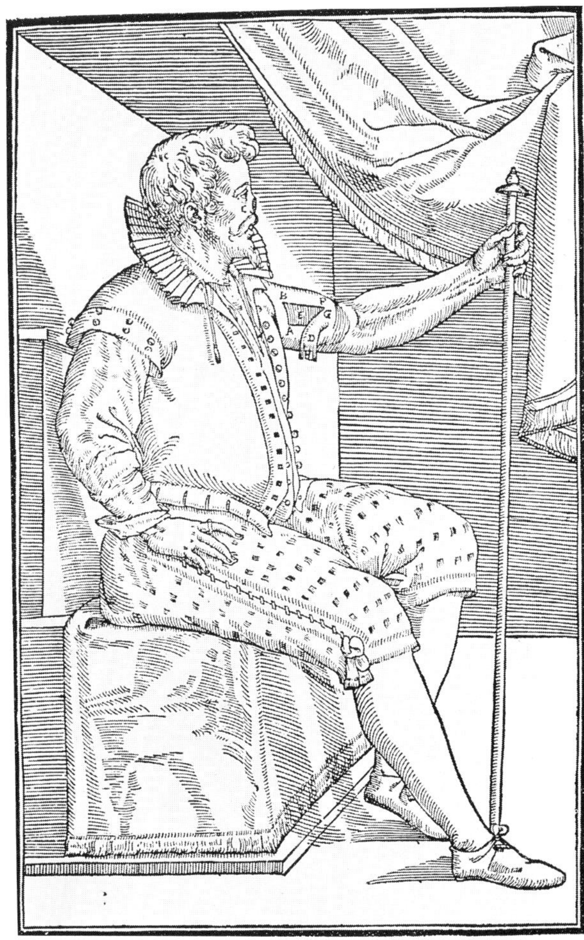

b

Fig. 2.14 Reproductions of Plates from the 'De Curtorum per Insitionem' by Gaspare Tagliacozzi (1597). **a.** The method of delaying the flap by parallel incisions with a piece of lint (marked B) inserted beneath the bipedicle flap in order to prevent its reattachment to its bed. **b.** The proximal pedicle has been divided prior to its transfer to the nose. One wonders whether the growth of the moustache and beard is supposed to indicate the length of the delay or perhaps the two illustrations show different patients!

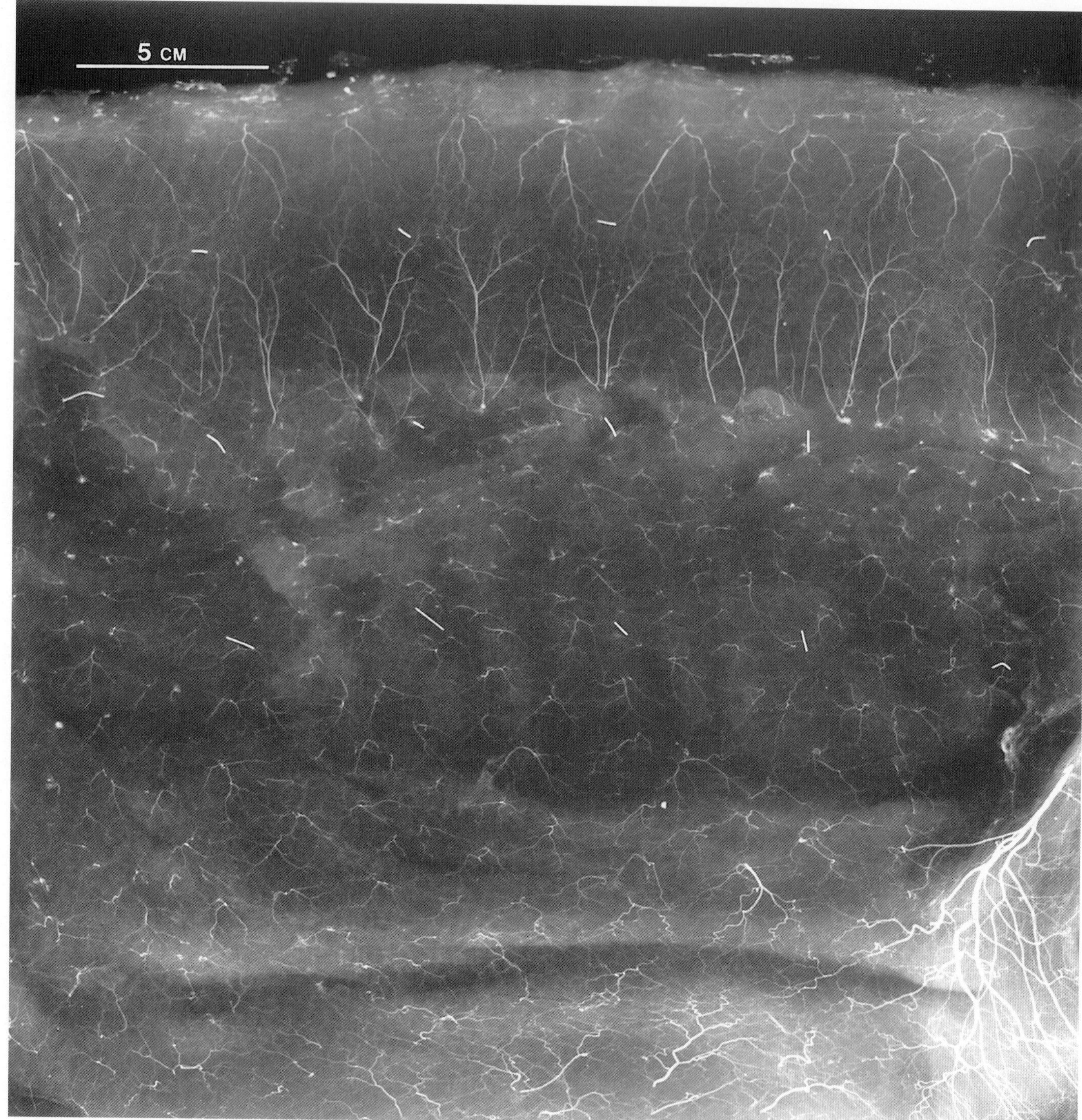

Fig. 2.15 Radiograph of barium sulphate injected pig skin. The presence of axial vessels perpendicular to the dorsal midline appears to have been ignored by some of the earlier experimental flap work which assumed a random orientation of all the vessels. These vessels correspond to dorsal medial cutaneous and dorsal lateral cutaneous arteries emerging at the medial and lateral edges of the paraspinal musculature. The other musculocutaneous perforators have an axiality with a predominantly ventral orientation. Opaque markers are pins 5 cm apart. See also Figure 2.17.

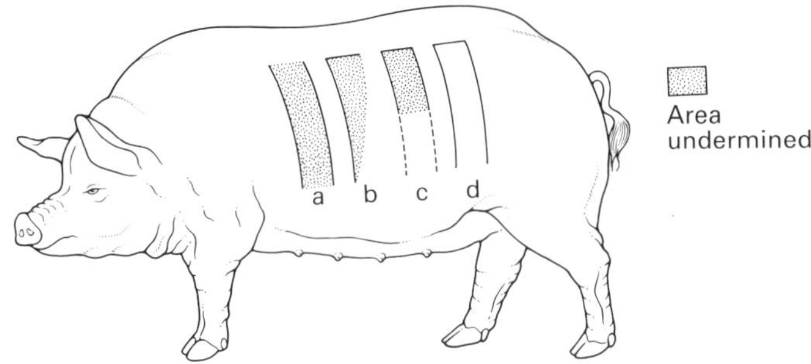

Fig. 2.16 Milton's experimental flap delays which he performed on the pig: **a**. bipedicle; **b**. undermining via an L-shaped incision; **c**. elongation; **d**. incision of margins. (From Milton S., Thesis, Oxford University)

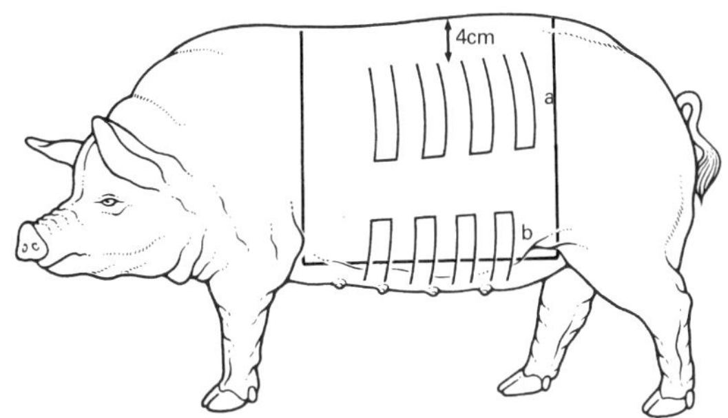

Fig. 2.17 Other classical experimental flaps raised on the pig: **a**. dorsal; **b**. ventral. The outlined rectangle shows area from which the skin was taken for the radiograph Fig. 2.15.

number of arteries in experimental animal flaps, but did not improve the efferent circulation and did not augment overall survival (DeHaan & Stark, 1961). Velander (1964) maintained that delay was the result of a non-specific inflammatory reaction, but Myers & Cherry (1969) disproved this in experiments on rabbits which compared paired 'delayed' pedicles identical in the amount of wounding but different in the amount of blood supply remaining after the first operation. These experiments appeared to show that for a delay procedure to improve the survival of a pedicle at a later date, the blood flow must be decreased at the first operation. This was interpreted by Myers & Cherry as indicating that ischaemia acted as the stimulus for the development of the delay phenomenon. McFarlane et al (1965) suggested that delay conditioned the tissues to hypoxia but any such effect is of secondary importance and does not explain the improvement in vascularity over the delay period.

Sympathectomy → vasodilatation hypothesis

In the 1970s interest centred on the role of the sympathetic nervous system and its control of basal vascular tone as the mediator of the delay phenomenon. It was thought that the denervation occurring during the delay procedure could produce a reduction in basal tone and thereby a vasodilatation. This vasodilatation hypothesis of delay had been first advanced by Hynes in 1951 but supporting evidence was slow to accumulate. A look back on previous experiments showed that the possible role of neural influences had been minimised and earlier work was open to reinterpretation. For example, the studies quoted above in which paired 'delayed' flaps were compared for their subsequent ability to enhance survival where each flap of a pair was equal in terms of wounding but differed in the degree of its blood supply. These experiments were interpreted as showing that ischaemia, and not inflammation, was the stimulus for the development of the delay phenomenon, but this ignored the fact that division of the vessels on three sides of a flap also divides the sympathetic nerves running with the arteries and an alternative explanation for the improved survival of the fully delayed flap might rest on the effects of denervation. This concept appeared to be supported by studies (Myers & Cherry, 1968) on acute dorsal skin flaps in the rat which suggested that the alpha-adrenergic blocking drug phenoxybenzamine, when either injected subcutaneously into the flap or applied topically in DMSO, produced an immediate improvement in flap circulation, although this was nowhere near as marked or as consistent as the improvement which followed a delay. However, early experiments with this flap model should be considered as inconclusive since the pattern of necrosis in the control flaps varied greatly. This was later shown to be due to the ability of parts of dorsal rat flaps to survive as free grafts and subsequent studies utilising polythene sheeting between the flap and its bed, and between surrounding skin and the flap edges, produced a much more consistent pattern of necrosis in control flaps varying from 61 to 70% (Körlof & Ugland, 1966; Dibbell et al, 1979; Griffiths et al, 1981).

Similarly, another paper which at the time appeared to support the sympathetic denervation concept was one by Finseth & Adelberg (1978). This appeared to show significant increases in acute flap survival compared to untreated controls when rats were treated for 15 days preoperatively and 7 days postoperatively with a vasodilator agent (isoxuprine, guanethidine, hydralazine or phenoxybenzamine). However, the experimental model was an abdominal flap based on one groin neurovascular bundle with the treatment groups receiving intraperitoneal injections through the flaps, and was largely discredited by the fact that the control animals received no injections. Furthermore, this particular model does not really reproduce the delay phenomenon, but at the time it was thought to support the sympathectomy → vasodilation hypothesis. Further criticisms of this overly simple concept are based on the time course of events – if sympathectomy is immediate why does the delay phenomenon only begin to appear after a minimum period of about 48 hours and why does it take 2 weeks to achieve its maximum effect?

Intraflap shunting hypothesis

In answer to these criticisms, an alternative theory based on the effects of sympathectomy postulated that the effect of sympathetic denervation was to dilate AV shunts more than precapillary sphincters. It was thought that in an acute flap this would produce a significant degree of intraflap shunting of blood away from the nutrient capillary bed. In the distal part of an acute flap, blood flow would already be reduced to a critical level and this shunting would be great enough to produce cell death. Initially, cell death would be remote from the shunts but would progressively extend to the cells around the shunts until they too became involved with resulting occlusion of the shunts themselves after 24–36 hours. Full tissue necrosis would then have occurred in the distal end of the flap.

This hypothesis was developed by Reinisch (1974) on the basis of experiments on pig dorsal and ventral skin flaps. He demonstrated that the fluorescein test was an accurate predictor of necrosis in these acute flaps and went on to make four observations:

1. The area beyond the fluorescein penetration that was doomed to necrosis, showed an unexpectedly high temperature incompatible with a 'no-flow' situation.

2. When ^{51}Cr-labelled red cells were injected intravenously and their presence at intervals along the flap measured 2 and 9 hours after flap elevation, it was found that there were considerable levels of radioactivity beyond the fluorescein marker indicating flow into this area. At 19 hours the level of radioactivity was found to decrease progressively distal to the marker, and at 24 hours there was little radioactivity.

3. When ^{85}Sr-labelled microspheres (15 μD) were injected into the aorta at the same time as the tagged red cells were injected intravenously, it was found that their distribution differed markedly from that of the cells, there being very few beyond the fluorescein marker. Since microspheres impact in the first capillary bed they enter, this suggested that beyond the fluorescein marker there was either no flow or arteriovenous shunting. Taken in conjunction with the red cell findings the suggestion was that shunting occurred in the distal region.

4. Intravenous ^{99}Tc was administered and the flaps scanned with a gamma camera. Activity was observed in the area of the flap beyond the fluorescein dye marker.

Reinisch suggested that a bipedicle delay procedure did not reduce the blood flow enough to endanger nutrient flow but that the division of sympathetic nerve fibres did produce some shunting. This shunting then returned to normal levels during the course of the 2-week delay period as the AV shunts resumed normal tone. The aetiology of the acquired tone was not known but was presumed to be a developing denervation hypersensitivity to endogenous circulating catecholamines. In this hypothesis it was envisaged that when the delayed flap was finally elevated, the potentially injurious shunting would not occur and the flap would exhibit increased viability and safety.

To some extent this concept of the delay phenomenon was borne out by the work of Myers & Cherry (1968) who found excellent post-mortem angiographic filling of vessels in the non-fluorescein-staining distal ends of their flaps at 24 hours (and occasionally at 36 hours) after elevation. They concluded that in the living animal these vessels must have been in spasm, opening only after the animal's death, but these findings could also be explained by blood flowing only through non-nutritive AV shunts in the area distal to the limit of fluorescein staining since to be seen, fluorescein must diffuse into the interstitial fluid through capillary vessels. Reinisch further postulated that if his theory was correct then induction of shunt closure in acute flaps by chemical means might be a mechanism for augmenting survival. He suggested that dilute noradrenaline in a concentration between 1:4 000 000 and 1:10 000 000 might selectively constrict AV shunts and gave anecdotal support to this by claiming to have produced an improvement in one out of three failing pig flaps infiltrated with 1:5 000 000 noradrenaline at a late stage. No satisfactory experimental evidence, however, exists to back this up. In a further experiment, Reinisch & Myers (1974) showed that noradrenaline 1:200 000 did not affect acute flaps, but adversely affected delayed pig flaps reducing their surviving length to 60% of that of the untreated but delayed controls – an observation that Wu et al (1978) had made by accident in patients and later confirmed in the rat using 1:400 000 noradrenaline. These results did not give much support to the shunting hypothesis even if the effects of noradrenaline on delayed flaps were attributed to denervation hypersensitivity.

Acceptance of the shunting theory poses other problems. Although the presence of flow distal to the eventual line of flap necrosis is taken as evidence for opening of AV shunts secondary to the sympathectomy, the measurements are in fact more indicative of a reduction of flow rather than an increase. More significantly, other workers have shown that division of adrenergic nerves results in the release of stored catecholamines from the ends of the transected sympathetic nerve fibres with a loss of the ability to inactivate them through a reuptake mechanism (Malmfors & Sachs, 1965). In the early period after elevation of a flap a hyperadrenergic state therefore exists within it (Palmer, 1970). This tends to affect precapillary sphincters and reduces nutrient capillary flow.

The hyperadrenergic state

The hyperadrenergic state resulting from transection of the sympathetic nerves is maximal over the first 16–30 hours after elevation of a flap and causes small vessel constriction which may result in necrosis if the blood flow has also been reduced to a critical level by the severing of multiple arterial in-flow channels. Evidence for this state of affairs in acute flaps comes from a number of sources.

Braithwaite et al, as far back as 1951, measured ^{24}Na clearance from intradermal sites on tube pedicles of patients, and showed the initial fall in perfusion on performing the delay procedure with subsequent progressive improvement during the delay period.

Barisoni & Veall (1969) measure ^{22}Na absorption from tubes/flaps and normal skin both with and without thymoxamine treatment (an alpha-adrenergic blocker). Although only a preliminary communication and lacking in rigorous methodology and analysis this work is of interest because it is one of the few studies with thymoxamine which have been carried out on patients. Thymoxamine intravenously or subcutaneously produced no change in ^{22}Na absorption from normal forearm skin. In 9 tubes and flaps in which initial clearance was low, thymoxamine produced a striking increase in the clearance rate when administered either intravenously or subcutaneously into the base of the flap. The effect on flaps, but lack of effect on normal skin, suggested a degree of alpha-adrenoceptor mediated vasoconstriction in the acutely raised bipedicle flap.

Hendel et al (1983) studied the blood flow in acute longitudinal abdominal rat flaps based on the inferior epigastric artery compared with adjacent normal skin. By administering various agents and observing the effect on xenon clearance they found that there was an increase in vasospastic tone in acute flaps. The agent responsible seemed to possess two characteristics. Firstly, it appeared to be working at the receptor-site level, and secondly, it caused flap vessels to be more sensitive to systemic alpha-agonists than was control skin. These findings were consistent with the existence of a naturally occurring vasoconstrictor confined to the flap such as serotonin, catecholamine, or a prostaglandin. By a further study, in which preoperative depletion of the sympathetic nerve terminals produced an increase in flap survival, they showed that noradrenaline released from sympathetic nerve endings was the most likely suspect.

Kay & Le Winn (1981) showed that when 12 cm × 2 cm acute dorsal rat flaps were prepared in such a way that no sympathetic denervation occurred, they survived better than when they were denervated. The innervated flap survived completely in all cases while the denervated flap survived to only 70% of its original length. This difference disappeared when a high dose (100 ng/kg) of 6-OH dopamine was given intraperitonealy 2 hours preoperatively. They concluded that an intact sympathetic nerve supply allowed a better control of the microvasculature in the flap. A better explanation is provided by the hyperadrenergic state concept which also explains the observation that in another experiment the administration of 6-OH dopamine in rats in half the dose that Kay used, given 24 hours preoperatively, increased rather than decreased experimental acute flap survival (Jurell & Jonsson, 1976). High doses of 6-OH dopamine lead to degeneration release of noradrenaline and with a 24-hour time interval between drug administration and operation, the adrenergic nerves are already well depleted of their noradrenaline by the time of flap elevation.

Aarts (1980) has developed a method of producing regional sympathetic blockade with guanethidine in the rabbit ear. This allows treated flaps to be compared with control flaps in the same animal thereby eliminating systemic factors as a cause of differences between the two flaps and has the further advantage that the vascular pattern in rabbit ears is constant and symmetrical in pattern and size. After intravascular injection, guanethidine is rapidly fixed in the tissues and selectively blocks the peripheral sympathetic nervous system for a relatively long period of at least 5 days in the rabbit ear. A paediatric size pneumatic tourniquet around the ear base with a rubber ball in the external auditory canal for counterpressure, allows isolation of the vascular supply of the ear. One ear was injected intra-arterially with guanethidine, the control with saline, and 24 hours later 1:6 width-to-length ratio flaps were elevated through all layers of the ear (Fig. 2.18). Flap survival was significantly better in flaps pretreated with guanethidine than it was in control flaps. On a further group a delay procedure was carried out by raising a 1:3 width-to-length flap and 2 weeks later

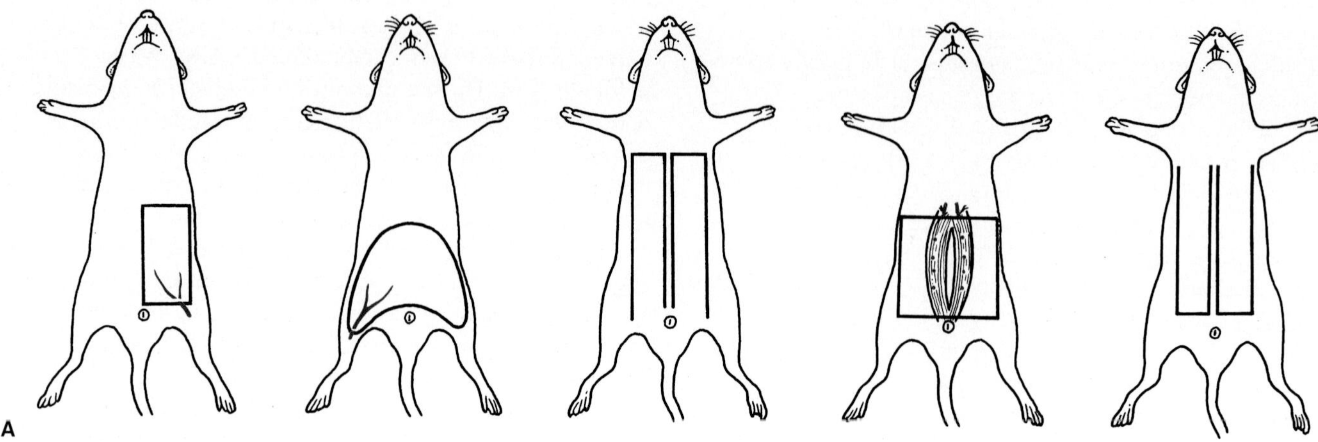

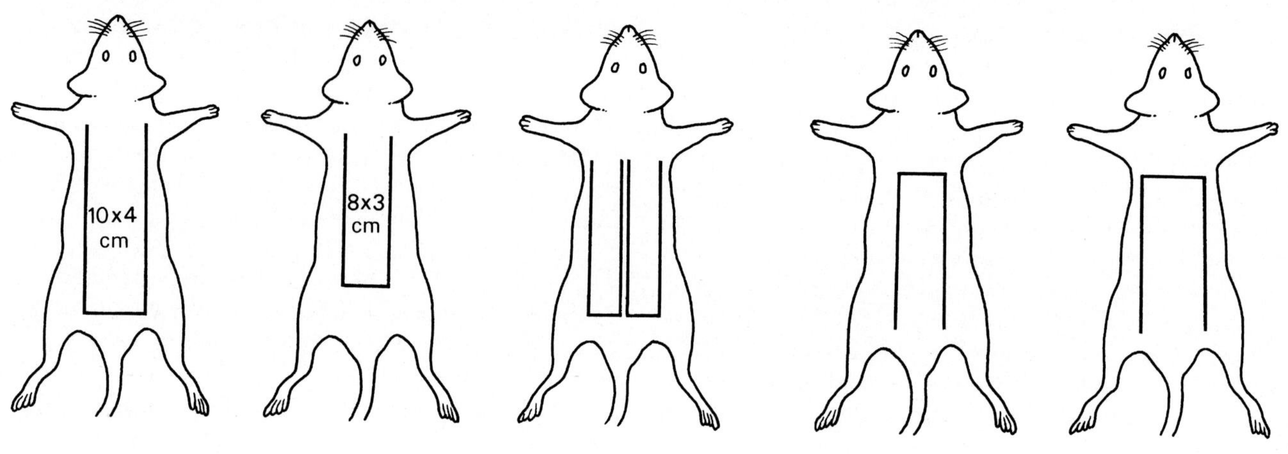

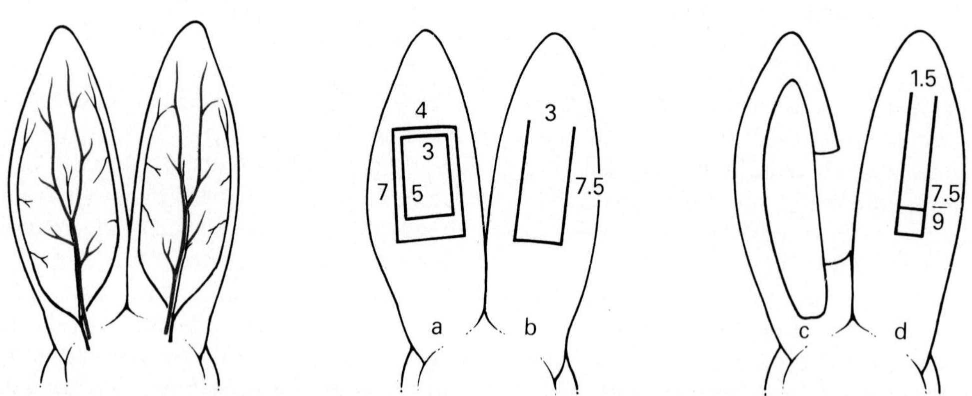

Fig. 2.18 **A**. Various designs of experimental rat flaps referred to in the text. **B**. Rabbit ear flaps: **a**. island flap or free flap of variable dimensions; **b**. pedicle flap of 2.5:1 length-to-width ratio; **d**. pedicle flaps of 5:1, 6:1 and 7:1 length-to-width ratios.

extending it to a 1:6 width-to-length ratio flap. At the same time a similar 1:6 flap was created in a guanethidine pretreated ear. Predictably enough, delayed flaps showed better survival than non-delayed controls but interestingly, guanethidine-pretreated non-delayed flaps showed significantly better survival than the delayed flaps.

The combined weight of evidence, therefore, indicates that a hyperadrenergic state initially exists in the acutely elevated flap. This concept is compatible with data on the effects of various sympatholytics on experimental flap survival – pretreatment of rats with systemic reserpine (Jurell & Jonsson, 1976); 6-OH dopamine (Wexler et al, 1975; Reinisch, 1974); propranolol (Finseth & Adelberg, 1978; Reinisch, 1974; Jonsson et al, 1975); guanethidine (Finseth & Adelberg, 1978; Aarts, 1980) and phentolamine (Jonsson et al, 1975) has increased flap survival. However, such statements must not be taken at face value and one must study each experiment in detail since other workers have failed to demonstrate any improvement in blood flow or flap survival with some of these agents (Kennedy et al, 1979; Pearl, 1981; Kerrigan & Daniel, 1982).

The design and execution of studies testing the effect of drugs on flap survival is also very complex. The following are all important variables: whether or not the treatment was commenced preoperatively; method of administration; production of toxicity; the animal; the anaesthetic agent; the variation between controls; use of placebo injections; the use of polythene interposition sheeting; when the baseline fluorescein tests were carried out; the time interval between injection and measurement of fluorescein penetration; variables in the measurement of drug-induced changes in blood flow etc. Many flap studies have not been reproduced in the literature and new models are constantly being introduced. There is certainly a need for the adoption of some basic guidelines for future pharmacological studies, and some have been suggested by Kerrigan & Daniel (1982). Many studies on experimental flap viability have utilised different criteria for measuring the degree of flap necrosis or survival. This also creates difficulties when comparing results from different studies and a consistent method of area measurement using a digitiser and a microcomputer would reduce some of these difficulties in the future (Nichter et al, 1984; Cormack & Lamberty, 1986).

Unifying theory of the delay phenomenon

Pearl (1981) has attempted to draw together some of the separate observations on acute and delayed flaps and to present a unifying theory of the delay phenomenon. This probably represents the 'best fit' hypothesis to date and envisages a situation where elevation of a pedicled skin flap produces a hyperadrenergic state within it lasting between 18 and 30 hours. This results in a vasoconstriction which affects particularly the precapillary sphincters and reduces flow in the nutrient capillary bed. Since maximum ischaemia time after which recovery is unlikely is probably at most 24 hours, any influences that decrease vascular flow for even one day can cause irreversible tissue necrosis.

In a *random acute flap* this may happen in the terminal part of the flap where the perfusion pressure has been reduced to the greatest degree by the division of multiple arterial in-flow channels.

By contrast, in the *bipedicle delayed flap* the vascular inflow has not been decreased as much, the arteriolar pressure is higher, nutrient capillary flow is maintained throughout the flap, and the vessels and tissues are able to survive the hyperadrenergic state. Recovery from the hyperadrenergic state follows over the next few days. Thus, when the flap is finally elevated, adverse vasoconstriction is avoided and a more reliable flap results.

The unifying theory is supported by Finseth & Cutting's work (1978) which was originally explained as supporting the sympathectomy → vasodilation hypothesis. They designed a rat skin flap model consisting of a 9 × 9 cm abdominal neurovascular island flap pedicled on one groin neurovascular bundle (Figs. 2.18 & 2.19). This in effect creates an axial pattern flap on the side of the pedicle with a random pattern flap on the other side of the midline which is entirely dependent on the axial pattern portion. A consistent, reproducible pattern of necrosis occurs in the random portion of the flap, and can be varied by delay procedures effected only on this side 6 weeks prior to elevation of the whole island flap. The delay procedure may take one of 5 forms:

1. division of artery, vein and nerve
2. division of nerve and 'skeletonising' of artery and vein
3. division of artery and vein with preservation of adventitia as much as possible
4. division of artery alone (adventitia preserved)
5. division of vein alone (adventitia preserved).

Finseth & Cutting found that compared to control acute flaps all five experimental delays produced increases in survival of the random portion of the flap. These increases were greatest in group 1 and least in group 5. They commented that these were 'curious observations' and suggested that the effects of these manipulations might have a common final pathway in vasodilation. On this basis both denervation and ischaemia were seen as

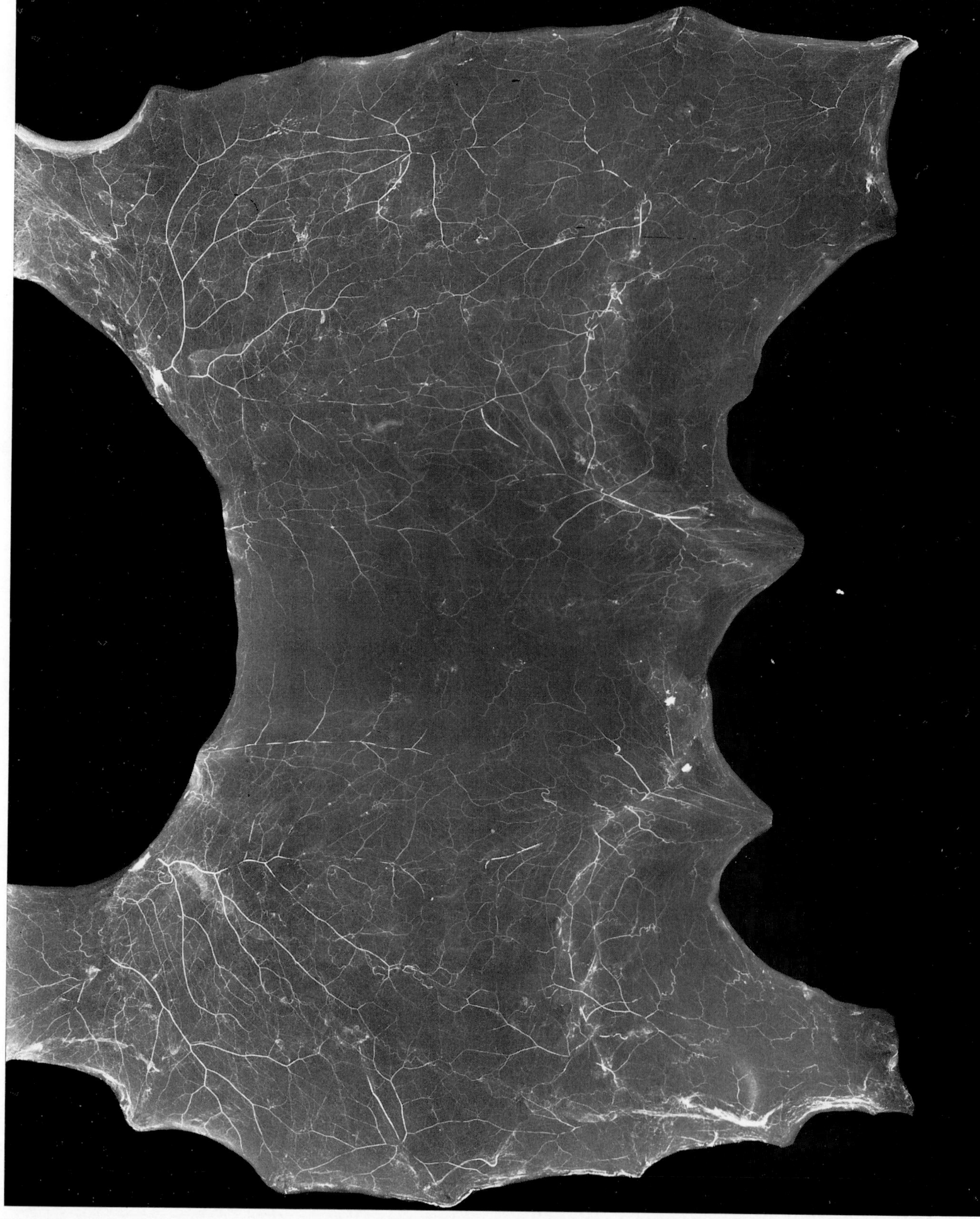

Fig. 2.19 Life size reproduction of injected rat skin preparation which shows how some of the 'random' experimental rat flaps may have included axial vessels. Male Sprague Dawley rat weighing approximately 350 g. Micropaque injection via right carotid artery. Dorsal midline incision, cephalic end on left but head not included, candal on right but tail not included.

contributing to the delay phenomenon. However, another interpretation may be based on the fact that the increase in flap survival is directly related to the degree of denervation produced by the delay procedure. The greater the denervation brought about by the delay, the smaller was the area of necrosis when the flap was finally elevated. This is perfectly in keeping with our concept of the hyperadrenergic state as bringing about flap necrosis, and of the delay period as enabling a recovery from this state to occur.

These and most other experimental studies of the delay phenomenon have used pedicled flaps but Pearl (1981) has carried out some studies using the rat abdominal flap as a free flap, which effectively divides all sympathetic nerves to the flap including the ones in the adventitia around the arteries. These studies were in effect an attempt to duplicate Finseth & Cutting's work using a free flap. At the initial procedure he elevated the whole ventral abdominal wall skin on both groin pedicles and divided either the artery or the vein or the nerve on one side only. After a delay period of 6 weeks the whole flap was re-elevated with complete division of both neurovascular bundles. The flap was then reattached by microvascular anastomoses of the vein and artery on the previously unoperated side. Survival of the 'random' half of the flap was measured 7 days later and found to be the same (differences present but not significant at 0.05 confidence level) for all three experimental groups as that of control acute flaps raised on the artery and vein of one groin pedicle in which the nerve was divided. It was postulated that the explanation for the lack of any effect of the so-called 'delays' on survival was provided by the division of the sympathetic nerves on the side of the microvascular anastomosis. Dividing these nerves created a hyperadrenergic state despite the previous 'delays' on the opposite side and neatly complemented Finseth & Cutting's work on delayed flaps by showing that disruption of sympathetic nerves can adversely affect flap survival.

The second element of the delay phenomenon

Recovery from the hyperadrenergic state is not the sole event taking place during the delay period. Other influences are also bringing about an increase in vascularity, and these events appear to have a longer time course of development than does the recovery from the hyperadrenergic state. This second element of the delay probably involves vasodilatation of the microcirculation from causes other than changes in the sympathetic system. Hendel et al (1983) have suggested that these changes in blood flow commence at the base of the flap and progress as an advancing wave front down the length of the flap. Five factors may theoretically be involved in this second element:

1. regression of inflammation and oedema caused by the initial surgery
2. loss of a second vasoconstrictor system
3. sensitisation of the beta-receptors
4. a direct smooth muscle action of an unknown agent
5. a change in the vascular architecture.

Furthermore, it has been suggested that the cells of the flap may adjust their metabolism to a lower rate of blood flow. These various possibilities will be considered in turn.

Regression of inflammation and/or oedema

This would fit in with the time course of the delay phenomenon. Hurvitz (1983) has investigated the effect of intraperitoneal hyaluronidase on acute 4 × 12 cm proximally based dorsal skin flaps with polythene interposition in the rat and found a minor degree of increased flap survival when hyaluronidase was started 6 days preoperatively ($0.05 < p < 0.1$). Hyaluronidase depolymerises the mucopolysaccharides of the ground substance, thereby decreasing the viscosity of the ground substance and increasing its permeability. Such augmentation of interstitial diffusion may aid the resolution of oedema as well as diffusion of nutrients to the cells in acute flaps. (An effect of hyaluronidase on perfusion may be considered unlikely, and DeHaan & Stark have demonstrated the hyaluronidase does not affect the rate of clearance of ^{51}Cr from tubed pedicles.) If so, similar regression of inflammation and oedema over time, may be contributing to the increased reliability of delayed flaps.

Anderson & Zarem (1977) have suggested that a delay procedure opens alternative pathways, possibly lymphatico-venous communications, for the egress of lymph from flaps. Their experimental model was not a true delay and there is no direct experimental evidence that this is the case. However, there seems to be a relationship between lymphatic tone and neural mechanisms of control, and Threefoot (1967) has shown that hexamethonium (a ganglion blocker) increases the incidence of demonstration of lymphatico-venous communications. Furthermore, Aarts' demonstration that pretreatment of rabbit ears with guanethidine reduces postoperative oedema may be related although mechanisms other than the effect of denervation on lymphatics may be involved; for example, changes in capillary blood pressure could have resulted in reduced oedema formation. The subject of oedema in flaps requires a lot more investigation.

Loss of a second vasoconstrictor system

The evidence from a series of studies by Hendel et al (1983) suggests that the active vasodilator element of the delay phenomenon does *not* involve loss of a second vasoconstrictor mechanism. In rats 3-week delayed ventral abdominal flaps on one side were compared with acute flaps on the other side (both based on the inferior epigastric systems). All sympathetic terminals were destroyed by 6-hydroxydopamine 24 hours before elevation of the acute flaps. Blood flow was measured by xenon clearance and found to be higher in the delayed flaps indicating that changes occurring in the sympathetic terminals are not the only mechanism at work in the delayed flap. It is possible that the delay period could have resulted in some persistent change in vessel diameter perhaps through prolonged stretch and atrophy of the precapillary vascular smooth muscle resulting in increased capillary flow. However, the nature of any second component of the delay phenomenon which might account for the increased xenon clearance was sought by administering terbutaline, a pure beta$_2$-agonist, from about 2 hours after elevation of the acute flaps, in increasing doses to these same rats which had had their sympathetic terminals destroyed. It was found that terbutaline increased the flow in control skin and in acute flaps at all doses (0.05, 0.1 and 0.15 mg/kg). The absence of an initial dip or lag in response suggests that there is *no* vasoconstrictor mechanism remaining to be overcome after elimination of the sympathetic terminals. The delayed flaps were less responsive than the acute flaps suggesting that the dilation in the delayed flaps was not the result of sensitisation of the beta-receptors. Rather it appears to be a mechanism acting beyond the level of the beta-receptor at the smooth muscle or vascular architecture level.

Direct smooth muscle action of unknown agent

It is possible that an as yet unidentified or little understood vasodilator may be acting directly on smooth muscle and thereby bypassing the beta-receptors. Likely candidates for such a substance are the prostaglandins, particularly those of the E series (e.g. PGE_2) and prostacyclin (PGI_2). Alternatively, the trauma of flap elevation may cause the release of prostaglandins with a vasoconstrictor action (e.g. $PGF_2\alpha$) or of thromboxane. Many authors have suggested a vasodilator role for locally generated PGE_2 in the vascular wall and other have suggested that PGE_1 is released. There is little evidence that PGE_1 is a naturally occurring prostaglandin in the cardiovascular system of mammals. In contrast prostacyclin is the major product of arachidonic acid metabolism in all vessel tissue so far studied. Prostacyclin is synthesised by arterial and venous intimal cells from precursors probably brought to the cells by blood platelets. It is a potent platelet anti-aggregation agent and causes vasodilatation (Fig. 2.20).

Given intravenously to the anaesthetised rabbit or rat, prostacyclin causes a fall in blood pressure and is four to eight times more potent than PGE_2, and at least 100 times more potent than 6-oxo-PGF_1 (Vane & Moncada, 1980). Since it is not inactivated by the pulmonary circulation, prostacyclin is equipotent as a vasodilator when given either intra-arterially or intravenously in the rat, rabbit or dog. In this respect prostacyclin is different from PGE_2 which, because of pulmonary metabolism, is much less active when given intravenously.

The many possible factors and mechanisms which may be involved in enabling the vascular endothelium to maintain its normal non-thrombogenic surface are listed below. Perhaps the most important is the ability to produce prostacyclin from arachidonic acid.

— electrostatic repulsion
— surface ADPase
— heparans-proteoglycans
— plasminogen activator
— thrombin binding
— prostacyclin

It is believed that there is a physiological thromboxane A_2 (TXA_2) which is generated in the blood platelets. For example, when the endothelium is damaged, local prostacyclin activity falls with the result that locally the balance is swung towards thromboxane-mediated aggregation of platelets and adhesion to the

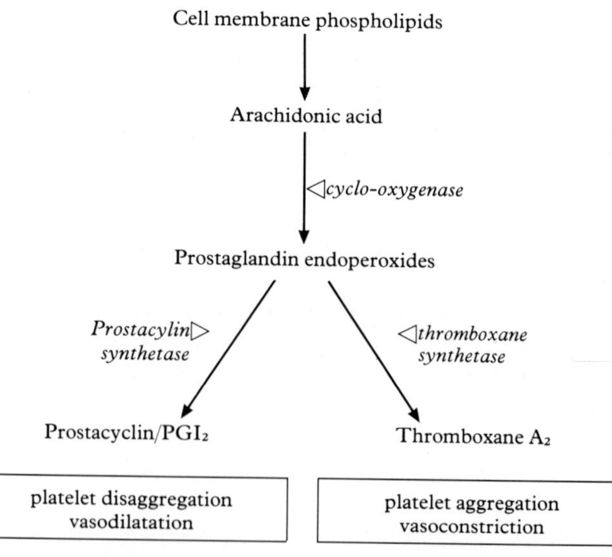

Fig. 2.20 Prostacyclin and thromboxane production from arachidonic acid.

vessel wall, such that a local platelet thrombus forms over the damaged area. The balance of this system, if it is correct to describe it as such, is open to pharmacological manipulation. Aspirin in low doses inactivates cyclo-oxygenase which has the effect of blocking thromboxane formation in platelets and prostacyclin formation in the vessel wall. The inhibition of cyclo-oxygenase in platelets is irreversible and is brought about by acetylating the active site of the enzyme. Since the platelets are unable to synthesise new protein and therefore cannot replace the cyclo-oxygenase, the effect on those platelets in circulation at the time of aspirin administration lasts throughout their life span of approximately 10 days, whereas the effect of aspirin on production of prostacyclin by the vessel wall is rapidly overcome within about 24 hours because endothelial cells can regenerate cyclo-oxygenase and can thereby synthesise prostacyclin. The net effect of aspirin administration is that the balance is swung towards prostacyclin mediated platelet disaggregation. Other agents, including non-steroidal anti-inflammatory agents, may act in such a way as to influence this balance, and have a potential role in the future development of methods of pharmacological manipulation of the failing flap.

The effect of administered prostacyclin on survival of caudally based dorsal flaps in the rat has been investigated and it was found that if treatment was begun at the commencement of the operation and continued afterwards, a significant improvement in viability over that predicted by dye penetration and over that of controls was obtained (Emerson & Sykes, 1981). Treatment with prostacyclin prior to raising the flaps did not improve their survival. The effects of prostaglandins and prostaglandin synthesis inhibitors on acute flap survival and blood flow have also been studied in the rat ventral abdominal neurovascular island flap (Sasaki & Pang, 1981). Blood flow in the flap was measured by the labelled microspheres technique. Treating the rats with prostaglandin synthesis inhibitors (indomethacin, ibuprofen) increased blood flow, and treatment either with inhibitors alone or in combination with exogenous PGE_2 significantly increased skin flap survival. Skin survival was greatest in rats receiving indomethacin and PGE_2 by subcutaneous injection twice daily for 3 days before and 3 days after skin flap construction. Similar treatment with ibuprofen alone also enhanced survival and ibuprofen injected once only before surgery increased the penetration of fluoresceind and microspheres into the flap when measured 15 minutes after surgery. Ibuprofen did not significantly alter mean arterial pressures in the treated rats and may therefore have improved flow by some means other than peripheral vasodilation. For example, ibuprofen might, by inhibiting TXA_2 formation, have reduced platelet aggregation.

These experiments suggest that certain kinds of arachidonic acid metabolites are important in determining the blood flow in acute flaps, and that blocking their production by synthesis inhibitors could significantly increase skin viability. Although no experiments have established a role for these agents in the delay phenomenon it is conceivable that their effect on vascular smooth muscle could be important, as also could be their effects on platelet aggregation.

Changes in the vascular architecture

It is accepted that some element of general vessel dilatation occurs in the delay phenomenon but in addition there may be changes in the orientation of certain vessels such that the predominating axiality of the vascular bed becomes aligned with the long axis of the flap. Alternatively some new vessel formation may occur, again predominantly aligned along the length of the flap. Such processes have been referred to as 'collateralisation', a term which suggests the opening up of pre-existing vessels of a particular orientation in a similar manner to that in which occlusion of a major limb vessel at a joint may result in enlargement of the collateral circulation.

Changes in vascular architecture during the delay phenomenon have been little studied but attention has recently been refocused on this by the fact that tissue expansion with the Radovan-type of inflatable expander has been observed to produce an increase in vascularity of the expanded skin. This has been a non-quantitative observation arising from use of the expander in patients but Cherry et al (1983) have stated that 'tissue expansion can be viewed as a form of delay' and have shown an increase in vascularity on angiograms of expanded pig skin compared with control skin in one animal. In five pigs the surviving lengths of dorsally-based flank flaps raised in skin expanded for 5 weeks using a 250 cm^3 rectangular Radovan-type tissue expander were compared with the surviving lengths of flaps elevated in: (1) tissue in which a similar prosthesis had not been expanded; (2) bipedicle flaps delayed for 5 weeks; and (3) control acutely raised random-pattern flaps. The expanded flaps had a mean increase in surviving length of 117% over control flaps, which was statistically significant. The delayed flaps had an increase in survival of 73% over control flaps, which was also statistically significant. There was no significant difference in survival between flaps raised from expanded skin and delayed skin. We have been able to confirm the increased vascularity of expanded skin demonstrated by Cherry et al but have also shown a significant degree of realignment of vessels (Cormack

& Lamberty, 1986). It was found that in pig skin overlying a hemispherical expander dilatation occurs specifically in vessels directed from the periphery radially towards the centre of the expanded area. Clearly any long flap raised through the centre of the expanded area, as in Cherry's experiments, will therefore possess a vascular network with a marked axiality along the length of the flap. We feel that it is in respect of collateralisation that 'expansion can be viewed as a form of delay' rather than in respect of general vascularity since the stimuli for angiogenesis in delay and in expansion are unlikely to be comparable.

Metabolic adaptation of flap tissue to hypoxia

This idea has been in circulation for a long time but has lacked supporting experimental evidence until relatively recently. Hoopes et al (1980) have measured hexokinase activity in dorsal guinea pig flaps. Hexokinase and certain other glycolytic enzymes (pyruvate kinase, lactate dehydrogenase, and glucose-6-phosphate dehydrogenase) showed increased activity in the distal ends of bipedicled dorsal flaps during varying delay periods. Values were twice as high as normal on day 3 but gradually returned towards normal levels. These increases occurred without alterations in enzymes of the tricarboxylic acid cycle (isocitrate dehydrogenase, malate dehydrogenase), indicating that glycolysis plays an important role in the energy metabolism of flap tissue experiencing ischaemia. Flaps raised after a delay period of 7–12 days showed continued elevation of enzyme activities. By contrast, flaps raised after only a 3-day 'delay' showed drastic decreases in enzyme activities at 24 hours following flap elevation, with low glucose levels (less than 20% of normal). Undelayed flaps exhibited distal necrosis with complete derangement of enzyme activities in that part.

These findings suggest that in flap tissues energy production from glucose is shifted to an emphasis on glycolysis and the pentose phosphate pathway. One might postulate that this occurs in order to minimise the consequences of a decreased oxygen supply and that the delayed flap is already 'prepared' in this way but much more work needs to be done.

TREATMENT OF THE FAILING FLAP

If the unified theory is correct, what implications does it have for pharmacological manipulation of the failing acute flap and is there any possibility of being able to bring about a pharmacological delay?

Pharmacological delay implies that the active agent is given for some time before the flap is elevated with the objective of overcoming the hyperadrenergic state with its adverse consequences. Skin vessels are assumed to be innervated largely (~ 95%) by alpha-adrenergic receptors and these therefore constitute an obvious target for therapy. The beneficial effect of beta-adrenergic blockade on ischaemic tissue is still open to speculation, but may be related to antagonism of beta-adrenergic stimulation of oxygen consumption, as has been reported for subcutaneous tissue (Fredholm & Karlsson, 1970).

Various agents capable of interfering with the formation of noradrenaline or its action on alpha-adrenergic receptors have been tried experimentally including phenoxybenzamine, reserpine, thymoxamine, 6-hydroxydopamine, guanethidine, bretylium, phentolamine and methyl-p-tyrosine-methyl ester.

Adrenergic neurone blocking drugs

Guanethidine (and bretylium). Guanethidine is an adrenergic neurone blocking drug acting on post-ganglionic sympathetic nerve fibres or terminals. It is taken up into the nerves where it then reduces noradrenaline release. It has a long half-life (~ 9 days) and is rapidly fixed in the tissues. Aarts (1980) has shown that following administration in the rabbit ear after 30 seconds and 10 minutes, 64% and 80% respectively of the dose was 'fixed' in the tissues. In the rabbit ear guanethidine causes a relatively long and reversible vasodilatation of at least 5 days. Using regional intra-arterial infusion and localising the guanethidine to the ear by the inflation of a pneumatic tourniquet round the base of the ear, Aarts has studied the effect of sympathetic blockade on the survival of distally based pedicled flaps cut through the full thickness of the rabbit ear (skin-cartilage-skin). Both ears were isolated by tourniquet for 10 minutes: the treated ear received 2.5 mg guanethidine into the central ear artery, the control ears received 0.9% NaCl. A day later distally based flaps 1.5 cm × 9 cm were elevated and resutured in both ears of 7 animals. Flap survival in these 1:6 width-to-length ratio pedicled flaps was found to be significantly better in the pretreated ears. In a further 4 animals delayed flaps were compared with acute flaps. The delay was performed by elevating a 1:3 flap and, 2 weeks later, lengthening it to 1:6 when a similar acute 1:6 flap was raised in the other ear. Delayed flaps showed better survival than non-delayed controls but guanethidine pretreated non-delayed flaps showed significantly better results.

Guanethidine treatment also has beneficial effects on peripheral neovascularisation and flap oedema (see p. 45) and Aarts' conclusion from both experimental and clinical experience was that regional intravascular sympathetic block with guanethidine was a safe and effective means of obtaining a 'pharmacological delay' in human extremities. It has been used on patients to produce regional sympathetic blockade for reimplantation surgery (Davies, 1976), and relief of Sudek's atrophy (Hannington-Kiff, 1977, 1984; Kay et al, 1977).

Alpha-adrenoceptor blockers

Phenoxybenzamine. This is a haloalkylamine with peak blockade about 1 hour after administration and a $t_{\frac{1}{2}}$ of 24 hours. Its position with regard to treatment of the acute flap remains equivocal. Myers & Cherry (1968) produced increased survival of dorsal rat flaps with the local use of phenoxybenzamine, but were unable to reproduce this effect in pigs. Their rat model was in any case suspect since no interposition film was used and Griffiths et al (1981) using such an improved model were unable to show any effect with phenoxybenzamine. Finseth & Adelberg (1978) appeared to produce an increase in survival with phenoxybenzamine in rats by intraperitoneal injection for 22 days starting 15 days preoperatively. This result in discredited by the fact that the controls did not receive sham intraperitoneal injections through the flap in the way the experimental group did. Wexler et al (1975) found an increase in survival with local injection into rat flaps. Smith et al (1980) administered phenoxybenzamine to rats for 1 week preoperatively and 5 days postoperatively and found no increase in survival. Kerrigan & Daniel (1982) were unable to demonstrate either increased survival lengths of pig flaps or increased blood flow by the microsphere technique after phenoxybenzamine i.v. postoperatively. Alpha-blockade was probably incomplete in these pigs since when challenged with noradrenaline the pigs responded with an increase in blood pressure. Pearl (1981) has recently suggested that phenoxybenzamine in low doses can increase flap survival, but in high doses can decrease survival. This is explained by the difference between its local and systemic effects. In low doses it may reverse the hyperadrenergic state; in high doses the systemic blood pressure falls with a consequent decrease in flap perfusion and survival.

Phentolamine. Jonsson et al (1975) have increased the survival of dorsal rat flaps with intraperitoneal phentolamine starting 1 day preoperatively and continuing for 5 days. The effect was dose dependent between 1 and 5 mg/kg per 24 hours and was statistically significant when compared with controls only at the dose level of 5 or 10 mg/kg per 24 hours.

Norberg & Palmer (1969) have presented evidence that the beneficial effect of alpha-adrenergic blockade is due to improved nutrition circulation in the flap.

Thymoxamine (4- (2-dimethylaminoethoxy)-5-isopropyl-2-methylphenyl acetate). This is an alpha-adrenergic-receptor blocker which also has a weak antihistaminic action but no beta-blocking action. It has a short half-life in vivo. It has been in clinical use for conditions due to vasospasm such as Raynaud's and acrocyanosis, and has been used intravenously during surgery for arterial disease and to counteract vasospasm on withdrawing a needle or catheter. Barisoni & Veall (1969) demonstrated that subcutaneous infiltration of thymoxamine in normal human skin had no effect on the blood flow as measured by ^{22}Na clearance. By contrast in the denervated skin of acutely raised tube pedicles and flaps there was an increased rate of clearance. Patel et al (1982) have studied the effects of thymoxamine on caudally based dorsal rat flaps. Treatment was by intraperitoneal injection 4-hourly or 8-hourly. Flow in the flap was assessed by Disulphine Blue penetration both after elevation of the flap, but before the commencement of thymoxamine treatment, and 3 days later when the course of injections was completed. It was found that thymoxamine 4-hourly increased the dye penetration over the treatment period and significantly increased final flap length over that of sham injected controls ($p < 0.001$).

Noradrenaline depletion

Reserpine. This blocks noradrenaline uptake into storage granules and consequently leads to a depletion of the noradrenaline stores in the adrenergic nerve endings. Jurell & Jonsson (1976) found that reserpine 1 mg/kg injected intraperitoneally for 3 days before and 1 day after elevation of a cranially based dorsal rat flap produced a 75% increase in survival as compared to control rats injected with saline. No further data is given concerning the experimental animals which may be significant in view of the fact that Cutting et al (1978) thought their apparent increases in flap survival with 2 weeks of reserpine pretreatment were actually due to other factors. The dose of reserpine they administered produced systemic toxicity with diarrhoea, failure to eat and weight loss of 20%. The resultant hypoproteinaemia was probably the cause of the enhanced flap survival (Cutting, 1978). On the other hand, in the study of Kennedy et al (1979) high doses of reserpine (5 mg/kg) produced toxicity but did not increase the survival of skin flaps in rats. The effect of reserpine on rat flaps therefore remains uncertain.

Beta-adrenoceptor stimulators

Beta-receptors are important in causing the vasodilatation of blood vessels in skeletal muscle and beta-agonists can increase muscle blood flow in animals and man. In the walls of skin blood vessels as many as 95% of the adrenergic receptors may be of the alpha-type and the effect of a beta-agonist on skin blood flow is likely to be negligible. Nevertheless, isoxuprine for a time was considered to have potential as a treatment for failing flaps.

Isoxuprine is similar chemically to the sympathomimetic amines and has often been described as a beta-receptor agonist but in fact it also appears to act as a direct vascular smooth-muscle relaxant, since its effects are not entirely abolished by prior treatment with beta-receptor antagonists. Isoxuprine was championed by Finseth & Adelberg (1978, 1979) but many other workers have been unable to demonstrate any effect with it on rat skin (Griffiths et al, 1981; Sasaki & Harii, 1980; Griffiths & Humphries, 1981) or pig skin (Kerrigan & Daniel, 1982; Cherry, 1979) although its ability to dilate vessels in muscles is not in dispute.

Zide et al (1980) using a slightly larger rat abdominal neurovascular island flap (9 cm × 9 cm) than that used by Finseth & Adelberg (8 cm × 8 cm) appeared to show that daily intraperitoneal injections of isoxuprine had to be given for at least 13 days preoperatively and 7 days postoperatively to achieve their full effect in enhancing survival. However, the controls did not receive placebo injections through their flaps and therefore there was no way of assessing the effects of needle punctures on the flap and the 'stress' of daily intraperitoneal injections. In a controlled study, Griffiths & Humphries (1981) were unable to produce increased survival in either the placebo injected or the isoxuprine treated group compared with untreated controls. Since there was no augmentation of survival in the sham injected group it becomes difficult to explain Finseth & Adelberg's results but the type of anaesthesia and the method of measuring the area of necrosis both varied between these studies. This shows that isoxuprine does not consistently produce increased skin flap survival in rats and further illustrates the general difficulty of reproducing results in experimental animals.

Beta-adrenoceptor blockers

Propranolol. The precise mechanism by which beta-blockade enhances flap viability is unknown but probably relates to an alteration of metabolism. Sympathetic nerve activity leads to accelerated metabolism, as evidenced by increased fatty acid mobilisation, glycerol production, oxygen consumption and carbon dioxide production (Fredholm et al, 1976). All these metabolic effects are antagonised by beta-adrenergic receptor blockers such as propranolol. Jonsson et al (1975) studied the effect of propranolol on the survival of rat dorsal flaps. Treatment at three dose levels by intraperitoneal injection 12-hourly was started 1 day preoperatively and continued for 5 days. In control rats receiving injections of saline, 38% of the flap survived. In rats receiving propranolol, 5 or 10 mg/kg per 24 hours, flap survival was 56% and 59% respectively which was a significant difference ($p < 0.02$ and 0.01 respectively). Jurell et al (1983) studied the noradrenaline, ATP and cyclic AMP changes in dorsal rat flaps treated with propranolol. Propranolol did not affect noradrenaline levels but did reduce cAMP, and although cAMP is affected by many factors, in this context it was taken to be a marker for cell metabolism. This suggests, but is not conclusive evidence for, an inhibition of beta-adrenoceptor-stimulated metabolism by propranolol.

Modulators of flap metabolism

Only recently have investigators begun to understand the roles of polyamines in numerous biological processes including ribosome stabilisation, nucleic acid and protein synthesis and cellular proliferation. An attack on polyamine synthesis may be a mechanism for slowing down the synthesis of these macromolecules and thereby also cell metabolism and the demand for substrate delivery. The result of a reduction in metabolism and overall energy demand may be beneficial in an ischaemic flap and the effect of substances which may bring about this effect have been studied in rat hearts and the rat ischaemic abdominal flap model.

Difluoromethylornithine (DFMO) is a specific irreversible 'suicide' inhibitor of ornithine decarboxylase (ODC) which catalyses the initial reaction in the biosynthesis of certain polyamines. Gelman et al (1987) have shown that pretreatment for 7 days in the rat model can inhibit ODC activity and protein synthesis, and can improve survival of rat skin flaps. Perona et al (1990) have shown that acute administration of systemic DFMO in the rat abdominal island flap model increases flap survival from 71 to 92%.

Prostaglandins and/or thromboxane

The possible roles of prostaglandin and thromboxane A_2 in flaps and the delay phenomenon have been outlined on page 58. Clinically the prostaglandins E_1 and I_2 have been found useful in peripheral vascular disease (Pardy et al, 1980; Clifford et al, 1980).

Prostacyclin. * The effects of exogenous prostacyclin (PGI_2) on flap survival in the dorsal cephalic-based rat flap have been studied (Zachary et al, 1982). It was found that rats given PGI_2 had significantly greater flap survival than controls and it was suggested that the effect might be mediated through its antiplatelet and vasodilating properties which would tend to overcome the effects of endogenously released thromboxane.

Pentoxifylline, although not a prostaglandin, affects prostacyclin levels. In addition to its viscosity lowering actions it also has an action on vascular endothelial cells which may be relevant to the treatment of the failing flap. Pentoxifylline increases production of prostacyclin and decreases production of thromboxane A_2, with an overall swing of the balance in favour of vasodilation and decreased platelet aggregation. In the treatment of ulcers in legs with peripheral vascular disease, the European literature reports response rates of 44–87% using pentoxifylline. Reports of benefit in experimental failing flap models are mixed (see p. 42).

Dipyridamole modifies platelet function by enhancing prostacyclin effect through a strong inhibition of phosphodiesterase and mild stimulation of adenyl cyclase formation. It has been shown to inhibit the formation of thromboxane A_2.

Ibuprofen and indomethacin inhibit the synthesis of arachidonic acid metabolites and appear to augment flap survival in rats (Sasaki & Pang, 1981).

*When initially discovered at the Wellcome laboratories in 1976 this substance was named PGX. Later it became PGI_2. It is now officially named epoprostenol and is marketed as Flolin.

Free radical 'scavengers' and production inhibitors

A number of extremely active and generally short lived, unstable chemical species known as 'free radicals' are formed during oxygen metabolism in all living cells and of these the superoxide anion radical ($O_2^{\dot{-}}$) is capable of generating H_2O_2 especially in the presence of transition metal ions when hydroxyl radicals ($OH^{\bullet}$) are also formed. To protect the cellular components from the destructive effects of free radicals, various natural scavenging mechanisms have evolved consisting of enzymatic control systems, physiological metal chelators and antioxidant compounds. Superoxide dismutases (SOD), catalase (CAT), and glutathione peroxidase (GSH-Px) are the major enzymatic control systems known today, and there are probably others still undiscovered. These mechanisms are backed up by the action of antioxidants such as ceruloplasmin, vitamin E, glutathione, betacarotene, vitamin A, lactoferrin, certain trace elements (e.g. Se, Mn) and some thiol-containing amino acids (Arfors, 1984).

Under certain conditions, the controlled production of free radicals appears to be important (e.g. synthesis of prostaglandins) or even essential (e.g. bacterial destruction) but increasing evidence indicates that superoxide radicals are involved in the injury of the microcirculation in metabolic disorders, inflammatory disease states, hyperoxia and ischaemic reperfusion injury.

Allopurinol. One of the sources of the superoxide radical in skin flaps is the xanthine oxidase system. In normal cells xanthine oxidase exists in the form of a dehydrogenase. Ischaemia triggers the conversion of xanthine dehydrogenase (D) to the oxygen radical producing xanthine oxidase (O). Skin has not been as fully studied in this respect as some other tissues but it is known that only 60 seconds of tissue hypoxia is required

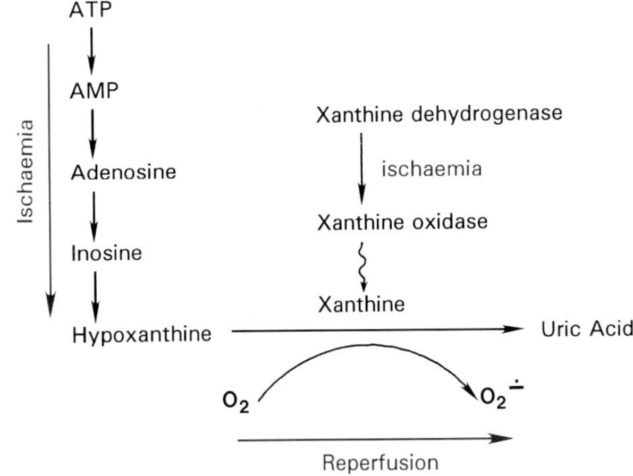

Fig. 2.21 The proposed mechanism for ischaemia/reperfusion induced production of superoxide radicals. The xanthine oxidase action is inhibited by allopurinol in the pathway marked 'Reperfusion'.

for complete D to O conversion in the intestine while the heart and kidneys require 10 minutes and 60 minutes respectively for complete conversion. (Fig. 2.21). Allopurinol, a xanthine oxidase inhibitor, offers one means of reducing the formation of free radicals by this pathway.

Superoxide dismutases (SOD) have been tried in experimental flaps. SOD administration has been shown to diminish reperfusion injury in several organs and species, notably the heart and lung, but evidence for an effect on human skin is lacking.

Mercaptoproprionylglycine (MPG), a synthetic amino acid derivative, has been reported to be a scavenger of superoxide radicals. It has also been used on experimental flaps. In addition to the superoxide radicals produced in endothelial cells and which are the principal mediators of reperfusion injury there are also systems for the production of superoxide radicals and hypochlorous HOCl radicals in granulocytes. Since granulocytes obstruct microvessels during ischaemia these cells could have a significant role in ischaemic flaps, although this possibility has been relatively under-represented in the literature.

AICA riboside (5-aminoimidazole-4-carboxamide) a naturally occurring by-product of purine biosynthesis is considered a naturally occurring anti-inflammatory mediator and inhibitor of superoxide generation by granulocytes. Engler (1987) has demonstrated that AICA riboside protects the myocardium during acute ischaemia and reperfusion. It is thought that it inhibits superoxide radical generation by ischaemia-stimulated granulocytes by the medium of adenosine released from endothelial cells which then occupies granulocyte A_2 receptors. When injected into rats before and after raising dorsal flaps, AICA reduced flap necrosis, but not quite at a statistically significant level when compared to controls (Salerno et al, 1991).

With regard to flaps there are three possible situations in which free radicals may be contributing to flap failure: (1) the globally ischaemic flap undergoing reperfusion; (2) the distally ischaemic flap; (3) the flap compromised by underlying haematoma . These are worth considering separately.

1. In the flap which has been ischaemic and is undergoing reperfusion free radicals are undoubtedly generated. In experimental studies of island flaps rendered ischaemic by venous occlusion there was no depletion of intracellular scavenger enzymes, but on reperfusion there were rapid falls in SOD and CAT tissue levels which then increase again in surviving flaps with duration of reperfusion. These changes have been demonstrated in rabbit island flaps subjected to venous occlusion (Goossens et al, 1990) and to rat island flaps subjected to arterial occlusion (Granger & Parks, 1983). Exactly what the explanation is for this fall is unknown; it is often assumed that naturally occurring enzyme activity is simply overwhelmed by the formation of oxygen free radicals during the reperfusion but the effects of washout and loss of intracellular enzymes due to increased permeability of damaged membranes may also be contributory. Also unanswered are questions concerning precisely where these changes are occurring; for example, does a 30% fall in tissue SOD activity mean that all the cells lose 30% of their SOD activity or do 30% of cells (e.g. mainly endothelial cells) lose 100% of their activity?

Nevertheless, from this simple understanding of the processes involved it seems reasonable to target both free radical production and scavenger availability to reduce damage in skin flaps undergoing reperfusion. Manson et al (1983) have shown in rat island flaps venous-occluded for 8 hours, that the administration of SOD into the artery of the flap immediately before or shortly after commencement of reperfusion, increased the number of surviving flaps compared to control injections. Sagi et al (1986) have demonstrated similar benefit with SOD after 10 and 11 hours of arterial and venous occlusion. Kim et al (1990) used MPG on the venous-occluded rat island flap model where they administered it systemically intravenously prior to commencement of flap ischaemia and again at the time of reperfusion. They found that flap survival was improved from 22% to 71% with MPG. As well as its action of reacting directly with intracellular oxygen free radicals a further action has been postulated based on its contained sulfhydryl group. It is thought that this enables MPG to prevent the conversion of xanthine dehydrogenase to oxidase by acting as a thiol agent, hence the benefit of administering MPG at the onset of ischaemia as well as the time of reperfusion.

2. In the distally ischaemic flap, and the clinically encountered situation of a failing skin flap which is showing early changes of ischaemia at its margins there may also be free-radical induced damage. If the concept of the hyperadrenergic state following flap elevation is correct then in partially ischaemic areas the hyperadrenergic state may result in not just reduction in flow but total shut down. When the hyperadrenergic state wears off, flow may resume in these partially ischaemic areas while more distal areas beyond perfusion will remain totally ischaemic. However, in the partially ischaemic areas a zone of injury mediated by oxygen free radicals may occur. If this were true, the injury might be substantially ameliorated by superoxide scavengers and the effect would be most seen in the transition zone. Evidence to support this concept comes from the work of Im et al (1985) using the rat abdominal 8 × 8 cm acute island flap model with its contralateral random component. Both SOD and allopurinol administration

increased the viable area within the random portion of the island skin flap. Approximately 10–30% of the random portion of the flap appeared receptive to such therapeutic manipulation.

In pedicled rat flaps with predictable distal necrosis, SOD administration has been attempted by various routes; either topically, or by injection into the artery of the flap, or by systemic administration. Topical administration was only effective if given under occlusive dressings or if applied directly to the undersurface of the flap (Suzuki et al, 1991); injection into the vessels of the flap was effective (Im et al, 1985); systemic administration was effective if given pre-operatively (Suzuki et al, 1989).

3. In the flap compromised by haematoma, it is the traditional view that there is a direct compression effect on the microcirculation by the haematoma but recent evidence indicates that the haematoma may also promote free-radical induced injury. Mulliken & Healey (1979) showed that even when there was apparently adequate tissue perfusion, an underlying haematoma was capable of compromising a flap and a high molecular weight compound released from haemolysed red cells was suggested as responsible. Studies using ischaemic and non-ischaemic rat flap models (Angel et al, 1986) showed that blood under ischaemic flaps significantly increased necrosis compared to controls with equivalent volumes of plasma beneath them, and furthermore when desferrioxamine was mixed with the blood there was significantly decreased necrosis compared to the blood-only flaps. Desferrioxamine, as well as being a free radical scavenger by a mechanism not totally understood at this time, is also a powerful specific iron chelator. From this and allied findings it was postulated that haemoglobin (by virtue of its iron) was able to catalyse the formation of hydroxyl radicals, and that these highly reactive cytotoxic species were responsible for bringing about flap necrosis. Ischaemic tissue, for reasons that are not clear, seems more susceptible to free radical damage and it may be that tissue damaged by haematoma-derived free radicals may then produce additional free radicals, establishing a positive-feedback loop that leads on to total necrosis. Clearly in such a situation measures need to be taken to counteract and eliminate the cause of the radicals, namely free blood under the flap.

CONCLUSIONS

In conclusion it may be said that despite many years of investigation uncertainty still persists regarding the mechanisms of the delay phenomenon. Some would argue that further investigation in this field is not justifiable because of the greatly diminished role that this procedure presently has in the plastic surgery armamentarium now that so many reliable flaps of large surface area can be successfully raised in one stage. Nevertheless, a study of the delay phenomenon provides an opportunity for concentrating attention on the biochemical and physiological basis of flap behaviour and has also increased our knowledge of the actions of various pharmacological agents on the acute flap.

Aside from the delay phenomenon, it is also the case that the technical abilities of surgeons have improved greatly from the early days of free flap surgery and so the extrinsic causes of flap failure, such as pedicle torsion and poor anastomotic repairs have become much less common, while the intrinsic sources of flap failure continue to be troublesome. Similar considerations apply in replantation surgery and this will continue until the biochemical events underlying the no-reflow and related phenomena are better understood.

At present some promising approaches to the problem of the failing flap, such as modification of cellular metabolism, are still in the early stages of being developed. Of the many other approaches that have been under investigation for longer, two broad themes emerge which appear to offer pathways by which the survival of acute flaps may be improved.

1. The first of these involves the action of pharmacological vasodilators, and is explained on a vascular basis: vasodilation sustains nutritional blood supply to the flap area in the transitional zone otherwise destined to undergo necrosis. The concept of the hyperadrenergic state indicates a mechanism by which this susceptible area is particularly subject to damaging vasoconstriction and therefore pretreatment with vasodilators may exert a beneficial effect by preventing initial adrenergic induced vasoconstriction.
2. If vasoconstriction in the transitional zone becomes established and is later followed by relief of vasoconstriction (reperfusion), then oxygen free radicals may act as mediators for the development of skin flap necrosis by their damaging action on endothelial cell membrane components and capillary basement membrane. The second line of approach therefore involves the use of allopurinol and superoxide radical scavengers to prevent this damage.

The precise clinical application of these agents and their derivatives, either alone or in combination, remains to be worked out but holds promise for the future.

References

Aarts H F 1980 Regional intravascular sympathetic blockade for better results in flap surgery: an experimental study of free flaps, island flaps and pedicle flaps in the rabbit ear. Plastic and Reconstructive Surgery 66: 690–698

Allen L 1938 Volume and pressure changes in terminal lymphatics. American Journal of Physiology 123: 3–4

Amato J J, Billy L J, Gruber R P, Lawson N S, Rich N M 1970 Vascular injuries: an experimental study of high and low velocity missile wounds. Archives of Surgery 101: 167–174

Anderson D K, Zarem H A 1977 The lymphatics in experimental flaps. Plastic and Reconstructive Surgery 59: 264–268

Angel M F, Narayanan K, Swartz W, Ramasastry S S, Basford R E, Kuhns D B, Futrell J W 1986 The etiologic role of free radicals in haematoma-induced flap necrosis. Plastic and Reconstructive Surgery 77: 795–801

Angel M F, Ramasastry S S, Swartz W M, Narayanan K, Kuhns D B, Basford R E, Futrell J W 1988 The critical relationship between free radicals and degrees of ischaemia: evidence for tissue intolerance of marginal perfusion. Plastic and Reconstructive Surgery 81: 233–239

Arfors K-E 1984 Symposium on free radicals in the microcirculation. Third World Congress for Microcirculation, Oxford, England

Austad E D, Pasyk K A, McClatchey K D, Cherry G W 1982 Histomorphologic evaluation of guinea pig skin and soft tissue after controlled tissue expansion. Plastic and Reconstructive Surgery 70: 704–710

Awwad A M, White R J, Lowe G D O, Forbes C D 1983 The effect of blood viscosity on blood flow in the experimental saphenous flap model. British Journal of Plastic Surgery 36: 383–386

Awwad A M, White R J, Webster M H C, Vance J P 1983 The effect of temperature on blood flow in island and free skin flaps: an experimental study. British Journal of Plastic Surgery 36: 373–382

Barisoni D M, Veall N 1969 Effect of thymoxamine on circulation in flaps and in denervated skin. Lancet: 400–401

Barnhill R K, Bader D, Ryan T J 1983 The effects of uniaxial tension on the superficial dermal microvasculature. Abstract. Journal of Investigative Dermatology 80: 382

Barsky S H, Rosen S, Geer D E, Noe J M 1980 The nature and volution of portwine stains: a computer-assisted study. Journal of Investigative Dermatology 74: 154–157

Bayliss W M 1902 On the local reactions of the arterial wall to changes in internal pressure. Journal of Physiology 28: 220–231

Blocker T G Jr, Smith J R, Dunton E F, Protas J M, Cooley R M, Lewis S R, Kirby E J 1959 Studies of ulceration and oedema of the lower extremities by lymphatic cannulation. Annals of Surgery 149: 884–896

Bollinger A, Butti P, Barras J-P, Trachsler H, Siegenthaler W 1974 Red blood cell velocity in nailfold capillaries of man measured by a television microscopy technique. Microvascular Research 7: 61–72

Boggon R P, Palfrey A J 1973 The microscopic anatomy of the human lymphatic trunks. Journal of Anatomy 114: 389–405

Brain S D, Tippins J R, Williams T J 1988 Endothelin induces potent microvascular constriction. British Journal of Pharmacology 95: 1005–1007

Braithwaite F 1951a Preliminary observations on the vascular channels in tube pedicles. British Journal of Plastic Surgery 3: 40–46

Braithwaite F 1951b Some observations on the vascular channels in tubed pedicles – II. British Journal of Plastic Surgery 4: 28–37

Braithwaite F, Farmer F T, Herbert F I 1951 Observations on the vascular channels of tubed pedicles using radioactive sodium. III. British Journal of Plastic Surgery 4: 38–47

Brånemark P-I 1968 Rheological aspects of low flow states. In: Shepro D, Fulton G P (eds) Microcirculation as related to shock. Academic Press, New York, p 161–180

Braverman I M, Fonferko E 1982 Studies in cutaneous ageing. II. The microvasculature. Journal of Investigative Dermatology 78: 444–448

Braverman I M, Keh-Yen A 1981 Ultrastructure of the human dermal microcirculation III. The vessels in the mid- and lower dermis and subcutaneous fat. Journal of Investigative Dermatology 77: 297–304

Braverman I M, Yen A 1977 Ultrastructure of the human dermal microcirculation II. The capillary loops of the dermal papillae. Journal of Investigative Dermatology 68: 44–52

Briedenbach W C, Terzis J K 1983 Vascularised nerve grafts. Plastic Surgical Forum 6: 131–133

Brown I A 1973 A scanning electron microscope study of the effects of increased tension on human skin. British Journal of Dermatology 89: 383–393

Brownlee G 1966 The use and abuse of vasodilator drugs. Angiology 17: 186–191

Burton A C 1939 The range and variation of the blood flow in the human fingers. American Journal of Physiology 127: 437–453

Casley-Smith J R 1977 Lymph and lymphatics. In: Kaley G, Altura B M (eds) Microcirculation Vol. I University Park Press, Baltimore

Cherry G W 1979 The differing effects of isoxuprine on muscle flap and skin flap survival in the pig. Plastic and Reconstructive Surgery 64: 670–672

Cherry G W, Austad E, Pasyk K, McClatchey K, Rohrich R J 1983 Increased survival and vascularity of random-pattern skin flaps elevated in controlled expanded skin. Plastic and Reconstructive Surgery 72: 680–685

Clarke R S J, Hellon R F, Lind A R 1958 Vascular reactions of the human forearm to cold. Clinical Science 17: 165–179

Clifford P C, Martin M F R, Sheddon E J, Kirby J D, Baird R N, Dieppe P A 1980 Treatment of vasospastic disease with prostaglandin E. British Medical Journal 281: 1031–1034

Clodius L 1977 Lymphoedema. Thieme, Stuttgart

Copley A L 1960 Apparent viscosity and wall adherence of blood systems. In: Copley A L, Stainsby G (eds) Flow properties of blood and other biological systems. Pergamon, London

Cormack G C, Lamberty B G H 1986 Measurement of geometric parameters in plastic surgery research. British Journal of Plastic Surgery 39: 307–311

Cutting B 1978 Letter to Editor of Plastic and Reconstructive Surgery 62: p 442

Cutting C B, Robson M C, Koss N 1978 Denervation supersensitivity and the delay phenomenon. Plastic and Reconstructive Surgery 61: 881–887

Davies K H 1976 Guanethidine sympathetic blockade; its value in reimplantation surgery. British Medical Journal 1: 876–877

DeHaan C R, Stark R B 1961 Changes in the efferent circulation of tubed pedicles, and in transplantability of large composite grafts produced by histamine iontophoresis. Plastic and Reconstructive Surgery 28: 577–583

Dibbell D G, Hedberg J R, McCraw J B, Rankin J H G, Souther S G 1979 A quantitative examination of the use of fluoresceine in predicting viability of skin flaps. Annals of Plastic Surgery 3: 101–105

Douglas B, Weinberg H, Song Y, Silverman D G 1987 Beneficial effects of ibuprofen on experimental microvascular free flaps: pharmacological alteration of the no-reflow phenomenon. Plastic and Reconstructive Surgery 79: 366–371

Earle A S, Fratianne R B, Nunez F 1974 The relationship of haematocrit levels to skin flap survival in the dog. Plastic and Reconstructive Surgery 54: 341–344

Edwards J M, Kinmonth J B 1969 Lymphovenous shunts in man. British Medical Journal 4: 579–581

Ellis R A 1958 Ageing of the human male scalp. In: Montagna W, Ellis R A (eds) The biology of hair growth. Academic Press, New York, 469–485

Emerson D J M, Sykes P J 1981 The effect of prostacyclin on experimental random pattern flaps in the rat. British Journal of Plastic Surgery 334: 264–266

Engler R 1987 Consequences of activation and adenosine mediated inhibition of granulocytes during myocardial ischaemia. Federation Proceedings 46: 2407–2412

Finseth F, Adelberg M G 1978 Prevention of skin flap necrosis by a course of treatment with vasodilator drugs. Plastic and Reconstructive Surgery 61: 738–743

Finseth F, Adelberg M G 1979 Experimental work with isoxuprine for prevention of skin flap necrosis and for treatment of the failing flap. Plastic and Reconstructive Surgery 63: 94–100

Finseth F, Cutting C 1978 An experimental neurovascular island flap for the study of the delay phenomenon. Plastic and Reconstructive Surgery 61: 412–420

Fredholm B, Karlsson J 1970 Metabolic effects of prolonged sympathetic nerve stimulation in canine subcutaneous adipose tissue. Acta Physiologica Scandinavica 80: 567–576

Fredholm B B, Linde B, Prewitt R L, Johnson T C 1976 Oxygen uptake and tissue oxygen tension during adrenergic stimulation in canine subcutaneous adipose tissue. Acta Physiologica Scandinavica 97: 48–59

Fujino T 1969 Contribution of the axial and perforator vasculature to the circulation in flaps. Plastic and Reconstructive Surgery 39: 125–137

Ganzer H 1943 Die Kriegsverletzungen des Gesichts und Gesichtsschaedels. Barth, Leipzig, p 226

Gelman J, Bartolome J V, Jenkins S, Serafin D, Schauberg S M, Klitzman B 1987 Reduced cell death in skin flaps in rats treated with difluoromethylornithine. FASEBJ 1: 474–477

Gillies H D 1920 The tubed pedicle in plastic surgery. New York Medical Journal 111: 1

Gillies H D, Fraser F R 1935 Treatment of lymphoedema by plastic operation. British Medical Journal 1: 96–98

Gillies H D, Fraser F R 1950 The lymphatic wick. Proceedings of the Royal Society of Medicine 2: 78

Goossens D P, Rao V K, Harms B A, Starling J R 1990 Superoxide dismutase and catalase in skin flaps during venous occlusion and reperfusion. Annals of Plastic Surgery 25: 21–25

Graham J M, Keatinge W R 1975 Responses of inner and outer muscle of the sheep carotid artery to injury. Journal of Physiology 247: 473–482

Granger D N, Parks D A 1983 Role of oxygen radicals in the pathogenesis of intestinal ischaemia. Physiologist 26: 159–164

Greenfield A D, Shepherd J T, Whelan R F 1951 The part played by the nervous system in the response to cold of the circulation through the finger tip. Clinical Science 10: 347–360

Griffiths R W, Humphries N L 1981 Isoxuprine and the rat abdominal pedicle flap: a controlled study. British Journal of Plastic Surgery 34: 446–450

Griffiths R W, Hobby J A E, Humphries N L, Trengrove-Jones G 1981 The influence of postoperative pharmacological vasodilator agents on the pattern of necrosis in a standardised rat skin flap. British Journal of Plastic Surgery 34: 441–445

Guttman L, Silver J, Wyndham C H 1958 Thermoregulation in spinal man. Journal of Physiology 142: 406–419

Hale A R, Burch G E 1960 The arterio-venous anastomoses and blood vessels of the human finger. Medicine 39: 191–240

Hannington-Kiff J G 1977 Relief of Sudeck's atrophy by regional intravenous guanethidine. Lancet 1: 1132

Hannington-Kiff J G 1984 Pharmacological target blocks in hand surgery and rehabilitation. The Journal of Hand Surgery 9B: 29–36

Hendel P M, Lilien D L, Buncke H J 1983 A study of the pharmacologic control of blood flow to acute skin flaps using xenon washout. Parts I & II Plastic and Reconstructive Surgery 71: 387–407

Henriksen O 1976a Effects of chronic sympathetic denervation upon local regulation of blood flow in human subcutaneous tissue. Acta Physiologica Scandinavica 97: 377–384

Henriksen O 1976b Local nervous mechanisms in regulation of blood flow in human subcutaneous tissues. 97: 385–391

Hertzman A B 1953 Some relations between skin temperature and blood flow. American Journal of Physiological Medicine 32: 233–251

Hibbs R G, Burch G E, Phillips J H 1958 The fine structure of the small blood vessels of normal human dermis and subcutis. American Heart Journal 56: 662–670

Hodgson R S, Brummett R E, Cook T A 1987 Effects of pentoxifylline in experimental skin flap survival. Archives of Otolaryngology, Head and Neck Surgery 113: 950–952

Hoopes J E, Chi-Tsung S U, Im M J 1980 Enzymatic responses to skin flap elevation following a delay procedure. Plastic and Reconstructive Surgery 66: 369–372

Hurvitz J S 1983 Efficacy of hyaluronidase augmented interstitial diffusion (AID) for the treatment of ischaemic flaps. Plastic Surgical Forum VI: 96–98

Hynes W 1951 The blood vessels in skin tubes and flaps. British Journal of Plastic Surgery 3: 165–175

Im M J, Shen W-H, Pak C J, Manson P N, Bulkley G B, Hoopes J E 1984 Effect of allopurinol on the survival of hyperaemic island skin flaps. Plastic and Reconstructive Surgery 73: 276–278

Im M J, Manson P N, Bulkley G B 1985 Effects of superoxide dismutase and allopurinol on the survival of acute island skin flaps. Annals of Surgery 201: 357–359

Jacobsson S, Kjellmer K 1964 Flow and protein content of lymph in resting and exercising skeletal muscle. Acta Physiologica Scandinavica 60: 278–285

Jones B M, Sanders R, Greenhalgh R M 1983 Interstitial fluid pressure as a circulatory monitor in skin flaps. British Journal of Plastic Surgery 36: 358–362

Jonsson C-E, Jurell G, Nylen B, Pandeya N 1975 Effects of phentolamine and propranolol on the survival of experimental skin flaps. Scandinavian Journal of Plastic and Reconstructive Surgery 9: 98–100

Jurell G, Jonsson C E 1976 Increased survival of experimental skin flaps in rats following treatment with antiadrenergic drugs. Scandinavian Journal of Plastic and Reconstructive Surgery 10: 169–172

Jurell G, Jhemdahl P, Fredholm B B 1983 On the mechanism by which antiadrenergic drugs increase survival of critical skin flaps. Plastic and Reconstructive Surgery 72: 518–523

Kay N N S, Woodhouse N J Y, Clarke A K 1977 Post-traumatic reflex sympathetic dystrophy syndrome (Sudeck's atrophy). Effects of regional guanethidine infusion and salmon calcitonin. British Medical Journal 1: 1575–1576

Kay S R, Le Winn L R 1981 Neural influences on experimental flap survival. Plastic and Reconstructive Surgery 67: 42–48

Keatinge W R 1964 Mechanism of adrenergic stimulation of mammalian arteries and its failure at low temperature. Journal of Physiology 174: 184–205

Kennedy T J, Pistone G, Miller S H 1979 The effect of reserpine on microcirculatory flow in rat flaps. Plastic and Reconstructive Surgery 63: 101–110

Kerrigan C L, Daniel R K 1982 Pharmacologic treatment of the failing skin flap. Plastic and Reconstructive Surgery 70: 541–548

Kiehn C S, Des Prez J D 1960 Effects of local hypothermia on pedicle flap tissue. I. Enhancement of survival of experimental pedicles. Plastic and Reconstructive Surgery 25: 349–359

Kim Y S, Im M J, Hoopes J E 1990 The effect of a free-radical scavenger, N-2-Mercaptopropionylglycine, on the survival of skin flaps. Annals of Plastic Surgery 25: 18–20

Kinmonth J B 1982 The lymphatics; surgery, lymphography and diseases of the chyle and lymph systems. Edward Arnold, London

Kinmonth J B, Hadfield G J, Connolly J E, Lee R H, Amoroso E C 1965 Traumatic arterial spasm. Its relief in man and in monkeys. British Journal of Plastic Surgery 44: 164–171

Kloner R A, Braunwald E, Maroko P R 1978 Long-term preservation of ischemic myocardium in the dog by hyaluronidase. Circulation 58: 220–226

Körlof B, Ugland O 1966 Flaps and flap necrosis. Improving the circulation in skin flaps with Complanin and with Dicoumarol: animal experiments. Acta Chirurgica Scandinavica 131: 408–412

Landis E M 1930 Microinjection studies of capillary blood pressure in human skin. Heart 15: 207–228

Lang J 1962 Über die Textur und die Vascularisation der Fascien. Acta Anatomica 48: 61–94

Lansman J B, Hallam T J, Rink T J 1987 Single stretch-activated ion channels in vascular endothelial cells as mechanotransducers? Nature 325: 811–813

Levick J R, Michel C C 1978 The effects of position and skin temperature on the capillary pressures in the fingers and toes. Journal of Physiology 274: 97–109

Lewis T 1927 The Blood Vessels of the Human Skin and their Responses. Shaw & Sons, London

Lewis T 1930 Observations upon reactions of vessels of human skin to cold. Heart 15: 177–208

Lowe G D O, Forbes C D (eds) 1981 Clinical Aspects of Blood Viscosity and Cell Deformability. Springer-Verlag, New York

Lowe G D O, Morrice J J, Forbes C D, Prentice C R M, Fulton A J, Barbenel J C 1979 Subcutaneous ancrod therapy in peripheral arterial disease: improvement in blood viscosity and nutritional blood flow. Angiology 30: 594–599

McFarlane R M, Heagy F C, Rodin S, Aust J C, Wermuth R E 1965 A study of the delay phenomenon in experimental pedicle flaps. Plastic and Reconstructive Surgery 35: 245–262
McGregor I A 1980 Fundamental techniques of plastic surgery, 7th edn. Churchill Livingstone, Edinburgh
McGregor I A, Jackson I T 1970 The extended role of the deltopectoral flap. British Journal of Plastic Surgery 23: 173–185
Malmfors T, Sachs C 1965 Direct studies on the disappearance of the transmitter and changes in the uptake-storage mechanisms of degenerating adrenergic nerves. Acta Physiologica Scandinavica 64: 211–223
Manson P N, Anthenelli R M, Im M J, Bulkley G B, Hoopes J E 1983 The role of oxygen free radicals in ischaemic tissue injury in island skin flaps. Annals of Surgery 198: 87–90
Milton S H 1965 The effects of 'delay' on the survival of experimental pedicled skin flaps. British Journal of Plastic Surgery 22: 244–252
Milton S H 1972 Experimental studies on island flaps. II. Ischaemia and delay. Plastic and Reconstructive Surgery 49: 444–447
Moncada S 1983 Prostacyclin, thromboxane and leukotrienes. British Medical Bulletin 39
Monteiro D T, Santamore W P, Nemir P 1986 The influence of pentoxifylline on skin-flap survival. Plastic and Reconstructive Surgery 77: 277–281
Moretti G, Ellis R A, Mescon H 1959 Vascular patterns in the skin of the face. Journal of Investigative Dermatology 33: 103–112
Müller R, Musikic P 1987 Hemorheology in surgery: a review. Angiology 38: 581–591
Mulliken J B, Healey N A 1979 Pathogenesis of skin flap necrosis from underlying haematoma. PRS 63: 540–545
Myers M B, Cherry G 1967 Design of skin flaps to study vascular insufficiency – failure of dextran 40 to improve tissue survival in devascularised skin. Journal of Surgical Research 7: 399–405
Myers M B, Cherry G 1968 Enhancement of survival in devascularised pedicles by the use of phenoxybenzamine. Plastic and Reconstructive Surgery 41: 254–260
Myers M B, Cherry G 1969 Mechanism of the delay phenomenon. Plastic and Reconstructive Surgery 44: 52–57
Myers B, Cherry G W 1971 Differences in the delay phenomenon in the rabbit, rat and pig. Plastic and Reconstructive Surgery 47: 73–78
Needleman P, Moncada S, Bunting S, Vane J R, Hamberg M, Samuelsson B 1976 Identification of an enzyme in platelet microsomes which generates thromboxane A_2 from prostaglandin endoperoxides. Nature 261: 558–560
Nichter L S, Sobieski M W, Morgan R F, Rodeheaver G, Edlich R F 1984 Quantitation of skin-flap survival: A computer-based method. Plastic and Reconstructive Surgery 73: 684–686
Nielson R W, Parkin J L 1976 Skin flap survival: influence of infection, anaemia and tubing. Archives of Otolaryngology 102: 727–728
Nomina Anatomica, 5th edn 1983 Williams and Wilkins, Baltimore. (A revision by the International Anatomical Nomenclature Committee, approved by the Eleventh International Congress of Anatomists in Mexico City, 1980)
Norberg K A, Palmer B 1969 Improvement of blood circulation in experimental skin flaps by phentolamine. European Journal of Pharmacology 8: 36–38
O'Brien B M, Black M J M, Fogdestam I 1978 Role of microlymphaticovenous surgery in obstructive lymphoedema. Clinics in Plastic Surgery 5: 293–304
Oden B 1960 Microlymphangiographic studies of experimental wounds healing by second intention. Acta Chirurgica Scandinavica. 120: 100–114
Oden B 1961 Microlymphangiographic studies of experimental skin autografts. Acta Chirurgica Scandinavica 121: 219–232
Östergren J, Fagrell B 1984 Capillary blood cell velocity: normal values and provocation tests. International Journal of Microcirculation 3: 492
Palmer B 1970 Sympathetic denervation and reinnervation of cutaneous blood vessels following surgery. Scandinavian Journal of Plastic and Reconstructive Surgery 4: 93–99
Pang C Y, Forrest C R, Morris S F 1989 Pharmacological augmentation of skin flap viability: a hypothesis to mimic the surgical delay phenomenon or a wishful thought. Annals of Plastic Surgery 22: 293–306
Pardy B T, Lewis J D, Eastgott H H G 1980 Preliminary experience with prostaglandins E_1 and I_2 in peripheral vascular disease. Surgery 88: 826–832
Patel C, Marsili A, Sykes P J 1982 Augmentation of flap survival by thymoxamine. British Journal of Plastic Surgery 35: 88–91
Pearl R M 1981 A unifying theory of the delay phenomenon – recovery from the hyperadrenergic state. Annals of Plastic Surgery 7: 102–112
Pearl R M 1983. Discussion of paper by Jurell et al. 'On Mechanisms by which antiadrenergic drugs increase survival of critical skin flaps.' Plastic and Reconstructive Surgery 72: 524–525
Pearl R M, Johnson D 1983 The vascular supply to the skin: an anatomical and physiological reappraisal. Part I. Annals of Plastic Surgery 11: 99–105
Perona B P, Bartolome J V, Sepka R S, Serafin D, Klitzman B 1990 Acute difluoromethylornithine treatment increases skin flap survival in rats. Annals of Plastic Surgery 25: 26–28
Prothero J, Burton A C 1962 The pressure required to deform erythrocytes. Biophysics Journal 2: 213–222
Reinisch J F 1974 The pathophysiology of skin flap circulation. Plastic and Reconstructive Surgery 54: 585–598
Reinisch J, Myers B 1974 The effect of local anaesthesia with epinephrine on skin flap survival. Plastic and Reconstructive Surgery 54: 324–327
Rhodin J 1967 The ultrastructure of mammalian arterioles and precapillary sphincters. Journal of Ultrastructural Research 18: 181–223
Rhodin J 1968 Ultrastructure of mammalian venous capillaries, venules and small collecting veins. Journal of Ultrastructural Research 25: 452–500
Roberts A H N 1985 A study of spasm in peripheral arteries. D M Thesis, Oxford University
Robson M C, Murphy R C, Heggers J P 1984 A new explanation for the progressive tissue loss in electrical injuries. Plastic and Reconstructive Surgery 73: 431–437
Ruberg R L, Falcone R E 1978 Effect of protein depletion on the surviving length in experimental skin flaps. Plastic and Reconstructive Surgery 61: 581–588
Rusznyak I, Foldi M, Szabo G 1967 Lymphatics and Lymph Circulation; physiology and pathology. Pergamon Press, Oxford
Ryan T J 1973 In: Jarret A (ed) The physiology and pathophysiology of the skin, Vol 2. Academic Press, London
Ryan T J, Barnhill R L 1983 Physical factors and angiogenesis. In: Development of the vascular system. Ciba Foundation Symposium 100. Pitman, London, p 80–94
Ryan T J, Kurban A K 1970 New vessel growth in the adult skin. British Journal of Dermatology 82: Suppl 5, 92–98
Sagi A, Ferder M, Levens D, Strauch B 1986 Improved survival of island flaps after prolonged ischaemia by perfusion with superoxide dismutase. Plastic and Reconstructive Surgery 77: 639–642
Salerno G M, McBride D M, Bleicher J M 1991 The use of S-aminoimidazole-4-carboxamide riboside (AICA riboside) to improve random skin flap viability in the rat model. Annals of Plastic Surgery 26: 544–550
Sasaki A, Harii K 1980 Lack of effect of isoxuprine on experimental random flaps in the rat. Plastic and Reconstructive Surgery 66: 105–108
Sasaki G H, Pang C Y 1981 Experimental evidence for involvement of prostaglandins in viability of acute skin flaps. Effects on viability and mode of action. Plastic and Reconstructive Surgery 67: 335–340
Sawhney C P 1980 The role of heparin in restoring the blood supply in ischaemic skin flaps: an experimental study in rabbits. British Journal of Plastic Surgery 33: 430–433
Schmid-Schönbein H 1981 Interaction of vasomotion and blood rheology in haemodynamics. In: Lowe G D (ed) Clinical aspects of blood viscosity and cell deformability. Springer-Verlag, New York
Smith D J 1952 Constriction of isolated arteries and their vasa vasorum produced by low temperatures. American Journal of Physiology 171: 528–537
Smith T W, Conway H 1962 Selection of appropriate surgical procedure in lymphoedema. Introduction of the hinged pedicle. Plastic and Reconstructive Surgery 30: 10–31

Smith G, Weeks P M, Wray C 1980 Pharmacological delay of neurovascular island skin flaps in rats. Paper presented at the 25th Annual Plastic Surgery Research Council Meeting, Hershey, Pennsylvania
Spalteholz W 1893 Die Vertheilung der Blutgefässe in der Haut. Archive für Anatomie und Physiologie (Anatomishe Abtheilung) 1–54
Squier C A 1980 The stretching of mouse skin in vivo: effect on epidermal proliferation and thickness. Journal of Investigative Dermatology 74: 68–71
Stark R B, DeHaan C R 1959 Vascular augmentation of pedicled tissues demonstrated by arteriography and injection mass. Plastic and Reconstructive Surgery 24: 19–23
Ström G 1960 Central nervous regulation of body temperature. Handbook of Physiology I, Neurophysiology II, pp 1131–1162, pp 1173–1196
Sundell B W, Patterson T J S 1963 The direct measurement of arterial, venous and tissue pressure in experimental skin flaps. Transactions of the 3rd International Conference of Plastic Surgery. International Conference Series 66: 348
Suzuki S, Miyachi Y, Niwa Y, Isshiki N 1989 Significance of reactive oxygen species in distal flap necrosis and its salvage with liposomal SOD. British Journal of Plastic Surgery 42: 559–564
Suzuki S, Matsushita Y, Isshiki N, Hamanaka H, Miyachi Y 1991 Salvage of distal flap necrosis by topical superoxide dismutase. Annals of Plastic Surgery 27: 253–257
Takayanagi S, Ogawa Y 1980 Effects of pentoxifylline on flap survival. Plastic and Reconstructive Surgery 65: 763–767
Threefoot S A 1970 The clinical significance of lymphaticovenous communications. Annals of Internal Medicine 72: 957–958
Threefoot S A, Kent W T, Hatchett B F 1963 Lymphaticovenous and lymphaticolymphatic communications demonstrated by plastic corrosion models of rats and by postmorten lymphangiography in man. Journal of Laboratory and Clinical Medicine 61: 9–22
Threefoot S A, Kossover M F, Kent W T 1967 Factors stimulating function of lymphatico-venous communications. Angiology 18: 682–698
Tooke J E 1984 Capillary pressure and flow velocity in diabetes. International Journal of Microcirculation 3: 494
Tsuchida Y, Tsuya A 1978 Measurement of skin blood flow in delayed deltopectoral flaps using local clearance of Xenon-133. Plastic and Reconstructive Surgery 62: 763–770
Tsuchida Y, Tsuya A, Uchida M, Kamata S 1981 The delay phenomenon in types of deltopectoral flap studied by Xenon-133. Plastic and Reconstructive Surgery 67: 34–41
Vane J R, Moncada S 1980 Prostacyclin. In: Blood cells and vessel walls; functional interactions. Ciba Foundation Symposium 71 (new series) Excerpta Medica, Elsevier, Amsterdam, p 7997
Vanhoutte P M, Shepherd J T 1970 Effect of temperature on reactivity of isolated cutaneous veins of the dog. American Journal of Physiology 218: 187–190
Velander E 1964 Vascular changes in tubed pedicles. Acta Chirurgica Scandinavica, Suppl 322
Ward A, Clissold S P 1987 Pentoxifylline: a review of its pharmacodynamic and pharmacokinetic properties, and its therapeutic efficacy. Drugs 34: 50–97
Wexler M R, Kalisman M, Yeschua R, Neuman Z 1975 The effect of phenoxybenzamine, phentolamine, and 6-hydroxydopamine on skin flap survival in rats. Journal of Surgical Research 19: 83–87
Whitmore R L 1968 Rheology of the circulation. Pergamon, Oxford
Wiedeman M P 1981 An introduction to microcirculation. Academic Press, New York
Wiederhielm C A 1968 Dynamics of transcapillary fluid exchange. Journal of Genetics and Physiology 52: 29–63
Willms-Kretschmer K, Majno G 1969 Ischaemia of the skin; a light and electron microscopic study. American Journal of Pathology 54: 327–353
Wu G, Calamel P, Shedd D 1978 The hazards of injecting local anaesthetic solutions with epinephrine into flaps. Plastic and Reconstructive Surgery 62: 396–403
Yen A, Braverman I M 1976 Ultrastructure of the human dermal microcirculation: the horizontal plexus of the papillary dermis. Journal of Investigative Dermatology 66: 131–142
Zachary L S, Heggers J P, Robson M C, Leach A 1982 Effects of exogenous prostacyclin on flap survival. Surgical Forum 33: 588–589
Zide B, Buncke H J, Finseth F 1980 A study of the treatment time necessary for the vasodilator drug isoxuprine to prevent necrosis in a skin flap. British Journal of Plastic Surgery 33: 383–387
Zweifach B W 1961 Functional behaviour of the microcirculation. Charles C. Thomas, Illinois

The direct cutaneous system of vessels

3

The principles of the direct cutaneous system of vessels

Clinical development of the axial pattern flap

Basic requirements for planning an axial pattern flap

The advantages and disadvantages of axial pattern flaps in practice

Reverse axial pattern flaps

3

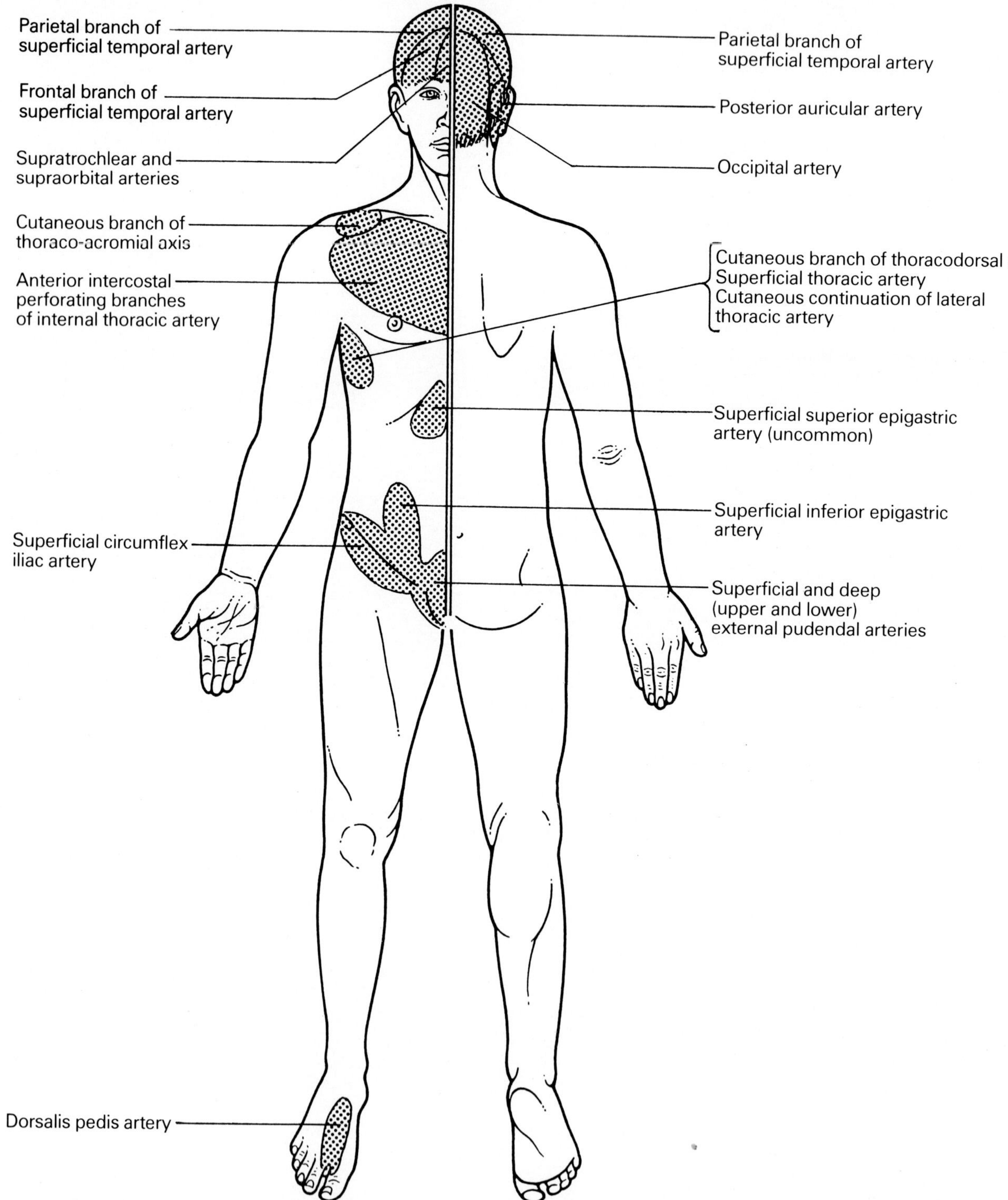

Fig. 3.1 Areas suitable for the raising of axial pattern flaps based on direct cutaneous arteries are shown. Proportions of flaps will differ from the shaded areas shown.

THE PRINCIPLES OF THE DIRECT CUTANEOUS SYSTEM OF VESSELS

In anatomical terms the direct cutaneous system of vessels consists of certain specific arteries, usually accompanied by veins, which run in the subcutaneous fat parallel to the skin surface and are confined to certain specific sites on the body (Figs 3.1 & 3.2).

These direct cutaneous arteries tend to run in a linear direction for some considerable distance, and when incorporated in a skin flap allow much greater length to breadth ratios to be achieved than would be possible in random pattern flaps. Such flaps, based on vessels of the direct cutaneous system, are traditionally known as *axial pattern flaps*. These flaps were originally conceived as pedicled skin flaps, but they have subsequently also been used as island flaps and as free microvascular transfers. In certain instances it may also be possible to include bone with these flaps (e.g. groin flap and iliac crest, dorsalis pedis flap and second metatarsal), with the bone deriving its blood supply by branches from the same vessel(s). In the normal anatomical arrangement the periosteal blood supply would come from deeper vessels (e.g. iliac crest from deep circumflex iliac artery) but in the osteocutaneous flap the anastomotic channels between the superficial and deep systems allow a reversal of this situation.

The concept of the skin being supplied solely by 'axial' and 'random' pattern vessels with the latter derived from underlying muscles was useful for a time but now requires modification as a result of the discovery of the fasciocutaneous system and of our increased understanding of cutaneous vascular anatomy. Three factors in particular must be taken into account:

1. Several flaps that were previously regarded as axial pattern flaps based on vessels of the direct cutaneous system are now known to be fasciocutaneous flaps, for example the medial arm flap.
2. The concept of axiality is now known to apply not only to the direct cutaneous vessels but also to the vessels of the fasciocutaneous system lying at the level of the deep fascia (see Ch. 5).
3. Musculocutaneous perforators in some locations possess a distinct axiality which may be exploited in the creation of musculocutaneous flaps, for example paraumbilical musculocutaneous perforators through rectus abdominis tend to radiate away from the umbilicus.

For these reasons the concept of skin being supplied solely by axial and random pattern vessels must be modified by a classification which takes into account our new knowledge of the blood supply to skin.

In the classification of cutaneous vascular anatomy here being advanced by the authors, all the vessels which supply the skin are either direct cutaneous vessels exhibiting the anatomical arrangement described in the first paragraph, or musculocutaneous perforators or fasciocutaneous perforators. In this classification there is no place for so-called 'random pattern' vessels although a *flap* may still be 'random' in orientation, i.e. raised in a direction that takes no account of local cutaneous vascular anatomy. In some situations where there is no predominating axiality of the vasculature a flap will inevitably be largely random whatever its orientation, but it is probably inappropriate to describe the vascular anatomy as 'random' because this is mainly an admission of ignorance. This book is not concerned with random flaps but when the term is used it will

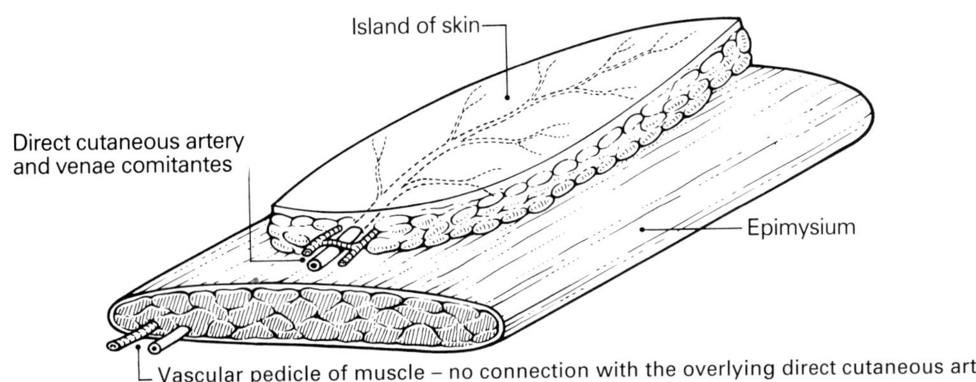

Fig. 3.2 Schematic diagram illustrating the anatomical principles of the blood supply to skin from direct cutaneous arteries.

refer to a flap which is raised in such a way that it does not intentionally exploit any existing axiality of the local vessels; such pedicled skin flaps are usually limited in their maximum dimensions to length-to-breadth ratios of 1:1 or, in the well vascularised area of the face 3:1.

The division of cutaneous vessels into three anatomical categories does not entirely solve the problems of flap nomenclature. Flaps based on the direct cutaneous system will inevitably continue to be known as axial pattern flaps, but this raises problems of terminology when it comes to describing fasciocutaneous flaps based on vessels forming a deep fascial plexus with a predominating orientation in one direction (Cormack & Lamberty, 1984). This also is a form of vessel axiality and a flap based on such an arrangement could legitimately be called axial pattern. To avoid confusion with axial pattern flaps based on a direct cutaneous vessel we have suggested a way of classifying the different arrangements of axial vessels in a fasciocutaneous flap by describing three flap TYPES (A to C). This is covered in Chapter 5 and may serve until an alternative formula for describing axiality in fascial flaps evolves.

CLINICAL DEVELOPMENT OF THE AXIAL PATTERN FLAP

As mentioned in Chapter 1, it was the publication of a letter describing the Indian rhinoplasty which prompted Carpue's development of the forehead flap method. In the early 19th century other European surgeons, notably the Italian Petrali (1842), the Germans Dieffenbach (1845) and Blasius (1848), and the Frenchman Labat (1834) all used slightly different forms of a pedicled vertical forehead flap folded on itself for the total reconstruction of noses. Their flaps were approximately triangular in shape with the apex situated over the medial end of one eyebrow and adjacent base of the nose. These flaps must have included the supratrochlear arteries and on occasions the supraorbital vessel of one side and constituted some of the first axial pattern flaps. Thereafter many other surgeons used axial pattern flaps, without perhaps fully appreciating the reasons for their improved survival.

Dunham, in 1893, described a laterally based forehead flap which included the anterior branch of the superficial temporal artery. This flap successfully survived with a 5:1 length-to-breadth ratio.

In the Lancet of 1917 Aymard described a medially based flap from the anterior chest which possessed length-to-breadth proportions well in excess of those that were customary at that time; this was the forerunner of the present deltopectoral flap. Joseph described a similar flap in 1931. Esser reported his experiences in 1934 and stated that 'The name "Artery Flaps" is added to establish the place of the "Biological Flaps" as their arteries are easy to find and feel and as their territory indicates the form and the size of the flaps'. Shaw & Payne (1946) described the hypogastric flap based on the superficial inferior epigastric artery for resurfacing the hand and their names are commonly associated with this flap although Wood had used a lower abdominal flap based on the superficial inferior epigastric artery in 1862 for release of a post-burn scar contracture of the forearm and wrist (Wood, 1863) and later used the flap in eight cases of ectopia vesicae (Khoo Boo-Chai, 1977). Its anatomy had also been reported earlier when Salmon (1936) wrote concerning the lower abdominal skin:

> 'Because of these multiple vascular anastomoses the surgeon may make curved or angulated incisions without fear of producing skin necrosis. On the other hand he must be aware of the general direction of the arteries when raising grafts of the Italian kind (pedicled flaps) on the abdominal skin. One should avoid basing flaps on the boundary line between vascular territories. When using the lateral abdominal skin it is preferable to place the base of a pedicled flap laterally. When the lower abdominal skin is used the pedicle must contain the subcutaneous abdominal artery (superficial inferior epigastric artery) as recommended by Lambret.' [Translation; author's interpretations in brackets]

Bakamjian (1965) used a deltopectoral flap to reconstruct the upper oesophagus and did much to popularise this flap so that his name became associated with it: McGregor & Jackson described this flap extensively (1970) and went on to design the groin flap based on the superficial circumflex iliac artery (1972).

The term 'axial pattern' to describe these flaps was coined by McGregor & Morgan in 1973. Their seminal paper 'Axial and random pattern flaps' clarified the distinction between these two types of flap and is often quoted as a significant milestone in the history of plastic surgery. At the same time equally important contributions to the understanding of these flaps were made by Milton (1970) and by Smith (1973). Milton (1970) raised vertical flaps on the sides of pigs and interpreted his results as indicating that flaps made under the same conditions of blood supply would all survive to the same length regardless of their width, which was a radical departure from the constraints of the traditionally taught length-to-breadth ratios. However it must be said that certain aspects of Milton's work were disadvantaged in their extrapolation to the patient by the model used, and some of his interpretations are not accepted in many quarters (Stell, 1977; Stell & Green, 1979). Smith raised longitudinal flaps on the flanks of rabbits – a site which normally contains longitudinally running vessels formed by an anastomosis of vessels from the forelimb region with vessels from the hindlimb region. As long as flaps incorporated these axial vessels they could be raised with length-to-breadth proportions of 8:1 with complete reliability and safety. When the base of the flap was situated just in front of the hindlimb then the vessels from the forelimb region had to be severed at the tip of the flap. When this was done the cut ends in the tip of the flap were observed to bleed indicating that there had been a reversal in the direction of flow in the anterior vessels. This bleeding was created by blood from the posterior vessels which had flowed through the anastomotic connections between the two systems into the anterior vessels. By contrast, the random pattern control flaps which Smith elevated at the same time necrosed until an approximately 1:1 ratio of viable flap remained. If the artery in the axial pattern flap was ligated at the base of the flap then only a small part survived; if, however, the ligation was performed further distally, then necrosis did not occur at that point but at the level of a 1:1 flap beyond the level of ligation. This indicated that the area beyond the point of ligation was a random flap being sustained by the axial pattern flap. In a similar way some axial pattern flaps may be raised to extend beyond the vascular territory of the vessel concerned without showing necrosis. In other words the dynamic territory is larger than the anatomical territory. This finding correlated well with McGregor and Morgan's concept of the existence of a vascular equilibrium or 'watershed' between adjoining anatomical vascular territories which might undergo a 'shift' if the intravascular pressure in one territory fell below that of the other.

In further experiments Smith showed that the distal end of an axial pattern flap was able to sustain a wider 'pancake' of tissue on the end of the flap if a prior delay procedure had been carried out. Here we see how the potential territory is the largest of all but precisely how large this may be has not yet been clearly defined.

At about the same time as the experiments of McGregor & Morgan – together with those of Milton and those of Smith – were clarifying the haemodynamic aspects of flap circulation, Behan & Wilson were concentrating rather more on the question of how separate anatomical territories could link up to form dynamic territories. They proposed in 1973, the term *angiotome* for 'any area of skin that can be cut as a flap which is supplied by an axial vessel but may be extended by its communication with branches of an adjacent vessel' (Behan & Wilson, 1973, 1976). They described the angiotome concept in detail as it pertained to the superficial temporal artery based forehead flap. By injecting radio-opaque media into one superficial temporal artery in the isolated forehead skin of cadavers they showed that the medium was able to move across the anatomical territories of the supraorbital and supratrochlear arteries and fill the contralateral superficial temporal artery. The principal vessel supplying the flap was termed the prop artery which is in accordance with the dictionary definition of 'axis' as the central prop which supports any system. The dynamic territory of the forehead flap when supported by the prop artery, i.e. a single superficial temporal artery, was seen to be made up of four separate angiotomes.

The angiotome concept may be represented diagrammatically as demonstrated in Figure 3.3. This indicates how the classical *deltopectoral* flap is made up of 2 or 3 prop arteries – the perforating branches of the internal mammary vessels – which supply the skin up to a point just medial to the deltopectoral groove. Here a second angiotome is vascularised by cutaneous branches of the thoracoacromial axis and extends onto deltoid. The third angiotome is made up of musculocutaneous perforators through deltoid but cannot reliably be appended onto the other two parts without a prior delay procedure. Using the angiotome terminology does not readily identify this fact and uncertainty frequently exists as to whether 'angiotome' refers to an anatomical or a dynamic territory. The authors therefore favour the use of the terms anatomical, dynamic and potential to

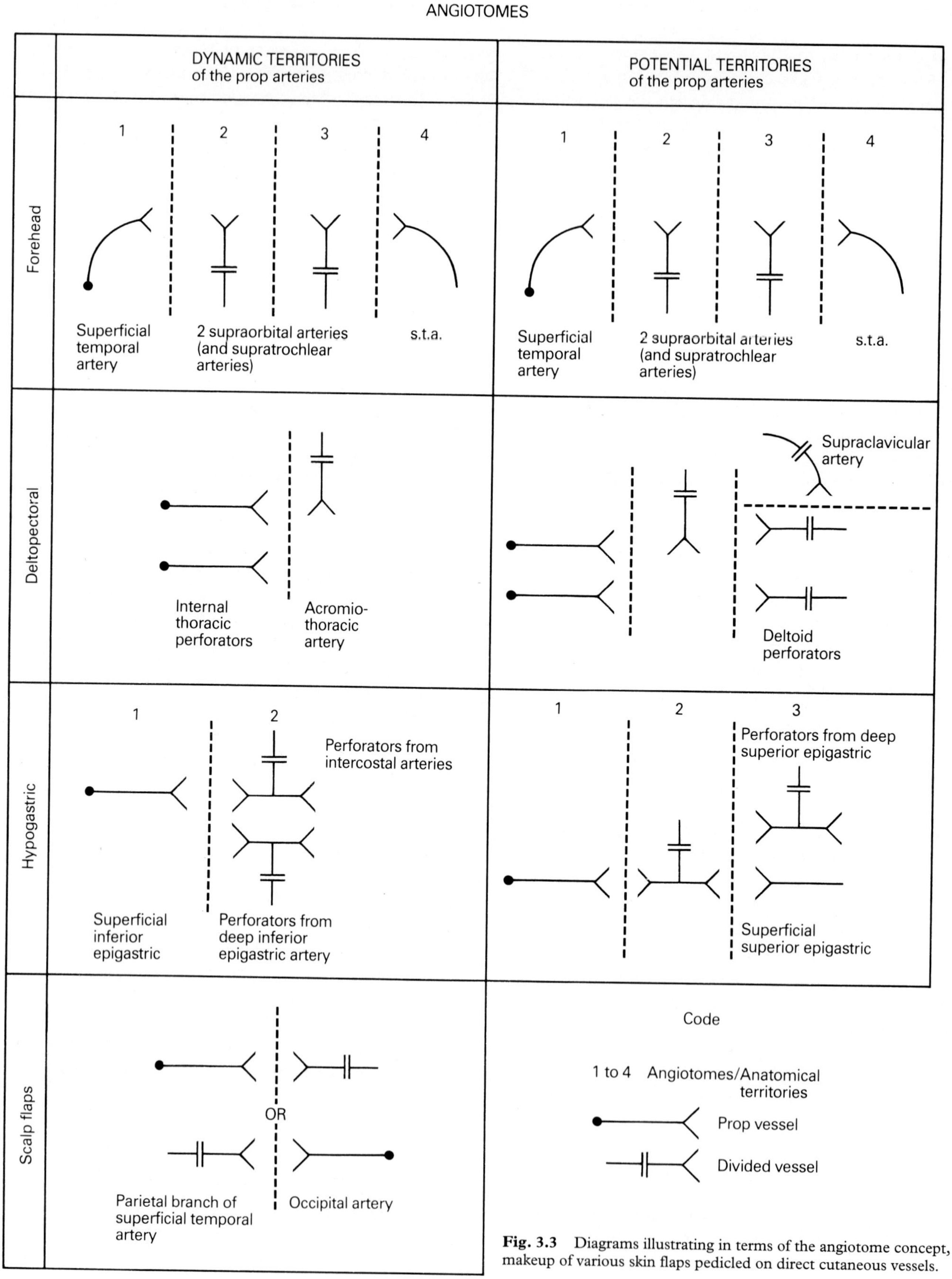

3

ANGIOTOMES

	DYNAMIC TERRITORIES of the prop arteries	POTENTIAL TERRITORIES of the prop arteries
Forehead	1 2 3 4 Superficial temporal artery; 2 supraorbital arteries (and supratrochlear arteries); s.t.a.	1 2 3 4 Superficial temporal artery; 2 supraorbital arteries (and supratrochlear arteries); s.t.a.
Deltopectoral	Internal thoracic perforators; Acromio-thoracic artery	Supraclavicular artery; Deltoid perforators
Hypogastric	1 2 Superficial inferior epigastric; Perforators from intercostal arteries; Perforators from deep inferior epigastric artery	1 2 3 Perforators from deep superior epigastric; Superficial superior epigastric
Scalp flaps	Parietal branch of superficial temporal artery; OR; Occipital artery	

Code

1 to 4 Angiotomes/Anatomical territories

Prop vessel

Divided vessel

Fig. 3.3 Diagrams illustrating in terms of the angiotome concept, the makeup of various skin flaps pedicled on direct cutaneous vessels.

describe the various types of territories. Furthermore 'angiotome' has for many years been defined in medical dictionaries (Dorland, 1965) as 'Any one of the segments of the vascular system of the embryo; called also vascular segment and intersegment', and it seems inappropriate to introduce the word in another context. It might be thought a logical term to use for a cutaneous vascular territory since it is superficially similar to dermatome – a cutaneous territory innervated by nerves originating from a single spinal segment. However, the word is in fact derived from the Greek words *angion* – a vessel (in the sense of a container but now established in medical terminology to indicate a blood vessel) and *tome* – to cut, whereas dermatome is derived from the Genitive of *derma* alone with no contribution from *tome* so the words are not comparable. Indeed, if one were looking for a word to denote the anatomical territory of a vessel, classicists assure us that angiotope, a combination of angios with topos (– a place or locality) would be the appropriate choice.

SUMMARY OF DIRECT CUTANEOUS VESSELS

Following these publications yet further axial pattern flaps were described (Table 3.1). In 1973 O'Brien & Shanmugan suggested the use of the thin, supple skin on the dorsum of the foot supplied by the *dorsalis pedis* artery, as a possible free flap. In 1975 McCraw & Furlow reported the clinical application of the dorsalis pedis flap in island and pedicled forms and Leeb et al (1977) used it as a free flap.

The use of *postauricular* skin as a free flap supplied by the postauricular artery was described by Fujino in 1975.

The development of flaps extending from the axilla onto the lateral chest wall was pursued by French surgeons from about 1974. Ricbourg (1975) described a flap based on the *lateral/superficial thoracic* artery, while the possibility of a nearby flap based on direct cutaneous branches of the *thoracodorsal* artery was investigated anatomically by De Coninck et al (1975) and used clinically by Baudet et al (1976).

Subsequently several other flaps were described which were thought to be supplied by vessels of the direct cutaneous system, e.g. the horizontal scapular, the parascapular, the saphenous artery and the medial arm flap. However, as has become evident only more recently, these flaps are in fact all based on branches of the fasciocutaneous system of vessels.

Table 3.1 The direct cutaneous system of vessels

Direct cutaneous vessel	Axial pattern flap
1. supraorbital artery	
2. frontal branch of superficial temporal artery	forehead flap
3. supratrochlear artery	Indian rhinoplasty flap
4. parietal branch of superficial temporal artery	hair-bearing flap
5. occipital artery	hair-bearing flap
6. postauricular artery	postauricular flap
7. 2nd and 3rd perforating branches of internal thoracic artery	deltopectoral flap
8. cutaneous branch of thoracoacromial axis	
9. lateral thoracic artery	external mammary flap
10. cutaneous branch of thoracodorsal artery	thoracodorsal axillary flap
11. superficial superior epigastric artery	
12. superficial inferior epigastric artery	hypogastric flap
13. superficial circumflex iliac artery	groin flap
14. superficial external pudendal artery	SEPA flap and penile flaps
15. dorsalis pedis artery	dorsalis pedis flap

3

BASIC REQUIREMENTS FOR PLANNING AN AXIAL PATTERN FLAP

The principal questions concern the proposed axial vessel:

1. Where is it?
2. What is the extent of its anatomical territory and to what extent does it interconnect with surrounding territories – i.e. what are the dynamic and even the potential territories?
3. What is the venous drainage of the area?

Where is the vessel?

This question must take into consideration all matters affecting the variability of the vessel, its size and location. Descriptions of the course of a vessel should as far as possible be related to prominent bony points. Ideally parameters of distance should be related to some feature of the individual that varies in proportion to overall size and build, e.g. finger breadths, but this is rarely done and measurements tend to be given in centimetres for a standard 'physiological' male. Appropriate allowances may therefore have to be made when transferring measurements from somebody else's written account onto one's patient. The sex of the patient may affect the size of the vessels, for example perforators from the internal thoracic artery are larger in the female since these vessels also contribute to the blood supply of the breast skin. Increasing age of the patient is associated with an increase in peripheral vascular disease which affects some vessels more than others; for example it frequently leads to occlusion of the dorsalis pedis artery. Not only may an artery itself be variable in size and location, but it may participate to a variable extent in the perfusion of vital areas other than the skin – in which case this must be detected before that vessel is operated on. For example retrograde flow of blood may take place through the supraorbital vessels into the circle of Willis in the presence of internal carotid artery stenosis or occlusion; the dorsalis pedis may, via the first web space, be the principal supply of blood to the plantar compartment of the foot when the posterior tibial artery is occluded. These situations can normally be detected by clinical examination perhaps aided by Doppler ultrasound flowprobes.

The wisdom of using arteriography in determining the size and position of the vessel has been repeatedly discussed in view of the deleterious effects of the radio-opaque medium on the endothelial lining of the arteries and veins in question – possibly predisposing to thrombotic occlusion of that vessel in the event of it being used as the basis of a free flap. Some authors recommend an interval of at least 14 days between arteriography and the transfer of a free flap, to allow for reversal of any such injury (Franklin et al, 1979). Doppler ultrasound has been found variously efficacious in tracing out the course of the artery of interest and requires an experienced operator.

What are the territories of the vessel?

The *anatomical territories* of these axial direct cutaneous arteries generally coincide with the limits of the ramifications depicted for those vessels in classical anatomical texts. Most such territories have been defined on the basis of dissection studies of vessels injected with latex or other solidifying material in fresh and fixed cadavers, supplemented with radiographs of suitably prepared material. Anatomical territories are probably also demonstrated by the area of cutaneous flushing produced by prostaglandin E_1 injection in the intact patient. PGE_1 is injected into the vessel whose territory is of interest after it has been cannulated via the transfemoral Seldinger technique and identified by arteriography under image intensifier control (Nakajima et al, 1981).

Dynamic territories can, to some extent, be simulated by dye injection studies in cadavers (e.g. methylene blue, Indian ink) and at certain sites they have been studied by intra-arterial fluorescein injection at the time of surgery (McGregor & Morgan, 1973). In the cadaver the extent of the skin discoloration following such a procedure is partly dependent on volume of dye used and on the pressure and speed of injection. A further significant limitation of these injection studies is that dye injected into an artery which supplies skin will follow the path of least resistance. Generally, this means that it will spread into adjoining anatomical territories only until it reaches the main stems of the arteries feeding those territories and the dye will then return into the larger arteries. This means that the injected dye will tend not to traverse the small vessels of several linked anatomical territories, and results in a dynamic territory which is, in many instances in the cadaver, much smaller than the territory which may be raised clinically as a flap based on that vessel. Such *potential territories* are only learnt through clinical experience.

It is, therefore, clear that illustrations of cutaneous vessels as they appear in some standard anatomical texts, are not sufficient as a guide to the true territorial limits of direct cutaneous vessels. Reliance on such information is likely to provide a safe flap but not necessarily a very useful one since it is generally true to say that the longer the flap, the more versatile it becomes. The anatomical territories of the various direct cutaneous arteries are described in Chapter 6 and their potential territories in Chapter 7.

What is the venous drainage of the area?

Details concerning the venous drainage are obviously important but many questions, particularly those relating to the importance of the valves in the veins, have remained largely uninvestigated until recently (see Chapter 5). Superficial veins on the trunk and limbs tend to drain towards the axillae and groins where they then pierce the deep fascia to meet up with the deep veins. Since several of the direct cutaneous arteries emerge from the groins or axillae a situation naturally arises in which arteries and veins supplying and draining skin tend to run countercurrent to each other. With flaps based at these sites (e.g. groin, hypogastric and thoracodorsal axillary flaps) the network of subcutaneous veins therefore tends to be the primary route for drainage of the flap. In addition, the arteries themselves will be accompanied by small venae comitantes which constitute a secondary drainage system. In areas where the subcutaneous network drains away from the base of the flap, for example, in the deltopectoral flap these venae comitantes form the only route for venous drainage.

Much less work has been done on the topographical arrangement of the subcutaneous venous system than has been done on the arteries. This is partly because of its greater variability and partly because it is often possible to see subcutaneous veins through the skin and very easy to demonstrate them on the limbs by proximal occlusion of the drainage system. This is also possible on the head – a method for revealing the veins using 'un garrot circulaire' below the level of the ears was described in 1959 (Dufourmentel & Mouly, 1959). Smith (1978) and Myers & Cherry (1967) have drawn attention to the importance of adequate venous drainage in axial pattern flaps. The key to this is that in many regions of the integument the anatomical territories of individual arterial perforators are matched by corresponding territories of valved veins and between adjoining venous territories there are valve-free veins. Detailed studies of the orientation and distribution of these valves have been carried out both in the integument (Taylor et al, 1990) and in muscles (Waterson et al, 1988).

THE ADVANTAGES AND DISADVANTAGES OF AXIAL PATTERN FLAPS IN PRACTICE

It is particularly difficult to draw general conclusions here since the flaps are so diverse, and since a quality that may be an advantage at one recipient site may be a disadvantage at another. However, it is possible to identify the following six factors, listed in no particular order, which vary from flap to flap.

Flap thinness. Some flaps based on direct cutaneous arteries are much thinner than others (e.g. dorsalis pedis v. groin flap). This will be viewed either as an advantage or disadvantage depending on the requirement for bulk.

Colour. The colour of the flap may be important – in general the nearer the donor site is to the recipient site the better will be the colour match.

Hairiness. This is an obvious consideration but it must be remembered that a free groin flap transferred in a child will later develop pubic hair at its medial end and the amount of the flap which will be affected by such hair development cannot be accurately predicted.

Donor defect. In the short-term, increased morbidity and possible prolongation of hospitalisation through difficulty in obtaining healing of the donor site may occur at some sites (e.g. dorsum of foot) more often than in others. In the long term, cosmetic and functional disability are paramount considerations. The forehead flap has largely fallen out of favour because of the unsatisfactory nature of the split skin graft on the forehead although it should be noted that in this case it is often advisable to remove all the forehead skin since a total replacement with a graft is less obvious than an isolated patch of graft above one eyebrow.

Reliability of the 'prop' vessel is crucial. Possible variations in size and course must be known.

Dependency. In a pedicled flap transfer to, for example, the hand, the position of immobilisation which will be necessary for approximately 3 weeks may be an important consideration. It may well be preferable to choose a donor site where there will be less dependency of the hand, e.g. deltopectoral flap, than a donor site such as the groin where dependency and consequently oedema will be greater.

Clearly all these factors additional to considerations of vascular anatomy must be weighed up for their advantages and disadvantages when choosing a flap based on a direct cutaneous vessel. It should be noted however that since this book is concerned with vascular anatomy and does not aim to guide the reader in the choice of the most suitable flap for any given defect it is felt to be inappropriate to deal with this topic in greater depth, particularly as several notable texts approach reconstructive problems from this viewpoint.

3

REVERSE AXIAL PATTERN FLAPS

This concept has not been touched on in the foregoing text to avoid possible confusion, but once the concept of flaps based on orthograde flow in one or more direct cutaneous arteries has been mastered it will be apparent that various possibilities exist for flaps based on these same vessels but with retrograde flow. The principles of three different types of direct cutaneous artery based reverse flaps are illustrated in Figure 3.4.

In this diagram the skin and subcutaneous fat are represented in cross-section and in all three cases a direct cutaneous artery enters the area from the right-hand side. The skin ± fat has been divided so as to create a flap which is represented by the stippled area. The arrows denote the direction of the flow of blood after raising the flap.

In Figure 3.4a an island flap is illustrated. These flaps are generally small in size, are used as local flaps only, and have very limited applications. The concept was probably first formalised in the report by Bostwick et al (1976) of a reverse-flow temporal artery island flap (Fig. 3.5a – see also under 'Superficial temporal artery' in Ch. 7). The key feature here is the island of skin carried on a fairly skeletonised pedicle in which there is reverse flow.

In Figure 3.4b the skin element of the flap has been divided to create an island on a pedicle of subcutaneous fat although this could equally have been drawn with an intact bridge of skin. This form of reverse-flow flap has a pedicle with multiple small, or not so small, choke vessel connections. This principle has probably been in use for many years; for example, the acromiothoracic tube pedicle used by McIndoe and by Gillies for nasal reconstruction had elements of a reverse-flow deltopectoral flap (Fig. 3.5b). However, this axiality was not appreciated at the time and the positioning of the base of the flap over the acromion rather than over the deltoid, whilst bringing the attachment closer to the nose, did not achieve the maximum potential inflow of blood into the base of the flap which consequently needed to be delayed for safety. The inverted superficial temporal artery scalp flap of Orticochea also conforms to this type of reverse-flow flap (Fig. 3.5c – see also Ch. 7). Recently established flaps such as the lateral calcaneal have been used with a retrograde flow design. The lateral calcaneal flap is based on the terminal part of the peroneal artery which runs in the fat over the lateral aspect of the calcaneus and then anastomoses deep to the tendon of peroneus brevis with lateral tarsal artery branches and possibly lateral plantar branches. These distal anastomoses are able to feed a reverse-flow distally-based flap (Fig. 3.5d).

The last type of reverse-flow flap (Fig. 3.4c) is one that depends on anastomoses with vessels from deep to the subcutaneous layer and is characteristically small, subcutaneously pedicled and uses the anastomoses with a direct cutaneous artery to produce a flap with length-to-breadth proportions of up to 6:1. The actual feeding vessels of these deeply vascularised flaps which are in general concentrated around the head and neck, are small and are not formally identified at operation. The branch

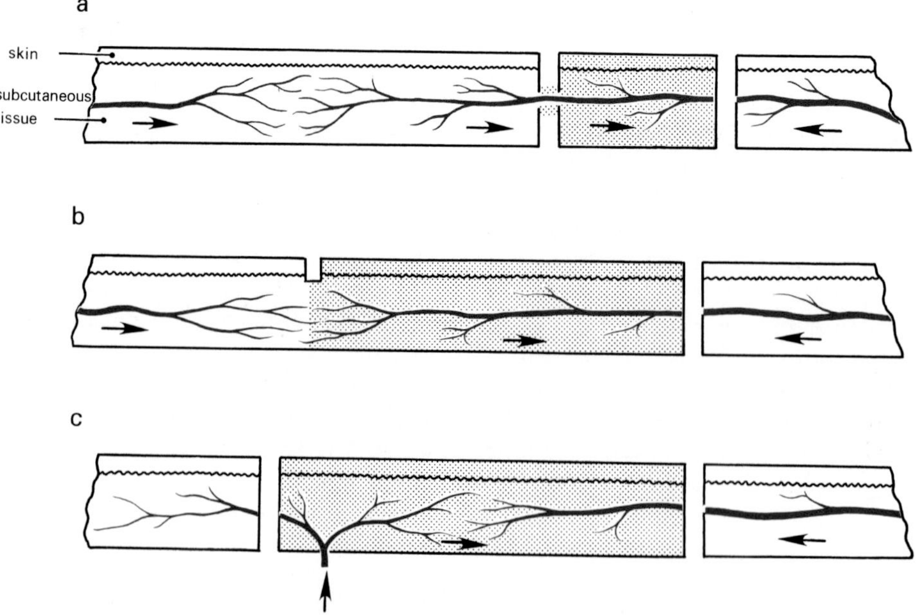

Fig. 3.4 Schematic view of the three main ways in which flaps may include the principle of reverse flow in a direct cutaneous artery. See text for explanation. The direct cutaneous artery enters the subcutaneous tissue on the right side of the diagram.

of the transverse cervical artery that runs vertically upwards in the neck may be used to produce a skin flap with a superior base extending down from the jawline with length-to-breadth ratios of 4:1. This vessel is not visualised in the dissection but is likely to be included if the flap is centred over the external jugular vein (which is left in place on the neck (see Ch. 7 – the 'Transverse cervical artery'). On the face a long vertical flap from the malar area can be raised on a subcutaneous pedicle and may be used for lower eyelid reconstruction/ectropion correction. The reliability of this flap is based in part on inclusion of the premasseteric branch of the facial artery which runs vertically upwards to make terminal anastomoses in the malar area (Fig. 3.5f).

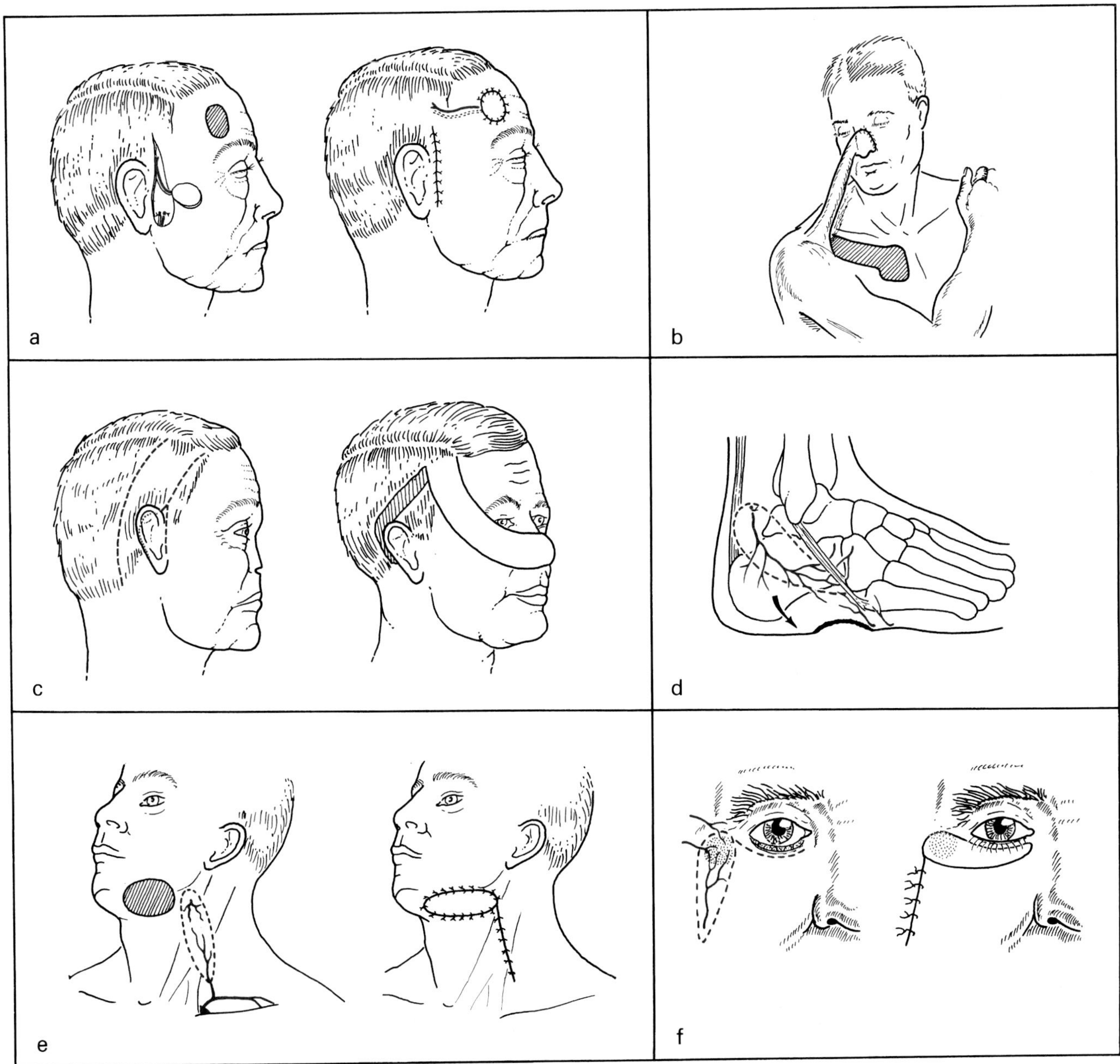

Fig. 3.5 a. Reverse-flow islanded flap on skeletonised superficial temporal artery pedicle as described by Bostwick. **b.** Acromiopectoral tube pedicle with elements of reverse flow in branches of the internal thoracic artery perforators (after Gillies & Millard, 1957). **c.** Reverse-flow superficial temporal artery flaps as designed by Orticochea. **d.** Distally-pedicled reverse-flow lateral calcaneal flap. **e.** Neck flap with reverse flow in ascending branch of the transverse cervical artery. **f.** Subcutaneously pedicled malar flap with reverse flow in premasseteric branch of facial artery.

References

Aymard J L 1917 Nasal reconstruction; with a note on nature's plastic surgery. Lancet 2: 888–891

Bakamjian V Y 1965 A two stage method of pharyngo-oesophageal reconstruction with a primary pectoral skin flap. Plastic and Reconstructive Surgery 36: 173–184

Baudet J, Guimberteau J C, Nascimento E 1976 Successful clinical transfer of two free thoracodorsal axillary flaps. Plastic and Reconstructive Surgery 58: 680–688

Behan F C, Wilson J S P 1973 The vascular basis of laterally based forehead island flaps, and their clinical applications. Presented at the Second Congress of the European Section of the International Confederation of Plastic and Reconstructive Surgery. Madrid 1973. Published by the Bernard Sunley Foundation, through the Institute of Basic Medical Sciences of the Royal College of Surgeons of England

Behan F C, Wilson J S P 1976 The principle of the angiotome – a system of linked axial pattern flaps. In: Marchac D, Hueston J T (eds) Transactions of the VIth International Congress of Plastic and Reconstructive Surgery, Paris, 1975. Masson, Paris, p 6

Blasius E 1848 Beiträge zur praktischen Chirurgie. Forstner, Berlin, p 157

Bostwick J, Briedis J, Jurkiewicz M J 1976 The reverse flow temporal artery island flap. Clinics in Plastic Surgery 3: 441–445

Cormack G C, Lamberty B G H 1984 Fasciocutaneous flap nomenclature. Letter to the Editor. Plastic and Reconstructive Surgery 73: 996

Daniel R K, Williams H B 1973 The free transfer of skin flaps by microvascular anastomoses. An experimental study and a reappraisal. Plastic and Reconstructive Surgery 52: 16–31

Corso P F 1971 Variations of the arterial, venous and capillary circulation of the soft tissues of the head by decades as demonstrated by the methyl methacrolate injection technique, and their application to the construction of flaps and pedicles. Plastic and Reconstructive Surgery 27: 160–184

De Coninck A, Boeckx W, Vanderlinden E, Claessen G 1975 Autotransplants avec microsutures vasculaires. Anatomie des zones donneuses. Annales de Chirurgie Plastique 20: 163–170

Dieffenbach J F 1845 Die operative Chirurgie. Brockhaus, Leipzig, Vol 2, p 331

Dorland's Illustrated Medical Dictionary. 1981. 26th Edition. Saunders, Philadelphia

Dufourmentel C, Mouly R 1959 Chirurgie plastique. Flammarion, Paris

Dunham M T 1893 A method for obtaining a skin-flap from the scalp and a permanent buried vascular pedicle for covering defects of the face. Annals of Surgery 17: 677–679

Esser J F S 1936 Biological or arterial flaps: general observations and techniques. Institute Esser de Chirurgie Structive, Monaco

Franklin J D, Withers E H, Madden J J Jr, Lynch J B 1979 Use of the free dorsalis pedis flap in head and neck repairs. Plastic and Reconstructive Surgery 63: 195–204

Gillies H D, Millard D R Jr 1957 Principles and art of plastic surgery. Little Brown, Boston

Jolly J 1901 Grundriss der indo-arischen Philologie und Alterstumskunde. Medicin

Joseph J 1931 Nasenplastik und Sonstige Gesichtsplastik. Kabitzch, Leipzig, p 673

Khoo Boo-Chai 1977 John Wood and his contributions to plastic surgery: the first groin flap. British Journal of Plastic Surgery 30: 9–13

Labat L 1834 De la rhinoplastie, art de restaurer ou de refaire complétement le nez. Ducessois, Paris

Leeb D, Ben-Hur N, Mazzarella L 1977 Reconstruction of the floor of the mouth with a free dorsalis pedis flap. Plastic and Reconstructive Surgery 59: 379–381

McCraw J B, Furlow L T Jr 1975 The dorsalis pedis arterialized flap. A clinical study. Plastic and Reconstructive Surgery 55: 177–185

McGregor I A, Jackson I T 1970 The extended role of the deltopectoral flap. British Journal of Plastic Surgery. 23: 173–185

McGregor I A, Jackson I T 1972 The groin flap. British Journal of Plastic Surgery 25: 3–16

McGregor I A, Morgan G 1973 Axial and random pattern flaps. British Journal of Plastic Surgery 26: 202–213

Milton S 1970 Pedicled skin flaps: The fallacy of the length : width ratio. British Journal of Surgery 57: 502–508

Myers M B, Cherry G 1967 Necrosis due to venous inadequacy: an experimental model in the skin of rabbits. Surgical Forum 18: 513–515

Nakajima H, Maruyama Y, Koda E 1981 The definition of vascular skin territories with prostaglandin E_1 – the anterior chest, abdomen, and thigh inguinal region. British Journal of Plastic Surgery 34: 258–263

O'Brien B, Shanmugan M 1973 Experimental transfer of composite free flaps with microvascular anastomoses. Australian and New Zealand Journal of Surgery 43: 285–288

Petrali N 1858 Due parole sull'arte di rifare i nasi. Gazzetta di Mantova 85: 5

Ricbourg B, Lassau J P, Violette A-M, Merland J J 1975 A propos de l'artère mammaire; Origine, territoire et intérêt pour les transplants cutanés libres. Archives d'Anatomie Pathologique 23: 317–322

Salmon M 1936 Artères de la peau. Masson, Paris

Schmid E 1952 Über neue Wege in der plastichen Chirurgie der Nase. Beiträge zur Klinischen Chirurgie 184: 385–412

Shaw D T, Payne R L 1946 One stage tubed abdominal flaps. Surgery, Gynaecology and Obstetrics 83: 205–209

Smith P J 1973 The vascular basis of axial pattern flaps. British Journal of Plastic Surgery 26: 150–157

Smith P J 1978 The importance of venous drainage in axial pattern flaps. British Journal of Plastic Surgery 31: 233–237

Stell P M 1977 The pig as an experimental model for skin flap behaviour: a reappraisal of previous studies. British Journal of Plastic Surgery 30: 1–8

Stell P M, Green J R 1979 The study of comparable skin flaps in pigs. British Journal of Plastic Surgery 29: 16–18

Taylor G I, Caddy C M, Watterson P A, Crock J G 1990 The venous territories (venosomes) of the human body: Experimental study and clinical implications. Plastic and Reconstructive Surgery 86: 185–213

Watterson P A, Taylor G I, Crock J G 1988 The venous territories of muscles: anatomical study and clinical implications. British Journal of Plastic Surgery 41: 569–585

Wilson J S P 1967 The application of the two-centimetre pedicle flap in plastic surgery. British Journal of Plastic Surgery 20: 278–296

Wood J 1863 Case of extreme deformity of the neck and forearm from the cicatrices of a burn, cured by extension, excision and transplantation of skin, adjacent and remote. Medico-Chirurgical Transactions 46: 149

The musculocutaneous system of perforators

4

The principles of the musculocutaneous system

Historical development of the musculocutaneous concept

The vascular anatomy of muscles

The anatomy of musculocutaneous perforators

Musculocutaneous flap planning

Musculocutaneous flap refinements

Advantages of musculocutaneous flaps in clinical practice

4

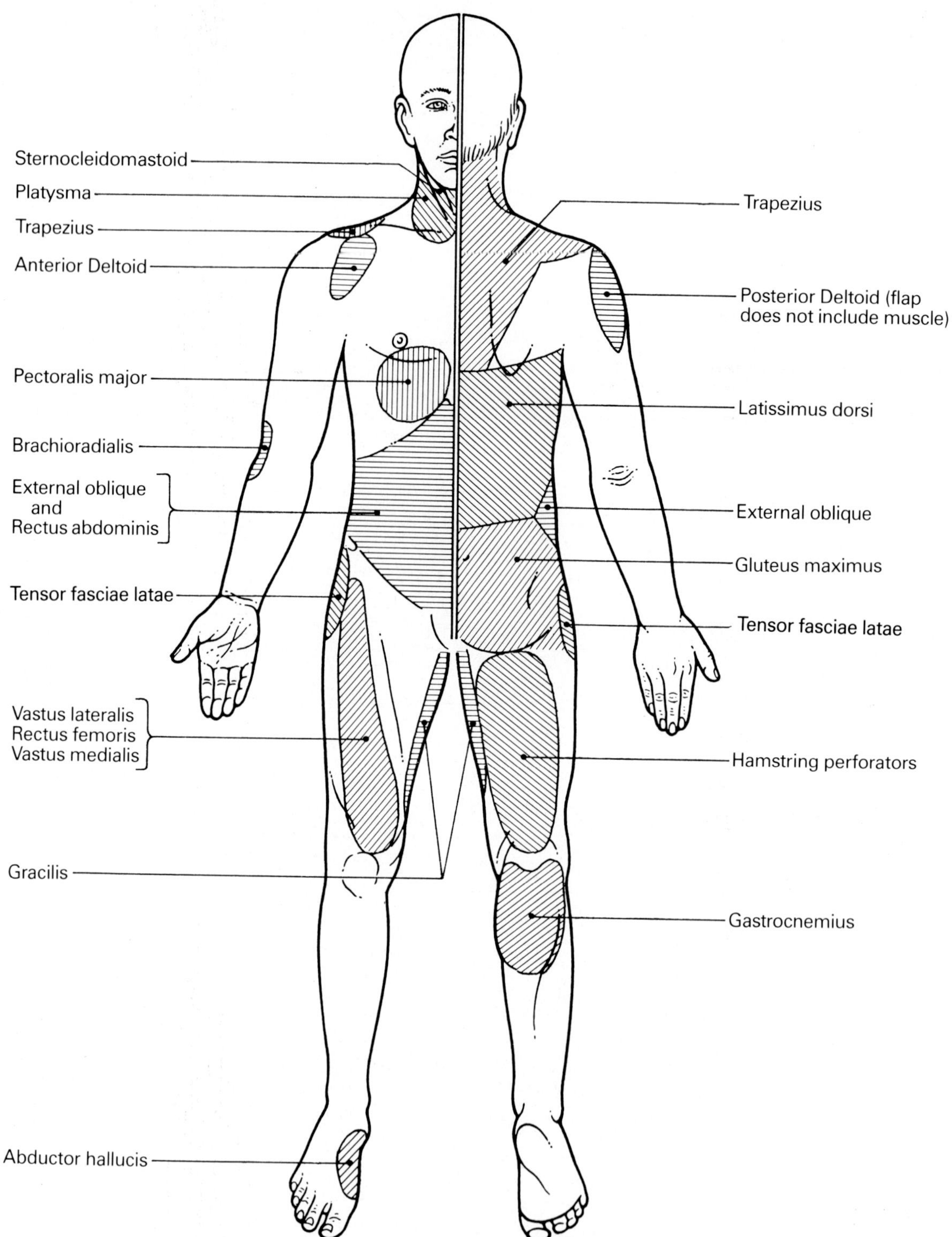

Fig. 4.1 Areas suitable for the raising of musculocutaneous flaps are shown. Proportions of actual musculocutaneous flaps will vary from the above.

THE PRINCIPLES OF THE MUSCULOCUTANEOUS SYSTEM

The musculocutaneous flap is a compound flap in which muscle, fascia, subcutaneous fat and skin are combined as one unit of tissue based on one or more vascular pedicles. The blood supply to this unit comes primarily from the supply to the muscle and reaches the skin by vessels which pierce the surface of the muscle, pass through the deep fascia and then spread out in the overlying subcutaneous tissues (Figs 4.1 & 4.2).

In a pedicled – as opposed to a free – musculocutaneous flap, the skin component may also be supplied by a secondary system of vessels coming in at the base of the skin flap. These vessels may be either direct cutaneous vessels entering the flap in an 'axial' manner or they may be fasciocutaneous vessels. In the latter case, the relationship of the axiality of the fascial vessels (see p. 119) to the orientation of the base of a given flap will determine the magnitude of this element of its blood supply. If the cutaneous component of the flap is 'islanded' or pedicled on the muscle alone then this creates a simpler situation in which only the vascular supply to the muscle supports the skin paddle. However, even in a pedicled musculocutaneous flap, the *essential* feature of the flap is that the *dominant* blood *supply* comes from the *muscle*. Any discussion of musculocutaneous flaps must therefore concentrate on the vascular anatomy of muscle but also on the question of *which* muscles give perforators to the overlying skin since McCraw et al's statement (1976) that 'the concept that skin is sustained primarily by its underlying muscle has not been clinically exploited' is too general. We now know that this should more properly read 'the concept that skin *in some areas* is sustained . . .' etc.

Similarly it is the ability of the skin to survive on the underlying muscle that characterises a musculocutaneous flap and not the merely random combination of muscle and skin. A second point of terminology concerns the slightly contentious issue of what a compound skin and muscle flap should be called. We shall adopt the convention of referring to these flaps as musculocutaneous although myocutaneous is also a popular term, having been introduced by McCraw (1980) for the sake of brevity and been accepted by the Editor of Plastic and Reconstructive Surgery 'after careful consideration of the pros and cons, and with no great sense of joy'. The purist will favour musculocutaneous since it is entirely Latin in derivation (musculus + cutis) whereas myocutaneous is half Greek and half Latin (mys + cutis). If brevity were the sole objective then myodermal which is all Greek (mys + derma) would be the obvious choice and although it is used occasionally it has not entered into widespread use.

As flap surgery has become more sophisticated this simple concept of the musculocutaneous flap as an entity in which muscle and skin coexist and are linked by blood vessels has inevitably been confronted by exceptions. Some surgeons have managed to dissect the vascular pedicle of a muscle free from its surrounding muscle fibres whilst still preserving the continuity of its perforators to overlying skin. In such a way it is possible to have a 'musculocutaneous' flap without any muscle in it. For example, the deep inferior epigastric artery may be dissected free of rectus abdominis whilst preserving one or two perforators to an island of tissue consisting only of periumbilical skin, fat and a patch of anterior rectus sheath. Nomenclature for this variant of the musculocutaneous flap has not been universally recognised (see Ch. 9) but examples are very few and are probably to be regarded as more a demonstration of technical skill than a significant advance in flap construction (muscle is spared but is it functional?).

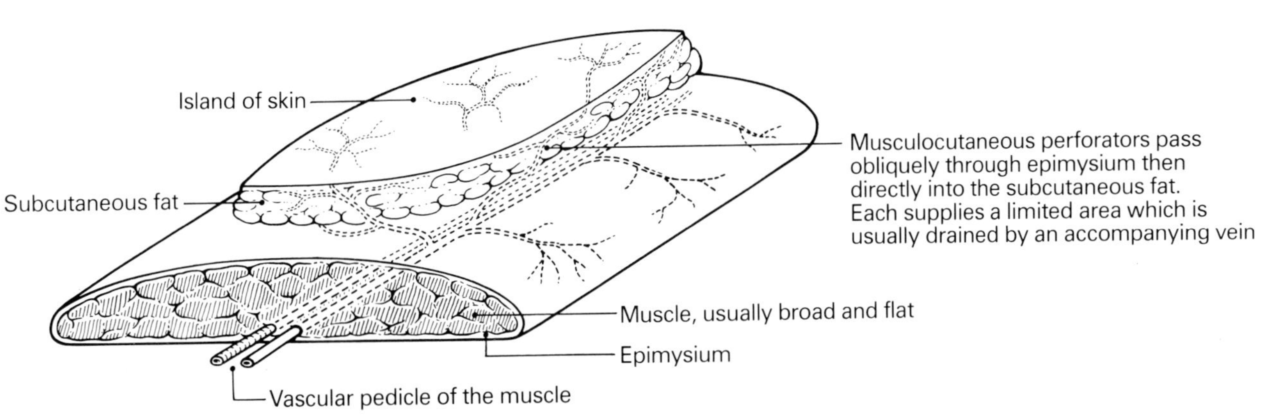

Fig. 4.2 Schematic diagram illustrating the anatomical principles of the blood supply to skin from musculocutaneous perforators.

4 HISTORICAL DEVELOPMENT OF THE MUSCULOCUTANEOUS CONCEPT

As with so much that is 'new' in reconstructive surgery, the history of the musculocutaneous flap can be traced back further in the literature than the rediscovery of the system during the early 1970s. It is to Tanzini in 1906 that the first report of a musculocutaneous flap is attributed. Tanzini had described the importance of the axial circulation to flaps, the musculocutaneous perforators in compound flaps, and the latissimus dorsi musculocutaneous unit. He had also appreciated many of the qualities of the latissimus flap which are today utilised in breast reconstruction; '. . . besides being assured of its viability, (the flap) is of a considerable thickness and succeeds in providing an even better repair of the loss of matter, (by) substituting latissimus dorsi muscle for the pectoralis major.' For some years between 1910 and 1920 'The method of Tanzini' – radical mastectomy with latissimus dorsi musculocutaneous flap wound closure – achieved some popularity in Europe and the procedure was published in many languages, including English (Purpura, 1908), in various journals around the world. However as Halsted's mastectomy with its use of thinned breast skin flaps became the standard method of management for this disease, Tanzini's method fell from favour. McCraw (1980) has pointed out that it is a sad reflection on the entrenched positions and attitudes of surgeons at that time (and since) that the magnitude of this discovery was not immediately realised and explored. As he pointed out 'had this been promptly done, the myocutaneous flap would have antiquated the tubed pedicle ten years prior to its conception!'

Less well recognised than Tanzini's work are the flaps of Snydacker and Morax. Snydacker described a flap in 1907 which was raised primarily from the mandibular angle to the clavicle and which measured 12 cm long by 2 cm wide. This flap was later modified by Morax who extended its length to below the clavicle and its width to between 5 and 7 cm. Filatov at the time commented that Snydacker's 'flap inspires fear as to the fate of the flap and pedicle because of the distance which the blood has to flow'. The flaps of Snydacker and Morax by their very length-to-breadth ratios behaved as either axial skin flaps or as musculocutaneous flaps. We know that there is no axial cutaneous vessel at that site in the neck and it is reasonable to assume that these flaps were raised so as to include the platysma muscle and received part of their blood supply from it, i.e. they were musculocutaneous. Bakamjian & Littlewood in 1964 reaffirmed the benefits of inclusion of the platysma muscle in cervical skin flaps to enhance their blood supply.

However, it was not until 1955 when Owens and later Bakamjian (1963) described the sternocleidomastoid musculocutaneous flap that we find further specific reference to the musculocutaneous system. The concept of the anatomical basis of the blood supply was still unrecognised although the concept of the muscle flap alone was also being developed (Ger, 1972, 1976). A further five years passed until, with the publications of Hueston & McConchie (1968) and DesPrez et al (1971) on respectively the pectoralis and latissimus dorsi musculocutaneous flaps, the full implications and potential of the musculocutaneous system began to be realised. They recognised independently that flat muscles could be used as the vascular support for the overlying skin but it was not until Orticochea's demonstration in 1972 that skin could be carried on a long thin muscle pedicle as 'an immediate and heroic substitute for the method of delay' that the vast potential of these flaps became apparent (Orticochea, 1972a, b).

At the same time McCraw's 'physiological dabbling' – as he described it – at Duke University led him, via the anatomy of muscles, into plastic surgery and to Atlanta under the aegis of Doctors Jurkiewicz and Woodward. Thus it was from Atlanta that so much of the anatomical description and clinical application of musculocutaneous flaps came (e.g. Vasconez et al, 1974; Mathes et al, 1974; McCraw et al, 1976, 1977, 1978, 1979).

Simultaneous expansion of the musculocutaneous concept continued in America and Europe with the development of the latissimus dorsi flap independently by Olivari (1976), Mühlbauer & Olbrisch (1977) and Maxwell et al (1978); the tensor fasciae latae flap (Nahai et al, 1978); and the pectoralis major flap (Ariyan, 1979; Arnold & Pairolero, 1979). The most significant contributions in the literature since then have been the classification of the vascular anatomy of muscles by Mathes & Nahai (1981) and their standard reference textbooks on the subject (1979, 1982).

In the 1980s we have seen a tendency towards refinement and modification of muscle and musculocutaneous flaps arising out of a better understanding of their vascular anatomy. This has taken three main forms:

1. There has been a trend towards using only a part of a muscle based on a knowledge of the patterns of division of the vessels and nerves within the muscle, e.g. the split latissimus dorsi flap or the gracilis neurovascular innervated subunit for reconstructing facial palsy.

2. There is a tendency to utilise part of a muscle so as to spare the rest for function or later use as a second flap, e.g. gluteus maximus musculocutaneous flaps for pressure sores.

3. Muscle combinations are evolving such as the latissimus dorsi with the serratus anterior, or the tensor fasciae latae with the gluteus medius and no doubt further advances in the musculocutaneous field lie ahead.

It is difficult, with hindsight, to see why so long a period elapsed between discovery and the realisation of the potential of these flaps. Perhaps as McCraw has observed (1980) surgeons were too preoccupied with the intricacies and vagaries of the tube pedicle; perhaps because surgeons tend towards conservatism; perhaps because surgeons were blinkered by the advent and growth of microsurgery in the 1960s and the quest for new free skin flap donor sites. Whatever the reason, the advances in our understanding of the musculocutaneous unit in the decade 1970 to 1980 have made up for 'the lost years'.

THE VASCULAR ANATOMY OF MUSCLES

The principal limb arteries run along flexor surfaces and avoid passing through muscular tissues which would compress them, but where they must pass through muscles, they do so through tendinous arches which protect them from pressure. The branches of supply to muscles are therefore given off outside the muscles and have an extra-muscular course which varies in length from muscle to muscle but in general the vessels pursue the most direct course. The angles which these arterial branches make with the stem vessel depends on haemodynamic factors; theoretically there is an optimum mathematical angle between branch and main stem which results in the least amount of energy loss by the circulating blood – the larger the branch, the smaller the angle. For example, branches of equal size to the remaining vessel should make an equal angle (i.e. a Y-shaped bifurcation) and branches so small that they hardly affect the size of the parent stem come off at a large angle (70–90°). Measurements show that in general terms, branching conforms to the mathematical expectations (Le Gros Clark, 1971).

The terminal distributing arteries communicate freely through numerous anastomoses which permit equalisation of pressure over vascular territories and provide alternative circulatory channels. In the limbs, there are many anastomoses around the joints which allow for free circulation when movement temporarily interferes with the flow through individual vessels. 'Free anastomoses' does not necessarily mean that under normal circumstances the blood flows along all channels open to it but these anastomoses are of particular importance in terms of the development of collateral circulations and in understanding the circulation in flaps. Developmentally, a small channel may become abnormally enlarged as an *anomaly* and as a result of this the main arterial supply to a given area, including muscle, may come from an *aberrant* vessel.

Accompanying these arteries are equivalent veins. Usually there are two such venae comitantes but large arteries are accompanied by only a single vein. The close relationship between arteries and veins arises as a secondary arrangement because in the early stages of development of the limbs, the main arteries are primarily axial while drainage is by superficial marginal veins. With limb differentiation it becomes mechanically disadvantageous for venous drainage to occur by only superficial veins and deep routes are developed along the same fascial planes as those used by arteries. The arrangement of the deep venous system in close physical proximity to the main arteries is important for the individual as a whole since it creates a countercurrent exchange system of heat transfer between the vessels

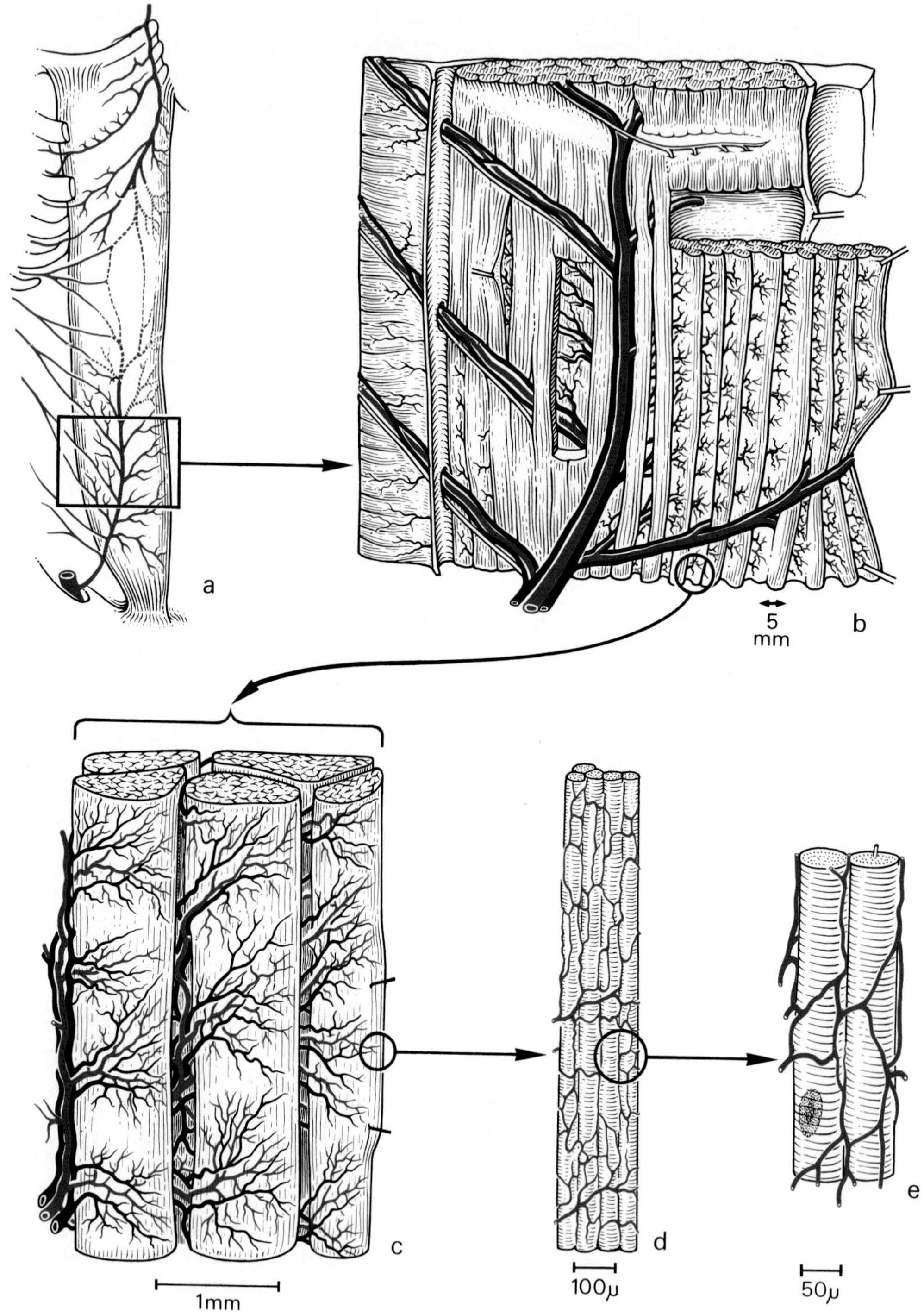

Fig. 4.3 Diagram showing the scheme of subdivision of arteries and veins between bundles of muscle fibres using rectus abdominis as the example. **a.** Posterior aspect of left rectus abdominis muscle with sheath removed showing the epigastric arcade and its connections with the intercostal arteries. **b.** On naked-eye examination the muscle is seen to be made up of parallel muscle bundles measuring approximately 5 mm in diameter. A musculocutaneous perforator is shown piercing the anterior rectus sheath. **c.** These first order bundles are made up of parallel bundles of the second order (only five are shown), each measuring about 0.8 mm in diameter. **d.** Each second order bundle is made up of parallel muscle fibres of an average diameter of 50 μ. **e.** Each muscle fibre is made up of a bundle of fibrils (each 1–2 μ in diameter surrounded by a sarcolemma sheath beneath which are situated the nuclei of the muscle fibres. The fibres are closely surrounded by capillaries. (Adapted from an original illustration by Max Brodel in Cullen & Brodel, 1937)

which aids conservation of the core temperature by raising the temperature of blood returning from cold peripheries. Furthermore the pulsation of an artery has a beneficial effect on the flow in the venae comitantes which lie in association with it, and this may be of value in a musculocutaneous flap. On the other hand the denervation accompanying flap transfer results in loss of the intermittent muscular contractions which, due to the venous valves, aid venous return. The persistence of the superficial system as a subcutaneous network may provide an important additional route for venous drainage in pedicled (but not islanded) musculocutaneous flaps.

Within the muscle, arteries and veins run together to the terminal arteriolar and venular level with most of these branches running *transverse* to the line of the muscle fibres (Fig. 4.3). Some of these transversely orientated vessels pass beyond the muscle through the epimysium to ramify in the capillary network at the subcuticular level. The transverse alignment of vessels in relation to muscle fibres goes some way towards explaining the structural dimorphism between musculocutaneous and fasciocutaneous perforators. In a musculocutaneous flap the arterioles passing from the muscle through the fascia to the skin are merely an extension of the arrangement of vessels seen in the muscle belly, that is vessels at right angles to the muscle fibres and at right angles to the plane of the skin. In a fasciocutaneous flap, the orientation of the arterioles is in the plane of the fascia and parallel to the plane of the skin.

As well as these general principles, a knowledge of the gross vascular anatomy is also an essential prerequisite to the raising of musculocutaneous flaps. Campbell & Pennefather (1919), Le Gros Clark & Blomfield (1945), Blomfield (1945), Edwards (1953), Jaya (1958) and finally Mathes & Nahai (1981) have all described the arterial patterns in some human muscles and Brash (1955) detailed the neurovascular hila of limb muscles with the emphasis on the nerves.

Campbell & Pennefather (1919) considered various examples of infarction of muscles following injury to their blood supply and classified muscles from the point of view of their vascular supply as follows:

1. Numerous sources of blood supply with good potential anastomoses, e.g. pectoralis major, deltoid, vastus lateralis
2. Two or three arteries of supply, potential anastomoses relatively few, e.g. sartorius, rectus femoris, hamstrings
3. Single artery of supply with practical absence of collateral channels, with almost total ischaemia if the artery is interrupted, e.g. gastrocnemius, gracilis, vastus intermedius.

Blomfield (1945) developed these ideas further with particular regard to the muscles of the lower limb and delineated five main types of intramuscular vascular patterns, namely:

1. A longitudinal anastomotic chain formed by separate vessels entering throughout length of muscle, e.g. peroneus longus
2. Longitudinal patterns of vessels derived from a single group of arteries arising from a common stem and entering one end of the muscle, e.g. gastrocnemius
3. A radiating pattern of collaterals arising from a single vessel entering the middle of the muscle, e.g. biceps brachii
4. Anastomotic loops throughout the length of a muscle and derived from a succession of entering vessels, e.g. tibialis anterior, extensor digitorum longus
5. An open quadrilateral pattern with sparse anastomotic connections. e.g. extensor hallucis longus.

Blomfield further suggested that the 'relative vulnerability of muscles to necrosis and clostridial infection' was related to several vascular factors in addition to the intramuscular pattern of its vessels; namely the site of entry and source of the main nutrient arteries, the number of arteries derived from independent sources, the efficiency of the intramuscular anastomoses and the relation between the size of the main nutrient vessels and the size of its anastomotic connections.

Almost precisely the same considerations are relevant to the raising of musculocutaneous flaps and many of them are incorporated in the classification devised by Mathes & Nahai (1981). This is concerned primarily with the *number* of vascular pedicles entering the muscle and their relative *dominance* within the muscle as assessed from the internal angiographic pattern. The *sources* of the pedicles entering the muscles and their *locations* in relation to the origin and insertion of the muscles then become important in determining the usefulness of the flap and the centre of its arc of rotation. Their classification of muscles into five types is shown in Table 4.1. Although derived from injection studies of cadavers its relevance to the clinical setting has been reliably demonstrated by its successful application to the design of numerous muscle and musculocutaneous flaps. In Table 4.1 muscles are indicated under a single type but some may exhibit any one of up to three different patterns and therefore Table 4.1 may differ slightly from the original classification of Mathes & Nahai since we have listed muscles in the category into which they appear to us to most commonly fall.

In looking at this scheme for some indication of an overall set of guiding principles one can only conclude that it is the physical proximity of parts of a muscle to major vessels which seems to govern the entry points of vascular pedicles. The avoidance of drag during contractions and movement does not seem to be a major consideration, nor does the need to enter where there is the maximum facility for even distribution. The latter requirement seems more to influence the points of entry of motor nerves and this perhaps accounts for why the arterial and nervous pedicles do not always enter at the same point, although in many muscles a neurovascular hilum exists in over 50% of cases, and in some in over 80%, and in three muscles (biceps brachii, latissimus dorsi and gastrocnemius) it has been recorded in over 90% of cases.

Because of the central importance of these vascular pedicles in the raising of flaps, the classification of Mathes & Nahai will now be described in greater detail. References in Chapter 6 in Roman numerals to muscle vascularisation patterns refer to this classification (Fig. 4.4).

Table 4.1 Classification of the vascular anatomy of muscles

Type I	*One vascular pedicle*		
	Gastrocnemius		
	Tensor fasciae latae		
	Anconeus		
	Vastus intermedius		
Type II	*One dominant vascular pedicle usually entering close to the origin or insertion of the muscle with additional smaller vascular pedicles entering the muscle belly*		
	Abductor digiti minimi	Peroneus longus	Sternocleidomastoid
	Abductor hallucis	Peroneus brevis	Temporalis
	Biceps femoris	Platysma	Trapezius
	Brachioradialis	Rectus femoris	Vastus lateralis
	Flexor digitorum brevis	Semitendinosus	
	Gracilis	Soleus	
Type III	*Two vascular pedicles, each arising from a separate regional artery (except orbicularis oris)*		
	Gluteus maximus		
	Rectus abdominis		
	Serratus anterior		
	Semimembranosus		
	Orbicularis oris		
Type IV	*Multiple pedicles of similar size*		
	Flexor digitorum longus	Extensor digitorum longus	
	Extensor hallucis longus	Flexor hallucis longus	
	Vastus medialis	Sartorius	
	External oblique	Tibialis anterior	
Type V	*One dominant vascular pedicle and several smaller secondary segmental vascular pedicles*		
	Pectoralis major		
	Latissimus dorsi		

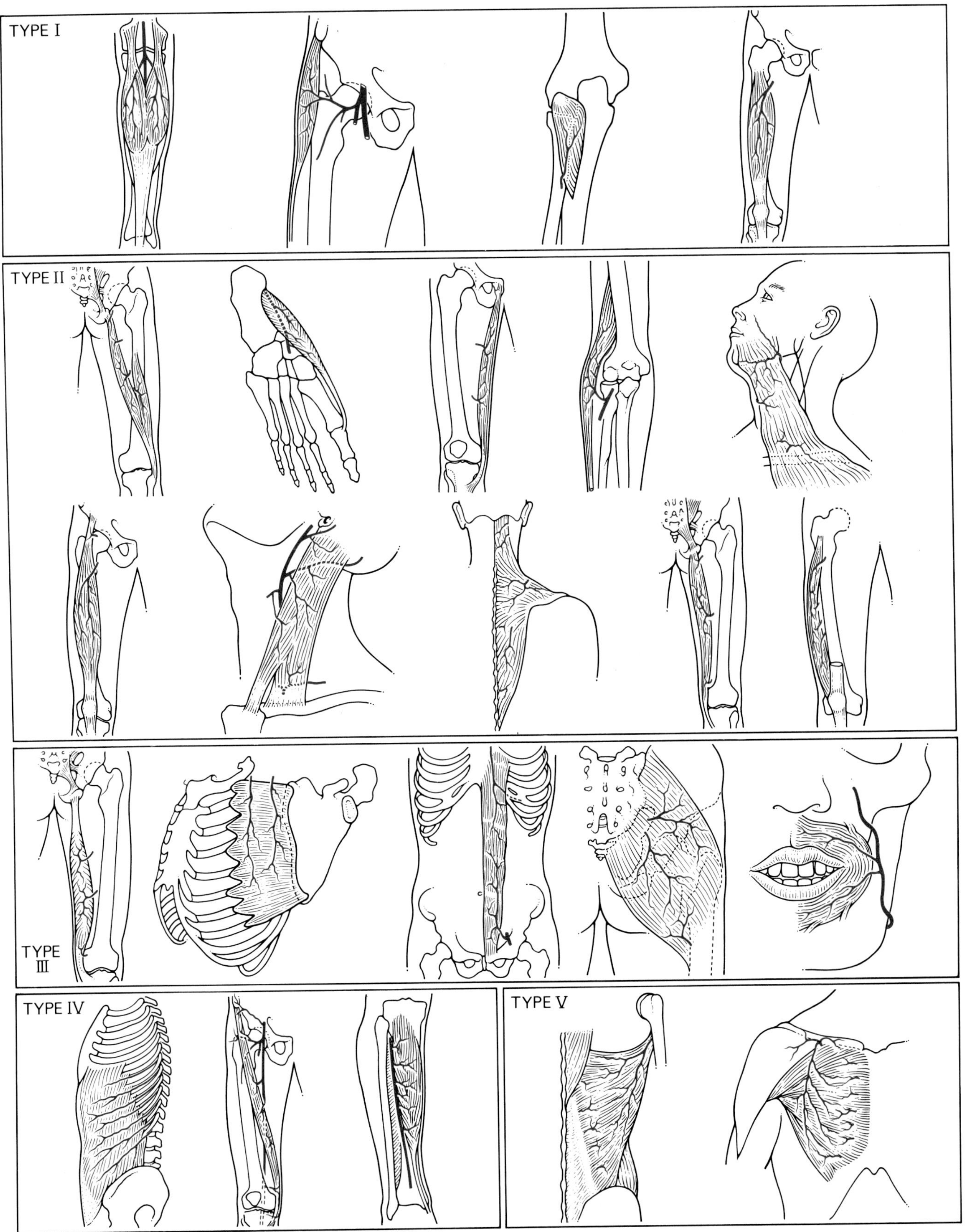

Fig. 4.4 Classification of the vascular anatomy of muscles after the system of Mathes & Nahai.

Type I

These muscles have a single vascular pedicle supplying the muscle belly although there may be other more minor vessels supplying the tendons of origin and insertion which are not considered in the classification. Well-known examples of this type which are commonly used as the basis of musculocutaneous flaps are the tensor fasciae latae, gastrocnemius and rectus femoris muscles. It is self-evident that with one vessel of supply all the skin overlying the muscle can be elevated with that muscle as a single musculocutaneous unit provided that there are musculocutaneous perforators from it to the overlying skin. A note of caution is appropriate with regard to the tensor fasciae latae flap; the perforators reach the skin, as with all musculocutaneous flaps, via the muscle and this does not include the fascia of the iliotibial tract which is in effect the tendon of the tensor. Blood vessels overlying the fascia are derived from the branches of the profunda perforators which emerge along the lateral intermuscular septum. The muscle is however able to support a distal extension of an overlying skin flap extending down the lateral aspect of the leg to within 15 or 20 cm of the knee joint by virtue of anastomoses with these vessels. This is discussed more fully on page 357.

Type II

These muscles have a single dominant vascular pedicle and several minor pedicles. Axial muscles tend to receive their predominant blood supply at their proximal end where they are fattest, before narrowing down to their tendon of insertion. It follows that the dominant pedicle tends to enter the muscle in the middle of the belly or nearer the origin, whilst the minor pedicles lie nearer the ends, particularly the distal one. Examples are biceps femoris, gracilis, vastus lateralis, semitendinosus, abductor digiti minimi, abductor hallucis, trapezius, sternocleidomastoid and platysma.

Depending on the degree of development of intramuscular anatomoses the dominant vascular pedicle may alone be able to support the whole muscle. The ability to reliably support a skin island overlying the muscle is greatest when the paddle overlies the part of the muscle supplied by the dominant pedicle. In a musculocutaneous flap served only by the dominant pedicle, the skin island becomes progressively less reliable as it is placed further away from this to overlie the territory of the minor pedicle – generally this means when it is placed further distally. The gracilis musculocutaneous flap demonstrates this very clearly. Secondly the muscle may be entirely supportable on a minor pedicle in which case it may be possible to carry a skin island, but not reliably so, situated over the territory of the dominant pedicle. For example, the first point is demonstrated by the sternocleidomastoid which can be raised entirely based on its dominant superior pedicle and may carry a distal skin island with some risk of loss. The opposite arrangement is also feasible, i.e. an inferior pedicle with a superior skin island, but is markedly less reliable, which demonstrates the second point.

It is necessary to have a detailed knowledge of the intramuscular vascular anatomy where several vessels are of relatively large diameter and, therefore, significance. This is exemplified by the various trapezius musculocutaneous flaps where skin islands may be carried on one of three distinct pedicles. The skin paddle must be designed specifically to correspond to the particular pedicle chosen and it is necessary to know which parts of the muscle are supplied by which pedicle.

The inclusion of platysma as a Type II muscle is debatable since the platysma is a muscular remnant of the panniculus carnosus and is therefore part of the cuticular rather than the skeletal muscular systems. It would, however, seem appropriate to classify flaps incorporating this muscle as musculocutaneous flaps since without doubt the survival of long length to breadth neck skin flaps is enhanced by inclusion of the platysma muscle and a skin island may even be carried on the muscle.

Type III

These muscles receive two separate dominant pedicles from two different regional arteries. Examples are gluteus maximus, receiving vessels from superior and inferior gluteal arteries, and rectus abdominis receiving the superior and inferior deep epigastric arteries. Whether or not filling of the whole muscle can be achieved from either vessel, so that the potential territory of each vessel becomes the whole of the muscle, depends on the adequacy of the anastomoses between the two vessels and on their relative sizes. This type of musculocutaneous flap can be very versatile, particularly in the case of rectus abdominis where an island of skin on either a long superiorly or inferiorly based muscle pedicle can be used.

Type IV

These muscles have multiple pedicles of similar size entering at multiple points along the belly of the muscle between origin and insertion. The pedicles are similar in size and each supplies roughly the same amount of muscle. The potential vascular territory which each pedicle alone can support will vary depending on the extent and size of the vascular anastomoses within the muscle belly which are generally poor or only moderately developed. In general terms, these muscles are of less use in reconstruction than the single or double pedicled muscles since their pedicles tend to be short and a single arterial pedicle is too small to be capable of providing a sufficient arterial input to supply the needs of the whole muscle. Examples are extensor digitorum longus, extensor hallucis longus, flexor digitorum longus, flexor hallucis longus, tibialis anterior and sartorius. It will be noted that these muscles fall within the category of long thin muscles rather than broad flat ones, and the skin overlying such muscles tends to be supplied by fasciocutaneous perforators rather than musculocutaneous ones. It follows that these muscles cannot be used as the basis of musculocutaneous flaps although the muscles may still have applications as purely muscle flaps (not covered by this book).

Type V

These vessels have one dominant vascular pedicle and multiple secondary *segmental* vascular pedicles. This arrangement applies to broad flat muscles and is seen in the latissimus dorsi and pectoralis major muscles. Each has a single large vascular pedicle entering near the muscle insertion and further segmental pedicles entering the muscle close to its origin. Characteristically the two systems anastomose extensively within the muscle. The segmental vessels are in fact branches of vessels passing through the muscle on their way to the skin and it is by the intramuscular anastomoses with these vessels that the dominant pedicle can supply the skin. These muscles are the basis of the most useful musculocutaneous flaps and can be used for reconstruction using either system of pedicles although the arc of rotation is much increased when the flap is based on the single pedicle. These flaps are unsuitable for free tissue transfer when based on their secondary pedicles since individually the arteries are too small.

THE ANATOMY OF MUSCULOCUTANEOUS PERFORATORS

The perforators which emerge from the surface of a muscle exhibit three features which are worth drawing attention to:

Firstly, they are accompanied by venae comitantes.

Secondly, there is often a slack length of the perforator lying at the level of the epimysium (Figs 4.5 & 4.6). This

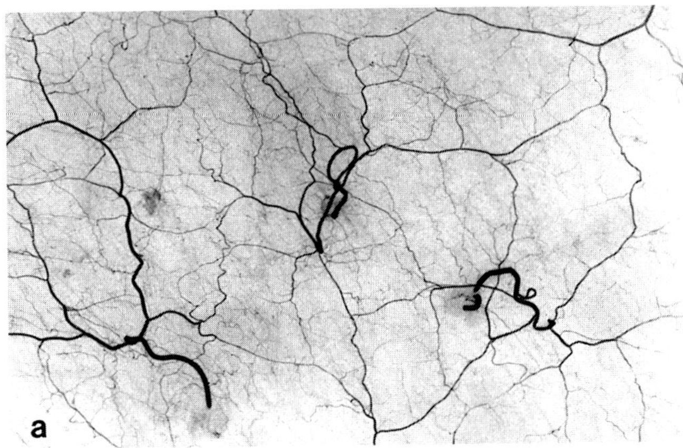

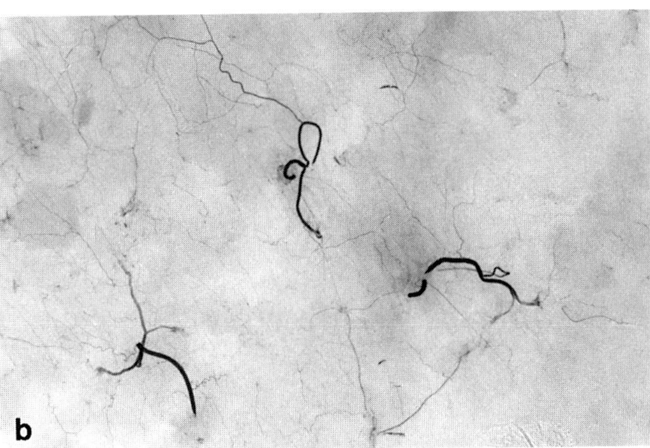

Fig. 4.5 Radiographs of injected cadaver tissue consisting of: **a.** skin, subcutaneous tissue and the epimysium over latissimus dorsi compared with **b.** epimysium only, showing the 'slack segments' of the musculocutaneous perforators.

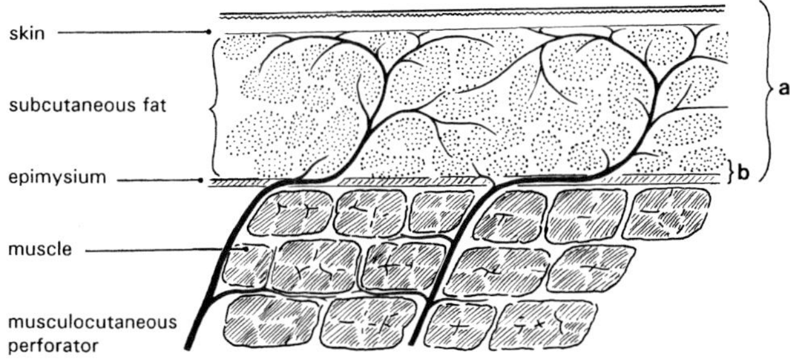

Fig. 4.6 Diagrammatic cross-section perpendicular to skin surface to illustrate the anatomy of the perforator responsible for the appearances of Fig. 4.5.

permits a limited amount of movement of the muscle beneath the overlying skin when the muscle contracts. It follows that the length of this 'slack segment' of the perforator will vary between different muscles depending on how great their excursion is beneath the skin. For example, with latissimus dorsi this segment is quite long over the upper third of the muscle. It is also notable that the 'slack segment' is generally characterised by an absence of significant branches and that musculocutaneous perforators enter the subcutaneous fat before they branch out to supply the tissues (note the difference from fasciocutaneous perforators which do branch at the level of the deep fascia).

Thirdly, there may be some axiality in the perforators. It has generally been assumed that musculocutaneous perforators emerge from the surface of a muscle and divide into branches which diverge equally in all directions in the subcutaneous tissues to supply the skin. A study of the morphology of distribution of musculocutaneous perforators in specimens of injected cadaver skin has shown that this is not always the case (Cormack & Lamberty, 1986). Many musculocutaneous perforators have a distinct axiality with the main stem of the perforator running in a particular direction and giving off smaller branches in a manner analogous to direct cutaneous arteries but on a smaller scale. Where certain perforators are concerned this is a consistent feature from individual to individual. Other musculocutaneous perforators diverge into two, three or more main branches which each supply their own small territory. When two equal branches are formed they may run in diametrically opposite directions thereby creating an axial territory. When three branches are formed they tend to diverge randomly so that the stem of the perforator lies approximately in the centre of its territory. Figure 4.8 is a histogram for D/L where D is the maximum dimension of the anatomical territory of blood supply of an individual perforator and L is the distance from the stem of the perforator to the most distant point of the anatomical territory which it supplies (Fig. 4.7). D/L can have any value between 1 and 2 and the more 'axial' the pattern of distribution of the perforator the closer the value of D/L will approach to 1. Figure 4.8 shows that many perforators show such axiality despite the fact that this method of assessing the 'axiality' of a perforator is biased towards non-axiality (the right in Fig. 4.8) because the branching arrangement described above, where one perforator divides into two stems which diverge in diametrically opposite directions, gives a value for D/L which approaches 2 but the overall territory may in fact be axial in type. Despite this bias it can be seen that many perforators exhibit an axial pattern. Figure 4.9 relates the *shapes* of the territories of supply of vessels on the trunk to their *areas* of supply and demonstrates that axiality is a property of musculocutaneous perforators supplying both large and small territories. For comparison are shown the direct cutaneous vessels on the trunk which are all axial and tend to supply larger areas than do individual musculocutaneous perforators. The knowledge that musculocutaneous perforators at some sites conform to an axial pattern may influence the design of certain flaps. For example, flaps may be designed with significant extension of the cutaneous component of the flap in a direction parallel to the axial vessels. If these vessels extend away from the muscle then the cutaneous component may similarly be extended beyond the edge of the muscle. An example of this is seen in the extended inferior epigastric flap designed by Taylor et al (1983). The skin island is based over the peri-umbilical part of the rectus abdominis and is fed by large perforators which emerge within 4 cm of the umbilicus and pass superolaterally towards the costal margin. This enables a skin island to be extended up to 15 cm in a similar direction beyond the lateral border of the muscle.

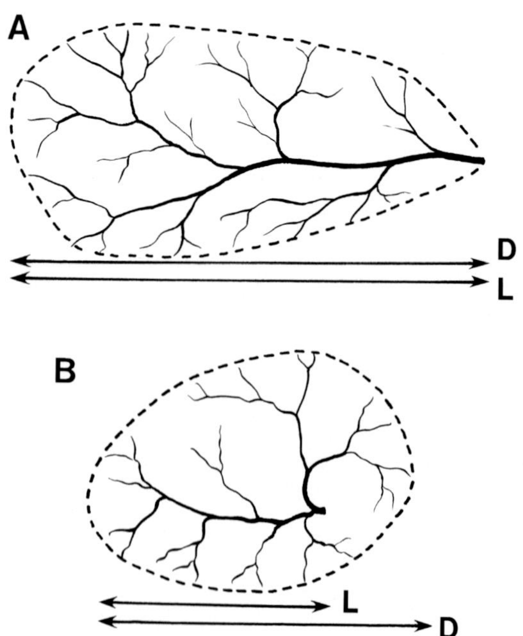

Fig. 4.7 The method of quantifying axiality of perforators in radiographs of injected skin (Dmax/L). Anatomical territory **A** has an axiality of 1, while territory **B** has an axiality of 1.4.

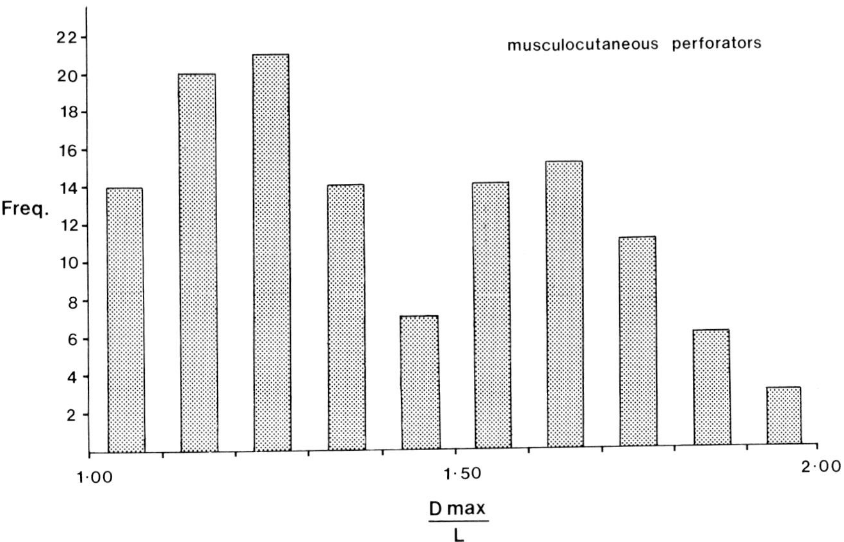

Fig. 4.8 Histogram of 10 classes of Dmax/L obtained from measurement of anatomical territories of musculocutaneous perforators on the trunk. Dmax is the maximum dimension of the anatomical territory of blood supply of an individual perforator. L is the distance from the stem of the perforator to the most distant point of the anatomical territory which it supplies.

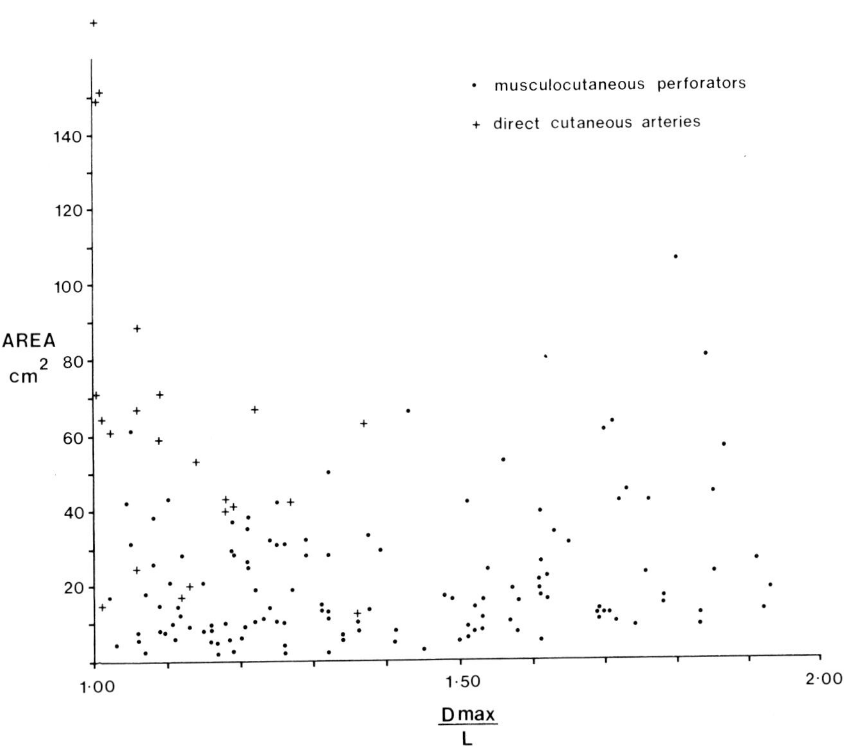

Fig. 4.9 Plot of areas of supply against 'axiality' as measured by Dmax/L. Musculocutaneous perforators can here be compared with direct cutaneous arteries.

MUSCULOCUTANEOUS FLAP PLANNING

The foregoing description of the vascular anatomy of muscles forms the basis for planning musculocutaneous flaps but other factors must also be taken into consideration. In particular the following four questions need to be answered:

1. Is the overlying skin supplied by musculocutaneous perforators and if so how large a skin paddle can be raised?
2. What is the vascular anatomy of the muscle and how much of the muscle is or can potentially be supplied by each pedicle? Are the vascular pedicles large enough and long enough to be used for free tissue transfer?
3. Is the muscle expendable?
4. What is the arc of rotation of the flap?

Is the skin supplied by perforators?

The answer to the first question is partly answered by the general statement that the skin over broad flat muscles tends to be well supplied by musculocutaneous perforators whereas that over long thin muscles is more likely to be supplied by fasciocutaneous perforators. Ignoring for the moment considerations relating to the vascular pedicles, and assuming that the muscle has in its entirety an adequate blood supply, it is self-evident that the skin paddle can be at least of the same area as the muscle itself. This brings us back to the fact that in general terms the most useful musculocutaneous units are those based on broad flat muscles rather than long thin ones – it is obvious that the latissimus dorsi can carry a larger skin island than the gracilis. If the skin paddle is smaller than the muscle which is raised with it, prudence dictates that the maximum number of perforating vessels to the skin should be preserved and this is aided by 'shelving' the subcutaneous tissues away from the skin edge towards the muscle to include as many perforators as possible. Lastly, the size of the skin paddle may be determined by factors other than the vascular anatomy. For example, a latissimus dorsi skin paddle may be restricted to a maximum of approximately 8 cm wide if direct skin closure of the donor site is to be obtained and cosmesis of the donor site may similarly be the primary consideration elsewhere when deciding whether the size of a skin paddle which can be raised at a certain site is large enough to meet the reconstructive requirements.

If the skin paddle is larger than the muscle, then the skin beyond the edges of the muscle is dependent for its blood supply on musculocutaneous perforators fanning out in the subcutaneous fat away from the muscle edge. In general terms, the 'overlap' of the skin beyond the muscle cannot exceed 3 cm unless there is a marked axiality of the musculocutaneous perforators away from the muscle, in which case a flap may be designed so as to exploit this directionality. For example, the deep inferior epigastric artery rectus abdominis musculocutaneous flap based on para-umbilical perforators may be extended obliquely up to the costal margin with the muscle component reduced to a small pad beneath the medial end of the flap (between the deep inferior epigastric artery and the skin flap; see p. 297).

What is the vascular anatomy of the muscle?

The general scheme has been described and the five broad groups outlined, but for each specific flap the details need to be known. These are described in Chapters 6 & 7.

Is the muscle expendable?

Expendability is commonly regarded as referring to motor function and it is surprising how muscles may often be removed with minimal overall functional impairment. In transferring a musculocutaneous flap the motor nerve to the muscle is generally divided but sometimes motor function must be preserved, e.g. when transferring a biceps femoris musculocutaneous flap to the anterolateral thigh with insertion of the tendon into the patella to restore active knee extension following a traumatic thigh injury, or transfer of a latissimus dorsi flap into the upper arm to replace biceps and restore elbow flexion in a traumatic injury to the flexor compartment. In paraplegics most functional considerations do not apply and one is at liberty to use muscles that one would otherwise be reluctant to use since in the adult once the musculocutaneous system of perforators has developed it persists despite denervation and atrophy of the muscle. It is an impression of the authors that the same may not hold true for denervation occurring in early childhood from, for example, poliomyelitis. With subsequent growth and development of the child the musculocutaneous supply to skin over affected muscles may fail to develop to the degree that would otherwise be the case and the skin may become more dependent on other (e.g. fasciocutaneous) systems – this however remains entirely speculative at the present time although suggested by the behaviour of some clinical cases.

What is the arc of rotation of the flap?

The arc of rotation is determined by the number of pedicles and the proximity of the dominant pedicle to one end of the muscle. The arc is increased if the flap is based on a single vascular pedicle which enters the muscle either at its origin or insertion. With multiply pedicled musculocutaneous units, the arc of rotation is inversely proportional to the number of pedicles which are required for the support of the flap. In other words, the arc of rotation is decreased as the 'base' of the flap is increased. In general terms, the arc of rotation of the flap is governed not only by the nature of the pedicles but also by the shape of the muscle itself.

Finally when considering a free tissue transfer it is necessary to ask whether or not the pedicles are long enough and large enough. It should be remembered that veins may in this respect also prove to be a limiting factor.

MUSCULOCUTANEOUS FLAP REFINEMENTS

During the 1970s the definition of musculocutaneous flap anatomy concentrated on the two fundamentals of the location of the vascular pedicle and the size of the skin island which it could support. During the 1980s the knowledge concerning the blood supply of musculocutaneous units progressed beyond these fundamentals to a level where a greater understanding of the intramuscular arrangement of the vessels and their connections with those of neighbouring muscles enabled at least three principal modifications of basic musculocutaneous flaps.

Splitting the muscle

A segmental morphology exists in several muscles and is reflected by a consistent branching of the neurovascular structures. This segmental anatomy enables each segment to be surgically separated from other segments by dissections along anatomic planes. The application of this is in creating small innervated muscle microvascular transfers in which only part of a muscle is transferred; for example, part of the gracilis or the serratus anterior muscle may be used for reanimation of the paralysed face. Another application is in creating two skin islands on one split muscle with the advantages of having only one vascular pedicle and one donor site defect.

The latissimus dorsi flap may be split to provide two flaps since the thoracodorsal artery undergoes a major intramuscular bifurcation approximately 9 cm from the point where the subscapular artery arises from the axillary artery. The upper branch passes between the bundles of muscle fibres parallel to the superior edge of latissimus while the lower branch passes parallel to the lateral edge of the muscle. Pectoralis major may also be split since it has three segmental subunits, two of which are fed by pectoral and clavicular subdivisions of the thoraco-acromial axis and the third one from a combination of the lateral thoracic artery and the lateral branches of the thoraco-acromial pectoral vessels (Tobin et al, 1981). Tobin et al (1982) have demonstrated how two flaps may be carried on pectoralis and used simultaneously to carry out pharyngoesophageal and oral mucocutaneous reconstructions.

Combining flaps on one pedicle

Greater knowledge of the details of muscle vascular anatomy has also enabled some combined units to be developed. For example, the gluteus medius–tensor fasciae latae flap based on the lateral circumflex femoral artery (Little & Lyons, 1983). In elevating a tensor fasciae latae flap vessels are encountered at the posterior aspect of the muscle which connect with those of gluteus medius and form part of the collateral circulation about the hip.

It is these vessels which provide an anastomotic connection between the superior and inferior rami of the deep branch of the superior gluteal artery with the terminal ascending branch of the lateral circumflex femoral artery, and enable a pedicled skin flap overlying gluteus medius to be supported by the vascular pedicle of tensor fasciae latae. Such flaps may be used as rotation advancement flaps for cover of trochanteric pressure sores. The ability to combine flaps is, of course, not confined to musculocutaneous flaps and can be carried out anywhere where the anatomy is suitable. When the majority of musculocutaneous flaps were defined in the 1970s many flaps, particularly fasciocutaneous ones, had not yet been discovered; subsequently developed flaps have, in specific instances, been combined with musculocutaneous ones to create large regional flaps. For example, the scapular flaps based on the branches of the circumflex scapular artery may be combined with the latissimus dorsi flaps to create a single large regional flap based on the subscapular artery (Mayou et al, 1982). The teres major muscle which lies between the two vascular pedicles must be divided to free the combined flap. Serratus anterior and latissimus dorsi, gastrocnemius and the superficial sural artery flap are further examples; indeed, it is likely that the skin in the conventional pedicled gastrocnemius musculocutaneous flap is partly dependent for its vascular support on the superficial sural vessels.

Preservation of function

Greater understanding of the intramuscular vascular anatomy has also helped in the design of musculocutaneous flaps which preserve the maximum possible amount of function in the muscle. This contrasts with the early flaps in which invariably far more of the muscle was transferred than was absolutely necessary for the support of the skin island. For example, a flap can be taken from the upper horizontal part of latissimus dorsi pedicled on the thoracodorsal vessels whilst preserving the major part of the muscle in continuity with the tendon of insertion and with an intact nerve supply. The remaining part of the muscle then receives its blood supply from the intercostal and lumbar artery perforators and remains functional (Elliot et al, 1989).

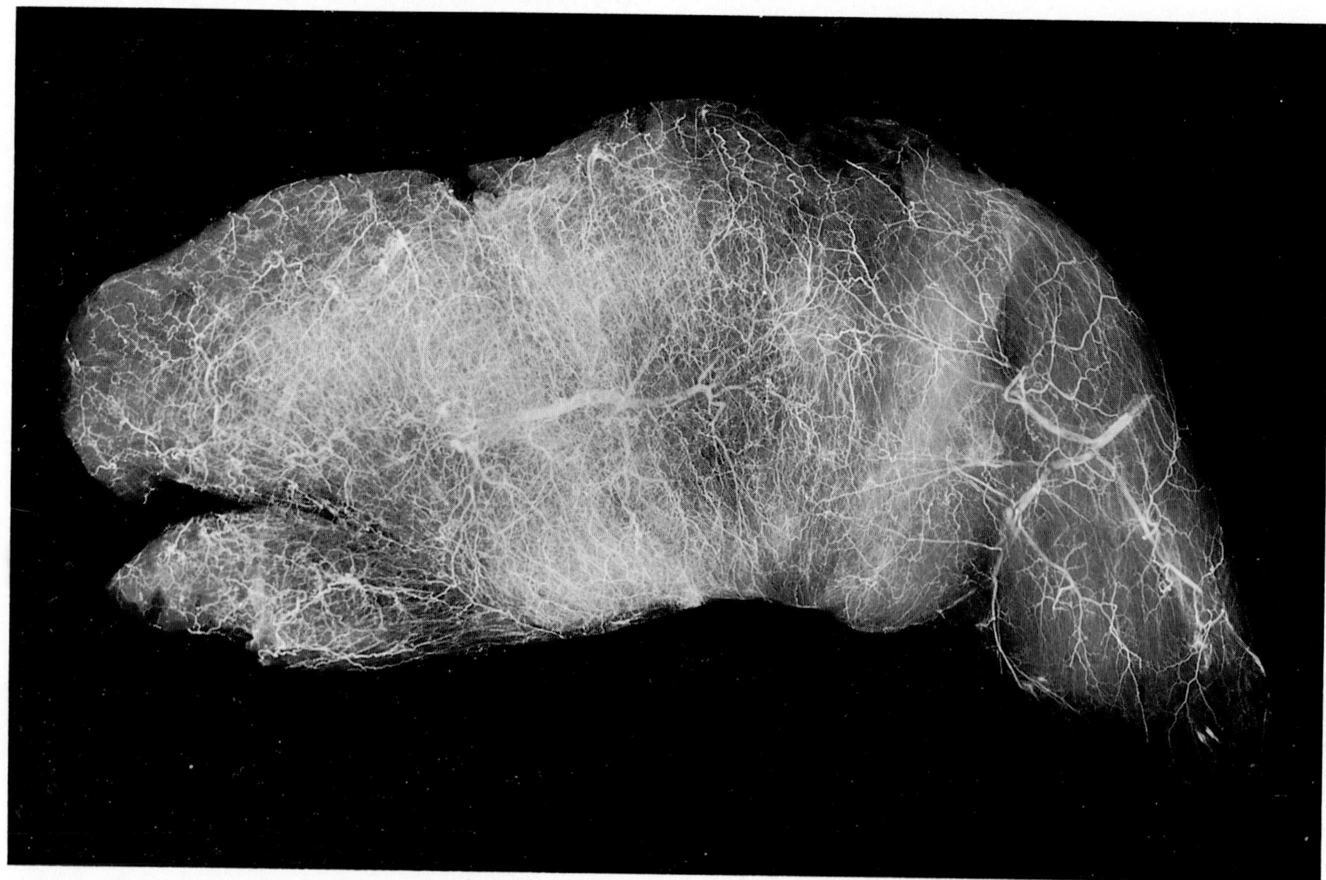

Fig. 4.10 Radiograph of injected gluteus medius and tensor fasciae latae muscles which were removed in continuity thereby preserving the anastomoses between the vessels of the two muscles. Tensor fasciae latae is on the right with its pedicle from the lateral circumflex femoral artery clearly visible. Gluteus medius is as the left and its pedicle from the superior gluteal artery is rather obscured by the high degree of small vessel opacification.

ADVANTAGES OF MUSCULOCUTANEOUS FLAPS IN CLINICAL PRACTICE

These flaps may be identified as having three particular qualities – good vascularity, bulk and the possibility of creating a reconstruction with motor function.

The last of these concerns the application of specific flaps in specific instances to unique problems and is not really a matter for discussion under the title of broad principles. However it should be noted that when the tendon(s) is reattached with the muscle in the new site, the new length of the muscle relative to the original is crucial to the proper functioning of the muscle. The use of a length of suture material attached at either end to the tendons of origin and insertion of the muscle should ensure that the resting length of the muscle after transposition is the same as it was before transposition. Animal studies have shown changes in the size of white and red fibres within the muscle if the resting tension and length of the muscle are reduced by tendon elongation (Frey et al, 1983). The same studies showed significant reductions in the twitch and tetanic tensions 6 months after tendon elongation.

The good vascularity of the muscle is responsible for the reliability and safety of these flaps with rapid healing and a high degree of resistance to infection. The latter feature was first pointed out by Orticochea (1972a): 'In addition the rich circulation can combat any infection around the exposed bones and tendons and such a flap represents the ideal biological dressing'. This has since been demonstrated in many clinical cases and proven experimentally in the laboratory by Chang & Mathes (1982) and by Feng et al (1983). They found that compared with relatively ischaemic skin flaps the musculocutaneous flaps demonstrated an ability to increase blood flow in response to infection, to produce effective mobilisation of leucocytes to specific sites of infection, and to effectively kill bacteria within a localised area involving fewer leucocytes. None of these features could be demonstrated with the 'ischaemic' skin flap. Two other papers often quoted in the literature on infection and flaps are those of Calderon et al (1986) and Gosain et al (1990). These studies are frequently used to support an argument that musculocutaneous flaps are more effective than fasciocutaneous flaps in inhibiting and eliminating bacterial growth. However, their model of anterior rectus sheath fascia with overlying skin as a 'fasciocutaneous flap' is not entirely appropriate. The anterior rectus sheath is the aponeurotic tendon of insertion of the external and internal oblique muscles, and as such does not possess the same degree of vascularity as, for example, lower leg fascia. Indeed we know that the perforators from the deep inferior epigastric artery pass straight through the fascia to supply the overlying skin and subcutaneous tissues, so this is not a well-vascularised structure. The case for muscle versus fascia is therefore unproven, all other factors being equal, but it is often the case that a piece of muscle is better able to plug a hole or conform to a very irregular surface, and in these circumstances, when infection is present, the muscle will obviously be superior as total obliteration of all dead space and close approximation of the flap to the defect are generally more effectively achieved with muscle than with a fasciocutaneous flap.

Neovascularisation of a muscle may occur to a limited extent from the base of the defect into which it is placed but this cannot be guaranteed, particularly since the bed for a flap is often poorly vascularised due to large areas of scar, cortical bone, irradiated tissue or prosthetic material. Experience has shown that late occlusion of the vascular pedicle to a muscle flap may be accompanied by necrosis of the muscle, but that this is less likely with a musculo-*cutaneous* flap due to the extra potential for vascular link ups between the dermal and subcutaneous plexi of the flap and the vessels of surrounding skin. In the event of late loss of flow through the vascular pedicle with development of necrosis on the surface of a free muscle flap, excision of the dead tissue should be carried out in a tangential fashion as the deepest layer may have become neovascularised and may accept a split skin graft.

The bulk conferred to the musculocutaneous flap by the muscle may be a great advantage when, for example, reconstructing pressure sores over bony prominences, while at other times it may be a great cosmetic problem. After transferring a muscle as a free flap a degree of oedema secondary to lymphatic interruption commonly occurs. This then settles and progressive shrinkage of the muscle due to atrophy also occurs. Several experimental studies have suggested that denervated skeletal muscle atrophies at the rate of approximately 1% per day for 60 days and then a plateau is reached (Knowlton & Hines, 1936; Tower, 1935; Sunderland & Roy, 1950). In these experiments various muscles in different animals gave similar results. In each experiment, muscle dry weight was used as the basis for comparison of the percentage atrophy, and denervated muscles were studied in situ rather than as free tissue transfers. Often, however, it can be observed clinically that 60% total volume reduction does not occur and this is commonly associated with transfer of the flap into a dependent position, where lymphatic drainage may be poor. To what extent partial reinnervation from the recipient bed occurs and if it maintains muscle bulk has not been established.

'Delay' by selective ligation of certain vascular pedicles can be effective in enhancing the reliability of skin paddles carried on certain muscles (Taylor et al, 1992). The mechanism is twofold: firstly, within the muscle there may be a dilatation of narrow anastomotic vessels linking pedicles supplying adjoining muscle segments with a secondary improvement in the circulation to the skin paddle. Secondly, there may be changes in the preferential routes of venous drainage within the muscle as a result of the selective ligations interrupting normal drainage routes and producing backpressure with regurgitant flow through valves towards the unligated pedicle(s). In the days following a 'delay' the backpressure element reduces and the new routes of venous drainage become established so that when the flap is finally elevated the congestion in the skin island is less than it would otherwise have been. Finally, attempts to improve circulation in musculocutaneous flaps by prior denervation have proved unsuccessful (Hagerty & Nahai, 1981).

References

Ariyan S 1979 The pectoralis major myocutaneous flap. Plastic and Reconstructive Surgery 63: 73–81

Arnold P G, Pairolero P C 1979 Use of pectoralis major muscle flaps to repair defects of the anterior chest wall. Plastic and Reconstructive Surgery 63: 205–213

Bakamjian V Y 1963 A technique for primary reconstruction of the palate after radical maxillectomy for cancer. Plastic and Reconstructive Surgery 31: 103–107

Bakamjian V Y, Littlewood M 1964 Cervical skin flaps for intraoral and pharyngeal repair following cancer surgery. British Journal of Plastic Surgery 17: 191–210

Blomfield L B 1945 Intramuscular vascular patterns in man. Proceedings of the Royal Society of Medicine 38: 617–618

Brash J C 1955 Neurovascular hila of limb muscles. E & S Livingstone, Edinburgh

Calderon W, Chang N, Mathes S J 1986 Comparison of the effects of bacterial inoculation in musculocutaneous and fasciocutaneous flaps. Plastic and Reconstructive Surgery 77: 785–792

Campbell J, Pennefather C M 1919 An investigation into the blood supply of muscles, with special reference to war surgery. Lancet 1: 294–296

Chang N, Mathes S J 1982 Comparison of the effects of bacterial innoculation in musculocutaneous and random pattern flaps. Plastic and Reconstructive Surgery 70: 1–9

Cormack G C and Lamberty B G H 1986 Cadaver studies of correlation between vessel size and anatomical territory of cutaneous supply. British Journal of Plastic Surgery 39: 300–306

DesPrez J D, Kiehn C L, Eckstein W 1971 Closure of large meningomyelocele defects by composite skin muscle flaps. Plastic and Reconstructive Surgery 47: 234–238

Dibbell D G 1974 Use of a long island flap to bring sensation to the sacral area in young paraplegics. Plastic and Reconstructive Surgery 54: 220–223

Edwards E A 1953 The anatomic basis for ischaemia localised to certain muscles of the lower limb. Surgery, Gynaecology and Obstetrics 97: 87–94

Elliot L F, Raffel B, Wade J 1989 Segmental latissimus dorsi free flap: clinical applications. Annals of Plastic Surgery 23: 231–238

Feng L J, Price D, Mathes S J 1983 Relationship of blood flow and leukocyte mobilization in infection. Plastic Surgical Forum 6: 128–130

Frey M, Gruber H, Freilinger G 1983 The importance of the correct resting tension in muscle transplantation: experimental and clinical aspects. Plastic and Reconstructive Surgery 71: 510–518

Ger R 1972 Surgical management of ulcerative lesions in the leg. Current Problems in Surgery 0: 1–52

Ger R 1976 The management of chronic ulcers of the dorsum of the foot by muscle transposition and free skin grafting. British Journal of Plastic Surgery 29: 199–204

Gosain A, Chang N, Mathes S J, Hunt T K, Vasconez L 1990 A study of the relationship between blood flow and bacterial inoculation in musculocutaneous and fasciocutaneous flaps. Plastic and Reconstructive Surgery 86: 1152–1162

Hagerty R, Nahai F 1981 Evaluation of strategic nerve section in myocutaneous flaps. Annals of Plastic Surgery 6: 283–286

Hagerty R, Bostwick J, Nahai F 1984 Denervated muscle flaps: mass and thickness changes following denervation. Annals of Plastic Surgery 12: 171–176

Hueston J T, McConchie I H 1968 A compound pectoral flap. Australian and New Zealand Journal of Surgery 38: 61–63

Jaya Y 1958 The arterial pattern of skeletal muscles. The Journal of the Anatomical Society of India 7: 30–34

Knowlton G C, Hines H M 1936 Kinetics of muscle atrophy in different species. Proceedings of the Society for Experimental Biology and Medicine 35: 394–398

Le Gros Clark W E 1971 The tissues of the body, 6th edn. Oxford University Press, Oxford

Le Gros Clark W E, Blomfield L B 1945 The efficiency of intramuscular anastomoses, with observations on the regeneration of devascularised muscle. Journal of Anatomy 79: 15–32

Little J W, Lyons J R 1983 The gluteus medius–tensor fasciae latae flap. Plastic and Reconstructive Surgery 71: 366–370

McCraw J B 1980 The recent history of myocutaneous flaps. Clinics in Plastic Surgery 7: 3–7

McCraw J B, Dibbell D G 1977 Experimental definition of independent myocutaneous vascular territories. Plastic and Reconstructive Surgery 60: 341–352

McCraw J B, Massey F M, Shanklin K D, Horton D E 1976 Vaginal reconstruction with gracilis myocutaneous flaps. Plastic and Reconstructive Surgery 58: 176–183

McCraw J B, Fishman J H, Sharzer L A 1978 The versatile gastrocnemius myocutaneous flap. Plastic and Reconstructive Surgery 62: 15–23

McCraw J B, Magee W P, Kalwaic H 1979 Uses of the trapezius and sternomastoid myocutaneous flaps in head and neck reconstruction. Plastic and Reconstructive Surgery 63: 49–57

McGregor I A, Jackson I T 1972 The groin flap. British Journal of Plastic Surgery 25: 3–16

McGregor I A, Morgan G 1973 Axial and random pattern flaps. British Journal of Plastic Surgery 26: 202–213

McMinn R M H, Vrbova G 1962 Morphological changes in red and pale muscles following tenotomy. Nature 195: 509

Mathes S J, Nahai F 1979 Clinical Atlas of Muscle and Musculocutaneous Flaps. C V Mosby, St Louis

Mathes S J, Nahai F 1981 Classification of the vascular anatomy of muscles: Experimental and clinical correlation. Plastic and Reconstructive Surgery 67: 177–187

Mathes S J, Nahai F 1982 Clinical applications for muscle and musculocutaneous flaps. C V Mosby, St Louis

Mathes S J, McCraw J B, Vasconez L 1974 Muscle transposition flaps for coverage of lower extremity defects. Anatomic considerations. Surgical Clinics of North America 54: 1337–1354

Mathes S J, Vasconez L O, Jurkiewicz M J 1977 Extensions and further applications of muscle flap transposition. Plastic and Reconstructive Surgery 60: 6–13

Maxwell G P, Stueber K, Hoopes J 1978 A free latissimus dorsi myocutaneous flap. Plastic and Reconstructive Surgery 62: 462–466

Mayou B J, Whitby D, Jones B M 1982 The scapular flap – an anatomical and clinical study. British Journal of Plastic Surgery 35: 8–13

Morax V 1908 L'autoplastie palpébrale ou faciale à l'aide de lambeau pédiculés empruntés à la region cervicale (procédé de Snydacker) et de l'autoplastie en deux temps avec utilisation du pédicule. Annales Oculist 89: 14–30

Mühlbauer W, Olbrisch R 1977 The latissimus dorsi myocutaneous flap for breast reconstruction. Chirurgia Plastica 4: 27–34

Nahai F, Silverton J S, Hill H L, Vasconez L 1978 The tensor fasciae latae musculocutaneous flap. Annals of Plastic Surgery 1: 372–379

Olivari N 1976 The latissimus flap. British Journal of Plastic Surgery 29: 126–128

Orticochea M 1972a The musculocutaneous flap method – an

immediate and heroic substitute for the method of delay. British Journal of Plastic Surgery 25: 106–110
Orticochea M 1972b New method of total reconstruction of the penis. British Journal of Plastic Surgery 25: 347–366
Owens N 1955 A compound neck pedicle designed for repair of massive facial defects: formation, development and application. Plastic and Reconstructive Surgery 15: 369–389
Pontén B 1981 The fasciocutaneous flap, its use in soft tissue defects of the lower leg. British Journal of Plastic Surgery 34: 215–220
Snydacker E F 1907 Lidplastik mit gesteiltem Lappen vom Halse. Klinisches Monatsblatt für Augenheilkunde 45: 71–76
Sunderland S, Roy L J 1950 Denervation changes in mammalian striated muscle. Journal of Neurology, Neurosurgery and Psychiatry 13: 159–177
Tanzini I 1906 Sopra il mio nuovo processo di amputatzione della mammella. Gazetta Medica Italiana 57: 141
Taylor G I, Corlett R, Boyd J B 1983 The extended deep inferior epigastric flap: a clinical technique. Plastic and Reconstructive Surgery 72: 751–764
Taylor G I, Corlett R J, Caddy C M, Zelt R G 1992 An anatomic review of the delay phenomenon: II. Clinical application. Plastic and Reconstructive Surgery 89: 408–416
Tobin G R, Schusterman M, Peterson G H, Nichols G, Bland K I 1981 Intramuscular anatomy of the latissimus dorsi muscle: the basis for splitting the flap. Plastic and Reconstructive Surgery 67: 637–641
Tobin G R, Spratt J S, Bland K I, Weiner L J 1982 One stage pharyngoesophageal and oral mucocutaneous reconstruction with two segments of one musculocutaneous flap. American Journal of Surgery 144: 489–493
Tower S S 1935 Atrophy and degeneration in skeletal muscle. American Journal of Anatomy 56: 1–44
Vasconez L, Bostwick J III, McCraw J B 1974 Coverage of exposed bone by muscle transposition and skin grafting. Plastic and Reconstructive Surgery 53: 526–530

The fasciocutaneous system of vessels

5

5

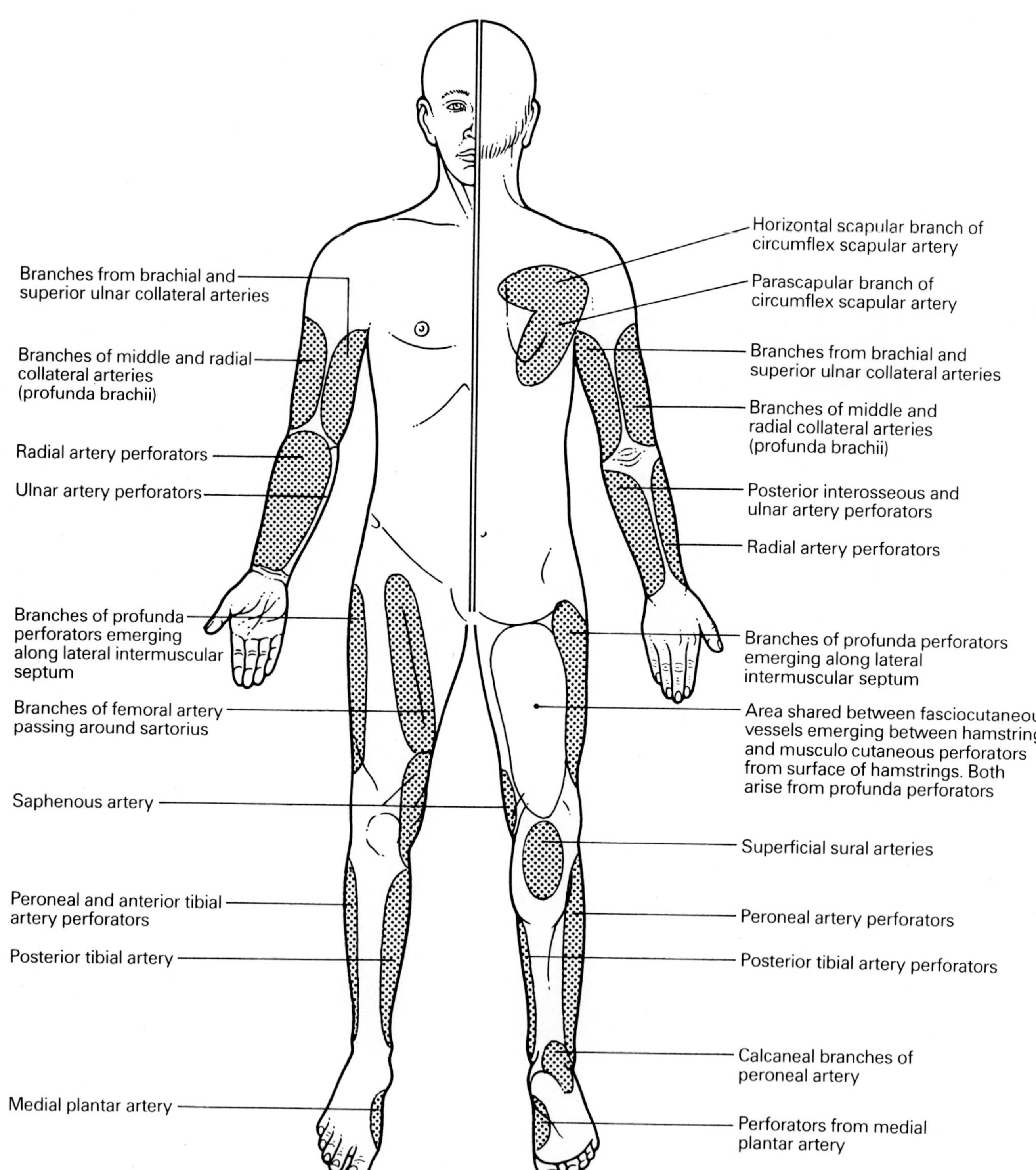
Branches from brachial and superior ulnar collateral arteries
Branches of middle and radial collateral arteries (profunda brachii)
Radial artery perforators
Ulnar artery perforators
Branches of profunda perforators emerging along lateral intermuscular septum
Branches of femoral artery passing around sartorius
Saphenous artery
Peroneal and anterior tibial artery perforators
Posterior tibial artery
Medial plantar artery
Horizontal scapular branch of circumflex scapular artery
Parascapular branch of circumflex scapular artery
Branches from brachial and superior ulnar collateral arteries
Branches of middle and radial collateral arteries (profunda brachii)
Posterior interosseous and ulnar artery perforators
Radial artery perforators
Branches of profunda perforators emerging along lateral intermuscular septum
Area shared between fasciocutaneous vessels emerging between hamstrings and musculo cutaneous perforators from surface of hamstrings. Both arise from profunda perforators
Superficial sural arteries
Peroneal artery perforators
Posterior tibial artery perforators
Calcaneal branches of peroneal artery
Perforators from medial plantar artery

Fig 5.1 Areas suitable for the raising of fasciocutaneous flaps are shown. Proportions of actual flaps will differ from the above.

THE PRINCIPLES OF THE FASCIOCUTANEOUS SYSTEM

The fasciocutaneous system consists of perforators which pass up to the surface along the fascial septa between adjacent muscle bellies and then fan out at the level of the deep fascia to form a plexus from which branches are given off to supply the overlying subcutaneous tissues and the dermis (Figs 5.1 & 5.2).

HISTORICAL DEVELOPMENT

Fasciocutaneous flaps based on this system of vessels are a relatively new concept largely attributable to the clinical work of Pontén who published his experiences with 23 lower leg fasciocutaneous flaps in 1981. These were all proximally based local flaps raised, without a prior delay procedure, to include the skin, subcutaneous fat and *deep fascia*. The impressive feature of these flaps was that they combined an average length-to-breadth ratio of 2.5:1, with a notable degree of reliability. Of his 23 flaps, he judged the results to be good in 17, fair in 3 and a failure in 3 of his cases. This was an impressive result when viewed in the context of classical teaching which held that all skin flaps below the knee were of the random kind and 'fraught with danger'. For several decades, many textbooks had advised against the use of local flaps below the knee yet Pontén demonstrated that lower leg fasciocutaneous flaps were simple, reliable and could be designed with dimensions of up to 18 cm × 8 cm with no problems. Indeed, his assistants were sufficiently impressed by the qualities of these flaps that they named them 'super flaps'.

Although Pontén made the essential and original clinical observations, he did not investigate the anatomical vascular basis of the 'super flap' in detail. Further work on the anatomical aspects was carried out by Haertsch (1981b) and later by Barclay et al (1982) who delineated the locations of the fasciocutaneous perforators. Haertsch also defined the surgical plane in the lower leg as lying beneath the deep fascia (Haertsch, 1981a). At the same time, the authors were working on the fascial plexus and were able to confirm the existence of a fascial plexus fed by perforators from the anterior tibial, posterior tibial and peroneal arteries. These perforators reach the deep fascia by passing from the anterior tibial artery along the anterior peroneal septum, from the peroneal artery along the posterior peroneal septum, and from the posterior tibial artery along the fascia between flexor digitorum longus and soleus (see Fig. 5.13). This basic pattern of cutaneous supply is augmented superomedially by the saphenous artery and posteriorly by the superficial sural arteries accompanying the sural nerves and by musculocutaneous perforators from the two muscle bellies of gastrocnemius. (The sizes and locations of all these perforators are described in greater detail in Chapter 6.)

In order to further define the anatomical vascular basis of the super flap in the lower leg we have measured the angles of vessels in the fascial plexus relative to the horizontal axis (Cormack & Lamberty, 1983a). In order to obtain data concerning the plexus of vessels at the level of the deep fascia, the following procedure was adopted on fresh cadavers. Undiluted Micropaque was injected into the popliteal artery at low pressure; the skin and deep fascia were elevated together

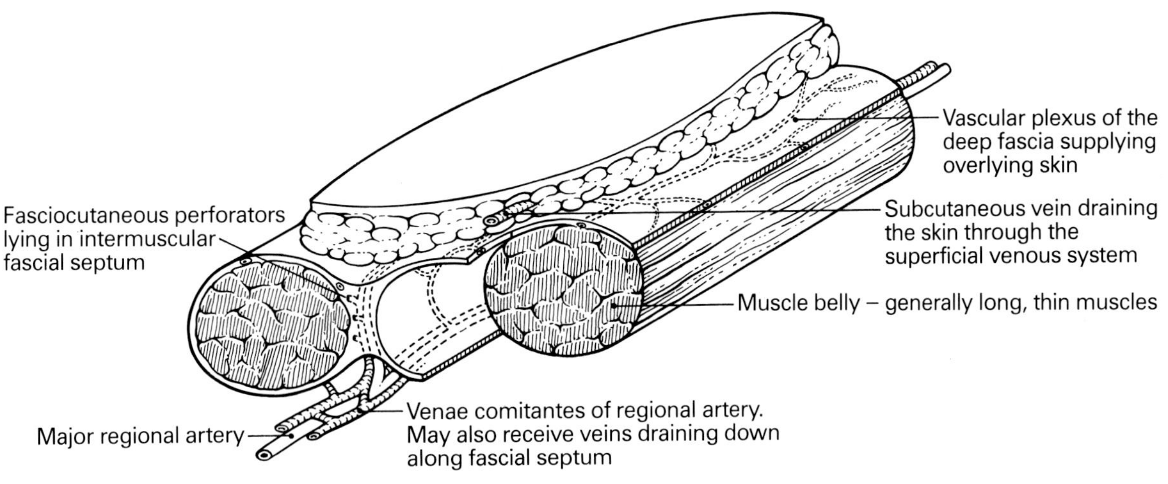

Fig 5.2 Schematic diagram illustrating the principal anatomical features of the blood supply to skin from perforators of the fasciocutaneous system.

from the underlying structures with ligation of feeding vessels; each vessel was numbered and its origin from the deeper structures recorded in writing and by photographs (Fig. 5.3); and radiographs were made of the detached specimen. The fascial surface was allowed to dry in order to facilitate its separation from the subcutaneous fat by sharp dissection. Separate radiographs were then made of the fascial and skin specimens followed by contact photographic prints of the fascial radiograph (Fig. 5.4). Vessel diameters were measured on the print using a dissecting microscope fitted with a calibrated eyepiece graticule, and vessels with an internal diameter of more than 0.1 mm were then traced out with a stylus on the print which was placed on the digitising tablet of a Kontron Videoplan image analyser. For each vessel, information was stored on a magnetic disc concerning its length, the distance between major branching points and the angle that a line between start and finish of its tracing made with the horizontal axis. The data were then analysed.

Figure 5.5, which is typical of the lower leg, is a computer generated histogram showing the frequency of 15 classes between 0° and 180° of angles of vessels (between major branching points) at the level of the deep fascia where 0° and 180° lie along the horizontal axis. The mode angle is 89.2° (median 92.5°, mean 96.7°), that is, along the long axis of the limb. Histograms were derived for the distance in a straight line between the major branching points of each vessel (Fig. 5.6). These two histograms can be combined to produce a three-dimensional plot which shows that most of the vessels in the fascial plexus lie in the region of 80–100° with a length of 5–20 mm (Fig. 5.7). However, these vessels are measured between major branching points, and a more functionally relevant method of

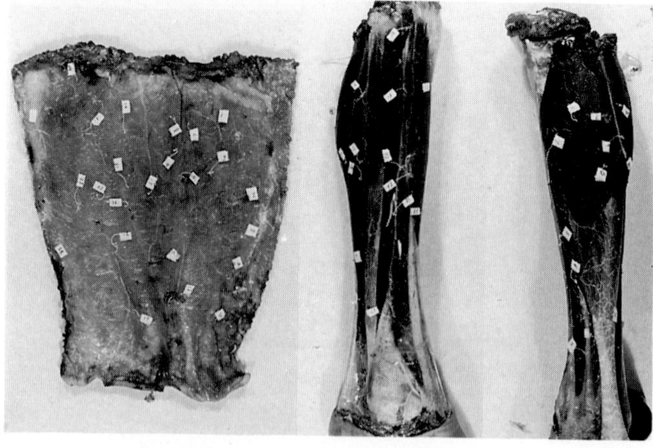

Fig 5.3 Photographs of a lower leg dissection with labelled perforators. Figures 5.4–5.8 relate to this specimen.

presenting this data is by adding together the lengths of all vessels falling within 45° angle sectors. Presented this way (Fig. 5.8) it can be clearly seen that in terms of functional length of vessels at the level of the deep fascia, the predominating direction is along the long axis of the limb.

The presence of the fascial plexus explains why a fasciocutaneous flap in the lower leg can be raised with greater safety and a much greater length-to-breadth ratio than an equivalent purely cutaneous flap in the same location. The clinical experience of Pontén (1981) and Barclay et al (1982) has also shown that the orientation of the flap is important; the 'super flap' is less reliable if raised obliquely or transversely. Our finding of a marked directionality of the fascial plexus explains this also.

In the past, new reports of flaps have been based on original theory without scientific quantification of the underlying vascular anatomy. This work demonstrates experimentally the basis for what is known to work clinically in the leg. This correlation between injection studies and the behaviour of living tissues appears to validate cadaver injection studies of this type and encourages their extension to other less well defined areas. However, before these other areas of the body are considered in terms of their fasciocutaneous vessels there are some further questions to be answered concerning the fascial plexus in the lower leg.

Questions regarding the location of the perforators can be explained in terms of their relationship to the fascial septa between long thin muscles, whereas it has already been seen how the skin over broad flat muscles tends to be supplied by musculocutaneous perforators. The perforators are feeding vessels and their branches form the fascial plexus, but at what level does this lie and why does the fascial plexus have a predominating axiality?

Haertsch (1981b) described the plexus as lying superficial to the fascia, but the fasciocutaneous perforators are passing obliquely through it giving off branches at all stages so that there are vessels present directly on the undersurface of the fascia, in the fascia, and directly on top of the fascia–principally the latter. Those on the undersurface of the fascia are much smaller and more delicate than those on its superficial surface. These facts had been reported in a the German anatomical literature several years before the clinical development of the fasciocutaneous concept but must have escaped the notice of the surgical world (Schäfer, 1975; Lang, 1962). The studies described above which analysed the direction of the fascial plexus concentrated on vessels greater than 0.1 mm ID which are present mainly in the upper/superficial part of the deep fascia. The vascularisation of the fascia itself comes from arterioles and capillaries smaller than 0.1 mm ID which lie in intimate relation to the bundles of collagen fibres which make up the deep fascia. These vessels lie both deep to and within the fascia.

The axiality of the fascial plexus was initially thought to be the result of the longitudinal pattern of growth of the limb although no studies have been carried out comparing the fascial plexus in the foetus, with that of the newborn, the child and the adult to establish this. Another possibility is that the fine structure of the deep fascia and the arrangement of the collagen fibres within it, may provide an explanation for the axiality of the fascial plexus not only in the lower leg but also in other regions.

Finally, the course of cutaneous nerves through, on, and then above the deep fascia has been recognised as important. Many of the larger branches of the perforators accompany these cutaneous nerves and since the nerves run longitudinally this influences the axiality of the vascular plexus.

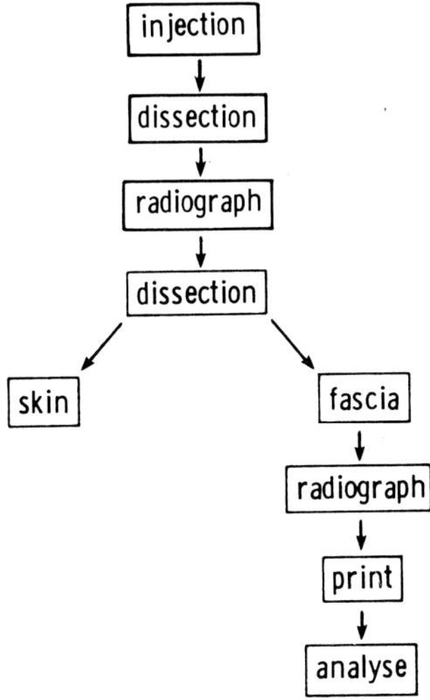

Fig. 5.4 Flow diagram to illustrate the procedure for obtaining radiographs of injected vessels at the level of the deep fascia.

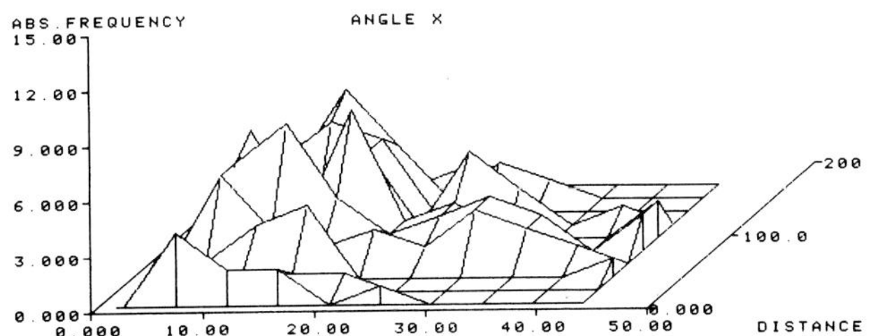

Fig. 5.7 Three-dimensional histogram combining angles and lengths of vessels.

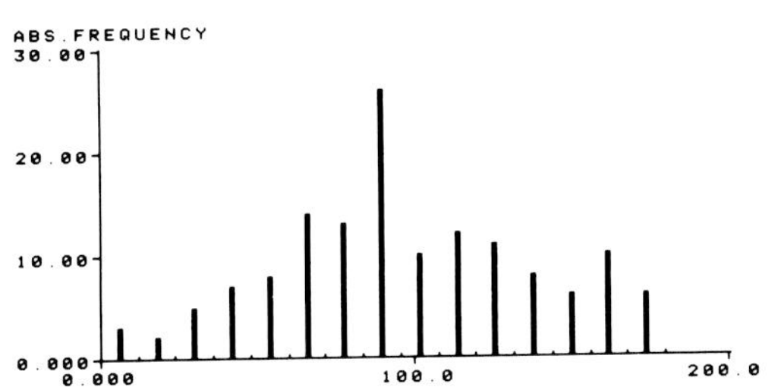

Fig. 5.5 Histogram for angles of fascial vessels (15 classes) relative to the horizontal axis.

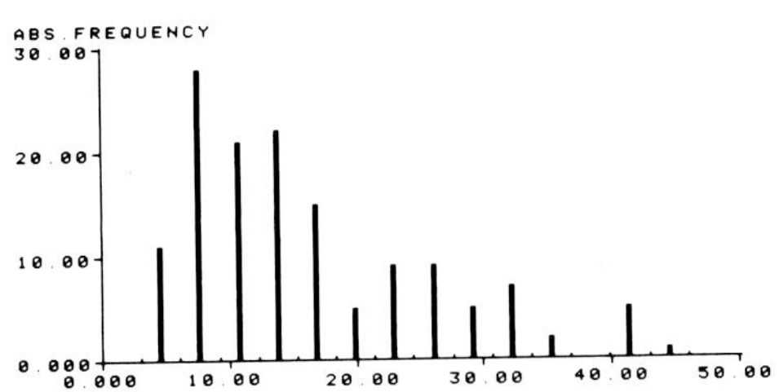

Fig. 5.6 Histogram for lengths of vessels (15 classes) between major branching points.

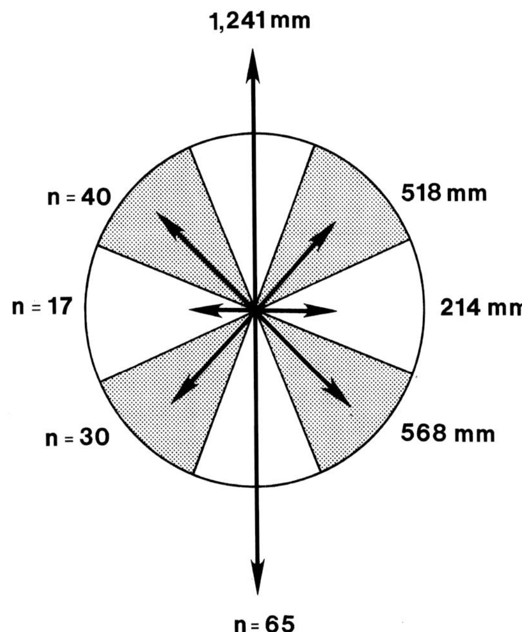

Fig. 5.8 A more functionally relevant way of presenting the data contained in Figure 5.7. The total lengths of all the vessels falling within 45° angle sectors are represented by the lengths of the arrows.

THE STRUCTURE OF DEEP FASCIA

The deep fascia is commonly regarded as a meshwork of collagen fibres with no particular structure or orientation except at certain sites where purely mechanical restraining functions are required such as across tendons on the flexural aspects of joints. Elsewhere highly ordered, thick, deep fascia is generally aponeurotic, that is it represents part of the origin or insertion of a fully functional muscle, e.g. the iliotibial tract which transmits the tension of tensor fasciae latae and part of gluteus maximus. The aponeuroses often referred to as 'fasciae' in the palm of the hand and the sole of the foot are protective layers that actually represent the degenerated remains of the expanded tendons of the palmaris longus and plantaris muscles which in man have undergone considerable phylogenetic degeneration. These are therefore not considered to be true deep fascia in the sense that is meant here. With these exceptions deep fascia is generally dismissed as being uniform in structure and of little interest. It is the commonly held view, summarised in 'Gray's Anatomy' (Williams & Warwick, 1980), that 'in the limbs, where the deep fascia is particularly well developed, many fibres are longitudinal in arrangement, while others encircle the limb, binding the longitudinal fibres together into a tough, inelastic sheath for the musculature'.

If it is indeed inelastic then one must ask how it is that the fascia can adapt to the changing shape of the muscle compartments during the phases of muscle contraction. In the lower leg, for example, plantar flexion is brought about by the plantar flexor muscles of the posterior compartment, and especially the combined mass of gastrocnemius and soleus whose muscle bellies can be observed on contraction to move proximally and increase the girth of the calf. Clearly during such a contraction the investing fascia must broaden out proximally whilst at the same time narrowing down in the more distal parts of the lower leg. Since the collagen fibres of which the deep fascia is composed are essentially inextensible there must be some subtle mechanism built into the fascial architecture to permit these changes to take place.

It can be easily demonstrated that in the lower leg the collagen fibres of the deep fascia are arranged in two lamellae (Lang, 1962) (Fig. 5.9). These fan out from the medial tibial plateau and from the head of the fibula in a posterior direction over the two heads of gastrocnemius. The fibres also incline distally and extend across the midline to pass round the sides of the lower leg and gain insertion into the anterior subcutaneous surface of the tibia. At their points of origin the bundles of collagen fibres lie heaped together but soon spread out into sheets which fan out over the calf.

On the lateral side the more anterior fibres pass downwards while the posterosuperior fibres pass over the two heads of gastrocnemius to form the lower part of the popliteal fascia. Between these two edges the fibres fan out, generally passing deep to those from the medial tibial condyle. This is particularly clearly seen in the midline between the two heads of gastrocnemius where the two lamellae enclose the superficial sural artery and the medial sural cutaneous nerve surrounded by a little fat. (By contrast the termination of the posterior cutaneous nerve of the thigh lies superficial to both lamellae of the calf fascia and the peroneal communicating branch of the lateral sural nerve, although initially deep to fascia, soon pierces it to lie above it.) The short saphenous vein generally lies above the deep fascia and pierces it below the popliteal crease but in 5–10% of cases it runs in the same tunnel as the medial sural nerve and the superficial sural artery between the lamellae of fascia. The fibres continue distally and medially and insert into the medial edge of the tibia. On the medial side the fan of fibres leaves the medial tibial plateau and passes both dorsally and distally to cross the calf and then the peroneal compartment where some of the fibres pass into the anterior and the posterior peroneal septa. The fibres

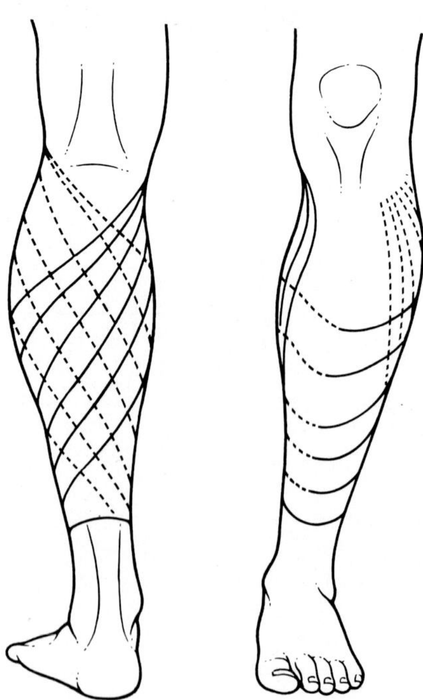

Fig. 5.9 The arrangement of the two lamellae which make up the deep fascia on the lower leg. One arises from the medial tibial condyle, the other from the area over the styloid process of the fibula. Both then fan out over the muscles of the leg and merge with the periosteum over the anterior subcutaneous surface of the tibia.

then cross over the anterior compartment and insert into the tibia. Considered together the fibres run in the form of multiple αs with the beginnings and ends attached to the fibular head and the medial tibial plateau. Over the calf muscles an anisotropic lattice web of rhomboids results. Although the angles at which the fibres intersect vary from place to place the majority of collagen fibres lie nearer the longitudinal axis than the horizontal axis of the limb. This architecture results in a fascial sheath which is able to accommodate both an increase in bulk in the proximal calf at the same time as a reduction in girth of the distal part.

Capillaries can be demonstrated between bundles of collagen fibres and also running between the lamellae. Vessels of each lamella anastomose with vessels in the other lamella and also with vessels above and below the fascia. These vessels are too small to be seen by direct vision but it appears that the orientation of vessels greater than 0.1 mm ID is also related to the architecture of the deep fascia.

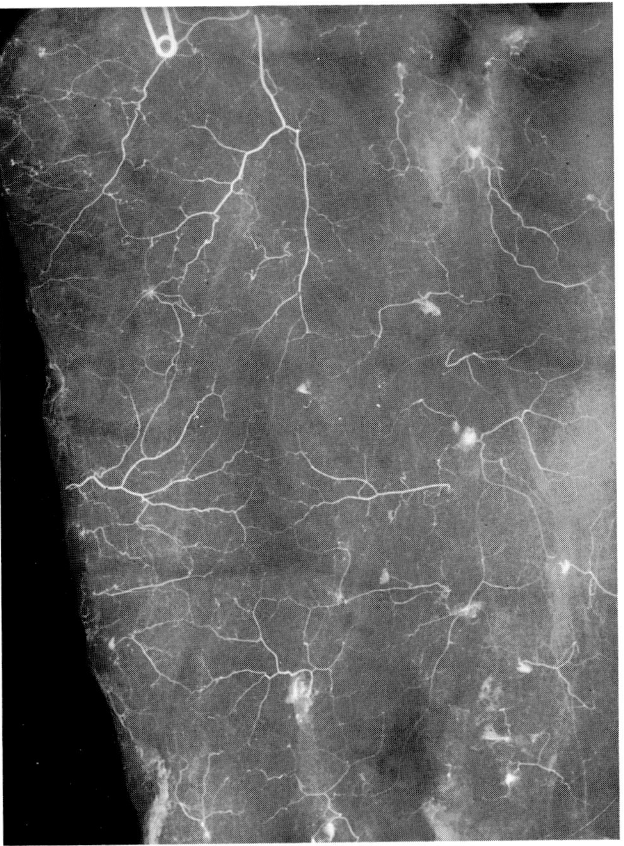

Fig. 5.10 Radiograph of injected volar forearm skin. The top of the specimen overlies the antecubital fossa (end of safety pin lies on the medial side of the anterior midline). Note the tendency towards a longitudinal arrangement of vessels in the proximal part and a more transverse orientation distally.

In the forearm the collagen fibres are arranged rather differently from the pattern in the lower leg. Over the proximal muscular part of the forearm both circular and longitudinal fibres occur while in the distal third of the forearm over the flexor tendons especially, the circular fibres predominate. The arrangement of the vessels of the fascial plexus follows the same pattern, namely the vessels are transversely orientated in the distal one-third and more longitudinally in the proximal two-thirds (Fig. 5.10). This reinforces the hypothesis that the direction of the collagen fibres is associated with the axiality of the facial plexus in the lower leg and tends to conflict with the view that the longitudinal orientation of the vessels simply results from the longitudinal growth pattern of the limb since if this were the case one would expect to see a longitudinal orientation of the fascial plexus throughout the length of the forearm. The arrangement of the collagen fibre bundles is also worth noting in regard to raised pressure in a compartment. The horizontal fibres over the anterior tibial compartment limit expansion and render this compartment prone to compression syndromes, and similarly the lack of extensibility of the fascia over the forearm flexor compartment may contribute to the generation of Volkmann's ischaemia; this explains why anterior fasciotomy is often necessary in severe hand and wrist injuries.

FASCIOCUTANEOUS FLAP PLANNING

This account of the clinical development of the lower leg fasciocutaneous flap and the subsequent elucidation of its underlying anatomical vascular basis, has served to draw attention to the three fundamental questions concerning the vascular anatomy which must be answered before a fasciocutaneous flap can be planned. These questions are:

1. Is there a significant fascial plexus at this site?
2. Where are the fasciocutaneous perforators located, and from which vessels do they arise?
3. What is the axiality of the fascial plexus?

The remainder of this chapter aims to give an overview of the fasciocutaneous system by answering these three questions in general terms for each of the major regions of the body. Specific details regarding locations of perforators can be found in Chapters 6 & 7.

The forearm

The pattern of blood supply to the skin of the forearm is in general principles similar to that of the leg below the knee. Although there are a few musculocutaneous perforators, most of the blood supply comes from fasciocutaneous perforators arising from the radial, ulnar, anterior and posterior interosseous arteries and reaches the surface by passing along the intermuscular fascial septa (Fig. 5.11). A significant plexus is formed by branches of these perforators at the level of the deep fascia.

Perforating arteries arise from the *radial artery* between brachioradialis and pronator teres in the proximal third of the forearm and between brachioradialis and flexor carpi radialis in the distal two-thirds of the forearm. Only one relatively large perforating vessel may arise proximally from the radial artery. This vessel is 0.5–1.5 mm in diameter and has been named by us the inferior cubital artery because of its origin in the lower part of the antecubital fossa. The *ulnar artery* gives off approximately five perforating arteries, which emerge between flexor carpi ulnaris and flexor digitorum superficialis. The *posterior interosseous artery* gives off multiple small perforating vessels at 1–3 cm intervals all the way down the forearm which emerge between extensor carpi ulnaris and extensor digitorum communis. Terminal small branches of the *anterior interosseous artery* pass around and between abductor pollicis longus and extensor pollicis brevis and supply the skin.

The fascial plexus on the anterior aspect is orientated predominantly along the longitudinal axis in the proximal two-thirds of the forearm and is orientated more transversely in the distal third (see Fig. 5.10). On the posterior aspect of the forearm the perforators from the posterior interosseous artery have an oblique or transverse orientation. This makes the posterior region unsuitable for the elevation of longitudinally orientated flaps.

The upper arm

With the exception of the area overlying deltoid, the blood supply of the upper arm is predominantly by the fasciocutaneous system, and not by musculocutaneous perforators from biceps and triceps despite their bulk (Fig. 5.12).

In the region overlying deltoid the skin is supplied by musculocutaneous perforators arising from the anterior and posterior circumflex humeral arteries, with one posterior perforator being particularly large. The remainder of the upper arm is supplied by fasciocutaneous perforators which emerge at the lower margins of deltoid and along the medial and lateral intermuscular septa. The fasciocutaneous arrangement is most striking; on the medial side there is a clear row of five or six vessels arising from the brachial artery, the biceps artery and/or from the superior ulnar collateral artery. In the upper or middle third of the arm there is usually one particularly large cutaneous branch up to 2 mm in diameter arising from one of these three named arteries. This vessel has not been formally named but will be referred to as the medial cutaneous artery. On the lateral side there is a similar row of fasciocutaneous perforators arising from the middle and radial collateral arteries (the terminal divisions of the profunda brachii artery) which descend respectively posterior and anterior to the origin of brachioradialis from the lateral intermuscular septum. We have found the middle collateral artery to be consistently the larger, and the more important of the two in supplying skin. There are no significant musculocutaneous perforators from the surface of the biceps muscle.

The fascial plexus on the upper arm is not orientated longitudinally. On the medial side the main branches of the perforators fan out either anteriorly or posteriorly and their finer offshoots anastomose longitudinally. In general, the main vessels incline obliquely distally. On the lateral side perforators tend to divide into two branches, one ascending obliquely, one descending obliquely.

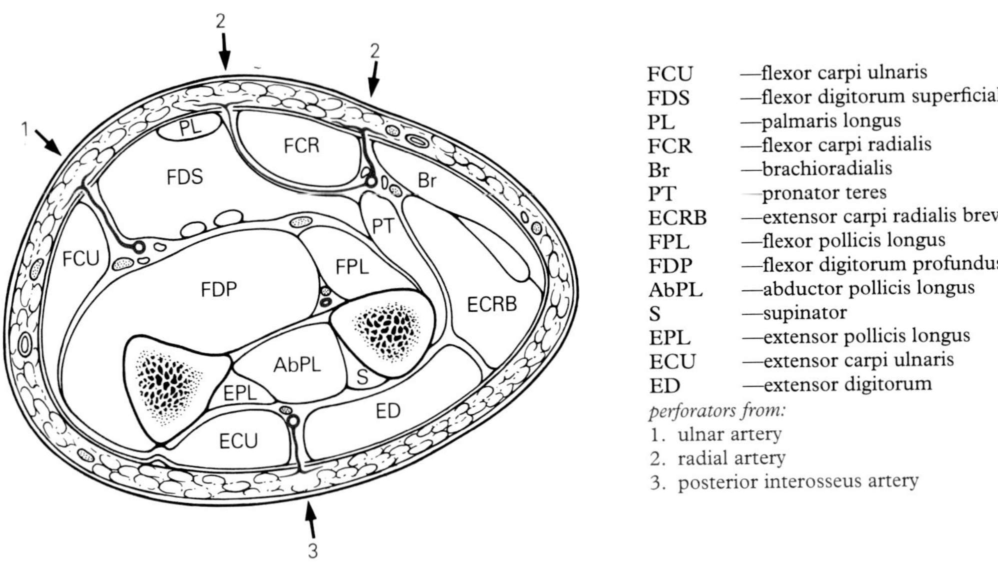

FCU —flexor carpi ulnaris
FDS —flexor digitorum superficialis
PL —palmaris longus
FCR —flexor carpi radialis
Br —brachioradialis
PT —pronator teres
ECRB —extensor carpi radialis brevis
FPL —flexor pollicis longus
FDP —flexor digitorum profundus
AbPL —abductor pollicis longus
S —supinator
EPL —extensor pollicis longus
ECU —extensor carpi ulnaris
ED —extensor digitorum

perforators from:

1. ulnar artery
2. radial artery
3. posterior interosseus artery

Fig. 5.11 Schematic transverse section through the mid-forearm showing locations of fasciocutaneous perforators.

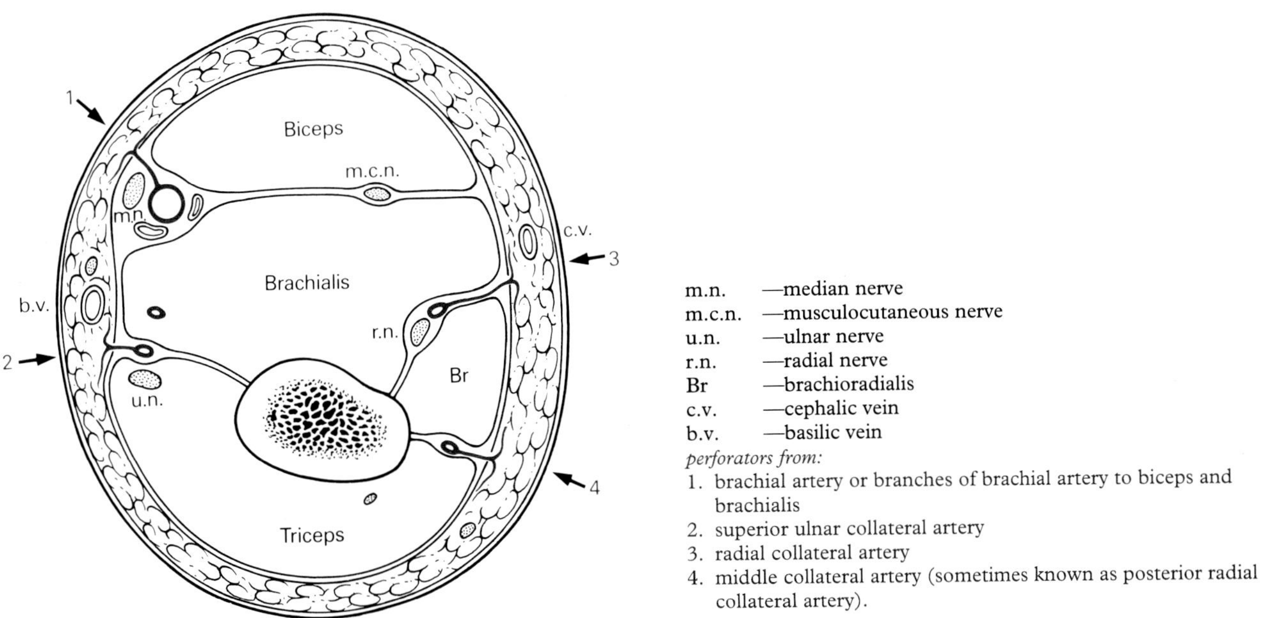

m.n. —median nerve
m.c.n. —musculocutaneous nerve
u.n. —ulnar nerve
r.n. —radial nerve
Br —brachioradialis
c.v. —cephalic vein
b.v. —basilic vein

perforators from:

1. brachial artery or branches of brachial artery to biceps and brachialis
2. superior ulnar collateral artery
3. radial collateral artery
4. middle collateral artery (sometimes known as posterior radial collateral artery).

Fig. 5.12 Schematic transverse section through the upper arm showing locations of fasciocutaneous perforators.

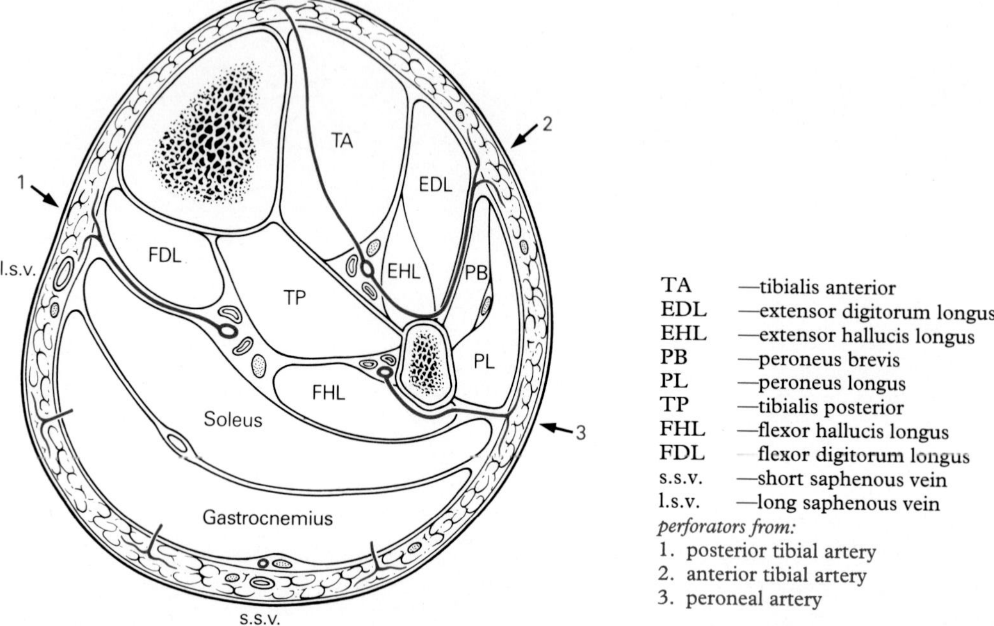

TA —tibialis anterior
EDL —extensor digitorum longus
EHL —extensor hallucis longus
PB —peroneus brevis
PL —peroneus longus
TP —tibialis posterior
FHL —flexor hallucis longus
FDL —flexor digitorum longus
s.s.v. —short saphenous vein
l.s.v. —long saphenous vein

perforators from:
1. posterior tibial artery
2. anterior tibial artery
3. peroneal artery

Fig. 5.13 Schematic transverse section through the mid-calf showing locations of fasciocutaneous perforators.

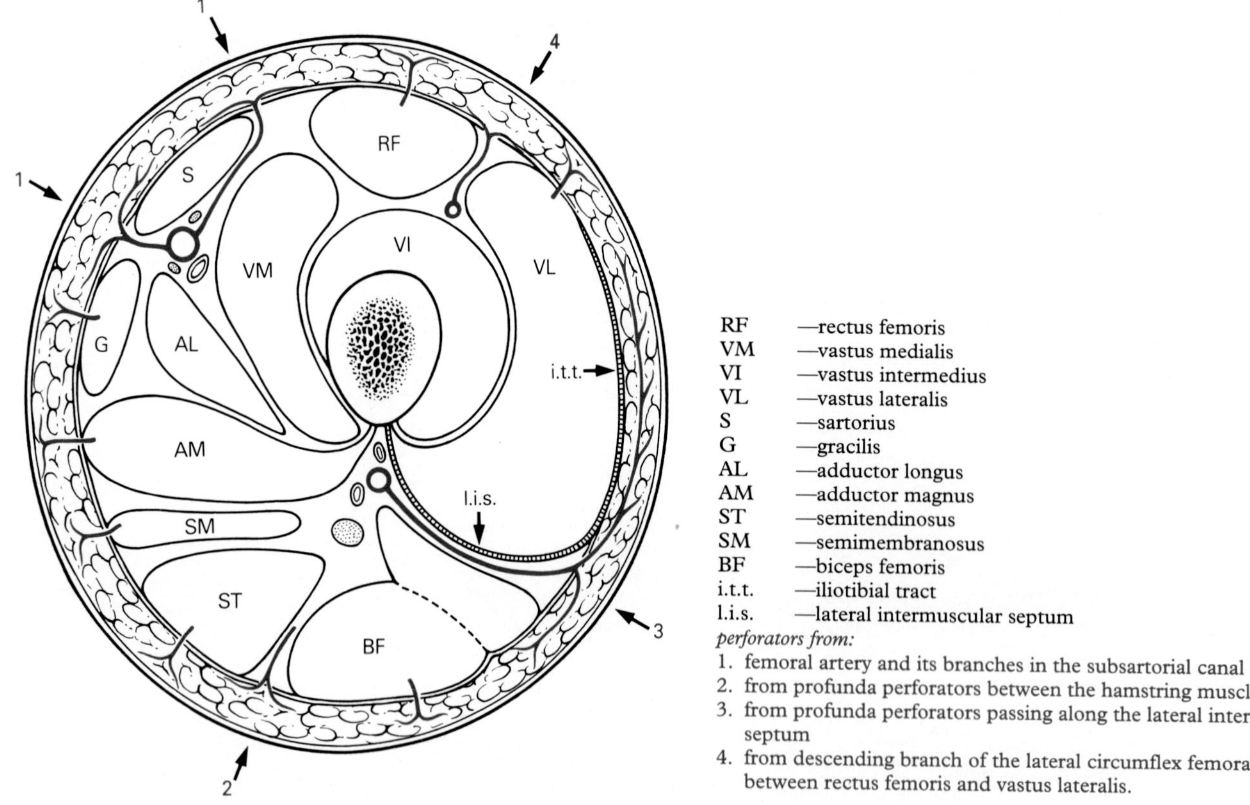

RF —rectus femoris
VM —vastus medialis
VI —vastus intermedius
VL —vastus lateralis
S —sartorius
G —gracilis
AL —adductor longus
AM —adductor magnus
ST —semitendinosus
SM —semimembranosus
BF —biceps femoris
i.t.t. —iliotibial tract
l.i.s. —lateral intermuscular septum

perforators from:
1. femoral artery and its branches in the subsartorial canal
2. from profunda perforators between the hamstring muscles
3. from profunda perforators passing along the lateral intermuscular septum
4. from descending branch of the lateral circumflex femoral artery between rectus femoris and vastus lateralis.

Fig. 5.14 Schematic transverse section through the mid-thigh showing locations of fasciocutaneous perforators.

The thigh

The blood supply to the thigh is shared between musculocutaneous and fasciocutaneous perforators.

The fasciocutaneous perforators are located in four main regions; anteromedially they lie along the edges of sartorius, posteriorly they emerge between the hamstring muscles, laterally they pass along the lateral intermuscular septum, and anterolaterally they emerge between rectus femoris and vastus lateralis at the anterior edge of the lower half of the iliotibial tract (Fig. 5.14).

1. The fasciocutaneous perforators passing round the anterior and posterior borders of sartorius have multiple sources of origin (see p. 230). The largest of these is the saphenous artery, which arises from the descending genicular artery, a branch of the superficial femoral just above the adductor hiatus.

2. and 3. The branches of the profunda perforators are of two types: posterior ones which supply hamstrings and the overlying skin by musculocutaneous and fasciocutaneous perforators; and lateral ones which head for vastus lateralis but give off fasciocutaneous vessels which run along the lateral intermuscular septum to emerge where it meets the iliotibial tract. There are six to ten of these lateral fasciocutaneous perforators along the length of the thigh, the upper ones being larger than the lower ones. The branch from the third profunda perforator appears to be consistently among the larger. In a study of these perforators by the authors, it was an unexpected finding that the branches of these perforators do not run closely applied to the surface of the iliotibial tract but just superficial to it in the lowermost part of the subcutaneous fat. The explanation may lie in the fact that the iliotibial tract is more in the nature of a tendon (of tensor fasciae latae) and a ligament (between the iliac crest and the tibia) than true deep fascia. It should be noted that, because the fascial perforators along the lateral intermuscular septum do not spread out at the level of the iliotibial tract, any attempt made to carry *islands* of skin on the tract in the expectation of the tract acting as a vascular pedicle are doomed to failure. There are a number of incidental reports of such failed flaps in the literature with no explanation given for their necrosis. From the foregoing description of the vascular anatomy it is easy to understand these flap failures.

At the lowermost part of the lateral thigh there may be a contribution from the superior lateral genicular artery.

4. The last group of perforators emerge between rectus femoris and vastus lateralis and arise from the descending branch of the lateral circumflex femoral artery. There may only be one or two of these perforators and they are unusual in that they may pass through the anterior muscle fibres of the vastus lateralis and therefore fall into a category of fasciocutaneous perforators perhaps best designated as septomuscular. Sometimes these vessels are deeply embedded in the vastus lateralis and more in the nature of musculocutaneous than fasciocutaneous perforators. This is probably related to the fact that the function of the descending branch is primarily to supply the lower anterior part of vastus lateralis. Note that these perforators do not pass through the iliotibial tract but lie anterior to it.

In Figure 5.15 the locations of the perforators on a typical thigh specimen are shown diagrammatically. The skin has been incised anteriorly, removed from the thigh and laid out flat. The vertical extent of the specimen is between horizontal planes passing through the lower end of the tensor fasciae latae muscle and through the patella. The crosshatched area overlies sartorius, the stippled area is over the iliotibial tract. Both musculocutaneous and fasciocutaneous perforators are shown by dots without distinguishing between them. The three rings beneath the iliotibial tract represent vessels from vastus lateralis which reach the undersurface of the tract, supplying it, but do not appear to penetrate through it to reach the overlying skin. Three regions have been distinguished and the direction of the subcutaneous vascular plexus analysed in each. The boundaries between the three regions, namely the anteromedial, anterolateral and posterior regions are: (1) a line between the anterior superior iliac spine and the patella; (2) the lateral intermuscular septum; and (3) a line between the pubis and the medial femoral condyle overlying the posterior edge of gracilis and often corresponding on the radiograph over its lower part to the course of the long saphenous vein.

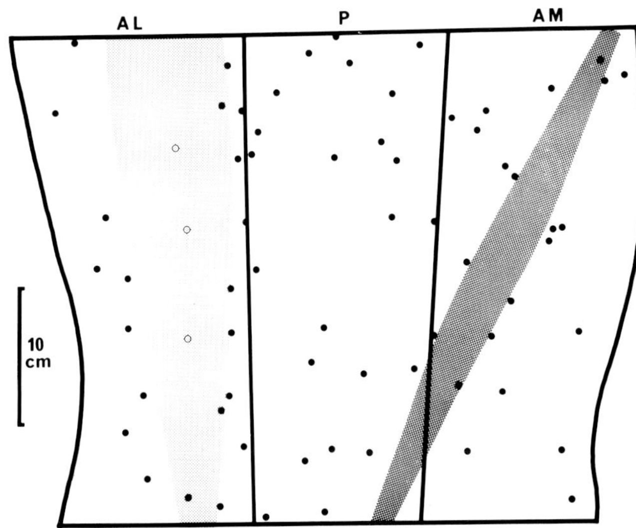

Fig. 5.15 Locations of principal perforators on the thigh. Stippled area indicates the region overlying the iliotibial tract, crosshatched area overlies sartorius.

Table 5.1 Data showing the total lengths of vessel segments (cm) and the number of branches in each 45° angle sector (B, C, D, A + E) for the three region of the thigh

	Anterolateral		Posterior		Anteromedial	
	length method	branches method	length method	branches method	length method	branches method
A	8	5	19	12	22	5
B	43	11	37	14	25	6
C	29	3	51	17	68	22
D	28	14	50	15	44	19
E	16	8	14	6	6	2
A+E	24	13	33	18	28	7

Table 5.2 A breakdown of the data relating to vessel lengths in Table 5.1. This reveals how the vessel length in each angle sector was made up in terms of numbers of vessels and their average lengths

	Anterolateral		Posterior		Anteromedial	
	average length (mm)	number of vessels	average length	number of vessels	average length	number of vessels
B	16	26	15	25	15	16
C	17	17	19	27	16	43
D	14	20	16	31	17	26
A+E	14	17	12	27	13	21

The axiality of the vascular plexus in these three regions has been analysed. The following text in small print describes the method but this may be passed over by the reader to reach the conclusions on page 117.

The subcutaneous plexus as a whole was analysed using the computer aided image analysis technique previously described for the fascia of the lower leg. By this method total lengths of vessels above 0.25 mm internal diameter falling within 45° angle sectors were derived for each of the three regions of the thigh. These data showed clear differences in the direction of the vascular plexus between the three regions. Figure 5.16 shows a typical example of a tracing from a radiograph of the injected vascular plexus (skin and fascia). Table 5.1 shows the figures obtained by this technique for one study but interpretation in easier by viewing Figure 5.17 which is a diagrammatic representation of the directionality of these vessels obtained by adding together the total length of vessels falling withing 45° angle sectors.

A second method of analysis was also applied to the same radiograph. In this a 2.5 cm radius circle was drawn around each perforator. A line was then drawn from the perforator to each point on the perimeter of the circle where it was crossed by a branch of that perforator (Fig. 5.18). It can be seen that both the total length method and the branches method indicate differences in the axiality of the vascular plexus between the three regions of the thigh. Table 5.1 constitutes a contingency table for the branches method data, with 3 columns (AL, P, AM) and four rows (B, C, D, A + E) available for statistical analysis. The hypothesis that the distribution of vessels in AL, P and AM regions is the same in each of the four angle sectors is rejected by a χ^2 statistic value of 234. This indicates a difference significant at better than the 99.9% level. In the anteromedial region the presence of a fascial plexus aligned with sartorius accounts for the predominance of the sector based on the long axis of the limb. Reference to Table 5.2 shows that in this sector (C) the increased total length of vessels is attributable to a greater number of vessels rather than greater individual length. There are also more vessels in the whole of the anteromedial region with an internal diameter of $\geqslant 0.25$ mm than there are in the anterolateral region (106:80).

For another case analysed by the total length method the results are presented diagrammatically in Figure 5.19. The figures are slightly based by the fact that the anterolateral area was slightly smaller than the others but again the trend is towards a longitudinal orientation for the plexus in the anteromedial region, transverse/oblique in the anterolateral region, and intermediate posteriorly.

The findings in a further case are presented differently in Figure 5.20. This again shows similar differences between the three areas.

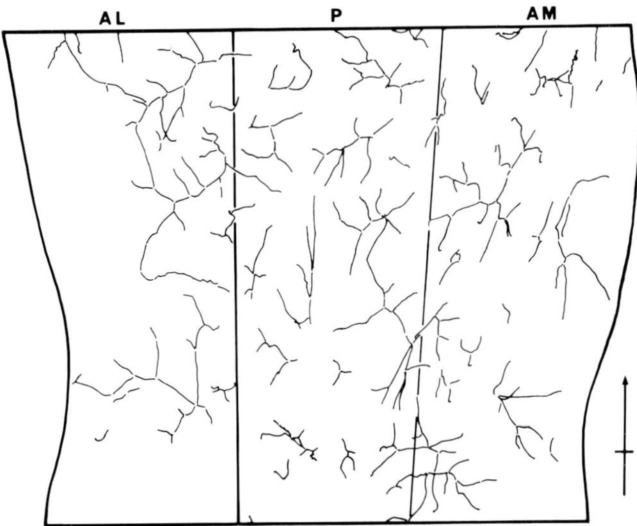

Fig. 5.16 Vessels with internal diameters greater than 0.25 mm.

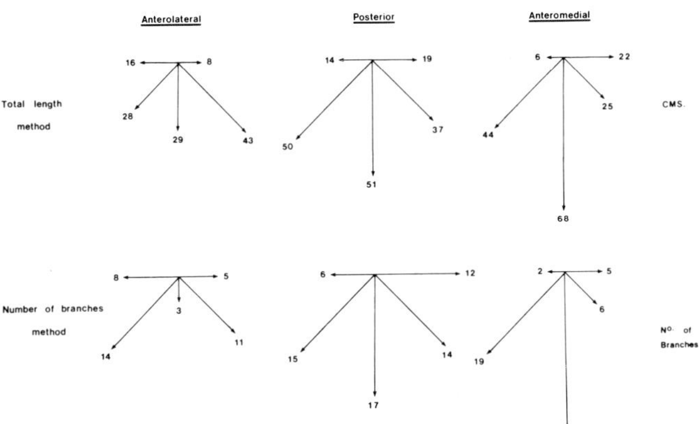

Fig. 5.17 Analysis of the three regions by two methods – the total length method corresponds to Figure 5.16, the radius method to Figure 5.18.

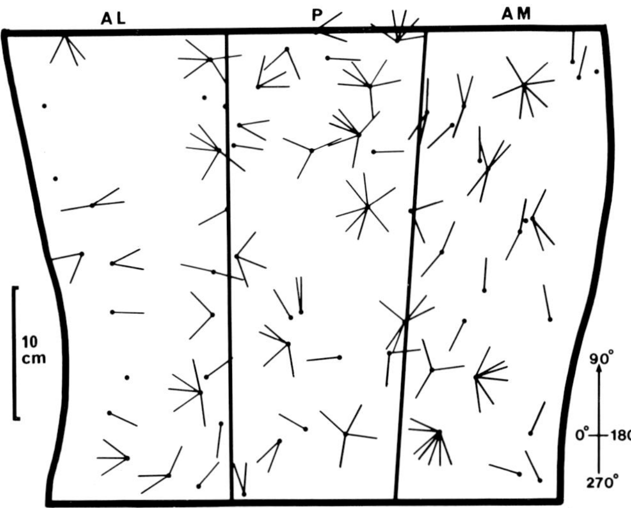

Fig. 5.18 Branches of each perforator that cross the perimeter of a 2.5 cm radius circle centred on that perforator.

The most striking feature about the vascular plexus in the three regions of the thigh is the variation in axiality. In the anteromedial region there is a well-developed fascial plexus with marked axiality aligned with sartorius. The posterior region has a fascial plexus that is moderately well developed. Its longitudinally directed component is mainly in the midline and is made up almost entirely of vessels running along the line of the posterior cutaneous nerve of the thigh. Superiorly a descending branch of the inferior gluteal artery runs at the level of the fascia with this nerve. Its diameter is variable and it would terminate very quickly were it not for the fact that it appears to act as a kind of 'relay vessel', being reinforced along its length by musculocutaneous and fasciocutaneous perforators arising from the profunda perforators. The other longitudinally directed element comes from the ascending branch of the popliteal artery. All the other fascial vessels in the posterior region run obliquely and horizontally. In the anterolateral region there are some large perforators but they run horizontally and obliquely although their smaller branches do anastomose longitudinally.

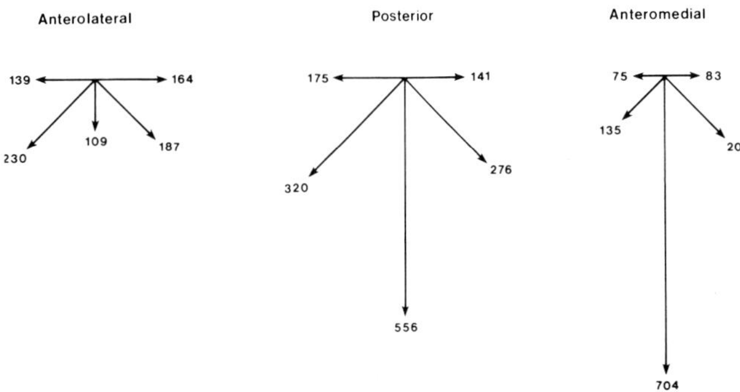

Fig. 5.19 Another case analysed by the total length method.

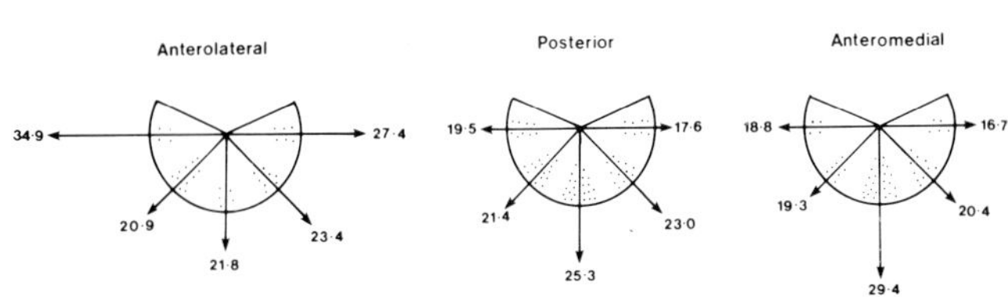

Fig. 5.20 Another case; arrows indicate average lengths of vessel segments between branching points, dots indicate the number of vessel segments.

The trunk

The examples of fasciocutaneous perforators given so far have all come from the limbs where muscles are generally long and thin with an abundance of fascial septa between them along which vessels may pass to the skin. It is a common misconception that the fascial plexus is ubiquitous, and some people consider that flaps depending primarily on a fascial plexus are an equally valid concept on the trunk. Classical anatomical teaching maintains that on the trunk there is no true deep fascia of the type forming intermuscular septa on the limbs, because the inextensibility of such a fascia would prevent the expansion of the chest and the distension of the abdominal viscera. There is a thin fascia of epimysium investing the muscles which is, of course, vascularised to some degree but there is no marked deep fascial plexus on the trunk and the blood supply of the skin is dependent on musculocutaneous perforators from underlying flat muscles, with supplementary direct cutaneous vessels at certain sites.

There is one place on the trunk, however, where fasciocutaneous perforators definitely do exist and that is where vessels emerge from between the muscles attaching to the lateral border of the scapula and run over the rather thicker fascia covering the infraspinatus muscle. These muscles belong, in evolutionary terms, to the upper limb rather than body wall musculature, and teres major and minor do approach the approximate dimensions of long thin muscles rather than broad flat ones. The vessels concerned are the cutaneous branches of the circumflex scapular artery. The circumflex scapular artery gives off two major fasciocutaneous branches which emerge along the 'space' bounded by teres minor above, teres major below, and the long head of triceps laterally. (Sometimes described in anatomical texts as one of the triangular spaces.) One branch runs over the posterior aspect of the scapula parallel to the scapular spine and has been named the horizontal branch, the other descends parallel to the lateral border of the scapula and has been named the parascapular branch. Of these two the parascapular branch is the more constant, although we have shown that it may emerge below teres major (Cormack & Lamberty, 1983b). By contrast, the horizontal branch may be very short or absent. Branches of both of these vessels travel at the level of the deep fascia.

Other fasciocutaneous perforators have been suggested on the anterior trunk. Reid & Taylor (1984) have described the branches of the thoraco-acromial axis in terms of direct cutaneous, musculocutaneous and fasciocutaneous vessels. They believe that the terminal twigs of the pectoral branch of the thoraco-acromial axis which turn round the infero-lateral border of pectoralis major are fasciocutaneous perforators.

Boyd et al (1984) have described the branches of the epigastric arcades which emerge from the rectus sheath along the linea alba and the linea semilunaris as fasciocutaneous perforators. However, these vessels do not fan out at the level of the anterior rectus sheath (see p.171) but run in the subcutaneous fat where they anastomose with adjacent musculocutaneous perforators and direct cutaneous vessels. Their diagrams also demonstrate that these vessels do not spread out at the level of the fascia, and it seems inappropriate to describe these branches as fasciocutaneous.

The conclusion is that on the trunk the only true fasciocutaneous perforators are those emerging between the teres major and minor muscles. These are the only vessels which lie in a fascial septum between muscles which are relatively long and thin, and which form a plexus at the level of the fascia. All other vessels on the trunk are either musculocutaneous or direct cutaneous in type.

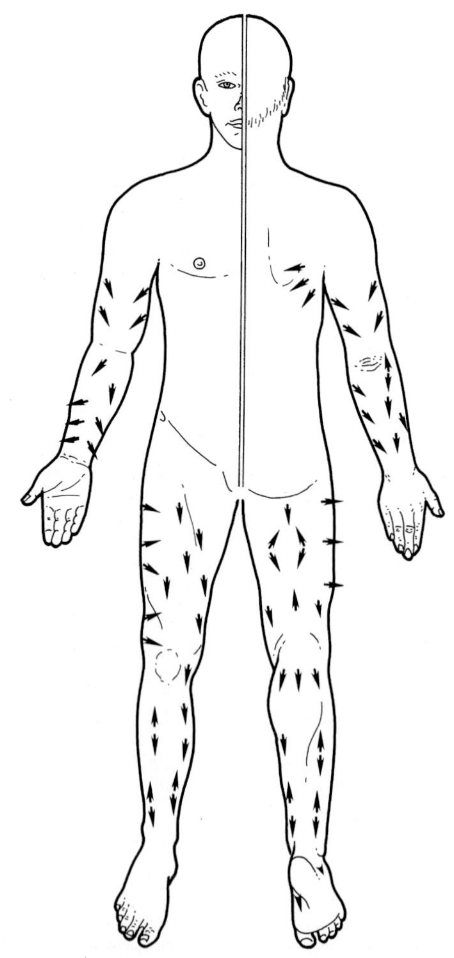

Fig. 5.21 An approximate guide to the axiality of the fascial plexus at sites throughout the body.

A CLASSIFICATION OF FASCIOCUTANEOUS FLAP TYPES (Fig. 5.24)

Equipped with these answers to the three questions posed earlier, namely:

1. Is there a significant fascial plexus at this site?
2. Where are the fasciocutaneous perforators located?
3. What is the axiality of the fascial plexus?

we are in a position to be able to establish the anatomical vascular basis of fasciocutaneous flaps. Combining clinical experience of these flaps with the anatomical observations has led the authors to suggest a simple classification of fasciocutaneous flaps. On the basis of their patterns of vascularisation fasciocutaneous flaps are divided into three types, designated A, B and C, although we do not see this as a rigid classification but rather as an anatomical basis on which to elaborate. It is also interesting to see how some established flaps – designed before the fasciocutaneous concept was established – fit into this scheme. The development of this classification has also proved useful in stimulating the search for further examples of the genre.

Type A flap

The Type A flap corresponds to the first recognised fasciocutaneous flap as described by Pontén on the lower leg. A Type A flap is dependent on multiple fasciocutaneous vessels entering its base and is orientated with the long axis of the flap lying parallel to the predominating direction of the arterial plexus at the level of the deep fascia (see Fig. 5.21).

Such a flap in the lower leg is generally proximally based and orientated longitudinally. Clinical work has shown that the flap does not attain the same degree of reliability and safety if it is raised obliquely or transversely. Used as a cross-leg flap, the longitudinal orientation is contrary to classical teaching which invariably described the random cross-leg flap as being elevated transversely on a broad pedicle. Another difference is that the greater length of the longitudinal fasciocutaneous flap facilitates positioning and allows greater mobility between the legs. An incidental point is that these cross-leg fasciocutaneous flaps do not require a preliminary division of the deep fascia before final division of the pedicle and insetting of the flap (Barclay et al, 1982).

Fasciocutaneous flaps raised on the medial side of the leg are clinically more reliable than ones based on the lateral side of the leg. This is in part due to the larger size of individual perforators on the medial side, in part to the continuation of the saphenous artery below the knee and in part probably due to the greater strength of the supplementary musculocutaneous supply likely to be entering the base of a flap raised on the medial side. These musculocutaneous perforators arise from the underlying gastrocnemius muscle and since the medial head is always larger and extends further distally than does the lateral head, there tend to be more perforators reaching skin on the medial side.

As well as the 'super flap' in the lower leg, there are examples on the thigh where a pedicled flap overlying sartorius conforms to the principles of a Type A flap, and on the upper arm where flaps based on the medial or lateral intermuscular septa will incorporate multiple perforators in their bases. Pedicled flaps overlying sartorius have little practical value but are mentioned here to draw attention to the pattern of perforators around the muscle in this part of the thigh, and to the fact that although the muscle may be raised with the overlying skin, the principal supply is not musculocutaneous but fasciocutaneous. (A Type B flap may be based on a single one of these perforators – see later.)

On the upper arm, flaps may be of Types A, B or C. Prior to 1980 upper arm flaps tended to be raised over the biceps muscle with no regard to the local pattern of blood supply. The classical Tagliacottian type of upper arm flap is actually created in the worst possible orientation as far as the blood supply is concerned

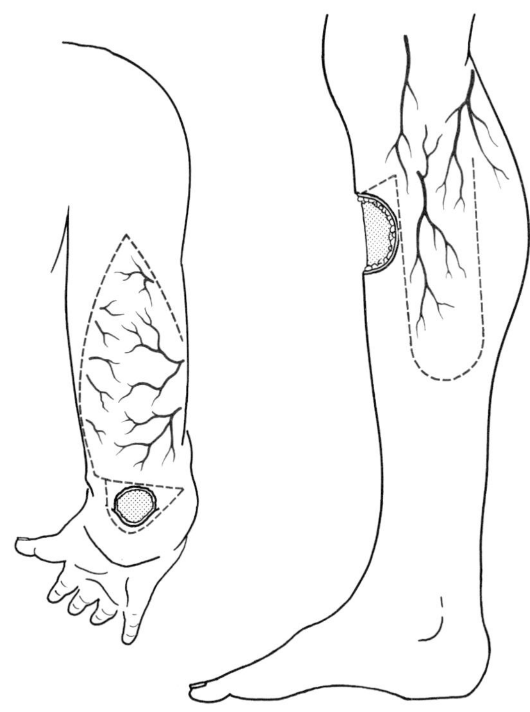

Fig. 5.22 The Type A fasciocutaneous flap has several vessels entering the base of the pedicle.

although it lies in a relatively convenient orientation for flap transfer. The Tagliacottian flap lies perpendicular to the direction of the larger vessels in the fascial plexus and fails to incorporate any perforators in its base, hence the need for a bipedicle delay procedure before this flap can be transferred with any degree of safety. In contrast, a flap which has its base on the lateral intermuscular septum can achieve a high degree of safety without a delay procedure, even if made fairly narrow. However, most of these flaps are in fact broadly based and used as rotation flaps, for example to close olecranon defects as shown in Figure. 5.22.

Type B flap

The Type B flap is based on a single fasciocutaneous perforator of moderate size, which is consistent both in its presence and its location. The flap may be used as a local pedicled flap or as a microvascular free flap and incorporates the territory supplied by this perforator. Venous drainage is by the subcutaneous system of veins or by the venae comitantes of the perforator, depending on the location of the flap and the way in which it is being used. Good examples are the medial arm flap (p. 455), the antecubital forearm flap based on the inferior cubital artery (p. 340), the saphenous artery flap (p. 428), and the scapular (p. 228) and parascapular flaps (p. 291). One of the perforators passing round the upper edge of sartorius at the junction of its upper and middle thirds is often large enough to support a Type B fasciocutaneous free flap (p. 333). The branch of the third profunda perforator emerging along the lateral intermuscular septum of the thigh is generally larger than the rest and may be used as the basis of a free flap – it is not necessary to include a portion of the iliotibial tract in this flap (p. 420).

Prior to the elucidation of the fasciocutaneous system, the vessels supplying these flaps were erroneously thought to be part of the direct cutaneous system of vessels. However, it is now clear that these vessels emerge along fascial septa and run at the level of the deep fascia.

A pedicled Type B flap need not necessarily include the skin in its base. The base of the flap may consist of subcutaneous fat and deep fascia incorporating the single perforator and carrying the blood supply to an island of skin situated some distance from the base of the flap. Such a flap has been designed on the lower leg with the island of skin situated over the upper part of gastrocnemius and the subcutaneous and fascial pedicle of about 5 cm width dissected *distally* to a point some 15 cm above the lateral malleolus where a particularly large perforator tends to emerge along the posterior peroneal septum, accompanied by two venae commitantes (p. 387). The flap may then be rotated downwards to reconstruct a defect over the Achilles tendon (Donski & Fogdestam, 1983). Distally based flaps supplied by individual posterior peroneal septal perforators demonstrate how a detailed knowledge of the axiality of the fascial plexus combined with accurate localisation of individual perforators can enable increasingly ingenious flaps to be elaborated from the four types of this simple classification.

When the authors first devised a classification of fasciocutaneous flaps a fifth type was included. In an endeavour to keep the classification as simple as possible this fifth type is now included as a modification of Type B. This type of fasciocutaneous flap is still fed by a single perforator but the essential characteristic of this flap is that the perforator is removed in continuity with

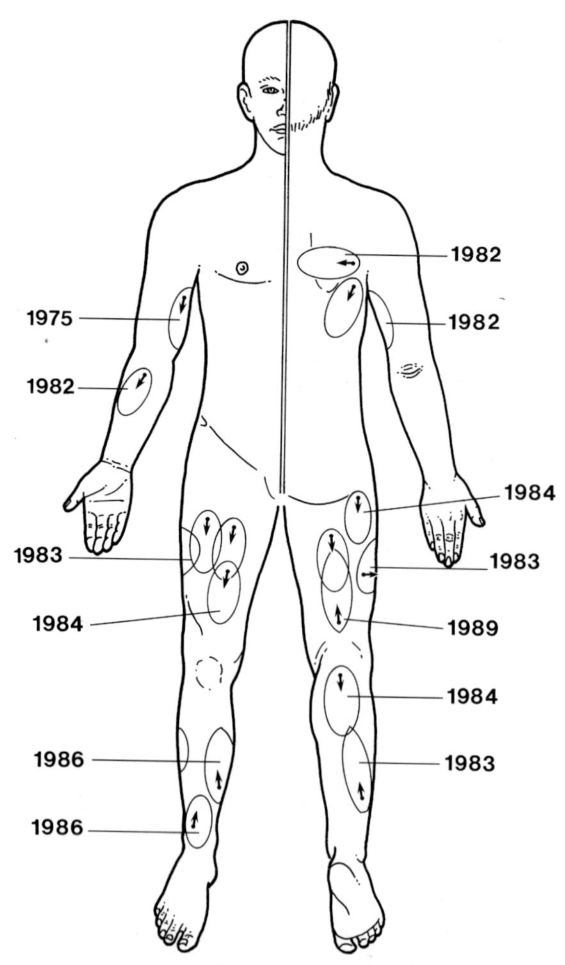

Fig. 5.23 The historical development of Type B fasciocutaneous flap donor sites. These are the dates when the descriptions were first published in English.

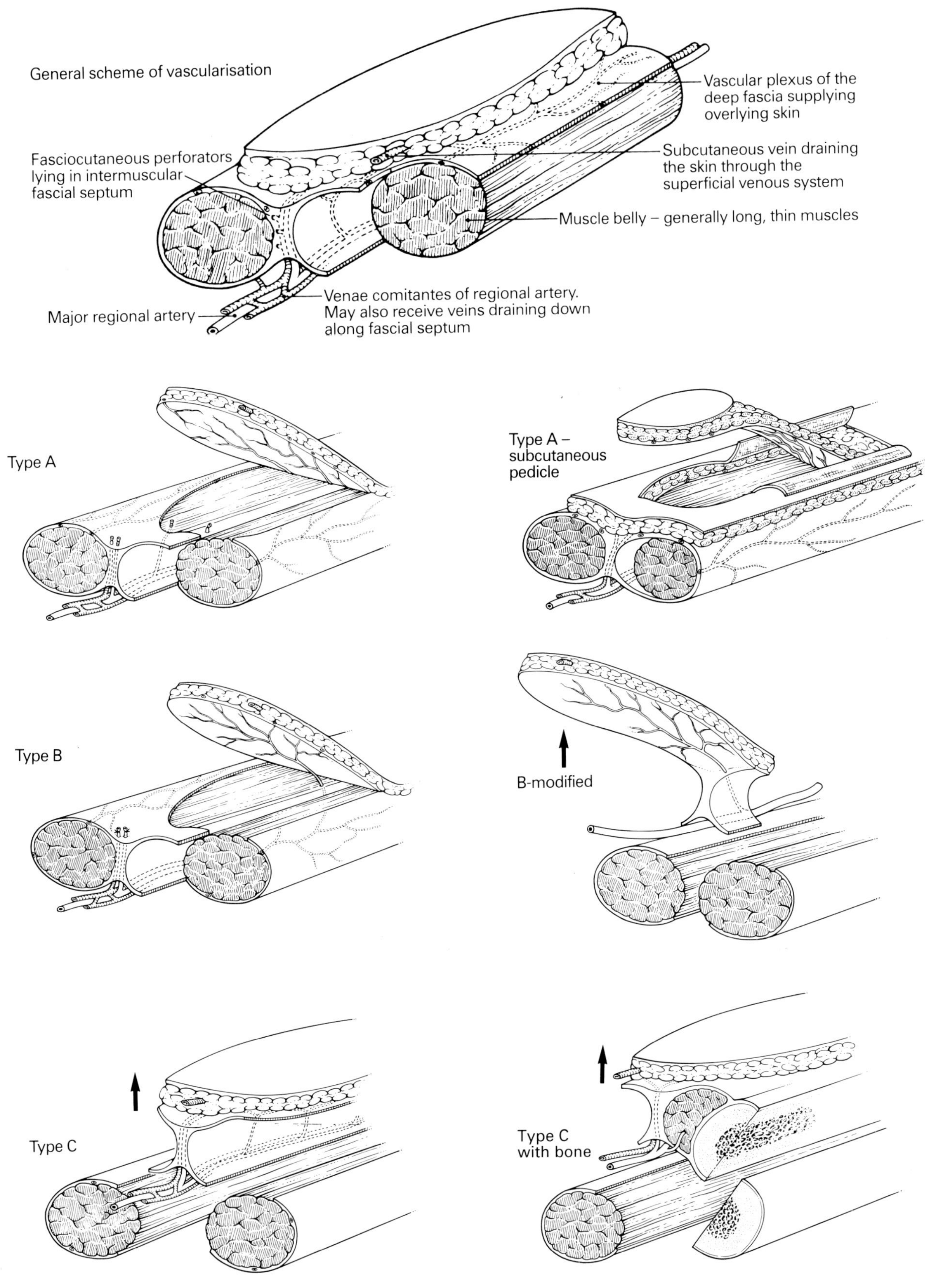
General scheme of vascularisation
Vascular plexus of the deep fascia supplying overlying skin
Fasciocutaneous perforators lying in intermuscular fascial septum
Subcutaneous vein draining the skin through the superficial venous system
Muscle belly – generally long, thin muscles
Venae comitantes of regional artery. May also receive veins draining down along fascial septum
Major regional artery
Type A
Type A – subcutaneous pedicle
Type B
B-modified
Type C
Type C with bone

Fig. 5.24 A classification of fasciocutaneous flaps.

the more major vessel from which it arises. There is in effect a T-junction on the single vessel at the base of the flap. The cross limbs of the T, being formed by a vessel rather larger than the perforator feeding the flap, are more suitable for microvascular anastomoses. The modified Type B flap is therefore intended for use as a free flap. These flaps appear to have certain haemodynamic advantages in a comparable way to the Type C flaps, and also, by virtue of the longer pedicle, allow greater versatility in flap orientation at the recipient site.

Examples of vessels which lend themselves to this modification would be the medial arm flap when the supplying perforator arises from the superior ulnar collateral artery, and the antecubital forearm flap supplied by the inferior cubital artery which can be removed in continuity with a segment of the radial artery. In the antecubital forearm flap the venous drainage is by the subcutaneous system draining into the cephalic vein. The cephalic vein may be dissected out proximally to match the length of the radial artery pedicle thereby obtaining a long flap and a long pedicle. There are various anatomical arrangements which would render this flap impossible (p. 340).

Type C flap

The Type C flap is supported by multiple small perforators along its length which reach it from a deep artery by passing along a fascial septum between muscles. It is used as a free flap by removing the skin, fascia and supplying artery in continuity. The arrangement may be likened to that of a ladder on its side. One longitudinal member represents the supplying artery, the other represents the fascial plexus, and the rungs of the ladder represent the separate perforators. The gaps between the rungs vary in size depending on the region and generally measure between 1 and 3 cm.

The first flap of this type to be described was a forearm flap incorporating the radial artery and the fascial septum between flexor carpi radialis and brachioradialis. This was developed by Doctors Yang Guofan, Chen Bao Qui, and Gao Yuzhi in 1978 and published in Chinese in 1981 (abstracted in English in Plastic and Reconstructive Surgery in 1982), and hence has come to be known as the Chinese forearm flap. In many early cases in which this flap was used, the radial artery was replaced by a reversed vein graft. With increasing experience it has become clear than careful patient selection and preoperative assessment can make a vein graft unnecessary in most cases as the hand may be adequately supplied with blood from the ulnar and interosseous arteries. The amount of skin carried on the radial artery varies, depending on need, from a small island overlying the flexor tendons above the wrist to the whole of the ventral forearm skin and may even be extended onto the lower quarter of the upper arm.

When the radial artery of this flap is anastomosed at both ends in the recipient site, a through-flow situation is created in the artery which may have certain haemodynamic advantages for the flap. Not only does brisk flow in the artery help maintain patency of the anastomoses but it can be envisaged that the perforators deliver adequate flow to the flap rather than too much as may occur in an end-vessel situation. Venous drainage of a Type C flap is generally through the subcutaneous system of veins although veins accompany the fasciocutaneous perforators. The latter system of veins drains into the venae comitantes of the major

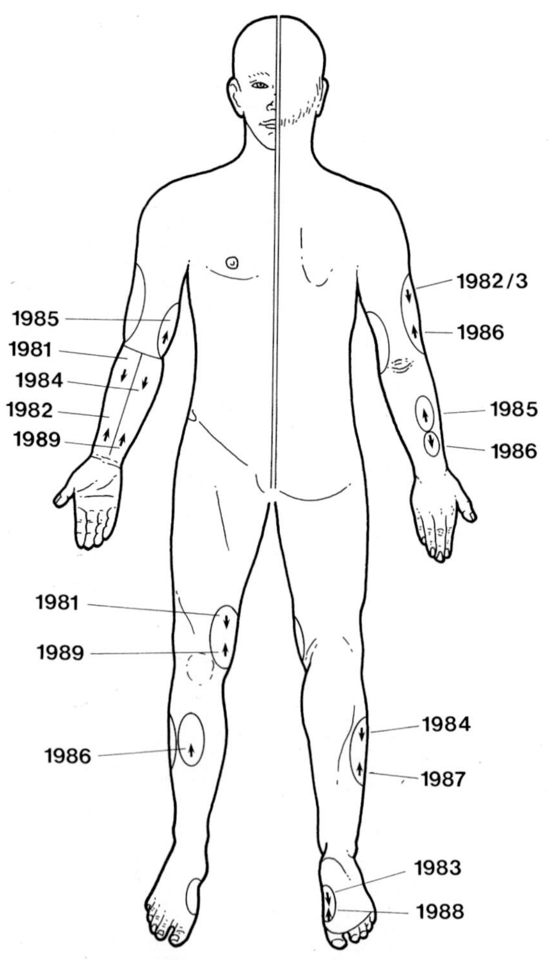

Fig. 5.25 The historical development of Type C fasciocutaneous flap donor sites. These are the dates when the descriptions were first published in English.

supplying artery. The venae comitantes of the radial artery contain values (Fig. 5.26) but reversal of flow in the veins appears to be possible. This may be due to the possibility of blood bypassing these valves through multiple collateral channels surrounding the artery (Fig. 5.27) (Lin et al, 1984) combined with valve incompetence as a result of excessive back pressure. Although these seem to us to be the most likely mechanisms accounting for the occurrence of reversed flow, the possibility of the valves becoming incompetent secondary to denervation of the veins has also been suggested (Timmins, 1984).

In the lower limb a Type C flap may be based on the peroneal artery (Yoshimura et al, 1983) and in the upper arm on the middle collateral branch of the profunda brachii artery.

Osteofasciocutaneous flaps

Originally called Type D flaps these are usually an elaboration of Type C flaps in which the skin flap and its supplying artery are removed in continuity with branches of the artery which run along the same septum down to bone. Separate designation as a Type D therefore seems unnecessary. The Chinese/radial forearm flap may be raised in this fashion to include half the cross-sectional diameter of the radius between the pronator teres and brachioradialis insertions. Two or three branches are given off by the radial artery to the periosteum in this area on the lateral aspect of the bone (Cormack et al, 1986). This flap may be used as a free tissue transfer (Soutar et al, 1983) or only the proximal end of the radial artery may be divided, the distal end left in continuity with the

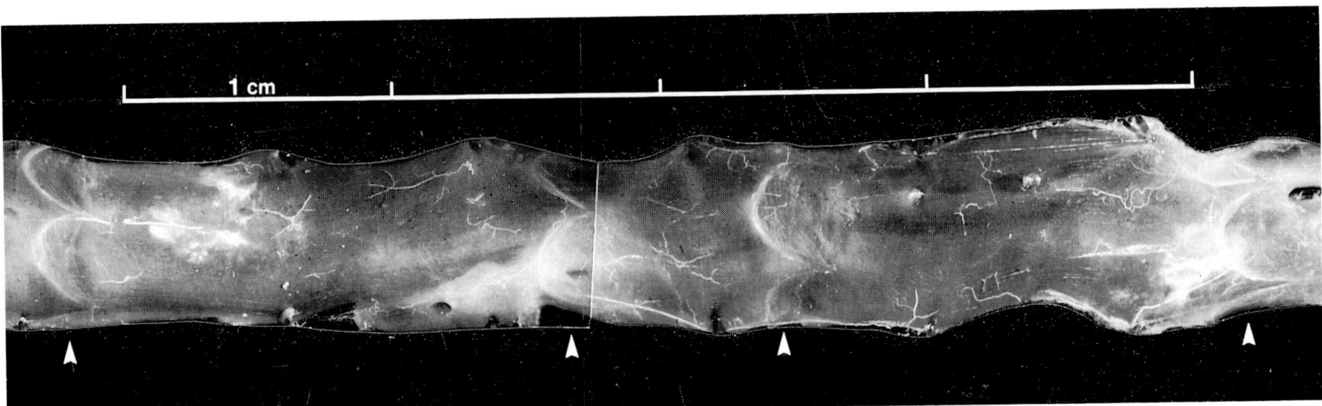

Fig. 5.26 Photograph of a 5 cm length of one of the venae comitantes of a radial artery. The vein has been incised longitudinally and pinned out flat with the luminal surface uppermost. 4 bicuspid valves can be seen. Valves are located at irregular distances apart but in a 15 cm length of vein there are usually approximately 6 valves giving a mean inter-valve distance of 2.5 cm. This specimen had previously been injected with barium sulphate suspension which accounts for the visualisation of the vasa vasorum.

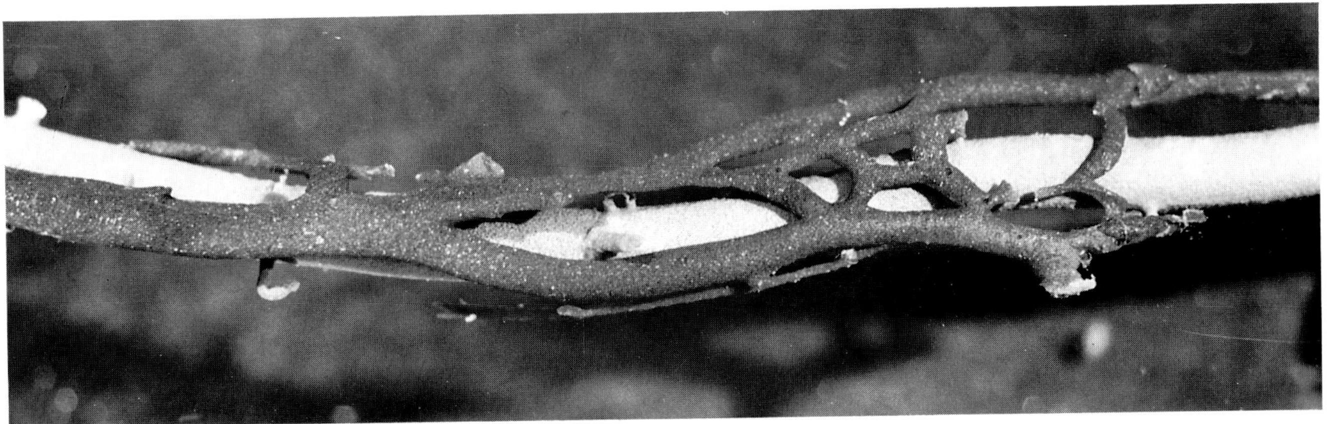

Fig. 5.27 Photograph of a resin corrosion cast in which the radial artery has been filled with a light coloured resin and its venae comitantes with a darker coloured resin. This demonstrates how the venae comitantes may be connected by a plexus of vessels, thereby possibly providing an explanation for how flow may be reversed in these veins despite the presence of valves. An impression left by a valve cusp may be seen on the vein in the top right-hand corner of this illustration.

palmar arch, and the tissue block swung on this arterial pedicle to reconstruct an amputated thumb (Biemer & Stock, 1983). Occasionally bone-containing fasciocutaneous flaps are osteo-*myo*-fasciocutaneous as shown in Figure 5.24 where the blood vessels to bone traverse a muscle attachment, for example, from the posterior interosseous artery through extensor pollicis longus to the ulna but this is a much less common version of the compound flap.

Other possible combinations are:

1. Lateral supracondylar ridge of humerus in association with lateral arm flap, both supported by middle collateral artery (Katsaros et al, 1984). This exploits fascioperiosteal vessels to bone passing from the middle collateral artery along the lateral intermuscular septum.

2. Fibular shaft and skin island over posterior peroneal septum both supported by peroneal artery (Chen & Yan, 1983). This exploits the nutrient artery of the diaphysis and also musculoperiosteal branches of the peroneal artery.

3. Segment of the ulna and overlying skin, both supported on posterior interosseous artery (Costa et al, 1988). This exploits the musculoperiosteal branches of the artery at the attachment of extensor pollicis longus to the bone.

4. Cortex of medial condyle of femur and saphenous flap (Hertel & Masquelet, 1989; Martin et al, 1991). This exploits the fact that the descending genicular artery has a musculo-articular branch before continuing as the saphenous artery.

5. Lateral border of scapula and scapular skin flap, both supported by branches of the circumflex scapular artery (Coleman & Sultan, 1991).

Reverse- or distally-pedicled variants

In the initial phase of development of the fasciocutaneous flaps all the flaps were designed with the base of the flap situated proximally or, in the case of the Type C flaps, with the flap orientated so that there was orthograde flow in the main artery. Clinical experimentation soon showed that fasciocutaneous flaps also survived when the base was situated distally or when there was retrograde flow in the main artery although because of impaired venous drainage these flaps were not always quite so reliable. This sequence of development of the fasciocutaneous flap concept is well demonstrated in Figure 5.25 where it can be seen that the first publication of each Type C flap was always orthograde, followed some years later by description of the same flap with retrograde flow. Reference to Figure 5.23 shows that among the Type B flaps described in the second half of the decade 1980–1990 were examples of islanded flaps based on a single perforator situated at the distal end of the flap. These distally pedicled arrangements have come to be known as 'reverse' flaps.

In summary therefore, the fasciocutaneous flaps Types A, B and C may be further subdivided on the basis of the direction of their blood supply as shown in Table 5.3.

Tabel 5.3 Fasciocutaneous flaps classified on the basis of their blood supply

Type	Original configuration	'Reverse' variants
A	Multiple independent perforators entering flap with a proximal base	Distally situated base
B	Solitary perforator at proximal end of islanded flap	Inflow through solitary vessel at the distal end of the islanded flap
C	Compartmental artery, septum containing several perforators and flap, all in continuity. Orthograde flow in main artery, when either locally pedicled or as a free flap	Retrograde flow through compartmental vessel. Either used as a loco-regional pedicled flap or as a free flap

ADVANTAGES OF FASCIOCUTANEOUS FLAPS IN CLINICAL PRACTICE

Although the impact of fasciocutaneous flaps has not been as dramatic as that of musculocutaneous and muscle flaps, it is nevertheless the case that they have gained an established and indispensable place in clinical practice. Like axial pattern direct cutaneous flaps and musculocutaneous flaps they do not require a preliminary delay procedure and can be raised with useful length-to-breadth ratios of generally about 3:1 with reliability and safety. Where cross-leg flaps are concerned this provides advantages of mobility and ease of positioning over the conventional random pattern cross-leg flap. Furthermore, preliminary division of the deep fascia in the base of a pedicled fasciocutaneous flap transfer before final division and insetting is not required, whereas with an axial pattern or direct cutaneous flap, such as the groin flap, a preliminary division of the axial vessels is recommended. Elevating these flaps is simple because the subfascial plane is easy to find and it is not difficult to dissect out an intermuscular septum. Split skin graft 'take' on the donor site does not constitute a problem. Preoperative location of perforators by angiography is never necessary whereas some axial pattern cutaneous flaps have such a variable pattern, e.g. dorsalis pedis, that this is often recommended. Neither is preoperative location of perforators with Doppler required, although this has been used on the lower leg when complex fasciocutaneous flaps with a very narrow pedicle incorporating only one perforator have been planned. Clearly in a Type C flap it is necessary to establish that the other major vessel(s) are fully developed and patent so that no impairment of blood supply to the distal part will occur.

Type C flaps may be useful in complex injuries of a limb where damage occurs to vessels as well as to skin. In this situation a Type C flap may be used to restore vascular continuity. For example, in an injury of the flexor aspect of the forearm in which skin, muscle, and segments of both the radial and ulnar arteries are lost, blood flow to the hand may be restored in conjunction with full thickness skin cover by transferring a Type C free flap from the opposite forearm. Anastomosis of the radial artery across a damaged segment would restore blood flow and if the injury also included bone loss then a composite tissue transfer might be appropriate. Applications in the treatment of lower leg injuries in which there is vessel damage can also be envisaged.

The vessel in a Type C flap may also be used as a 'conduit' for blood to a second flap, such as a Type B fasciocutaneous or a direct axial-pattern cutaneous flap, and the combination of two such flaps might enable large defects to be filled.

'Reverse' flaps have particular application in reconstructing defects in the distal parts of the extremities. A proximal position of the donor site on a forearm or leg also has an advantage since a donor site in the distal leg is likely to expose tendons and/or bone, and with a flap sited proximally over the muscle bellies a more satisfactory bed for a split skin graft is obtained.

Perhaps the greatest advantage lies in the many different ways in which the separate elements of the fasciocutaneous system can be combined at one site to create a variety of flaps. Consider, for example, the fasciocutaneous perforators which arise from the peroneal artery and reach the deep fascia along the posterior peroneal septum; the following nine different flaps may be based on these vessels and their longitudinally anastomosing ramifications at the level of the deep fascia:

1. Type A proximally-based pedicled flap, orientated longitudinally
2. Type A distally-based pedicled flap, orientated longitudinally
3. Type B pedicled or free flap based on a single perforator, either distally or proximally
4. Type B subcutaneous and fascial pedicle, skin island, based on a single perforator
5. Modified Type B free flap with a segment of the peroneal artery
6. Type C free flap
7. Type C flap pedicled on the proximal peroneal artery
8. Type C flap pedicled on the distal peroneal artery
9. Composite osteo-myo-fasciocutaneous free tissue transfer.

ALTERNATIVE TERMINOLOGY

Confusion between fasciocutaneous and septocutaneous

It may be argued that there are more appropriate terms than 'fasciocutaneous', both as it is applied to the anatomy of the perforators and to the classification of flaps, and some of the issues concerned merit discussion.

Firstly, is 'fasciocutaneous' a good term for the system of perforators passing between muscles to reach the deep fascia? Although widespread use of the term really only followed Pontén's use of the term in 1980, it should be noted that he used the words as descriptive of the tissue content of his lower leg 'super flaps'. Lamberty & Gilbert (1981) subsequently investigated flaps on the forearm and applied the term to the anatomical system of perforators. Professor Ruyao Song (1982) used the term 'septocutaneous' to describe his forearm and upper arm flaps, and then Y.G. Song et al use the same term to refer to the anatomical system of perforators in a paper published in 1984 entitled 'The free thigh flap: a new free flap concept based on the septocutaneous artery'. As a result it is not entirely clear what these terms now mean, particularly as they have come to be used interchangeably in the context of anatomy and in the context of flaps.

'Septocutaneous' as an anatomical term

In the context of anatomy there has been confusion as to what 'septocutaneous' refers to. Satoh (1990) has suggested that a distinction be made between the two sorts of intermuscular connective tissue in the limbs, namely on the one hand that which marks out a series of compartments containing separate muscle groups (with different actions, developmental histories and innervations), and on the other hand that which simply lies between muscles. Satoh feels that vessels (perforators to skin) lying in compartmental septa should be called 'septocutaneous vessels' and those lying in intermuscular septa should be termed 'intermuscular cutaneous vessels'. The equivalent flaps would then be termed septocutaneous flaps and intermuscular cutaneous flaps. Table 5.4 identifies some of these different septa. It is relevant to ask whether such distinctions are useful or not and if distinctions between different types of septa are going to be recognised then where does the process of 'splitting' stop? Why only identify two types of septa? Why, for example, not recognise those septa which serve to connect rather than separate muscles by virtue of the fact that muscles arise from both sides of them and call these intermuscular aponeuroses? Then there are the septa which are in fact degenerate variations of muscles, for example the fibrous tissue of the medial intermuscular septum in the arm represents the lower part of the coraco-brachialis muscle which has been lost during evolutionary development; why not call these atavistic septa? In practical terms these distinctions seem of little benefit with one possible exception and that is that the true intercompartmental septa are often well endowed with fascioperiosteal branches and are therefore appropriate for the raising of composite osteo-fasciocutaneous flaps. It is perhaps worth noting that the editors of 'Gray's Anatomy' seem content to designate all intermuscular and intercompartmental connective tissue fascia within the broad category of septa. We conclude that, on balance, there does not appear to be any great merit in reserving the term septocutaneous to describe a perforator along one specific type of septum as opposed to another.

If 'septocutaneous' is not to be used for vessels on one particular type of septum, should it instead be used for all vessels that reach skin by passing along fascial septa? These vessels are all part of the one anatomical fasciocutaneous system of perforators and there is no clear benefit from introducing another word for the same thing. This would only enhance the uncertainty over what each word means.

'Septocutaneous' as a surgical term for flaps

It has been argued by Satoh that the use of the term septocutaneous to describe flaps based on intercompartmental septa (Song R Y et al, 1982) and later to describe flaps based on intermuscular septa (Song Y G et al, 1984) sowed the seeds of confusion which were later propagated by others (e.g. Carriquiry et al, 1985; Satoh et al, 1988). In fact Song and Song were making, perhaps unconsciously, a useful *surgical* distinction. They used 'septocutaneous' to refer quite specifically to flaps which incorporated the septa containing the perforators in the sense that in raising the flap the septum had to be actively dissected out from its intermuscular position. These flaps were then clearly differentiated from Pontén's flaps of skin and deep fascia which did not require the septal vessels to be dissected out and these flaps are simply designated as fasciocutaneous. Chang for example has written that he does not regard the radial forearm flap as a fasciocutaneous flap, and fasciocutaneous is a term he confines to the Pontén-type flap (Chang, 1989). Song, therefore, far from creating confusion, was actually clarifying a distinction between two types of flap based on the one anatomical fasciocutaneous system; a distinction that is comparable to the differences between Type A and Type C flaps in our classification (Type B flaps may fit into either category depending on the details of anatomy of the vascular pedicle). Unfortunately this is a subtlety that has been lost on many authors and as a result fasciocutaneous and septocutaneous have come to be used interchangeably. However, there are several merits in confining the term septocutaneous to the description of flaps that require a specific surgical technique to elevate them. Used in this way the terms fasciocutaneous and septocutaneous become specific, discriminative and not interchangeable. A further advantage of this approach is that the surgical flap type can then be further qualified by anatomical terms so that one might have, for example, intercompartmental septocutaneous flaps and intermuscular septocutaneous flaps. Figure 5.28 attempts to show how these various ways of looking at fasciocutaneous flaps overlap.

Although we have advocated a fairly restrictive definition of fasciocutaneous flaps as those flaps specifically vascularised by vessels of the anatomical fasciocutaneous system of perforators, other have argued for a less restrictive interpretation which takes into account the tissue constituents of the flap to a greater extent. For example Tolhurst has included a whole variety of trunk flaps under the fasciocutaneous heading on the basis that '. . . if the deep fascia in the body of the flap is continuous with the fascia in the pedicle, one is still justified in naming this a fasciocutaneous flap' (in Hallock, 1992, p. 43). (Without wishing to get involved in this issue here, one must briefly repeat the point that although the epimysium on the trunk muscles and the deep fascia of the limbs are both known as fascia, they are

Table 5.4 Septa containing fasciocutaneous perforators: those in italics are intercompartmental septa, and the others are intermuscular septa

Region	Vessel of origin	Location of septum
Shoulder girdle	Circumflex scapular artery	Teres major / teres minor
	Middle collateral A – interosseous recurrent A	*Triceps lateral head / brachialis / brachioradialis*
	Radial collateral A – radial recurrent A	Brachioradialis / brachialis
	Superior ulnar collateral A – posterior ulnar recurrent A	*Coracobrachialis / triceps medial head*
Forearm	Radial A	Brachioradialis / flexor carpi radialis
	Ulnar A	Flexor carpi ulnaris / flexor digitorum superficialis
	Posterior interosseous A	Extensor carpi ulnaris / extensor digitorum communis
	Anterior interosseous A	Abductor pollicis longus / extensor pollicis brevis / extensor pollicis longus
Hand	Dorsal metacarpal A	Between extensor tendons
Thigh	Superficial femoral artery	Around sartorius
	Saphenous artery	Around sartorius
	Descending branch of lateral circumflex femoral A	Vastus lateralis / rectus femoris
	'Adductor' artery	Around gracilis
	Inferior gluteal A	Biceps femoris / semitendinosus
	Profunda femoris, lateral branches	*Vastus lateralis / biceps femoris*
	Profunda femoris, posterior branches	Biceps femoris / semitendinosus / semimembranosus
	Popliteal A	*Vastus lateralis / biceps femoris /* semitendinosus
Leg	Anterior tibial A	*Extensor digitorum longus / peroneus longus and brevis*
		Tibialis anterior / extensor hallucis longus
	Posterior tibial A	Flexor digitorum longus / soleus
	Peroneal A	Peroneus longus / soleus
Foot	Medial plantar A	Around abductor hallucis
	Lateral plantar A	Around abductor digiti minimi
	Dorsalis pedis A	Extensor hallucis longus / extensor digitorum, over 1st intermetatarsal space

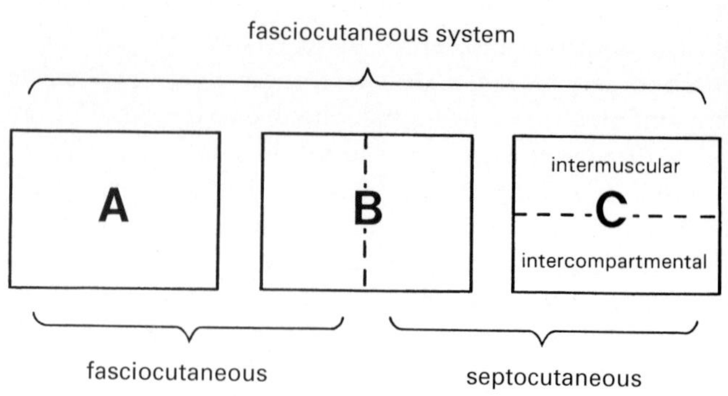

Fig. 5.28 Overlap of the anatomically and surgically defined sub-groups of flaps based on the fasciocutaneous system of perforators.

nevertheless rather different in structure and vascularisation.) Scalp fascial and fasciocutaneous flaps are another case in point. It is apparant from this that another advantage of the discriminative use of 'fasciocutaneous' and 'septocutaneous' is that it puts the septocutaneous (i.e. unarguably fasciocutaneous) flaps in a separate category where they are unlikely to be confused with flaps which have been more liberally interpreted on the basis of tissue constituents as being in the fasciocutaneous category (e.g. deltopectoral and groin flaps).

This approach to terminology solves several of the problems raised by Hallock in his excellent book on fasciocutaneous flaps (see Hallock, 1992, pp. 139–142).

This is an area of terminology that it is impossible to obtain universal agreement upon, and the continuing development of adipofascial and fascia-only flaps makes it even more complex. Certainly the last word has not yet been written on this subject but we would support any move towards restricting the use of 'septocutaneous' to any flap whose elevation involved dissecting out its vessel containing septum.

References

Barclay T L, Cardoso E, Sharpe D T, Crockett D J 1982 Repair of lower leg injuries with fasciocutaneous flaps. British Journal of Plastic Surgery 35: 127–132

Biemer E, Stock W 1983 Total thumb reconstruction: a one-stage reconstruction using an osteo-cutaneous forearm flap. British Journal of Plastic Surgery 36: 52–55

Bonnel F, Lesire M, Gornis R, Allieu Y, Rabischong P 1981 Arterial vascularization of the fibula. Microsurgical transplant techniques. Anatomia Clinica 3: 13–22

Boyd J B, Taylor G I, Corlett R 1984 The vascular territories of the superior epigastric and the deep inferior epigastric systems. Plastic and Reconstructive Surgery 73: 1–14

Carriquiry C, Costa M A, Vasconez L O 1985 An anatomic study of the septocutaneous vessels of the leg. Plastic and Reconstructive Surgery 76: 354–361

Chang S-M 1989 Classification of fasciocutaneous flaps. Letter to the Editor, British Journal of Plastic Surgery 42: 616

Chen Z-W, Yan W 1983 The study and clinical application of the osteocutaneous flap of fibula. Journal of Microsurgery 4: 11–16

Coleman J J, Sultan M R 1991 The bipedicled osteocutaneous scapula flap: A new subscapular system free flap. Plastic and Reconstructive Surgery 87: 682–691

Cormack G C, Lamberty B G H 1983a Fasciocutaneous Vessels. Presentation at the Annual Meeting of the American Society of Plastic and Reconstructive Surgeons, Dallas, Texas. November 1983. Winning Essay in Clinical Research Category of the 1983 Scholarship Awards of the Plastic Surgery Educational Foundation

Cormack G C, Lamberty B G H 1983b The anatomical vascular basis of the axillary fasciocutaneous pedicled flap. British Journal of Plastic Surgery 36: 425–427

Cormack G C, Lamberty B G H 1984 A classification of fasciocutaneous flaps according to their patterns of vascularisation. British Journal of Plastic Surgery 37: 80–87

Cormack G C, Duncan M J, Lamberty B G H 1986 The blood supply to the bone component of the compound osteo-fasciocutaneous radial artery forearm flap. British Journal of Plastic Surgery 39: 173–175

Costa H, Smith R, McGrouther D A 1988 Thumb reconstruction by the posterior interosseous osteocutaneous flap. British Journal of Plastic Surgery 41: 228–233

Donski P K, Fogdestam I 1983 Distally based fasciocutaneous flap from the sural region. Scandinavian Journal of Plastic and Reconstructructive Surgery 17: 191–196

Emerson D J M, Sprigg A, Page R E 1985 Some observations on the radial artery island flap. British Journal of Plastic Surgery 38: 107–112

Hallock G G 1992 Fasciocutaneous flaps. Blackwell Scientific Publications, Boston, Massachusetts

Haertsch P A 1981a The surgical plane in the leg. British Journal of Plastic Surgery 34: 464–469

Haertsch P A 1981b The blood supply to the skin of the leg: a post-mortem investigation. British Journal of Plastic Surgery 34: 470–477

Hertel R, Masquelet A C 1989 The reverse flow medial knee osteoperiosteal flap for skeletal reconstruction of the leg. Surgical and Radiological Anatomy 11: 257–262

Katsaros J, Schusterman M, Beppu M, Banis J C, Acland R D 1984 The lateral upper arm flap: anatomy and clinical applications. Annals of Plastic Surgery 12: 489–500

Lamberty B G H, Gilbert D A 1981 The anatomy of potential fasciocutaneous flaps in the forearm. British Association of Plastic Surgeons Research Group Meeting, October 1980 abstracted in British Journal of Plastic Surgery 34: 230–231

Lang J 1962 Über die Textur und die Vascularisation der Fascien. Acta Anatomia 48: 61–94

Lin S-D, Lai C-S, Chin C-C 1984 Venous drainage in the reverse forearm flap. Plastic and Reconstructive Surgery 74: 508–512

Martin D, Bitonti-Grillo C, De Biscop J, Schott H, Mondie J M, Baudet J, Peri G 1991 Mandibular reconstruction using a free vascularised osteocutaneous flap from the internal condyle of the femur. British Journal of Plastic Surgery 44: 397–402

Pontén B 1981 The fasciocutaneous flap: its use in soft tissue defects of the lower leg. British Journal of Plastic Surgery 34: 215–220

Reid C D, Taylor G I 1984 The vascular territory of the acromiothoracic axis. British Journal of Plastic Surgery 37: 194–212

Satoh K, Yoshikawa A, Hayashi M 1988 Reverse-flow anterior tibialis flap type III. British Journal of Plastic Surgery 41: 624–627

Satoh K 1990 Confusion of the use of the term 'septocutaneous'. Letter to the Editor, British Journal of Plastic Surgery 43: 632–633

Schäfer K 1975 Das subcutane Gefäss-System (untere Extremität): Micropräparatorische Untersuchungen. Gegenbaurs Morphologisches Jahrbuch, Leipzig 121: 492–514

Soutar D S, Scheker L R, Tanner N S B, McGregor I A 1983 The radial forearm flap: a versatile method for intraoral reconstruction. British Journal of Plastic Surgery 36: 1–8

Song R Y, Gao Y Z, Song Y G, Yu Y S, Song Y L 1982 The forearm flap. Clinics in Plastic Surgery 9: 21–26

Song Y G, Chen G Z, Song Y L 1984 The free thigh flap: a new free flap concept based on the septocutaneous artery. British Journal of Plastic Surgery 37: 149–159

Timmins M J 1984 William Harvey revisited; reverse flow through the valves of forearm veins. The Lancet ii: 394–395

Tolhurst D E, Haeseker B, Zeeman R J 1983 The development of the fasciocutaneous flap and its clinical application. Plastic and Reconstructive Surgery 71: 597–605

Williams P L, Warwick R 1980 Gray's Anatomy, 36th edn. Churchill Livingstone, Edinburgh, p 523

Yang Guofan, Gao Yuzhi 1981 Forearm free skin flap transplantation. Journal of the Chinese Medical Association 61: 139. Abstracted in Plastic and Reconstructive Surgery 69: 1041

Yoshimura M, Honda T, Uganji Y, Shimamura K, Yamauchi S 1983 Free peroneal flap in extremity reconstruction. 7th Symposium of the International Society for Reconstructive Microsurgery, New York

The blood supply to the skin by regions

6

Notes

1. The nerve supply to skin and muscles is well covered in conventional anatomy texts and is not repeated here.
2. Arteries are only described fully in so much as they supply skin. Nutrient vessels to bones are generally not described and branches to muscles are only described if they contribute to the blood supply of skin.
3. The correct Latin names for some of the vessels mentioned in the text are indicated by the *Nomina Anatomica* preceding the description of each area. This lists only those vessels directly or indirectly involved in the supply of skin and indicates by means of the layout the most common pattern of branching. The format is that adopted by the 5th Edition of *Nomina Anatomica* (1983, Excerpta Medica), a revision by the International Anatomical Nomenclature Committee and approved by the Eleventh International Congress of Anatomists in Mexico City, 1980.
4. Note that territories described in this section are anatomical. Dynamic and potential territories, as evidenced by clinical experience with flaps, are described in Chapter 7. At the end of the description of each region an outline of the possible flaps appropriate to that region is given. Further anatomical details concerning the relevant vessels and their territories may then be found on the pages indicated.

6 HEAD AND NECK

Nomina Anatomica of vessels reaching skin

ARTERIA CAROTIS EXTERNA

Arteria thyroidea superior
- Ramus infrahyoideus
- Ramus sternocleidomastoideus

Arteria facialis
- A. submentalis
- A. labialis inferior
- A. labialis superior
  - Ramus septi nasi
- Ramus lateralis nasi
- A. angularis

(*Truncus linguofacialis*)

Arteria occipitalis
- Rami sternocleidomastoidei
- Rami occipitales

Arteria auricularis posterior
- Ramus auricularis
- Ramus occipitalis

Arteria temporalis superficialis
- A. transversa faciei
- Rami auriculares anteriores
- A. zygomatico-orbitalis
- Ramus frontalis
- Ramus parietalis

Arteria maxillaris
- A. alveolaris inferior
  - A. mentalis
- A. infraorbitalis

ARTERIA CAROTIS INTERNA

Arteria ophthalmica
- A. lacrimalis
  - Aa. palpebrales laterales
- A. supraorbitalis
  - Aa. palpebrales mediales
- Arcus palpebralis superior
- Arcus palpebralis inferior
- A. supratrochlearis
- A. dorsalis nasi (A. nasi externa)†

ARTERIA SUBCLAVIA

Truncus thyrocervicalis
- A. thyroidea inferior
- A. suprascapularis
  - Ramus acromialis
- A. transversa cervicis*
  - Ramus superficialis (A. cervicalis superficialis)*
    - Ramus ascendens
    - Ramus descendens
  - Ramus profundus (A. dorsalis scapulae)
- A. dorsalis scapulae (A. scapularis dorsalis)*

* There is evidence of confusion in the literature regarding the nomenclature of these vessels. The authors favour the following scheme:

Transverse cervical artery (A. transversa cervicis)
In about 60% of cases it arises from the thyrocervical trunk and passes laterally over the trunks of the brachial plexus to reach levator scapulae. Here it divides into a superficial branch penetrating trapezius (ramus superficialis) and a deep branch going deep to levator scapulae (ramus profundus).

Dorsal scapular artery (A. scapularis dorsalis)
This term may be applied to the deep branch of the transverse cervical artery. It is better reserved, however, for those cases in which no transverse cervical artery is present. In these cases the dorsal scapular artery is the single trunk which arises from the subclavian artery and continues towards the superior angle of the scapula to pass with the dorsal scapular nerve deep to the rhomboids along the vertebral border of the scapula.

Superficial cervical artery (A. cervicalis superficialis)
This is reserved for the vessel which, when the transverse cervical artery is absent, arises as a well-developed and distinct vessel from the thyrocervical trunk to supply the territory of the absent superficial branch of the transverse cervical artery, i.e. chiefly the trapezius.

† More commonly the dorsal nasal is regarded as a branch of the external nasal. See page 141.

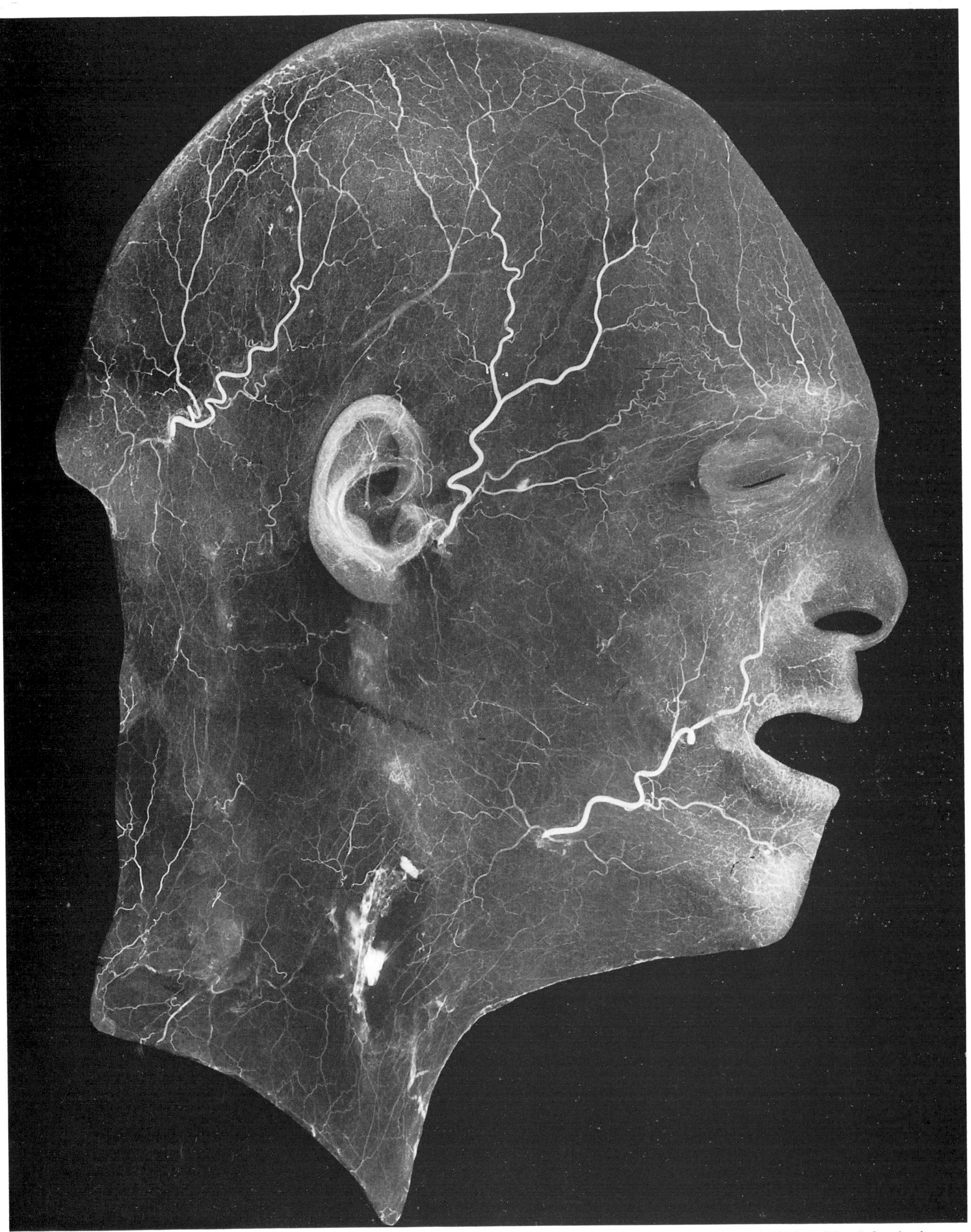

Fig. 6.1 Radiograph of injected skin of head and neck. The skin from the posterior neck overlying trapezius is not included. The defect in the neck represents the access site for injection into the common carotid artery.

6 HEAD AND NECK

The territories of those branches of the external carotid, internal carotid and subclavian arteries which reach the skin of the head and neck have been listed on page 132 as they appear in *Nomina Anatomica.* The vessels will be described in the same order, and the principles of the blood supply to each region will then be summarised, with an accompanying list of flaps and clinical applications.

EXTERNAL CAROTID ARTERY

The common carotid arteries divide at the upper border of the thyroid cartilage which is generally on a level with the upper border of the fourth cervical vertebra. At its origin, the external carotid is actually anteromedial to the internal but almost at once inclines superficially, the vessels becoming separated by stylopharyngeus and the glossopharyngeal nerve, the pharyngeal branch of the vagus and the styloid process

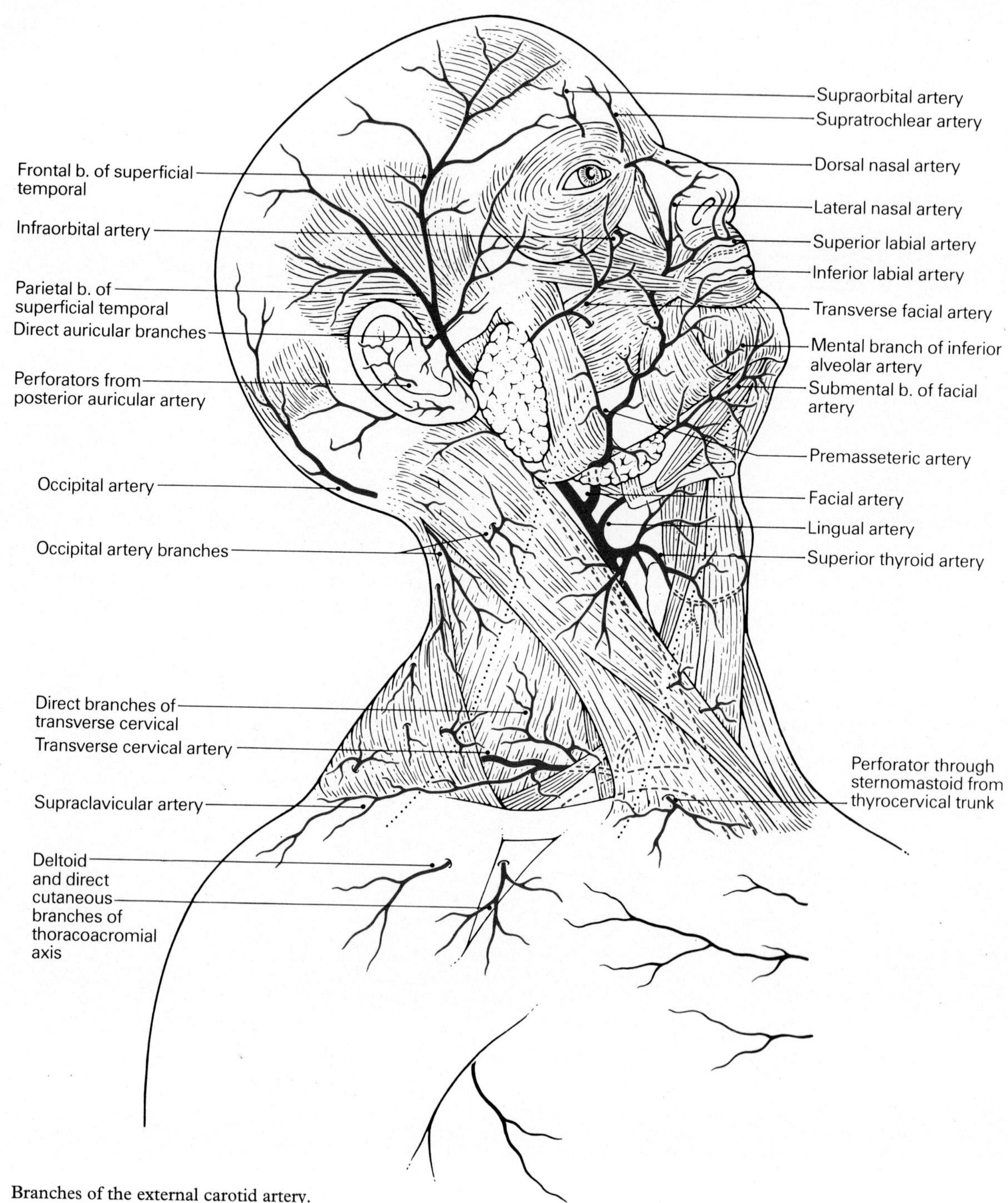

Fig. 6.2 Branches of the external carotid artery.

with styloglossus. The external carotid then passes through the parotid gland, deep to the retromandibular vein and branches of the facial nerve, emerging from the anteromedial aspect of the gland to divide into its terminal branches behind the neck of the mandible.

The superior thyroid artery

This is the first branch of the external carotid. It arises deep to sternomastoid at the level of the greater horn of the hyoid bone and has thyroid, infrahyoid, sternomastoid, superior laryngeal and cricothyroid branches. The sternomastoid branch may alternatively arise directly from the external carotid and is the only branch of interest as a source of blood supply to the skin. It arises within a centimetre of the origin of the superior thyroid artery and runs downwards and laterally across the carotid sheath. It divides into a muscular branch for the middle of sternomastoid which it enters on its deep surface, and a cutaneous branch for platysma and skin over the anterior triangle of the neck and the middle part of sternomastoid. Of the two, the cutaneous branch is the more important; the muscular branch forms the smallest of the three pedicles of sternomastoid (Fig. 6.3.).

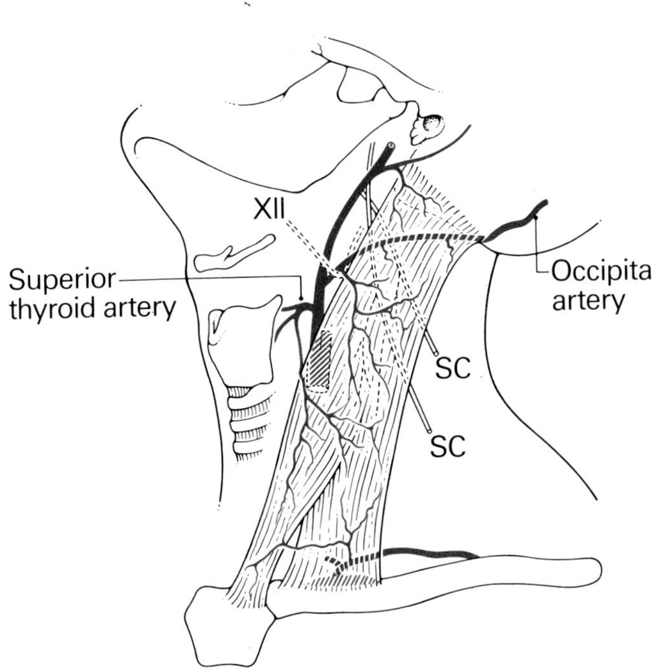

Fig. 6.3 Superior thyroid and occipital artery branches to sternomastoid and overlying skin.

The facial artery

This arises from the external carotid immediately above the greater horn of the hyoid bone. It runs upwards behind the submandibular gland deep to stylohyoid and the posterior belly of digastric. Above stylohyoid it turns downwards and forwards between the lateral surface of the submandibular gland and the medial pterygoid muscle to reach the lower border of the mandible which it hooks round to pierce the deep fascia in front of masseter, deep only to platysma. It then takes a very tortuous course towards the medial canthus lying under cover of the skin, the fat of the cheek, and, near the angle of the mouth, the platysma, risorius and zygomaticus major. It lies on buccinator and levator anguli oris, and passes either over or through the levator labii superioris. It usually runs through levator labii superioris alaeque nasi and, as the angular artery, approaches the medial canthus of the eye where it passes beneath the medial palpebral ligament and anastomoses with branches of the ophthalmic artery. Between the lower border of the mandible and the angle of the mouth, the facial artery can be mobilised with ease, unlike the portion of the artery above the angle of the mouth which is fixed and passes superficial to or through the facial muscles. The facial artery has a number of named cutaneous branches and many small unnamed ones, as follows:

The submental artery arises deep to the mandible and runs forwards on the surface of mylohyoid to supply adjacent muscles and glands and then turns round the lower edge of the mandible to end on the surface of the chin where it anastomoses with the mental artery and the inferior labial arteries. The submental artery gives off many small branches which form an important source of blood supply to platysma and the skin over the submental triangle.

Premasseteric branch. With the exception of Cunningham, contemporary texts ignore this vessel. Classic texts called it the masseteric branch. Toldt (1921) illustrated it but did not name it, and Adachi (1928) was the first to describe it accurately and name it the premasseteric branch. He found it to be as strong as or even stronger than the facial artery in 3% of cases, and to exist as a small vessel in an unspecified larger number than this. It arises at the lower border of the mandible from the facial artery and ascends along the anterior edge of the masseter in the company of the facial vein (Fig. 6.2). (The facial artery and vein lie together only at the edge of the mandible – they diverge as they ascend with the artery lying anterior to the vein.)

The inferior labial artery is given off by the facial artery near the angle of the mouth and passes upwards deep to depressor anguli oris where it penetrates orbicularis oris, to run a tortuous course in the lower lip between this muscle and the mucous membrane (Fig. 6.4). It anastomoses with the artery of the opposite side and with the mental branch of the inferior alveolar artery.

The superior labial artery is the next branch and follows a similar tortuous course along the edge of the upper lip between orbicularis oris and the mucous membrane. It gives off an alar branch and a nasal septal branch and anastomoses with the artery of the opposite side. The alar branch passes around the inferior aspect of the ala deep in the groove between the ala and the upper lip, and continues in the groove between nose and cheek where it divides into two branches, one of which passes superiorly and anastomoses with the external nasal, the other passes towards the tip of the nose. Alternatively, this vessel arises from the facial artery. A significant anastomosis between superior and inferior labial arteries occurs at the angle of the mouth.

The lateral nasal branch (or alar branch) is given off to supply dilator naris and the alar skin (see above). At this point, the facial artery may terminate (~ 80% of cases according to Mitz et al, 1973) or it may continue beyond levator anguli oris towards the medial canthus of the eye in which case it is renamed the angular artery.

The angular artery lies directly beneath skin to which it gives off a number of small but significant unnamed branches. The angular artery communicates with the infraorbital artery and sends branches over the side of the nose.

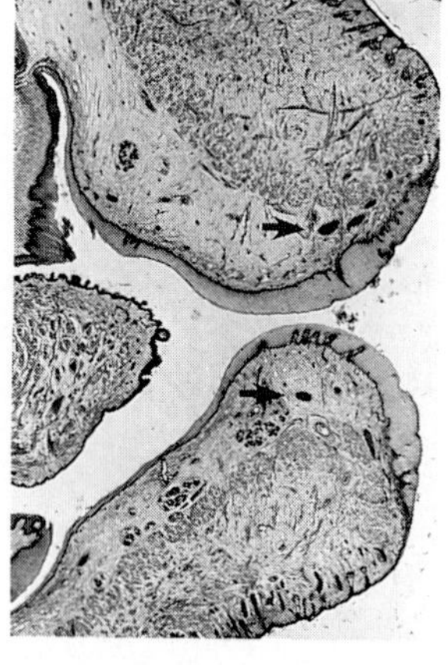

Sagittal section of foetal lips showing location of arteries

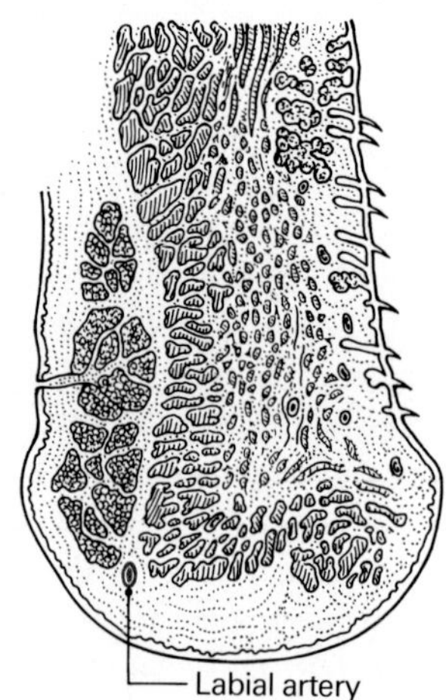

Fig. 6.4 Labial artery branches of the facial artery.

Variations (see Fig. 6.5): The facial artery may be weak – reaching only as far as the angle of the mouth and giving off only labial branches (~ 10%) – or may fail to reach the face at all, being represented only by the submental branch (1%). In all these cases the territory of the absent facial is 'taken over' by the contralateral facial and the ipsilateral transverse facial, sometimes aided by the infraorbital and buccinator arteries. In Adachi's study, 0.5% of 1000 + hemi-faces were found to have a very strongly developed transverse facial artery to the extent that it supplied the labial arteries and ended as the angular artery. Herbert (1978) has also described this finding.

The occipital artery

This arises from the posterior surface of the external carotid opposite the facial artery and runs posteriorly across the internal jugular vein, deep to the posterior belly of digastric, and comes to lie medial to the mastoid process in a groove on the temporal bone. Here it lies deep to sternomastoid, splenius capitis and longissimus capitis. Passing medially it emerges from beneath these muscles and pierces the fascia in the interval between sternomastoid and trapezius (Fig. 6.6). Here it divides into its tortuous terminal occipital branches which ramify in the superficial fascia of the scalp. (*Variation:* Occasionally, the occipital artery may have a superficial course lying superficial to the lateral part of sternomastoid or even lying superficial to the mastoid process as well (1%). More often, a weaker horizontal branch of the occipital artery follows this course while the main stem continues in the usual way.)

The occipital artery has a number of branches of which the following reach the skin:

The sternomastoid branches. Upper and lower sternomastoid branches supply the cephalic end of sternomastoid and may reach the skin over the upper half of the muscle via small musculocutaneous perforators (Fig. 6.3). The lower branch arises from the beginning of the occipital artery but sometimes directly from the external carotid and has the hypoglossal nerve hooking round it in a characteristic way. The upper branch arises from the occipital as it crosses the accessory nerve and runs postero-inferiorly to enter the deep surface of sternomastoid with the accessory nerve.

A small *auricular branch* may supply the back of the ear and anastomose with the posterior auricular artery.

A *trapezius branch* supplies the uppermost part of the muscle.

The terminal *occipital branches* lie between the skin and the occipital belly of occipitofrontalis. They are tortuous and ramify all over the occipital region right

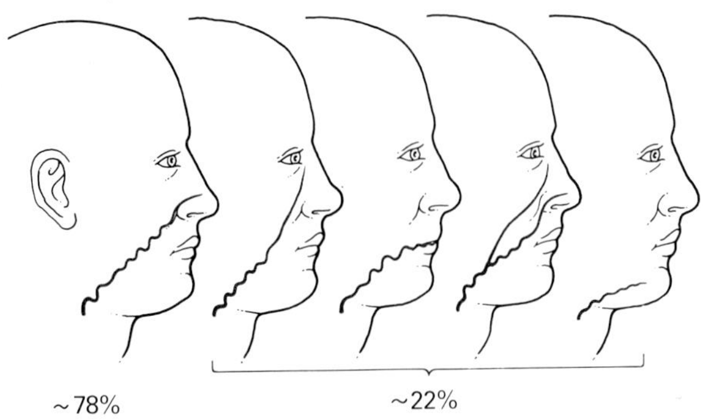

Fig. 6.5 Facial artery – variations.

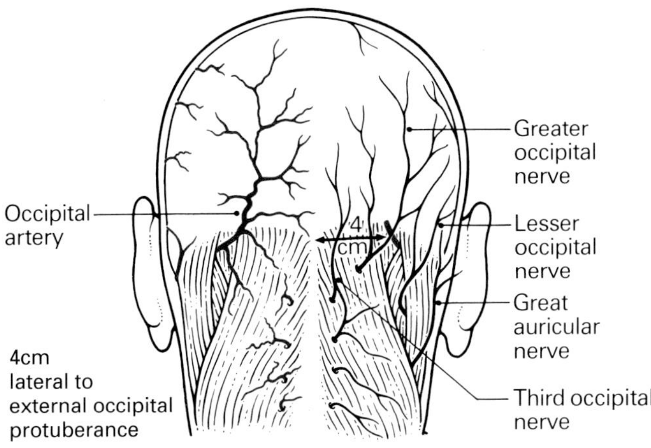

Fig. 6.6 Occipital artery (and nerves).

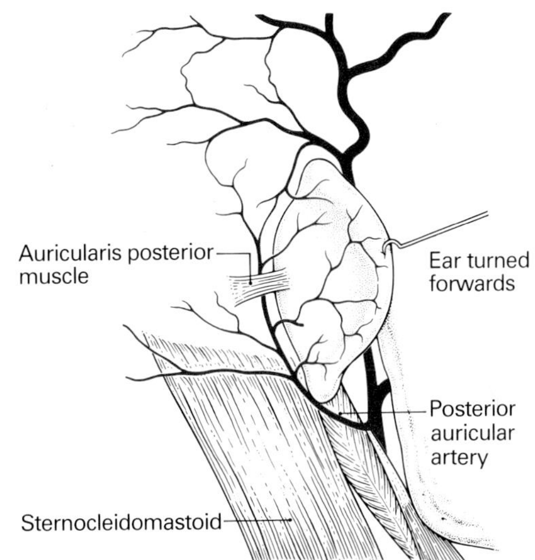

Fig. 6.7 Posterior auricular artery.

up to the vertex. They anastomose with posterior auricular and temporal vessels of their own side and with the opposite occipital branches. The main occipital vessel crosses deep to the greater occipital nerve about 4 cm lateral to the external occipital protuberance (Fig. 6.6).

Three or four *descending branches* arise from the horizontal part of the occipital artery which lies on semispinalis in the interval between trapezius and sternomastoid. As they descend, these pierce the overlying muscles and deep fascia and supply the skin, where they anastomose with branches of the transverse cervical artery (ascending branches of the ramus superficialis). These cutaneous branches are an important source of blood to the skin over the posterior neck. (These cutaneous branches are unnamed and are not to be confused with the ramus descendens of *Nomina Anatomica* which lies deep to splenius where it splits into a superficial branch supplying splenius and a deep branch which goes between the semispinales to anastomose with the vertebral artery.)

The posterior auricular artery

This arises from the posterior aspect of the external carotid (85%) immediately above the digastric and stylohyoid, or it arises in common with the occipital (14%) or superficial temporal (1%). It ascends over digastric between the cartilage of the ear and the mastoid process, pierces the deep fascia at, or just below, the level of the external auditory meatus, and divides into auricular and occipital branches (Fig. 6.7).

The auricular branch ascends deep to auricularis posterior and anastomoses with branches of the superficial temporal artery (posterior branch) over the lower fibres of temporalis. It gives off two or three sets of branches to the cranial surface of the ear and two small branches which pierce the cartilage to reach the external surface. (One pierces the concha near the crus of the helix, the other appears below the intertragal sulcus.) The branches to the cranial surface of the ear fan out, sometimes forming an arcade in the groove corresponding to the antihelix, and anastomose around the edge of the ear with vessels from its anterior surface. The most superior auricular branch anastomoses with branches of the superficial temporal.

The occipital branch runs back over the insertion of sternomastoid to supply the scalp behind the ear and the occipital belly of occipito-frontalis. At the anterior border of sternomastoid it gives off a small branch which enters the muscle. It anastomoses with occipital branches of the occipital artery.

The superficial temporal artery

This is the smaller terminal division of the external carotid. At its origin it measures about 2 mm in diameter (D) and lies deep to, or within, the parotid gland. In the first part of its course, measuring about 15 mm long, it ascends behind the neck of the mandible, then pierces the deep fascia 4 to 5 mm in front of the tragus (according to one study where it crosses a line between the upper part of the external auditory meatus and the middle of the supraorbital rim – Eustathianos, 1932). In the second, or superficial, part of its course it crosses the posterior part of the zygomatic process of the temporal bone, lying anterior to the auriculotemporal nerve and the superficial temporal vein and can be easily palpated. It may lie beneath auricularis anterior and may be tortuous (sometimes called the superficial temporal syphon) which is significant in that if 'released' it may increase the pedicle length of an island flap by up to 1.5 cm. Its middle temporal branch to the temporalis muscle is given off in this region. At a point between 2 and 4 cm above the zygomatic arch (range 0–5 cm) it divides into two or three terminal branches, the two larger of these being termed the frontal (anterior) and the parietal (posterior). A delayed division is commonly associated with a well-developed zygomatico-orbital branch from the main stem of the superficial temporal and occurs in 80% of cases (Ricbourg et al, 1975). (Alternatively the zygomatico-orbital arises from the frontal branch: see Fig. 6.9.) The frontal is generally larger (1.2 mm D) or the same size as the parietal (1.1 mm D).

The *frontal branch* runs tortuously upwards and forwards supplying all the layers of the scalp, and anastomoses with the corresponding vessel of the opposite side and also with the ipsilateral supraorbital and supratrochlear arteries.

The *parietal branch* continues in the direction of the main stem passing vertically upwards towards the vertex. In ~7.5% it may be double, with the two branches roughly parallel to each other. Its course lies within a 2 cm strip (Fig. 6.8) centred on the auditory meatus and passing upwards to the vertex. Within this band the artery inclines from the anterior to the posterior margins. The superficial temporal vein (~3.0 mm D) accompanies the artery, in front of it in ~30% and sometimes up to 3 cm distant from it. The parietal branch anastomoses with the opposite artery and with the posterior auricular and occipital arteries.

The superficial temporal gives off the following branches to the skin:

The transverse facial artery arises deep to the parotid gland and runs forwards over masseter. (A variation is that in 35% of cases it arises from the external carotid or its terminal bifurcation.) It runs forwards accompanied by branches of the facial nerve in the interval between the zygomatic arch and the parotid duct, often crossing the duct. It supplies the parotid gland and duct, masseter and the skin. A large branch constantly supplies cheek skin over masseter roughly at the point of intersection of a vertical line drawn 2 cm lateral to the lateral canthus with a horizontal line through the alar base. The transverse facial artery anastomoses superiorly with the lacrimal and infraorbital arteries, anteriorly with the premasseteric and facial arteries, and deeply with the buccal. It is mainly an artery supplying muscle but may also make a significant contribution to the blood supply of the skin over masseter and the parotid and to a lesser extent to the skin up to the infraorbital margin and nasolabial fold (see Figs 6.2 & 6.11). (*Variation:* The facial artery may be weak or absent in which case the transverse facial to a greater or lesser extent 'takes over' its territory – see facial artery variations above. In all those

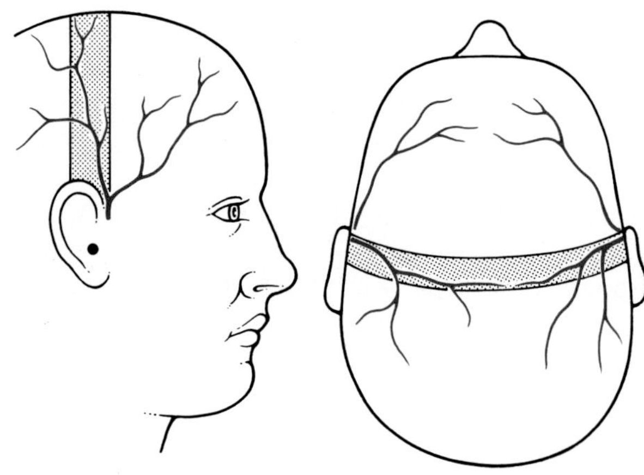

Fig. 6.8 Surface marking of parietal branch of superficial temporal artery.

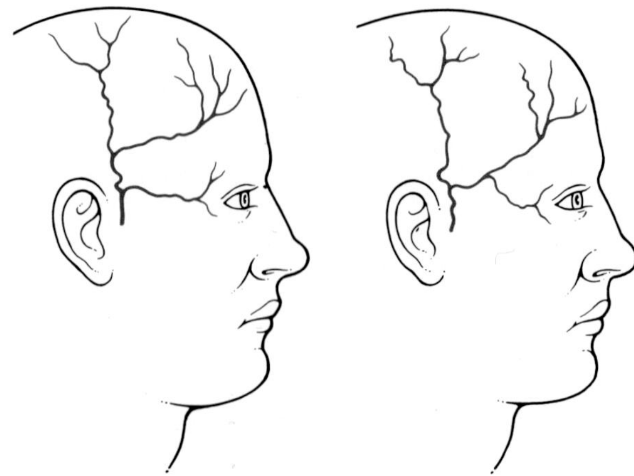

Fig. 6.9 Variation in origin of zygomatico-orbital branch.

cases in which the transverse facial artery has substituted almost entirely for the facial, it has been found to lie below the parotid duct).

The auricular branches are in three groups: firstly an inferior group supplies the lobule and tragus; secondly two or three branches in a superior group, often from a common trunk, run onto the upper part of the helix, its crura and triangular fossa, and follow the curve of the scaphoid fossa; thirdly the superficial temporal or its parietal terminal division gives off a small branch which runs down behind the ear for a short distance, supplies the uppermost part of the cranial surface of the ear, and anastomoses with the posterior auricular artery.

The zygomatico-orbital artery is generally a branch of the superficial temporal, its middle temporal branch or its frontal branch (Ricbourg et al, 1975) (Fig. 6.9). It runs along the upper border of the zygomatic arch between the two layers of the temporal fascia to the lateral angle of the orbit. It supplies branches to the orbicularis oculi, anastomoses with the lacrimal and palpebral branches of the ophthalmic artery, and completes the periorbital ring with the infra- and supraorbital vessels.

The maxillary artery

This artery is said to have at least 15 branches. Only two concern us because the others do not reach the skin.

The mental branch of the inferior alveolar emerges from the mental foramen, helps supply the chin, and anastomoses with the submental and inferior labial vessels.

The infraorbital branch enters the orbital cavity through the inferior orbital fissure and leaves via the infraorbital canal. It emerges deep to levator labii superioris onto the face. Some branches ascend to the medial angle of the eye and the lacrimal sac, anastomosing with the terminal branches of the facial artery; others run towards the nose, anastomosing with the external nasal branch of the ophthalmic artery; others descend between the levator labii superioris and levator anguli oris, and anastomose with the facial, transverse facial and buccal arteries.

THE INTERNAL CAROTID

From its point of origin the internal carotid passes directly upwards in front of the glossopharyngeal and accessory nerves and enters the carotid canal in the base of the skull. It curves forwards through the petrous temporal bone, crosses the foramen lacerum and follows an S-shaped course upwards and forwards through the cavernous sinus. On leaving the sinus it gives origin to the ophthalmic artery which enters the orbit through the optic canal, before the internal carotid divides into its four terminal branches.

The ophthalmic artery is the only branch of the internal carotid which contributes to the blood supply of skin. Through its cutaneous branches to the forehead, significant anastomoses are created between the internal and the external carotid systems. These may become of great importance in providing a collateral circulation to the circle of Willis if the internal carotid is stenosed or occluded, for example in its course through the cavernous sinus. If such a block exists, then flow in the supraorbital artery will be reversed, but will cease completely or even reverse back to normal (if IC only stenosed) when the superficial temporal arteries are occluded by the examiner's fingers. The flow in the supraorbital artery can easily be detected by insonating the vessel at the supraorbital ridge with a single directional Doppler. This is the basis of the temporal artery occlusive test (TAOT) for internal carotid stenosis/occlusion but does have both false positive and false negative results (Brockenbrough, 1964).

The ophthalmic artery

This artery gives off many branches to the contents of the orbit including a lacrimal branch, then passes over or under the optic nerve and gives off a supraorbital artery before emerging below superior oblique where it divides into its two terminal branches, the supratrochlear artery and the dorsal nasal artery (Fig. 6.10). *Variation:* in 2% the ophthalmic artery arises from the middle meningeal (Gillilan, 1961).

The lacrimal branch runs forward at the junction of orbital roof and lateral wall, supplies the lacrimal gland and is then distributed to the eyelids and conjunctiva. The eyelid branches are called the lateral palpebral arteries; they run in the upper and lower eyelids (Fig. 6.11) and anastomose with the medial palpebral arteries. A small zygomatic branch appears on the cheek through the zygomaticofacial foramen and anastomoses with the transverse facial and zygomatico-orbital arteries. *Variation:* in 1% the lacrimal rises from the middle meningeal artery via the superior orbital fissure; in 2% it arises from an abnormal ophthalmic artery.

The supraorbital artery. This artery (0.5–0.75 mm D) runs between levator palpebrae superioris and the roof of the orbital cavity in the company of the supraorbital nerve. It passes through the supraorbital foramen or notch and divides into superficial and deep branches which variously supply skin, muscle and pericranium. The deep branch sends a vessel to the diploë of the

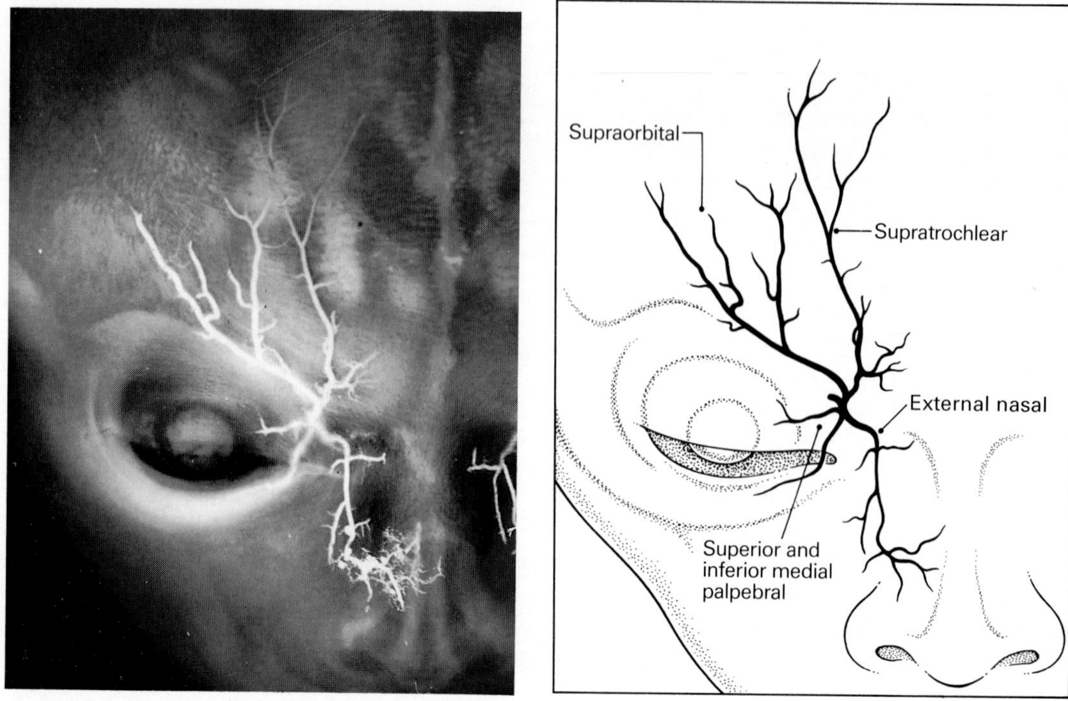

Fig. 6.10 Branches of the ophthalmic artery. Foetal specimen injected intra-arterially with latex and cleared by the glycerol-KOH technique. Terminal division of the ophthalmic artery in a trifurcation is shown in this specimen.

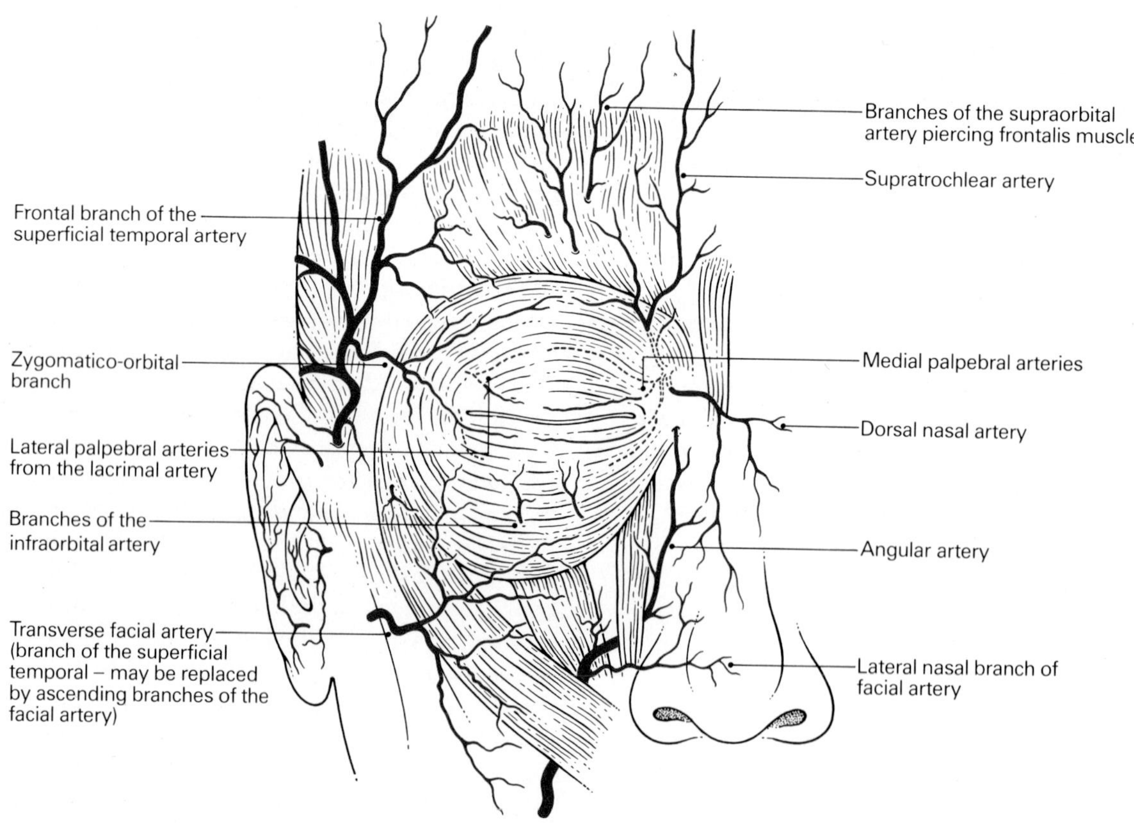

Fig. 6.11 Blood supply of the periorbital region.

frontal bone which probably also supplies the mucoperiosteum of the frontal sinus. It remains beneath the orbicularis oculi and frontalis muscles. The superficial branch is inversely related in size and distribution to the frontal branch of the superficial temporal, and is usually not a very large or long vessel, although the supraorbital nerve reaches right back to the vertex. The supraorbital artery gives off a branch (in ~50%) which runs horizontally in a lateral direction deep to the eyebrow and joins the zygomatico-orbital artery to help form the periorbital ring. The main stem of the supraorbital divides into two or three branches which fan out beneath the forehead skin and anastomose with the frontal branch of the superficial temporal, the ipsi- and contralateral supratrochlear arteries, and the other supraorbital artery.

The medial palpebral arteries. These two arteries, superior and inferior, are given off by the ophthalmic artery and enter the eyelids, where each divides into two branches running along the edges of the tarsal plates. Two arches are therefore formed in each eyelid. The superior palpebral artery anastomoses with a branch from the lacrimal artery and with the zygomatico-orbital artery. The inferior palpebral artery anastomoses with the transverse facial artery and a branch of the lacrimal artery.

The supratrochlear artery. This is one of the terminal branches of the ophthalmic artery. With the supratrochlear nerve it leaves the superomedial angle of the orbit and supplies a small area of the forehead adjacent to the midline. It anastomoses with the supraorbital artery and the artery of the opposite side so that the territory that may be based on it is in fact much larger than might be expected (see p. 461).

The external nasal artery. This is the other terminal branch of the ophthalmic artery. It emerges between the trochlea of the superior oblique muscle and the medial palpebral ligament and supplies the upper part of the nose. The external nasal is classically regarded as a separate branch of the ophthalmic but in many cases the ophthalmic trifurcates in giving origin to the nasal, the supratrochlear and a common trunk for the medial palpebral arteries. The external nasal branch runs forwards for a short distance onto the nose and then makes a characteristic right-angled turn inferiorly towards the ala. It runs towards the nostril overlying the frontal process of the maxilla rather than the nasal bone, and gives off branches to the side and bridge of the nose. That to the bridge and mid-line of the nose may be known as the dorsal nasal branch. These branches anastomose with the ipsilateral angular artery, the lateral nasal branch of the facial artery, the alar branch of the superior labial artery, and the contralateral external nasal artery.

THE SUBCLAVIAN ARTERY

The branches of the subclavian artery supply most of the skin of the neck, from the clavicles to the level of the chin. Much has been written about the branches of the subclavian artery during the past 100 years but changes of nomenclature and the great variability of the vessels in origin, course, branching and relationship to the brachial plexus, make this a difficult area. The authors have greatly simplified what can be made a very complicated subject.

The subclavian artery has only four principal vessels and trunks, namely the vertebral, internal thoracic, costocervical and thyrocervical. With regard to the blood supply of neck skin we are concerned only with the thyrocervical trunk which arises from the first part of the subclavian artery. (The subclavian is classically regarded as divided into three parts by scalenus anterior.) The thyrocervical trunk has four branches according to *Nomina Anatomica*. Minute descriptions of the various possible arrangements would convey a poor impression of the general scheme and it appears best to describe the variations in a graphic manner. Figure 6.12 is based on an anatomical study which gave 38 different arrangements (Thompson, 1891). The seven shown make up the most commonly found as borne out by subsequent studies (Bean, 1905; Huelke, 1958; Daseler & Anson, 1959). It should be noted that the dorsal scapular artery frequently arises directly from the subclavian.

The transverse cervical artery

This artery arises from the thyrocervical trunk in 75% of cases, often in common with the suprascapular artery (Fig. 6.12). It passes laterally beneath omohyoid and over the trunks of the brachial plexus to reach the lateral border of levator scapulae. A small branch is given off just beyond omohyoid to the supraclavicular fat pad, platysma and skin. At the lateral border of levator scapulae the transverse cervical artery may divide into a superficial or ascending branch (ramus superficialis) which supplies the middle part of trapezius, and a deep branch (ramus profundus) which has the course and distribution of the dorsal scapular artery which it replaces when that vessel does not have an independent origin from the subclavian. The superficial branch divides on the deep surface of trapezius (rami ascendens and descendens), with some branches running laterally between the muscle fibres which insert into the acromion and scapular spine (Fig. 6.13). Musculocutaneous perforators pierce the muscle to reach the overlying skin. Some branches also supply

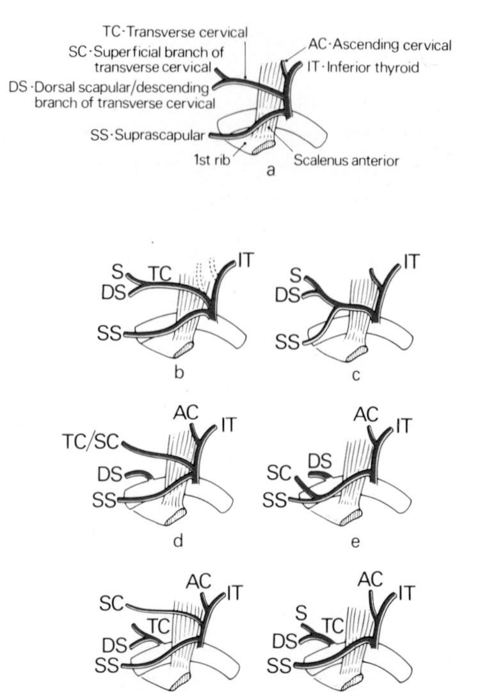

Fig. 6.12 Variations in the origins of the branches of the thyrocervical trunk.

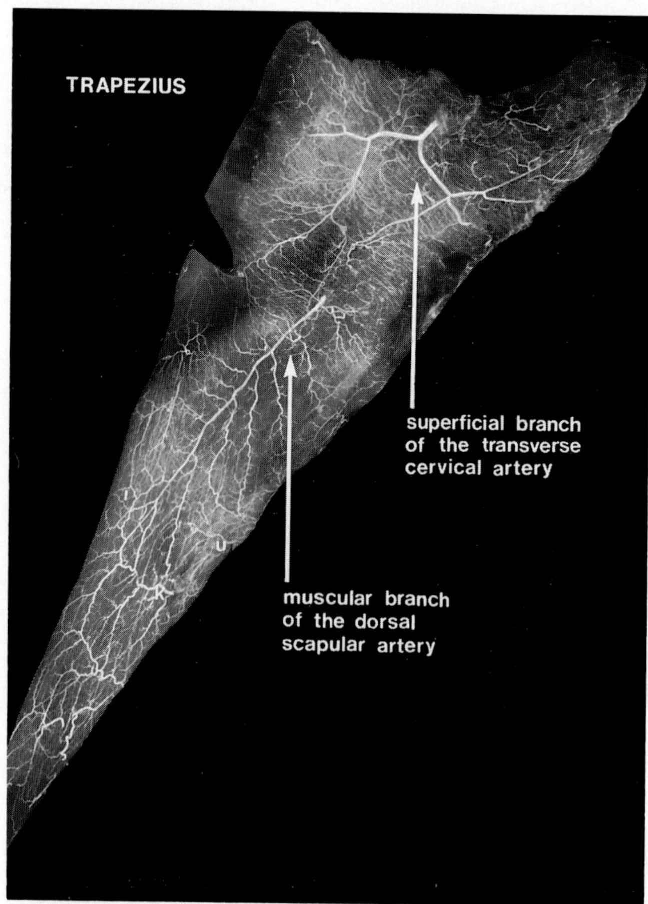

Fig. 6.13 Radiograph of injected trapezius muscle.

semispinalis capitis, and a fasciocutaneous branch may pass over the shoulder (see supraclavicular artery below). In 28% of one study, a branch of the transverse cervical passed upwards just beneath the anterior edge of trapezius to supply the upper one-third of the muscle which is usually supplied by the occipital artery (Huelke, 1958).

The dorsal scapular artery

This may be the name given to the deep branch of the transverse cervical artery or, in those cases in which no transverse cervical artery is present, it is the vessel that arises from the second or third part of the subclavian and passes with the nerve to the rhomboids along the vertebral border of the scapula (Fig. 6.14). Although traditionally considered a branch of the transverse cervical artery it actually has an origin more frequently from the subclavian (~66%) than from the transverse cervical (~30%). Other origins are rare.

The course of the artery is variable; when it arises directly from the subclavian it passes through the brachial plexus lying above or below the middle trunk, and runs lateral to scalenus medius and scalenus posterior although it may pass through or medial to either or both of them (26%). When the dorsal scapular artery arises from the transverse cervical artery, its origin is always near the superior border of the scapula; in this location the artery is posterior and superior to the brachial plexus and therefore it is never found passing through the plexus. Such arteries are always lateral to the scalene muscles and from the superior border of the scapula turn directly downwards along its medial border, deep to the rhomboids.

In the majority of cases (~90%) the dorsal scapular artery gives off a muscular branch to trapezius as it lies level with the base of the scapular spine. This branch runs for 1–3 cm medial to the vertebral border of the scapula, pierces one of the rhomboids or goes between rhomboideus major and minor, and reaches the deep surface of trapezius where it supplies the lower third of the muscle (Fig. 6.14). This muscular artery always arises from the dorsal scapular artery and never from the transverse cervical artery. Within the trapezius it anastomoses with branches of the medial and lateral posterior segmental cutaneous rami and may thereby reach the skin.

The dorsal scapular artery may also give off small twigs to the lower part of levator scapulae, a branch onto the surface of supraspinatus (in 2%), and an ascending branch which passes up just beneath the anterior edge of trapezius (in 5%).

The superficial cervical artery

This name, as used in *Nomina Anatomica*, is an alternative for the superficial branch of the transverse cervical artery. It may also be used for the distinct vessel arising from the thyrocervical trunk (see Fig. 6.12d, f) or suprascapular artery (see Fig. 6.12e), which supplies the territory of the superficial branch of the (absent) transverse cervical artery. Others consider it a separate vessel which ends beneath the lateral part of trapezius (Bean, 1905). It has significant branches to platysma and skin over the lower part of the posterior triangle of the neck.

The suprascapular artery

This artery arises from the thyrocervical trunk, or, more rarely, from the subclavian. It passes over the ligament of the suprascapular notch and supplies the supraspinatus and infraspinatus musculature. It may give off a muscular branch to sternomastoid and a branch to the subcutaneous tissues over the tip of the shoulder (ramus acromialis).

The supraclavicular artery

This cutaneous vessel arises in ~93% from the superficial cervical/transverse cervical artery and in ~7% from the suprascapular artery. It pierces the deep fascia anterior to trapezius, just above the clavicle, and runs over the lateral end of the clavicle. This branch of the suprascapular artery may be the ramus acromialis of *Nomina Anatomica* but the term supraclavicular artery applied to the vessel of this course and distribution, is preferable and clearly differentiates it from the ramus acromialis of the thoraco-acromial axis. The supraclavicular artery is worth identifying by name since it is the vascular basis of an axial pattern flap.

The inferior thyroid artery

This ascends along the medial border of scalenus anterior giving off branches to the deeper structures. It gives a branch to the lower part of sternomastoid but there are only a few small musculocutaneous branches from the lower third of the muscle to the skin.

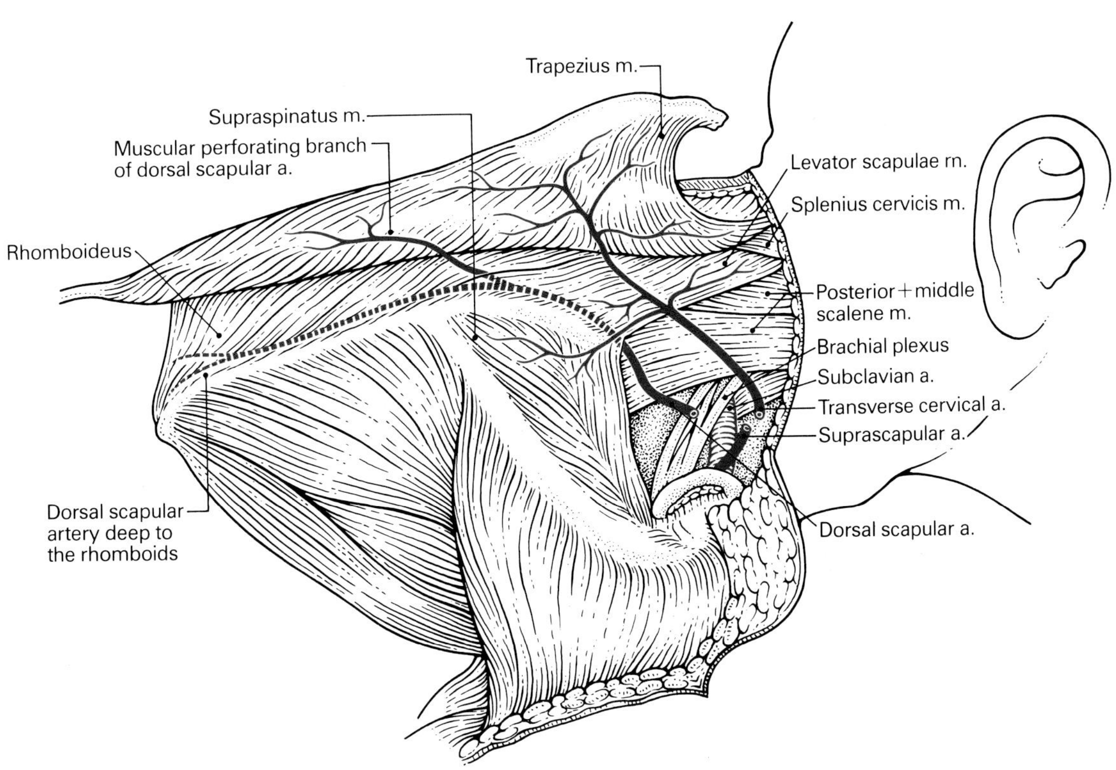

Fig. 6.14 Illustration showing how the superficial branch of the transverse cervical artery and the deep branch/dorsal scapular artery reach trapezius to supply the muscle and the overlying dorsal skin. Trapezius has been detached from the spine of the scapula and the acromion and has been reflected medially.

6 CUTANEOUS BLOOD SUPPLY OF HEAD AND NECK BY REGIONS

This is summarised in Table 6.1 and Figures 6.15 and 6.16.

Table 6.1 Summary of cutaneous blood supply by regions

Skin over	Supplied by
NECK	
submental triangle	– facial artery via submental branch
digastric triangle	– facial artery via direct branches
carotid triangle	– superior thyroid artery via infrahyoid and sternomastoid branches
muscular triangle	– superior thyroid artery inferior thyroid artery via very small musculocutaneous perforators
sternomastoid muscle	– upper part – posterior auricular artery via direct branches occipital artery via descending branches occipital artery via musculocutaneous perforators – middle part – superior thyroid artery – lower part – subclavian artery via direct branch
occipital triangle	– occipital artery via descending branches
omoclavicular triangle	– transverse cervical artery via direct branch supraclavicular artery
trapezius	– upper part – occipital artery and ascending ramus of superficial branch of transverse cervical artery – lateral part – supraclavicular artery and superficial branch of transverse cervical artery via musculocutaneous perforators
HEAD	
scalp – forehead	– supratrochlear artery, supraorbital artery } of ophthalmic artery frontal branch of superficial temporal artery
– temporo-parietal region	– frontal branch of superficial temporal artery parietal branch of superficial temporal artery
– occipital region	– occipital artery posterior auricular artery
periorbital region	– supraorbital artery supratrochlear artery lacrimal branch zygomatico-orbital branch of superficial temporal artery infraorbital branch of maxillary artery angular artery – the continuation of the facial artery
nose	– external nasal branch of ophthalmic artery and its dorsal nasal branch lateral nasal branch of facial artery collumellar and alar branches of superior labial artery
cheek	– infraorbital branch of maxillary artery branches of facial artery/angular artery premasseteric artery if present transverse facial branch of superficial temporal artery
lips	– superior labial artery inferior labial artery mental branch of inferior alveolar artery
chin	– mental branch of inferior alveolar artery submental branch of facial artery
ear – external surface	– anterior auricular branches of superficial temporal artery perforating branches of posterior auricular artery
– cranial surface	– unnamed branch of superficial temporal artery posterior auricular artery
nasolabial fold	– direct branches of facial artery terminal branches of infraorbital artery and transverse facial artery

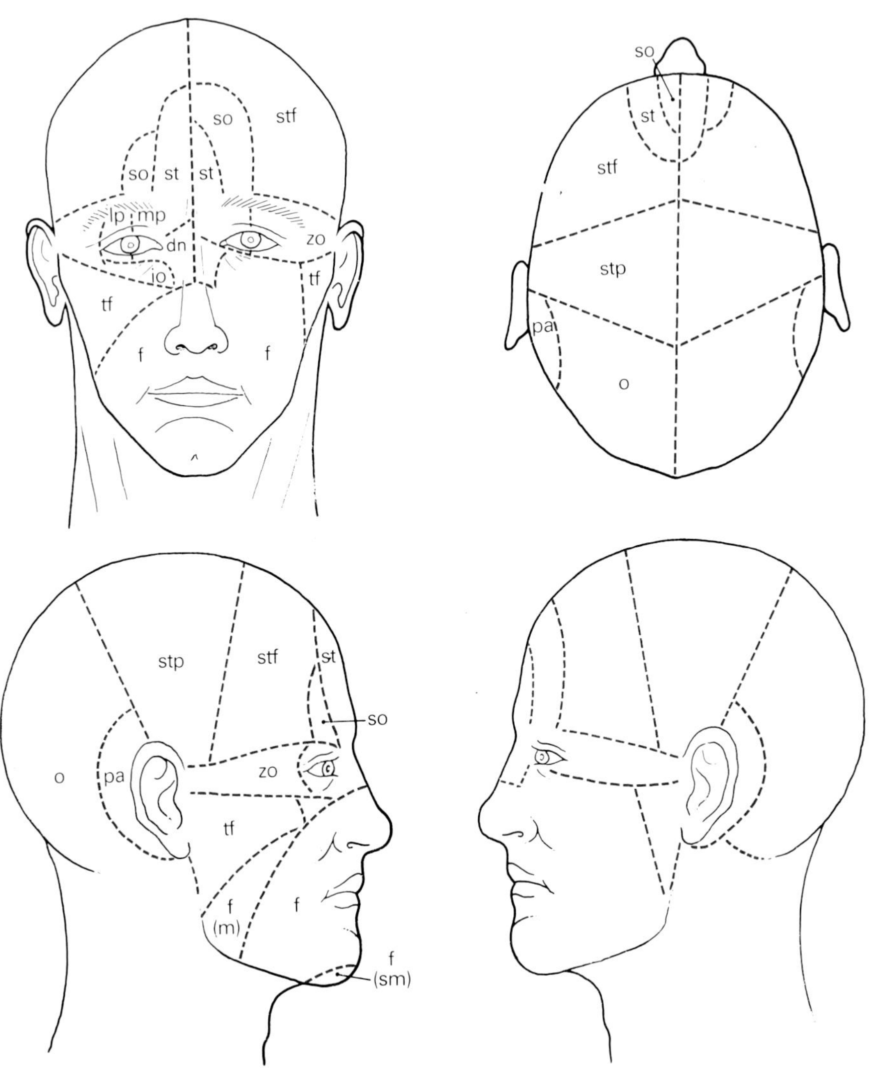

Fig. 6.15 Anatomical territories of cutaneous supply.

On the right side of the face the territories of moderately well-developed facial and transverse facial arteries are shown. On the left side the facial artery is well developed and reaches the medial canthal area; strong masseteric and ascending branches of the facial supply the anterior part of the cheek and compensate for a weak transverse facial artery.

On the right of the forehead the supratrochlear artery is better developed than the supraorbital (the usual situation) while on the left the situation is reversed. The lateral surface of the auricle is mainly supplied by the superficial temporal artery although the posterior auricular artery may send a few branches through the cartilage to the conchal area.

stf. superficial temporal – frontal branch, **stp.** superficial temporal – parietal branch, **zo.** zygomatico-orbital branch of superficial temporal, **lp.** lateral palpebral, **mp.** medial palpebral, **io.** infraorbital, **tf.** transverse facial, **f.** facial artery, **o.** occipital artery, **pa.** posterior auricular, **dn.** dorsal nasal.

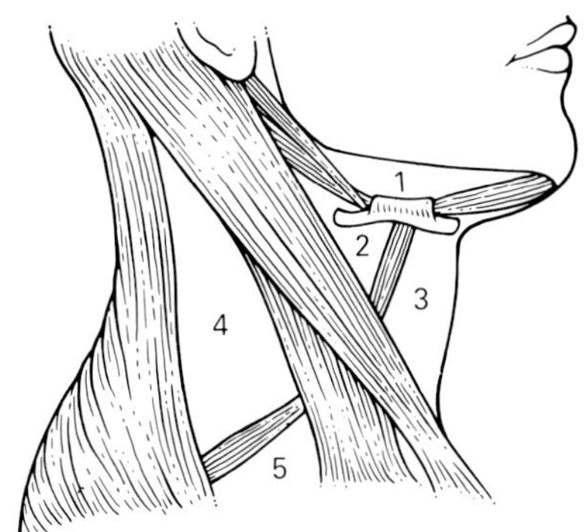

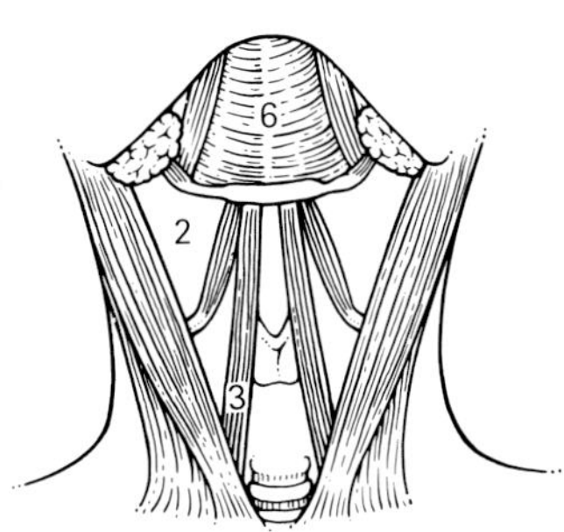

Fig. 6.16 Triangles of the neck referred to in the text:

1. Digastric triangle } anterior triangle
2. Carotid triangle } anterior triangle
3. Muscular triangle } anterior triangle
4. Occipital triangle } posterior triangle
5. Omoclavicular triangle } posterior triangle
6. Submental triangle

6

FLAPS IN THE NECK

Flaps in the neck may be divided into three categories – random cutaneous, musculocutaneous and fasciocutaneous. The platysma lies in the superficial fascia and might therefore be considered as being vascularised by direct cutaneous arteries. In this discussion, however, platysma based flaps are considered in the musculocutaneous category.

Random pattern cutaneous flaps

These have been used for many years, e.g. the lateral neck flaps of Mütter (1842) and Zovickian (1957). The 'apron flap' as originally designed was considered a random pattern flap (Ward & Hendrick, 1950), and the 'epaulette' flap (Kirschbaum, 1958), which was designed without due regard for the local blood supply, was noted to have a greater than expected length-to-breadth ratio. Although inexplicable at the time, with the more recent understanding of the principles of the musculocutaneous system of perforators and the details of the vascularisation of platysma, many neck flaps are now known to have a significant musculocutaneous element (Futrell et al, 1978). A random flap from the clavicular area incorporating the supraclavicular nerves has been used in a three-stage procedure for providing sensate reconstructions of the severely degloved hand (Sommerlad & Boorman, 1981). None of these flaps is described in greater detail in Chapter 7 since they are not based on specific vessels but the reader will find further information in the references indicated.

Musculocutaneous flaps

These flaps may be based on trapezius, sternomastoid and platysma.

Trapezius

There are three different musculocutaneous flaps based on the trapezius muscle: the upper, based on a branch of the occipital artery (see p. 382); the lateral, based on the superficial branch of the transverse cervical artery or the superficial cervical artery (see p. 484) (by including a segment of the acromion this may be made a myo-osteo-cutaneous flap); and the lower or posterior, which is not a neck flap, but is based on the dorsal scapular/deep branch of the transverse cervical artery (see p. 324).

Sternomastoid

There are two flaps based on the sternomastoid muscle. These are skin islands based over either the superior or inferior end of the muscle and pedicled about the opposite end. They are both discussed on page 380. Because of the feeble nature of the musculocutaneous perforators from the surface of the muscle to the overlying skin, and the poor anastomoses within the muscle, these flaps are rather unreliable.

Platysma

Platysma flaps have recently become better understood as details of the vascular anatomy have been elucidated. The original apron flap was modified in 1959 for use as intra-oral lining by de-epithelialising the proximal part, thereby in effect creating a distal skin island supported by the vascular plexus in platysma (DesPrez & Kiehn, 1959). More recently the muscle has been used as a pedicled carrier for an island of skin situated in the lower lateral neck over the posterior triangle. The vascular input comes superiorly from the submental and direct branches of the facial artery which anastomose within the platysma with the superior thyroid and tranverse cervical branches. As a further development, the flap has been reversed, with the skin island superiorly and the vascular pedicle inferiorly. These are described on page 330.

Fasciocutaneous flaps

These may be based on the supraclavicular artery and extend from the lower neck over the shoulder (p. 458). The cervico-humeral flap includes this vessel and also the musculocutaneous perforators through the lateral part of trapezius (p. 481).

Neurovascular free flaps

A neurovascular free flap from the lower part of the posterior triangle is possible and is described on page 487. It is based on the direct branch of the transverse cervical or superficial cervical artery which supplies the supraclavicular fat pad and overlying platysma/skin complex.

FLAPS ON THE HEAD AND FACE

This region is notable for its excellent blood supply and therefore many defects may be reconstructed with local flaps which have been raised without regard to local patterns of blood supply. Local flaps may exceed the constraints of the limited length-to-breadth ratios usually associated with random flaps and are excluded from the following list of flaps. Flaps based on identifiable vascular anatomy are considered in three groups – axial cutaneous, nasolabial and musculocutaneous. Flaps in the area of the nasolabial groove are here considered on their own because of the unusual way in which several vessels supply the skin in this area, thereby allowing a variety of permutations of flaps to be created, including subcutaneously pedicled sliding varieties.

Axial pattern flaps

These flaps are based on vessels of the direct cutaneous system. Although modifications in detail are numerous, they are all variations of basic patterns supported by the supraorbital, superficial temporal, occipital and posterior auricular arteries.

The supraorbital and/or supratrochlear arteries
These arteries can support flaps of forehead skin and have been used in India over several centuries for nasal reconstruction. Millard has developed a seagull-shaped or cruciform flap for nasal reconstruction based on these vessels (see p. 463).

The superficial temporal arteries
Forehead flaps based on the *frontal branch* of the superficial temporal artery and using the full width of the forehead were developed by Gillies for nasal reconstruction (see pp. 443 & 462).

The *parietal branch* of the superficial temporal artery can support various forms of hair-bearing flaps, generally used for reconstructing the frontal hairline. Many hair-bearing flaps are not specifically axial pattern; several require a preliminary delay (e.g. Juri). The short Elliot flap (see p. 447) sacrifices a temporal artery for a flap which supplies only one-half of the frontal hairline, but does so without the need for a prior delay. Stough has modified the flap by two delays so that in most cases it will cover three-quarters of the frontal hairline. The parietal branch of the superficial temporal artery may be incorporated in a large area of temporo-parietal scalp and used as the (temporary) pedicle for an area of non-hair-bearing skin from the skull behind the ear. This is the basis of the two-stage Waschio flap (see p. 452). Alternatively, the anastomosis of the parietal branch with the posterior auricular artery may be exploited to produce a one-stage island flap from the skin on the cranial surface of the ear and adjacent skull (see p. 453).

Island free flaps may be created on one superficial temporal artery for transfer to the other side of the head for treatment of localised temporal and sideburn alopecia. The superficial temporal artery has been used to transfer very small islands of skin from non-hair-bearing areas in front of the ear onto the surface of exposed areas of prosthesis in ear reconstructions.

The posterior auricular artery
This supplies an area of hair-free skin and has been successfully used as a free flap (see p. 402).

The occipital artery
This artery may support large areas of hair-bearing skin (see p. 448).

The transverse facial artery
This artery can support most of the skin of the cheek and the skin overlying the mandible and upper neck. This is the basis of the cervico-facial flap pedicled over the parotid gland, for advancement upwards into the orbit.

Nasolabial flaps

The 'spare' skin in the nasolabial fold is supplied in its lower part by direct branches of the facial artery and in its middle part by terminal branches of the infraorbital and transverse facial arteries, while the uppermost part is supplied by branches from the angular artery. The supply to this area is therefore unusual in being made up of many small branches directed perpendicular to the skin surface; there is no single axial vessel in the skin because the facial/angular artery lies at a deeper level passing through levator labii superioris. Nasolabial flaps may be based superiorly (commonly), inferiorly (such as Esser's flap for closing palatal fistulae) or may be subcutaneously pedicled island flaps. In the latter instance they must be based either on the cutaneous branches of the facial artery penetrating the subcutaneous tissues from below, or on the branches of the transverse facial artery entering from the lateral side (see p. 327).

Musculocutaneous flaps

There are no true musculocutaneous flaps on the face in the sense that the skin is not supplied by perforators from the underlying muscles. Rather, the vessels on the face give off branches to muscles and separate branches to skin. Flaps combining muscle and skin are possible round the mouth, being based on the superior and inferior labial arteries.

The Abbe V-lip-switch two-stage flap is a method of transferring a full thickness triangle of one lip, pedicled on the labial vessels of one side, into a V-shaped defect of the other lip. In the Abbe-Estlander V-fan-flap the defect lies near the oral commissure and the transferred flap is swung from the opposite lip so that the pedicle reconstructs the angle of the mouth (see p. 354).

Larger defects of part or all of the lower lip have traditionally been reconstructed with the Bernard procedure (1853) or variations on the Gillies fan flap (1957), which make use of the excess skin in the naso-labial region to close the defect. Modified versions of the former and latter procedures have been described. Fan flaps employ the full thickness of the cheek and muscle based on a narrow pedicle of upper lip which contains within it the superior labial vessels. They may be unilateral or bilateral (see p. 356).

Such flaps are without motor or sensory supply and this may become a significant disability when the whole lower lip is reconstructed with bilateral flaps. To overcome this disadvantage, Karapandžić has developed innervated musculocutaneous island flaps based on superior and inferior labial vessels (see p. 356).

Limited reconstruction of the vermilion of the lip may be brought about by raising the remaining lip margin including the respective labial artery and surrounding muscle fibres of orbicularis oris and 'stretching' the lip margin to reconstruct the defect. This is in effect a strip-like musculocutaneous flap incorporating a labial artery.

6 TRUNK

Nomina Anatomica of those vessels supplying skin, plus a few that do not

ARTERIA SUBCLAVIA
Arteria thoracica interna
  Rami sternales
  Rami perforantes
    Rami mammarii
  (Ramus costalis lateralis)
  Rami intercostales anteriores
  A. epigastrica superior
Truncus thyrocervicalis
  A. transversa cervicis*
    Ramus superficialis (A. cervicalis superficialis)
    Ramus profundus
  Arteria scapularis dorsalis*
  A. suprascapularis
    Ramus acromialis
Truncus costocervicalis
  A. intercostalis suprema
    A. intercostalis posterior prima
    A. intercostalis posterior secunda
      Rami dorsales
      Rami spinales

ARTERIA AXILLARIS
Rami subscapulares
A. thoracica superior
A. thoracoacromialis
  Ramus acromiale
    Rete acromiale
  Ramus clavicularis
  Ramus deltoideus
  Rami pectorales
A. thoracica lateralis
  Rami mammarii laterales
A. subscapularis
  A. thoracodorsalis
  A. circumflexa scapulae
(A. thoracica superficialis)†

PARS THORACICA AORTAE
Aa. intercostales posteriores
  Ramus dorsalis
    Ramus spinalis
    Ramus cutaneous medialis
    Ramus cutaneous lateralis
  Ramus collateralis
  Ramus cutaneus lateralis
    Rami mammarii
A. subcostalis
  Ramus dorsalis

PARS ABDOMINALIS AORTAE
Arteriae lumbales
  Ramus dorsalis

ARTERIA ILIACA INTERNA
Arteria iliolumbalis
  Ramus lumbalis
    Ramus spinalis
  Ramus iliacus
Arteriae sacrales laterales
Arteria glutea superior
  Ramus superficialis
  Ramus profundus
    Ramus superior
    Ramus inferior
Arteria glutea inferior
Arteria pudenda interna
  A. perinealis
  Rami scrotales posteriores
  Rami labiales posteriores
  A. dorsalis penis

ARTERIA ILIACA EXTERNA
Arteria epigastrica inferior
Arteria circumflexa ilium
  Ramus ascendens‡

ARTERIA FEMORALIS
Arteria epigastrica superficialis
Arteria circumflexa ilium superficialis
Arteriae pudendae externae
  Rami scrotales anteriores
  Rami labiales anteriores
  Rami inguinales

* See footnote to *Nomina Anatomica* of vessels in the Head and Neck (p. 132)
† This vessel is not officially in *Nomina Anatomica*, but we have included it here
‡ Ramus ascendens, formerly known as arteria epigastrica lateralis

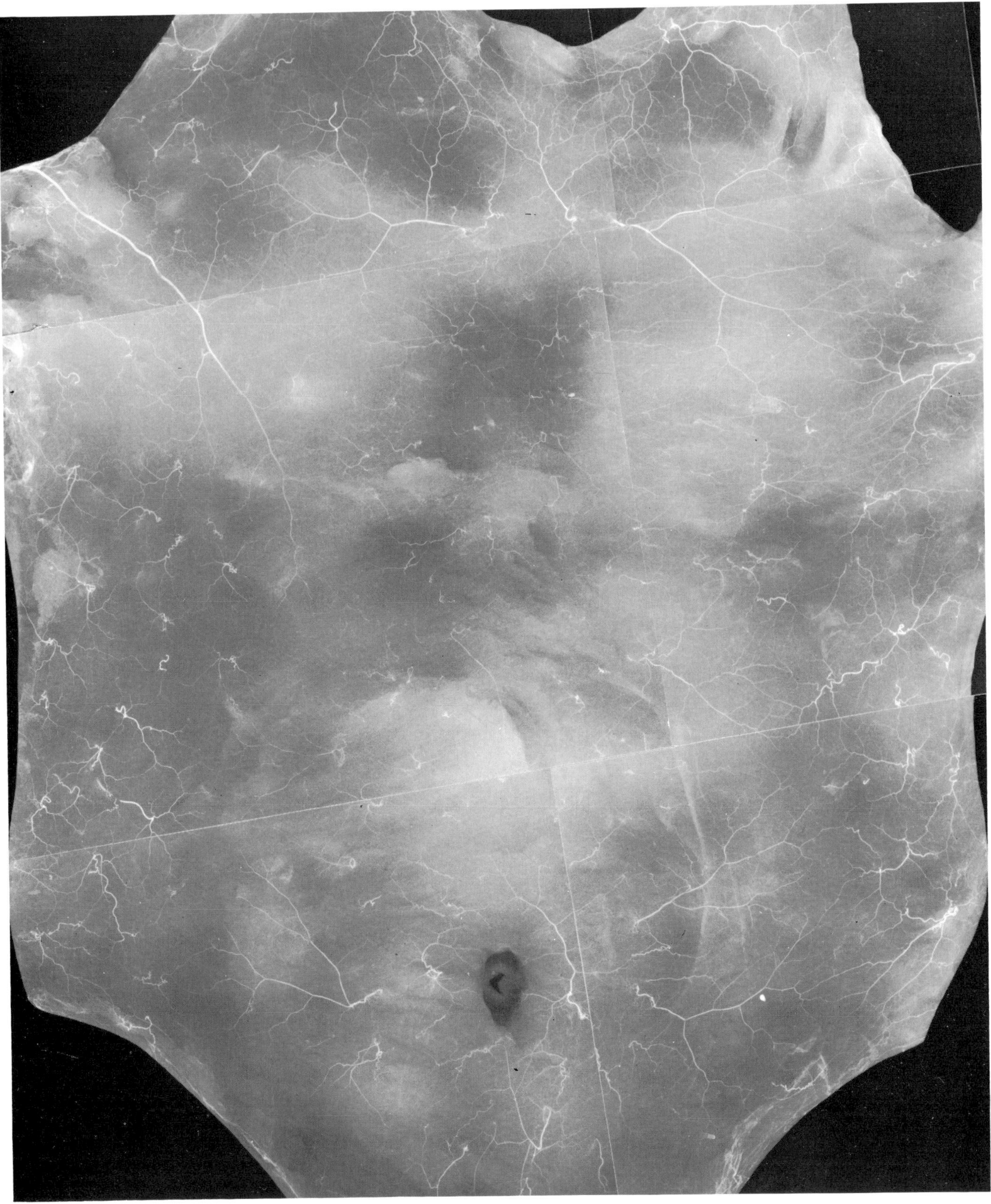

Fig. 6.17 Radiograph of anterior trunk skin and subcutaneous tissues extending round to the mid-lateral lines. Note the size of the perforating branches of the internal thoracic artery through the second intercostal space; the size of the musculocutaneous paraumbilical perforators and the absence of the superficial inferior epigastric artery which tends to vary inversely in size with the latter (contrast this with the arrangement in Fig. 6.38).

6

TRUNK

The major sources of blood supply to the skin of the trunk are: firstly, the musculocutaneous branches of the segmental intercostal, lumbar and sacral arteries; secondly, the musculocutaneous perforators arising from the abdominal muscles and also from the dominant vascular pedicles of the flat muscles attaching to the pectoral girdle; and thirdly, from direct cutaneous arteries on the anterior aspect of the thorax and abdomen. The buttocks are described with the thighs because the territory of the inferior gluteal artery often extends onto the upper thigh.

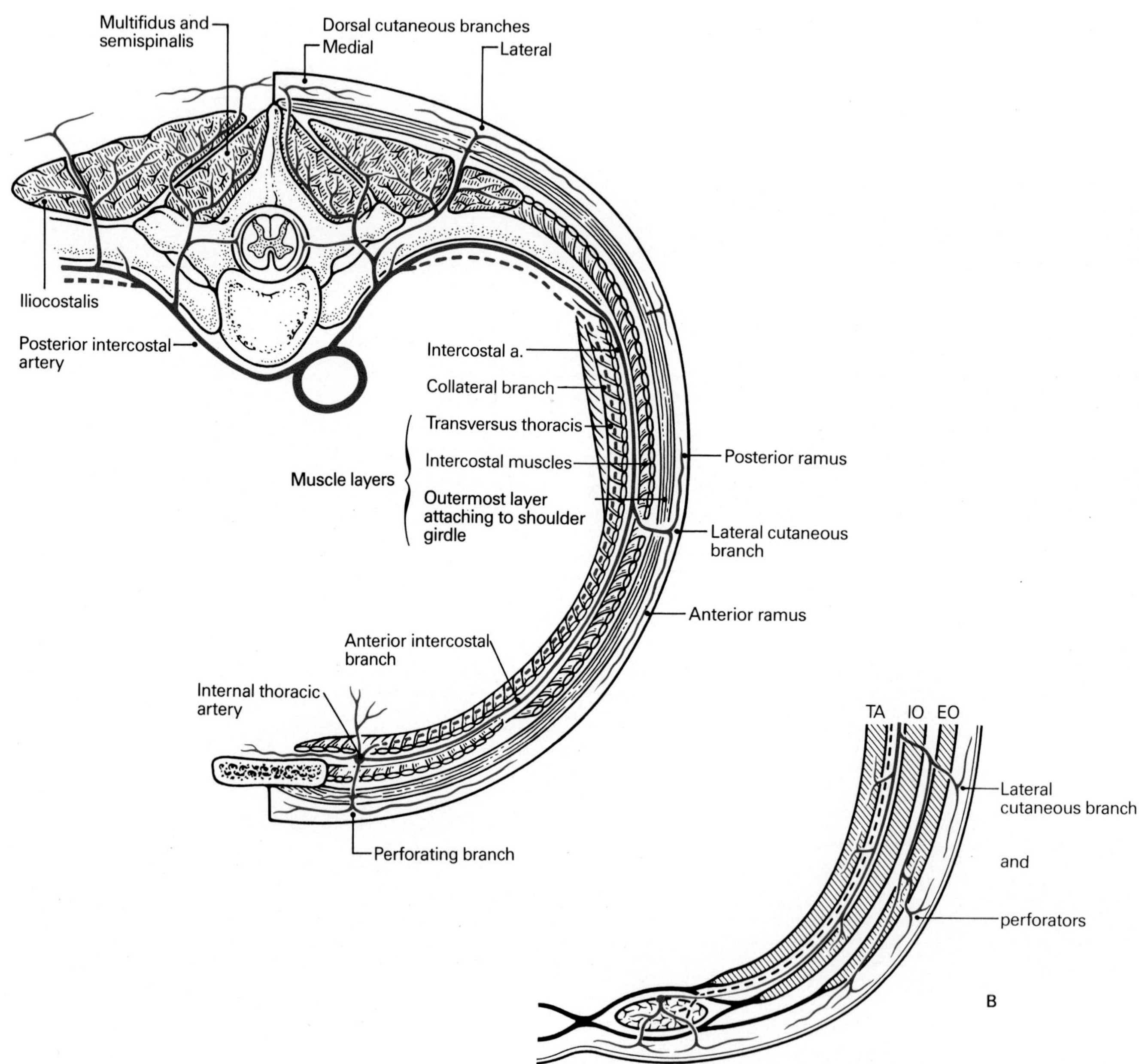

Fig. 6.18 **A.** Schematic oblique transverse section through one half of a lower intercostal space illustrating the branches of a typical intercostal artery. Alternative arrangements of the dorsal cutaneous branches are shown on either side of the spine. **B.** Schematic transverse section through the middle part of the abdominal wall showing the relationships of the segmental vessels and their branches to the three muscle layers and the rectus sheath. Anastomosis with the epigastric arcade is shown.

GENERAL SCHEME OF ARRANGEMENT OF INTERCOSTAL VESSELS

Figure 6.18 shows the intercostal vessels in a schematic cross-sectional diagram through the chest wall. There are usually nine pairs of intercostal arteries distributed to the lower nine intercostal spaces, the first and second spaces being supplied by the superior intercostal artery arising from the costocervical trunk of the subclavian artery.

In general each artery arises individually from the aorta and crosses its intercostal space obliquely towards the angle of the rib above. This is known as the 'vertebral segment' of the vessel and its oblique course is an important practical point in the dissection of free rib grafts or intercostal island flaps. Three or four branches arise in this segment. Each posterior intercostal gives off a dorsal branch which runs backwards through a space which is bound above and below by the necks of the ribs, medially by the body of a vertebra and laterally by a superior costotransverse ligament. This dorsal branch gives off a spinal branch which enters the spinal canal through the intervertebral foramen. The dorsal branch then passes over the transverse process with the dorsal ramus of the corresponding thoracic spinal nerve and divides into medial and lateral musculocutaneous branches. Often medial and lateral dorsal musculocutaneous rami do not arise from a common dorsal trunk but are given off separately (see Fig. 6.18 left side). A nutrient branch to the rib and a collateral branch are given off but are not concerned with the vascular supply to the skin. The collateral branch is variable, but when present runs in the lower part of the intercostal space with a collateral branch of the intercostal nerve.

Note that a spinal branch arising from one of the dorsal cutaneous branches given off by a lower intercostal or upper lumbar artery between T7 and L2 constitutes the principal blood supply to the thoracolumbar enlargement of the spinal cord. This vessel, named the artery of Adamkiewicz (arteria radiculo-medullaris magna) usually lies at T11 (Last, 1984) and is indispensable – its transection, during a correction of scoliosis or replacement of a thoracic aneurysm, has resulted in permanent paraplegia. This is a relevant consideration when harvesting vascularised rib grafts based on a posterior intercostal artery in this area.

The 'costal groove' segment of the intercostal artery lies in a plane between the internal intercostals and the sparse fibres of transversus thoracis. It extends round to the costal cartilages in the upper six spaces and in the lower (T7–T11) spaces extends to the origins of the abdominal wall muscles. In this segment a significant lateral cutaneous branch is given off which pierces the intercostal muscles and continues subcutaneously towards the lateral border of rectus abdominis, with a slight inferior inclination. When the lateral cutaneous branch of one space is absent it will be replaced by several long musculocutaneous perforators or by the lateral cutaneous branches of the intercostal spaces immediately above and below. This is described in greater detail below.

The 'intermuscular segment' extends from the origin of the abdominal musculature to the lateral border of rectus abdominis. The arteries and accompanying nerves lie in a plane between transversus abdominis and internal oblique, to which they give off many small branches.

The 'rectus segment' incorporates the width of the rectus abdominis muscles. Classical texts have indicated that the intercostal vessels terminate by becoming cutaneous at the lateral border of rectus abdominis. Recent studies have demonstrated that the vessels pass deep to the rectus and terminate by anastomosing with the epigastric system (Figs 6.18B & 6.36). Numerous musculocutaneous perforators arise from the epigastric system to supply rectus abdominis and the overlying skin.

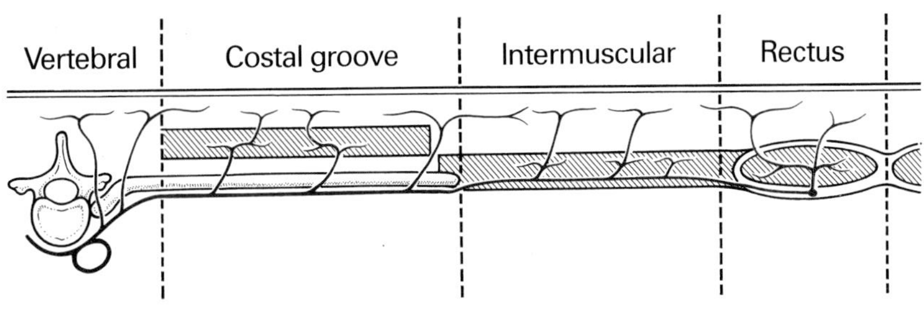

Fig. 6.19 Schematic representation of the various segments of a lower intercostal artery.

The following variations exist and are mentioned because they may be encountered when elevating island intercostal flaps (see p. 346). Although intercostal and lumbar vessels generally arise as single vessels from the aorta it may be found that: (1) left and right arteries at one level arise as a common trunk; and (2) on a single side intercostals to more than one space may arise from a common trunk. Figure 6.20 illustrates the prevalence of these different configurations. It can be seen that a single trunk supplying both sides at any level, whilst uncommon, is most likely to be encountered with the seventh and eighth intercostals, and in the lumbar region. The other variation is that two or three spaces may be supplied by division of a single branch off the aorta. Figure 6.20 shows that the third intercostal artery arises in this manner in approximately 40% of cases, such intercostals usually being branches of a parent trunk arising at a lower segmental level. This arrangement may be encountered among the lower intercostals (10–12) at which level dissection of the intercostal vessels is more likely to be required in flap elevation.

The designation of an intercostal as first, second, third, etc., is determined by the intercostal space in which it runs but this segmental level at which the vessel passes round the chest does not necessarily coincide with the vertebral level of origin from the aorta. This is illustrated diagrammatically in Figure 6.21. The first three intercostals, when not arising from the superior intercostal artery, arise as much as three vertebral segments lower. From T8 downwards the intercostals arise at the level of the disc below their respective vertebral body (i.e. the ninth intercostal from the disc between vertebral bodies 9 and 10). In the lumbar area the arteries arise more nearly opposite their own bodies. All the vessels effectively pass initially upwards from their point of origin before passing round the trunk. Finally, there is a tendency for intercostals on the left side to arise at a higher level than their counterparts on the right.

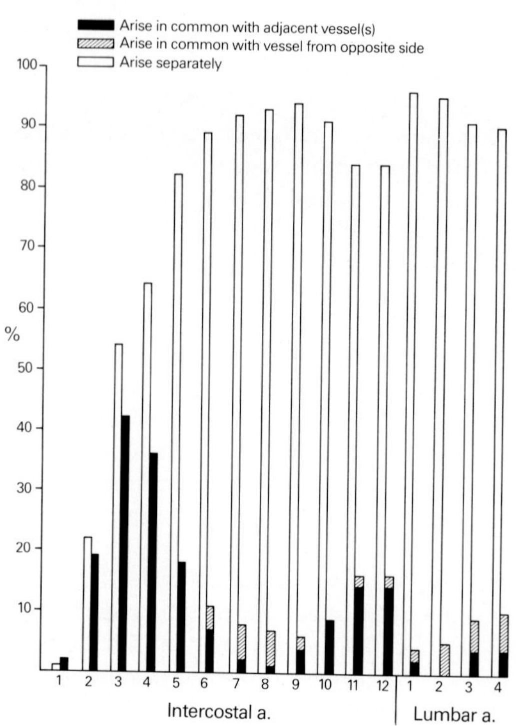

Fig. 6.20 Histogram to describe the manner in which intercostal and lumbar arteries at any given level arise from the aorta. Intercostal arteries arise either individually, or left and right sides arise together from a common trunk, or two or more vessels on one side arise from a common trunk. Where no origin is shown the arteries had an origin from some site other than the aorta. (After Adachi, 1928.)

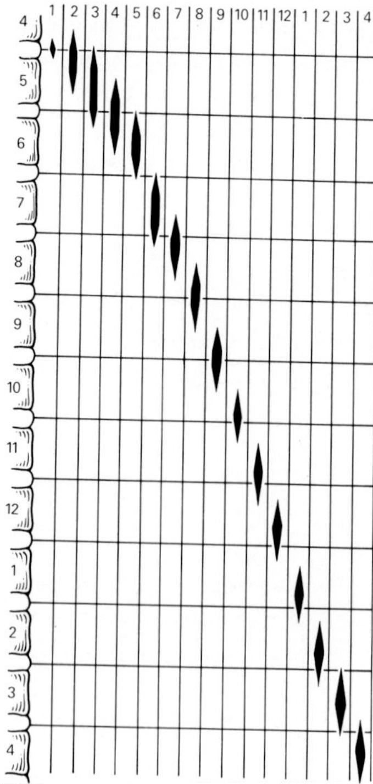

Fig. 6.21 Diagram illustrating the level of origin from the aorta of individual intercostal and lumbar arteries relative to vertebral bodies and intervertebral discs. The shape of each oblong also indicates the range of variation encountered in 30 hemithoraces. (Adachi, 1928.)

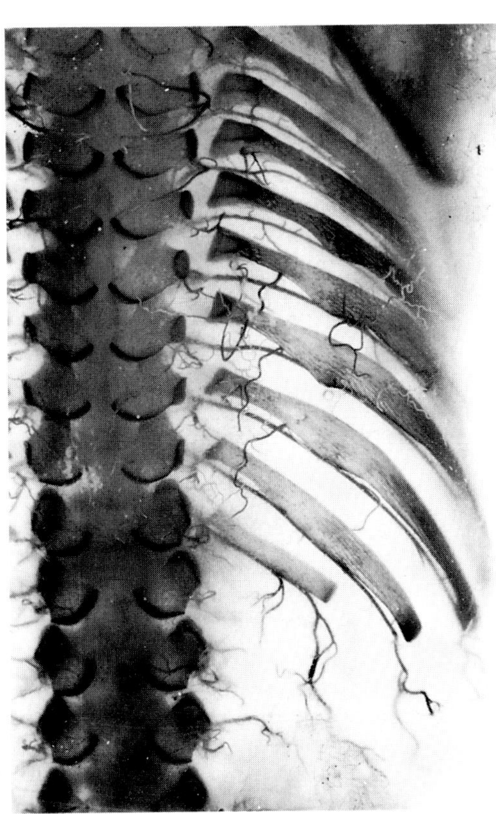

Fig. 6.22 Photograph of the dorsal aspect of an approximately 20-week gestation foetus in the lower thoracic and upper lumbar area. The vascular tree has been filled with red latex and the tissues cleared in potassium hydroxide and glycerol. Calcified structures have been stained with alizarin but cartilagenous structures are not visualised.

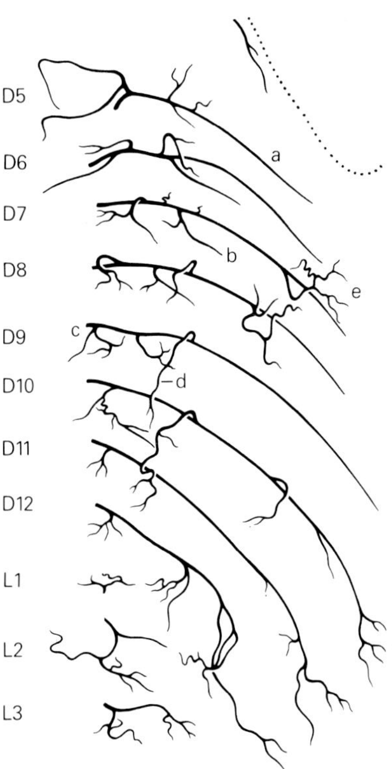

Fig. 6.23 A tracing of the vessels in Fig. 6.22. Representative vessels have been labelled and may be identified as follows: **a.** intercostal artery (fifth); **b.** collateral branch; **c.** medial dorsal cutaneous branch; **d.** lateral dorsal cutaneous branch; **e.** perforator to overlying trunk musculature.

DORSAL TRUNK (Fig. 6.24)

Consideration will first be given to the skin of the dorsal trunk reaching from the spine of C7 superiorly, to the iliac crests inferiorly, and extending to the midscapular line laterally.

Superiorly the deep branch of the transverse cervical artery/dorsal scapular artery (see Footnote to *Nomina Anatomica*, p. 132) supplies the lower part of the trapezius and contributes musculocutaneous perforators to the overlying skin. Inferiorly, below the level of T4 spinous process, the supply is from medial and lateral dorsal cutaneous branches of the intercostal and lumbar arteries, and musculocutaneous perforators through latissimus dorsi from the thoracodorsal artery.

The superficial cervical artery

This is one of the three vascular pedicles of the trapezius muscle and its cutaneous area of supply constitutes part of the potential territory of the lateral trapezius musculocutaneous flap. The approximate anatomical territory of this vessel is shown as area 8 in Figure 6.24. Musculocutaneous perforators pierce the muscle to reach overlying skin.

The dorsal scapular artery

This runs deep to levator scapulae and the rhomboids, supplying these muscles and the lower part of trapezius by small perforators. In just under 50% of cases a large branch is given off which passes inferomedially, supplies the inferior part of trapezius and, via perforators, supplies skin. The contribution of these perforators varies inversely to that of the intercostals in this region.

The intercostal arteries

The *medial* dorsal musculocutaneous rami supply spinalis and longissimus before reaching the skin just lateral to the vertebral spines. The calibre of these arteries does not diminish from above downwards in a regular way; indeed there are often very large arteries in the region of the eighth to tenth intercostal spaces. The territory of these medial dorsal cutaneous branches is indicated in Figure 6.24 as area 1.

The *lateral* dorsal musculocutaneous rami supply longissimus and iliocostalis before reaching trapezius and latissimus dorsi which they penetrate to reach the overlying skin. These cutaneous branches are best developed from T6 downwards and branches pierce the superficial muscles at a variable distance between 5 cm and 8 cm from the midline, often in company with a posterior perforating branch of the intercostal nerve and run inferolaterally at the level of the deep fascia for 0.5 or 1.0 cm before finally passing up to the skin in multiple divergent branches. The relationship between the perforating nerves and the cutaneous arteries is variable; the artery may lie above or below the nerve and there is often an accompanying vein present. Anastomoses in this region are well developed and the approximate territory of these lateral dorsal cutaneous branches is shown in Figure 6.24 as area 2.

The origin of the medial and lateral dorsal cutaneous branches from a common dorsal ramus, as outlined above, is in accordance with classical texts and *Nomina Anatomica*. This arrangement is shown on the right side of Figure 6.18. Frequently, instead of a single dorsal ramus, there are separate medial and lateral ones as illustrated on the left side in Figure 6.18.

The lumbar arteries

Four lumbar arteries arise on each side opposite the bodies of the upper four lumbar vertebrae in series with the posterior intercostal arteries. The lumbar branches of the iliolumbar arteries take the place of a fifth pair of vessels. The lumbar arteries run laterally into the gaps between adjacent transverse processes, and then continue into the abdominal wall, piercing the posterior aponeurosis of transversus abdominis at the lateral border of quadratus lumborum to pass forwards between transversus abdominis and internal oblique. They give off dorsal rami analogous with those of the intercostals which terminate in medial and lateral cutaneous branches. The lateral cutaneous branches are large and after supplying the paravertebral musculature, pierce the thoracolumbar fascia to reach overlying skin (area 4 in Fig. 6.24). Many of the cutaneous twigs run back medially to anastomose with the medial dorsal cutaneous branches (area 3 in Fig. 6.24).

The lateral sacral arteries

These, by their posterior branches, supply all the skin lying between the midline and an oblique line joining the posterior superior iliac spine and the coccyx. The medial branches are very small whilst the lateral ones are larger and lie along this oblique line.

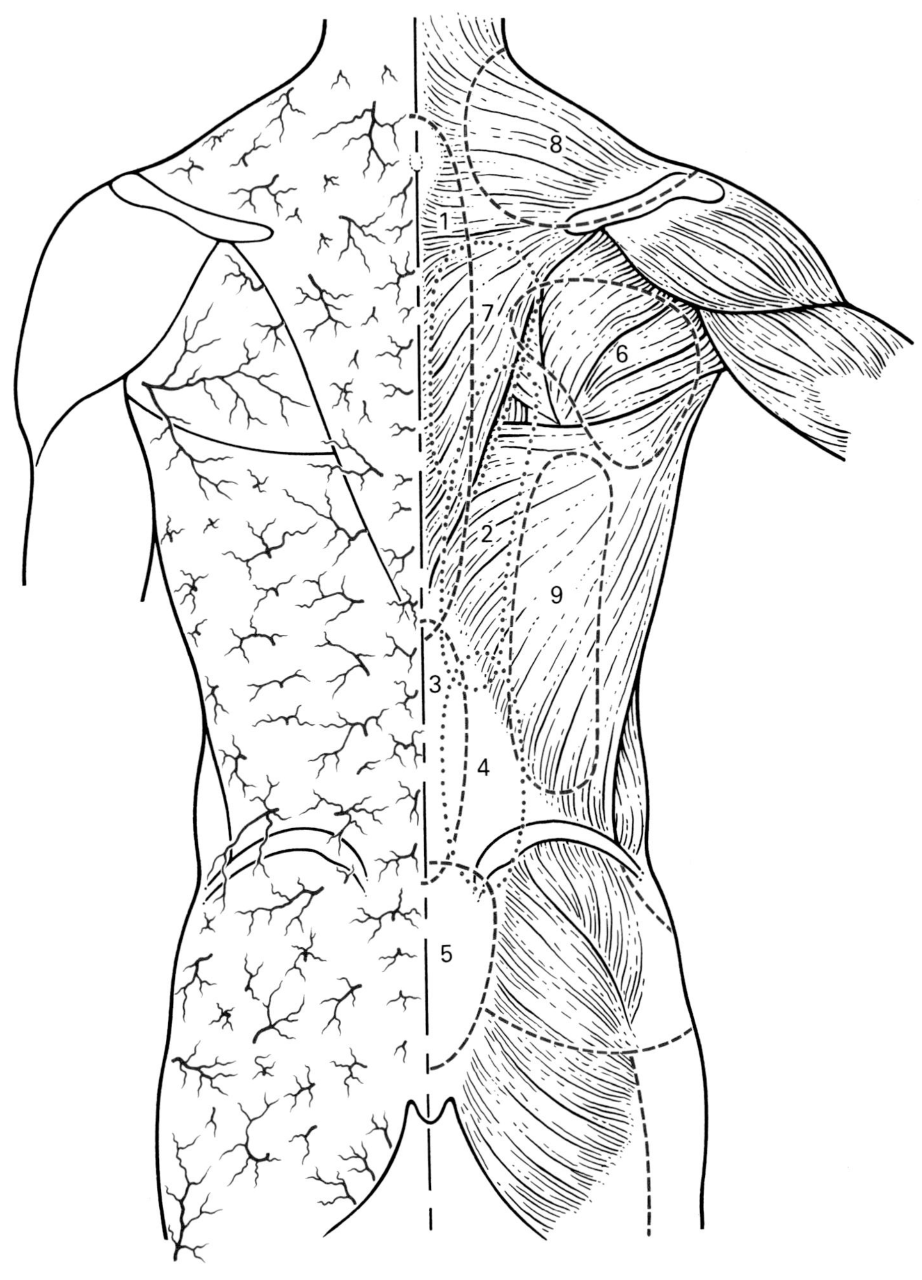

Fig. 6.24 Dorsal trunk – anatomical territories of cutaneous blood supply.
1. Intercostal arteries – medial dorsal cutaneous branches,
2. Intercostal arteries – lateral dorsal cutaneous branches,
3. Lumbar arteries – medial dorsal cutaneous branches,
4. Lumbar arteries – lateral dorsal cutaneous branches,
5. Sacral arteries,
6. Circumflex scapular artery – horizontal and parascapular branches,
7. Deep branch of transverse cervical artery/dorsal scapular artery,
8. Superficial branch of transverse cervical artery/superficial cervical artery,
9. Musculocutaneous perforators through latissimus dorsi arising from the intercostal and lumbar arteries.

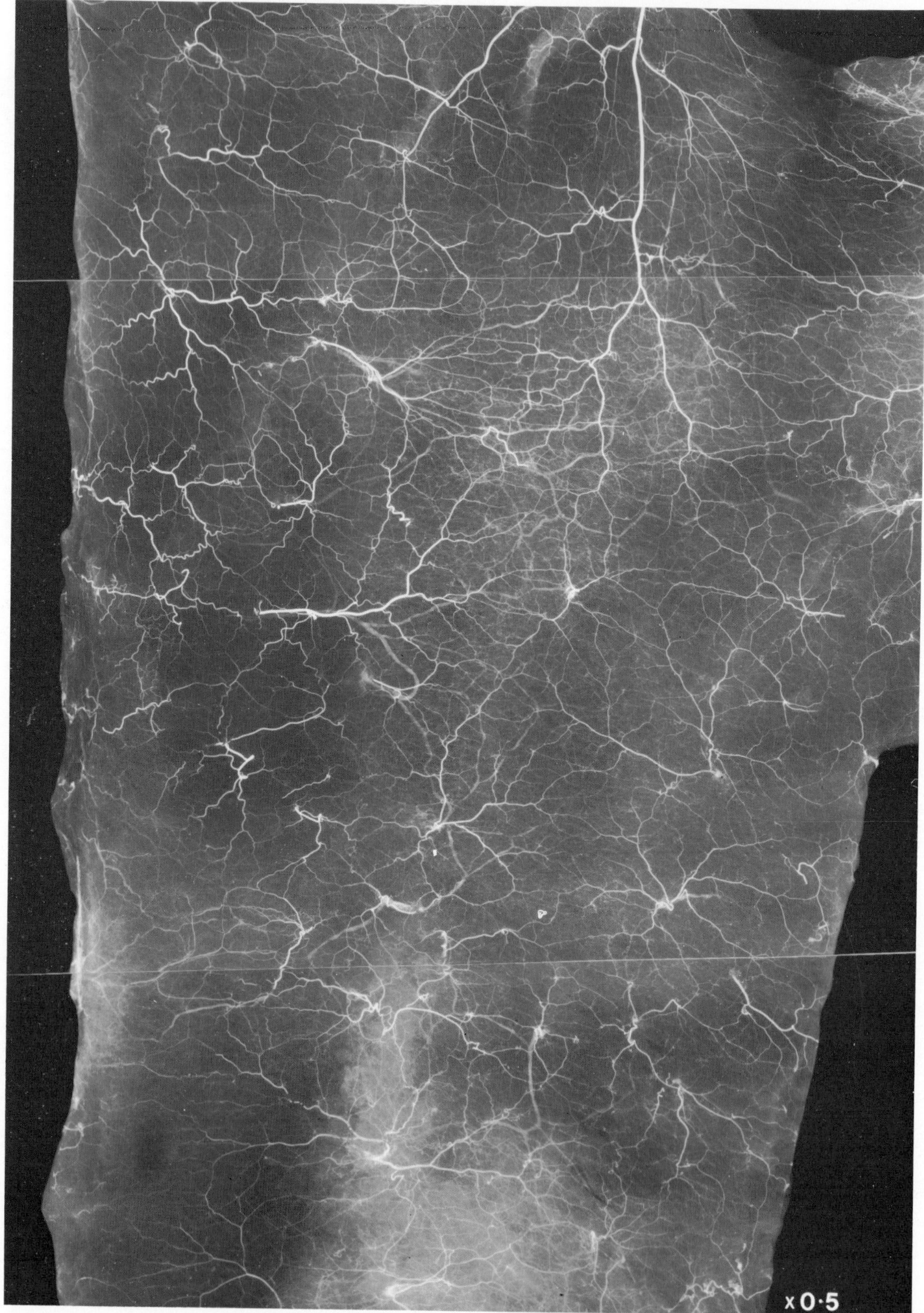

Fig. 6.25 Radiograph of skin and subcutaneous tissues from the right side of the dorsal trunk. Upper margin of the specimen lies approximately at the level of the scapular spine, lower margin at the level of the iliac crest. Left margin along midline overlying spinous processes. Note dorsal cutaneous branches of intercostal arteries and branches of circumflex scapular artery.

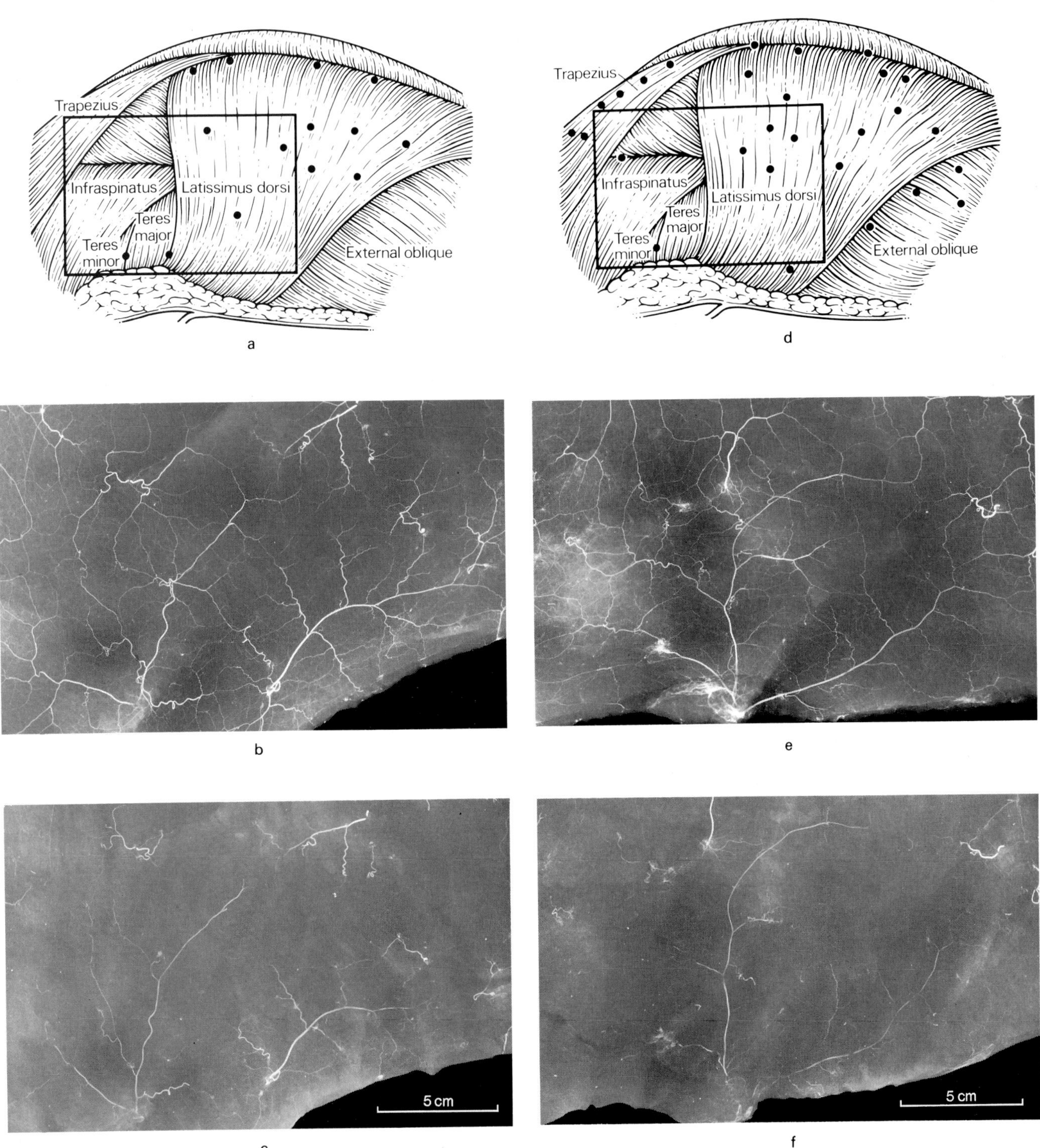

Fig. 6.26 **a.** Tracing of a photograph of the posterolateral chest wall of a cadaver after removal of the overlying tissues which are illustrated in b and c. Dots indicate the sites of major perforators. **b.** Radiograph of skin, fat and 'deep fascia' overlying the rectangle in a. Note the horizontal and parascapular branches of the circumflex scapular artery emerging above and below teres major. **c.** Radiograph of the deep fascia alone after it had been dissected off the specimen X-rayed in figure b. Note the vessels running at the level of the deep fascia. **d.** Tracing of a photograph of the posterolateral chest wall of a cadaver after removal of the overlying tissues which are illustrated in e and f. Dots indicate the sites of major perforators. **e.** Radiograph of skin, fat and deep fascia overlying the rectangle shown in d. This illustrates a more common pattern of vessels than that shown in b. **f.** Radiograph of the deep fascia after it had been dissected off the specimen X-rayed in figure e.

DORSO-LATERAL TRUNK (Figs 6.24–6.26)

This area lies between the mid-scapular and mid-axillary lines and reaches from acromion to iliac crest. It is supplied superiorly by the superficial branch of the transverse cervical artery/superficial cervical artery over the shoulder tip and inferiorly by musculocutaneous branches of the intercostals and by posterior branches of lateral intercostal and lumbar perforators. In between there is an area supplied by branches of the circumflex scapular artery, and by musculocutaneous branches of the thoracodorsal artery which pierce the surface of latissimus dorsi.

The superficial branch of the transverse cervical artery

This is the principal vessel of supply of the lateral part of trapezius and, via its musculocutaneous perforators, forms the vascular basis of the lateral trapezius musculocutaneous flap, with myo-osteo-cutaneous capability if a portion of the acromion is taken with the muscle. The posterior extent of this vessel's anatomical territory is indicated in Figure 6.24 whilst the potential territory of the flap is described on page 484.

Intercostal arteries

Both the intercostal artery and its collateral branch give off muscular branches to the intercostal muscles, and some branches penetrate the overlying latissimus dorsi. In the posterior part of the intercostal space the intercostal artery gives off a lateral cutaneous branch which runs forwards for 2 or 3 cm with the lateral cutaneous branch of the respective intercostal nerve below it, and a vein of similar diameter above it. Together both nerve and artery pierce the intercostal muscles, emerge between the interdigitations of serratus anterior and external oblique, and divide into anterior and posterior rami. This division frequently takes place beneath the deep fascia with the anterior and posterior branches diverging before piercing the deep fascia at points 2 or 3 cm apart. This situation is seen in Figure 6.30. The posterior branches contribute to the blood supply of the dorso-lateral region. Whilst this is the general scheme and is illustrated in Figures 6.27 to 6.31, there are a number of variations:

1. The lateral branches reaching skin in the third, fourth and fifth intercostal spaces may be so small as to be insignificant.
2. In the lower intercostal spaces the lateral branches are generally larger but one or more may be absent in which case the perforator of an immediately adjacent space compensates for its deficiency.

Circumflex scapular artery

In the upper part of the dorso-lateral area there are two significant cutaneous branches from the circumflex scapular artery. These emerge along the fascial space between teres major below, teres minor above and the long head of triceps laterally (the medial 'triangular space' of anatomical texts). The upper or horizontal branch, so named after its course, runs in a medial direction parallel to the spine of the scapula. The lower branch has been named the cutaneous parascapular artery after its course in an inferomedial direction parallel to the lateral border of the scapula. Both of these vessels may be up to 8 cm in length although the parascapular is the more constant of the two. Both fulfil the criteria for fasciocutaneous perforators as they reach the surface by passing up between adjacent muscle bellies and then fan out *at the level of the deep fascia*. This can be clearly seen by comparing radiographs of injected skin and fascia with radiographs of fascia alone from this area (Fig. 6.26). Occasionally the parascapular artery emerges from below teres major (e.g. Fig.6.26a–c). The terminal branches of these fasciocutaneous vessels anastomose at the subcuticular level with musculocutaneous perforators emerging from latissimus dorsi.

Thoracodorsal artery

This contributes to the supply of the dorsolateral area but is described fully below.

THE LATERAL TRUNK (Figs 6.27 & 6.28)

This region extends from the mid-scapular line to the anterior axillary line. Inferiorly it is bounded by the iliac crest. Down to the level of the fifth or sixth rib the skin is supplied by branches of the axillary artery, namely the thoracodorsal and lateral thoracic vessels, and below this level by intercostal and lumbar artery perforators.

The thoracodorsal artery

This arises where the subscapular artery divides, within 3–4 cm of its origin from the third part of the axillary artery, into thoracodorsal and circumflex scapular arteries. (The subscapular artery may arise from the axillary as a common trunk with the posterior circumflex humeral in about 30% of cases.) The thoracodorsal artery together with the thoracodorsal nerve forms the principal neuro-vascular pedicle of the latissimus dorsi muscle and the skin over the upper part of this muscle is supplied by musculocutaneous perforators arising from branches of the artery. It is a significant practical point that one of these branches lies in a constant position 2.5 cm behind the anterior border of the muscle and runs parallel to this free edge. The thoracodorsal artery, shortly before entering the latissimus, may send up to three branches to the serratus anterior. When present, these vessels are 1–2 mm in diameter and are usually accompanied by two veins. Flow rate measurements in the thoracodorsal artery and its branches to the latissimus dorsi and serratus anterior muscles have been carried out. Approximately 50 $cm^3.min^{-1}$ was the average flow in the thoracodorsal artery, 27 $cm^3.min^{-1}$ in the latissimus branch, and 22 $cm^3.min^{-1}$ in the serratus branch (Fisher et al, 1983). After division of the thoracodorsal artery, reverse flow in the serratus anterior branch has been observed with a flow rate into the latissimus of 25 $cm^3.min^{-1}$. This serratus anterior collateral may become significant in supplying blood to the latissimus muscle and its overlying skin when the thoracodorsal artery has been divided during the course of an axillary dissection carried out as part of a mastectomy. In 28 patients with a ligated thoracodorsal artery, who underwent latissimus musculocutaneous flap reconstructions of the breast with serratus collateral as the vascular support, one flap was lost and four flaps became ischaemic at the distal end. The authors attributed the ischaemic tips to incorrect orientation of the skin island which was either too horizontal or encroaching too far on thoracolumbar fascia, since, as indicated above, the main intramuscular vessels and the largest musculocutaneous perforators of the latissimus are orientated in the lateral region of the muscle. A further, but less significant, possible source of collateral supply to latissimus comes from the circumflex scapular and dorsal scapular vessels reaching teres major. No significant vessels have been noted entering latissimus through its tendon of insertion.

Whilst these details do not significantly affect the supply to the skin in the normal individual, they do become significant when considering post-mastectomy reconstruction with a local latissimus flap in the presence of a ligated thoracodorsal artery. Such a secondary procedure would need to be carried out after a sufficient time interval had elapsed to allow the collaterals to develop. Note also that in the presence of a ligated thoracodorsal artery the blood supply to the muscle from segmental posterior intercostal perforators would also be expected to increase, and significantly more skin would become dependent upon them for blood supply. This fact might account for the greater propensity of the horizontal skin islands described above to undergo ischaemic necrosis at their medial tip.

The serratus branches may also be of use in the construction of a latissimus free flap as they enable a short T-junction to be created at the end of the arterial pedicle which may be advantageous when anastomosing the flap pedicle onto the recipient vessels in certain sites. Double flaps, consisting of latissimus dorsi and part of serratus anterior – perhaps with an attached rib segment – may therefore be carried on a single pedicle.

Cutaneous branch of the thoracodorsal artery

This is present in about 75% of cases (Cabanié et al, 1980). Rowsell et al (1984) have also observed a cutaneous artery in this region in 81% of 100 cadaver dissections, but found that it arose from the thoracodorsal artery in only 47%; in the remainder it arose from the subscapular (27%) and axillary (7%) arteries. It lies just anterior to the lateral edge of latissimus dorsi, running parallel and posterior to the lateral thoracic artery with which it may make several communications (one proximally and often another one more distally). It arises either very close to the origin of the thoracodorsal artery, even from the subscapular, or, and more commonly, rather further distally. The distance to the point of origin, measured from the axillary artery, has been found to vary between 0.5 and 7.0 cm. When this cutaneous branch is absent the territory is taken over by extension of latissimus musculocutaneous perforators, by serratus anterior perforators and by the lateral thoracic artery.

The lateral thoracic artery

This artery arises in 40% of cases from the second part of the axillary artery and in 60% of cases in common with one of the other axillary branches, usually the subscapular or the thoraco-acromial. It follows the lateral border of pectoralis minor to the side of the thorax, and supplies pectoralis minor, pectoralis major, serratus anterior, subscapularis and skin. Note that it never runs, as has been illustrated in some texts, with the long thoracic nerve although it gives off a branch to the anterior part of serratus anterior which may accompany the nerve. The lateral thoracic artery generally runs no further than the fifth interspace and gives off several branches to the skin which pass round the lateral border of pectoralis major and contribute significantly to the blood supply of the female breast (rami mammarii laterales of *Nomina Anatomica*). Although this represents the classical description it is worth noting that there are numerous variations on this theme:

1. The lateral thoracic may be completely replaced by lateral perforating branches of the intercostals.
2. It may pierce the deep fascia in the region of the 4th rib and itself become cutaneous.
3. It may give off (12% of cases in one study), a major direct cutaneous branch which runs obliquely antero-inferiorly in the subcutaneous tissues.
4. This may communicate with a cutaneous branch of the thoracodorsal artery.

Confusion may occur with the superficial thoracic artery which is described below.

Several different 'axillary' flaps have been described but confusion is inevitable, given the many variations, and one is often uncertain as to precisely what the flap is based on. However, it is clear that the blood supply to the skin in this area is generous and exposure of the area may reveal a significant direct cutaneous vessel rather than multiple perforators from the lateral thoracic. Flaps in this area are described on pages 371 & 478.

It should be noted that this lateral thoracic artery is not the same as the one described by Quain, Tiedemann, Henle and other anatomists. Their vessel was an anomaly, derived from the internal thoracic close to its origin from the subclavian, and passing inside the chest between the parietal pleura and the ribs, sending branches into the first to fifth intercostal spaces, and sometimes reaching as far as the diaphragm. In 1905 Bean described five instances of this vessel in 25 cases (50 sides) in which it was looked for and the vessel was then ignored until 1951 (Kropp) and later 1982 when Nathan et al reported finding 13 examples of what they termed the *accessory internal thoracic artery* among a sample of 120 internal thoracic arteries dissected (10.8%). The importance of a knowledge of this vessel lies in correct interpretation of angiograms since on a PA view this vessel might be misinterpreted as a cutaneous branch of the internal thoracic.

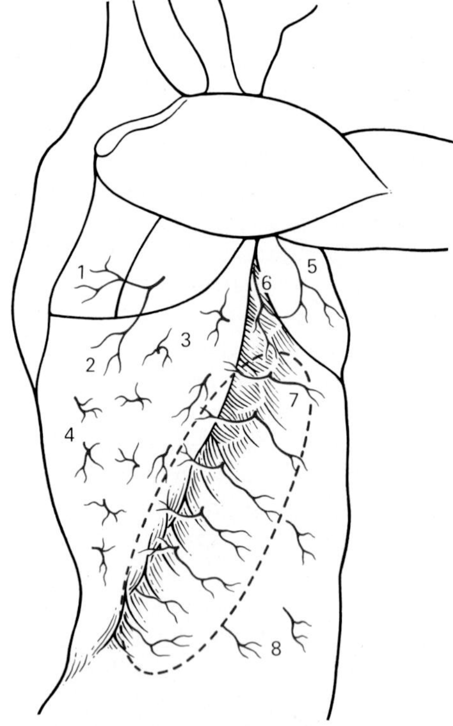

Fig. 6.27 The vessels of the lateral trunk:
1. Horizontal cutaneous branch of the circumflex scapular artery,
2. Parascapular cutaneous branch of the circumflex scapular artery,
3. Perforators from the thoracodorsal artery,
4. Perforators from intercostal arteries – lateral dorsal cutaneous branches,
5. Superficial thoracic artery or a cutaneous branch of the lateral thoracic artery,
6. Cutaneous branch of the thoracodorsal artery,
7. Lateral perforating branches of intercostal and lumbar arteries,
8. Cutaneous perforators from muscular branches of intercostal and lumbar arteries.

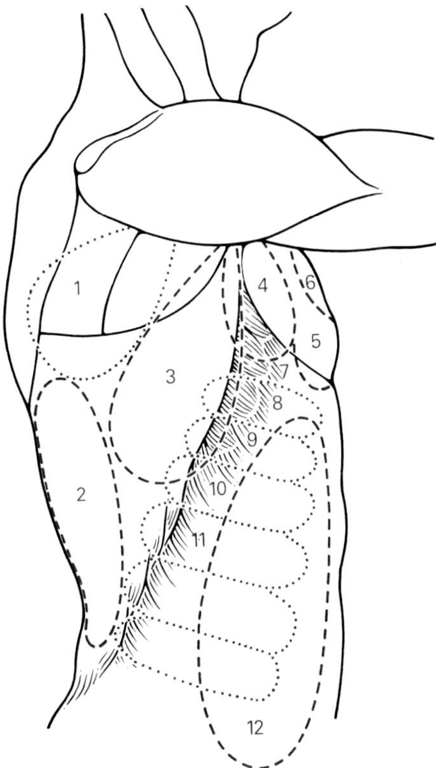

Fig. 6.28 Anatomical territories of cutaneous blood supply:
1. Circumflex scapular artery territory,
2. Musculocutaneous perforators from the 'costal groove' segment of the intercostals, and from lumbar arteries,
3. Thoracodorsal artery, muscular branch to latissimus dorsi,
4. Cutaneous branch of thoracodorsal and lateral thoracic arteries,
5. Thoraco-acromial axis,
6. Internal thoracic artery,

7–11. Lateral cutaneous branches of intercostal arteries,

12. Musculocutaneous perforators through external oblique from the intercostal arteries.

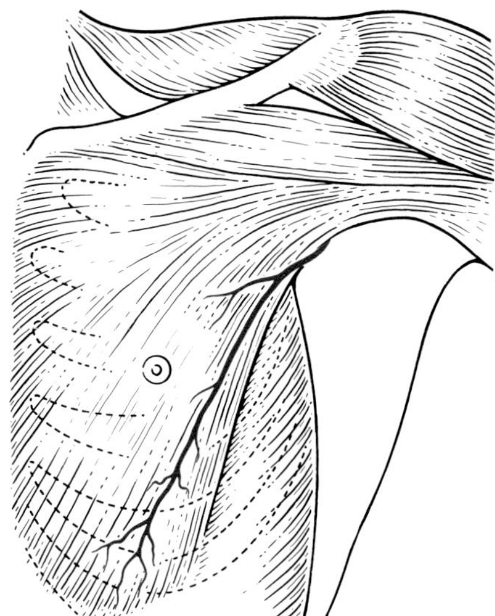

Fig. 6.29 A diagram to illustrate the position of the superficial thoracic artery which lies superficial to the lateral part of pectoralis major and supplies skin. This vessel should not be confused with the lateral thoracic artery which lies deeper and more posteriorly – it supplies the lateral chest wall, pectoralis minor and the anterior part of serratus anterior. An example of the superficial thoracic artery can be seen in Figure 6.17.

The superficial thoracic artery

This was named by Manchot (A. thoracica superficialis) and had been previously described under a variety of names. It is a cutaneous artery which lies in front of the lateral part of pectoralis major and may be the dominant vessel over the anterolateral chest in both males and females (Fig. 6.29). It occurs much more frequently than classical anatomy texts would suggest and is perhaps the cutaneous vessel found arising from the axillary artery by Rowsell et al (1984) in 7% of cases. It arises from the distal part of the axillary artery or proximal part of the brachial artery in the 5 cm segment related to the lower border of the tendon of insertion of pectoralis major. It may extend down to the sixth intercostal space. Figure 6.17 shows such a vessel with an internal diameter of 1.5 mm extending for 26 cm down the anterior chest wall. Salmon (1936) also described it arising from the lateral thoracic artery (probably variation 3 described above), or the subscapular, but does not seem to have encountered a specimen in excess of 8 cm in length. Our longest vessel of 26 cm is in accordance with the findings of some of the older anatomical texts. Contemporary texts either ignore this vessel or misrepresent it as the lateral thoracic artery.

The intercostal arteries

These arteries give off lateral cutaneous branches which have already been described in so far as their posterior branches contribute to the blood supply of the dorsolateral trunk. Their anterior branches are given off either before or after the lateral branch crosses the deep fascia and run antero-inferiorly, for a distance of 2–4 cm, along the direction of the fibres of external oblique in company with the lateral cutaneous nerves and then fan out in the subcutis. Although a general scheme is identifiable, it is rare for contiguous vessels to have equal-sized territories and great variation is normally seen. Indeed, the lateral cutaneous branch itself is inconsistent and is often replaced by several large musculocutaneous perforators. The territories shown in Figure 6.28 are therefore somewhat artificial. In the third, fourth and fifth interspaces the vessels are so small as to be insignificant. In the lower spaces the perforators are larger but one or more may be absent in which case the perforator in the immediately adjacent space above or below compensates for the deficiency. In addition, there are three or four musculocutaneous perforators through external oblique arising from intercostal, subcostal and lumbar arteries.

Nakajima et al (1981) studied the anatomical territories of the sixth to twelfth intercostal arteries using in vivo prostaglandin E_1 injection techniques. The vessels of adjacent territories were not interfered with and therefore the vascular equilibria were largely undisturbed although theoretically it is possible that the vasodilatation induced by the PGE_1 may have produced a slight shift in the location of the 'watersheds'. The territory of each intercostal artery was found, over the anterolateral trunk, to correspond in shape to the respective underlying intercostal space and, in addition, the anterior margin of the territory extended across the costal arch for a short distance. The territory of the sixth intercostal artery was overlapped by the area of supply of the thoracodorsal artery.

Badran et al (1984) have studied the territories of single intercostal arteries in the cadaver by the injection of dyes. (The collateral arteries and the nutrient arteries to the ribs had been ligated.) They found that the territories of the tenth and eleventh posterior intercostal arteries extended from the paravertebral line posteriorly to the lateral border of the rectus sheath anteriorly with an average width of 4.3 interspaces. The medial border occasionally extended over rectus abdominis and sometimes past the midline. The ninth intercostal artery had a slightly smaller territory (3.9 interspaces wide and a smaller incidence of dye extension beyond the semilunar line). The subcostal artery was absent in 5%, but was replaced by a branch from the eleventh intercostal artery. Its cutaneous territory did not reach the semilunar line in most cases, but descended to the anterior superior iliac spine. Selective dye injection of the lateral cutaneous artery stained a skin territory similar to that produced by injection of the posterior intercostal artery except that the posterior extent was less and its anterior extent always stopped at the lateral border of the rectus abdominis. Clearly, in these experiments dye penetrated well beyond the margins of the anatomical territories.

Rectangular flaps of skin (7 cm × 20 cm) orientated parallel to the fibres of external oblique and based on the lateral perforating branches of the intercostal, subcostal and lumbar arteries have been raised (Fisher, 1983). These flaps demonstrate good vascularity when raised right up to the lateral margin of rectus abdominis. Because these flaps also included the fascia they have been termed fasciocutaneous flaps but it should be noted that these lateral perforators pass

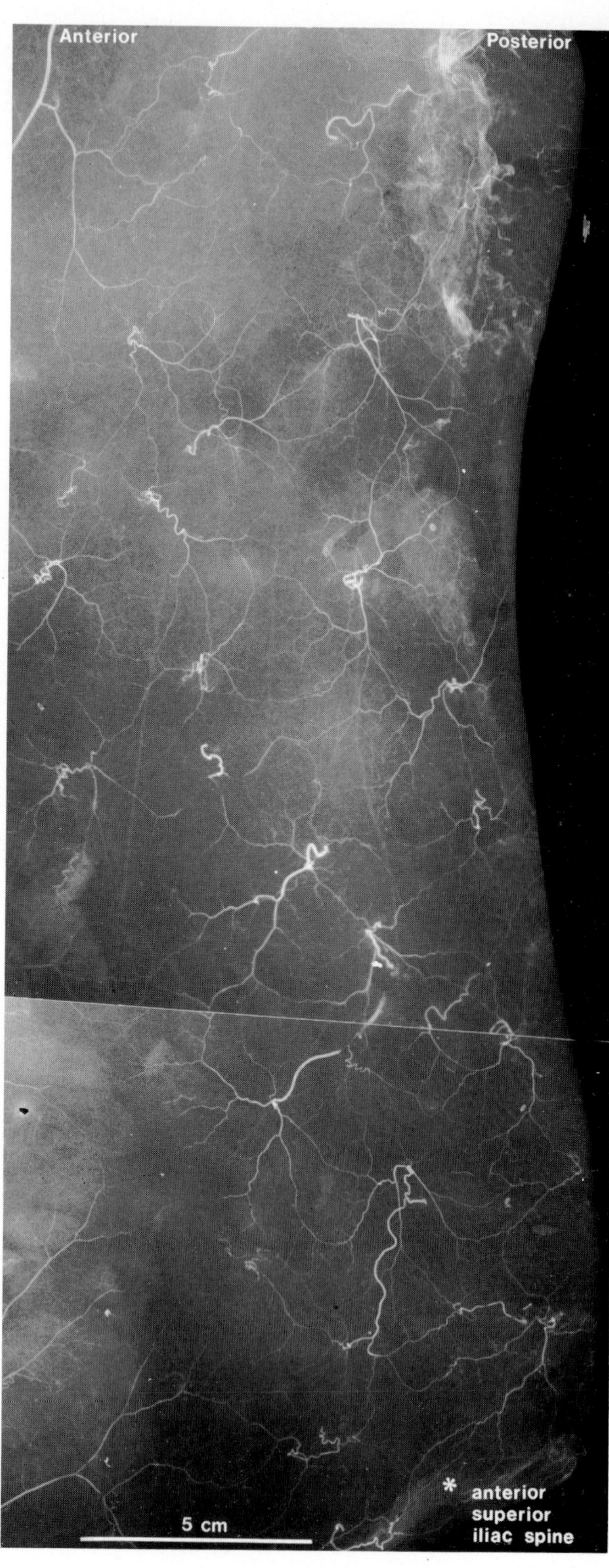

Fig. 6.30 Radiograph of lateral cutaneous branches. In this specimen the lateral cutaneous branches divided into anterior and posterior terminations whilst still lying deeply between the muscles so that they appear separated by 2 to 4 centimetres in the skin specimen.

obliquely through the fascia for only a couple of centimetres at the very most and continue their course in the subcutaneous tissues. Essentially it is musculocutaneous vessels which supply this flap but the muscle is not elevated.

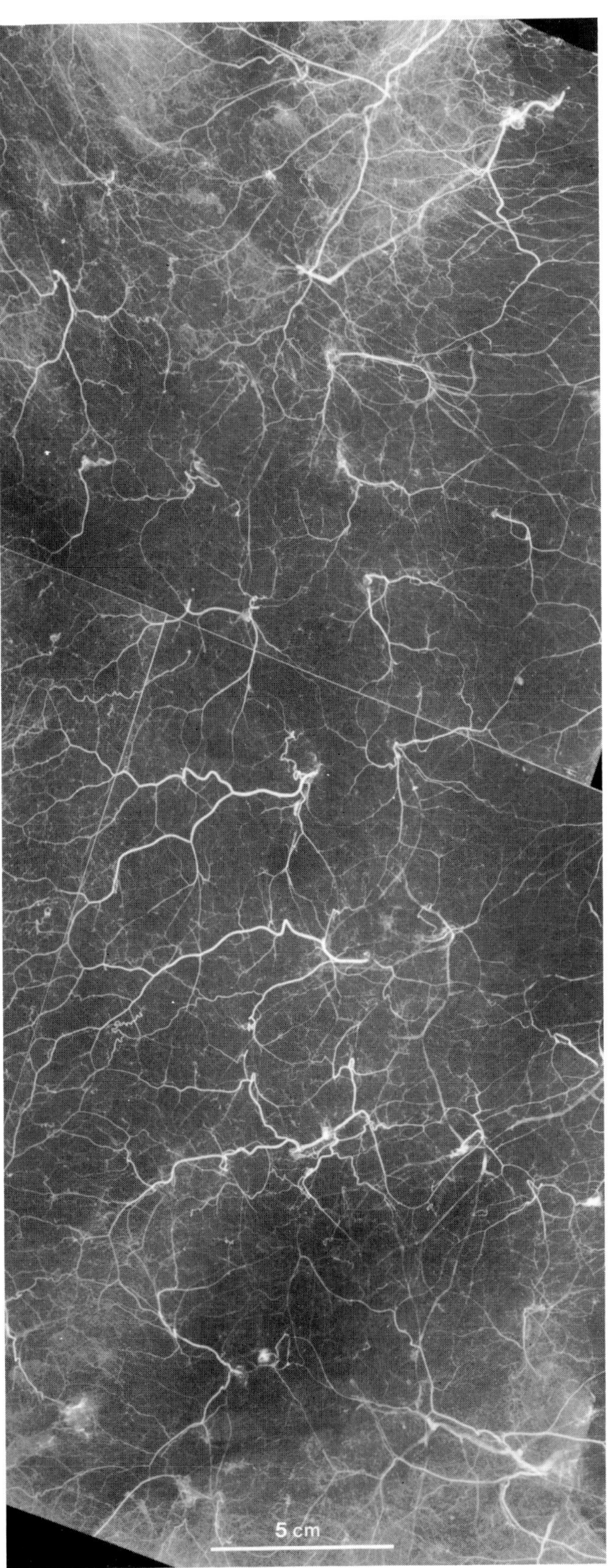

Fig. 6.31 Radiograph of lateral cutaneous branches.

ANTERIOR TRUNK

This region is defined superiorly by the clavicles, inferiorly by the inguinal ligaments and extends laterally as far as the anterior axillary lines. It may include the female breast.

Over the thorax the skin is supplied, on each side, by the thoraco-acromial axis, the lateral thoracic artery, the internal thoracic artery and the intercostal arteries. Over the abdomen the arteries involved are the deep superior and inferior epigastrics (together forming the epigastric arcade), the superficial superior and inferior epigastrics, the superficial and deep circumflex iliacs, and abdominal branches of the superficial external pudendal artery. The vessels will be described in this order.*

The thoraco-acromial axis

This arises from the second part of the axillary artery, passes round the medial margin of pectoralis minor tendon, pierces the clavipectoral fascia and divides classically into four branches – acromial, clavicular, deltoid and pectoral. These supply the anterior part of deltoid, pectoralis minor, pectoralis major and the skin in the region over the clavipectoral fascia (Figs 6.33 & 6.34). The pectoral branch is the largest and sends a small vessel to pectoralis minor before continuing on the deep surface of pectoralis major within its epimyseal sheath. The vessel penetrates the muscle and anastomoses within it with branches of the perforators of the internal thoracic artery which have passed through the medial ends of the intercostal spaces. Anastomoses may also occur with branches of the lateral thoracic artery. Musculocutaneous perforators are given off which supply overlying skin. Additionally, in up to approximately 60% of cases, the acromial or deltoid branches of the thoraco-acromial axis have been found to give off a major direct cutaneous vessel which spreads out in the subcutaneous fat for a variable distance but rarely more than 10 cm across the chest and 7.5 cm below the clavicle. Its branches anastomose with those

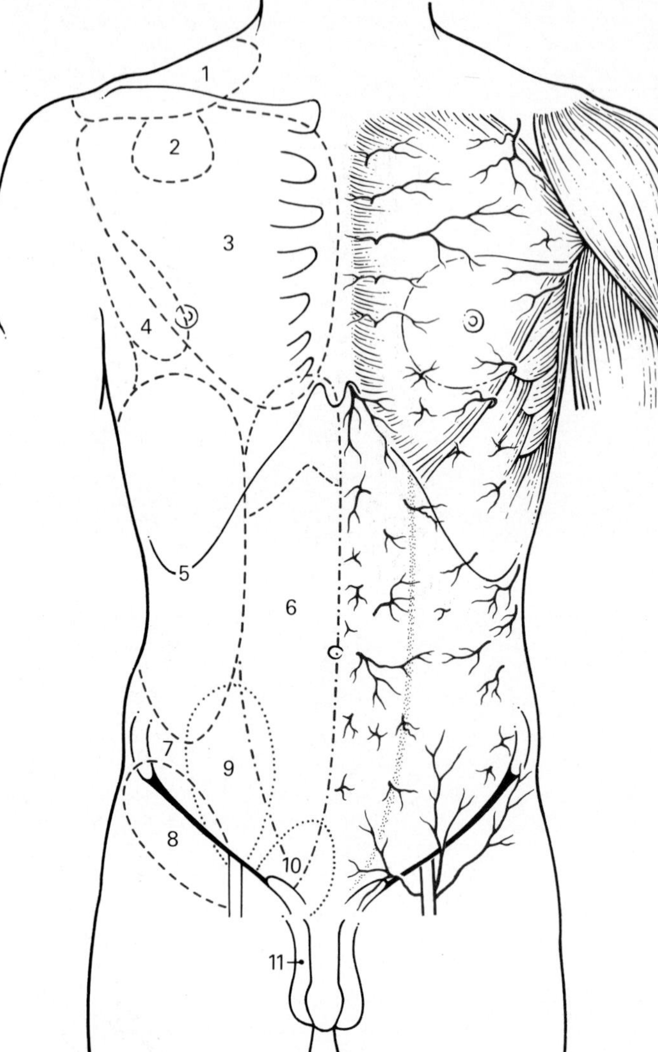

Fig. 6.32 Anterior trunk – anatomical territories of cutaneous blood supply:

1. Transverse cervical artery,
2. Direct cutaneous branch of the thoraco-acromial axis,
3. Anterior perforators from the internal thoracic artery,
4. Superficial thoracic artery,
5. Intercostal perforators,
6. Perforators from the epigastric arcades (the small subdivision at the upper end of this territory is for the infrequently occurring superficial superior epigastric artery),
7. Possible contribution from deep circumflex iliac artery,
8. Superficial circumflex iliac artery,
9. Superficial inferior epigastric artery,
10. Superficial external pudendal artery,
11. Deep external pudendal artery.

Note: In this area more than in any other there exists the greatest range in development of vessels between individuals. The territories of the direct cutaneous vessels are particularly subject to variation and the figure above represents a hypothetical situation in which these vessels show moderate development. In some instances the vessels are absent and in others they are particularly well developed.

* A scheme of division of the anterior abdominal wall into three zones has been used by certain authors. These zones are:
Zone I – Xiphoid to pubis between the lateral borders of both recti; supplied by the epigastric arcades.
Zone II – The area defined superiorly by a line between the anterior superior iliac spines, and inferiorly by the groin and pubic creases; supplied by the superficial inferior epigastrics, the external pudendals and the deep inferior epigastrics.
Zone III – The lateral abdomen and flanks; supplied by lumbar, subcostal and intercostal branches.
This scheme has no particular merits and is not used here.

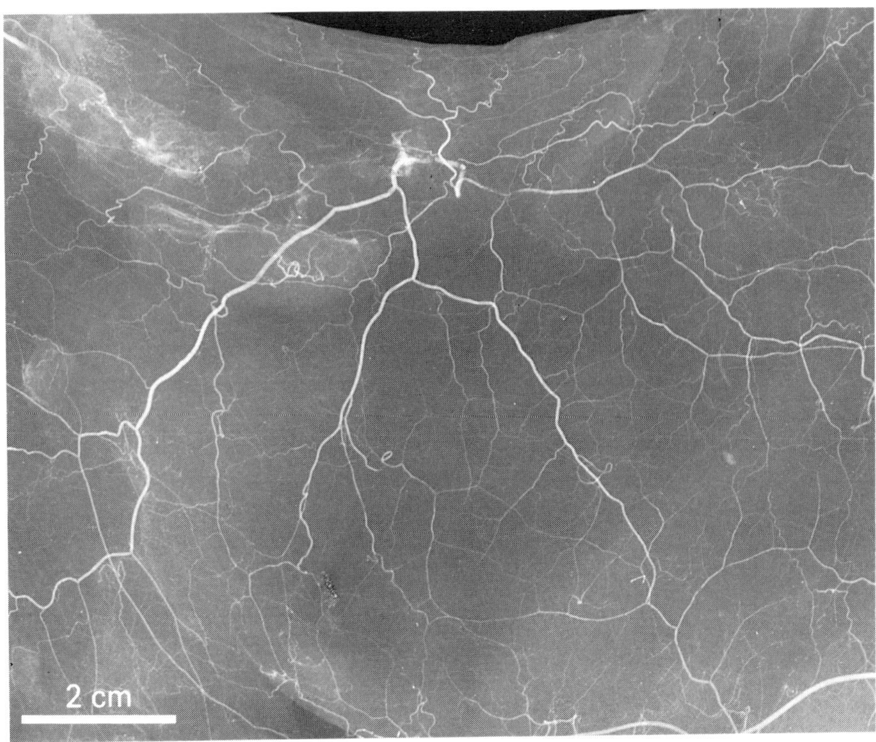

Fig. 6.33 Radiograph of direct cutaneous branch of the thoraco-acromial axis.

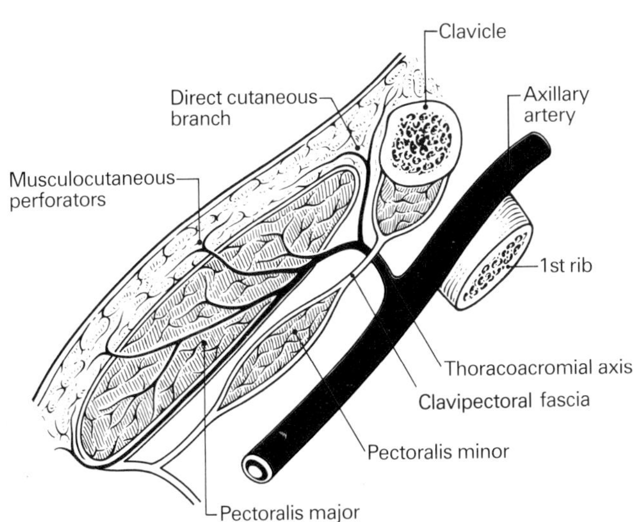

Fig. 6.34 A schematic view of the thoraco-acromial axis and its relationship to the clavipectoral fascia. It pierces the fascia and divides into its four terminal branches of which only the pectoral branch is shown. The pectoral branch is the principal vessel of supply to pectoralis major and sends musculocutaneous perforators to the overlying skin, its terminal branches turn round the lower lateral border of pectoralis major. The thoraco-acromial axis may also send direct cutaneous branches to the skin over the infraclavicular fossa as shown.

of the second and third intercostal perforators from the internal thoracic artery. Variation in the manner of branching of the thoraco-acromial axis has been studied by Reid & Taylor (1984) in over 100 cadavers (see pp. 467 & 470).

The lateral thoracic artery

This arises from the second part of the axillary artery, turns round the lateral margin of the tendon of pectoralis minor and follows the lateral border of the muscle for 4 or 5 cm before running along the undersurface of pectoralis major. Here it communicates with the pectoral branch of the thoraco-acromial artery and via perforators which pass round the lateral border of pectoralis major contributes the major blood supply to the lateral part of the female breast. In cadaver injections of the thoraco-acromial axis some of the medium may pass along the anastomoses between the pectoral branch and the lateral thoracic artery, filling the cutaneous branches of the latter.

The internal thoracic artery

This generally arises alone from the first part of the subclavian artery (or from the thyrocervical trunk in 5–10%), and passes down inside the chest approximately 1.5 cm lateral to the edge of the sternum (Table 6.2). Intercostal branches are given off to the intercostal spaces usually as single vessels which divide to send one branch to the superior part and another to the inferior part of each space. Alternatively the anterior intercostal branches arise posterior to the costal cartilages, sending one branch above and the other below the adjacent rib, or there may be two separate intercostal branches given off by the internal thoracic to each space. Any two or all three of these arrangements may be found on one side of a subject, and the chances of the internal thoracic giving off one branch or two are about equal. These branches anastomose with corresponding posterior intercostal arteries and their collateral branches in each space. The internal thoracic gives off pericardiacophrenic, mediastinal, pericardial and sternal branches as well as the perforating branches which are so important in the supply of skin. These perforating branches emerge through the upper five or six intercostal spaces, in the company of the anterior cutaneous branches of the corresponding intercostal nerves. They enter pectoralis major, supplying the muscle and anastomosing with ramifications of the pectoral branch of the thoraco-acromial axis within the muscle. They then pierce the surface of pectoralis major and run laterally in the subcutaneous fat as direct cutaneous arteries. The perforator in the second space is large in both sexes, but in the female the perforators in the third and fourth spaces are also large since they contribute significantly to the blood supply of the breast.

The internal thoracic artery bifurcates at the sixth space with the *musculophrenic branch* continuing obliquely inferolaterally behind the seventh, eighth and ninth costal cartilages to perforate the diaphragm near the ninth costal cartilage, and end opposite the last intercostal space. It gives off intercostal branches to the seventh, eighth and ninth spaces in a similar way to the internal thoracic, anastomosing with posterior intercostal arteries in these spaces. It also supplies the abdominal muscles and anastomoses with the ascending branch of the deep circumflex iliac artery (the lateral epigastric artery). The other terminal branch is the *deep superior epigastric artery* (vide infra).

Table 6.2 Distance of internal thoracic artery and its anterior perforators from the edge of the sternum (in millimetres). (Adapted from: Adachi; Sandemann; Poirier & Testut)

Intercostal space	Japanese		Europeans	
	mean	*range*	*mean*	*range*
I	8	0→16	11	6→20
II	13	6→19	15	10→20
III	13	5→18	16	10→21
IV	12	6→16	15	8→25

The blood supply of the female breast (Fig. 6.35)

It is obvious that all the vessels on the anterior chest participate in the supply of this structure, but a little further explanation of their relative contributions is desirable. The classical view is that the internal thoracic is the main artery of supply via perforators through the second, third and fourth intercostal spaces. A principal vessel passes through the second or third space and divides into two branches with the superior branch supplying the upper inner quadrant and the other branch passing to the areolar area, both giving off many tortuous branches to the superficial fascia and skin. The adjacent smaller perforators supply the glandular tissue. An equally significant contribution comes from branches of the lateral thoracic artery or from the superficial thoracic artery directly off the axillary. These enter the breast in the upper outer quadrant or when single divide into two branches, superior and inferior, which run superficially within the gland giving branches to the skin. Superiorly there may be an additional contribution from the cutaneous branches of the thoraco-acromial axis. Perforators from the pectoral branch of the thoraco-acromial leave the surface and lateral edge of pectoralis major to supply the glandular tissue. The posterior intercostals do not contribute.

From this description it can be seen that there is a clear correlation between routes of blood supply to the breast and the rather better known routes of lymphatic drainage away from the breast.

The deep epigastric arcade

This is formed within the rectus sheath by the superior and inferior deep epigastric arteries.

The deep superior epigastric branch of the internal thoracic descends between the costal and xiphoid origins of the diaphragm, anterior to the lower fibres of the transversus thoracis and the upper fibres of the transversus abdominis. It enters the sheath of the rectus abdominis usually lying behind the medial third of the muscle (Fig. 6.36). Initially it lies behind the muscle, but then perforates and supplies it. Approximately half-way between xiphoid and umbilicus it anastomoses with the inferior epigastric artery.

The two superior epigastric arteries may communicate superiorly by a small vessel passing in front of the xiphoid process. Some small twigs are also given off superiorly to the diaphragm and into the falciform ligament. The majority of branches, however, either pierce the surface of the muscle or pass round its lateral edge to penetrate the anterior rectus sheath and supply the skin.

The deep inferior epigastric artery leaves the external iliac immediately above the inguinal ligament, ascends obliquely along the medial margin of the deep inguinal ring, and runs forwards in the extraperitoneal tissue (forming the lateral umbilical fold). In passing medially it pierces the transversalis fascia and enters the rectus sheath. Above the level of the umbilicus its terminal divisions form an anastomosis with branches of the superior epigastric artery. This anastomosis varies in its degree of development. The unequal role of the superior and inferior vessels in the supply of rectus abdominis and overlying skin is also demonstrated by the discrepancy in size between the two vessels: the superior epigastric artery averages 1.6 mm in external diameter at its point of origin whereas the inferior measures 3.4 mm. The veins show a similar discrepancy (Boyd et al, 1984).

The vertical channel so formed is termed the epigastric arcade. It lies medial to the points where the lower intercostal nerves penetrate the posterior wall of the rectus sheath to innervate rectus abdominis. Terminal branches of the posterior intercostal arteries accompany these nerves and may anastomose with the epigastric arcade. These anastomoses have a segmental arrangement in that the superior epigastric may give off one or two branches for the seventh and eighth segments which are analogous to the anterior intercostal branches given off by the internal thoracic artery, while the inferior epigastric artery may give off similar branches to the lower four segments (McVay & Anson, 1940). The lateral branches of the epigastric arcades pass through the fibrous semilunar lines into the plane between transversus abdominis and internal oblique. These arteries are accompanied by two veins and lie with the respective intercostal nerve enclosed in a ribbon of fat and connective tissue. In 160 rectus muscle dissections Milloy et al (1960) found that there were 541 arteries leaving the epigastric arcade in a lateral direction, the number per muscle ranging from 0 to 6. Of these 3% did not go beyond the linea

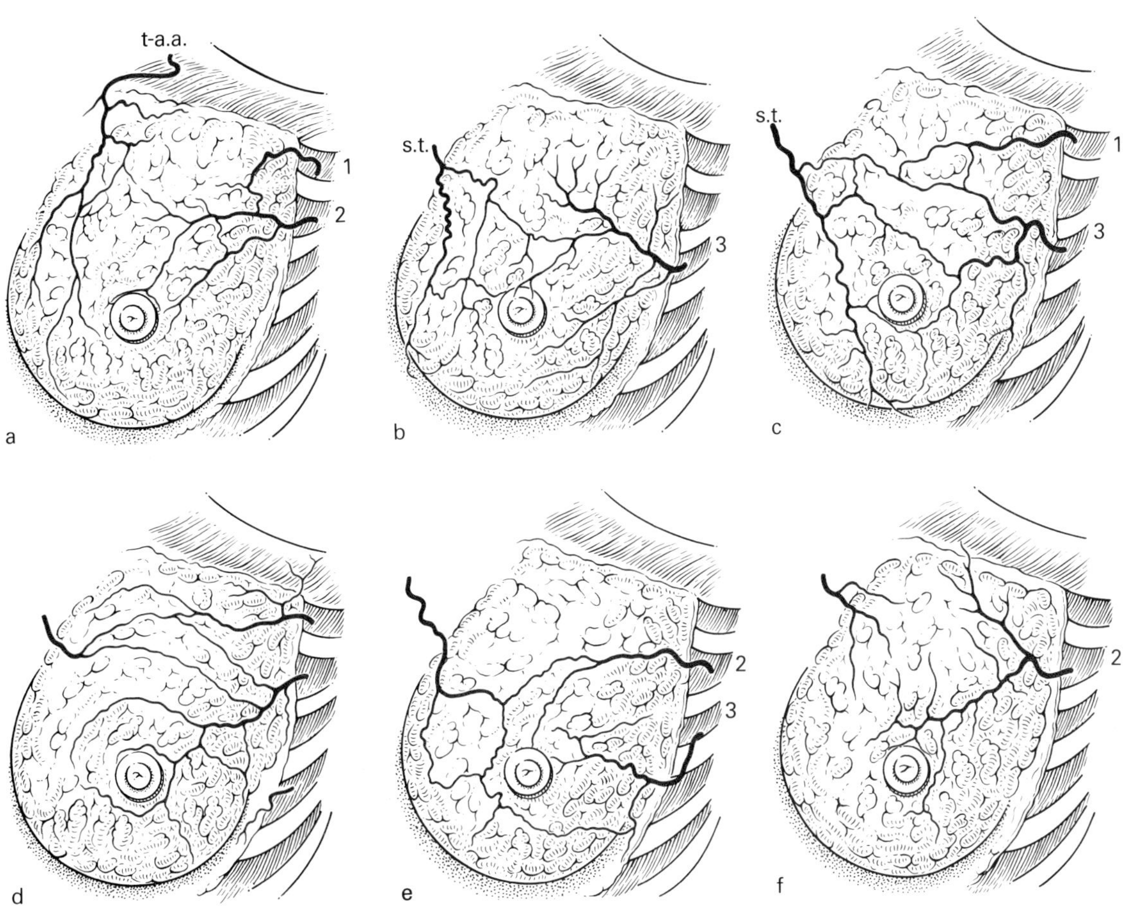

Fig. 6.35 Blood supply of the female breast: **a, b, c, e & f** after Carr et al, 1942. **d** after Anson et al, 1939. t–a.a. thoraco-acromial axis; s.t. superficial thoracic artery.

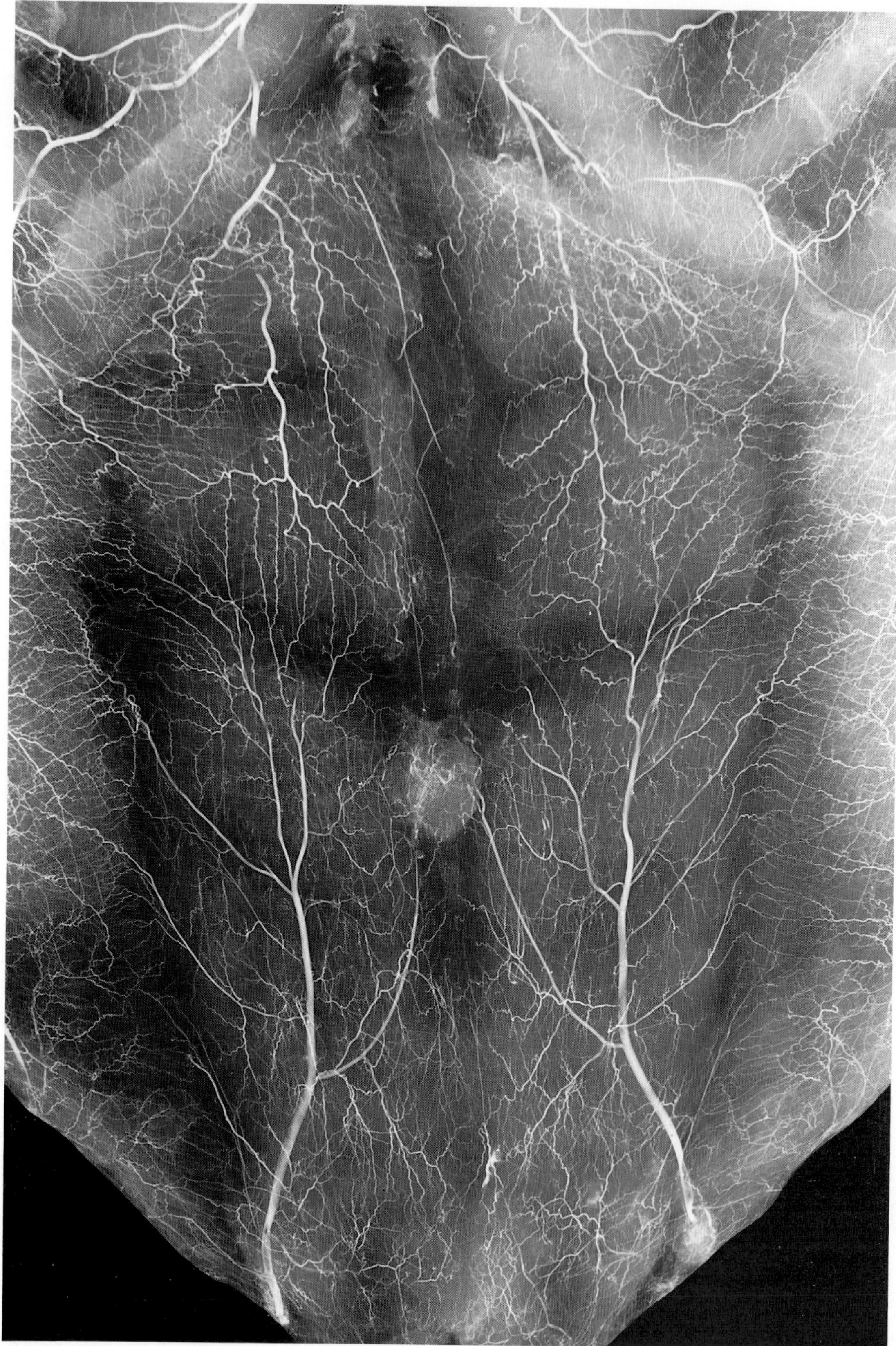

Fig. 6.36 Radiograph of rectus abdominis muscles. The specimen included the entire musculature of the anterior abdominal wall. All overlying tissues and the peritoneum were removed. Note particularly the anastomoses between superior and inferior epigastric arteries and between the epigastric arcades and the intercostal and lumbar vessels at the lateral margins of the rectus sheaths.

semilunaris, 48% passed through the linea semilunaris and entered the lateral abdominal musculature but did not macroscopically anastomose with intercostal arteries, and 15% anastomosed with their respective intercostal arteries or the deep circumflex iliac artery.

Figure 6.37 further amplifies these findings but as can be clearly seen in Figure 6.36, there are numerous anastomoses between vessels too small to see in a dissection. These small vessels have not previously been demonstrated. In these illustrations the arteries have been classified as lying with the fibres of a specific spinal nerve in most instances (although by this stage in the abdominal wall the nerves are beginning to spread out and form a plexus). Figure 6.37a shows that the macroscopic lateral branches from the epigastric arcade were most common in the T10, T11 segments, i.e. at and just below the umbilicus. Figure 6.37b shows what happens to these arteries. Only a small percentage of the T10, T11 segmental arteries actually anastomose in the lateral abdominal wall, whereas all of those lying in the T7 segment do. The vessels which anastomosed with their respective intercostal arteries or the deep circumflex iliac artery, constituted only 15% of the 541 macroscopic lateral branches, indicating that the majority of lateral branches either do not go beyond the linea semilunaris (37%) (these are the cutaneous perforators) or passed through the linea and entered the abdominal musculature (48%). Of the ones that ended in the lateral abdominal musculature the majority had a course of less than 2 cm, whereas the remainder could be followed for 3–6 cm before they terminated in the muscles. The great majority of these vessels radiated from the sheath in a course parallel to that of the nerves at an angle of 45–60° to the midline. These observations are relevant to the raising of posterior intercostal neurovascular island flaps and of extended rectus abdominis musculocutaneous flaps.

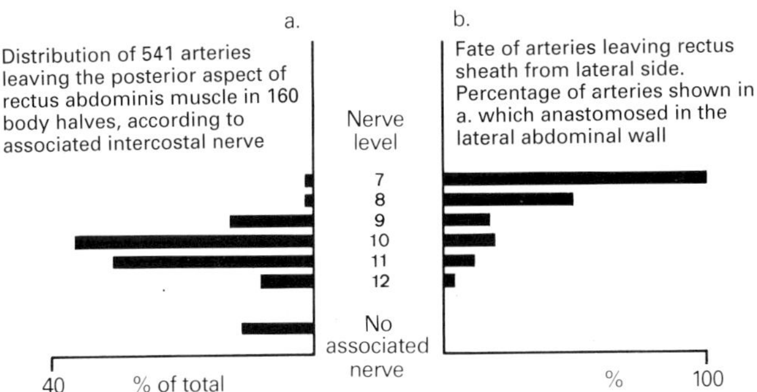

Fig. 6.37 See text for explanation.

The musculocutaneous perforators from the epigastric arcade reaching skin over the recti are a mixture of small and large vessels, with the largest having an internal diameter of up to 1.5 mm. The larger vessels characteristically lie at the level of the umbilicus but large perforators are also to be found below this level. The anastomoses of these perforators are important and are of two kinds: firstly, perforators of the two epigastric arcades definitely communicate across the midline, as can be seen in Figure 6.17. Secondly, perforators overlying the lateral parts of the recti tend to run in a lateral direction where they form significant anastomoses with musculocutaneous perforators of intercostal, subcostal and lumbar vessels passing through the external oblique muscle.

External oblique is supplied mainly by the eighth to twelfth posterior intercostal arteries and by the lateral branches of the epigastric arcades. Salmon (1936) maintained that the ninth and tenth intercostals did not play a major part in this. In his dissections, the eleventh and twelfth intercostals were larger and split into a set of deep branches running between internal oblique and transversus abdominis, and a superficial set on the deep surface of external oblique which might pierce the muscle to reach the skin.

Clinical experience with the lower rectus abdominis musculocutaneous flap bears out these findings. The horizontal ellipse in a lower abdominal dermolipectomy can survive if completely isolated except for its attachments to both underlying recti. If the perforating vessels from one rectus abdominis muscle are then divided, the skin island still has an adequate blood supply over four-fifths of the flap, but will show vascular stasis in one-fifth, i.e. the end of the ellipse on the side separated from its rectus muscle. Alternatively one lateral half of the dermolipectomy ellipse (i.e. a triangle) may be pedicled on the ipsilateral external oblique muscle, leaving the rectus abdominis intact (p. 348). The vascular support of this triangle of skin, fat, external oblique aponeurosis and anterior rectus sheath, is by segmental intercostal, subcostal and lumbar segmental vessels and their anastomoses in the subcutaneous tissues with branches of the lateral rectus musculocutaneous perforators.

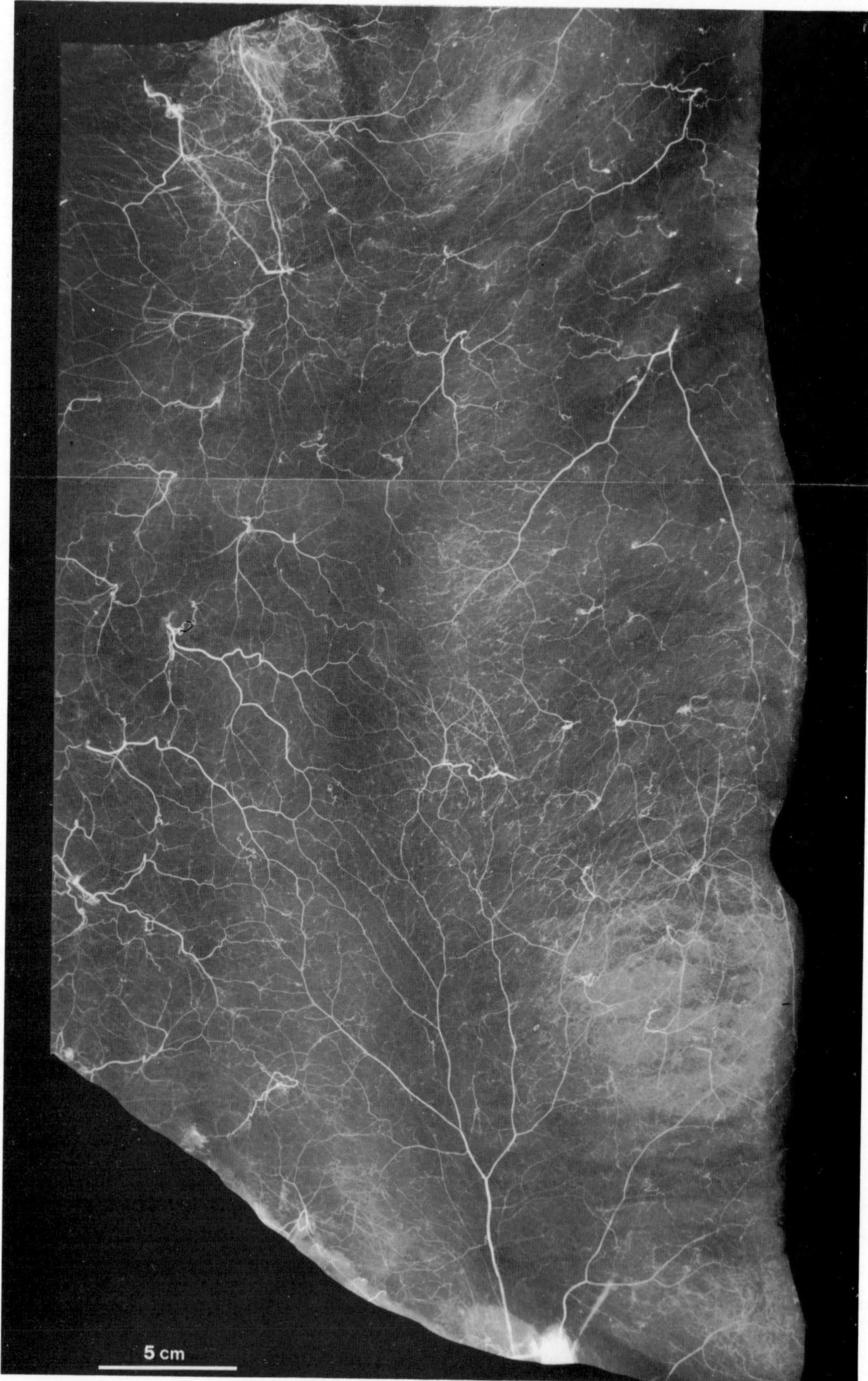

Fig. 6.38 Radiograph of skin and subcutaneous tissues from the right side of the anterior abdominal wall from a specimen showing well-developed superficial superior and inferior epigastric arteries. The superior margin of the specimen corresponds to a horizontal line around the chest at the level of the floor of the axilla.

The superficial superior epigastric artery

This artery is ignored in conventional anatomy texts. Manchot (1889) identified it and described it as a considerable vessel which ran down to the level of the umbilicus where it anastomosed with the superficial inferior epigastric artery. The vessel is inconstant but in about 25–30% of cases it arises from the deep superior epigastric artery (occasionally the musculophrenic), pierces the origin of rectus near the xiphoid, and runs obliquely inferolaterally, usually as two equal branches (Fig. 6.38). These vessels run in the subcutaneous tissue with the lateral one following the costal margin and anastomosing with vessels over the chest. The medial branch is more vertical and both anastomose with musculocutaneous perforators from the deep superior epigastric artery. It is very rare indeed for branches to descend as far as the umbilicus, as Manchot described.

The superficial inferior epigastric artery (SIEA)

This is a constant direct cutaneous vessel arising either directly from the medial side of the femoral artery or via a common trunk with the superficial circumflex iliac. The origin of the vessels lies 2–5 cm below the inguinal ligament and its diameter is between 2 and 3 mm. It pierces the cribriform fascia a finger's breadth beneath the inguinal ligament and ascends in the subcutaneous tissues for up to 15 cm. Its course is vertical or laterally inclined from the vertical; its medial branches anastomose with musculocutaneous perforators from the epigastric arcade, and its lateral branches anastomose with intercostal arteries. Manchot emphasised this vessel and placed the common trunk with the superficial circumflex iliac artery above the inguinal ligament, as well as giving emphasis to the abdominal branches of the superficial external pudendal artery. The venous drainage of this system is mainly through the superficial inferior epigastric vein but when it is small the venae comitantes of the SIEA may substitute.

Table 6.3 Origins of the superficial circumflex iliac artery

Author	Number of cases studied	SCIA independent origin	SCIA + SIEA common origin
Lipshutz, 1916	83	35%	65%
Adachi, 1928	39	38%	61%
Smith, 1972	14	93%	7%
O'Brien, 1973	100	50%	50%
Taylor, 1975		26%	74%
Harii, 1979	87	50%	30%

The superficial circumflex iliac artery (SCIA)

This artery encroaches on the abdomen and is described here. The vessel arises either independently from the femoral artery, or from a common trunk with the superficial inferior epigastric artery (Table 6.3). Exceptionally, it may arise independently from the profunda.

It can be noted that in the common origin situation it is arguable whether in fact the SIEA is present at all, as this pattern may be interpreted as an early branching of the SCIA. This probably explains the discrepancies in the figures in Table 6.3 and reference to the original articles will clarify these points.

The point of origin lies between 0 and 8 cm (mode 3 cm) below the mid-inguinal point. The vessel is less than 2 mm in diameter. The main stem of the SCIA usually divides into equal-sized superficial and deep branches in its first 2 cm. This is not mentioned in

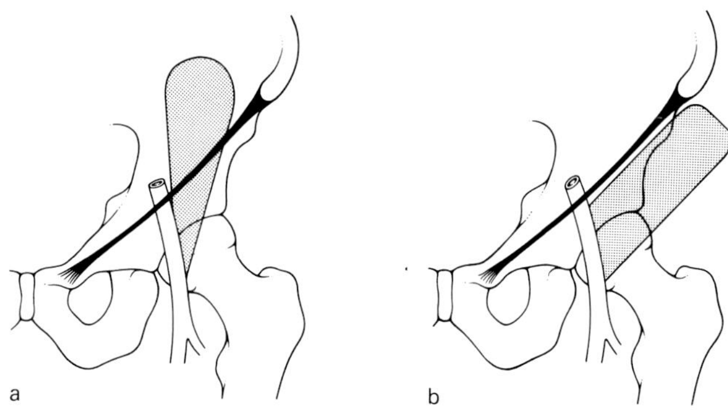

Fig. 6.39 **a.** Surface marking of the area within which the superficial inferior epigastric artery commonly lies. **b.** Surface marking of the area within which the superficial circumflex iliac artery commonly lies.

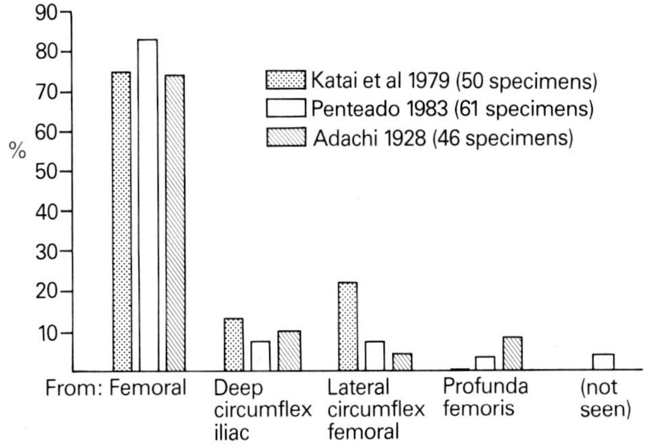

Fig. 6.40 Sites of origin of the superficial circumflex iliac artery.

anatomical texts and has received little attention in published papers. The superficial branch mentioned by Smith et al (1972) is tortuous and supplies lymph nodes and skin. The deep branch runs a straighter course beneath the deep fascia, parallel to the inguinal ligament, giving off branches to the muscles in the femoral triangle. The deep branch passes up through the deep fascia at a point about 2 cm below the anterior superior iliac spine (between 2 and 5 cm lateral to the femoral artery) and then continues in the subcutaneous fat becoming more superficial as it crosses the anterior superior iliac spine where it divides into terminal twigs. It should be noted however that:

1. The superficial branch may be absent or may expend itself early on in supplying inguinal lymph nodes, fat etc., so that it makes no significant contribution to the blood supply of the skin.
2. The deep branch may expend itself completely in muscle branches and make no significant contribution to the blood supply of the skin.
3. The deep branch may stay beneath the deep fascia giving off only small cutaneous perforators through the deep fascia.

In summary, the territory of the superficial circumflex iliac artery may be supplied entirely by the superficial branch, entirely by the deep branch or equally by both. In the small proportion of instances in which the SCIA is absent on one side it does not automatically follow that it will be absent on the other side. The anatomical territory is based on the femoral artery medially and covers the area reaching 5 cm above and below an axis running 3 cm below and parallel to the inguinal ligament. The distal extent of this anatomical territory coincides with the lateral edge of the anterior superior iliac spine (Fig. 6.32). Veins in this area are particularly large and numerous with the superficial circumflex iliac vein lying superficial to the artery throughout its course. Medially this is often joined by the superficial inferior epigastric vein. In addition there are deeper veins in the form of venae comitantes of the artery itself.

The superficial external pudendal artery (SEPA)

This has an upper branch which supplies suprapubic skin and therefore it is described in this section. In approximately 80% of instances the SEPA possesses both an upper and a lower branch, which arise from the femoral artery either separately or as one common trunk (one-third and two-thirds of cases respectively). The main trunk of the artery or its branches penetrate the cribriform fascia medial or lateral to the saphenous bulb. The surface marking of this area lies 1 cm medial and 5 cm distal to the point where the femoral artery emerges from beneath the inguinal ligament.

The upper branch runs along an axis from the point of origin as defined above to the pubic tubercle. It has abdominal, pubic, anterior scrotal/vulval and some inguinal branches. The territory lies along the axis indicated and the abdominal branch overlies the lowermost part of rectus abdominis and pyramidalis. This immediately suprapubic area is generally not served by musculocutaneous perforators from the underlying muscles. This may be related to the fact that the deep inferior epigastric artery approaches the lateral border of rectus approximately 7 cm above the pubic crest.

See 'External genitalia and perineum' (p. 270) for further details concerning these vessels, and the deep external pudendal artery.

The deep circumflex iliac artery

This artery arises from the lateral side of the external iliac artery or from the femoral artery and passes laterally between transversus abdominis and the transversalis fascia towards the anterior superior iliac spine where the vessel divides into two branches. The lower branch continues laterally in the line of the parent artery towards the anterior superior iliac spine lying behind transversus abdominis. It pierces the transversalis fascia and passes along the crest of the ilium supplying iliacus. When this vessel is large it penetrates transversus abdominis at about the middle of the iliac crest and continues posteriorly between this muscle and internal oblique, to anastomose with the iliolumbar and superior gluteal arteries. The other branch of the main stem is the *ascending branch*, formerly known as the *lateral epigastric artery*, which immediately, or after a short course, pierces the transversus abdominis and ascends in the plane between this muscle and the internal oblique (Figs 6.41 & 6.42). It anastomoses with lumbar arteries, inferior intercostals and the musculophrenic artery. The relative sizes of these two branches has been assessed visually by the authors in preserved cadavers and the continuation of the deep circumflex iliac artery has generally been found to be larger (60%) or the same size (25%) as the lateral epigastric.

Manchot (1889) drew attention to the contribution of the deep circumflex iliac artery to the blood supply of skin by small branches reaching the skin over the anterior superior iliac spine. Some anatomical injection studies (Allieu et al, 1980; Penteado, 1984) have tended to suggest that the contribution from the deep circumflex iliac artery to the skin is insufficient to support a skin flap.

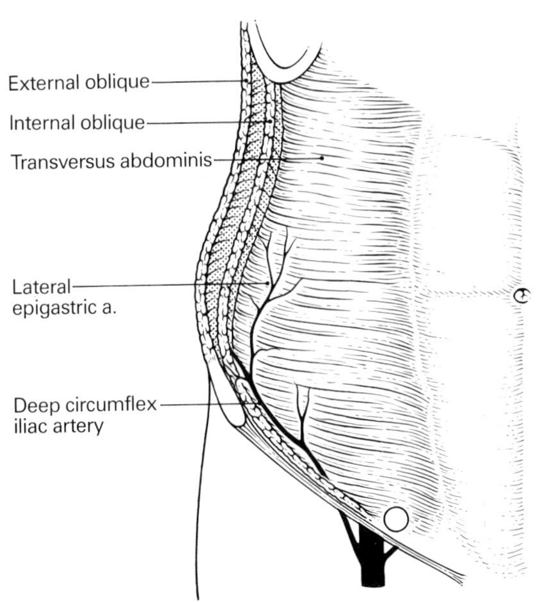

Fig. 6.41 External oblique and internal oblique have been cut away to reveal the deep circumflex iliac artery and its lateral epigastric branch.

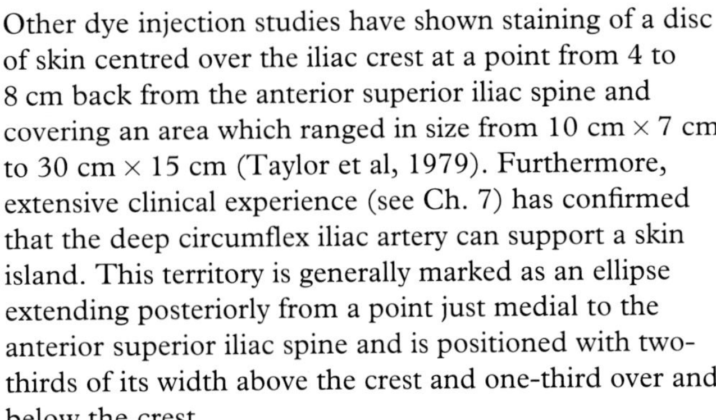

Other dye injection studies have shown staining of a disc of skin centred over the iliac crest at a point from 4 to 8 cm back from the anterior superior iliac spine and covering an area which ranged in size from 10 cm × 7 cm to 30 cm × 15 cm (Taylor et al, 1979). Furthermore, extensive clinical experience (see Ch. 7) has confirmed that the deep circumflex iliac artery can support a skin island. This territory is generally marked as an ellipse extending posteriorly from a point just medial to the anterior superior iliac spine and is positioned with two-thirds of its width above the crest and one-third over and below the crest.

The ascending branch anastomoses with branches of the intercostal vessels which may perforate the overlying muscles to reach skin but it is not itself directly a source of blood supply to the skin. The relevance of this rather neglected vessel to the making of abdominal incisions has been pointed out by some surgeons (von Mihalik, 1967). Muscle flaps have been based on this vessel but not skin flaps (Ramasastry et al, 1984).

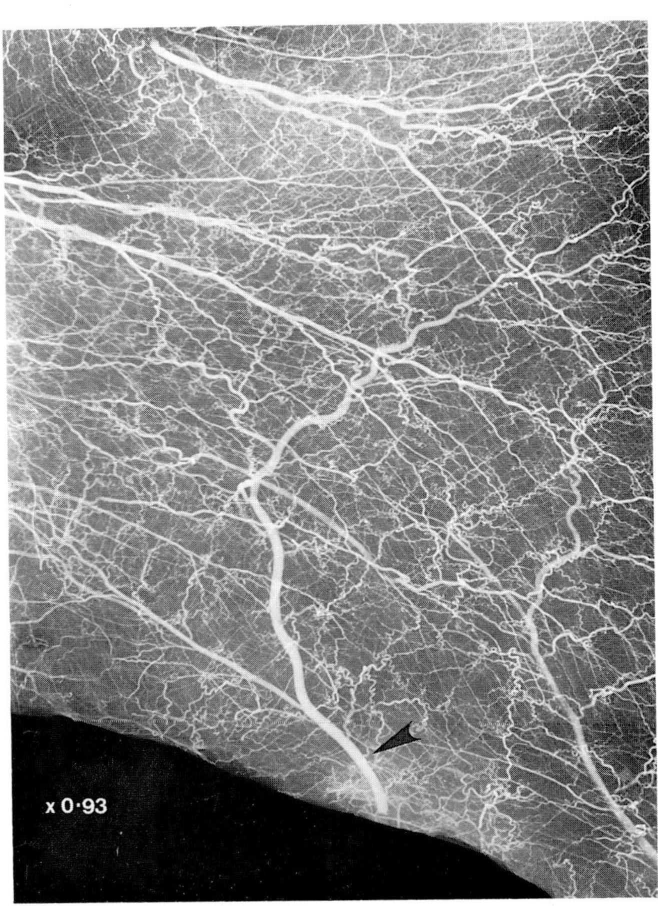

Fig. 6.42 This shows all three muscle layers of the abdominal wall in the area of the lateral epigastric artery which is indicated by an arrow.

BLOOD SUPPLY TO TRUNK MUSCLES

This is summarised in Table 6.4.

Table 6.4 Summary of blood supply to trunk muscles

Muscle	Supplied by
MUSCLES ATTACHING TO THE SHOULDER GIRDLE	
Pectoralis major	– pectoral branch of thoraco-acromial axis – clavicular branch of the thoraco-acromial axis – deltoid branch of the thoraco-acromial axis – segmental branches of the internal thoracic artery – lateral thoracic artery
Pectoralis minor	– highest thoracic artery (first branch of axillary) – lateral thoracic artery
Rhomboids	– deep branch of transverse cervical artery or – dorsal scapular artery
Serratus anterior	– thoracodorsal artery – perforating branches of posterior intercostal as.
Trapezius – upper part	– occipital artery branches
– middle, lateral part	– superficial branch of transverse cervical artery
– lower part	– deep branch of transverse cervical artery or dorsal scapular artery
CHEST AND ABDOMINAL WALL MUSCLES	
External and internal intercostals	– posterior intercostal arteries and their collateral branches
External oblique	– eighth to twelfth posterior intercostal arteries – lumbar arteries – lateral branches of the epigastric arcade
Internal oblique	– as for external oblique plus: – lateral epigastric artery – deep circumflex iliac artery
Transversus abdominis	– seventh to twelfth posterior intercostal arteries – lateral epigastric artery – deep circumflex iliac artery
Rectus abdominis	– deep inferior epigastric artery – deep superior epigastric artery

SUMMARY OF FLAPS ON THE TRUNK

Flaps which can be elevated on the trunk fall into the three categories of axial cutaneous, musculocutaneous and fasciocutaneous. The anterior abdominal wall has traditionally been the site chosen for the creation of delayed tube pedicles but these are not included here since they are basically random pattern flaps although a few, such as the thoracoepigastric tube pedicle of Webster (1937), bear some relation in their planning to the general direction of the cutaneous vascular plexus. Further details of specific vessels are given on the pages indicated.

Axial pattern flaps based on vessels of the direct cutaneous system are possible on the front and sides of the trunk; see Table 6.5.

Musculocutaneous flaps. There are numerous such flaps possible on the trunk as might be expected from the general principle of the skin overlying broad flat muscles being supplied by musculocutaneous perforators; see Table 6.5.

Fasciocutaneous flaps. The only truly fasciocutaneous flaps are those based on the branches of the circumflex scapular artery. The vessels emerging around the lateral border of pectoralis major from the pectoral artery and the vessels emerging through the linea semilunaris have been described as fasciocutaneous but in fact they are musculocutaneous perforators which fan out at the subcutaneous level and not at the level of the deep fascia; see Table 6.5.

Table 6.5 Summary of flaps on the trunk

Flap	Principal vessels	Page number
AXIAL PATTERN FLAPS		
Deltopectoral flap	second and third perforating branches of the internal thoracic artery	350
External mammary flap	cutaneous branches of the lateral thoracic artery/the superficial thoracic artery	371
Groin flap	superficial circumflex iliac artery	431
Hypogastric flap	superficial inferior epigastric artery	437
Infraclavicular flap	cutaneous branches of the thoraco-acromial axis	467
Lateral chest and abdominal flaps	lateral cutaneous branches of the posterior intercostal arteries	346
Suprapubic flap	superficial external pudendal artery	434
Thoracodorsal axillary flap	cutaneous branch of the thoracodorsal artery	478
MUSCULOCUTANEOUS FLAPS		
External oblique	posterior intercostal and lumbar arteries	346
Latissimus dorsi	thoracodorsal artery	473
(Reversed latissimus dorsi)	lateral dorsal branches of posterior intercostal and lumbar arteries	343
Pectoralis major – sternocostal head	pectoral branch of thoraco-acromial axis	470
Rectus abdominis – upper	deep inferior epigastric artery	296
Rectus abdominis – lower	deep superior epigastric artery	300
Trapezius – lateral	transverse cervical artery	484
Trapezius – lower	dorsal scapular artery	324
FASCIOCUTANEOUS FLAPS		
Horizontal scapular flap	horizontal branch of the circumflex scapular artery	288
Parascapular flap	parascapular branch of the circumflex scapular artery	291
Vertical ascending flap	vertical ascending branch of the circumflex scapular artery	295

6 UPPER LIMB

Nomina Anatomica

ARTERIA AXILLARIS
A. circumflexa humeri anterior
A. circumflexa humeri posterior

ARTERIA BRACHIALIS
(A. brachialis superficialis)*
A. profunda brachii
Ramus deltoideus
A. collateralis media**
A. collateralis radialis
A. collateralis ulnaris superior
A. collateralis ulnaris inferior

ARTERIA RADIALIS
A. recurrens radialis
Ramus carpeus palmaris
Ramus palmaris superficialis
Ramus carpeus dorsalis
Rete carpale dorsale
Aa. metacarpales dorsales
Aa. digitales dorsales
A. princeps pollicis
A. radialis indicis
Arcus palmaris profundus
Aa. metacarpales palmares
Rami perforantes

ARTERIA ULNARIS
A. recurrens ulnaris
Ramus anterior
Ramus posterior
A. interossea communis
A. interossea anterior
A. comitans nervi mediani
A. interossea posterior
A. interossea recurrens
Ramus carpalis dorsalis
Ramus carpalis palmaris
Ramus palmaris profundus
Arcus palmaris superficialis
Aa. digitales palmares communes
Aa. digitales palmares propriae

* A variant of the A. brachialis.

** Frequently referred to in the plastic surgery literature as the posterior radial collateral artery.

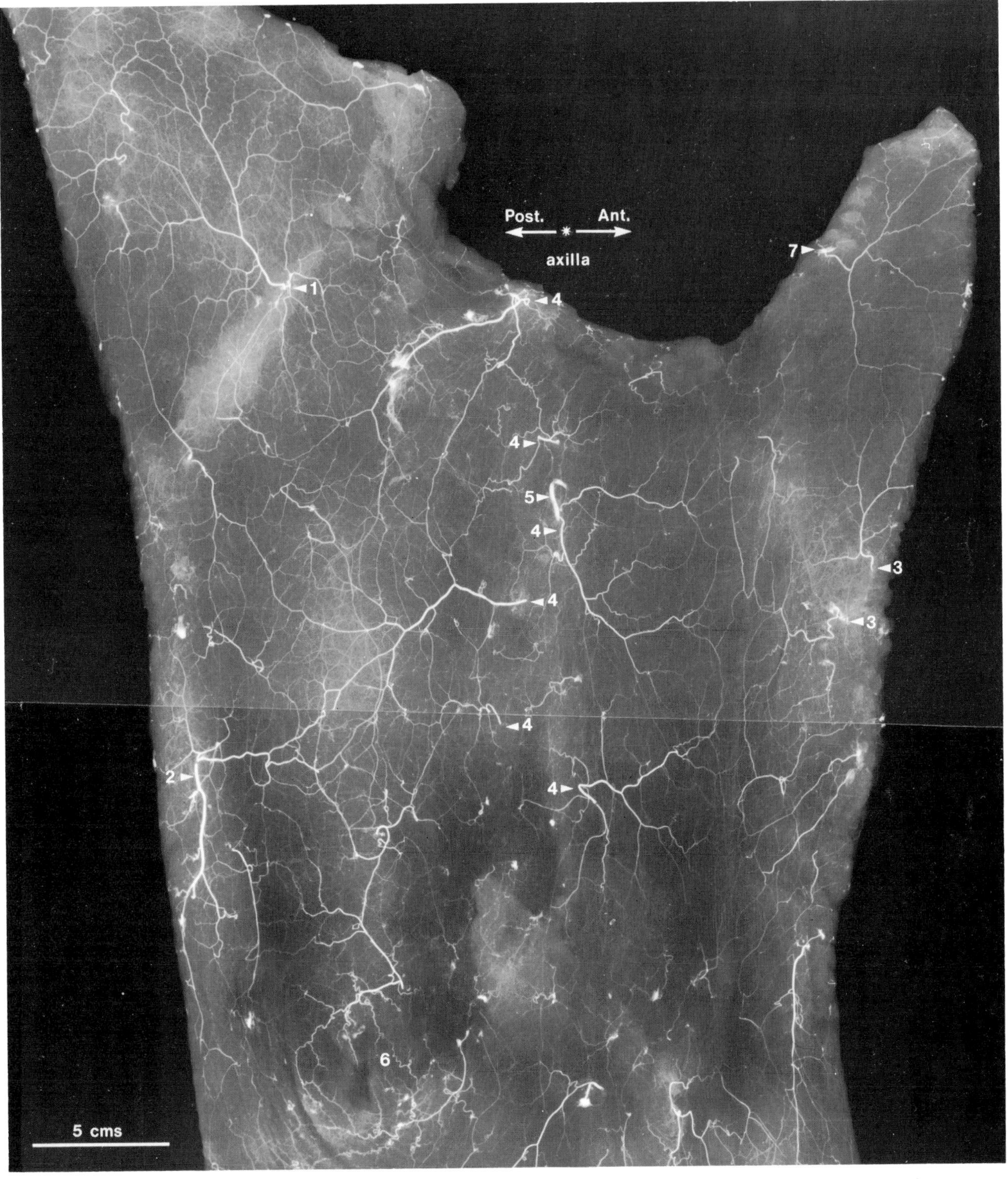

Fig. 6.43 Radiograph of upper arm and shoulder skin including the subcutaneous tissues and the deep fascia. The upper margin of the specimen resulted from an incision which passed vertically downwards from the tip of the acromion on anterior and posterior aspects of the shoulder and then crossed the lateral part of the floor of the axilla. A longitudinal incision was made from the acromion down the lateral aspect of the upper arm immediately anterior to the lateral intermuscular septum. The lower edge of the specimen lies immediately distal to the elbow joint. **1.** posterior subcutaneous artery arising from the posterior circumflex humeral artery and passing round the posterior edge of deltoid. **2.** terminal portion of the middle collateral artery. **3.** fasciocutaneous perforators from the proximal part of the middle collateral artery. **4.** fasciocutaneous perforators emerging along the medial intermuscular septum (various origins). **5.** segment of the superior ulnar collateral artery giving off branches to the skin. **6.** plexus of tortuous vessels around the olecranon region. **7.** musculocutaneous perforator through the anterior part of deltoid probably arising from the deltoid branch of the thoracoacromial axis.

6

UPPER ARM

The blood supply to the skin overlying deltoid and the upper arm is described in this section. The region over the olecranon is also dealt with but the region in front of the elbow is described with the forearm in the next section.

The floor of the axilla is conveniently considered here. It is moderately well supplied by vessels reaching it from its periphery, especially its medial and lateral sides. Laterally there are two small branches from the axillary artery, and medially branches from the chest wall and intercostals. A variable branch of the second intercostal artery that accompanies the intercostobrachial nerve and runs onto the medial aspect of the upper arm is one of these contributors (Figs 6.43 & 6.49).

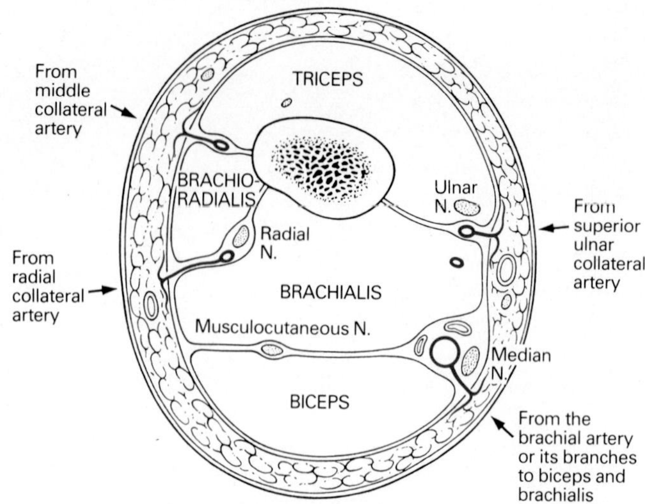

Fig. 6.44 Transverse section through the upper arm. Location of fasciocutaneous perforators indicated by arrows. These perforators lie on the superficial aspect of the deep fascia. Note their relationship to cephalic and basilic veins and to cutaneous nerves; perforators from the superior ulnar collateral artery lie near the medial cutaneous nerve of the arm, and those from the middle collateral artery close to the lateral cutaneous nerve of the arm and the posterior cutaneous nerve of the forearm.

THE BLOOD VESSELS OF THE UPPER ARM – CLASSICAL DESCRIPTION

The axillary artery, which is divided into three parts by the tendon of pectoralis minor, gives off *anterior and posterior circumflex humeral arteries* and the subscapular artery in its third part. The axillary artery becomes *the brachial artery* at the lower border of teres major. The brachial artery, covered only by skin and fascia, then crosses in turn the long and medial heads of triceps and the insertion of coracobrachialis, passes on to brachialis, inclines to the front of the arm and, now medial to biceps, passes deep to the bicipital aponeurosis in front of the elbow. The brachial artery, accompanied by the two brachial veins, is lateral to the basilic vein but separated from it below by deep fascia before being crossed by the median cubital vein on the bicipital aponeurosis. The brachial artery supplies the muscles on the front of the upper arm by three or four muscular branches and those on the back of the arm by the profunda brachii artery, which it gives off just below teres major. *The profunda brachii* accompanies the radial nerve posteriorly to the spiral groove, gives off the main nutrient artery to the humerus, supplies deltoid and the three heads of triceps, and under the lateral head of triceps divides into posterior and anterior branches. *The posterior descending or middle collateral branch*, running behind the lateral intermuscular septum and epicondyle, and *the anterior descending or radial collateral branch* piercing the septum to reach the front of the epicondyle

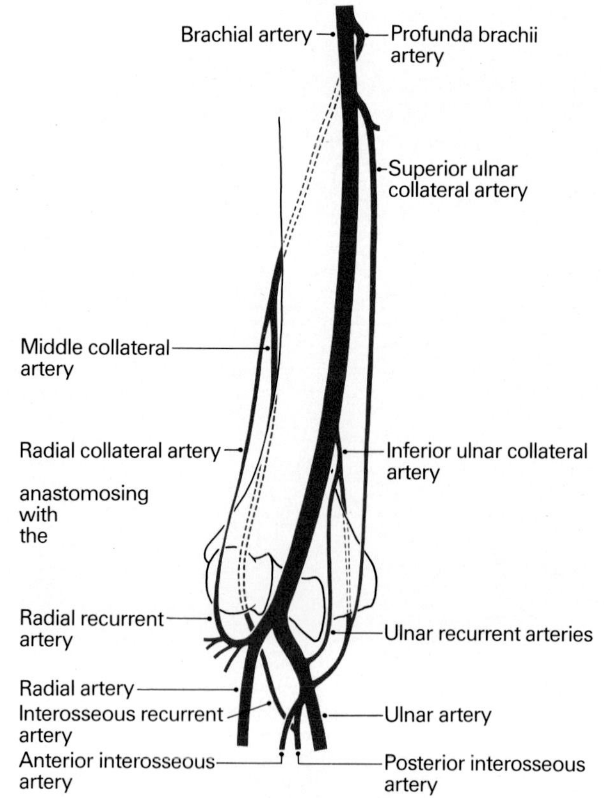

Fig. 6.45 Arrangement of collateral arteries participating in the anastomosis around the elbow joint. Branches given off by the arteries to supply muscles and skin have been omitted.

in the groove between brachioradialis and brachialis, take part in the anastomosis around the elbow. The brachial artery meanwhile gives off the superior and inferior ulnar collateral arteries. *The superior ulnar collateral artery* arises from the medial side of the brachial artery near the insertion of coracobrachialis and accompanies the ulnar nerve backwards through the medial intermuscular septum to the back of the medial epicondyle. *The inferior ulnar collateral altery*, arising approximately 5 cm above the elbow joint, runs medially over brachialis behind the median nerve, pierces the medial intermuscular septum and curves behind the humerus towards the medial epicondyle close to the bone.

Variations

McCormack et al (1953) have studied arterial patterns in the upper arm and found variations from the 'norm' in 18%.

A common variant of the brachial artery recognised in *Nomina Anatomica* is the *Arteria brachialis superficialis*. During embryological development the upper limb is supplied by two vessels, the superficial of which usually regresses leaving the deeper as the brachial artery supplying blood to the forearm. However, in approximately 25% of cases the superficial vessel persists as the superficial brachial artery, either in the presence of a normal brachial artery or in the presence of a greatly reduced brachial. If the brachial artery is rudimentary then the superficial brachial, after giving branches to biceps, may either end as the radial artery, or anastomose with the radial artery, or become the Arteria antebrachialis volaris superficialis. If the superficial brachial is large it may form the main source of inflow into the radial artery; the ulnar and common interosseous then arise from the brachial artery and the appearance is that of what is commonly termed a 'high division of the brachial artery'.

Two basic types are recognised depending on whether the origin of the superficial brachial is lateral or medial to the ulnar nerve. In the former case the vessel crosses the median nerve, in the latter it crosses both median and ulnar nerves. These two patterns are designated A. brachialis superficialis lateralis and A. brachialis superficialis medialis. Further variation occurs in how far distally the origin lies. A superior origin is one in the axilla, a middle origin lies between the upper quarter and the upper third of the humerus, an inferior origin is between the upper third and the midpoint of the humerus. Adachi (1928) studied this subject in immense detail and found that of the six possible types the A. brachialis superficialis lateralis inferior is the most common form, occurring in 65% of cases in which an A. brachialis superficialis was present.

There are other possible causes for the presence of two major vessels instead of a single brachial artery. These are:

1. An abnormally high origin of the ulnar artery.
2. An abnormally high origin of the radial artery.
3. The presence of an accessory brachial. This term is given to a branch of the brachial given off in the proximal arm which runs down parallel to it to rejoin it in the antecubital fossa where it may form additional anastomoses with other vessels.

The important main branches of the axillary and brachial arteries supplying the skin, and the ways in which these vessels arise either separately or in various combinations are indicated in Table 6.6 which has been abstracted from the data of Adachi (1928).

Table 6.6 The five main branches of the axillary and brachial arteries

subscapular	○	○│	○	○	○│	○	○│	○	○│	○│	○	○	○│	○│	○│	○
posterior circumflex humeral	○	○	○│	○│	○	○	○│	○	○	○│	○│	○│	○│	○│	○	○
radial collateral	○│	○│	○│	○	○│	○	○│	○│	○	○│	○│	○	○	○	○	○
middle collateral	○	○	○	○	○│	○	○│	○│	○	○	○│	○│	○	○│	○│	○│
superior ulnar collateral	○	○	○	○	○	○	○	○	○	○	○	○	○	○	○	○
number of cases (out of 533)	124	102	78	43	34	30	21	19	18	15	13	11	10	6	6	3

○ arise individually

○│○ ○│○│○ two or three vessels arise from common trunks

○│○ ○│○ } vessels arising in common, two separate trunks

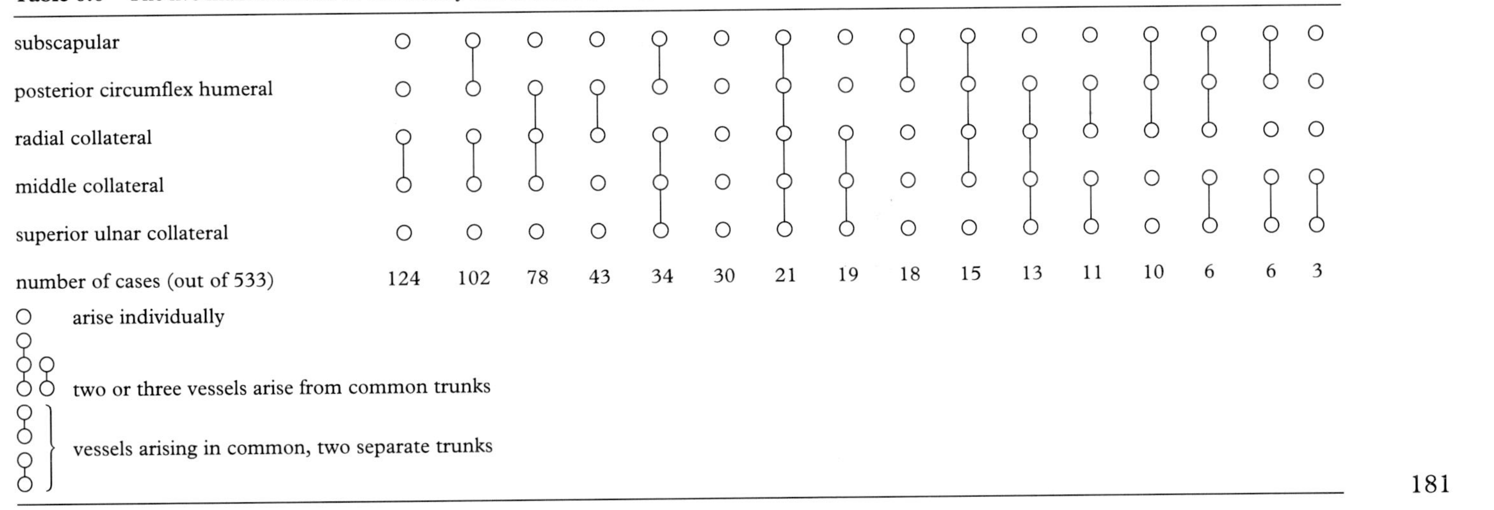

6 CUTANEOUS BLOOD SUPPLY OF THE UPPER ARM

The blood supply to the skin of the upper arm has a very simple arrangement. Essentially, there are three regions with separate supplies; the region overlying deltoid with a musculocutaneous supply, and medial and lateral regions based on the intermuscular septa with fasciocutaneous supplies. These will be described in turn under the headings:

The deltoid region
The medial side of the upper arm
The lateral side of the upper arm
The olecranon region

THE DELTOID REGION

The posterior circumflex humeral artery (PCHA)

This arises independently from the third part of the axillary artery and passes through the 'quadrangular space' with the axillary nerve in 70% of cases. A number of variations shown as c to f in Figure 6.46 make up most of the remaining 30%. These are illustrated because they may be encountered when raising the 'deltoid' free flap. The PCHA winds round the surgical neck of the humerus, anastomoses with the invariably much smaller anterior circumflex humeral, and supplies the deltoid muscle and overlying skin by multiple musculocutaneous perforators.

Anteriorly, its branches anastomose with deltoid and acromial branches of the thoraco-acromial axis. This may be related to the fact that the anterior fibres of deltoid have a similar action to the clavicular fibres of pectoralis major and share a common blood supply. Therefore, the territory of the thoraco-acromial axis, via its deltoid and acromial branches, extends onto the anterior part of the shoulder.

Posteriorly, a descending branch of the PCHA (less commonly a branch of the profunda brachii) runs down to the deltoid insertion supplying it and the skin over the lowermost part of the muscle. A more constant and

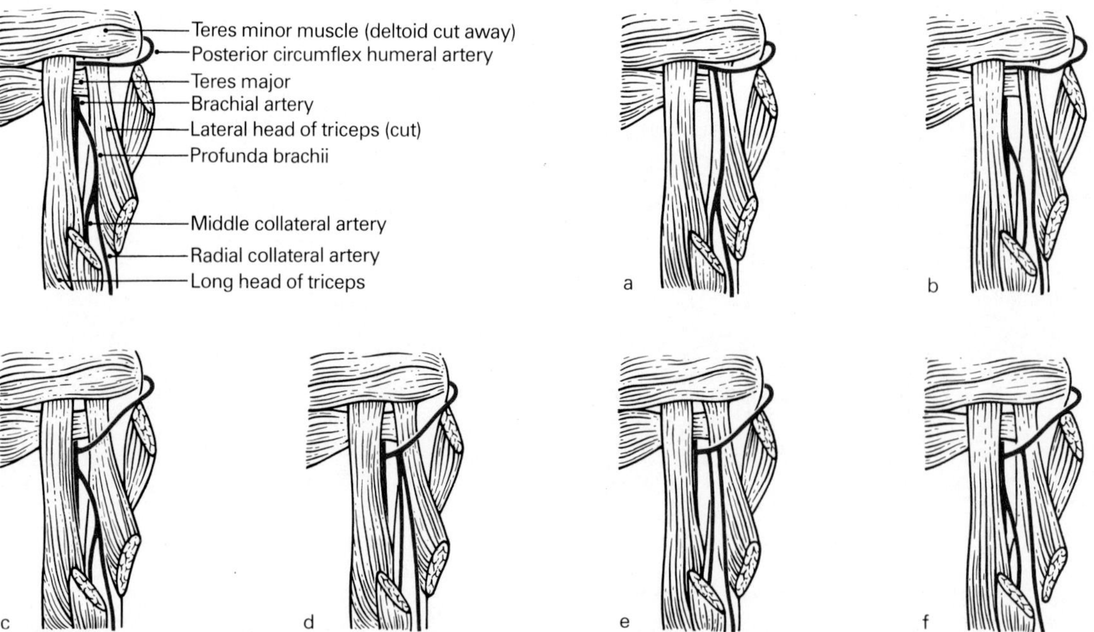

Fig. 6.46 Schematic view of the posterior aspect of the right upper arm showing the origin and course of the posterior circumflex humeral artery in relation to the tendon of teres major, and the origins of the middle and radial collateral arteries. (After Adachi, 1928.)

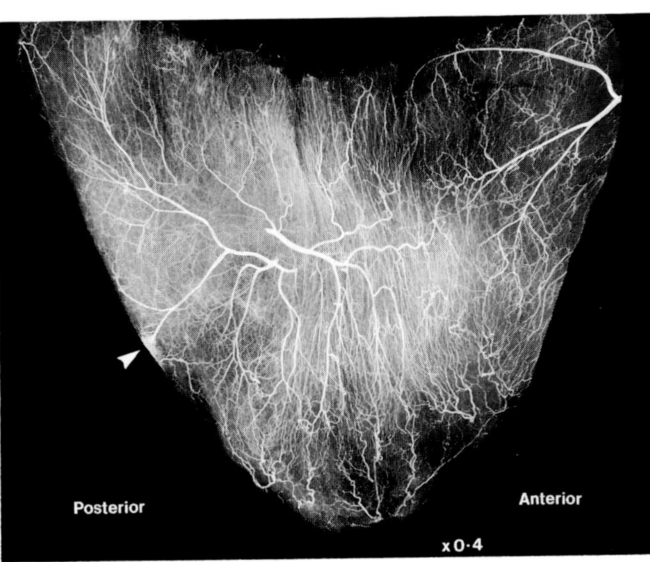

Fig. 6.47 Radiograph of injected deltoid muscle. The muscle is supplied mainly by the posterior circumflex humeral artery but also in its anterior part by the deltoid branch of the thoraco-acromial axis (and to a minor degree by the anterior circumflex humeral artery). Overlying skin is supplied by musculocutaneous perforators from these vessels. Note the large branch of the posterior circumflex humeral artery at the lower one-third of the posterior margin of the muscle – it appears to end abruptly where it becomes cutaneous as the posterior deltoid subcutaneous artery.

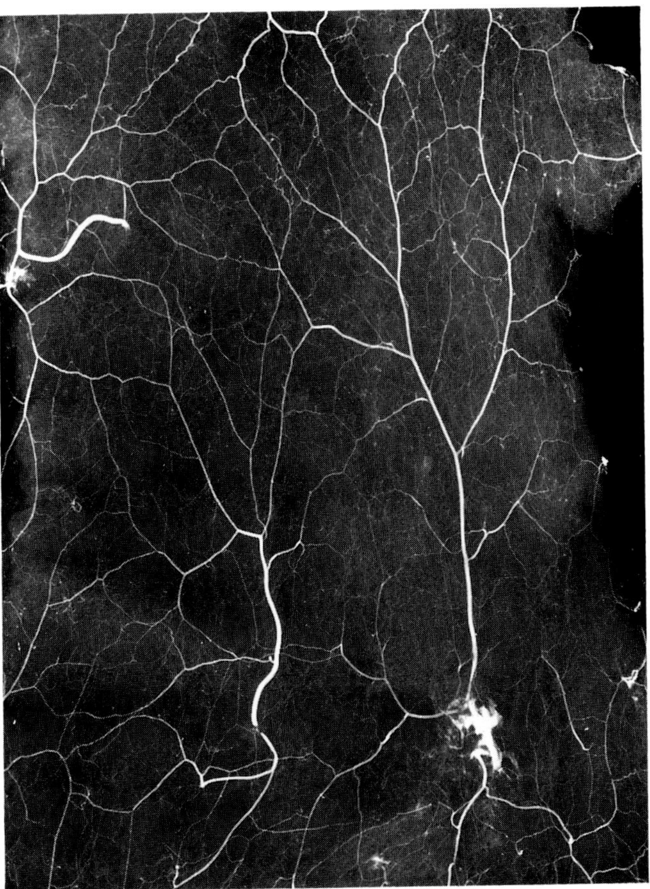

Fig. 6.48 Radiograph of the arteria deltoidea subcutanea posterior.

significant branch is the ascending one given off beneath the posterior edge of deltoid. Usually this vessel arises independently from the PCHA but it may share a common trunk with the descending branch. This ascending branch, named the *arteria deltoidea subcutanea posterior* by Manchot, is constant although variable in size and is shown in Figures 6.47 & 6.48. Sometimes this vessel pierces the edge of the muscle in its course to the skin and it would be reasonable to call it a musculocutaneous perforator. It behaves as a musculocutaneous perforator in that it passes through the deep fascia to fan out at the subcutaneous level and anastomoses with adjacent perforators. However, in the distance which it travels and the marked directionality it possesses, it approaches the characteristics of a direct cutaneous artery. Whichever it is, it is worth noting that it runs predominantly in a superior direction towards the acromion and not transversely as was described by Salmon (1936). The radiograph on page 179 and the further illustrations on page 404 which describe the 'deltoid flap' based on this vessel, show this clearly. The vessel may be closely related at its origin to the upper posterior cutaneous nerve of the arm, a branch of the axillary nerve, which runs more horizontally across the deltoid muscle.

THE MEDIAL SIDE OF THE UPPER ARM

This region is supplied by a row of five or six perforators which pass along the medial intermuscular septum to spread out in the deep fascia (Figs 6.49 & 6.50). These fasciocutaneous perforators arise from three sources: the brachial artery, the superior ulnar collateral artery and the artery to biceps. The artery to brachialis has also been reported as supplying skin but we have not observed this. After running for up to 1.5 cm these perforators divide into branches which descend obliquely either posteriorly over triceps or anteriorly over biceps to join in a fascial plexus with the vessels above and below and with those from the opposite side. Note that there are virtually no musculocutaneous perforators through biceps or triceps despite the large fleshy nature of these muscles. The internal diameter of these vessels ranges from 0.2 mm to 1.2 mm. Of these six perforators, two tend to be more important than the others and are large enough for microvascular anastomosis. They also supply significantly large areas of skin but it is impossible to predict in any individual precisely where such a vessel arises and in which direction, anteriorly or posteriorly, it fans out over the upper arm. The variability of the arterial pattern in the upper arm adds further difficulty to describing a simple scheme for this area. The following four paragraphs describe in greater detail the origin of the perforators. Fasciocutaneous perforators can arise from the following four arteries:

The biceps artery

The blood supply to biceps may be from a single large vessel (muscle vascularisation classification Type I, 35%) or by multiple widely separated arteries (Type IV, 40%), or the pattern may be intermediary (Types II and III). In a Type I blood supply the vessel generally arises from the brachial artery at the midpoint of the upper arm, runs laterally on a horizontal or slightly descending course, passes behind the median nerve (sometimes in front) and divides into ascending and descending branches which enter the biceps muscle. This artery, which is less than 2 cm long, gives off one or two cutaneous branches early in its course which measure 0.5–1.5 mm ID. However, a single biceps artery may alternatively arise from the superior ulnar collateral artery, the subscapular artery, the axillary artery, the ulnar artery in cases of a high brachial division, the profunda or the arteria brachialis superficialis, in which case the branches tend to be anterior to the median nerve. In a Type IV supply there are six or seven separate branches from the brachial artery supplying the muscle and these tend not to give off branches to the skin. With Type II and III patterns of supply to the muscle the presence of cutaneous branches is unpredictable.

The superior ulnar collateral artery

This may be a considerable vessel with a diameter of 2–3 mm or alternatively it may be absent. It usually arises from the brachial artery at about the midpoint of the upper arm or slightly lower, and runs down in the posterior compartment supplying the medial head of triceps. Other origins are indicated in Table 6.6. Although mainly muscular in destination it gives off one (or two) fasciocutaneous perforators but in general the size of such a vessel is inversely proportional to that of the perforator from the biceps artery, i.e. one or other is always dominant. Its diameter ranges from 0.5 to 1.5 mm. The area supplied on the medial aspect of the upper arm by this single vessel averages 7 cm × 10 cm and venous drainage is by paired venae comitantes which form a single 2 mm vein prior to entering the brachial vein.

The middle ulnar collateral artery

If present, this arises from the brachial between the superior and inferior ulnar collaterals and passes down in front of the medial epicondyle to anastomose with ulnar recurrent vessels. It gives off branches of supply to triceps which also send small fasciocutaneous perforators along the medial intermuscular septum to the skin.

The inferior ulnar collateral artery does not supply skin directly but its anastomoses with the anterior ulnar recurrent may give branches to the antecubital fossa.

The brachial artery

This artery may itself give off several sizeable cutaneous branches of up to 1.5 mm diameter but these vessels are very variable.

In summary, vessels emerging along the medial intermuscular septum supply skin in an anatomical territory reaching to the midline of the upper arm both anteriorly and posteriorly.

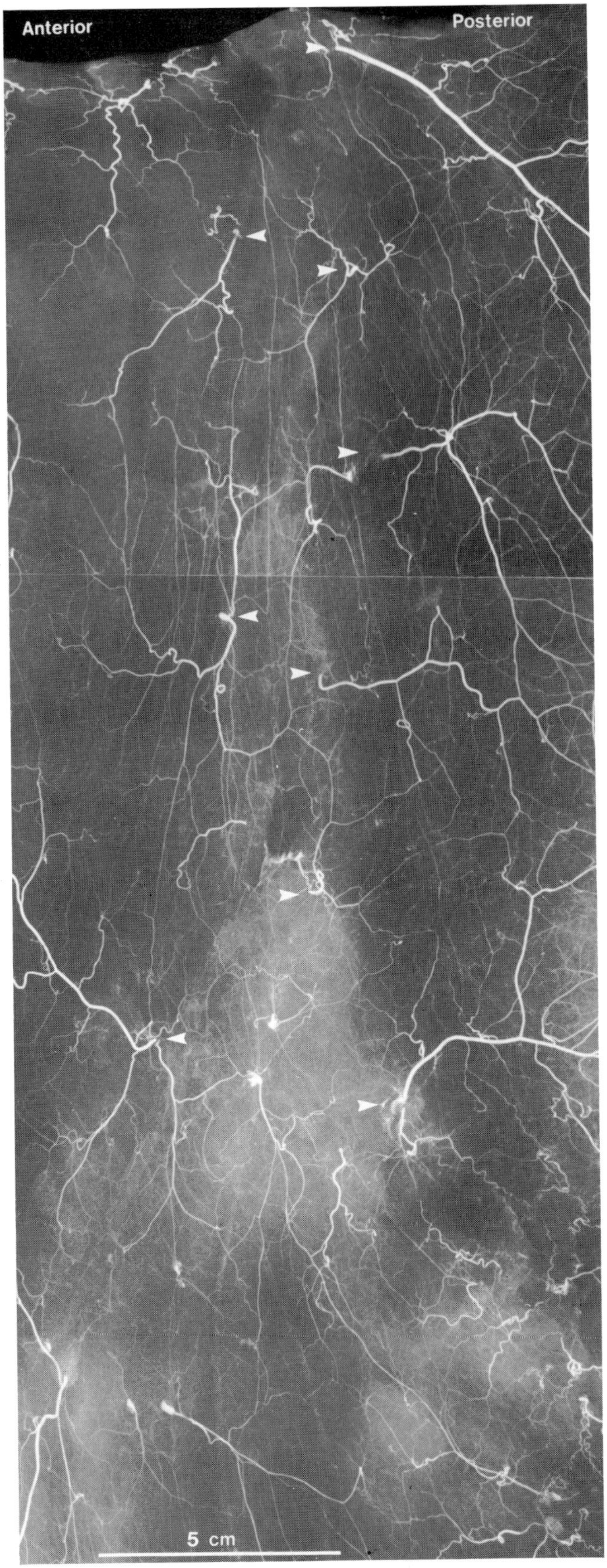

Anterior Posterior

5 cm

Fig. 6.49 The radiograph is of a 12 cm wide strip of skin, subcutaneous tissue and deep fascia from the area directly overlying the medial intermuscular septum. The upper end of the specimen lay at the level of the floor of the axilla while the lower end was at the level of the medial epicondyle of the humerus. Multiple fasciocutaneous perforators which have emerged along the medial intermuscular septum can be seen spreading out in anterior and posterior directions. A further example of this arrangement can be seen in Figure 6.43.

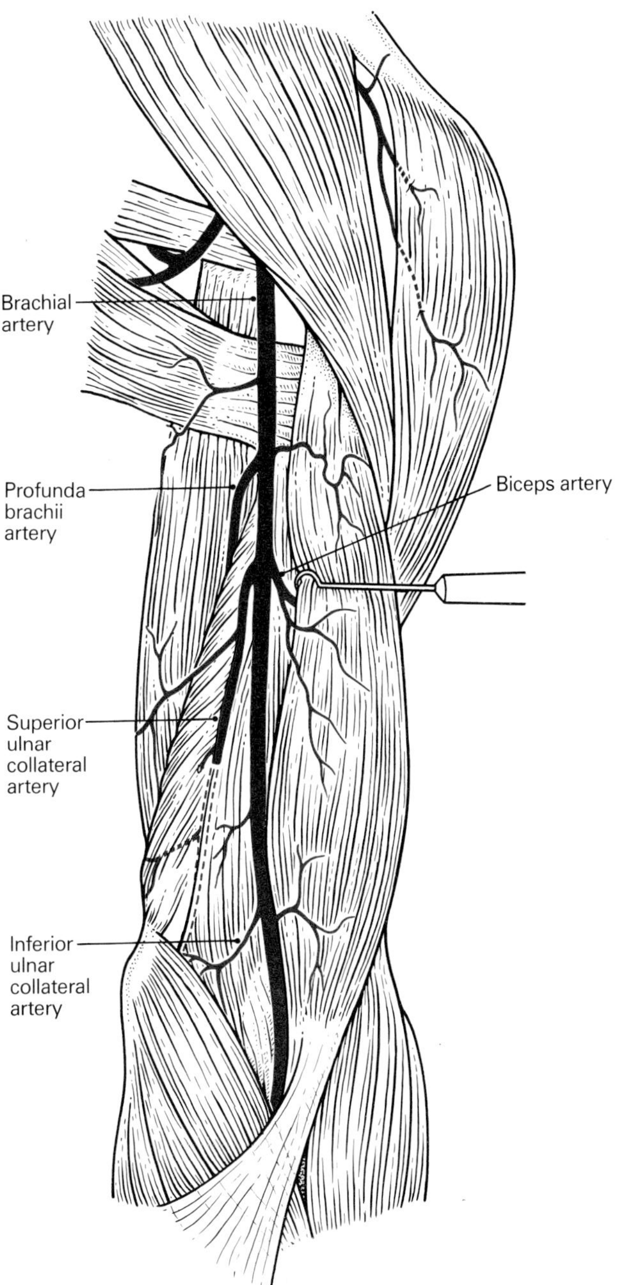

Fig. 6.50 In the diagram of the anteromedial aspect of the upper arm the origins of the cutaneous branches have been displayed but the branches to muscles have been largely omitted.

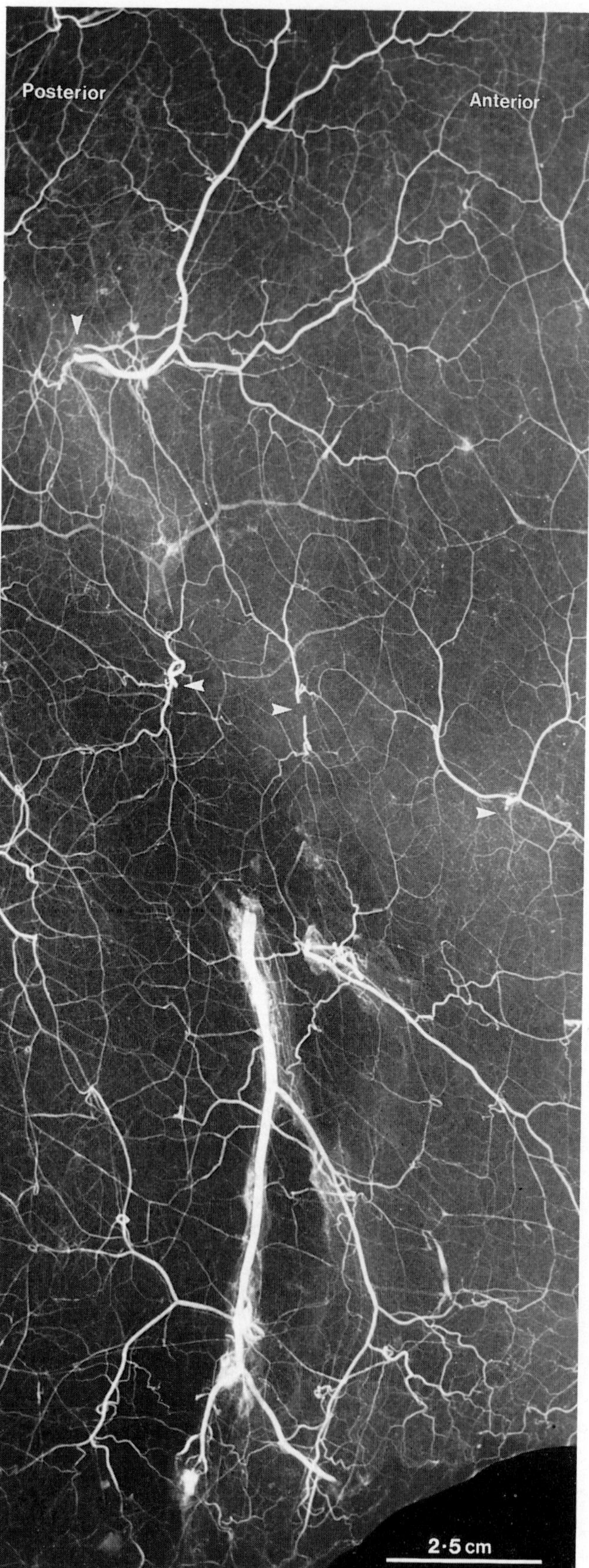

Fig. 6.51 The radiograph is of a 9.5 cm wide strip of skin, subcutaneous tissue, and deep fascia which in its lower part includes the portion of the lateral intermuscular septum containing the middle collateral artery. The upper end of the specimen lay at the mid-deltoid level while the lower end was immediately proximal to the lateral epicondyle of the humerus. The posterior deltoid subcutaneous artery can be seen at top left with three smaller perforators below it lying at the level of the deltoid insertion. The large vessel with substantial cutaneous branches in the lower half of the specimen is the middle collateral artery. The portion of this vessel that lay above the level of the deltoid insertion was not dissected out.

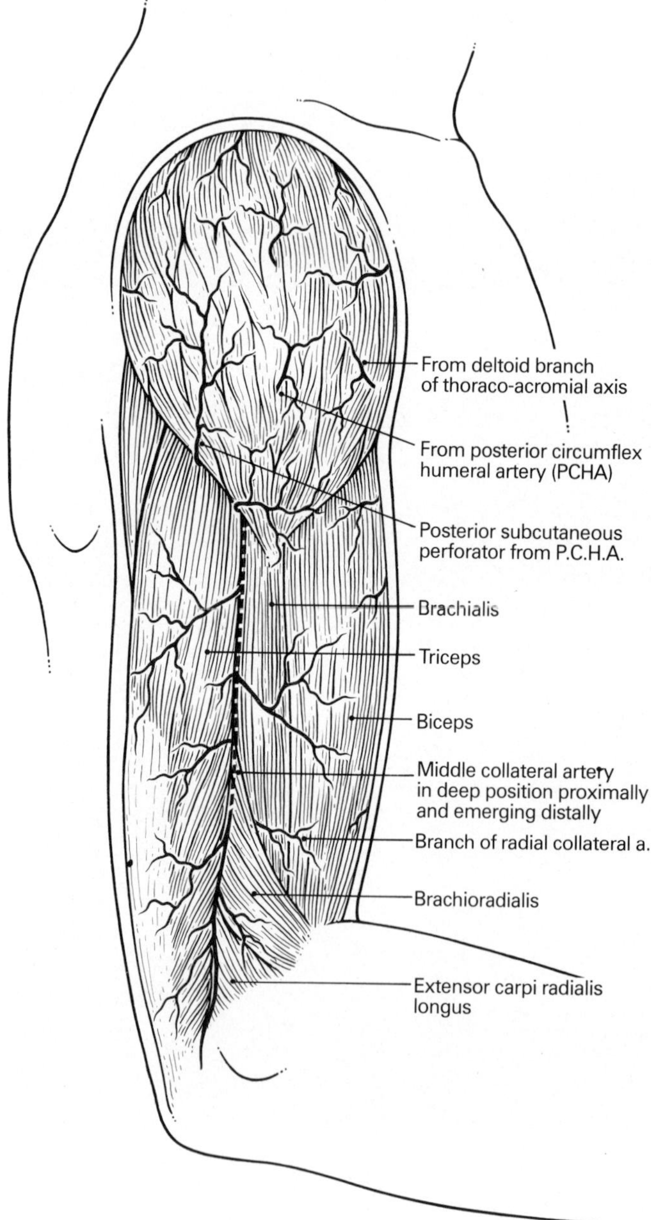

Fig. 6.52 In the diagram of the lateral aspect of the upper arm and shoulder the cutaneous branches are shown and the position of the deep-lying proximal part of the middle collateral artery is indicated by an interrupted line.

THE LATERAL SIDE OF THE UPPER ARM

This region is supplied superiorly by the posterior circumflex humeral artery as already outlined and below deltoid by the middle and radial collateral arteries which usually arise as terminal divisions of the profunda brachii. Figure 6.46 and Table 6.6 show variations in the manner of origin of these vessels. The radial collateral artery descends in the company of the radial nerve in the space between brachioradialis and the anterior compartment. The middle collateral artery descends along the lateral intermuscular septum behind brachioradialis in the company of the lower lateral cutaneous nerve of arm and lateral cutaneous nerve of forearm (Fig. 6.44). Both vessels give off fasciocutaneous perforators which pass along the intermuscular septa to reach the overlying skin where they then fan out over biceps and triceps to anastomose at the level of the deep fascia with vessels from the opposite side (Figs 6.51 & 6.52).

The middle collateral artery

This runs down the posterior surface of the lateral intermuscular septum. It gives off approximately five small branches to the skin on the lateral side of the arm and may itself pierce the deep fascia or alternatively it may remain deep to the fascia all the way down to the elbow joint. The distance below the deltoid insertion of the point at which the middle collateral artery gives off its last fasciocutaneous perforator or itself becomes cutaneous varies between 7 and 12 cm (Fig. 6.35). The vessel ranges in diameter from a maximum of 2.4 mm at its upper end to 0.6 mm at its lower end. At the level of the elbow joint it may anastomose behind the lateral epicondyle with the interosseous recurrent branch of the posterior interosseous artery (Fig. 6.45) and sends branches to the anastomosis around the olecranon.

The radial collateral artery

This gives few branches to the skin of the upper arm. It is mainly concerned with supplying brachialis, brachioradialis and the radial nerve before anastomosing in front of the lateral epicondyle with the radial recurrent artery. Twigs are given off to skin in front of the elbow joint.

THE OLECRANON REGION

This is covered by a plexus of many small vessels which appear tortuous on Figure 6.43 because the skin is in the relaxed, elbow extended, position. Clearly when the elbow is flexed, and the skin is stretched over the olecranon, these vessels straighten out. The plexus is supplied on its medial side by several small twigs arising from the posterior ulnar recurrent and superior ulnar collateral arteries which accompany the ulnar nerve. The inferior ulnar collateral may also contribute to this plexus by branches passing round or through the edge of the medial head of triceps. On the lateral side the supply is from the middle collateral and posterior interosseous recurrent arteries. The interosseous recurrent arises from the first part of the posterior interosseous and passes up through supinator to lie behind the lateral epicondyle deep to anconeus. It anastomoses with the middle collateral branch of the profunda brachii and gives off small branches to the skin which anastomose around the olecranon with the posterior ulnar recurrent and the ulnar collateral arteries. All these anastomoses make for a very good plexus which on radiographs of the area appears to be arranged in a circular manner around the olecranon.

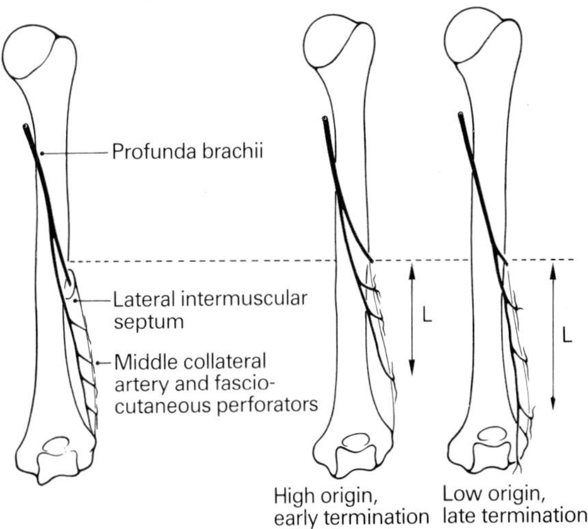

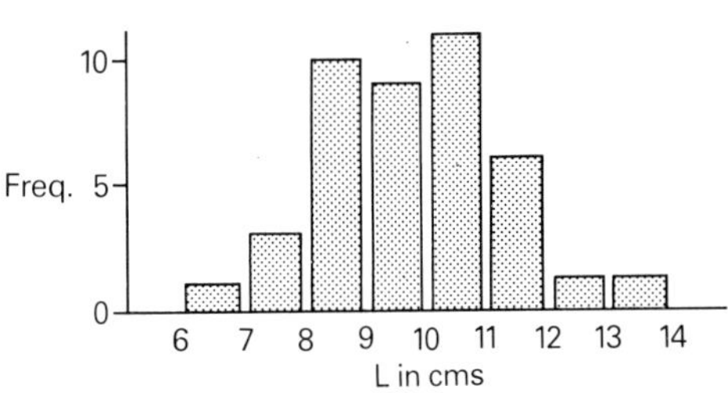

Fig. 6.53 Data relating to the artery passing down the posterior aspect of the lateral intermuscular septum – the middle collateral artery.

SUMMARY OF BLOOD SUPPLY TO MUSCLES IN THE UPPER ARM

Biceps. The pattern of vascularisation of this muscle may fall in any category from Type I to Type IV. In Types I and II the brachial artery gives off a large branch (2 to 3 mm diameter) in the middle of the upper arm (the bicipital artery) which runs laterally, behind the median nerve, and joins the bicipital branch of the musculocutaneous nerve to enter the deep surface of the muscle near its medial side. Branches supply both bellies and one ascends in the short head. Variations in origin of this artery have been noted above. The second smaller vessel in Type II arises from the brachial a short distance below the major pedicle and runs up inside the long head all the way to the tendon.

In Type III there are two equal sized vessels of supply from the brachial.

In Type IV there are from four to eight separate branches arising from the brachial artery and running to the muscle like the horizontal rungs of a ladder.

Some of the arteries to biceps may also give branches to brachialis.

Coracobrachialis. It receives one or more branches from the axillary artery and possibly from the anterior circumflex humeral. A small artery frequently accompanies the musculocutaneous nerve and passes through coracobrachialis without supplying it. It ends in brachialis and biceps.

Brachialis. This has a Type III vascularisation with a superior pedicle from the brachial artery just below the origin of the superior ulnar collateral, and an inferior pedicle (which may be small – Type II), from the superior ulnar collateral or less commonly the brachial. There are several connections between the arteries of brachialis and biceps.

Triceps. Its blood supply is derived principally from the profunda brachii and the superior ulnar collateral artery with an additional supply from the posterior circumflex humeral.

The medial head of triceps has a variable source of blood supply. The profunda, shortly after its origin, gives off a large branch from its medial side which passes in front of the radial nerve and enters the posterior surface of the medial head of triceps. When the profunda arises from the posterior circumflex humeral then this artery to triceps tends to arise from the brachial artery. In addition the medial head of triceps receives on its anterior surface two or three branches from the superior ulnar collateral artery. The long head of triceps receives a branch from the posterior circumflex humeral on its posterior surface and receives two arteries on its anterior surface. One of these arises from the axillary artery in front of the tendon of latissimus dorsi; the other arises from the brachial artery or the superior ulnar collateral. (These two anterior branches of supply may be combined as a common trunk coming off the brachial.)

The lateral head receives a branch of the posterior circumflex humeral at its upper end which anastomoses with an ascending branch of the profunda brachii. This probably explains the frequent occurrence of a profunda arising from the PCHA. All the other branches to the lateral head come from the profunda. It is worth noting that one of these branches may pass through the upper part of the lateral head to reach the deltoid insertion where it contributes to the blood supply of the skin.

SUMMARY OF ANATOMICAL TERRITORIES OF CUTANEOUS SUPPLY

The area overlying deltoid is supplied by the anterior and posterior circumflex humeral arteries, mainly the latter, augmented anteriorly by the deltoid branch of the thoraco-acromial axis.

The remainder of the upper arm is divided into medial and lateral territories by ventral and dorsal axial lines. The lateral territory is supplied by the radial and middle collateral arteries from the profunda brachii; the medial territory is supplied by perforators arising directly from the brachial artery or from its branches to muscles.

FLAPS

The branch of the second intercostal artery that accompanies the intercostobrachial nerve and runs onto the medial aspect of the upper arm can support a flap. Budo et al have reported the use of fasciocutaneous flaps raised on the inner aspect of the upper arm which probably incorporated this artery in their base (p. 457).

A posterior brachial flap has been described based on the cutaneous continuation of an unnamed branch of the brachial artery which supplies the medial head of triceps (Masquelet & Rinaldi, 1985).

The arteria deltoidea subcutanea posterior is the axis of the deltoid flap developed by Franklin (p. 404).

On the medial side of the upper arm, Type B fasciocutaneous flaps and neurovascular free flaps may be based on a single large fasciocutaneous perforator, whether it arises from the biceps artery or the superior ulnar collateral artery. These are described on page 455. Distally pedicled flaps based on the posterior ulnar recurrent artery and its anastomoses with the superior ulnar collateral artery have been described (p. 494).

On the lateral side of the upper arm, a Type C fasciocutaneous flap may be raised on the middle collateral artery (p. 377).

Anconeus local musculocutaneous flaps are theoretically possible but of limited practical relevance (p. 353).

6 FOREARM

From the elbow flexure to the wrist joint the skin is supplied by fasciocutaneous perforators arising from the radial, ulnar, anterior and posterior interosseous arteries. Figures 6.54 & 6.55 show how the perforators reach the skin by passing along the intermuscular fascial septa. The directions taken by the ramifications of these perforators are predominantly along the long axis of the forearm in the proximal part and transverse in the distal part of the forearm. This is seen in Figure 6.56.

THE BLOOD SUPPLY OF THE FOREARM – CLASSICAL DESCRIPTION

The classical anatomical texts describe the brachial artery as dividing into radial and ulnar arteries 1 cm below the elbow joint. The *radial artery* lies deep to brachioradialis and gives off the radial recurrent artery. It lies on supinator and continues down the forearm crossing in turn the insertion of pronator teres, the lateral part of flexor digitorum superficialis, flexor pollicis longus and pronator quadratus. In the lower two-thirds of the forearm it lies beneath skin and deep fascia between the tendons of flexor carpi radialis and brachioradialis. It gives off a superficial palmar branch and passes beneath the tendons of abductor pollicis longus and extensor pollicis brevis to reach the dorsum of the carpus. It is accompanied throughout its course by venae comitantes. The *ulnar artery* gives off anterior and then posterior ulnar recurrent arteries and passes deep to pronator teres where it gives off the common interosseous artery. It continues towards the medial side of the forearm where it lies beneath flexor carpi ulnaris on top of flexor digitorum profundus. The artery continues down the forearm beneath skin and deep fascia, between flexor carpi ulnaris and flexor digitorum superficialis. It is accompanied by two venae comitantes with the ulnar nerve medial to the lower two-thirds of the artery. It crosses into the palm lying in the canal of Guyon lateral to the pisiform and above the main part of the flexor retinaculum. The *common interosseous artery* is a short trunk passing backwards to the upper border of the interosseous membrane where it divides into anterior and posterior interosseous arteries. The *anterior interosseous artery* descends with the anterior interosseous nerve in front of the membrane, overlapped by flexors digitorum profundus and pollicis longus, giving off near its origin the slender median artery which accompanies the median nerve but may be large and reach the palm. It gives branches to the bones and adjacent muscles and, at the upper border of pronator quadratus, sends a branch deep to the muscle to the palmar carpal network before piercing the interosseous membrane to reach the back of the forearm where it

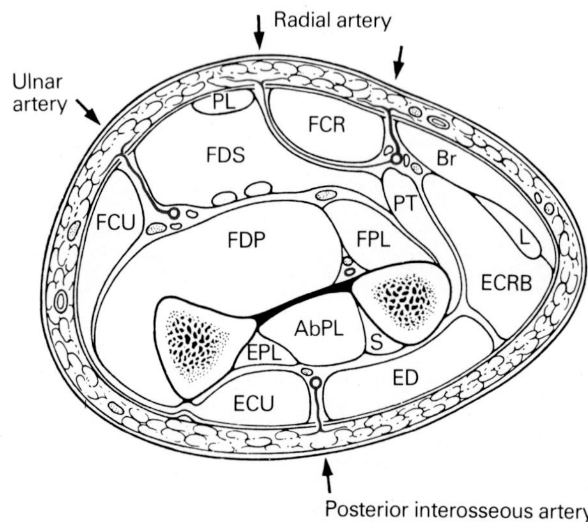

Fig. 6.54 Schematic transverse section through the middle region of the forearm to demonstrate the positions of the principal vessels and the courses taken by their fasciocutaneous perforators to reach the overlying skin. Occasionally there are also small musculocutaneous perforators from the surfaces of brachioradialis and flexor carpi ulnaris but they are not shown in this figure.

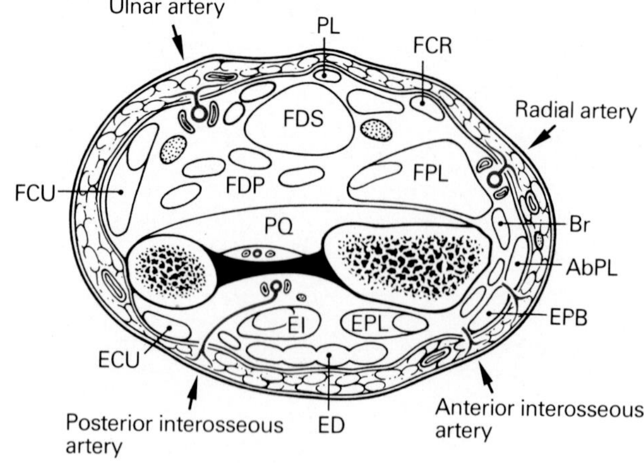

Fig. 6.55 Schematic transverse section through the distal part of the forearm showing the superficial positions of the radial and ulnar arteries and their fasciocutaneous perforators. The terminal branches of the anterior interosseous artery pass through the interosseous membrane to reach the posterior compartment where they incline laterally and emerge around extensor pollicis brevis and abductor pollicis longus.

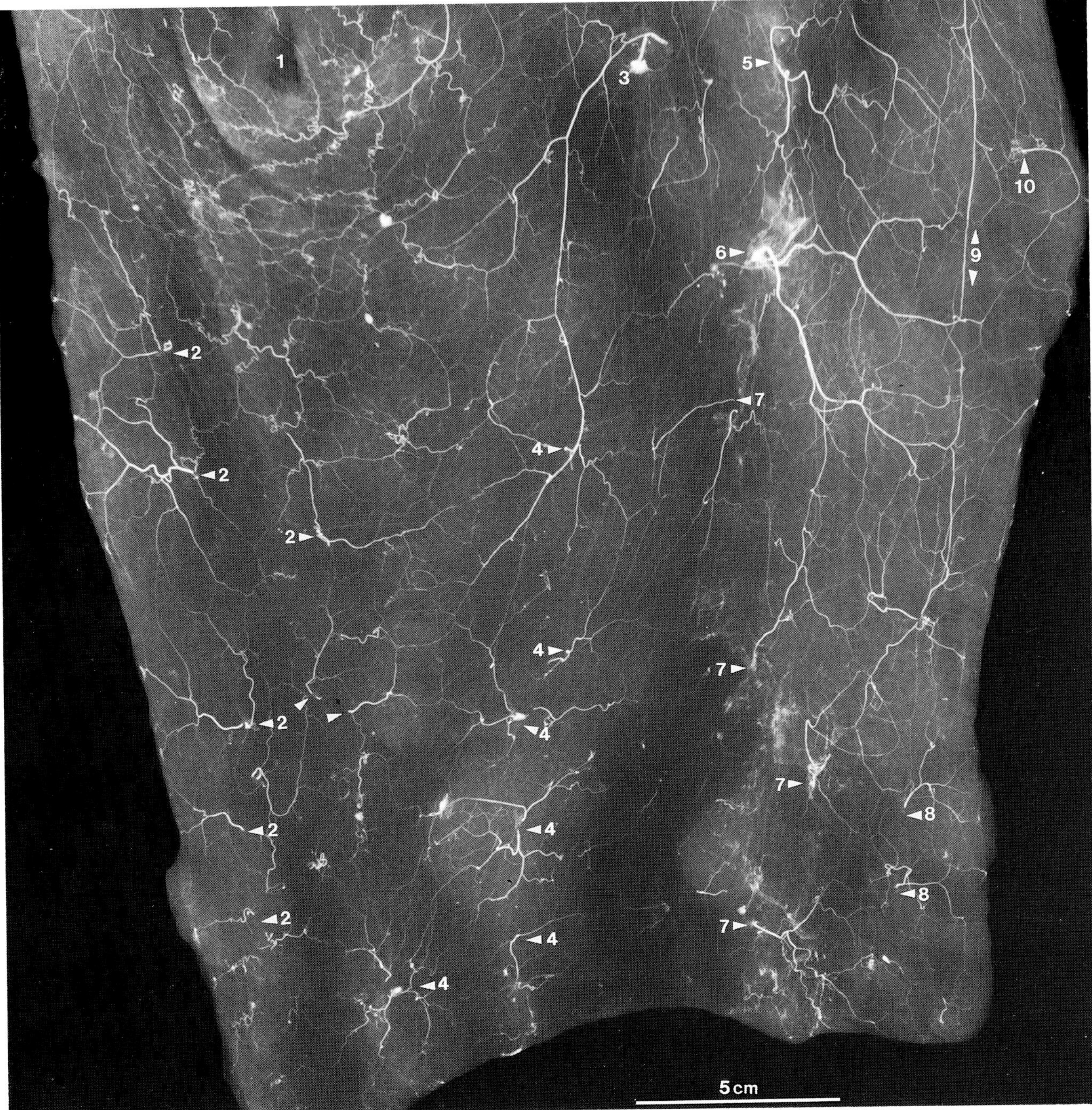

Fig. 6.56 Radiograph of forearm skin. To remove the specimen and enable it to be laid out flat, a longitudinal incision was made which passed obliquely across the extensor aspect of the forearm between the lateral epicondyle of the humerus and the ulnar styloid process. The upper end of the specimen lay at the level of the epicondyles while the lower end coincided with the wrist joint. This radiograph is the distal continuation of Fig. 6.43.

1. Circular anastomosis of tortuous vessels around the olecranon,
2. Fasciocutaneous perforators from the posterior interosseous artery,
3. Unusual perforator of uncertain origin,
4. Ulnar artery perforators mostly emerging between flexor carpi ulnaris and flexor digitorum superficialis but the most distal and posterior perforator emerges posterior to flexor carpi ulnaris,
5. Perforator arising from the radial recurrent artery and emerging between brachialis and brachioradialis,
6. Fasciocutaneous perforator arising from the radial artery and emerging in the distal part of the antecubital fossa (the inferior cubital artery),
7. Fasciocutaneous perforators arising from the radial artery and emerging between branchioradialis and flexor carpi radialis,
8. Two fasciocutaneous perforators arising from the anterior interosseous artery and emerging around abductor pollicis longus and extensor pollicis brevis,
9. Longitudinal anastomosis of vessels along the line of the posterior cutaneous nerve of the forearm,
10. Musculocutaneous perforator emerging from brachioradialis.

joins the dorsal carpal arch. The *posterior interosseous artery* appears on the back of the forearm below the lower border of supinator, gives an interosseous recurrent artery to the anatomoses around the elbow and, accompanied for a short distance by the posterior interosseous nerve, descends between the superficial and deep extensor muscles, where it breaks up into small muscular branches and branches which anastomose with the terminal part of the anterior interosseous artery.

Variations

These are frequent in the forearm and may either be the result of abnormal vascular arrangements in the upper arm or may arise independently. The arteries of the forearm develop from plexi which come together in the region of the major nerves to form the principal vessels. The intervening mesh of vessels normally regresses but may persist in various forms. Abnormal vessels in the proximal part of the forearm frequently assume the normal anatomical arrangement in the distal part. Conversely, variations may occur only in the lower part of the forearm and have effects on the vascular anatomy of the hand. There are several basic variations from normal in the forearm:

1. The radial artery may arise from the superficial brachial.

2. The radial artery may give off a superficial branch which crosses superficial to brachioradialis, extensor pollicis brevis, abductor pollicis longus and the extensor retinaculum in the company of the superficial radial nerve. It enters the first web space and continues in the normal manner of the radial artery. This superficial artery varies in size but may replace the radial artery which meanwhile is reduced to 1 or 2 mm in diameter. Many isolated cases are recorded in the literature but few have attempted to quantify its prevalence. Adachi found this vessel in 1.1% of 698 arms and named it the A. antebrachialis dorsalis superficialis. It seems reasonable to call this the superficial dorsal radial in English. It is best regarded as an additional vessel to the radial rather than an abnormal course of the radial artery. It may be encountered when raising the radial forearm flap and many an anaesthetist has inadvertently cannulated this artery when mistaking it for the cephalic vein.

3. The radial artery may be greatly weakened by giving off the common interosseous or median arteries. This is unlikely to be bilateral.

4. The ulnar artery may be replaced by a superficial vessel. This vessel may be regarded as either a consequence of a superficial brachial artery, or the result of an abnormally high origin of the ulnar artery (but see also note 7b below). It runs superficially over the forearm flexor musculature (except for palmaris longus which it may cross either over or under) and may be at risk in elevating the radial forearm flap (Fatah et al, 1985; Thoma & Young, 1992).

5. Any one of the principal arteries may be greatly enlarged and the others correspondingly weaker, in which case it will take over part of the territory of the adjacent vessels.

6. The median artery is occasionally a large vessel and contributes to the superficial palmar arch. It may arise from the superficial brachial as a variation on the arrangement described above.

7. The arteria antebrachialis volaris superficialis is an uncommon vessel occurring in less than 3% of cases. It is a superficial vessel running from the level of the elbow joint down to the mid-forearm or even the wrist. Its existence is always associated with the presence of a superficial brachial artery in the upper arm and may take one of three forms:

a. When the superficial brachial is large and feeds the radial artery then the arteria antebrachialis volaris superficialis may arise from it at the level of the elbow joint and proceed as a fairly strong vessel down the midline of the forearm to the wrist.

b. When the brachial artery ends in the upper arm and the superficial brachial is the main source of supply to the forearm then the arteria antebrachialis arises from the superficial brachial at the level of the elbow joint, runs superficially down the anteromedial aspect of the forearm, and assumes the function of the 'absent' ulnar artery. In this situation the vessel is – if being pedantic – the arteria antebrachialis superficialis ulnaris and has the appearance of what is commonly termed a 'superficial ulnar artery'.

c. The arteria antebrachialis superficialis may be the terminal continuation of the superficial brachial, in which case it is small and ends in the proximal forearm.

THE CUTANEOUS BLOOD SUPPLY OF THE FOREARM

The skin overlying the *antecubital fossa* and its adjacent margins is supplied by branches of the descending radial collateral, ascending radial recurrent, brachial and anterior ulnar recurrent arteries. On the lateral side there is no single large cutaneous branch but rather a series of small perforators from the radial collateral artery in the groove between brachioradialis and biceps and also some small perforators through the brachioradialis muscle from the radial recurrent artery. A brachioradialis musculocutaneous flap based inferiorly on these vessels and pedicled on the radial recurrent artery has been used to provide skin cover over the elbow joint (Lai et al, 1981; Lendrum, 1980). On the medial side of the biceps tendon the anastomosis between the inferior ulnar collateral artery and the anterior ulnar recurrent artery provides some branches to the skin. A further variable contribution comes from a branch of the brachial artery which has been much misunderstood since described by Gruber in 1852 as the arteria plicae cubiti superficialis. This constant vessel has no name in the English literature but we have drawn attention to it and pointed out that the designation 'superficial' is incorrect (Lamberty & Cormack, 1982). Manchot (1889) quoting Gruber, described the vessel as cutaneous and represented it in his diagrams as superficial to the bicipital aponeurosis, but Salmon (1936) correctly described this vessel (as the artère du pli du coude) and was in agreement with our findings that this vessel lies deep to the deep fascia over most of its course, before ending in the groove between flexor carpi radialis and palmaris longus by dividing into mainly muscular branches with a few cutaneous twigs. The vessel is shown in Figure 6.57 lying beneath the fibres of the lacertus fibrosus and supplying flexor muscles. It is therefore not available as the basis for an axial pattern skin flap, although its terminal branches may become cutaneous to anastomose with the most proximal of the ulnar artery fasciocutaneous perforators. Although usually arising from the brachial artery it may arise from the anterior ulnar recurrent or the radial artery.

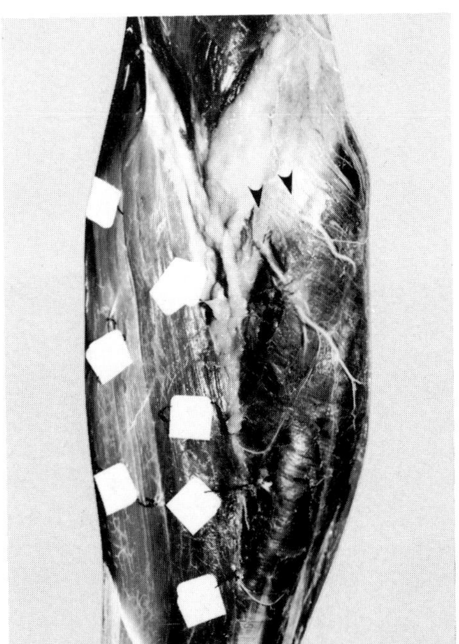

Fig. 6.57 Photograph of injected 'arteria plicae cubiti superficialis' which is in fact not superficial but lies beneath the deep fascia and supplies muscle. It should not be confused with the inferior cubital artery.

The inferior cubital artery

In the lowermost part of the antecubital fossa there is a perforator of variable size which we have called the inferior cubital artery. When large this vessel may, in the past, have been interpreted as the A. antebrachialis volaris superficialis or A. antebrachialis superficialis mediana. The essential criterion for these, and also the A. antebrachialis superficialis ulnaris, is that they run all the way down the forearm from elbow to wrist lying superficially or crossed, at most, by one tendon. These are all very rare (<1%) and are ignored here.

The inferior cubital artery arises from the radial artery or the radial recurrent and reaches the deep fascia by passing up to the surface in the apex of the antecubital fossa, between brachioradialis and pronator teres. It lies lateral to the tendon of biceps in the fork of the inverted V formed by the median cubital vein and its deep branch given off to communicate with the deep venae comitantes of the radial artery. This is shown in Figures 6.58 & 6.59. The vessel then fans out over the proximal anterior forearm, lying at the level of the deep fascia, and some good examples of it are shown in Figures 6.60–6.62. At its distal end it anastomoses with perforators arising from radial and ulnar arteries. Injection studies suggest that the territory of this vessel is larger than that of any other single perforating cutaneous vessel in the forearm. Including the small perforating branches of the radial artery emerging between brachioradialis and flexor carpi radialis or flexor digitorum superficialis with which it anastomoses, the ramifications extend distally in the forearm for up to 15 cm. Conventional pedicled fasciocutaneous flaps and various forms of fasciocutaneous free flap have been based on this vessel.

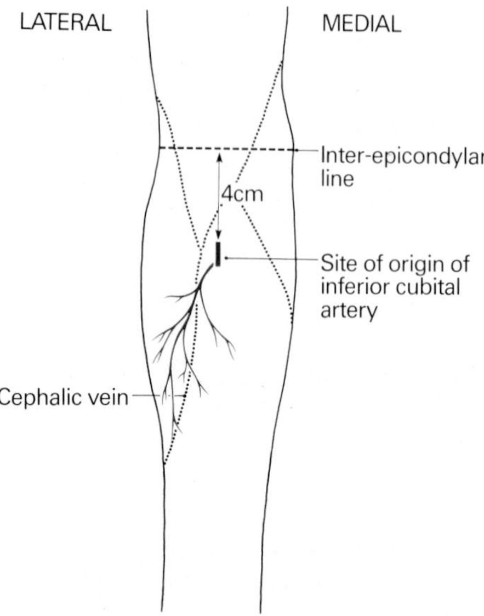

Fig. 6.58 Surface marking of the site of origin of the inferior cubital artery in the lowermost part of the antecubital fossa.

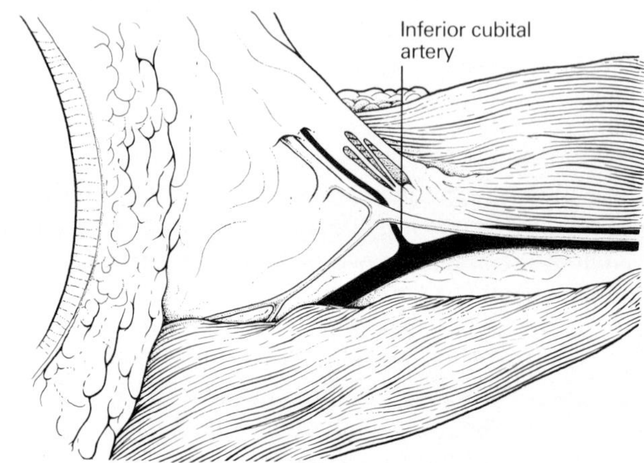

Fig. 6.60 Diagram illustrating the principal features of Fig. 6.61 which shows an inferior cubital artery.

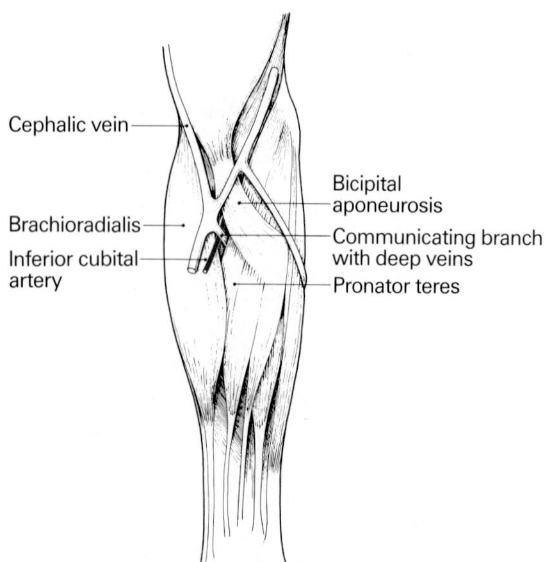

Fig. 6.59 The inferior cubital artery emerges in the fork of the inverted V formed by the cephalic vein and its deep branch given off to communicate with the venae comitantes of the radial artery.

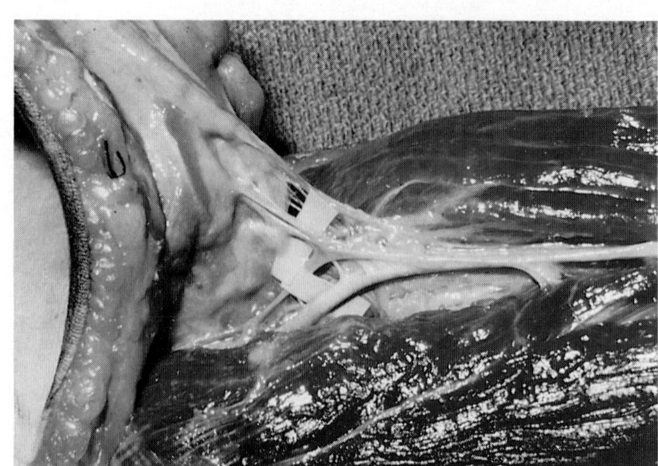

Fig. 6.61 View from the medial side of an inferior cubital artery.

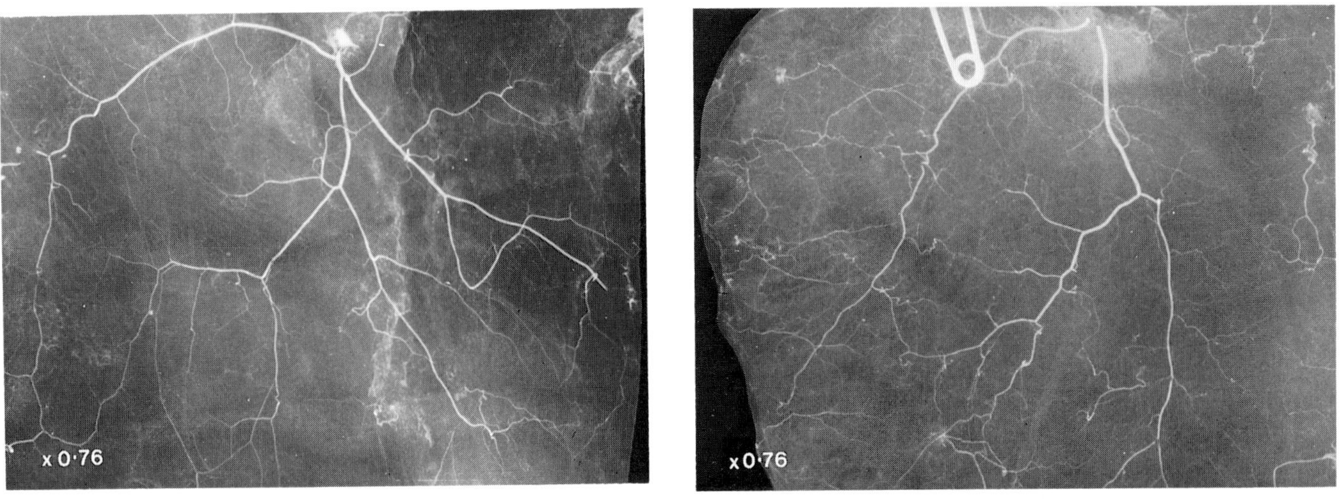

Fig. 6.62 Radiographs at reduced size showing particularly well-developed inferior cubital arteries.

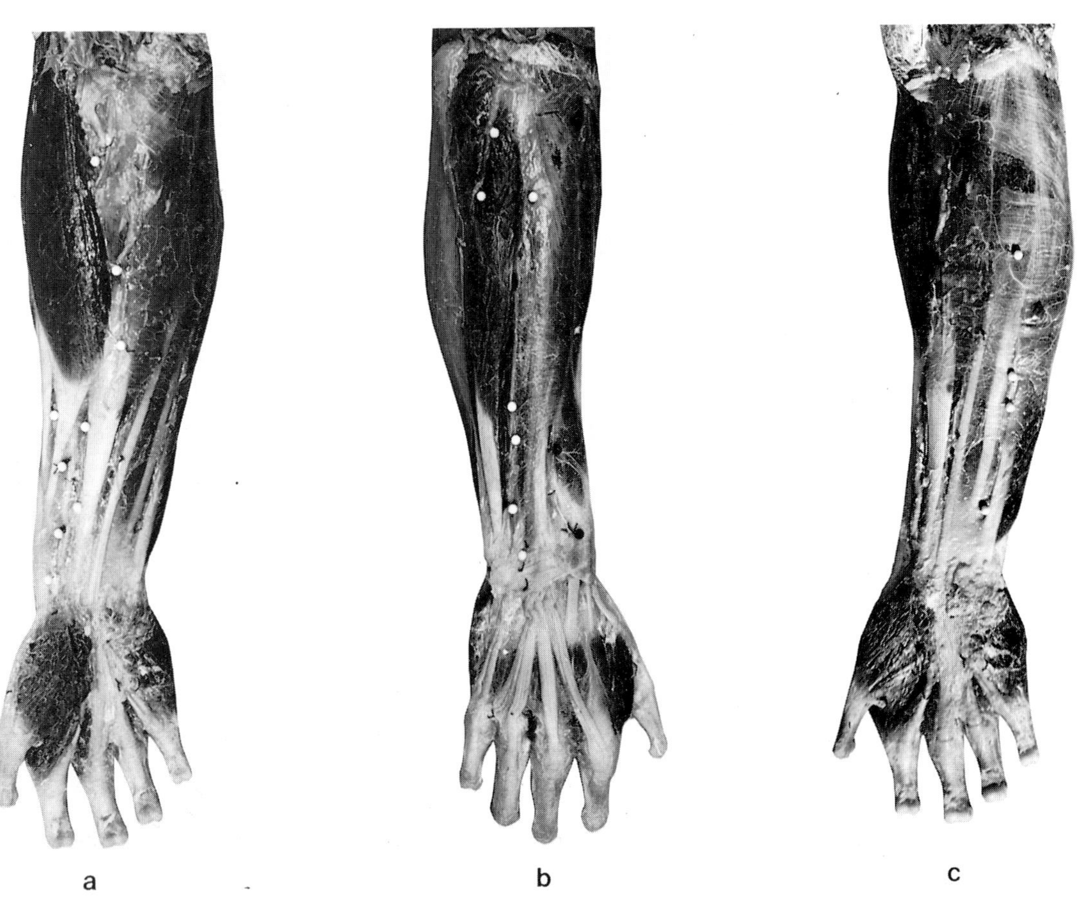

Fig. 6.63 Dissections of a forearm showing typical locations of fasciocutaneous perforators which have been marked with pins: **a.** from radial artery, **b**. from posterior (white) and anterior (black) interosseous arteries, **c.** from ulnar artery.

The radial artery

This gives off in addition to the inferior cubital artery, a series of smaller perforators. In the proximal third of the forearm these emerge between brachioradialis and pronator teres. In the distal two-thirds they emerge between brachioradialis and flexor carpi radialis or flexor digitorum superficialis. In the distal part of the forearm the branches of these perforators run transversely to anastomose with ulnar perforators medially and anterior interosseous or posterior interosseous branches laterally. Adjacent radial perforators also anastomose longitudinally. There are on average six of these smaller perforators with an internal diameter less than 0.5 mm, but the proximal ones are generally larger than the distal ones. These findings are relevant to the design of the Chinese radial forearm free flap.

The superficial radial nerve in the early part of its course lies beneath brachioradialis and becomes superficial in the lower third of the forearm where it runs over abductor pollicis longus and extensor pollicis brevis. Throughout its length it receives branches from the radial artery and sometimes there is a significantly sized vessel running along its medial border (Breidenbach's Type II pattern of nerve vascularisation making it suitable for free grafting) (Taylor & Ham, 1976; Breidenbach & Terzis, 1983). This may be seen on injected specimens of forearm skin.

In summary, the territory of the radial artery comprises the lateral half of the anterior surface of the forearm and the lateral border except for an area over the lower part of extensor pollicis brevis and abductor pollicis longus which is supplied by the anterior interosseous artery (vide infra). The boundary between radial and ulnar territories varies and depends on the size of the inferior cubital artery but in general it overlies palmaris longus. The lateral boundary between radial and posterior interosseous territories corresponds to the lateral edge of extensor digitorum communis.

The ulnar artery

This artery gives off anterior and posterior ulnar recurrent vessels which give off small branches to the skin respectively in front of and behind the elbow. The anterior ulnar recurrent lies between brachialis and pronator teres and anastomoses with the inferior ulnar collateral artery in front of the medial epicondyle. In the absence of significant branches from the brachial artery to this area (such as the a. plicae cubiti superficialis mentioned above) this anastomosis gives off a number of small vessels which reach the skin. Both anterior and posterior ulnar recurrent arteries supply the proximal parts of the forearm flexor muscles.

The remainder of the ulnar territory is supplied by a series of about five or six perforators which reach the surface by passing along the fascial septum between flexor carpi ulnaris and flexor digitorum superficialis (Fig. 6.64). Generally these perforators pass in front of the ulnar nerve as shown in Figure 6.54, rather than behind it. Their branches tend to fan out in all directions rather than being mainly transversely orientated and they tend to anastomose longitudinally. A few small musculocutaneous perforators may pierce flexor carpi ulnaris which receives its blood supply by three vascular pedicles from the ulnar artery, but the blood supply to skin is largely fasciocutaneous. Sometimes there are very few perforators and the ulnar territory is partly taken over by radial and posterior interosseous perforators. The posterior margin of the ulnar territory is marked by the posterior subcutaneous border of the ulna.

The anterior interosseous artery

This arises from the common interosseous and runs down the forearm on the anterior surface of the interosseous membrane which it pierces at the level of the upper border of pronator quadratus to reach the posterior compartment. Classical anatomical texts do not describe the vessel beyond this point but it does in fact go on to supply skin over the lower lateral border of the forearm. It does this by sending about three perforating branches to the small area overlying abductor pollicis longus, extensor pollicis brevis and the tendon of

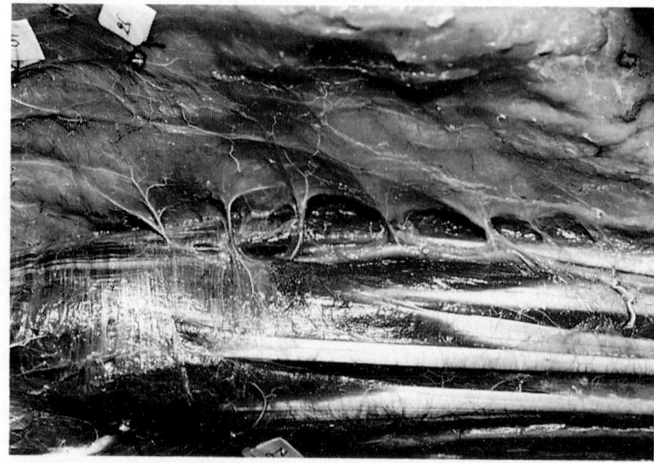

Fig. 6.64 Perforators arising from the ulnar artery are seen emerging between flexor carpi ulnaris and flexor digitorum superficialis.

extensor pollicis longus. The upper branch lies at the superior edge of abductor pollicis longus, the middle one between this muscle and extensor pollicis brevis.

The median artery

This arises from the ulnar artery, the common interosseous or the origin of the anterior interosseous to run with, and supply, the median nerve. It averages about 2 mm in diameter and is soon spent in supplying nearby flexor muscles but in ~8% it is enlarged and runs all the way down to the wrist. In such a case it may give off one or two minor perforators emerging between flexor carpi radialis and palmaris longus to the skin in the distal third of the forearm. Manchot greatly misrepresented the territory of this vessel.

The posterior interosseous artery

This passes backwards over the free upper edge of the interosseous membrane to appear on the back of the forearm between supinator and abductor pollicis longus. Here it gives off the interosseous recurrent branch which ascends towards the elbow beneath extensor carpi ulnaris and runs on the deep surface of anconeus in which it ends. (When absent this artery is replaced by a branch of the radial recurrent which passes around the neck of the radius beneath the extensor muscles.) The main stem of the posterior interosseous descends between the superficial and deep layers of muscles lying on abductor pollicis longus accompanied by the deep branch of the radial nerve. The posterior interosseous gives off a large branch which passes laterally and runs down the back of the radius in the gap between supinator and abductor pollicis longus; it supplies the periosteum of the radius, the adjacent muscles and often sends a branch to the skin. As the posterior interosseous artery runs down to the wrist in the depths of the groove between extensor carpi ulnaris and extensor digitorum communis it gives off muscular branches and two groups of fasciocutaneous perforators. The first group are given off mainly in the proximal part and reach the surface between flexor carpi ulnaris and extensor carpi ulnaris. The second group are given off in the lower two-thirds and pass along the fascial space between extensor carpi ulnaris and extensor digitorum communis (Fig. 6.65). Their branches tend to fan out equally in all directions or are more transversely orientated. The territory of the posterior interosseous artery therefore extends from the lateral edge of extensor digitorum communis where it abuts on radial territory, to the posterior subcutaneous border of the ulna where it abuts on ulnar territory.

The distal anastomoses of the posterior interosseous artery are classically described as being with the anterior interosseous artery and the dorsal carpal network. The anastomosis between the two interosseous arteries is by a connecting vessel that lies beneath the tendon of extensor indicis proprius at the level of the head of the ulna.

The posterior interosseous artery is subject to three variations which are significant from the point of view of raising flaps (see Penteado et al, 1986):

1. The interosseous recurrent branch may be absent in up to 20% of cases.
2. The artery may give off large branches in a radial direction to muscles and be rapidly dissipated in the proximal part of the posterior compartment. The distal part is then supplied by a large branch of the anterior interosseous artery which perforates the interosseous membrane half-way down the forearm and takes over the distal territory of supply. This may occur in up to 6% of cases.
3. The terminal anastomosis of the posterior interosseous artery with the anterior interosseous artery on the back of the distal radius, although described as consistent in anatomical texts, has been reported as absent in up to 2% of cases.

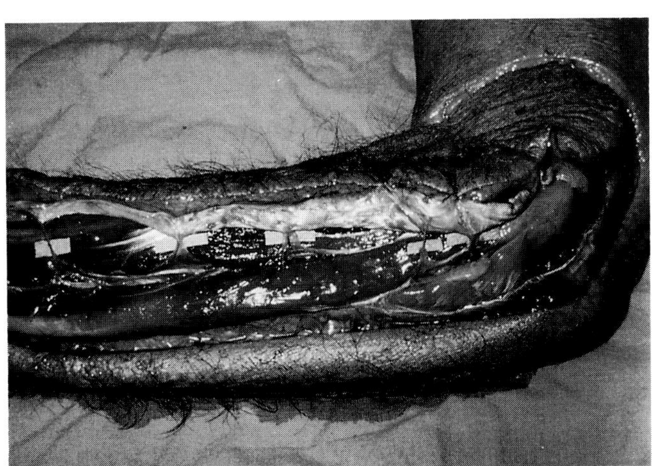

Fig. 6.65 Perforators arising from the posterior interosseous artery are seen emerging between extensor digitorum and extensor carpi ulnaris.

SUMMARY OF BLOOD SUPPLY OF FOREARM MUSCLES

Although forearm muscles are generally not involved in the blood supply of the overlying skin, their blood supply is described here because it may be affected by the elevation of certain types of flap e.g. radial artery Type C fasciocutaneous flap. Considerations of muscle vascular anatomy may also be relevant to tendon and muscle transfers.

Superficial flexor group

These muscles are supplied at their origin by the inferior ulnar collateral artery and in the proximal forearm by the anterior ulnar recurrent artery. These vessels anastomose outside the muscles in about a third of cases, and in all cases send multiple branches to the muscles and the median and ulnar nerves. In the middle part of the forearm the superficial flexors are supplied by the ulnar and radial arteries.

Flexor carpi radialis (FCR). This is supplied by a single dominant proximal pedicle and several accessory branches. The main pedicle is formed by a branch of the ulnar recurrent which passes deep to pronator teres and enters the deep surface of FCR in the company of its supplying nerve. Within the muscle this artery divides into a small ascending branch and a larger descending branch which anastomoses with the most proximal of a series of six to eight small branches (~0.3 mm diameter) of the radial artery which enter the muscle on its anterolateral side. The proximal of these cross the anterior surface of pronator teres (supplying it). The distal branches run for 1–2 cm in the fascial septum between brachioradialis and FCR before entering the muscle or supplying its tendon.

Pronator teres. This is variously supplied by all the arteries in the area. The superior head is supplied by the ulnar recurrent, the coronoid head from the common interosseous, the middle of the muscle by the ulnar, and the insertion by the radial. The median artery, when well developed, may also be involved.

Palmaris longus. The muscle belly receives a small branch from the ulnar recurrent artery. The tendon may receive one or two branches from the median artery when it is well developed.

Flexor digitorum superficialis. On its anterior surface it is supplied by three or four branches from the radial artery and a similar number from the ulnar artery. The dominant blood supply, however, is through the posterior surface. The median artery tends to enter the muscle about half-way down the forearm and a branch accompanies the inferior nerve of supply. Accessory supplies are derived from the ulnar artery which gives three or four branches to the deep surface, the anterior ulnar recurrent which supplies the humeral head, and the radial artery which supplies a strip along the lateral border of the muscle.

Flexor carpi ulnaris (FCU). This has a small supply from the inferior ulnar collateral artery at its origin and then has three main pedicles. The posterior ulnar recurrent artery passes obliquely upwards and medially between the deep and superficial flexors and then passes posteriorly between the humeral and ulnar heads of FCU, where it gives off a branch which turns distally into the muscle as the superior pedicle. The middle pedicle arises from the ulnar artery at the junction of upper and middle thirds and enters the muscle. The inferior pedicle is larger and arises from the ulnar artery just below the middle pedicle or in common with it, and then passes down the forearm almost to the point where muscle fibres run into tendon, before entering the muscle.

Deep flexor group

These muscles are supplied at their origin by the inferior ulnar collateral and by the ulnar recurrent arteries. In the forearm they are supplied mainly by branches from the ulnar and the anterior or common interosseous arteries.

Flexor digitorum profundus (FDP). Origin – as above. The main pedicle arises from the ulnar artery or sometimes from the anterior interosseous. This branch passes distally and medially for about 3 cm with the nerve of supply to FDP and supplies the middle third of the muscle. Sometimes this pedicle is made up of two vessels, one arising from the ulnar and the other from the interosseous with an accessory pedicle from the median artery. The anterior interosseous artery, and three to four branches of the ulnar artery supply the distal third.

Flexor pollicis longus. The anterior interosseous artery gives off four to six branches which supply the medial half of the muscle, while the lateral part receives two or three branches from the radial. Of these, the one lying at the junction of the middle and lower thirds of the forearm tends to be the largest. These vessels may contribute to the blood supply of the radial bone component of an osteo-myo-fasciocutaneous forearm flap. If the median artery is unusually large it may also support the muscle.

Pronator quadratus. The principal supply is through its posterior surface by the anterior interosseous artery just before that vessel passes through the interosseous membrane. On its anterior surface it receives one or two small branches of the radial and the ulnar arteries.

Extensor compartment muscles

The proximal and lateral group of extensors arising from the lateral supracondylar ridge of the humerus are supplied by the radial recurrent artery. Classically this is described as giving one or two branches to brachioradialis, and one branch each to the radial extensor of the carpus and one to supinator but this is an oversimplification. The other extensor muscles arise from the common extensor origin in the posterior compartment and are supplied by the posterior interosseous artery aided in the distal part of the forearm by the perforating terminal branch of the anterior interosseous artery. On passing through the interosseous membrane and reaching the posterior compartment, the posterior interosseous artery gives off its posterior recurrent branch.

Brachioradialis. This is supplied mainly by the radial recurrent artery with supplementary supplies from the radial collateral branch of the profunda brachii and the radial. The most common pattern is for the radial recurrent to give off two branches which pass in front of the posterior interosseous and superficial branches of the radial nerve (supplying them) and then pierce the posteromedial surface of brachioradialis. Within the muscle these arteries anastomose with branches from the radial collateral artery. The radial artery usually gives a few small branches to the distal part of the muscle belly and to the tendon.

Extensor carpi radialis longus (ECRL). The principal pedicle is a single branch from the radial recurrent. Accessory supplies come from the same vessels as are mentioned above as supplying brachioradialis.

Extensor carpi radialis brevis. The blood supply is the same as that of ECRL except that there are usually two principal pedicles, the second arising from the radial artery about a third of the way down the forearm.

Supinator. The superficial part of the muscle is supplied by the radial recurrent artery and the deep part by the posterior interosseous artery and its recurrent branch.

Anconeus. Classical texts state that anconeus is supplied by the middle collateral artery but we have certainly never seen this in 40 dissections of that artery. The muscle is supplied by the posterior interosseous recurrent artery. It is moderately vascular and the artery gives off one or two perforators to the overlying skin.

Extensor carpi ulnaris. Proximally it receives a few branches from the radial recurrent and sometimes a large branch from the posterior interosseous at its point of bifurcation into ascending and descending branches. Further distally it is supplied by several branches from the posterior interosseous.

Extensor digitorum communis. The proximal third is supplied by the radial recurrent artery and the lower two-thirds by the posterior interosseous artery; in addition the lower third may receive a perforating branch of the anterior interosseous artery through the interosseous membrane.

Abductor pollicis longus. This is supplied superiorly by a lateral branch of the posterior interosseous artery which runs between supinator and abductor pollicis longus. Further distally it is supplied on the medial side by a perforating branch of the anterior interosseous.

Extensor pollicis brevis. This is variably supplied by contributions from the posterior interosseous artery, the proximal perforators of the anterior interosseous and the terminal perforating branch of the anterior interosseous artery.

Extensor pollicis longus and extensor indicis. These are supplied on their superficial surfaces by the posterior interosseous artery and on their deep surfaces by the perforators from the anterior interosseous artery.

It therefore seems that removal of the radial or the ulnar artery as part of a flap will not seriously compromise the blood supply of forearm muscles provided that the proximal branches (common interosseous and the various recurrent arteries) given off within 4 cm of the antecubital flexion crease are preserved intact. This is in accordance with the observations of Parry et al (1988) on 440 cadaver muscles who concluded that use of a radial or ulnar artery as the recipient vessel for a free tissue transfer to the forearm would not jeopardise the blood supply of any muscle in the forearm (see also Revol et al, 1991).

6

SUMMARY OF ANATOMICAL TERRITORIES OF CUTANEOUS SUPPLY

The five anatomical territories which may be distinguished are shown in Figure 6.66.

1. The radial artery supplies the major part of the anterior surface of the forearm between the elbow and the wrist. Its anatomical territory covers the lateral two-thirds of the anterior surface and – with the exception of the area over the extensor pollicis brevis and abductor pollicis longus tendons – the lateral border and the lateral one-quarter of the posterior surface.

2. Within the territory of the radial artery can be defined the area of its largest fasciocutaneous perforator, namely the inferior cubital artery; although this perforator is variable in size and distribution its territory lies approximately parallel to the cephalic vein and extends distally from the apex of the antecubital fossa for a distance not exceeding 10 cm.

3. The territory of the ulnar artery abuts on that of the radial on the anterior surface, passes round the medial border of the forearm and extends onto the posterior surface as far as the subcutaneous border of the ulna. It extends from olecranon to wrist.

4. The territory of the posterior interosseous artery extends from the lateral edge of extensor digitorum communis where it abuts on radial territory, to the posterior subcutaneous border of the ulna where it abuts on ulnar territory.

5. The terminal perforating branches of the anterior interosseous artery supply a small area over the tendons of extensor pollicis brevis and abductor pollicis longus.

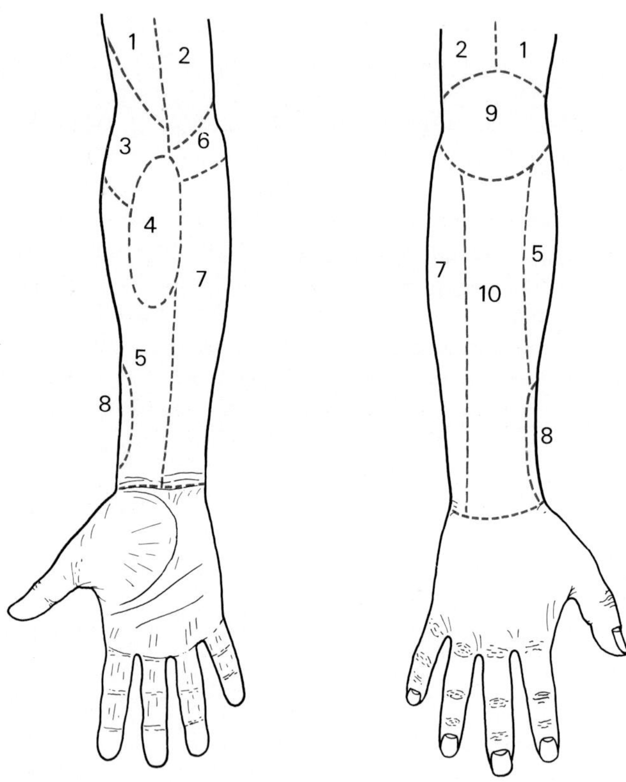

Fig. 6.66 Anatomical territories of cutaneous blood supply on the forearm:
1. Middle and radial collateral arteries
2. Superior ulnar collateral and brachial arteries
3. Radial recurrent artery } radial artery
4. Inferior cubital perforator } radial artery
5. Radial artery } radial artery
6. Anterior ulnar recurrent } ulnar artery
7. Ulnar artery } ulnar artery
8. Anterior interosseous artery
9. Olecranon anastomosis
10. Posterior interosseous artery.

Because of the extensive anastomoses between the vessels of adjacent anatomical territories, the potential territories are radically different and it has on occasion been possible to elevate the whole forearm skin supported only by the perforators of the radial artery.

FLAPS

Since the blood supply to forearm skin is largely by fasciocutaneous perforators, flaps also tend to be fasciocutaneous in type, although an inferiorly-based musculocutaneous brachioradialis pedicled flap has been described (p. 426).

The inferior cubital artery Type B flap may be transposed to cover an elbow joint and is a less bulky alternative to a musculocutaneous flap (p. 440).

Type C fasciocutaneous (i.e. septocutaneous) flaps based on the radial artery with or without a segment of radius, are well established. These may be used as proximally or distally pedicled loco-regional flaps, or as free flaps (p. 423). Ulnar artery flaps on similar principles are an alternative (p. 490). Islanded flaps on the posterior interosseous artery, whilst a difficult dissection, are feasible and may be distally based for reconstructions on the dorsum of the hand (p. 407).

Recurrent flaps around the elbow based on the posterior ulnar recurrent artery (p. 494), or the radial recurrent artery (p. 426) rely on the anastomoses around the elbow joint which are described on the next page.

UPPER ARM AND FOREARM

Anastomoses between the two

In the preceding pages the blood supply of the upper arm and of the forearm have been discussed separately as though they were separate regions. Thereby insufficient emphasis has been given to the multiple anastomoses that occur between the vessels of these two regions. This section is intended to correct this deficiency and at the same time draw attention to anastomoses that have clinical significance.

The classical description of the anastomoses around the elbow joint conforms to the pattern shown in Figure 6.45, i.e. anastomoses are between:

proximal	*distal*
middle collateral A.	interosseous rec. A.
radial collateral A.	radial rec. A.
superior ulnar collateral A.	posterior ulnar rec. A.
inferior ulnar collateral A.	anterior ulnar rec. A.

The extent of the interconnections between proximal and distal vessel groups has traditionally been classified into two types. Either the anastomosis occurs by one or more macroscopically identifiable vessels ('choke vessels' – Taylor & Palmer, 1987; 'anastomoses par inosculation' – Salmon, 1939) or by multiple small precapillary arterioles not identifiable with the naked eye ('anastomoses rétiformes' – Salmon). Variation also occurs in the location of the point of this anastomosis which in the case of a direct communication between proximal and distal vessels may be defined as the point of minimum diameter of the communicating vessel concerned.

Around the elbow most of the anastomoses are of the choke vessel type, with the exception of the middle collateral artery – interosseous recurrent artery anastomosis. The latter is rarely identifiable by the naked eye, as the middle collateral artery consistently terminates at the level of the deep fascia immediately proximal to the lateral epicondyle.

The other three anastomoses have been documented in a series of 16 cadaver dissections by Hayashi & Maruyama (1990). Their findings are summarised with the site of the anastomosis measured with reference to the inter-epicondylar line where + is a measurement proximal to it and – a measurement distal to it.

These findings are relevant to the raising of retrograde flow reverse-pedicled flaps around the elbow and suggest that the axis of preference on the lateral side should be the radial recurrent A. (the reverse lateral upper arm flap p. 426) and on the medial side the posterior ulnar recurrent A. (the reverse medial upper arm flap p. 494).

Table 6.7 (Adapted from Hayashi & Maruyama, 1990)

		IUCA-AURA	SUCA-PURA	RCA-RRA
Choke vessel	No. of cases	10	11	10
	Mean calibre	0.3	0.4	0.3
	Range (mm)	0.2 to 0.5	0.2 to 0.8	0.2 to 0.5
Microscopic	No. of cases	6	5	6
	Mean site of anastomosis	– 17	+ 10	+ 34
	Range (mm)	–39 to +20	– 10 to + 35	+ 15 to + 65

6 WRIST AND HAND

It has been pointed out that variability in the size of the major vessels occurs frequently in the forearm. It follows that the relative contributions to the vascularity of the hand made by the radial and ulnar arteries also vary, both normally and in disease. In 1929 Allen described a clinical test for determining ulnar artery patency in patients with thromboangiitis obliterans. More recently this has become a standard procedure for evaluating the patency of the radial and ulnar arteries and for assessing the completeness of the superficial and deep palmar arches (Gelberman & Blasingame, 1981).

The timed Allen test

The test is performed by the examiner occluding the patient's radial and ulnar arteries with two fingers just above the wrist (11 or more pounds of pressure are required to occlude the vessels reliably, and this degree of pressure causes discomfort in most patients). The hand is meanwhile exsanguinated by the patient making three tight fists. The patient then opens the hand to a resting position in which hyperextension at the wrist and finger joints is avoided. The radial or the ulnar artery is then released and the time taken from artery release to the appearance of a vascular flush on the volar aspect of the distal part of the middle finger is recorded. Any suggestion of delayed vascular filling of any part of the hand is also recorded. In about 1% of cases a revascularisation end point may not be obtained because of the normal pallor of the skin. The remaining cases will fall into one of the following three groups listed in Table 6.8.

In a study of 774 hands of normal volunteers in whom normal skin pallor did not prevent the test, it was found that 9% of hands showed delayed or absent filling through one artery. 48% of subjects with delayed or absent fill in one hand had delayed fill in the other, and hand dominance, age and sex were not related to the hand revascularisation times (Table 6.9). In studies comparing the findings of Allen's test with those on arteriography, it was concluded that when the test was performed correctly, no false positives resulted (Hirai & Kawai, 1980; Hirai, 1980).

THE WRIST

The wrist and carpal area has been defined in the past as the area extending 2 cm above and below the apex of the radial styloid. The blood supply of this area will be considered on its dorsal and palmar aspects and then the blood supply of the hand and fingers will be described.

The dorsal aspect of the wrist

The dorsal aspect is supplied by branches of the radial, ulnar and both interosseous arteries. Of these the radial is classically regarded as the most significant and its contribution to the dorsal carpal arch is formally named the dorsal carpal branch. However, this vessel arises deep to the extensor tendons of the thumb, passes beneath the other extensor tendons and sends only very small branches back to the skin in the wrist area defined above, its major supply being to the skin of the back of the hand over the metacarpals. The skin over the dorsum of the wrist proper is supplied by a plexus on the extensor retinaculum classically known as the rete carpi dorsale which is also regarded as the property of the radial artery (*Nomina Anatomica*). We have found, however, that this plexus is supplied mainly by the anterior interosseous artery aided by the posterior interosseous and reinforced laterally by radial twigs ('recurrent') and medially by twigs from the dorsal carpal branch of the ulnar. (This dorsal carpal branch arises from the ulnar artery proximal to the pisiform bone and turns posteriorly above or below the tendon of flexor carpi ulnaris to divide into the dorsal carpal branch which completes the carpal arch, and a small artery to the ulnar side of the fifth metacarpal.) This arrangement of the dorsal carpal network (rete) is shown in Figure 6.68 but the arrangement is variable.

Table 6.8 Definition of filling rates used in Allen Test

Rapid fill	—revascularisation in less than 6 seconds
Delayed fill	—revascularisation in 6→15 seconds
Absent fill	—failure of revascularisation, unchanged for 15 seconds

Table 6.9 Radial and ulnar arterial filling rates

	Through radial artery	Through ulnar artery
Rapid fill	98%	93%
Delayed fill	1.4%	3.7%
Absent fill	0.6%	3.3%

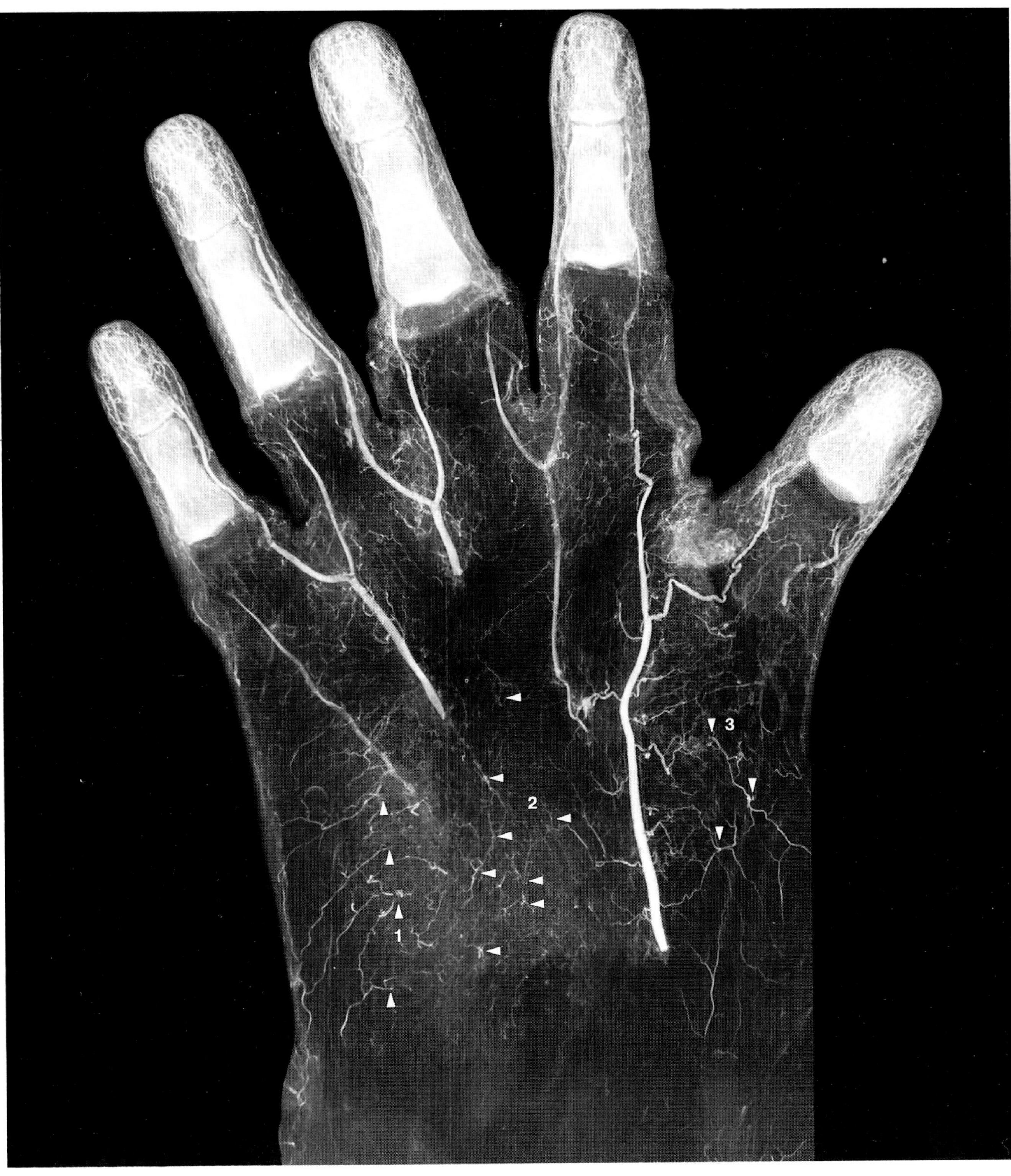

Fig. 6.67 Radiograph of injected skin of the palm of the hand and the volar wrist. The distal phalanx of the thumb has been preserved with the nail bed and terminal pulp intact, and on the other fingers the middle and distal phalanges with their covering volar and dorsal skin have been preserved. In this case the superficial palmar branch of the radial artery was a well-developed vessel which passed superficially over flexor pollicis brevis to supply the index finger and the thumb – its connection with the 'superficial arch' was very small. The apparent tortuosity of the princeps pollicis artery is due to the folding of the slack skin of the first web space. Note: **1.** Perforators arising from the ulnar artery and emerging between flexor digiti minimi and abductor digiti minimi, **2.** Multiple very small and fine vessels which have pierced the palmar aponeurosis, **3.** Perforators through abductor pollicis brevis and flexor pollicis brevis.

The flexor aspect of the wrist

The flexor aspect is supplied by branches of the radial and ulnar arteries with very occasionally a contribution from the median artery when it is large enough to reach the level of the wrist. The anterolateral border of the wrist is supplied by an unnamed vessel which arises from the lateral side of the radial artery and runs distally over the tendon of brachioradialis supplying skin. Once again there is a carpal arch closely related to the bones and joints but there is no palmar network comparable to the rete dorsale. Instead, fine perforators lie on either side of the palmaris longus tendon and also pierce the palmar aponeurosis. On the radial side, these arise from the superficial palmar branch of the radial artery as two or three separate twigs. On the ulnar side, there is a constant unnamed vessel arising from the ulnar artery or its deep branch which turns round the pisiform bone and runs medially and distally into the hypothenar muscles. It gives off several small twigs which join two or three other fine branches from the ulnar to supply the skin over the wrist. The division between radial and ulnar territories lies along the palmaris longus tendon and the middle of the palmar aponeurosis except for those cases in which a median artery exists. Radiographs show that the cutaneous branches are small, run horizontally across the wrist, and that the fine dermal network arising therefrom lies longitudinally.

THE DORSAL ASPECT OF THE HAND AND FINGERS

The radial artery reaches the back of the wrist by turning posteriorly between the lateral radiocarpal ligament and the tendons of abductor pollicis longus and extensor pollicis brevis. It passes across the floor of the 'anatomical snuff box', beneath the tendon of extensor pollicis longus, and disappears between the two heads of the first dorsal interosseous to re-emerge in the palm between the oblique and transverse heads of adductor pollicis. On the dorsum of the hand the radial artery gives off small twigs to the rete dorsale, a larger branch to the dorsal carpal arch, and cutaneous branches to the dorsal aspects of the first and second metacarpals via the first dorsal metacarpal artery.

In 95% of cases the radial artery conforms to this standard pattern as shown in Figure 6.69 but in the remainder it passes between the tendons of extensor carpi radialis longus and brevis. It may then enter the palm between the second and third metacarpals instead of the first and second. These variations are shown in Figure 6.68.

Other variations affecting the radial artery are:

1. The area normally supplied by the radial artery may be taken over by a very large anterior interosseous artery which pierces the interosseous membrane in the usual way and then continues on to the dorsum of the wrist and hand. This is very rare.

2. The dorsal carpal branch of the radial artery is generally represented in European texts as a prominent transversely running vessel. However, it may be almost entirely spent in forming a second dorsal metacarpal artery and only a very small vessel then continues across the carpus. It follows from this that the third and fourth dorsal metacarpal arteries may be fed almost entirely by perforators from the palmar arches and not by the dorsal carpal arch.

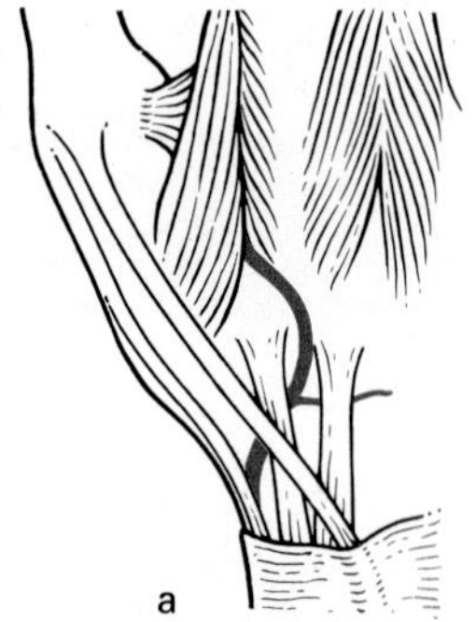

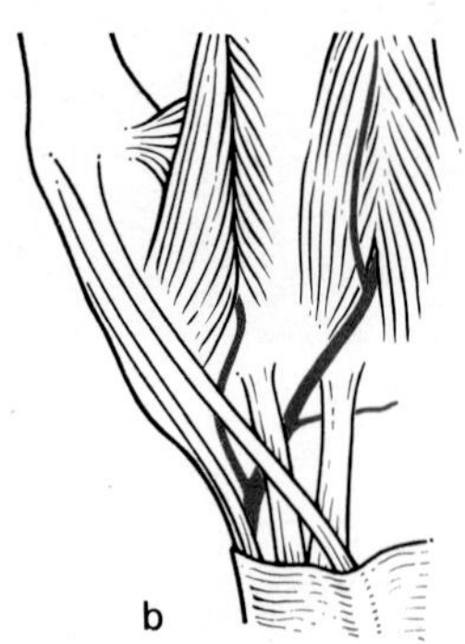

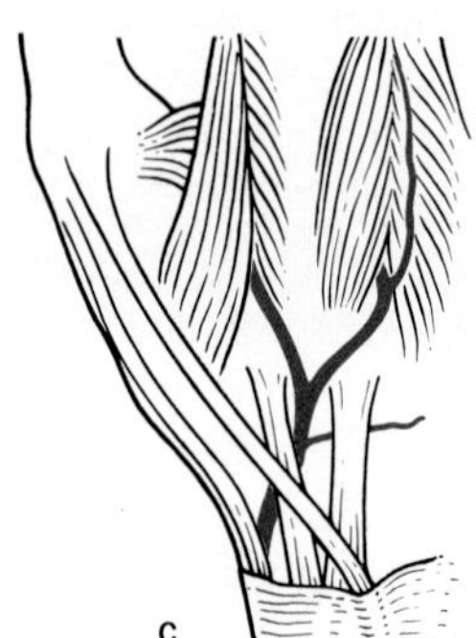

Fig. 6.68 Variations in the course of the radial artery occurring in up to 5% of cases.

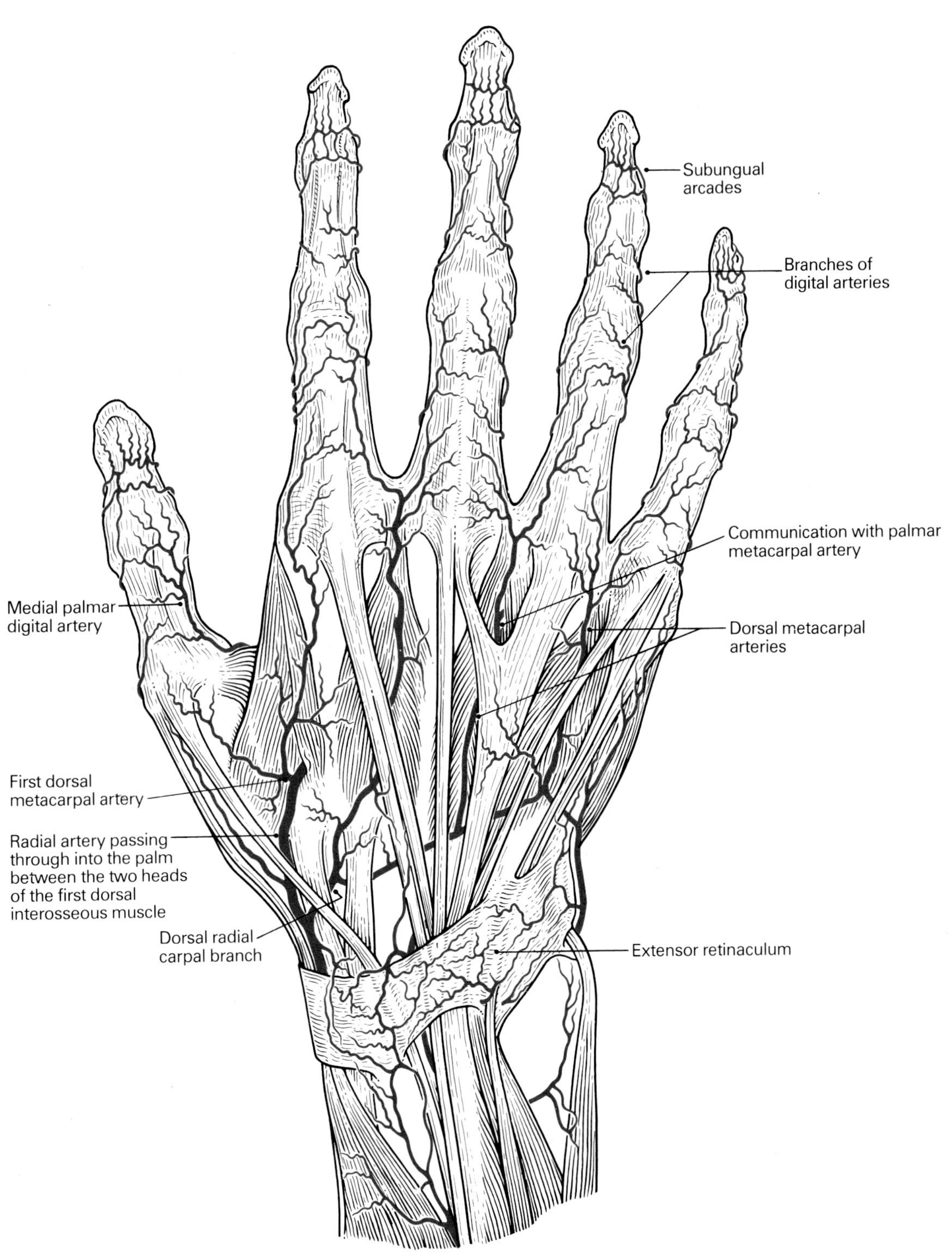

Fig. 6.69 Blood supply to the skin on the dorsum of the hand and wrist.

Branches to the dorsum of the thumb

Over the dorsum of the metacarpal there is usually a small direct branch of the radial artery lying radial to the extensor pollicis longus tendon and a branch of the first dorsal metacarpal artery lying ulnar to the tendon although this ulno-dorsal artery may alternatively arise directly from the radial artery as shown in Figure 6.71b. Terminology for this vessel and the first dorsal metacarpal artery are often confused. The first dorsal metacarpal artery is strictly only the short vessel that divides into the ulno-dorsal artery of the thumb and the radio-dorsal artery of the index. However, in the surgical literature the term first dorsal metacarpal artery is often applied to the vessel that runs along the index metacarpal.

Dorsal metacarpal arteries

The dorsal carpal arch lies deep to the extensor tendons across the distal row of carpal bones and may be completed medially by the dorsal carpal branch of the ulnar artery. This dorsal carpal branch arises from the ulnar artery whilst still proximal to the pisiform, and gives off a small branch which runs along the ulnar side of the fifth metacarpal down to the metacarpophalangeal joint, before passing back across the carpus to complete the dorsal arch. Classically the dorsal metacarpal arteries are described as arising from this dorsal carpal arch.

In fact they have four possible sources of origin: from the radial artery, from the dorsal carpal arch, from the deep palmar arch and from another dorsal metacarpal artery. In moving across the dorsum from radial to ulnar the origins follow this sequence.

In general terms all the arteries lie deeply in the fascia over the dorsal interosseous muscles between the extensor tendons and are accompanied by venae comitantes. Each artery, in its course towards the corresponding web space, may give off four or five extremely small cutaneous twigs which make longitudinal rows overlying the interosseous spaces but any one such row may be completely absent. At points approximately 1 cm proximal to the metacarpal heads the second, third and fourth arteries give off larger branches to the skin. The metacarpal arteries then run onwards to the web spaces where they divide into dorsal digital branches for adjacent sides of the proximal phalanges of the index,

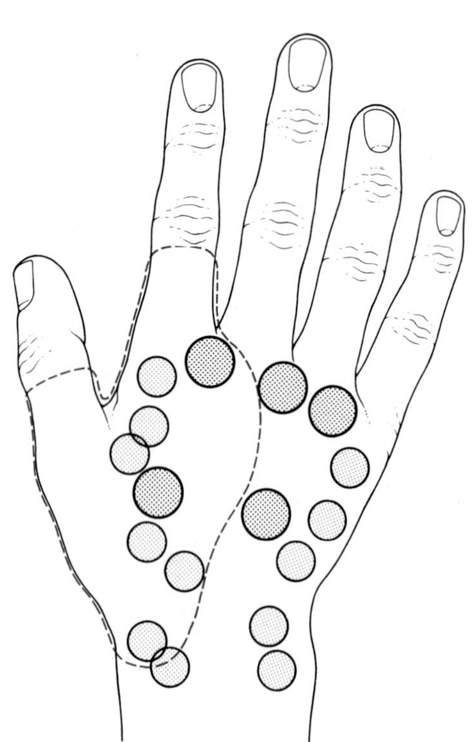

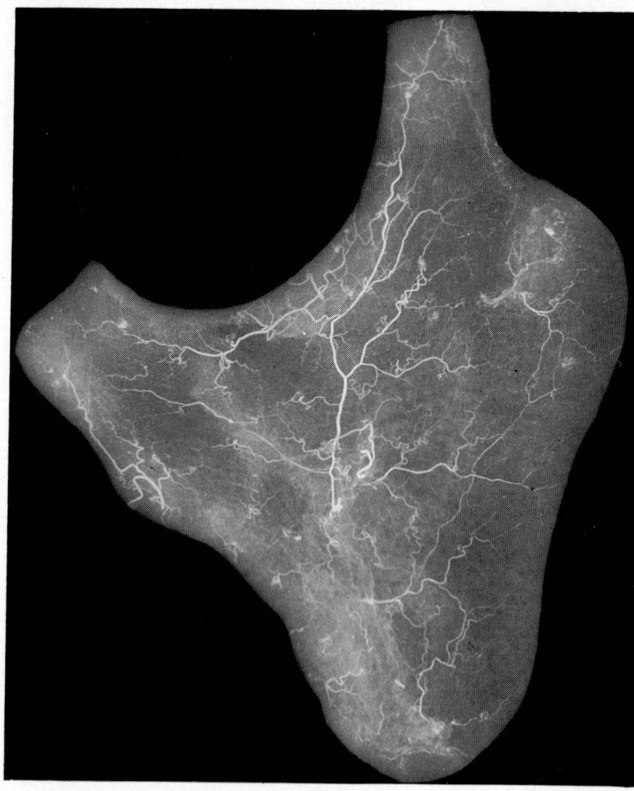

Fig. 6.70 The diagram shows the commonest locations of the major branches to skin on the dorsum of the hand. The larger circles indicate the sites of the larger branches. (The circles over the second, third and fourth webs have perhaps been drawn a little further distally than they should have been.) The interrupted red outline shows the boundaries of the skin specimen in the accompanying radiograph. This shows the first dorsal metacarpal artery and a branch of the second dorsal metacarpal artery which has emerged proximal to the metacarpal heads (corresponding to circle over second web).

middle, ring and little fingers. These branches do not extend much beyond the bases of the proximal phalanges and anastomose with dorsal branches of the palmar digital arteries beyond this. The second to fourth arteries may have deep connections in the proximal part of each intermetacarpal space with the deep arch and in the distal part of each space with the corresponding common palmar digital artery.

This general scheme is illustrated in Figures 6.69 and 6.70, but variations apply to individual dorsal metacarpal arteries as follows:

First dorsal metacarpal artery. For the purposes of this description the term first dorsal metacarpal artery will be taken to include the branch to the radio-dorsal aspect of the index proximal phalanx. The typical course of the FDMA is within the fascial layer overlying the first dorsal interosseous muscle where it runs parallel to the index metacarpal, becoming more superficial and branching into smaller vessels as it approaches the metacarpophalangeal joint. It then runs onto the proximal phalanx to supply skin over its proximal part. This arrangement is shown in Figure 6.71a & b. However, in the remaining cases the FDMA has a deep course within the substance of the first dorsal interosseous muscle (Fig. 6.71c) and in only half these cases does the artery then emerge at the level of the metacarpal head. In up to 30% of cases superficial and deep forms of the DMCA may coexist and this is in addition to a direct branch of supply from the radial artery to the first dorsal interosseous muscle. A further complication is that at the level of the neck of the second metacarpal the terminal branches of the FDMA may either become cutaneous or may disappear deeply beneath the extensor tendon expansion or round the neck of the metacarpal to join with the palmar metacarpal artery. This has been termed the 'second metacarpal sink'. In this situation the FDMA does not contribute to the blood supply over the index proximal phalanx. Detailed studies of the 'fascial' and 'muscular' variants have been described (Earley, 1986; Earley & Milner, 1987; Dautel et al, 1989).

Second dorsal metacarpal artery. The anatomy of this vessel is more consistent than that of the FDMA. It is also generally larger than the dorso-radial index branch of the FDMA because it has to contribute to the supply of both index and middle fingers. In 80% of cases it arises from the dorsal carpal arch and in the remainder from various sources: radial artery, deep palmar arch, or FDMA. Once it has passed beyond the index extensor tendons its course becomes predictable, as it lies within the fascia over the second dorsal interosseous muscle, heading for the index/middle web space. A branch to skin is a consistent finding approximately 1 cm proximal to the metacarpal heads. A proximal deep communication with the deep palmar arch is common, but communication at the level of the metacarpal heads with the palmar common digital artery is much less common.

Third dorsal metacarpal artery. Contrary to the classical description, this dorsal metacarpal artery may arise more commonly from the deep palmar arch than from the dorsal carpal arch. It may on occasion arise from the SDMA. Its branches to skin are restricted by the overlying extensor tendons to the distal part of the area over the third intermetacarpal area.

Fourth dorsal metacarpal artery. This is larger than the third. As well as the branch in the distal part of the intermetacarpal space it also gives off branches more proximally. In many case, perhaps the majority, rather than a single artery there are really proximal and distal branches from different sources which include the deep palmar arch.

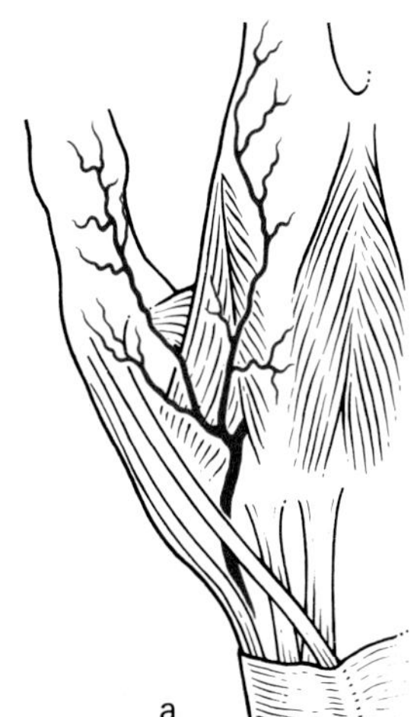

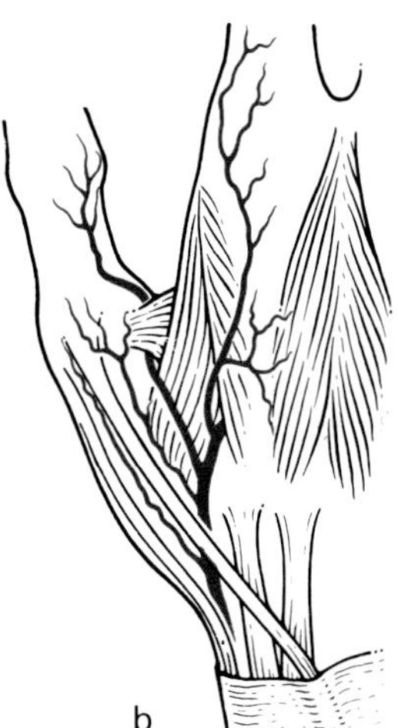

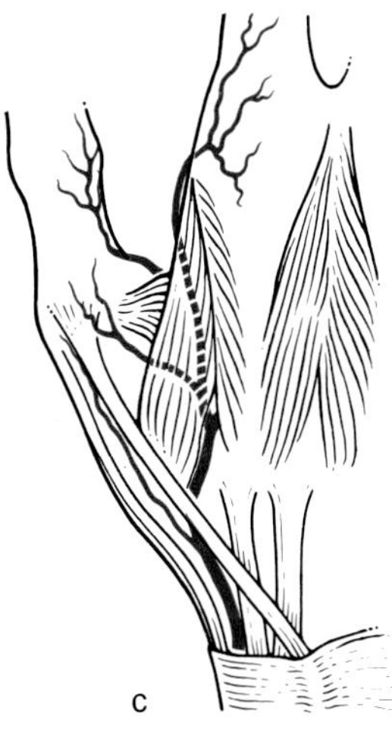

Fig. 6.71 Variations in the arrangement of the first dorsal metacarpal artery and its branches.

Dorsal aspects of the fingers

The blood supply to the backs of the fingers may be considered in four parts:

1. The region over the web and metacarpal head is supplied by cutaneous perforators from the ends of the dorsal metacarpal arteries.
2. The backs of the proximal phalanges are supplied over their bases by the dorsal digital arteries. This represents the distal limit of the territory supplied by the dorsal metacarpal arteries. The remainder of the proximal phalanx is supplied by branches of the palmar digital arteries which run obliquely dorsally and distally. However, these are not necessarily symmetrical on the two sides of a finger.
3. The dorsum of the middle phalanx is supplied by one or two small branches of the palmar digital arteries.
4. The dorsum of the distal phalanx is covered by three (or more) arcades.

Arcades over the dorsum of the distal phalanx

The most proximal of these lies in the subcutaneous tissue over the base of the distal phalanx just distal to the distal interphalangeal (DIP) joint. This superficial arcade is fed from either side by a vessel originating from the digital artery much more proximally in the finger. These feeding vessels arise from the middle segments of the digital arteries and run obliquely distally and dorsally (Fig. 6.72). In addition, terminal branches of the digital arteries contribute to the superficial arcade. The second arcade lies over the waist of the distal phalanx and the third over the base of the ungual process. Both of these subungual arcades are fed by vessels from the cruciate anastomosis on the volar aspect of the phalanx. These feeding vessels turn dorsally around the base between it and an interosseous ligament. All these arcades are interconnected and form a particularly rich vascular bed (Flint, 1956).

The thumb

The thumb is different in that over the metacarpal the arteries lie deeply and supply the skin by multiple small twigs. Occasionally the ulnar dorsal branch is large and runs on to the distal phalanx (Fig. 6.71a), but over the dorsum of the proximal phalanx the supply is usually by branches from the princeps pollicis (Fig. 6.71c). The distal phalanx resembles in its blood supply that of the other fingers.

Subungual arcades
Superficial arcades
Terminal branch
Middle branch
Digital artery

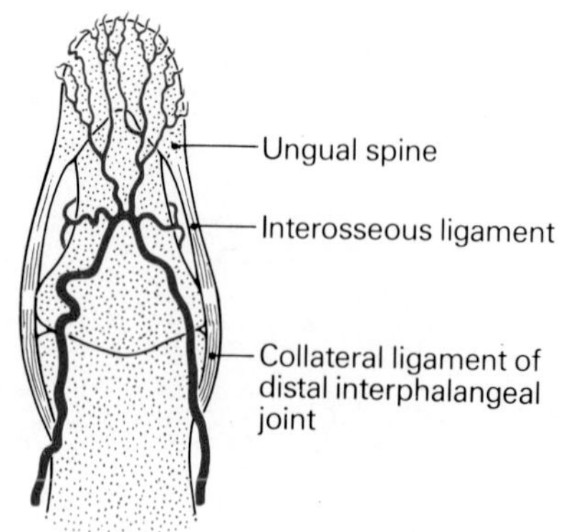

Palmar aspect of the terminal phalanx showing cruciate anastomosis and branches to the subungual arcades.

Fig. 6.72 Diagrams to show the dorsal arcades and the branches of the digital arteries which arise in the middle segment and pass both dorsally and distally. (Copied from Flint 1956, with permission.)

FLAPS

On the dorsum of the hand the dorsal metacarpal arteries provide the basis for three different types of flap:

1. Islanded skin flaps isolated on a first or second dorsal metacarpal artery pedicle and raised from the dorsum of the proximal phalanx of the second or third finger, or from contiguous sides of the second web. Innervation may be provided by incorporation of branches of the radial nerve. These flaps are particularly useful for skin cover on the injured thumb.

2. Distally based island flaps from the back of the hand incorporating the second, third or fourth dorsal metacarpal artery in a manner analogous to the Type C septocutaneous flaps. The point of rotation is in the web space and the flap is useful for cover on the dorsum of a finger.

3. Distally based island flaps from the back of the hand positioned so that the distal end of the flap overlies the main branch to skin 1 cm proximal to the metacarpal head. These flaps are useful for rotation onto the dorsum of an injured proximal phalanx or PIP joint. A distally based flap from the fourth web may be useful for scar release on the ulnar border of the fifth finger. These flaps are all described on page 316.

The difference between the longitudinal blood vessels on the dorsum of the thumb and the multiple branches to the dorsal aspects of the fingers has implications for the raising of palmar skin advancement flaps to resurface tip injuries. On the thumb such a procedure is reasonable (p. 309) but on the other fingers it is highly likely to result in necrosis of dorsal skin unless steps are taken to preserve the dorsal branches given off by the palmar digital arteries opposite the middle phalanges. Even then it is not a recommended procedure on the fingers.

Dorsal finger flaps include oblique flaps for tip reconstruction, cross-finger flaps with a traditional lateral base or an even distal base, and distally based flaps for homodigital pulp reconstruction. All these are dependent on branches of the digital arteries with the cross-finger flap and the oblique dorsal flap for homodigital finger pulp reconstruction being based on the middle segment branches of the palmar digital arteries (pp. 306–310).

The anastomoses between the vascular arcades supplying the nail bed suggest the possibility of raising the nail complex as a flap based on the dorsal branch of the palmar digital artery which ends in the superficial arcade. This enables the nail to be relocated more proximally in those cases where fingertip amputation or pulp injury with scar formation have resulted in a 'parrot-beak' deformity of the nail.

On the sides of the fingers flaps may be pedicled for local transposition or islanded for transfer to a more distant location. Local transposition flaps from the side of a finger to cover, for example, a short length of exposed flexor tendon are based on branches of a digital artery and need not interrupt it. Islanded flaps raised from the side of the proximal phalanx require division of a digital artery and may be used on a proximal pedicle to fill small defects in the distal palm and on a distal reverse-flow pedicle for fingertip reconstruction. In this situation the fact that both digital arteries to a finger are not invariably present is important and it is essential to know whether a digital artery exists on the other side of the finger capable of supplying the distal part of the finger (pp. 308 – 314).

Various other designs of flap from the distal part of a finger based on branches of a single digital artery and designed for fingertip reconstruction are described on page 305.

6

THE PALMAR ASPECT OF THE HAND AND FINGERS

The blood supply of the palm – classical description

It has been customary to regard the arteries of the hand as a series of arches from which terminal branches emerge to supply the fingers. There is tremendous variability in these arches and several extremely accurate morphological classifications were devised many years ago which still form the basis of modern studies and discussions. It is not proposed to describe these in detail and only the traditional scheme as enshrined in the format adopted by *Nomina Anatomica* will be described.

RADIAL ARTERY
- superficial palmar branch
- princeps pollicis artery
- radialis indicis artery
- deep palmar arch
  - palmar metacarpal arteries
  - posterior perforators

ULNAR ARTERY
- deep palmar branch
- superficial palmar arch
  - common palmar digital arteries
    - palmar digital arteries

The palm and fingers are supplied by the radial and ulnar arteries via superficial and deep arches. The superficial arch is formed mainly by the ulnar artery and completed by the superficial palmar branch of the radial artery. It lies immediately beneath the palmar aponeurosis at the level of the web of the extended thumb and is further protected on the ulnar side by lying beneath palmaris brevis. It lies anterior to the branches of the median nerve and gives off a palmar digital artery to the ulnar side of the fifth finger and three common palmar digital arteries which run to the three web spaces between the fingers. As they pass distally on the lumbricals these common palmar digital arteries come to lie dorsal to the digital nerves. Approaching the metacarpal heads they receive anastomotic palmar metacarpal branches from the deep palmar arch. In the web spaces they divide, usually more distally than the common digital nerves, into palmar digital arteries for the adjacent sides of the fingers.

The deep arch is formed mainly by the radial artery and is completed by the deep palmar branch of the ulnar artery. On passing through the first dorsal interosseous and arriving in the palm, the radial artery gives off the princeps pollicis and the radialis indicis arteries and passes medially deep to adductor pollicis. The deep arch gives off three palmar metacarpal arteries which run distally on the palmar interossei of the second, third, and fourth spaces. They give off posterior perforators which join the dorsal metacarpal arteries before themselves joining with the common palmar digital arteries from the superficial arch. In addition, the deep arch gives off a branch to the hypothenar muscles and recurrent branches to the carpal network.

Recently this classical terminology has been challenged and an alternative description devised in terms of arterial systems supplying well-defined territories with four constant vascular systems – the radial, the ulnar, the thenar, and the hypothenar – being recognised (Barreiro & Valdecasas, 1976).

Edwards (1960) has shown that digital arteries are not all the same size. In particular the digital artery to the ulnar side of the index finger, the ulnar side of the thumb, and the radial side of the little finger are usually much larger than the other vessels to the same fingers. Variations can occur in any finger and it is unwise to rely on two fully effective digital arteries.

Variations

These are extremely common.

1. Coleman & Anson (1961) found that the superficial arch had the classic form in only 34% of 650 specimens. In 37% the arch was incomplete and was formed by the ulnar artery alone.
2. The deep arch is much more constant than the superficial and is absent in only 4% of cases.
3. The radialis indicis has the traditional origin from the deep arch or princeps pollicis artery in less than 50% of cases. It arises from the superficial arch in 13% and in the remainder from both. It may supply only the radial side of the index finger but in 75% it gives off a communicating branch to the common digital artery of the second web space, and in some of these cases is the main or only supply to that space.
4. There are a number of variations in the arrangement of the two branches of the princeps pollicis. The most common is that the princeps pollicis, rather than arising from the deep palmar arch, arises from the radial artery on the dorsum of the first web space and passes over (or under) the lateral head of the first dorsal interosseous to reach the palmar aspect of the thumb by passing through between adductor pollicis and the first metacarpal (Fig. 6.71b). The classical description is that the princeps pollicis divides into two branches which run along the medial and lateral palmar aspects of the thumb (the medial and lateral palmar digital arteries). These vessels may alternatively arise

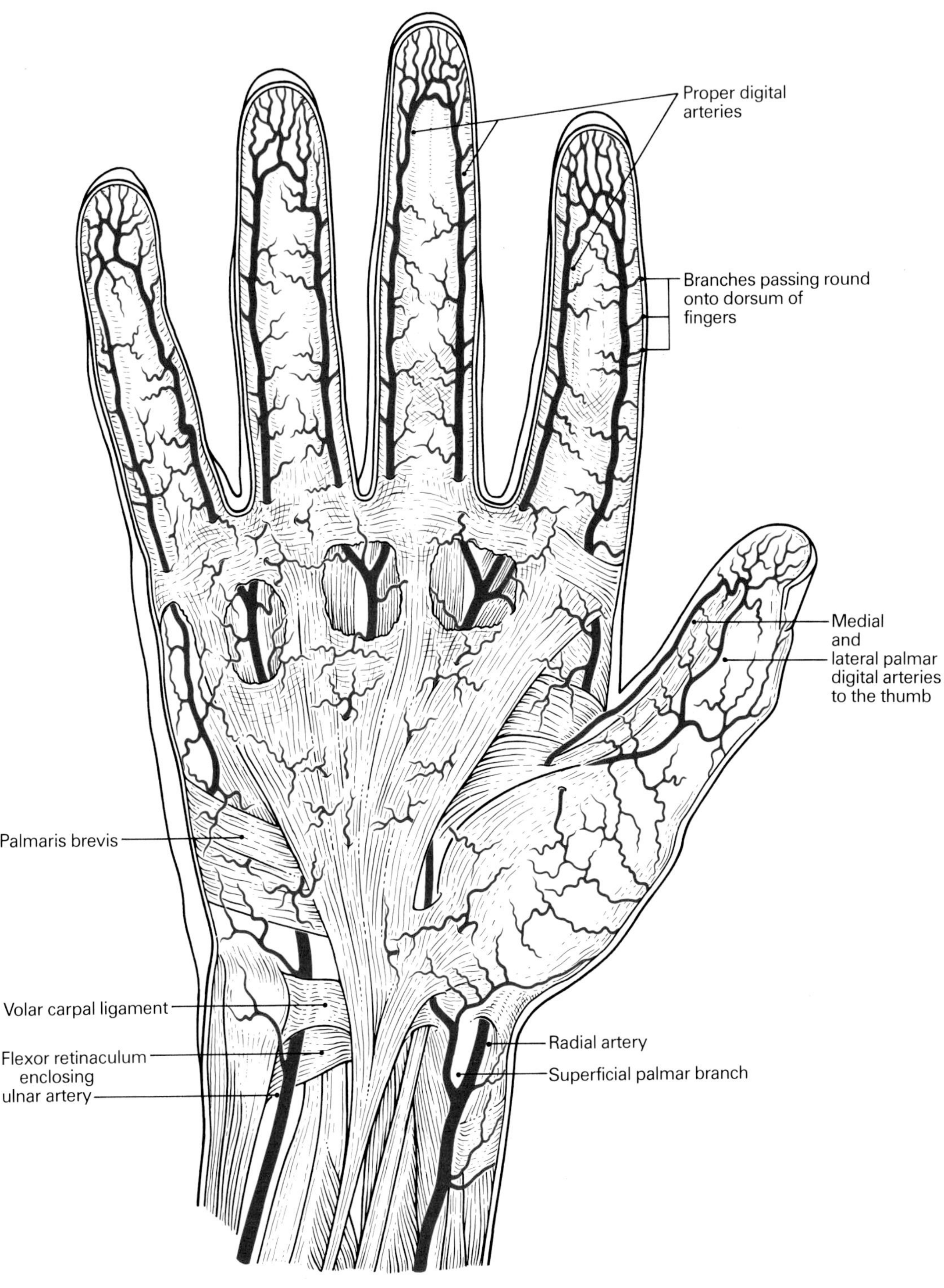

Fig. 6.73 Blood supply to the skin on the palmar aspect of the hand and wrist.

from the superficial arch or even, in the case of the medial palmar digital artery, from the first dorsal metacarpal (Fig. 6.74c). Representative findings in a series of 100 hands are shown in Table 6.10.

5. The palmar digital arteries are regarded as arising from the common palmar digital arteries off the superficial arch. This is largely true for the middle, ring and little fingers where only 5–10% of digital arteries have an alternative origin from a palmar metacarpal artery (deep arch). However, in the index finger the digital arteries may arise from the deep arch in 30% of cases. Very occasionally a dorsal metacarpal artery may be the principal supply to a palmar digital vessel.

6. It is also the case that the two hands are rarely identical in terms of these variations.

Various authors have studied variations in digital vessels. In addition to those mentioned above we have consulted Eaton, 1968; Nicoletis & Morel-Fatio, 1968; Popoff, 1934; Weathersby, 1954; Ikeda et al, 1988; Leslie et al, 1987; and Libersa et al, 1982.

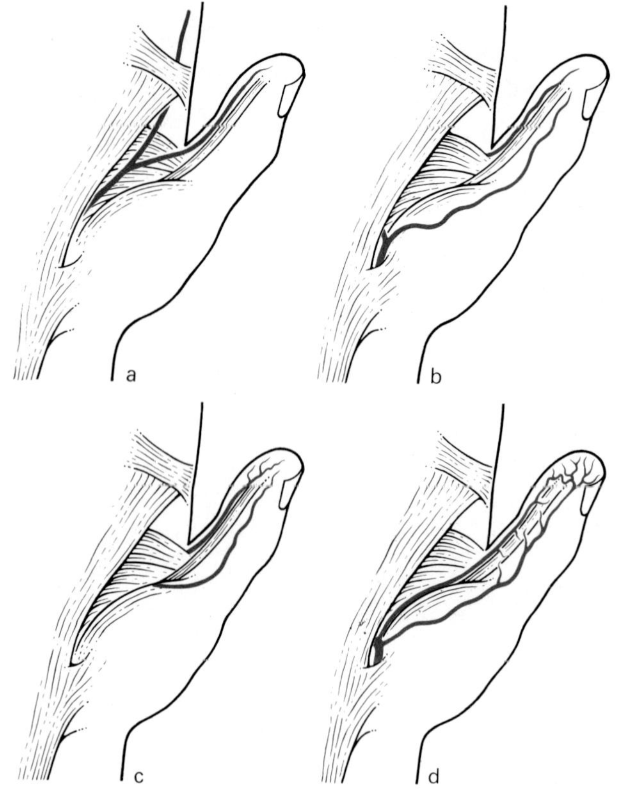

Fig. 6.74 Variations in the origin of the palmar digital arteries of the thumb.

Table 6.10 Origins of palmar digital arteries of the thumb

Origin	Lateral palmar digital artery of thumb	Medial palmar digital artery of thumb	Radialis indicis
From superficial arch (mainly ulnar) or superficial palmar branch of radial	21[1]	24[2]	31[3]
From a single princeps pollicis (i.e. deep palmar arch)	74[4]	28[4]	29[4]
From a dorsal metacarpal artery	0	42[5]	25
Others, including those unidentifiable because destroyed by student dissectors	5	6[6]	15[6]

[1] See Fig. 6.74a; [2] see Fig. 6.74d; [3] see Fig. 6.74b; [4] see Fig. 6.73, main illustration; [5] see Fig. 6.74c; [6] 13 cases of an origin from a palmar metacarpal artery.

CUTANEOUS BLOOD SUPPLY TO THE PALM OF THE HAND AND FINGERS

The superficial palmar branch

This branch of the radial artery passes through and supplies the muscles of the thenar eminence. It gives off a number of twigs to the skin over the proximal parts of abductor and flexor pollicis brevis.

The princeps pollicis

This runs along the first metacarpal deep to adductor pollicis. Its lateral branch emerges at the base of the proximal phalanx between the insertions of adductor pollicis and flexor pollicis brevis. Here it generally divides into two branches which pass along the ulnar and radial sides of the flexor surface of the thumb. These vessels supply the skin of the thumb from the metacarpophalangeal joint distally, but early branches of the princeps pollicis aid in the supply of the skin over the thenar eminence. These vessels have no particular direction but are in general longer and slightly larger than the multiple small perforators through the palmar aponeurosis.

The radialis indicis artery

This passes distally between the first dorsal interosseous and the overlying adductor pollicis to emerge at the distal border of this muscle. Here it may communicate with the princeps pollicis and the superficial palmar arch. Small branches supply skin over the radial border of the palm. It runs along the radial border of the index finger to its tip supplying half the palmar surface and sending branches around on to the backs of the phalanges.

The common palmar digital arteries

These arise from the superficial arch. There are three, and one palmar digital artery to the ulnar side of the little finger. These give off numerous small twigs which pierce the overlying palmar aponeurosis to reach the skin of the palm. All these perforators are equally small and have a random distribution. The common palmar digital arteries communicate with the palmar metacarpal arteries from the deep arch and divide into the palmar digital arteries proper.

The ulnar artery

As it enters the palm the ulnar artery gives off small branches to the skin over palmaris brevis and the hypothenar muscles. These are somewhat larger than the perforators through the palmar aponeurosis.

The palmar digital arteries

These are the main blood supply to the digits. In the web space short dorsal branches are given off to the dorsal web skin. The arteries run dorsal to the digital nerves and range in diameter from 1.0 mm at the proximal end of the finger to 0.5 mm at the level of the distal interphalangeal joint. Each artery gives off three small branches, which run onto the dorsum of each phalanx to anastomose with the branches from the other side. Edwards (1960) has named two other anastomosing branches – the proximal and distal transverse digital arteries which lie across the necks of proximal and middle phalanges respectively. They run close to the bone, deep to the tendons and are closely related to the proximal parts of the interphalangeal joints. Over the middle phalanx segment of its course each digital artery gives off a branch which runs distally and dorsally to form the superficial arcade over the base of the distal phalanx (Fig. 6.72). The digital arteries run on, and opposite the base of the distal phalanx each gives off a terminal branch which runs dorsally and divides into two limbs; one limb contributes to the superficial arcade, the other limb forms a proximal subungual arcade (Flint, 1956). The palmar digital arteries themselves carry on to converge in the pulp beneath the distal phalanx in a cruciate or an H-shaped anastomosis. At the point of confluence two vessels arise, one to each side of the finger. Each vessel passes dorsally round the waist of the distal phalanx to form the distal subungual arcade. All arcades are interconnected and supply the subungual corium whilst from the cruciate anastomosis many branches fan out to supply the finger pulp. With age, vessels become increasingly unequal and dominant ones appear particularly associated with a dominant digital artery.

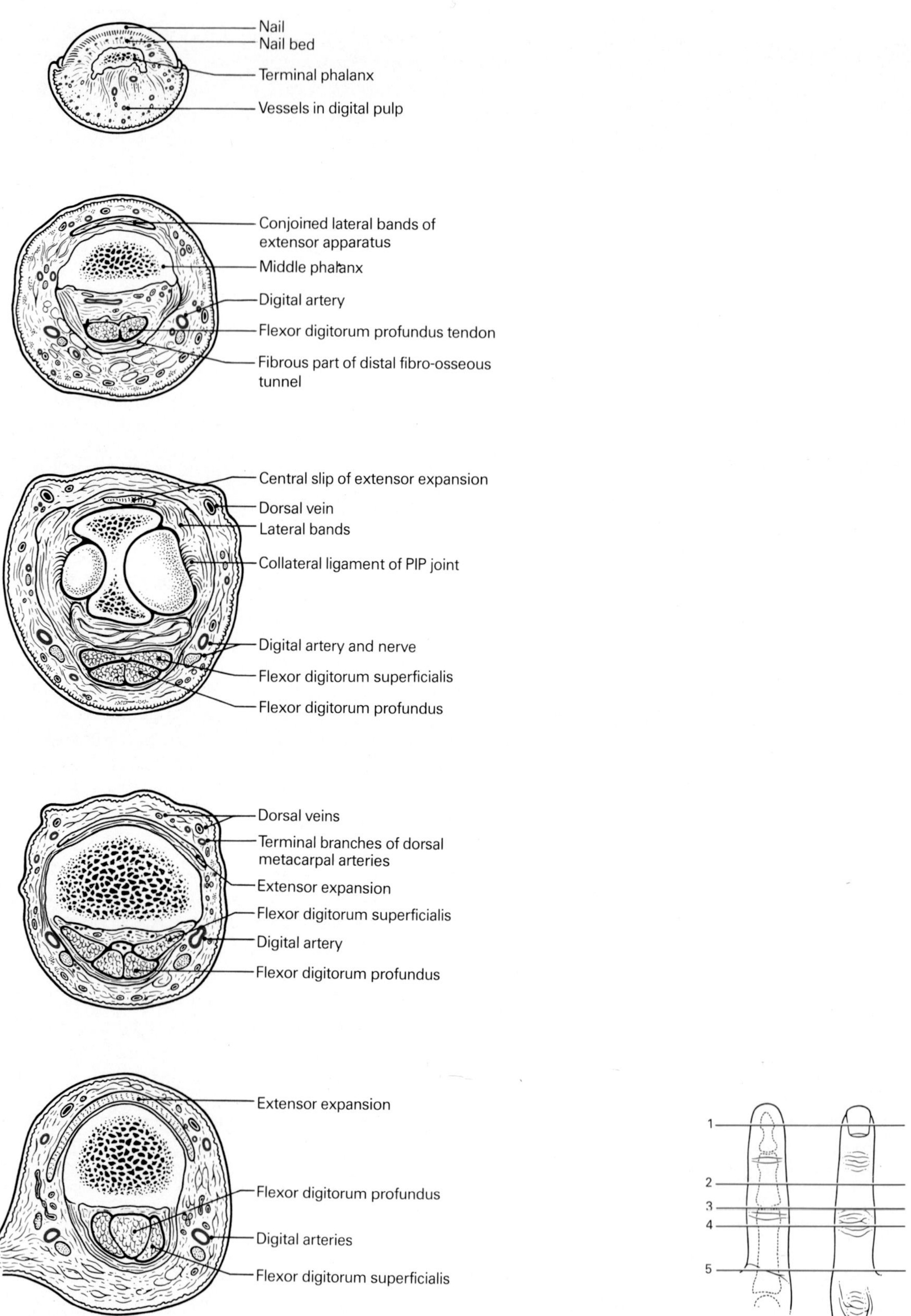

Fig. 6.75 Cross-sections through an index finger at various levels to show the positions of the digital arteries and nerves relative to other structures.

The venous drainage of the fingers

This is a matter of great importance in the construction of finger flaps, in digital replants and transfers, and in the transfer of neurovascular island flaps. Whereas almost everywhere else in the body one can presume that there are venae comitantes accompanying the arteries, in the finger this is not necessarily the case. Usually the digital artery is the only vessel running with the digital nerve, while the veins drain to a plexus over the dorsum of the finger which runs proximally to join the superficial dorsal venous arch on the hand. Deep digital veins may be present but are complicated relative to the digital arteries, often being small and multiple with thin walls. Kaplan (1965) has shown that there may occasionally be a single large digital vein running with the artery or there may be a pattern of closely related venae comitantes – but only rarely. The palmar venous network consists of small superficial veins over the palmar surfaces of the fingers which turn proximally and dorsally. These veins tend not to cross the flexion creases opposite the interphalangeal joints, and instead there are large transverse anastomoses. These all drain into the large veins on the dorsal surfaces of the fingers. These lie mainly along the borders of the fingers and anastomose with each other, particularly around the joints where there are large transverse linkages. The dorsal veins pass back in the grooves between the metacarpal heads to reach the back of the hand, and again have transverse anastomoses at this point. On the back of the hand the arrangement is so variable as to defy description (Lucas, 1984).

FLAPS

Palmar flaps of one kind or another are an old concept. These are all random pattern in type but are either of the pedicled variety, e.g. fingertip reconstruction with a thenar flap, or sliding variety, e.g. V-Y advancement, Z-plasty, trapezoid flap. Neurovascular pedicled island flaps were developed in the early 1960s and are well established as a means of providing sensate skin reconstructions of the damaged index or thumb tip. For these it is clearly necessary to have digital arteries arising from common palmar metacarpal arteries and some knowledge of the variations that might be encountered is useful. Digital replantation is now an established technique. Replantations through the palm also require an understanding of the inter-relationships between palmar vessels.

THE DIGITAL NERVES

Because of the importance of providing sensory reconstructions of the damaged finger tip and pulp, increasing use is nowadays being made of neurovascular flaps. A detailed knowledge of the course, depth and distribution of the digital nerves is, therefore, as important as an understanding of the blood supply in the planning of many finger flaps. The following is a brief account of the innervation of the thumb and fingers based on current anatomical teaching. No comprehensive investigation into the variability of all of the digital nerves appears to have been published although Wallace & Coupland (1975) have studied variations in the nerves of the thumb and index fingers.

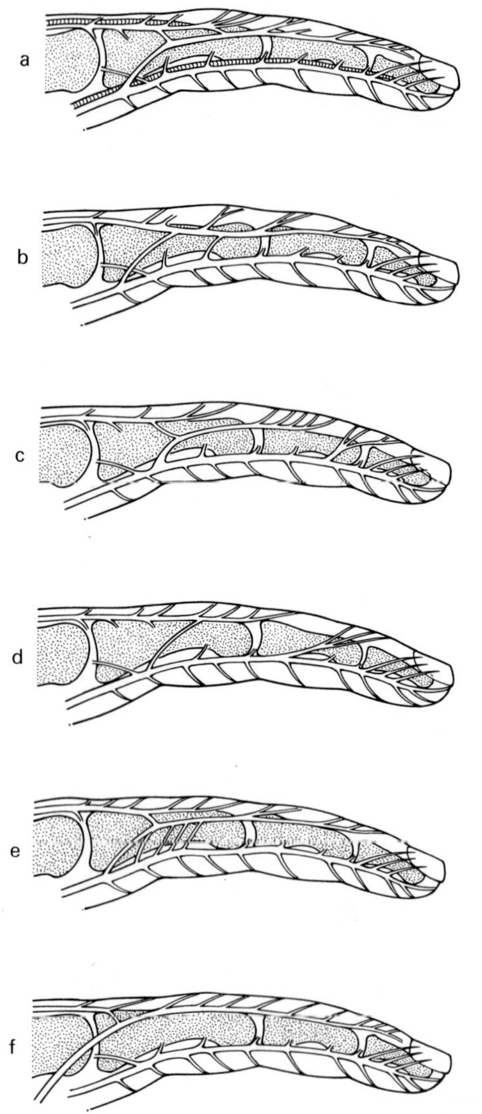

Fig. 6.76 Arrangement of the digital nerves in the index finger – see text for explanation. (Copied from Wallace & Coupland, 1975 with permission.)

Fingers

The proper palmar digital nerves pass between the superficial and deep transverse metacarpal ligaments to enter the fingers. Here they lie on the sides of the long flexor tendons in the plane of the volar surfaces of the phalanges, immediately anterior to the digital arteries which they accompany. Just beyond the base of the proximal phalanx, each palmar digital nerve gives off a dorsal branch which turns obliquely distally and dorsally to supply branches to the skin over the back of the middle and distal phalanges. A little beyond the base of the distal phalanx, the digital nerve gives off a branch which passes dorsally to supply the nail bed, while the main nerve divides into about three branches which supply the skin of the terminal part of the digit and the pulp.

The proximal part of the dorsum of each finger not supplied by branches of the palmar digital nerves, is supplied by dorsal digital nerves. On the little finger the dorsal digital nerves extend as far as the base of the distal phalanx, on the ring and middle fingers as far as the base of the middle phalanx. There are from two to four branches per finger.

Dankmeijer & Waltman (1950) concluded that where dorsal and ventral nerves are found together, innervating respectively the dorsal and volar side of a phalanx, the line formed by the terminations of the papillary ridges indicates the boundary between the regions and constitutes the only place on the human skin surface where an external configuration indicates a frontier between nervous territories.

Index

In a study of 50 palmar digital nerves in index fingers, Wallace & Coupland (1975) found much variation in the detailed anatomy. The most common pattern occurred in 37 of the nerves, with a dorsal branch being given off just proximal to the proximal digital crease. This branch passed either deep (20 cases) or superficial (17 cases) to the digital artery, pierced Cleland's ligament and, after anastomosing with the dorsal digital nerve, supplied the skin over the dorsum of the middle and distal phalanges but not the nail bed (Fig. 6.76a).

In five palmar digital nerves no large dorsal branch was found, but one or two small twigs did communicate with the dorsal digital nerve (Fig. 6.76b). Figures 6.76c, d, e show other patterns of variation relating mainly to the supply of the dorsum of the finger and in one case (Fig. 6.76f) the dorsal branch of the palmar digital nerve was given off proximally within the palm and passed into the digit as a quite separate nerve, to supply virtually all of the dorsum of the finger.

It is clear, therefore, that the cutaneous supply to the dorsum cannot be defined accurately, particularly because of the variable nature of the communication between the dorsal digital nerve and the palmar digital nerve (usually through its dorsal branch). It does appear, however, that in the index finger this variation is more marked on the ulnar side. On the radial side pattern 'a' occurred 23 times and pattern 'c' the other two times. On the ulnar side the commonest pattern was seen 14 times and other patterns in the remaining 11.

Wallace & Coupland also counted the number of endoneurial tubes in one case and found that of about 5000 endoneurial tubes entering the finger, about 3000 passed beyond the distal digital crease, carrying fibres which terminated in the pulp and nail bed. The endoneurial tubes within the finger were found to be symmetrically placed in position and number on either side of the digit. On dissection no evidence of cross-over innervation of the pulp was apparent. The cross-sectional area of a palmar digital nerve was measured, and found to change little in size as it passed from the palm to the distal digital crease. In this part of its course its diameter was between 1 and 1.5 mm.

Thumb

The pattern of distribution of nerves to the thumb is more constant. Two palmar digital nerves, derived from the median nerve, pass distally on the radial and ulnar sides of the thumb lying palmar to the digital arteries. At the level of the distal digital crease each nerve divides into three or four branches to supply both the pulp and the nail bed. Wallace & Coupland found that in no case did the palmar nerves give off a dorsal branch, but in eight cases out of 25 a short lateral cutaneous branch from the radial palmar digital nerve supplied the skin over the radial side of the first metacarpophalangeal joint. In 25 dissections they found no evidence of cross-over of nerve fibres from the digital nerves to the opposite side of the thumb. The dorsal digital nerves to the thumb all arise from the radial nerve and the number of branches varies from two to five.

6 BUTTOCK

Nomina Anatomica

ARTERIA ILIACA INTERNA

Arteria iliolumbalis
  Ramus lumbalis
  Ramus iliacus

Arteriae sacrales laterales

Arteria obturatoria
  Ramus pubicus
  Ramus anterior
  Ramus posterior

Arteria glutea superior
  Ramus superficialis
  Ramus profundus
    Ramus superior
    Ramus inferior

Arteria glutea inferior
  A. comitans nervi ischiadici

Arteria pudenda interna
  A. perinealis
  Rami scrotales/labiales posteriores
  A. dorsalis penis/clitoridis

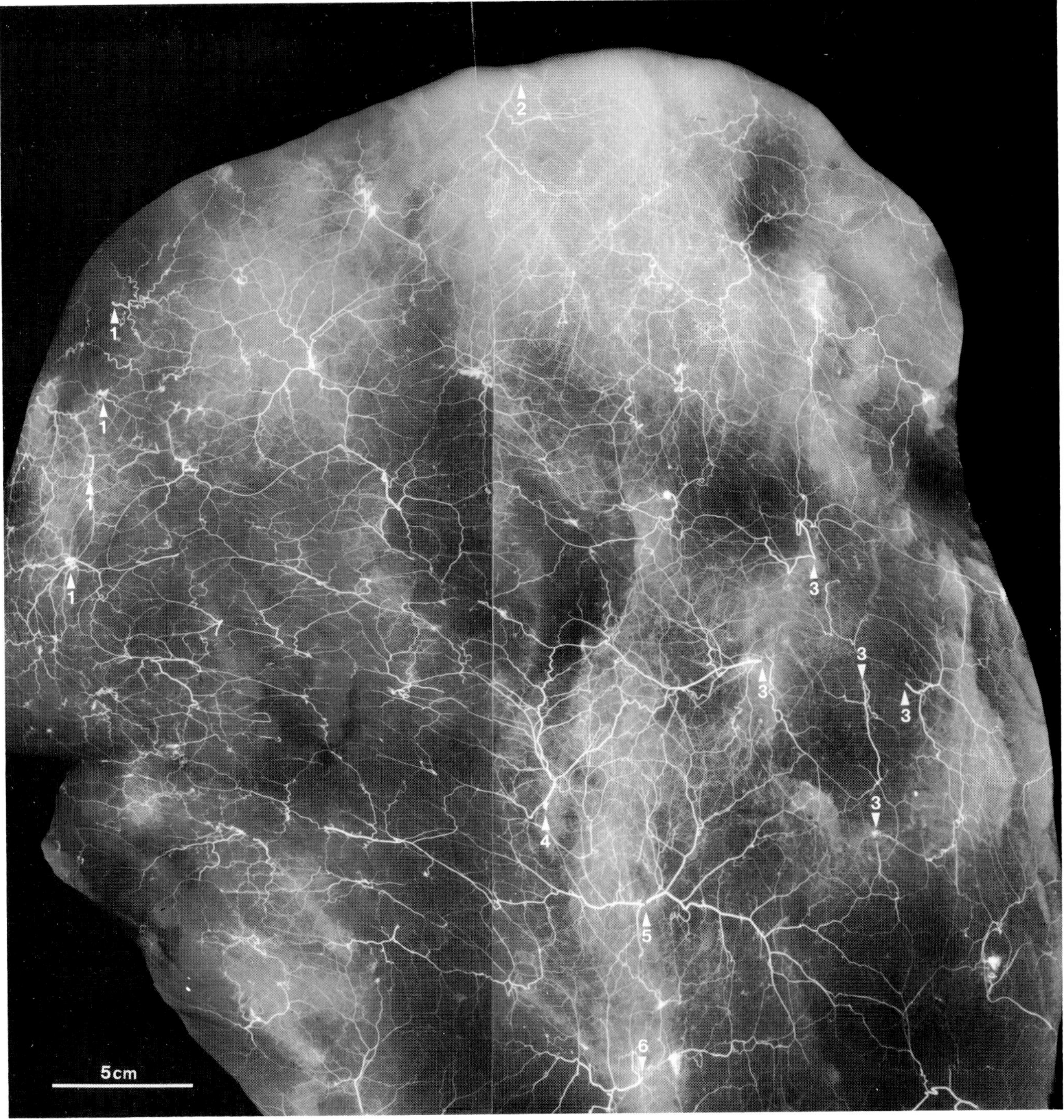

Fig. 6.77 Radiograph of injected skin and subcutaneous tissue from the region overlying the buttock and uppermost part of the thigh. The boundaries of the specimen are: posteriorly, the midline; superiorly, the crest of the ilium; anteriorly, a line passing from the anterior superior iliac spine towards the patella; and inferiorly, a horizontal line round the thigh at a level immediately distal to the insertion of gluteus maximus into the iliotibial tract. (This radiograph is continuous with that of thigh skin shown in Fig. 6.84.)

1. Perforators from the lateral sacral arteries,
2. A branch of a lumbar segmental artery passing over the iliac crest,
3. Perforators through tensor fasciae latae,
4. Branch of the first profunda femoris perforator piercing the insertion of gluteus maximus,
5. Branch of first profunda femoris perforator which has passed along the lateral intermuscular septum and on reaching the deep fascia has divided into two branches, one directed posteriorly and the other anteriorly across the iliotibial tract,
6. Branch of the second profunda perforator emerging at the posterior edge of the iliotibial tract.

All other unlabelled vessels are musculocutaneous perforators arising from the superior and inferior gluteal arteries and piercing the surface of gluteus maximus.

6

BUTTOCK

For the purposes of description the buttock may be considered as the region falling within the following boundaries: medially, the midline; laterally, a line between the anterior superior iliac spine and the greater trochanter; superiorly, the iliac crest; and inferiorly, the buttock fold extended laterally and upwards to the greater trochanter. The general scheme is simple with most of the skin being supplied by perforators from the superior and inferior gluteal arteries. In addition, there is a small area around the anal canal supplied by the internal pudendal artery, an area medial to the posterior superior iliac spine supplied by iliolumbar and sacral branches and an area over the inferolateral part of gluteus maximus supplied by the first perforator arising from the profunda femoris. The region is therefore mainly supplied by multiple small musculocutaneous perforators which measure approximately 0.5 mm ID and supply areas of 15–20 cm^2.

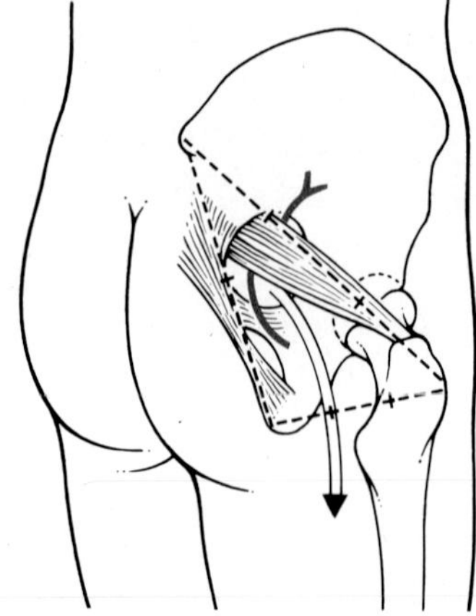

Fig. 6.78 Surface markings related to bony points.

The superior gluteal artery

This arises from the internal iliac artery in the majority of cases as the continuation of its posterior trunk. In ~27% it may arise from a common stem (truncus gluteалis) with the inferior gluteal. The superior gluteal artery enters the buttock in the company of the superior gluteal nerve lying above piriformis in the greater sciatic notch. The vessel measures 5 mm in diameter at this point and can be marked out on the surface by a point lying one-third of the way along a line drawn from the posterior superior iliac spine to the top of the greater trochanter (Fig. 6.78). The veins in this area tend to be particularly numerous, large and thin-walled, and generally lie superficial to the arteries. The main stem of the superior gluteal artery gives off a nutrient vessel to the ilium and then divides into a superficial and a deep branch.

The superficial branch

This further subdivides in the plane between gluteus maximus and gluteus medius into three ramifying branches which are not designated in *Nomina Anatomica* but may be called posterior, intermediate and anterior.

The posterior branch is closely applied to the undersurface of gluteus maximus and gives off numerous branches of supply to its superior half which, after further division, pierce the surface of the muscle to reach the overlying skin. Some of these vessels anastomose with branches of the inferior gluteal artery and others perforate the tendinous origin of the muscle to anastomose with posterior branches of the lateral sacral arteries and supply skin over the sacrum.

The intermediate branch runs directly upwards and at the posterior gluteal line (the posterior limit of the gluteus medius origin), passes off gluteus medius onto the periosteum of the posterior iliac crest. Ink injection of this vessel in cadavers has demonstrated consistent staining over the posterior iliac bone, and the adjacent muscles as well as an area of overlying skin measuring up to 10 cm × 14 cm. This vessel, and its accompanying veins, have been described as the basis of an osteo-myo-cutaneous free flap consisting of a mono-cortical bone block (8 cm × 13 cm) with a thick cancellous component covered by muscle and skin. This has been named the posterior iliac flap (Mialhe & Brice, 1985).

The anterior branch runs between the gluteus maximus and the gluteus medius supplying them both. Terminal branches may emerge at the supero-lateral edge of the gluteus maximus to pierce the deep fascia and supply skin. This cephalic edge of gluteus maximus can be marked on the surface by a point starting on the iliac crest one hand's breadth anterior to the posterior iliac spine and curving towards the greater trochanter.

At this edge the muscle becomes continuous with the deep fascia over gluteus medius which is in fact the upper part of the iliotibial tract. It is along this edge that the 'question-mark incision' of Henry (1957) passes for exposure of the gluteal vessels and sciatic nerve. This arrangement of vessels passing round the edge of the muscle is analogous to that described for the pectoral artery whose terminal branches pass round the lateral edge of pectoralis major to reach skin. They behave like musculocutaneous perforators. From the cephalic edge of gluteus maximus forwards to tensor fasciae latae, the skin overlying the tract is supplied by a few perforators through gluteus medius from the deep branch of the superior gluteal artery.

The deep branch of the superior gluteal artery

This spreads out between gluteus medius and gluteus minimus, applied more closely to the former, and runs laterally supplying both. The deep branch has superior and inferior divisions which are hidden beneath gluteus medius in Figure 6.79. The superior runs along the upper border of gluteus minimus towards the anterior superior iliac spine anastomosing here with a branch of the lateral circumflex femoral artery and the superficial circumflex iliac artery. The inferior division crosses and supplies gluteus minimus, supplies the hip joint and anastomoses with the inferior gluteal artery, the medial circumflex and the lateral circumflex femoral arteries. It does not supply skin.

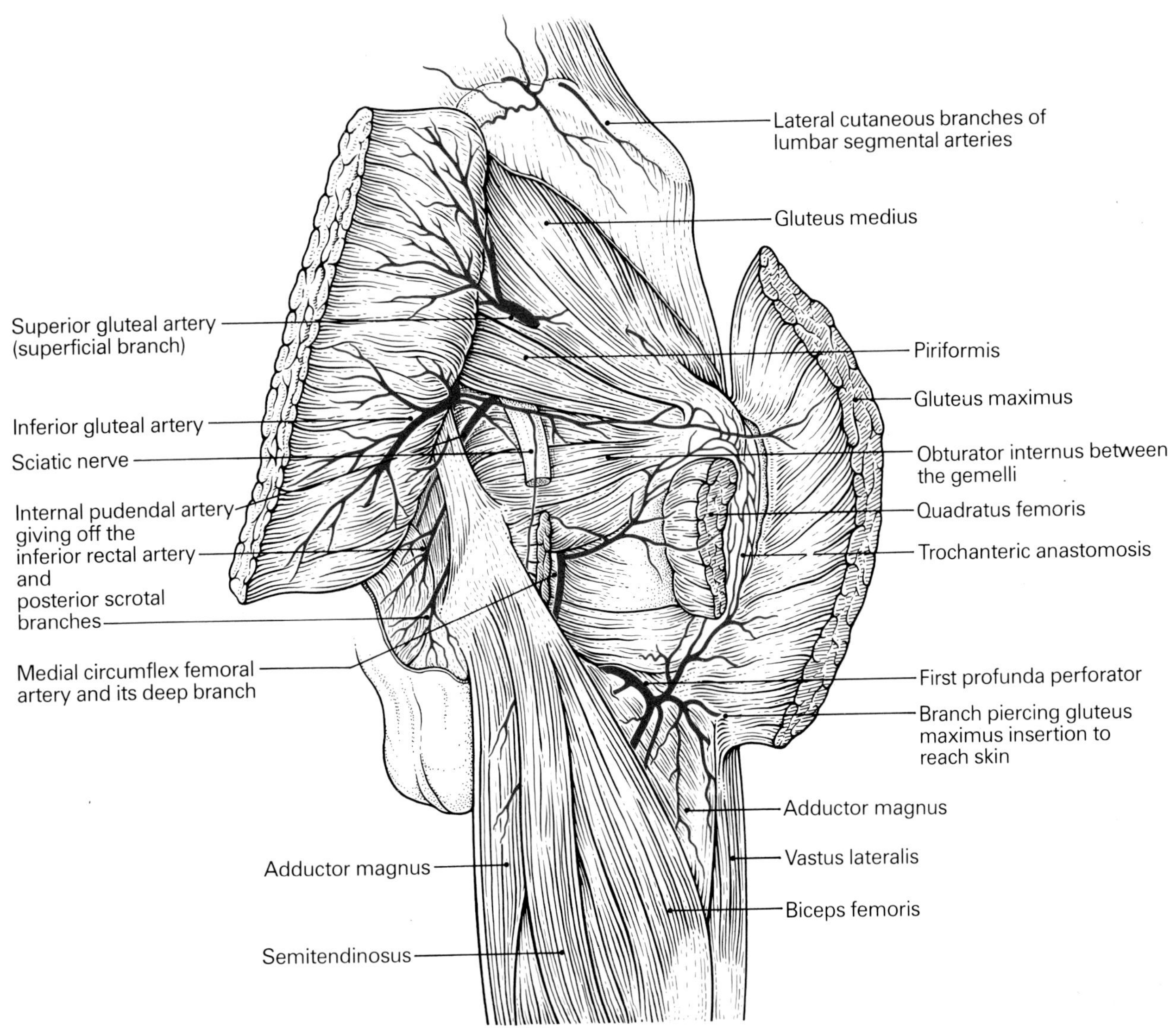

Fig. 6.79 Deep vessels of the buttock region. Gluteus maximus has been divided to reveal the superior and inferior gluteal arteries and the first profunda perforator.

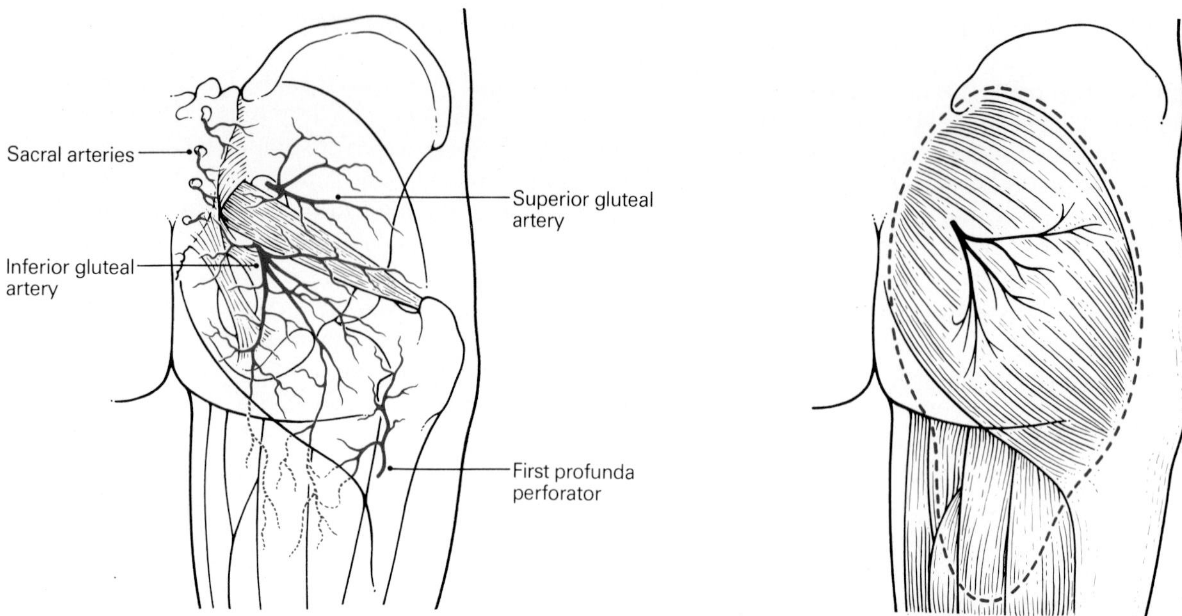

Fig. 6.80 Distribution of the gluteal arteries and branches of the first profunda perforator within gluteus maximus.

Fig. 6.81 Total anatomical area of cutaneous blood supply under the dependency of gluteus maximus outlined by broken red line. The distribution of the inferior gluteal nerve has been superimposed on the muscle.

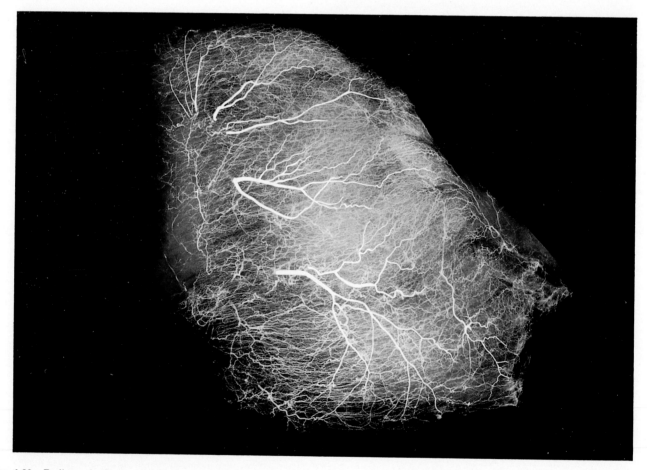

Fig. 6.82 Radiograph of injected right gluteus maximus muscle.

The inferior gluteal artery

This is usually a terminal branch of the anterior trunk of the internal iliac but may arise with the superior gluteal from a common trunk. It enters the buttock with the inferior gluteal nerve by passing through the greater sciatic notch. Here it lies below piriformis closely related to the internal pudendal vessels medially and the sciatic nerve laterally. Occasionally it may pass through piriformis. At this point it measures 3.5 mm in diameter and can be marked on the surface by a point half-way along a line drawn from the posterior superior iliac spine to the ischial tuberosity. Figure 6.79 shows the inferior gluteal dividing into two main branches, medial and lateral, with a branch to the sciatic nerve which is classically regarded as the remains of the embryonal continuation of the main trunk.

The inferior gluteal artery is the major blood supply to the lower two-thirds of gluteus maximus and sends many perforators through the muscle to supply the overlying skin. The medial division is large and sends branches both superiorly and inferiorly on the undersurface of gluteus maximus right up to the sacral origin of the muscle. These vessels anastomose with branches of the superior gluteal whilst the lateral division supplies the short rotator muscles of the hip, the upper parts of the hamstrings, and the lower lateral part of the gluteus maximus. Here it anastomoses with the first profunda perforator and the medial circumflex femoral artery.

Not shown in Figure 6.79 is a branch of the inferior gluteal which accompanies the posterior cutaneous nerve of the thigh. Under gluteus maximus the nerve gives off two sets of branches, inferior clunial nerves curving below the muscle and turning round its inferior border to supply the lower buttock skin as far laterally as the greater trochanter, and perineal branches which curve medially over the hamstrings, below the ischial tuberosity to supply the skin of the anal region and of the posterior scrotum or labium majus. Some fine branches of the inferior gluteal artery accompany these nerves for a short distance but a more major vessel lies with the posterior cutaneous nerve of the thigh itself just below the deep fascia of the thigh.

All the musculocutaneous perforators given off by the gluteal vessels have a random distribution in the subcutaneous tissues. Manchot's statement (1889) that all the vessels converge towards the greater trochanter has some truth in so far as the upper vessels of this region fan out anteriorly, and the medial ones run laterally, as a glance at the radiograph in Figure 6.77 will show, but perhaps this assertion ascribes more order to the vessels than is warranted. Subdermal anastomoses are particularly large and numerous.

The first profunda perforator

This pierces adductor magnus close to the linea aspera and sends a branch upwards which enters the insertion of gluteus maximus. This anastomoses within the muscle with the inferior gluteal artery and sends a few musculocutaneous perforators to the overlying skin. Branches also emerge along the lateral intermuscular septum through the insertion of gluteus maximus, thereby continuing the line of perforators along the lateral side of the thigh. The uppermost of these cutaneous branches of the profunda perforators generally reaches skin about 32 cm above the line of the knee joint, and fans out both anteriorly over the iliotibial tract and posteriorly over the gluteus maximus insertion.

The medial circumflex femoral artery

This does not contribute to the supply of the skin of the buttock directly but it may take part in the blood supply of gluteus maximus. The deep branch (ramus profundus) of the medial circumflex femoral appears in the buttock beneath quadratus femoris and divides into ascending and descending branches. The ascending branch is distributed to the short rotators and the trochanteric anastomosis; the descending branch regularly gives branches to the lowermost part of gluteus maximus and ends in the hamstrings.

The internal pudendal artery

This artery is classically regarded as the other terminal branch of the anterior trunk of the internal iliac artery, although in 50% of cases it shares a common stem in the sciatic notch with the inferior gluteal (truncus pudendo-glutealis inferioris). It passes over the ischial spine, re-enters the pelvis through the lesser sciatic foramen and passes in the pudendal canal along the medial side of the inferior pubic ramus to the perineum. Its inferior rectal branch is given off above the ischial tuberosity. This crosses the ischiorectal fossa as a number of branches which supply the skin of the anal region. One or two branches turn round the lower edge of gluteus maximus to supply the infero-medial part of the buttock. (The perineal branch is considered in the section dealing with the perineum.)

The lumbar and sacral arteries

These contribute to the supply of skin over the superior and medial borders of the buttock. The fourth lumbar artery pierces external oblique and in the company of the cutaneous branch of the posterior primary ramus of L1 crosses the crest of the ilium around its midpoint. This is not a constant vessel but it generally sends a few twigs to the skin.

The iliac branch of the iliolumbar artery runs along the iliac crest and supplies abdominal and gluteal muscles. It anastomoses with the superior gluteal artery and indirectly contributes to the supply of skin.

The lateral sacral arteries enter the anterior sacral foramina, emerge through the posterior foramina and are distributed to the skin over the sacrum. They anastomose laterally with branches of the superior gluteal.

Variations occur:

1. In the manner of origin of the superior gluteal, inferior gluteal and internal pudendal arteries as outlined above.
2. In the manner of division of the inferior gluteal artery – medial or lateral branch may be dominant.
3. In the extent to which the superior and inferior gluteal arteries share the supply of gluteus maximus.
4. In the degree to which the superficial circumflex iliac artery extends beyond the anterior superior iliac spine to encroach on the buttock region.
5. In the contribution of the medial circumflex femoral to the blood supply of the inferior part of gluteus maximus and thereby the overlying skin (usually minimal).
6. In the degree to which branches of the inferior gluteal artery extend inferiorly with the posterior cutaneous nerve of the thigh and supply skin over the posterior thigh.

SUMMARY OF TERRITORIES

Classically the buttock has been divided by a line from sacral tip to greater trochanter into upper and lower zones each of which is supplied by a number of vessels. From a practical point of view it is more useful to first define a midline zone and then look at the lateral part. The skin nearest the midline is closely applied to the underlying structures, has little mobility and is supplied by numerous small, short vessels. Superiorly (area 1 in Fig. 6.83) these vessels are medial dorsal cutaneous branches of the lumbar arteries. Below this, and within the buttock region, this midline area is supplied by the lateral sacral arteries, (area 4 in Fig. 6.83). Inferiorly, two or three branches of the internal pudendal, which are exceptionally difficult to find in the ischiorectal fat, supply skin over gluteus maximus (area 7). This midline area has little use for surgeons wishing to raise flaps; indeed flaps from the buttock region are often being raised for transfer into this area.

The area lateral to this is much better vascularised and although the boundary between superior and inferior gluteal territories varies depending on the size of the vessels, the best guide is a line between the middle of the sacrum and the tip of the greater trochanter (i.e. different from the classical line). Above this, and covering the upper fibres of gluteus maximus, lies the territory of the superior gluteal artery. The area beyond the supero-lateral edge of gluteus maximus is shared between perforators from the deep branch of the superior gluteal artery which pass through gluteus medius (not differentiated in Figure 6.83 from the remainder of the superior gluteal territory) and branches of lumbar and iliolumbar arteries which come over the iliac crest. The superficial circumflex iliac artery may extend beyond the anterior superior iliac spine to come onto this territory. Laterally the territory of the superior gluteal artery ends 2 cm behind the posterior edge of tensor fasciae latae.

The lower area is mainly inferior gluteal territory and this can be regarded as the principal vessel of supply to gluteus maximus. The inferior gluteal territory may extend inferiorly for a variable distance depending on the length of the branches accompanying the posterior cutaneous nerve of thigh (area 10 in Fig. 6.83). Laterally, the territory adjoins that of the first perforator which supplies the insertion of gluteus maximus and the overlying skin. Note that although these are the anatomical territories, the dynamic and potential territories are markedly different. For example, the entire gluteus maximus muscle with overlying skin may be advanced vertically based only on the inferior gluteal artery.

FLAPS

The great vascularity of the muscle forms the basis for the good blood supply to the skin of this area. Flaps based on gluteus maximus are of essentially four types, depending on blood supply, and may be further subdivided on the basis of whether they are used as free flaps, or local muscle flaps carrying an island of skin. Flaps may be based on:

1. Superior gluteal artery, superficial branch.
2. Inferior gluteal artery.
3. Inferior gluteal artery extended onto thigh by deep fascial branch.
4. First profunda perforator.

Further details of these flaps are given on page 336.

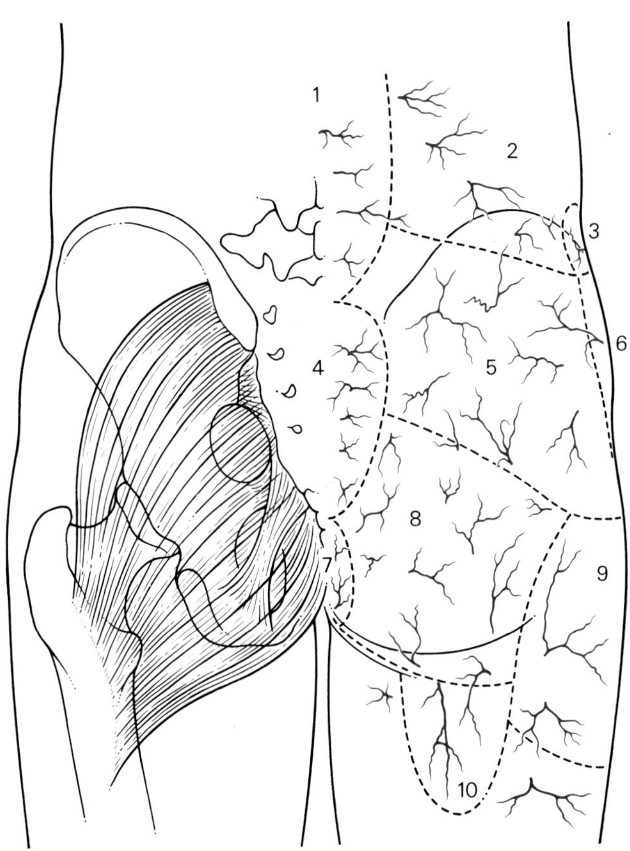

Fig. 6.83 Anatomical territories of cutaneous blood supply in the buttock region:
1. Medial dorsal cutaneous branches of lumbar arteries,
2. Lateral dorsal cutaneous branches of lumbar arteries and the iliolumbar artery,
3. Superficial circumflex iliac artery,
4. Lateral sacral arteries,
5. Superior gluteal artery,
6. Perforators from the lateral circumflex femoral artery emerging from the surface of tensor fasciae latae,
7. Internal pudendal artery,
8. Inferior gluteal artery,
9. First profunda perforator,
10. Inferior extension of the inferior gluteal artery at the level of the deep fascia with the posterior cutaneous nerve of the thigh.

6 LOWER LIMB

Nomina Anatomica

ARTERIA ILIACA INTERNA
Arteria iliolumbalis
Ramus lumbalis
Ramus iliacus
Arteriae sacrales laterales
Arteria obturatoria
Ramus pubicus
Ramus anterior
Ramus posterior
Arteria glutea superior
Ramus superficialis
Ramus profundus
Ramus superior
Ramus inferior
Arteria glutea inferior
A. comitans nervi ischiadici
Arteria pudenda interna
A. perinealis
Rami scrotales/labiales posteriores
A. dorsalis penis/clitoridis

ARTERIA FEMORALIS
Arteria epigastrica superficialis
Arteria circumflexa iliaca superficialis
Arteriae pudendae externae
Rami scrotales/labiales anteriores
Rami inguinales
Arteria descendens genicularis
Ramus saphenus
Rami articulares

ARTERIA PROFUNDA FEMORIS*
A. circumflexa femoris medialis
Ramus profundus
Ramus ascendens
Ramus transversus
A. circumflexa femoris lateralis
Ramus ascendens
Ramus descendens
Ramus transversus
Aa. perforantes

ARTERIA POPLITEA
A. superior lateralis genus
A. superior medialis genus
A. media genus
Aa. surales
A. inferior lateralis genus
A. inferior medialis genus
Rete articulare genus
Rete patellae
Arteria tibialis anterior
A. recurrens tibialis anterior
(A. recurrens tibialis posterior)
A. malleolaris anterior lateralis
A. malleolaris anterior medialis
Rete malleolare laterale
Arteria dorsalis pedis
A. tarsalis lateralis
Aa. tarsales mediales
(A. arcuata)
Aa. metatarsales dorsales
Aa. digitales dorsales
A. plantaris profundus
Arteria tibialis posterior
Ramus circumflexus fibularis
Rami malleolares mediales
Rami calcanei
Arteria plantaris medialis
Ramus profundus
Ramus superficialis
Arteria plantaris lateralis
Arcus plantaris profundus
Aa. metatarsales plantares
Rami perforantes
Aa. digitales plantares communes
Aa. digitales plantares propriae
(Arcus plantaris superficialis)
Arteria fibularis [peronea]
Ramus perforans
Ramus communicans
Rami malleolares laterales
Rami calcanei
Rete calcaneum

*The arrangement of the branches of this artery is subject to much variation. The arrangement adopted here is merely the most common. The origin of the circumflex femoral branches is particularly variable.

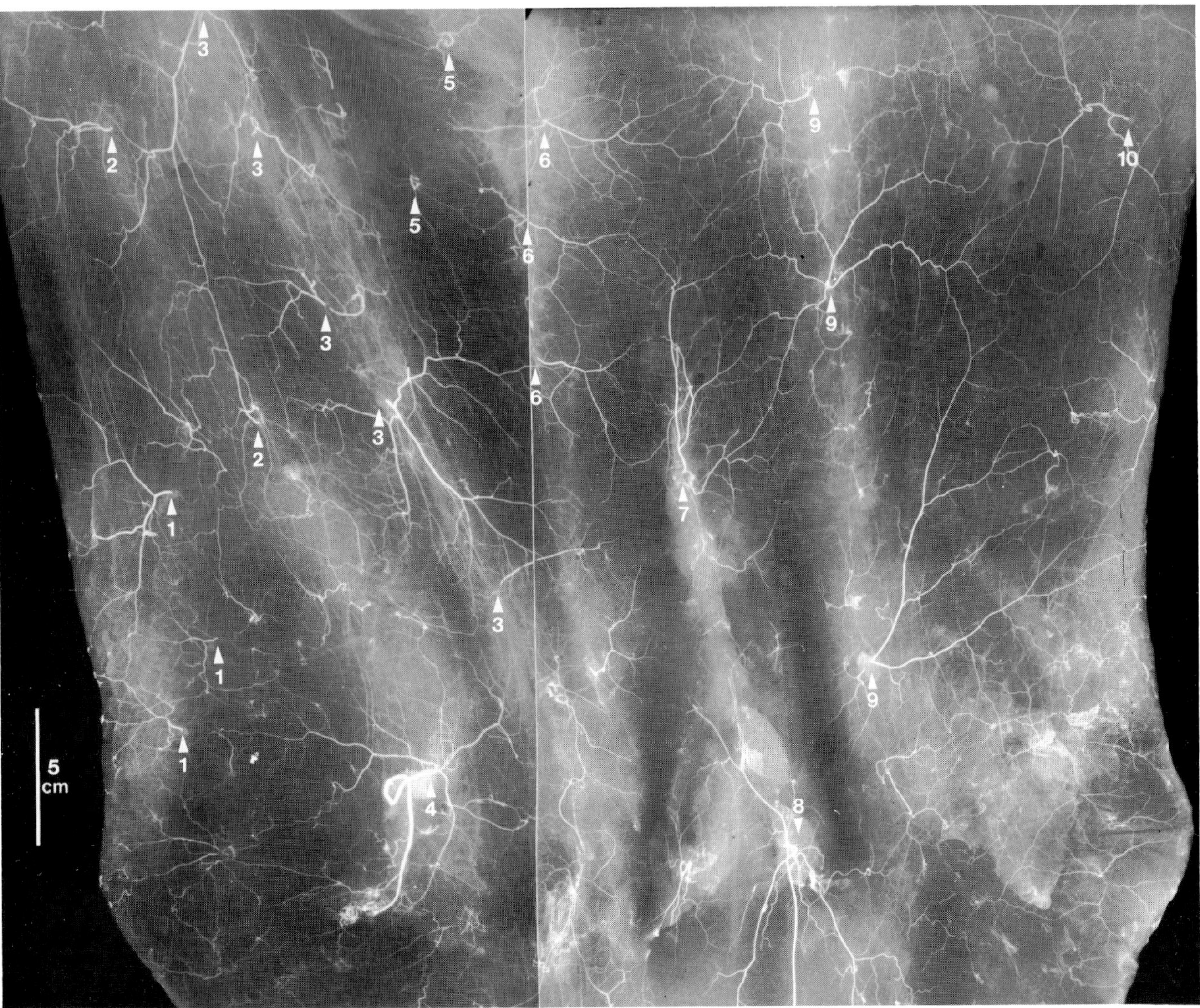

Fig. 6.84 Radiograph of injected thigh skin, subcutaneous tissue and deep fascia. The posterior part of the radiograph is continuous with that of the buttock region in Fig. 6.77. The upper margin of the specimen lies at the level of the perineum, and the lower margin at the level of the knee joint. The specimen has been opened out by a vertical incision passing between the anterior superior iliac spine and the middle of the patella.

1. Musculocutaneous perforators arising from the three branches of the femoral artery which supply vastus medialis, and emerging from the surface of the muscle,
2. Fasciocutaneous perforators arising from the femoral artery and emerging along the anterior edge of sartorius,
3. Fasciocutaneous perforators arising from the femoral artery and emerging along the posterior border of sartorius. Sartorius therefore underlies the skin in the area between rows 2 and 3,
4. Saphenous and articular branches of the descending genicular artery. (The convoluted appearance of the artery is due to the fact that this segment of the vessel was lying free on top of the specimen and became displaced),
5. Musculocutaneous perforators emerging from the surface of gracilis. The muscle receives a major pedicle from the profunda femoris in its upper part and from the femoral artery in its lower part,
6. Musculocutaneous perforators from semimembranosus and semitendinosus (branches of the profunda femoris perforators),
7. Perforator in the upper part of the popliteal fossa passing vertically upwards in the midline,
8. Superficial sural arteries arising from the popliteal or sural arteries and emerging between the two heads of gastrocnemius,
9. Terminal lateral branches of the profunda femoris perforators emerging along the lateral intermuscular septum,
10. Branch of the descending branch of the lateral circumflex femoral artery either emerging from the surface of vastus lateralis in front of the anterior margin of the iliotibial tract, or emerging in the interval between rectus femoris and vastus lateralis.

6 THIGH

From the inguinal ligament and gluteal fold down to the upper pole of the patella, the skin of the thigh is supplied largely by two major vessels, namely the femoral and the profunda femoris, with lesser contributions from the popliteal, the obturator and the inferior gluteal arteries. The *femoral artery* enters the thigh midway between the anterior superior iliac spine and the symphysis pubis, runs down the thigh in the subsartorial canal, and ends at the adductor hiatus where it becomes the *popliteal artery*. The *profunda femoris artery* arises from the lateral side of the femoral artery about 3.5 cm below the inguinal ligament and gives off the *medial and lateral circumflex femoral arteries* before ending as a series of perforating arteries which pass through the adductor muscles to reach the posterior compartment. The *obturator artery* enters the thigh through the obturator foramen to supply the adductor compartment. In addition, the *inferior gluteal artery* may contribute to the blood supply of the upper posterior thigh. The branches of each of these vessels will be described in turn in so far as they contribute to the cutaneous vascularisation.

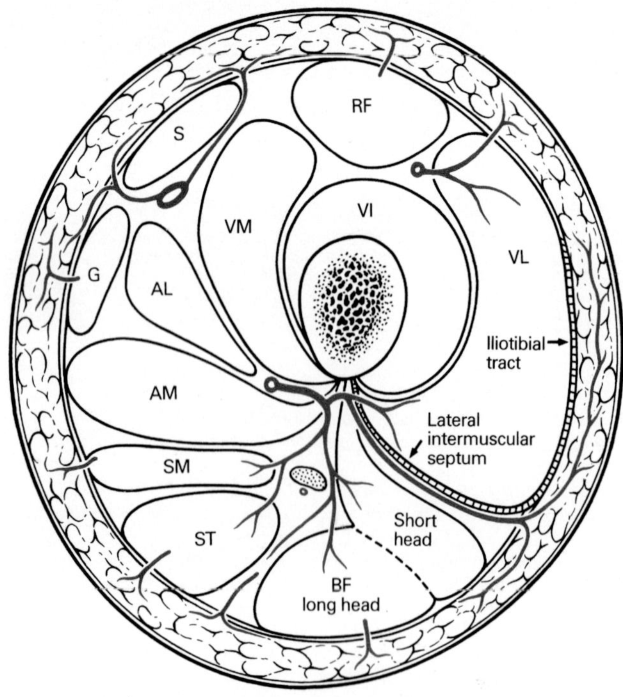

Fig. 6.85 Schematic transverse section through the mid-thigh showing the locations of the principal vessels and their musculocutaneous and fasciocutaneous perforators.

THE FEMORAL ARTERY

The femoral artery passes from a point beneath the inguinal ligament midway between the anterior superior iliac spine and the symphysis pubis to the adductor hiatus. In the first 3 or 4 cm of its course it lies in the femoral sheath but then emerges into the area of the femoral triangle which is bounded by the inguinal ligament, sartorius and the medial edge of adductor longus where it gives off four large *direct cutaneous arteries* and a number of smaller vessels to the skin. The femoral artery then enters the subsartorial canal (Hunter's canal) where it gives off branches principally to sartorius and to vastus medialis, and supplies the skin overlying these muscles by *musculocutaneous* and *fasciocutaneous perforators* just before it passes through the adductor hiatus. The femoral artery gives off a particularly large fasciocutaneous vessel, the descending genicular artery, which supplies a significant area over the medial side of the knee and extends for a variable distance onto the lower leg.

DIRECT CUTANEOUS ARTERIES

The four major cutaneous vessels are the superficial circumflex iliac, the superficial inferior epigastric and the superficial and deep external pudendal arteries. The epigastric artery is described in the section dealing with the anterior abdominal wall, and the pudendal vessels are described in greater detail in the section on the perineum and external genitalia.

The superficial circumflex iliac artery

The SCIA arises either independently from the femoral artery, or from a common trunk with the superficial inferior epigastric artery. Occasionally (<10%) the vessel is double, and then is too small for microvascular anastomosis. Exceptionally, it may arise independently from the profunda, the lateral circumflex femoral or the deep circumflex iliac artery. The point of origin lies between 0 and 8 cm (mode 3 cm) below the mid-inguinal point. The main stem of the SCIA is about 2 mm in diameter and passes laterally towards the anterior superior iliac spine on a course parallel to the inguinal ligament. In approximately 80% of cases it divides within its first 3 cm into equal-sized superficial and deep branches – a fact which is generally not mentioned in anatomical texts. In ~ 50% it also gives off, near its origin, a descending branch (Fig. 7.231). The superficial branch is tortuous and supplies mainly lymph nodes but also overlying skin. The deep branch runs a straighter course beneath the deep fascia, parallel to the inguinal ligament, giving off branches to the muscles in the femoral triangle. It then passes up through the deep fascia on a level about 2 cm below the anterior superior iliac spine (between 2 and 5 cm lateral to the femoral artery) and then continues in the subcutaneous fat becoming more superficial as it crosses the anterior superior iliac spine where it divides into terminal twigs. Note however that:

1. the superficial branch may be absent or may expend itself early on in supplying inguinal lymph nodes, fat etc., so that it makes no significant contribution to the blood supply of the skin
2. the deep branch may expend itself completely in muscle branches and make no significant contribution to the blood supply of the skin
3. the deep branch may stay beneath the deep fascia giving off only small cutaneous perforators through the deep fascia.

In summary, the territory of the superficial circumflex iliac artery may be supplied entirely by the superficial branch, entirely by the deep branch or equally by both. In the small proportion of instances in which the SCIA is absent on one side, it does not automatically follow that it will be absent on the other side.

The anatomical territory is based on the femoral artery medially and covers the area reaching 5 cm above and below an axis running 3 cm below and parallel to the inguinal ligament. The distal extent of this territory coincides with the lateral edge of the anterior superior iliac spine where the superficial circumflex iliac artery anastomoses with the deep circumflex iliac, the superior gluteal and the ascending branch of the lateral circumflex femoral artery. Veins in this area are particularly large and numerous with the superficial circumflex iliac vein lying superficial to the artery throughout its course. Medially this is often joined by the superficial inferior epigastric vein. In addition there are deeper veins in the form of venae comitantes of the artery itself.

Deep external pudendal artery

This arises from the femoral artery and passes medially on a horizontal course in front of the femoral vein but behind the great saphenous vein (hence *deep* external pudendal artery although its branches are superficial ones to skin and subcutaneous tissues). As it passes medially this vessel gives off branches to a small area over the upper medial part of the femoral triangle. Often a distinct descending branch may be given off which may sometimes arise directly from the femoral and be designated as a third external pudendal artery (Fig. 6.128). Salmon (1936) recorded a case in which a descending branch reached 12 cm below the genito-thigh fold but usually the vessel is much shorter than this.

MUSCULOCUTANEOUS BRANCHES

The femoral artery gives off small branches of supply onto the anterior surface of adductor longus, occasionally to rectus femoris, and always to sartorius and vastus medialis. The branches to sartorius give off fasciocutaneous perforators (vide infra) which pass in the fascia round the sides of the muscle to overlying skin. The branches to vastus medialis penetrate the surface of the muscle to reach skin.

Vastus medialis. The femoral artery gives three large vessels of supply to this muscle, which may be termed its superior, middle and inferior pedicles after their positions. The superior pedicle arises from the femoral, occasionally from the profunda femoris or even in common with the medial pedicle of vastus intermedius. It passes beneath the saphenous nerve and the nerve to vastus medialis and enters the muscle at the junction of its upper and middle thirds in the company of nerve branches. The middle artery arises from the femoral in the subsartorial canal, sometimes by a common trunk with the superior artery, and forms the main vascular pedicle of the muscle. It may run downwards in the subsartorial canal for up to 3 cm before entering the muscle. The inferior artery arises from the femoral, sometimes by a common trunk with the descending genicular artery, and after a short course enters the muscle in its lower part. (Accessory vessels of supply come from the lateral circumflex femoral and the descending genicular arteries.) All three principal arteries lie superficially within the muscle and send musculocutaneous perforators to the overlying skin (Fig. 6.86).

FASCIOCUTANEOUS BRANCHES

Sartorius is mainly supplied by multiple branches of the femoral artery which may be divided for descriptive purposes into superior, middle and inferior groups. Accessory supplies are also found superiorly at the origin of the muscle where an inconstant branch of the superficial circumflex iliac, often supplemented by a branch of the lateral circumflex femoral, supplies the muscle. The superior pedicle has a variable origin which may be from any of the large vessels in the area but is characterised by lying in close relationship to the proximal nerve to the muscle. The middle group of arteries, of which there may be two or three, arises mainly from the femoral but one vessel may arise in common with a branch of the femoral going to adductor longus or to vastus medialis. The inferior group arises from the femoral and the descending genicular arteries. All these vessels are similar in giving branches to the muscle which enter it on its deep surface, usually near its medial border. As they pierce the muscle these arteries give off branches which pass both medially and laterally across the posterior surface of sartorius to then turn around its borders frequently passing between the fibres at the very edge of the muscle. In this manner the vessels reach the investing deep fascia of the thigh and spread out, in the manner of fasciocutaneous perforators, at the fascial level. Some of these perforators are larger than others and a consistently large vessel emerges round the medial border of the muscle in the apex of the femoral triangle. In 50 cadaver dissections, the authors consistently found this significantly sized perforator between 21 and 30 cm above the plane of the knee joint. A large perforator much less commonly emerges on the lateral side of sartorius in the interval between rectus femoris, sartorius and vastus medialis.

In a study of these fasciocutaneous perforators by the authors it has been shown that the plexus of vessels at the level of the deep fascia has a marked directional axiality which is aligned with the muscle and falls within the 45° angle sector orientated upon the longitudinal axis of the lower limb. This is described in detail on page 116.

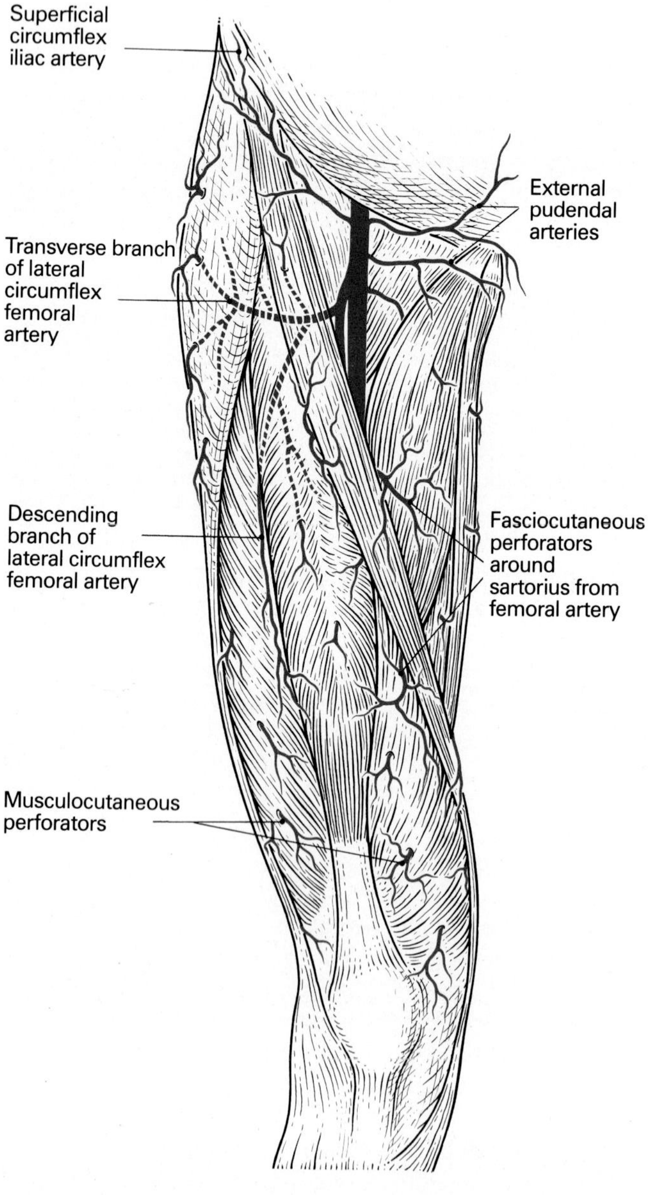

Fig. 6.86 Anterior aspect of thigh showing the principal branches to the skin.

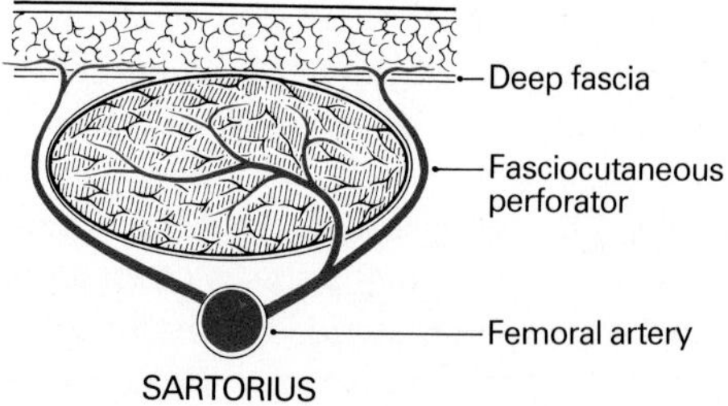

Fig. 6.87 Schematic diagram to illustrate arrangement of fasciocutaneous perforators in relation to sartorius.

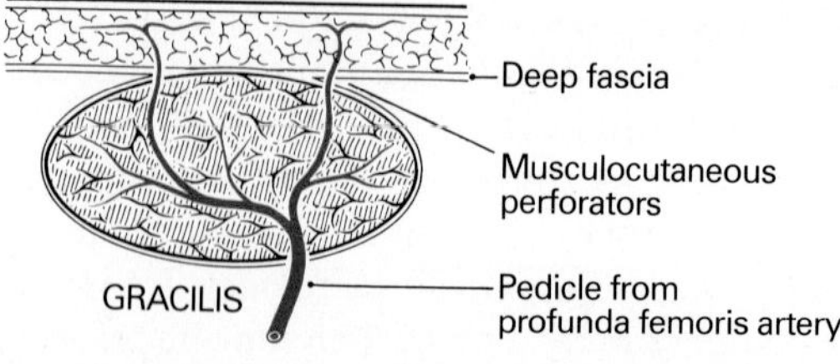

Fig. 6.88 Schematic diagram to illustrate arrangement of musculocutaneous perforators in relation to gracilis.

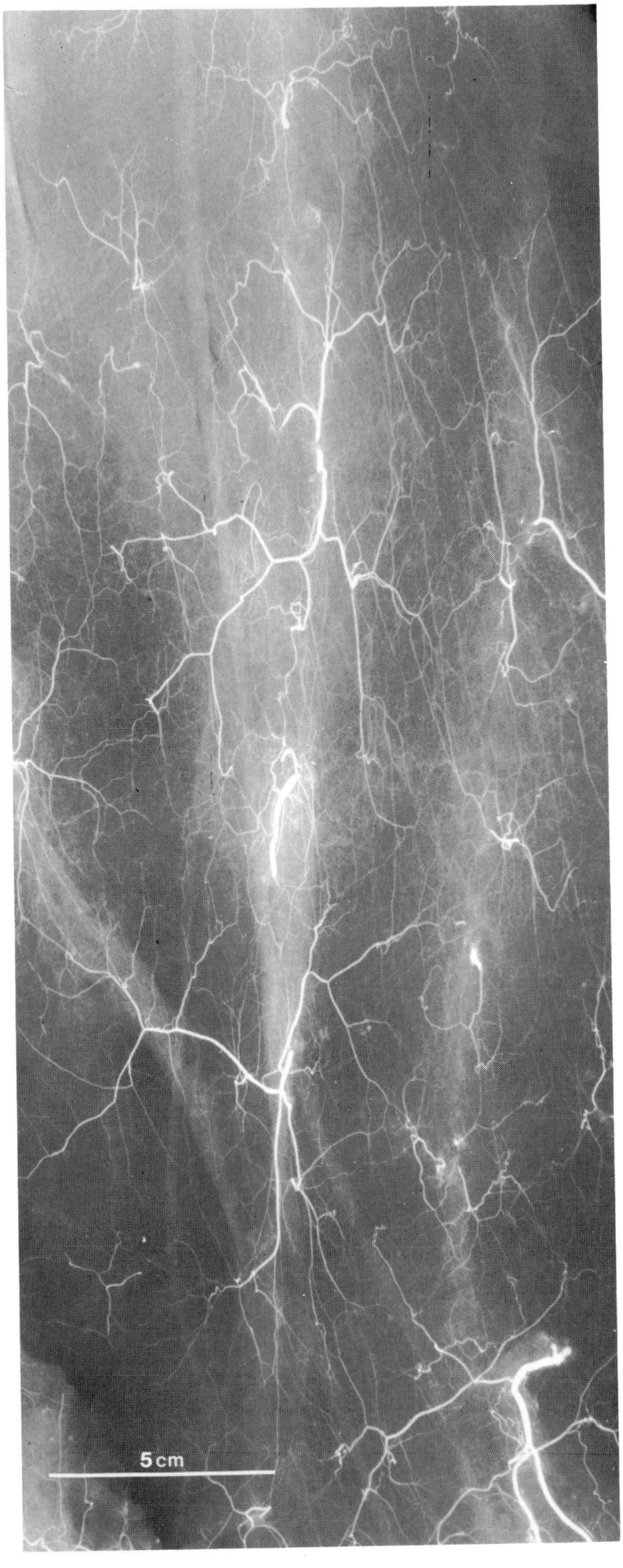

Fig. 6.89 Radiograph of skin and deep fascia overlying sartorius.

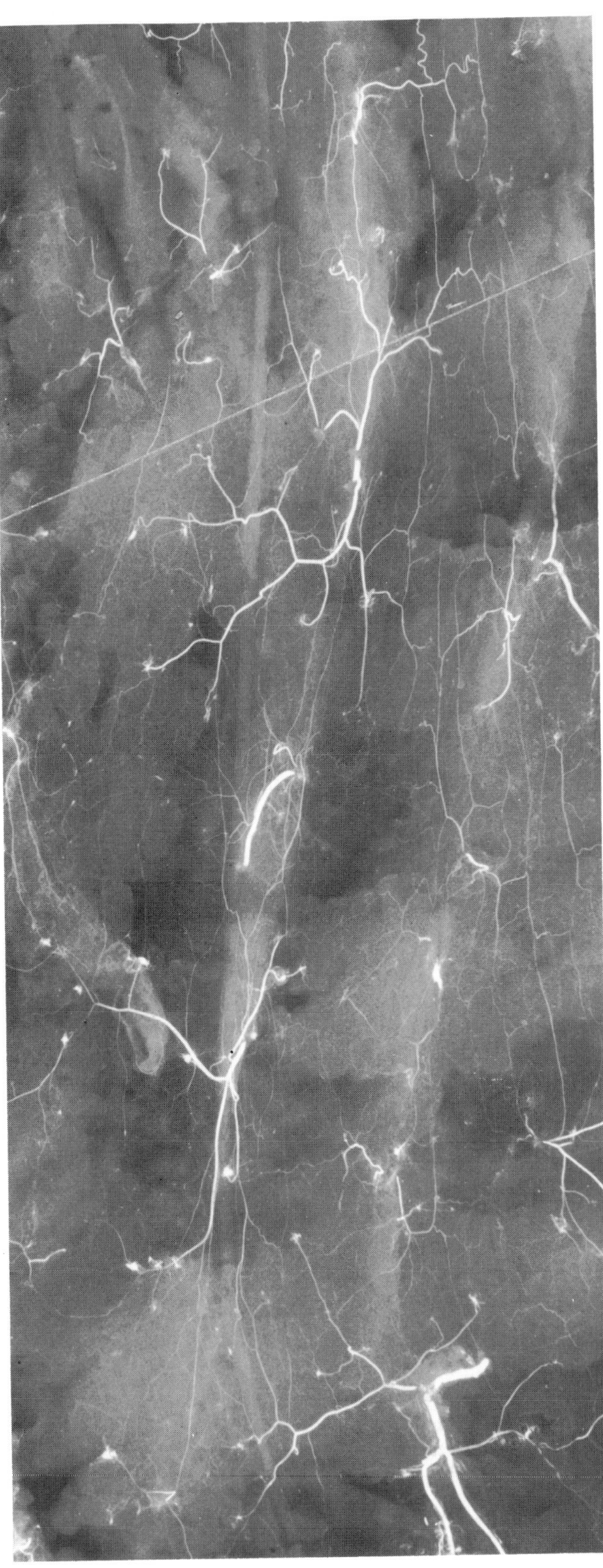

Fig. 6.90 Radiograph of deep fascia alone from specimen in Fig. 6.89.

THE PROFUNDA FEMORIS

The profunda femoris arises from the lateral side of the femoral artery between 2 and 5 cm below the inguinal ligament and gives off the medial circumflex femoral and the lateral circumflex femoral arteries. These vessels, their branches and the continuations of the profunda give off a large number of musculocutaneous and fasciocutaneous perforators which supply most of the skin over the thigh.

In the classical description of these vessels the lateral circumflex femoral artery arises from the lateral side of the profunda and the medial circumflex arises from the posteromedial aspect of the profunda femoris. Variations in the manner of origin of these vessels occur frequently, such that the conventional form only occurs in about 60% of cases. Table 6.11 shows the variations and their frequencies compiled from published Japanese and European studies totalling over 1000 cases (Adachi, 1928; Dubreuil-Chambardel, 1926; Williams et al, 1934).

The profunda perforators

The profunda femoris passes back between pectineus and adductor longus and continues distally between adductor longus and adductor magnus. It gives off three perforating arteries before ending as the fourth perforator (variation – perforators may number between two and six). These profunda perforators pierce the insertion of adductor magnus to reach the posterior compartment of the thigh. In the posterior compartment they give off three sets of vessels; anastomotic branches which unite successive perforators; muscular branches to the hamstrings; and fasciocutaneous branches between the hamstrings (Figs 6.85, 6.91 & 6.92). Each profunda perforator finally ends by dividing into two branches at the point where the lateral intermuscular septum meets the shaft of the femur. One branch pierces the septum and enters the posterior part of vastus lateralis to supply it. The other branch passes along the lateral intermuscular septum and pierces the deep fascia where it then spreads out anteriorly and posteriorly to supply skin (Figs 6.93 & 6.94).

The first profunda perforator. As it passes back between pectineus and adductor brevis it gives off a large branch, 2 or 3 mm in diameter, which may be regarded as the main artery to the adductors. This vessel may alternatively arise directly from the profunda femoris but pursues the same course passing medially, with a slight distal inclination deep to adductor longus across the front of adductor magnus. Deep to adductor longus it gives off branches which enter adductor brevis on its anterior surface and adductor longus on its posterior surface. The main stem of this adductor artery then ends by supplying adductor magnus and by forming the principal vascular pedicle of gracilis. It enters the deep surface of gracilis at the junction of its upper and middle thirds and divides into branches which ascend and descend within the muscle giving off musculocutaneous perforators to the overlying skin. The 'adductor artery' may also supply the skin of the upper inner aspect of the thigh by a direct branch which passes superficial to adductor longus and over the origin of gracilis.

The first profunda perforator gives off two or three branches to *adductor magnus* which ascend within the muscle and give off musculocutaneous perforators to the overlying skin. The first perforator then pierces adductor magnus close to the femur and appears in the posterior compartment. Here it gives off an ascending stem which supplies the insertion of gluteus maximus and the inferolateral portion of the muscle within which it anastomoses with the inferior gluteal artery; branches from the same stem participate in the trochanteric anastomosis and further branches become cutaneous where the gluteus maximus inserts into the iliotibial tract. The largest of these cutaneous perforators divides into two cutaneous vessels about 1 mm ID. One of these fans out anteriorly over the iliotibial tract and superiorly over the greater trochanter, the other is directed posteriorly. Distally these anastomose with the lateral cutaneous branch of the second perforator.

The main trunk of the first profunda perforator passes distally and medially deep to the long head of biceps femoris which receives small branches direct from the main trunk at the junction of its upper and middle thirds. The first perforator continues medially deep to the sciatic nerve and divides into medial and lateral terminal divisions. The medial division supplies semitendinosus and semimembranosus and in 30% of cases gives off a recurrent branch to biceps femoris. The lateral division enters the middle of the long head of the biceps after branching into two or more secondary

Table 6.11 Variations in origin of profunda femoris, medial circumflex femoral and lateral circumflex femoral arteries

	Prevalence %
classical form, truncus profundo-circumflexus perfectus	51–63
truncus profundo-circumflexus lateralis	15–20
truncus profundo-circumflexus medialis	13–15
all three vessels arise separately	4–5
profunda alone arises separately	1
descending branch of lateral circumflex femoral is independent	2
medial circumflex femoral is absent	0.3

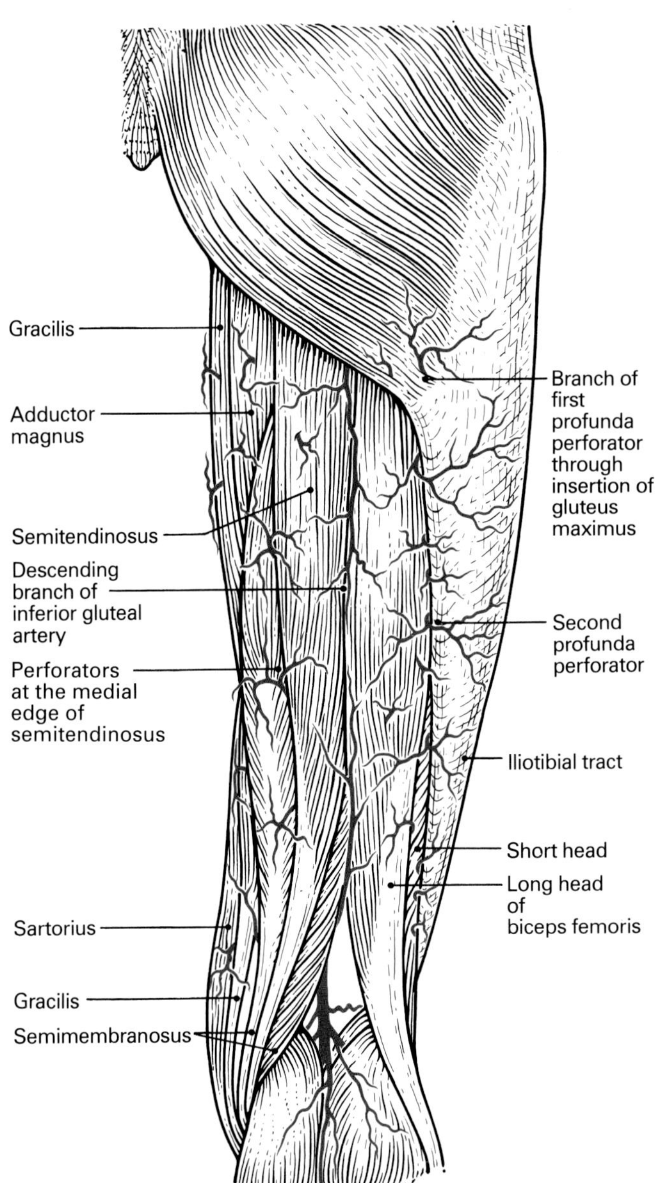

Fig. 6.91 Diagram showing cutaneous branching over the posterior thigh. Note longitudinal vessels in the midline, fasciocutaneous perforators laterally, and a combination of musculocutaneous and fasciocutaneous perforators medially. The areas of skin directly overlying the tendons of the hamstrings are poorly vascularised. Although the vessels are shown lying on the surfaces of the muscles they in fact lie largely on the superficial surface of the deep fascia although the descending branch of the inferior gluteal artery (not always present) may lie directly beneath it.

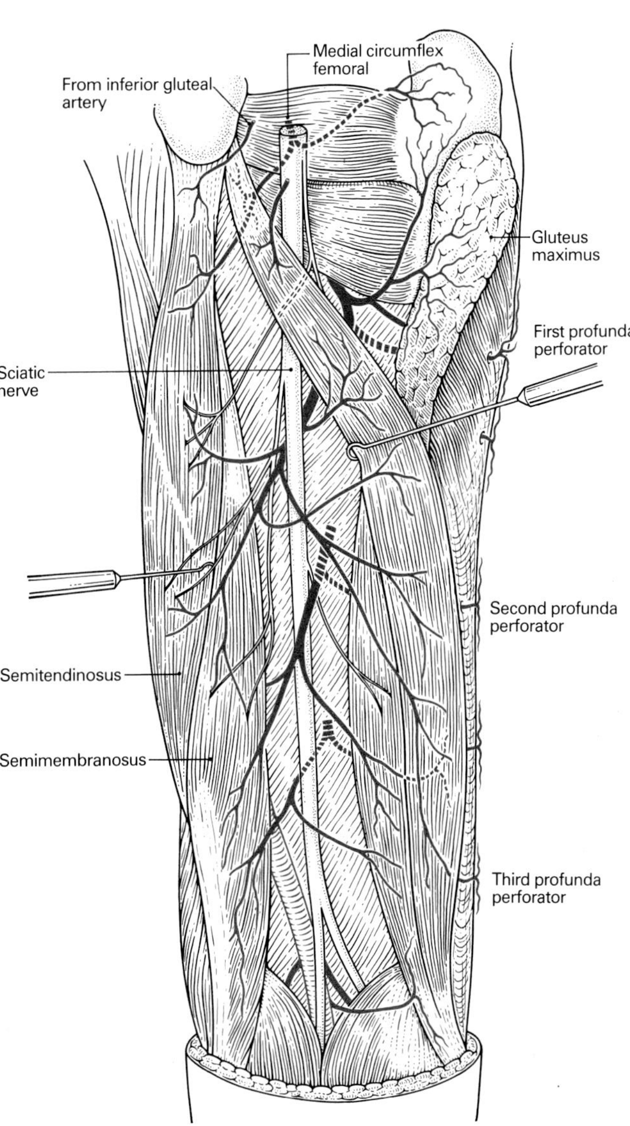

Fig. 6.92 Schematic illustration of the arrangement of the lateral and posterior branches of the profunda femoris perforators as revealed by retraction of biceps femoris laterally and semitendinosus and semimembranosus medially. The vessels are subject to considerable variation (see text). Musculocutaneous and fasciocutaneous perforators have not been shown with the exception of those emerging along the lateral intermuscular septum.

twigs. In 50% of cases this lateral division gives off a long artery which descends on the deep surface of the long head of biceps. This vessel is present particularly when the second perforator is a small vessel, but in Figure 6.92 we have shown both a long artery and a second perforator branch both going to the long head. When the second perforator is large it may replace this lateral division and be the principal supply to biceps femoris.

The principal pedicle of adductor magnus. This arises from the profunda just distal to the origin of the first perforator and enters the middle part of the muscle. Two musculocutaneous perforators leave the posteromedial edge of the upper part of the muscle which lies subcutaneously. These perforators lie on average 21 cm and 26 cm above the line of the knee joint, and may arise from this pedicle or from the two or three branches supplied by the first perforator.

The second perforator. This may be larger than the first. It pierces the insertions of adductor brevis and adductor magnus. It supplies semimembranosus and the lower half of both long and short heads of biceps femoris. A large branch continues from the trunk of the perforator, curves round the back of the femur and passes through the lateral intermuscular septum to supply vastus lateralis. As it pierces the septum it gives off a branch which passes laterally to emerge where the lateral intermuscular septum meets the iliotibial tract about 2 cm below the insertion of gluteus maximus. This fasciocutaneous perforator is generally the largest of those in the row emerging along the lateral intermuscular septum and measures up to 1.5 mm D. This point lies about 26 cm up from the plane of the knee joint (~65% of the distance between knee joint and tip of greater trochanter).

The third perforator. This starts below adductor brevis and pierces adductor magnus. It supplies semimembranosus and the lower part of the short head of biceps femoris. The latter vessel or the branch to vastus lateralis, gives off a perforator which passes along the lateral intermuscular septum to supply skin. This perforator measures up to 1 mm in diameter at the point where it reaches the subcutaneous tissues. This point often lies about half-way between the tip of the greater trochanter and the plane of the knee joint. Again it sends branches predominantly anteriorly but also posteriorly.

The fourth perforator. This name is sometimes given to the terminal perforating branch of the profunda femoris which, when present, behaves in a similar way to the other perforators. Any of the profunda perforators may give off fasciocutaneous branches along the fascial septa between the hamstring muscles. These are in fact less common than might be expected and cannot be relied upon, except for one fairly constant perforator in the upper part of the popliteal fossa. This emerges through the fat between semimembranosus and biceps femoris to reach skin about 11 cm above the plane of the knee joint and is surrounded by multiple branching veins which are passing between the deep and superficial systems. This vessel may arise from the lowermost profunda perforator in which case it is small, or from the popliteal artery in which case it may ascend in the midline for up to 11 cm as originally described by Manchot. The main source of blood supply to the skin comes from musculocutaneous perforators from the hamstrings. Rather than piercing the flat, subfascial surfaces of the hamstrings, these perforators tend to emerge along the posterolateral edge of semimembranosus and along the posteromedial edge of biceps femoris. In 50 cadaver thighs studied by the authors, the existence of significantly sized fasciocutaneous perforators between semimembranosus and semitendinosus was uncommon, and perforators between semimembranosus and biceps femoris were occasionally present. This finding contrasts with some published diagrams which indicate constant fasciocutaneous branches from each profunda perforator between semimembranosus and biceps femoris.

The cutaneous perforators passing along the lateral intermuscular septum are unusual in that they appear to be fasciocutaneous vessels in their course along a fascial septum but they do not fan out at the level of the deep fascia. Instead they spread out in the subcutaneous fat, perhaps because the iliotibial tract is more in the nature of a tendon (of tensor fascia latae) and a ligament (between the iliac crest and the tibia) than true deep fascia. A comparison of radiographs of iliotibial tract alone with radiographs of the skin and iliotibial tract combined shows the location of these cutaneous vessels and the fact that they do not run (in an individual with adequate subcutaneous fat) directly on the tract.

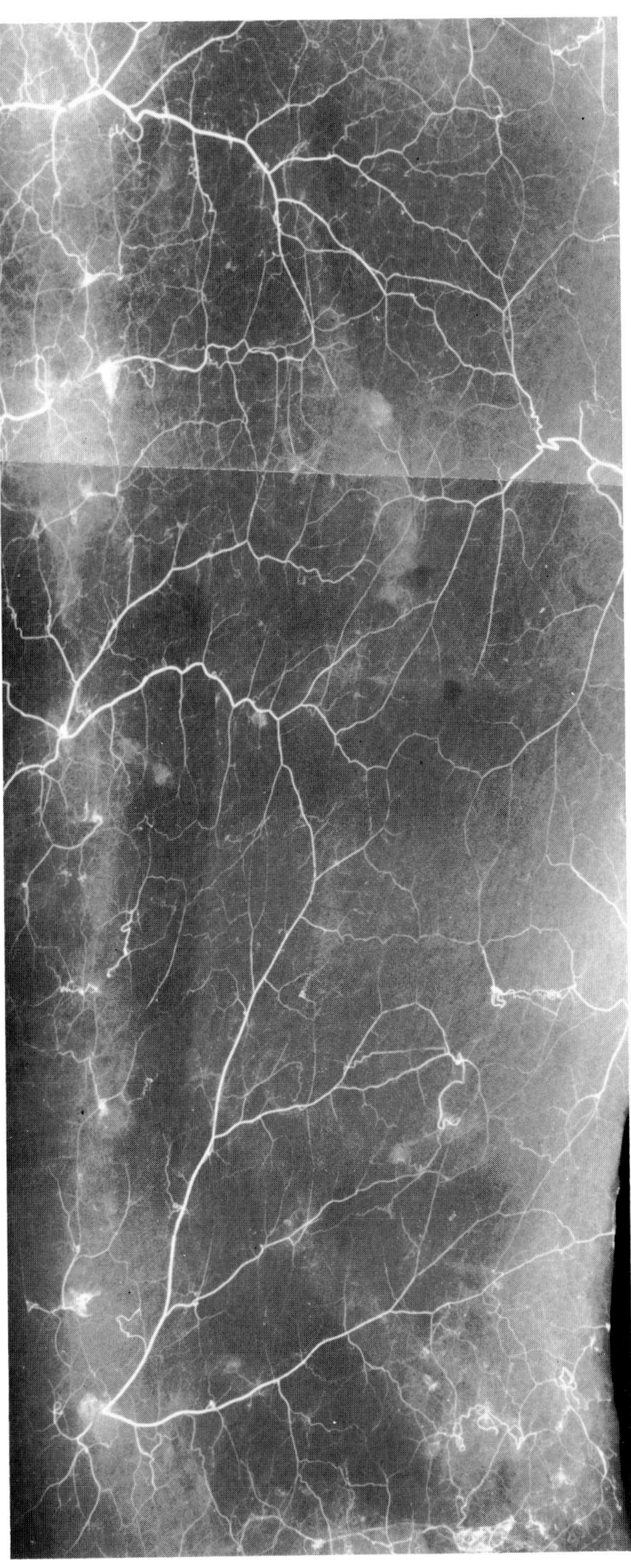

Fig. 6.93 Radiograph of skin, subcutaneous tissue and iliotibial tract from the lateral side of the thigh. The lateral intermuscular septum lies along the left-hand side of the radiograph and the rest of the specimen is from the area anterior to this. Multiple small branches emerge along the line of the septum and three large branches are seen fanning out over the tract.

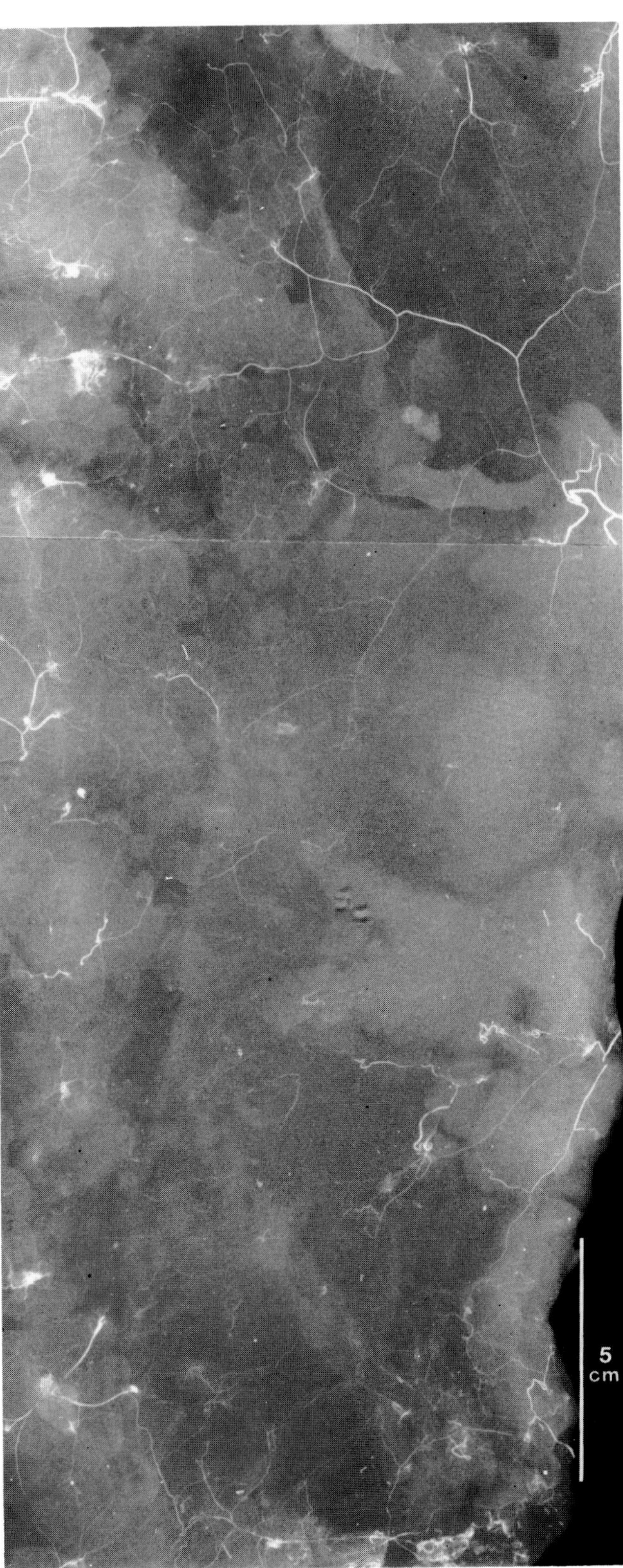

Fig. 6.94 Radiograph of the iliotibial tract alone after removal of the overlying structures. It is apparent that the majority of the large vessels seen in Fig. 6.93 are not lying directly on the tract but in the superficial fascia above it. Therefore free flaps raised on these vessels may be elevated superficial to the iliotibial tract which may be left intact.

6

The medial circumflex femoral artery

This arises from the posteromedial aspect of the profunda or, less commonly, from the femoral artery (see Table 6.11). It gives off a small superficial branch which passes anterior to pectineus and supplies adductors longus and brevis (Fig. 6.86) while the main trunk (ramus profundus) passes back between psoas and pectineus, and between obturator externus and adductor brevis, to lie beneath the femoral neck. It supplies adductor muscles and sends a branch to the origin of gracilis which may reach skin as a musculocutaneous perforator. Deep to quadratus femoris it divides into an ascending branch and a so-called 'transverse' part. The ascending branch passes above quadratus femoris and joins the trochanteric anastomosis (Fig. 6.92). It also links up with the inferior gluteal artery and it is conceivable that it might contribute to an insignificant extent to the blood supply of the skin through gluteus maximus musculocutaneous perforators. The 'transverse' part is really the continuation of the parent vessel and supplies the most proximal parts of semitendinosus and the long head of biceps femoris (Fig. 6.92). It may make a small contribution to the skin over the proximal parts of these muscles.

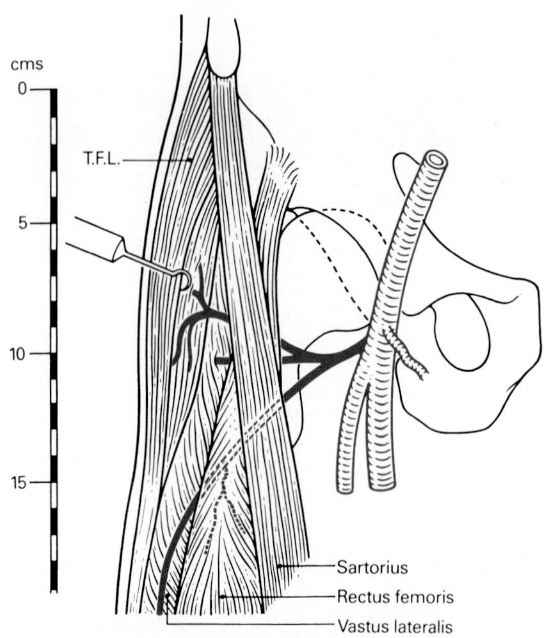

Fig. 6.95 Course of the lateral circumflex femoral artery and approximate positions of its points of division into ascending, transverse and descending branches relative to bony points such as the pubic symphysis and the anterior superior iliac spine.

The lateral circumflex femoral artery

This artery is important in the context of flaps because it sends musculocutaneous and fasciocutaneous perforators to the antero-lateral part of the thigh. It will be described in some detail.

The lateral circumflex femoral is larger than the medial circumflex and arises from the profunda femoris in 75% of cases, and from the femoral in the remainder. It passes laterally, usually lying posterior to the divisions of the femoral nerve, to run behind sartorius and rectus femoris where it divides into ascending, transverse and descending branches (ascending and transverse generally together). This point of division lies about 12 cm from the midline and 5 cm below the top of the symphysis pubis.* The ascending branch supplies the gluteals, tensor fasciae latae, and the upper part of vastus lateralis. The transverse branch supplies vastus lateralis and participates in the cruciate anastomosis. The descending branch runs down behind rectus femoris and supplies vastus intermedius, rectus femoris, and vastus lateralis.

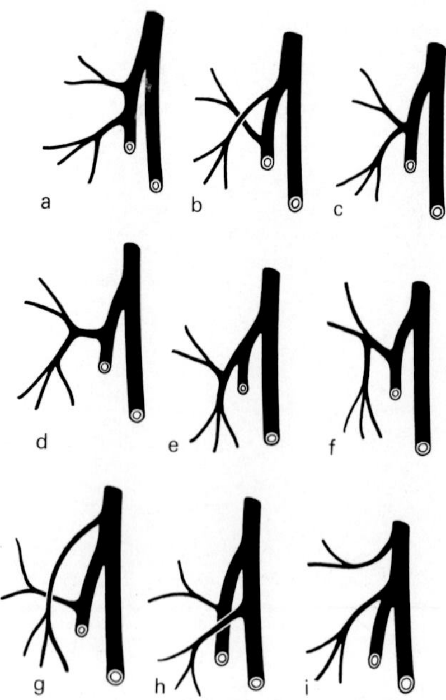

Fig. 6.96 Variations in the manner of branching of the lateral circumflex femoral artery. The descending 'branch' often arises separately on its own from the profunda or from the femoral artery (see text for details).

*This reference point was chosen because these and subsequent measurements referring to this point were obtained from femoral angiograms on which the a.s.i.s. often did not appear but the symphysis invariably did (Armenta & Fisher, 1981).

French anatomists have traditionally described the descending branch autonomously as the 'quadriceps artery' despite the fact that it does not supply vastus medialis but only the three other muscles of the quadriceps group. The manner of its origin is highly variable but is simplified by classification into three types:

Type 1. The quadriceps artery arises independently from the profunda femoris, usually at a point distal to the origin of the lateral circumflex (Fig. 6.96a). Less commonly, proximal to (b) or at the same level as (c) the lateral circumflex.

Type 2. The quadriceps artery arises by a common trunk with the lateral circumflex. This is the form described by English anatomists. The common trunk may lie horizontally (d), descend (e), or ascend (f).

Type 3. The quadriceps artery arises from the femoral artery, either above the origin of the lateral circumflex (g), or (rarely) below it (h). Dubreuil-Chambardel (1926) gave the following figures:

Type 1
a—31
b— 9 } 42%
c— 2
Type 2 44%
Type 3
a—11 } 14%
b— 3

Salmon also found Type 2 to be the most common (62%).

The 'quadriceps artery' gives off the following:
—the principal pedicle of rectus femoris
—the inferior pedicle of vastus lateralis
—the inferior pedicle of vastus intermedius
—a small branch to vastus medialis.
The branch to vastus lateralis is the most constant and the largest of these.

The ascending branch
The ascending branch of the lateral circumflex femoral passes between iliacus and rectus femoris and, at a point about 13.5 cm from the midline and 4 cm vertically below the top of the symphysis pubis, gives origin to a vessel which supplies the proximal parts of vastus lateralis, sartorius, and rectus femoris. The ascending branch continues to curve upwards and, about 14 cm from the midline and 3 cm vertically down from the symphysis, it gives off the branch which supplies tensor fasciae latae. The ascending branch continues as a much smaller vessel which follows the intertrochanteric line to supply the head and neck of the femur.

The branch to tensor fasciae latae enters the deep surface of the muscle half-way between its anterior and posterior borders about 8 or 9 cm below the anterior superior iliac spine. Within the muscle it divides into mainly ascending and descending branches which give off five to seven perforators through the surface of the muscle to the overlying skin (Fig. 6.77). These contribute the most important component to the blood supply of the upper lateral thigh. In the proximal part of the tensor muscle, anastomoses may occur with the deep branch of the superior gluteal artery. Also from the proximal part of the muscle, vessels pierce the iliac crest. In addition some small branches are given off by the lateral circumflex femoral artery before it pierces tensor fasciae latae and these enter gluteus medius. This completes the system of anastomoses on the lateral thigh between the gluteal vessels posteriorly and the femoral vessels anteriorly. The cutaneous anatomical territory supplied by tensor fasciae latae is confined to the area overlying the muscle and an area 2–3 cm wide all round it. These perforators do not in fact extend down the lateral aspect of the thigh as has so often been stated. It would indeed be extraordinary for musculocutaneous perforators to behave in such a way. It is, however, possible to create a tensor fasciae latae musculocutaneous flap with a cutaneous extension down the lateral aspect of the thigh and the anatomical basis for such a dynamic territory is the existence of large diameter anastomoses between separate lateral intermuscular septum perforators as is explained on page 358.

The transverse branch
This branch commonly arises from the ascending branch and is the smallest of the three. It lies on vastus intermedius and passes laterally beneath the anterior edge of vastus lateralis. It pierces and supplies vastus lateralis and winds posteriorly round the femur below the greater trochanter where it forms the cruciate anastomosis with the medial circumflex femoral, the inferior gluteal and the first perforator arteries. It may give off a fasciocutaneous perforator just before it disappears beneath vastus lateralis. This perforator emerges between the adjoining edges of tensor fasciae latae and rectus femoris, just as they diverge to expose vastus lateralis, and supplies skin.

The descending branch
This branch ('quadriceps artery') gives branches to vastus intermedius, rectus femoris, sometimes sartorius, and continues as a large vessel along the anterior border of vastus lateralis in the company of the nerve to that muscle. It may give origin to fasciocutaneous perforators in the interval between tensor fasciae latae and rectus femoris. Branches to vastus Cateralis may pierce the anterior part of the muscle to reach skin.

Branches to muscles from the lateral circumflex femoral artery

Vastus intermedius has two principal vascular pedicles (medial and lateral) which in 60% of cases enter the muscle with the nerve supply. This is usually double, one main branch from the nerve to vastus lateralis and a subsidiary branch from the proximal nerve to vastus medialis. The lateral pedicle arises from the descending branch of the lateral circumflex, often as a common trunk with the artery to rectus femoris, and the medial pedicle arises from the profunda femoris. The long artery to vastus lateralis also gives branches to vastus intermedius. Vastus intermedius does not contribute to the blood supply of skin.

Rectus femoris has a minor vascular pedicle proximally and a dominant pedicle further distally at the junction of its proximal and middle thirds (Type II). The proximal artery is from the ascending branch of the lateral circumflex femoral artery where it crosses the deep surface of rectus femoris. This artery may anastomose within the muscle with the deep branch of the superficial circumflex iliac artery given off to pass deep to sartorius. The distal pedicle is larger and generally divides into a superior and an inferior branch. It arises from the descending branch of the lateral circumflex femoral artery and after descending for about 8 cm enters the muscle in common with the nerve supply (in 85%) deep to the medial border, at the junction of the upper and middle thirds of the muscle. Its superior branch divides into ascending and descending parts lying within the muscle nearer its posterior surface. The inferior branch runs axially downwards in the muscle nearer its anterior surface giving off musculocutaneous perforators and may anastomose at the lower end with the long artery of vastus medialis. Sometimes this vessel may lie on the posteromedial surface of the muscle rather than within it, in which case the cutaneous branches may not be musculocutaneous ones passing through the muscle but fasciocutaneous perforators passing round its medial side. Variations include branches from vastus lateralis and/or vastus medialis to rectus femoris inferiorly, and also branches direct from the femoral artery. The anatomical territory supplied by the muscle conforms to its general outline. (The area that may be carried on the muscle is larger; p. 358.)

Vastus lateralis has multiple arteries from the descending branch, a small contribution from the transverse, and profunda perforators supplying it. The descending branch continues downwards lying either along the anterior edge of vastus lateralis (10%) or within the muscle (90%). In the latter case the artery tends to enter the muscle about 25 cm above the knee joint (Cormack & Lamberty, 1984). This artery gives off up to ten branches which penetrate the deep surface of the proximal and middle thirds of the muscle in the company of supplying nerves. These branches run perpendicular to the direction of the muscle fibres, lie nearer the anterior than the posterior surface of the muscle, and give off a few musculocutaneous perforators to the skin over the anterior part of the muscle. Within the muscle these branches have fine anastomotic connections with the third source of supply to vastus lateralis, namely the terminal branches of the profunda perforators which reach vastus lateralis by piercing the lateral intermuscular septum close to the femur. It is, therefore, clear that the territory of the lateral circumflex femoral artery includes the anterior part of vastus lateralis and its overlying skin, whilst the posterior part of the muscle under cover of the iliotibial tract is supplied by the perforators from the profunda femoris.

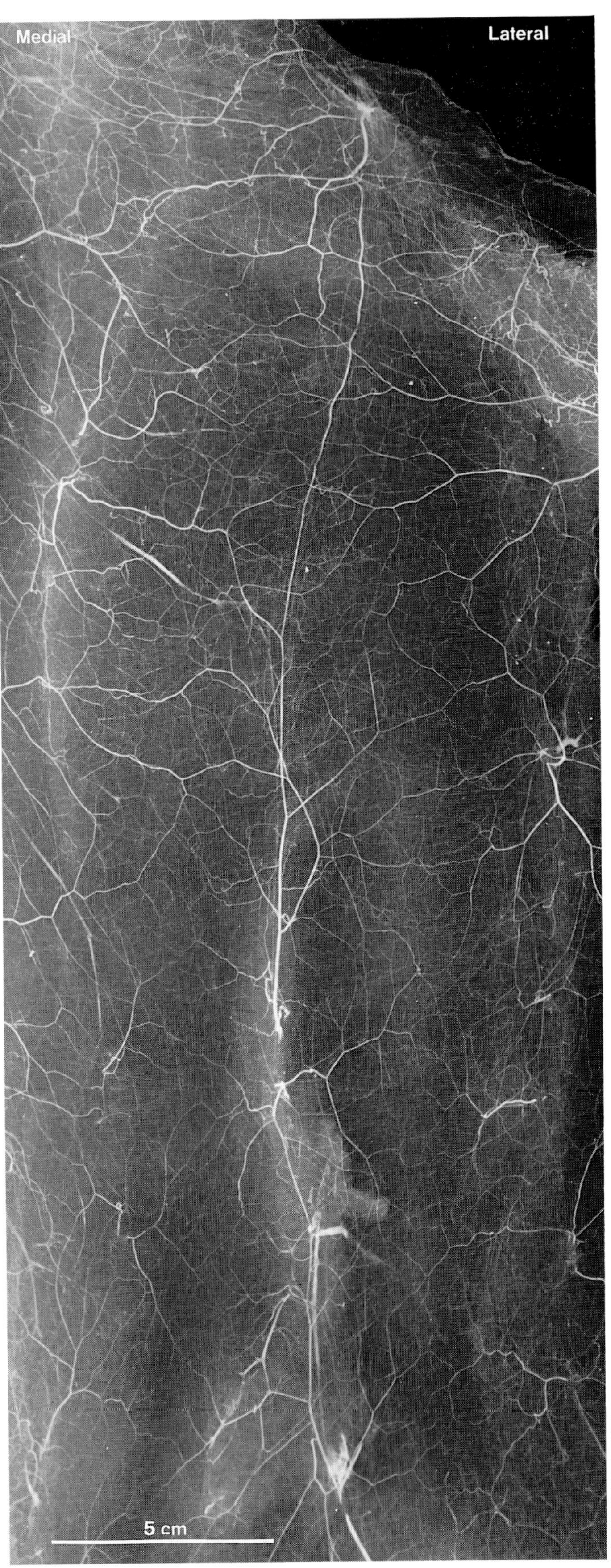

THE OBTURATOR ARTERY

After arising from the internal iliac or inferior epigastric arteries, the obturator artery passes through the obturator foramen and reaches the thigh where it divides into anterior and posterior branches. The anterior branch runs downwards and forwards to lie between adductor longus and adductor brevis where it anastomoses with branches of the medial circumflex femoral artery. It gives off branches to obturator externus, pectineus, adductors and gracilis. It does not supply skin.

The posterior branch runs posteriorly and then turns forwards on the ischium where it supplies the muscles arising from the tuberosity and anastomoses with the inferior gluteal artery. When the posterior branch is very well developed it supplies a small area of skin on the upper medial thigh just below the thigh-perineal skin crease.

THE INFERIOR GLUTEAL ARTERY

This usually branches off the anterior trunk of the internal iliac and reaches the buttock by passing through the greater sciatic notch beneath piriformis. Its supply to the buttock has been described. It sends branches beneath the lower border of gluteus maximus which may extend for several centimetres down the posterior aspect of the thigh in close relation to the posterior cutaneous nerve of the thigh (Fig. 6.97).

Fig. 6.97 Radiograph of posterior thigh skin showing a longitudinally running vessel formed by an anastomosis between a descending branch of the inferior gluteal artery and an ascending branch from the popliteal fossa. This vessel is inconstant but when present lies with the posterior cutaneous nerve of the thigh and is reinforced along its length by branches of the profunda perforators. The artery lies at the level of the deep fascia and is the vascular basis for the gluteal thigh flap.

Table 6.12 Summary of blood supply to thigh muscles

Muscle	Classification	Vascular pedicles
Gracilis	II	1° (junction of proximal and middle thirds) from adductor branch of profunda femoris or its first perforating branch
		2° (distal third) superficial femoral
Adductor longus	II	1° (entering deep surface) from adductor branch of profunda femoris or its 1st perforator
		2° (at origin) medial circumflex femoral
		2° (on superficial surface) small branches from superficial femoral
Adductor brevis	II or IV	1° (on deep surface) from profunda femoris
		2° (on superficial surface) from superficial branch of medial circumflex femoral
		2° (middle third) from adductor branch of profunda femoris or its first perforator
		2° (on deep surface) posterior branch of obturator artery
Adductor magnus	IV	Anteriorly (upper third) from posterior branch of obturator artery and deep branch of medial circumflex femoral
		1° (middle third) from profunda femoris below 1st perforator, or from 1st perforator
		(lower third) from profunda femoris
		(adductor hiatus) branch of femoral going to gracilis
		(tendon) descending genicular
		Posteriorly (origin of muscle) descending branch of medial circumflex femoral
		(upper part) 1st perforator
		(middle part) 2nd perforator
		(lower part) popliteal artery
Pectineus	III	Anteriorly (upper part) branch of common femoral
		(middle part) medial circumflex femoral
Sartorius	IV	1° = (upper part) lateral circumflex femoral or profunda femoris or femoral
		2° = (upper part) superficial circumflex iliac
		1° = (middle part) femoral
		1° = (lower part) femoral
		2° = (lower part) descending genicular
Rectus femoris	III	1° = (upper part) lateral circumflex femoral
		1° = (lower part) lateral circumflex femoral
		2° (in 30%) superficial circumflex iliac
		2° (rarely) femoral, direct or from branches to vastus medialis
Vastus lateralis	II	2° (antero-superiorly) transverse branch of lateral circumflex femoral
		1° (middle & inferior parts) descending branch of lateral circumflex femoral
		2° (posterior) terminations of profunda perforators
Vastus medialis	II	2° (upper part) femoral } may have a common trunk
		1° (middle part) femoral } may have a common trunk
		2° (lower part) femoral
		2° (small variable contribution) lateral circumflex femoral
		2° (small variable contribution) descending genicular
Vastus intermedius	I	1° lateral and medial branches from a common trunk derived from lateral circumflex femoral
Tensor fasciae latae	I	ascending branch of lateral circumflex femoral
Semimembranosus	III	1° = medial terminal division of the 1st profunda perforator
		1° = 2nd profunda perforator
		2° (at origin) inferior gluteal
alternative arrangements	II	1° third or fourth profunda perforator
		2° (variable supply to lower end), branch of femoral piercing adductor magnus
		2° branch of popliteal (sometimes when adductor hiatus lies very high)
		2° (at origin) inferior gluteal
and variations between these two types		
Semitendinosus	II	1° (middle part) first profunda perforator
		2° (upper part) descending branch of medial circumflex femoral
		2° (at origin) inferior gluteal
		2° (at lower end) branch of popliteal
Biceps femoris, long head	II	1° (junction upper and middle thirds), from 1st profunda perforator directly and via lateral terminal division
		2° (lower part) long branch from lateral terminal division of 1st perforator
		2° (lower part) second profunda perforator
		2° (lower part) recurrent branch from medial terminal division of first perforator
		Accessory supplies, inferior gluteal, medial circumflex femoral, lateral superior genicular
short head		1° 2nd or 3rd profunda perforator
		2° superior lateral genicular artery

1° principal pedicle
1° = more than one principal pedicle of equal size
2° supplementary pedicle

SUMMARY OF BLOOD SUPPLY TO THIGH MUSCLES

A summary of the blood supply to the thigh muscles is given in Table 6.12.

SUMMARY OF ANATOMICAL TERRITORIES OF CUTANEOUS BLOOD SUPPLY

The territory of the *profunda femoris and its perforators* consists of the region overlying the insertion of gluteus maximus, the posterior thigh below the level of the buttock fold and the region overlying the iliotibial tract (Fig. 6.98). The territory extends medially over adductor magnus and the upper part of gracilis. This area is encroached on superiorly to a variable extent by the inferior gluteal artery and inferiorly by an ascending branch of the popliteal artery. To some extent these latter two vessels are inversely related to each other in size. Superomedially the territory includes that supplied by perforators from the underlying adductor magnus. This muscle is largely supplied by profunda perforators, but also by the medial circumflex femoral artery, the obturator and the superficial femoral. The main source in the majority of cases is a large branch from the profunda femoris which supplies all the central part of the muscle.

The cutaneous anatomical territory of supply of the *medial circumflex femoral artery* is difficult to define exactly but may include part of the upper inner aspect of the thigh.

The cutaneous anatomical territory supplied by the *lateral circumflex femoral artery* incorporates the areas over tensor fasciae latae muscle, the anterior part of vastus lateralis not covered by the iliotibial tract, and the area overlying the origin of sartorius. This is shown in Figure 6.99.

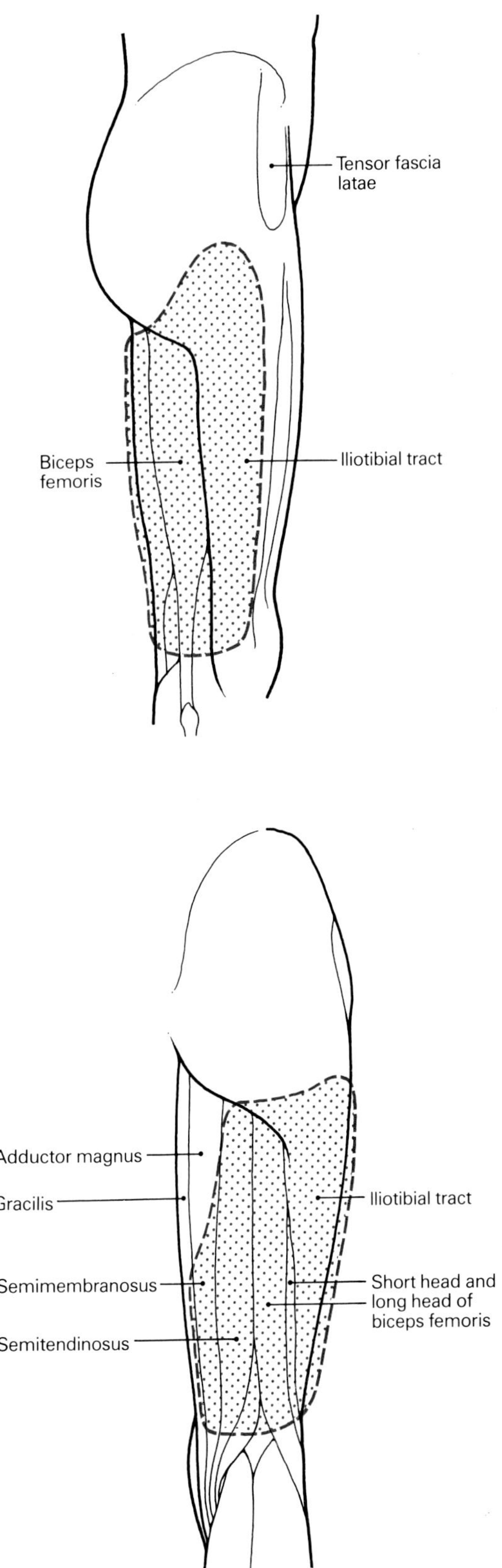

Fig. 6.98 Anatomical territories of cutaneous blood supply under the dependency of the profunda femoris perforators on the lateral and posterior aspects of the thigh.

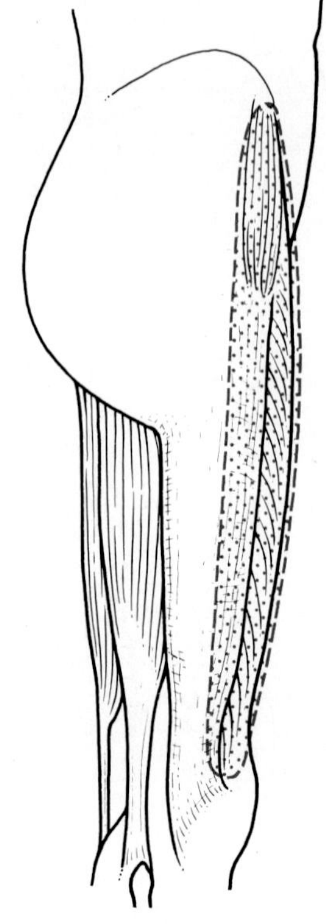

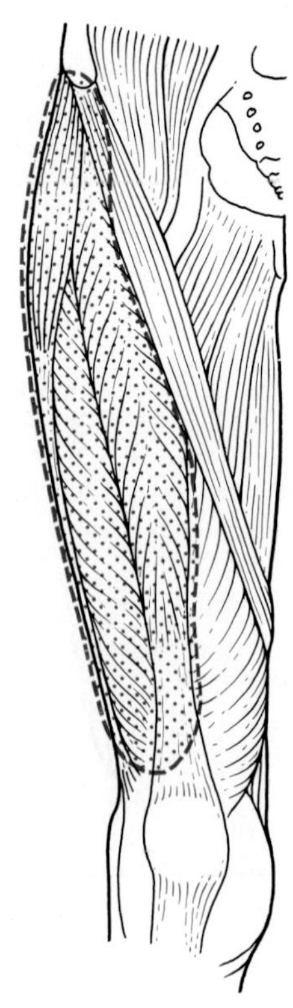

Fig. 6.99 Anatomical territory of cutaneous blood supply under the dependency of the lateral circumflex femoral artery on the lateral and anterior aspects of the thigh.

FLAPS

Anteromedial

The direct cutaneous vessels arising from the femoral are the basis of several traditional and some less well-known flaps: superficial circumflex iliac artery flap, page 431; superficial inferior epigastric flap, page 437; superficial external pudendal artery flap, page 434; deep external pudendal and penile flaps, page 434. Type A fasciocutaneous pedicled flaps may be based over the sartorius muscle and Type B fasciocutaneous free flaps may be based on the single perforator passing round sartorius in the apex of the femoral triangle. The fasciocutaneous perforators arising from the descending genicular artery and its terminal cutaneous branch, the saphenous artery, are the basis for a fasciocutaneous free flap. The descending genicular artery may also have a musculo-articular branch which supplies the periosteal vascular plexus on the medial condyle of the femur thereby permitting a composite flap to be raised (p. 504). The gracilis muscle is the main muscle or musculocutaneous flap available in this area (p. 413).

Anterolateral

The presence of musculocutaneous perforators from the lateral circumflex femoral system through the tensor fasciae latae and rectus femoris muscles has been appreciated for some time and their musculocutaneous flaps are well established. Their potential territories are described on pages 357–362. The TFL flap has also been combined with a segment of the iliac crest, supplied through the origin of the muscle from the bone, as a combined myo-osteo-cutaneous free tissue transfer.

The anastomoses between the lateral circumflex femoral system and the superior gluteal system have been exploited in a combined TFL gluteus medius musculocutaneous rotation flap for trochanteric cover (p. 100).

Vastus lateralis has been used as a sliding muscle flap for covering trochanteric sores for many years but only recently have the musculocutaneous perforators from its antero-inferior part been appreciated, resulting in the design of musculocutaneous flaps based on this part of the muscle.

Fasciocutaneous perforators from the descending branch of the lateral circumflex femoral artery may support a septocutaneous flap from the anterolateral surface of the thigh and the input into these perforators is so good that a large skin island can often be supported by just one perforator (p. 366).

Above the knee the lateral superior genicular artery can support a flap (p. 398).

The vessels arising from the profunda perforators which pass along the posterior surface of the lateral intermuscular septum and fan out above the iliotibial tract are the basis for several free flaps (p. 420).

Posterior

A variety of musculocutaneous flaps based on the hamstring muscles have been used for many years in reconstructing paraplegic pressure sores over the ischial tuberosity. These are either large, laterally based transposition flaps or island flaps advanced in a V-Y manner. It is clear that any fasciocutaneous perforators emerging between the hamstring muscles will also contribute to the supply of these hamstring musculocutaneous flaps (p. 416).

Island musculocutaneous flaps overlying the long head of biceps and pedicled on that muscle's neurovascular pedicle have been successfully used for reconstructing traumatic defects on the anterior and lateral aspects of the thigh as well as hip and perineal defects. In some cases these flaps have been combined with a functional reconstruction of the knee extensor mechanism by inserting the distal end of biceps femoris into the patella (p. 416).

Free flaps from the posterior thigh have been based on posterior cutaneous branches of the profunda perforators. When these are fasciocutaneous vessels, dissection of the pedicle is greatly facilitated whereas when the vessels pass through biceps femoris the covering muscle fibres must be divided so as to enable an adequate length of vascular pedicle to be dissected free from the muscle.

The posterior midline 'relay artery' accompanying the posterior cutaneous nerve of the thigh is fed superiorly by the inferior gluteal artery and inferiorly by the popliteal artery. This is the basis for the superiorly-based extended inferior gluteal flap (p. 336), and for the inferiorly-based popliteo-thigh flap (p. 398).

6 KNEE

The principal arteries of supply at the sides of the knee and over the patella are the genicular branches of the popliteal, the descending genicular branch of the femoral, and the anterior recurrent branch of the anterior tibial. Additional small vessels come from vastus medialis, semimembranosus and the short head of biceps femoris. The contribution of each of the major arteries will be described in turn.

The popliteal artery gives off superior and inferior genicular arteries which lie deeply and supply the capsule of the knee joint but also give off branches which reach the skin. (The middle genicular artery supplies the cruciate ligaments and synovium only.) Both superior genicular arteries are given off at approximately the level of the upper edge of the femoral condyles.

The medial superior genicular runs deep to semimembranosus and semitendinosus to reach the lowermost fibres of vastus medialis which it supplies. Here it anastomoses with the articular branch of the descending genicular artery (to which it is inversely related in size) and gives off branches to the skin superior and medial to the patella.

The lateral superior genicular runs deep to the tendon of biceps and gives a branch of supply to vastus lateralis. It sends branches across the upper pole of the patella to anastomose with the medial superior genicular, and it also sends branches to the skin along the lateral side of the patella which anastomose with the lateral inferior genicular artery. Both the inferior genicular arteries arise from the popliteal at a slightly variable level but approximately level with the joint line.

The medial inferior genicular runs deep to the medial head of gastrocnemius and the tibial collateral ligament. Here it gives off branches which fan out over and under the ligamentum patellae to join the vessels from the lateral side and also fan out upwards to anastomose with the descending genicular and medial superior genicular artery. It contributes to the cutaneous patellar plexus.

The lateral inferior genicular runs deep to the lateral head of gastrocnemius and the fibular collateral ligament and then gives branches to the skin inferolateral to the patella. A deep branch passes across the tibia behind the patellar ligament.

The anterior recurrent artery is given off by the anterior tibial immediately after it has traversed the

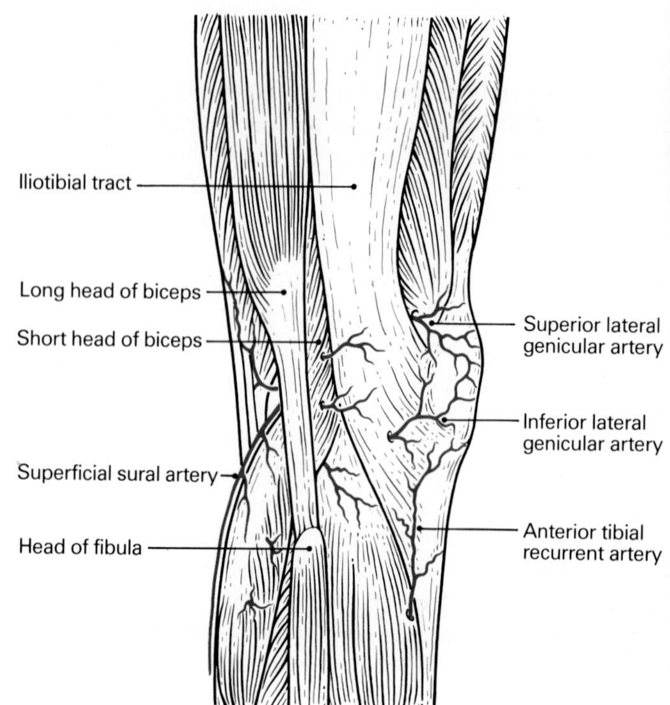

Fig. 6.100 Lateral aspect of the right knee showing principal branches of supply to the skin.

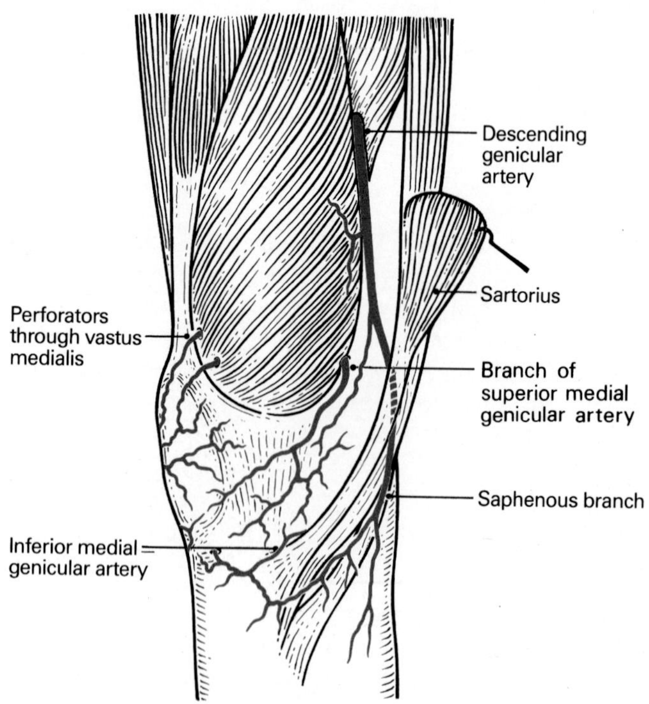

Fig. 6.101 Medial aspect of the right knee. Sartorius has been divided, the proximal part removed and the distal part turned outwards.

interosseus membrane and appeared in the anterior compartment of the lower leg. It pierces tibialis anterior to run upwards on the lateral side of the tibial tuberosity and anastomoses with the lateral inferior genicular and circumflex fibular arteries. It contributes to the capsular plexus and also to the cutaneous patellar plexus.

The descending genicular artery arises from the femoral artery just before that vessel passes through the adductor hiatus. It pierces the fascia between vastus medialis and adductor magnus in the company of the saphenous nerve and two venae comitantes. It usually divides within 3 cm of its point of origin into a deep musculoarticular branch and a superficial saphenous branch. The deep branch continues distally between vastus medialis and adductor magnus, supplying them, and ends as branches to the knee joint. The superficial branch accompanies the saphenous nerve and vein. It gives off a significant infrapatellar branch to the patellar anastomosis and a number of other branches to the skin as it continues on distally to reach the upper medial aspect of the lower leg.

Posteriorly there are several small unnamed vessels arising directly from the popliteal which send branches to the skin. One of these branches lies in the upper part of the popliteal fossa and ascends in the midline between semitendinosus and biceps femoris. It is inconstant and when present is of a variable size, but may reach an internal diameter of 0.8 mm and exceed 10 cm in length. The radiograph illustrated in Figure 6.97 shows an example of this vessel. Over the lowermost part of the popliteal fossa the skin receives branches from the popliteal artery and branches from the sural arteries. These run vertically downwards over gastrocnemius with one of the branches generally being much larger than the others. (Note that these cutaneous arteries are unnamed; the actual *sural* arteries are the ones supplying gastrocnemius, plantaris and soleus, and they may be an alternative origin for these cutaneous vessels which will be referred to as the superficial sural arteries.)

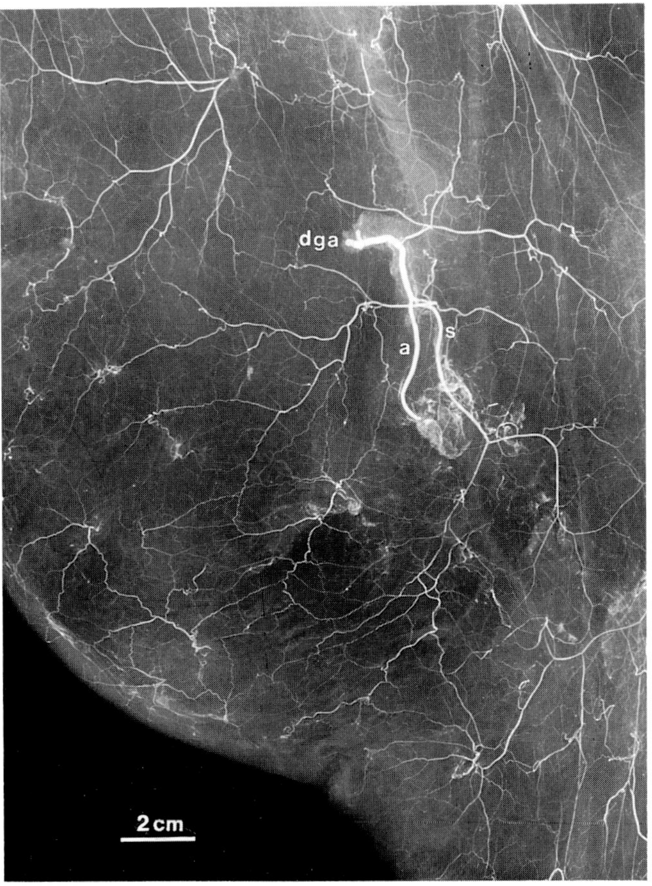

Fig. 6.102 Radiograph of the medial side of the knee showing the descending genicular artery (**dga**) dividing into saphenous (**s**) and articular (**a**) branches.

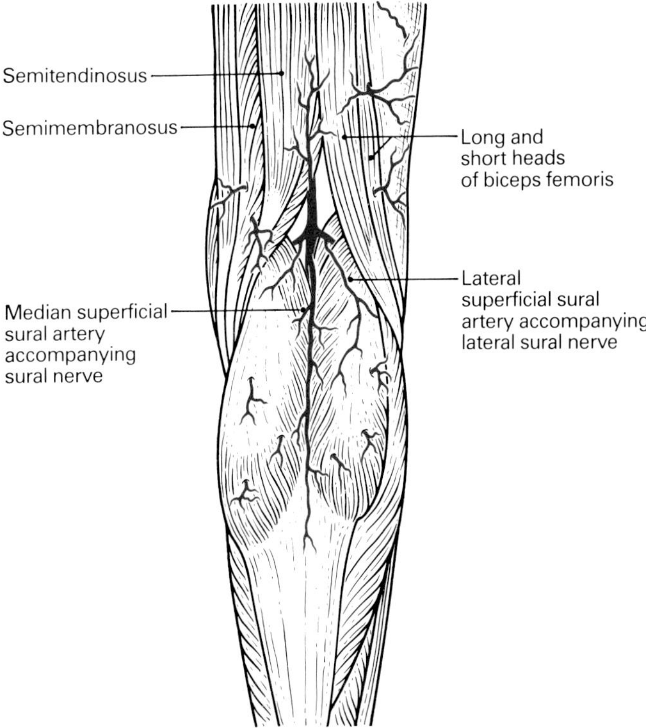

Fig. 6.103 Posterior aspect of the right knee. The arrangement of the superficial sural arteries is very variable. Examples of these vessels are shown in Figs 7.246 & 7.247. The size of the branch ascending in the midline is also very variable.

FLAPS

The principal flaps of this region are ones based on the descending genicular artery and its saphenous branch. By incorporating the saphenous nerve this can be made a neurovascular free flap. The detailed anatomy of the branches of the saphenous artery and the elevation of the flap are described on page 428.

Axial pattern fasciocutaneous flaps can be raised on the superficial sural artery accompanying the sural nerve and short saphenous vein. Free flaps based on this vessel are also possible (p. 440). The sural nerve has been investigated as a possible site for a donor vascularised nerve graft (Taylor & Ham, 1976; Franchinelli et al, 1981). Briedenbach had found the artery to be suitable in only 30% of cases studied (Briedenbach & Terzis, 1983).

The superior lateral genicular artery is the basis for a Type B distally pedicled fasciocutaneous flap described on page 398. The superior medial genicular artery has a cutaneous branch reaching the deep fascia in front of the sartorius tendon which may be the basis for a similar flap. Although not described in Chapter 7 this flap has been described by Hayashi & Maruyama (1990).

6

6 LOWER LEG

From the level of the tibial tuberosity to the ankle the lower leg is supplied by a combination of direct cutaneous, musculocutaneous and fasciocutaneous vessels. Figures 6.104–6.106 show how the anterior tibial, posterior tibial and peroneal arteries give off multiple fasciocutaneous perforators which reach the skin by passing along the intermuscular fascial septa. In addition there are musculocutaneous perforators from the surface of gastrocnemius and supplementary vessels superomedially where the saphenous artery extends below the knee, and posteriorly where cutaneous branches of the popliteal artery accompany the sural nerves. A further subcutaneous vessel, rarely named, is the artery accompanying the superficial peroneal nerve.

The relative contribution that each of the three main arteries makes to the blood supply of the lower limb becomes an important consideration when one of these vessels is going to be used as a donor or recipient vessel for a free flap. Palpation of the posterior tibial, anterior tibial and dorsalis pedis pulses may be useful in indicating the extent to which these vessels participate in the supply of the foot but is no guide to the anatomy of the three major vessels in the lower leg. For example, the posterior tibial artery may be absent and the 'posterior tibial pulse' may then be entirely due to a peroneal artery which in the terminal part of its course has passed medially behind the ankle joint and taken over the role of the posterior tibial in supplying the foot. Clearly some understanding of the possible variations in the principal arteries is desirable and these will be described.

THE BLOOD SUPPLY OF THE LOWER LEG: CLASSICAL DESCRIPTION

In 90% of cases the popliteal artery runs obliquely inferolaterally to the lower edge of popliteus where it divides into anterior and posterior tibial arteries. This course can be marked on the surface by a line drawn from the junction of the middle and lower thirds of the thigh 2.5 cm medial to the midline of the back of the limb, running downwards and slightly laterally to reach the midline between the femoral condyles. From here the course of the vessel continues inferolaterally along the same line to the level of the tibial tuberosity. The *anterior tibial artery* passes forwards between the tibial and fibular heads of tibialis posterior to pass over the upper edge of the interosseous membrane and reach the anterior compartment. It descends on the front of the interosseous membrane and gradually approaches the tibia to lie on it in the lower third of the leg. The anterior tibial artery is initially medial to the deep peroneal nerve, but descends behind it to lie once more medial to it at the ankle. Near the ankle it is crossed by the extensor hallucis longus tendon and the superior extensor retinaculum, and gives origin to the medial and lateral malleolar arteries before passing midway between the malleoli onto the dorsum of the foot as the dorsalis pedis artery. The *posterior tibial artery* is the larger and more direct terminal branch of the popliteal. It passes downwards in the posterior compartment separated from the interosseous membrane by tibialis posterior, and lying beneath soleus though separated from it by a fascial layer. It gives a nutrient branch to the tibia and continues downwards behind flexor digitorum longus and, becoming superficial, crosses the lower end of the tibia parallel to and 2.5 cm in front of the medial border of the Achilles tendon. At the ankle joint it passes deep to the flexor retinaculum, midway between the medial malleolus and the medial tubercle of the calcaneus and divides, deep to abductor hallucis, into the medial and lateral plantar arteries. The tibial nerve is medial to the origin of the artery, and crosses behind it at about the origin of the peroneal artery and thereafter descends on its lateral side, so that the artery at the ankle lies between the tibial nerve and the tendon of flexor digitorum longus. The *peroneal artery* arises from the posterior tibial artery 2.5 cm below the lower edge of the popliteus muscle. It inclines laterally to descend along the medial crest of the fibula deep to or in the substance of flexor hallucis longus and ends behind the tibiofibular syndesmosis. It sends a nutrient artery to the fibula, and is linked to the posterior tibial artery by a communicating branch which lies on average 6.5 cm above the tip of the fibular malleolus. Nearer the ankle (approximately 5 cm above the fibular tip) it gives off a perforating branch which pierces the interosseous membrane and descends in front of the tibiofibular syndesmosis to the anastomosis round the ankle.

Variations

1. Variations occur in the location and manner of branching of the popliteal artery. Persistence of the embryonic axial artery in the segment known as the deep popliteal artery results in the popliteal artery passing in front of the popliteus muscle. Other types of displacement of the popliteal artery usually coexist with faulty development of the gastrocnemius muscle

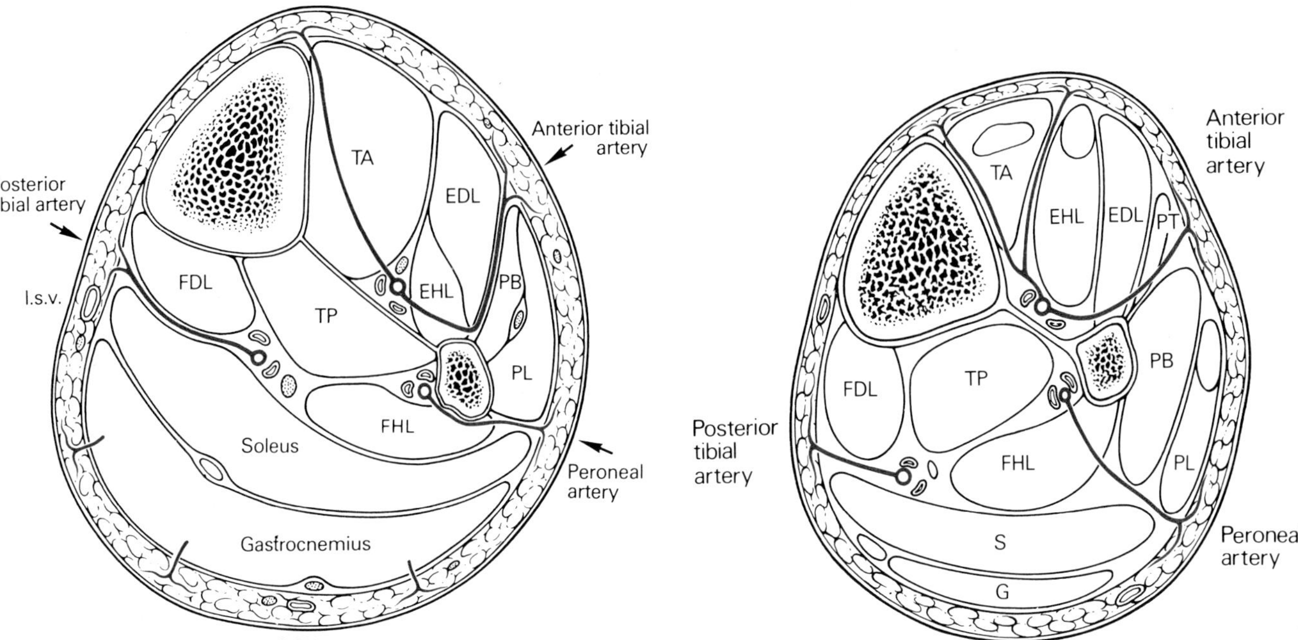

Fig. 6.104 Schematic transverse section through the upper third of the lower leg showing positions of the major vessels relative to the intermuscular septa. The principal fasciocutaneous and musculocutaneous perforators are shown.

Fig. 6.105 Schematic transverse section through the lower third of the lower leg.

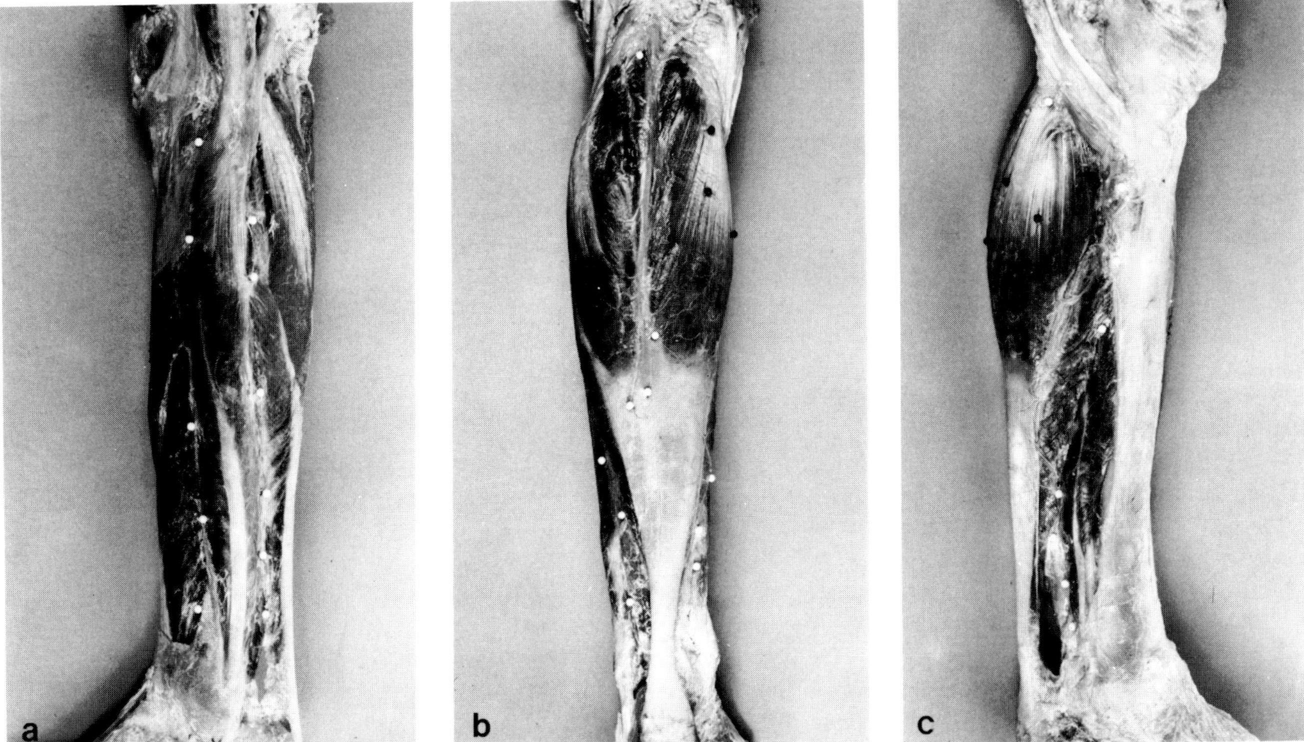

Fig. 6.106 Micropaque injected preparation of the lower leg showing (**a**) lateral, (**b**) posterior and (**c**) medial aspects. The fasciocutaneous perforators have been marked with white pins, the musculocutaneous perforators with black pins. In this particular case there were no perforators through the lateral head of gastrocnemius and the skin in this region was supplied by a particularly well-developed lateral superficial sural artery. A vessel lies deep in the groove between the two heads of gastrocnemius supplying the muscle by several branches and ending as two branches (marked by pins) piercing the deep fascia to reach skin – this is an unusual arrangement.

(Delaney & Gonzales, 1971). The classical description of the division of the popliteal is accurate in 90% of cases. The remainder show either a high division 5% (Fig. 6.107b, c, d), low division 1% (Fig. 6.107e), or a trifurcation 4% (Fig. 6.107f). All of these can logically be explained in terms of the embryological development of the vessels (Senior, 1919).

2. Because of the competitive pattern of development between the arteries with continuous formation and breakdown of 'ladder' anastomoses during development, variations from normal in the size of vessels may occur (Fig. 6.108). The *anterior tibial artery* is often diminished in calibre but never entirely absent. The middle portion may be greatly reduced in which case the perforating branch of the peroneal artery joins the distal portion (5% of 2458 cases). When greatly increased in size the anterior tibial supplies the plantar surface of the foot. The *posterior tibial* may reach only as far as the distal third of the leg where it is then reinforced by a large communicating branch from the peroneal. It may end as a nutrient vessel to the tibia or in supplying a muscle, or it may even be absent, in which case its territory is supplied by a particularly well-developed peroneal artery (peronea magna, in four studies totalling 886 cases the prevalence was 6.5%). Rarely it may be increased in calibre. The *peroneal artery* is never absent but is occasionally much reduced in size. Anatomically its size is inversely proportional to that of the other arteries in the leg, and as described above it may feed the distal parts of the anterior or posterior tibial arteries. Interestingly it is the vessel least affected by arteriosclerosis in the lower leg (Haimovici, 1967.) In one large series of patients with arteriosclerosis and diabetes, the peroneal artery was never found to be occluded.

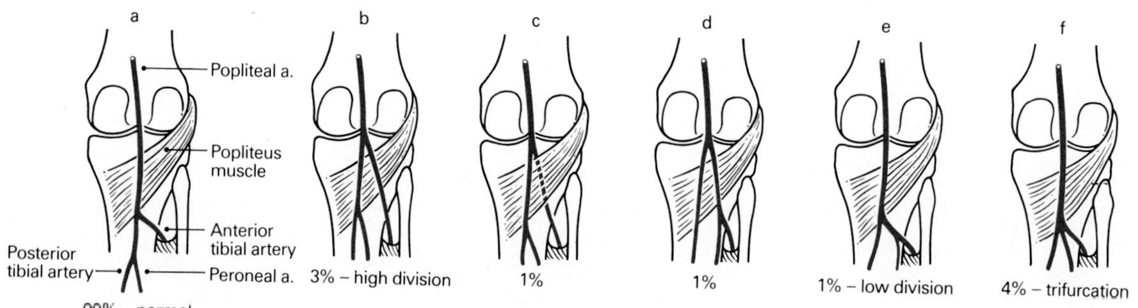

Fig. 6.107 Variations in the manner of division of the popliteal artery.

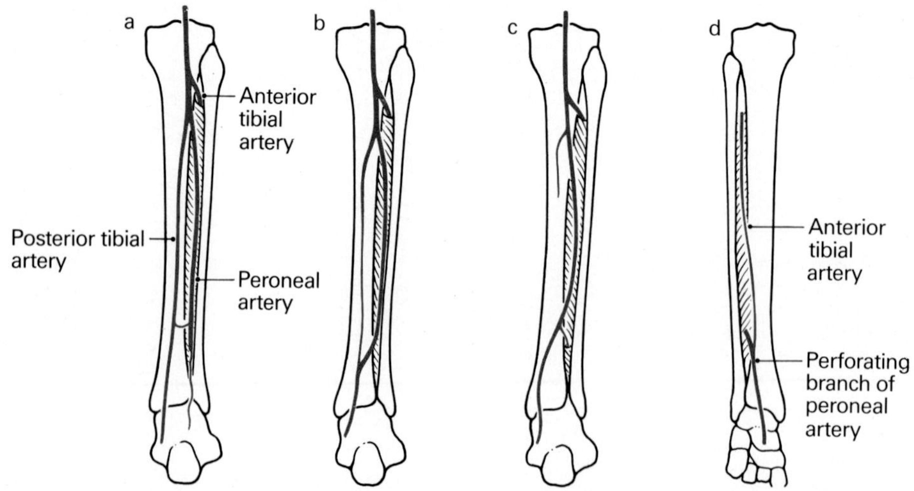

Fig. 6.108 Variations in the degree of development of the major vessels in the lower leg: **a.** normal situation; **b.** posterior tibial artery weak, the peroneal artery reinforces its lower part; **c.** posterior tibial artery fails, the peroneal takes over its distal territory (b and c together make up 5–10% of cases); **d.** the anterior tibial artery is weak, the peroneal artery reinforces it distally by its perforating branch (5–10% of cases).

BLOOD SUPPLY TO THE COMPARTMENTS

The problem with the classical account of the lower limb vessels is that it fails to give an adequate impression of the blood supply to each of the three separate compartments. The implication is that each of the three major vessels supplies one compartment but this is not entirely correct.

The blood supply to each of the three compartments will now be described.

The peroneal compartment

This is supplied by:
— the arteria comitans of the common peroneal nerve
— a superior artery from the anterior tibial to the peroneal compartment
— an inferior artery from the anterior tibial to the peroneal compartment
— branches of the peroneal artery.

1. The arteria comitans of the common peroneal nerve arises from a sural artery (72%), the popliteal artery (19%) or the superior lateral genicular artery (9%). It runs on the lateral side of the common peroneal nerve, passes round the neck of the fibula, and divides into two branches which follow the deep and superficial peroneal nerves. Usually this makes only a small contribution to the blood supply of the peroneal compartment.

2. The superior artery to the peroneal compartment arises from the anterior tibial immediately after it passes over the interosseous membrane (45%) or it arises by a common trunk with the anterior tibial recurrent (55%). It passes laterally, deep to extensor digitorum and pierces the anterior peroneal septum either alone or through the same opening as the deep peroneal nerve. In the peroneal compartment it inclines distally along the fibula and lies posterior to the superficial peroneal nerve deep to peroneus longus. It supplies the origin of peroneus longus and ends further distally within the muscle after giving off a branch which accompanies the superficial peroneal nerve.

3. The inferior artery to the peroneal compartment arises from the anterior tibial artery just above the midpoint of the leg. It supplies peroneus brevis but is inconstant, such that when absent the superior artery is larger and extends distally to supply peroneus brevis.

4. The peroneal artery sends two or three branches to the lower third of the peroneal compartment in 65% of cases. These branches arise within the belly of flexor hallucis longus and pass laterally around the fibula and through the posterior peroneal septum. They divide into ascending and descending branches which anastomose with the anterior tibial branches above and supply peroneus brevis. One of these peroneal branches may be large and replace the inferior branch of the anterior tibial, and in a minority of cases (~15%) these branches of the peroneal constitute the dominant blood supply of the peroneal compartment. All the vessels in the peroneal compartment anastomose freely.

The anterior compartment

This has a very simple scheme of vascularisation. The anterior tibial artery simply gives off 25 to 30 branches to the muscles, each branch being fairly small in diameter and running horizontally to a nearby muscle. Tibialis anterior is supplied by the anterior recurrent artery and by two sets of branches coming off the tibial artery on its anterior and medial sides often straddling the deep peroneal nerve. Some of these branches reach the deep fascia and supply skin. Extensor digitorum is supplied by branches which come off the anterior aspect of the tibial artery, sometimes in common with the branches to tibialis anterior. Several of these vessels pass along the lateral side of the muscle to emerge along the anterior peroneal septum. The extensor hallucis is supplied by four or five small branches of the anterior tibial artery but also by a branch of the peroneal artery which passes through the peroneal compartment, perhaps supplying peroneus brevis, to reach the front of the leg.

The posterior compartment

These muscles are vascularised by the popliteal, the posterior tibial and the peroneal arteries. Each muscle must be considered in turn. Each belly of gastrocnemius has its own neurovascular pedicle containing a sural artery and in addition there may be accessory supplies to the origins of the muscles from the popliteal or genicular arteries. The sural arteries are given off by the popliteal at a variable level which is either at a point on the plane of the tibial plateaus (61%), above them (31%) or below them (8%) with the medial sural artery usually arising a little higher than the lateral. The sural arteries divide into branches which run within the muscle and often end as musculocutaneous perforators to the overlying skin. The sural arteries may also give off cutaneous branches which accompany the medial and lateral sural cutaneous nerves.

Soleus has a much more variable pattern of vascularisation. The commonest pattern consists of two dominant pedicles (superior and inferior) and several accessory ones. The superior pedicle arises from the popliteal artery at the lower border of the popliteus and after running distally for a few centimetres enters the deep surface of the soleus near its lateral border in the company of the nerve of supply. Within the muscle the branches descend nearer to the anterior than the posterior surface. The inferior pedicle arises from the peroneal artery at its origin or from the posterior tibial artery (20%). It passes medially behind the tibial nerve and enters the muscle to descend within it nearer the posterior than the anterior surface. Accessory arteries are numerous: the lateral sural artery may give off a branch which passes posterior to plantaris and enters the superficial surface of soleus; the popliteal may give a few branches to the upper origin of the muscle; the posterior tibial gives off three or four branches from its posterior surface which enter the medial edge of soleus in its distal part; and the peroneal gives off two or three branches which may supply the lower lateral part of the muscle on their way to the skin. There are few, if any, significant anastomoses within the muscle between these inferior accessory arteries and the two principal pedicles.

Flexor digitorum longus is supplied on its posterior surface by seven to ten branches of the posterior tibial artery. One of these is particularly large; it usually supplies the middle part of the muscle and gives off a large fasciocutaneous perforator which reaches the deep fascia by passing between soleus and flexor digitorum longus.

Flexor hallucis longus is supplied by nine to ten branches of the peroneal artery. Many of these also supply tibialis posterior. Branches of the peroneal artery also pass through the flexor hallucis longus in order to get to the peroneal muscles and to give off fasciocutaneous perforators along the posterior peroneal septum. As they pass through the muscle they give off small branches of supply to it.

Tibialis posterior is supplied by multiple branches of both the posterior tibial and the peroneal arteries.

CUTANEOUS BLOOD SUPPLY OF THE LOWER LEG

Anterior tibial artery

The first cutaneous branch is the anterior tibial recurrent artery which is given off either anterior or posterior to the interosseous membrane and passes up through tibialis anterior to emerge between it and the tibia at the level of the upper border of the tibial tuberosity. There are usually two or three further perforators from the anterior tibial artery emerging in a row along the anterior border of the upper third of the tibia. Most of the perforators, however, pass along the anterior peroneal septum. There are on average six of these significantly sized fasciocutaneous perforators emerging between extensor digitorum longus and the peroneal compartment although in the lower two-thirds of the leg one or two may be displaced to lie between extensor digitorum longus and tibialis anterior. The uppermost perforator may arise from the lateral inferior genicular artery. One usually accompanies the superficial peroneal nerve and may run alongside it as far as the ankle (vide infra). The lower perforators are smaller, but just above the level of the ankle joint the anterior tibial artery gives off a larger malleolar branch which spreads out over the anterior aspect of the lateral malleolus at the level of the deep fascia.

Peroneal artery

About five fasciocutaneous perforators arise from the peroneal artery and run along the posterior peroneal septum to spread out and anastomose longitudinally at the level of the deep fascia (Figs 6.109 & 6.110). A perforating branch pierces the interosseous membrane to appear on the front of the leg, anterior to the peroneal tendons, immediately above the superior extensor retinaculum. The terminal part of the peroneal artery gives of a lateral malleolar branch and then lies on the os calcis giving off the lateral calcaneal branches. Occasionally the artery accompanying the superficial peroneal nerve arises from the peroneal artery.

Posterior tibial artery

The most proximal part of the medial side of the lower leg is supplied by the saphenous artery (Fig 6.111 & 6.112). Below this the posterior tibial artery gives off four large fasciocutaneous perforators which emerge between flexor digitorum longus and soleus, give off periosteal vessels to the anterior surface of the tibia, and divide into anterior and posterior branches. The anterior branches run inferiorly over the subcutaneous surface of the tibia and anastomose with perforators from the anterior tibial artery. The posterior branches pass obliquely upwards and downwards anastomosing with each other over the medial side of the leg and in the fascia surrounding the tendo calcaneus. Distally, the posterior tibial artery gives off malleolar and calcaneal branches which supply skin.

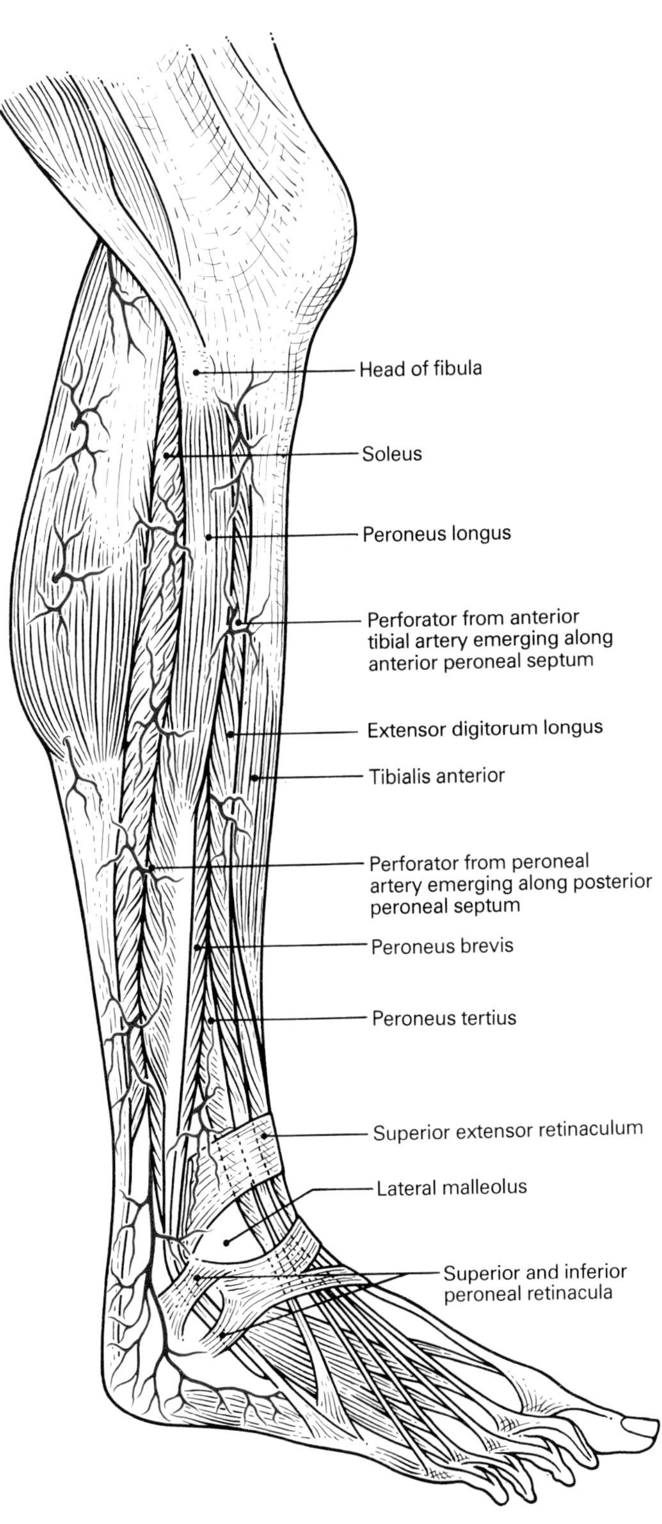

Fig. 6.109 Lateral aspect of lower leg. Although the deep fascia has been removed in order to display the muscles and the septa between the various compartments, the fasciocutaneous branches to the skin have been indicated as lying on the muscles. They would in fact have been lying on the superficial aspect of the deep fascia.

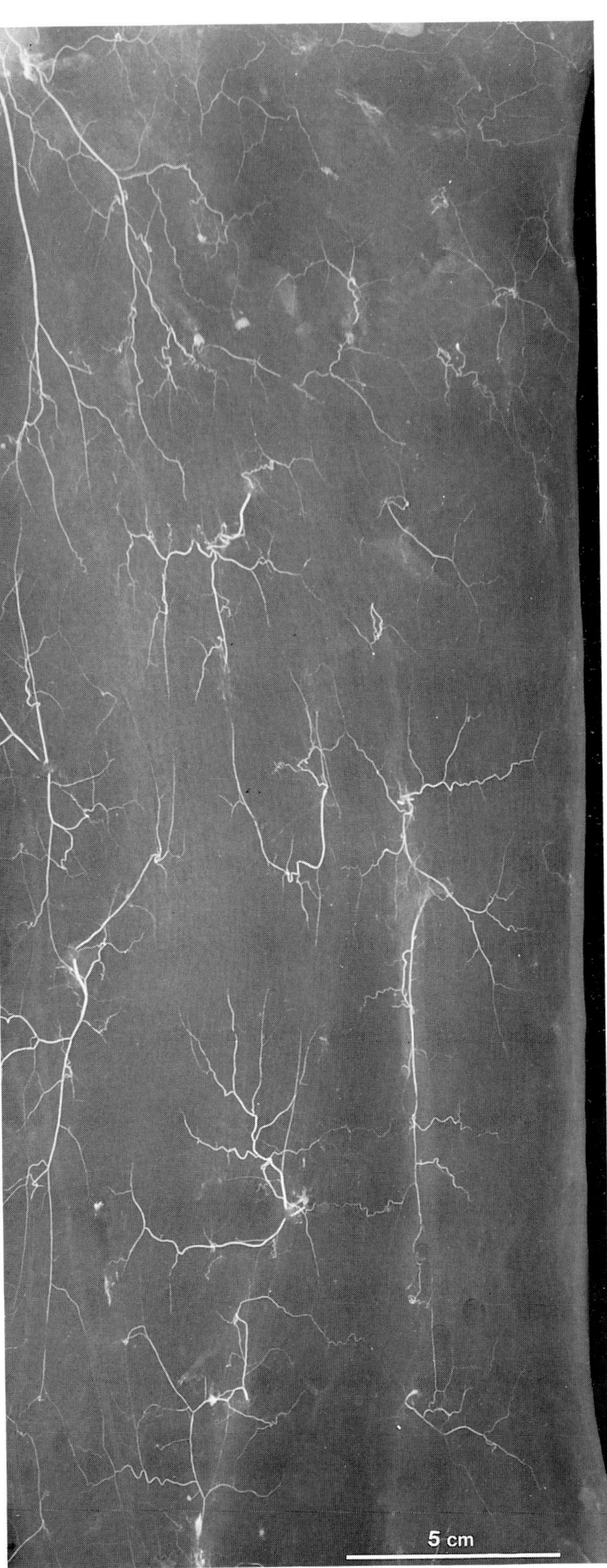

Fig. 6.110 Radiograph of skin showing rows of perforators overlying the peroneal septa. The right-hand edge of the specimen was created by an incision overlying the anterior subcutaneous border of the tibia.

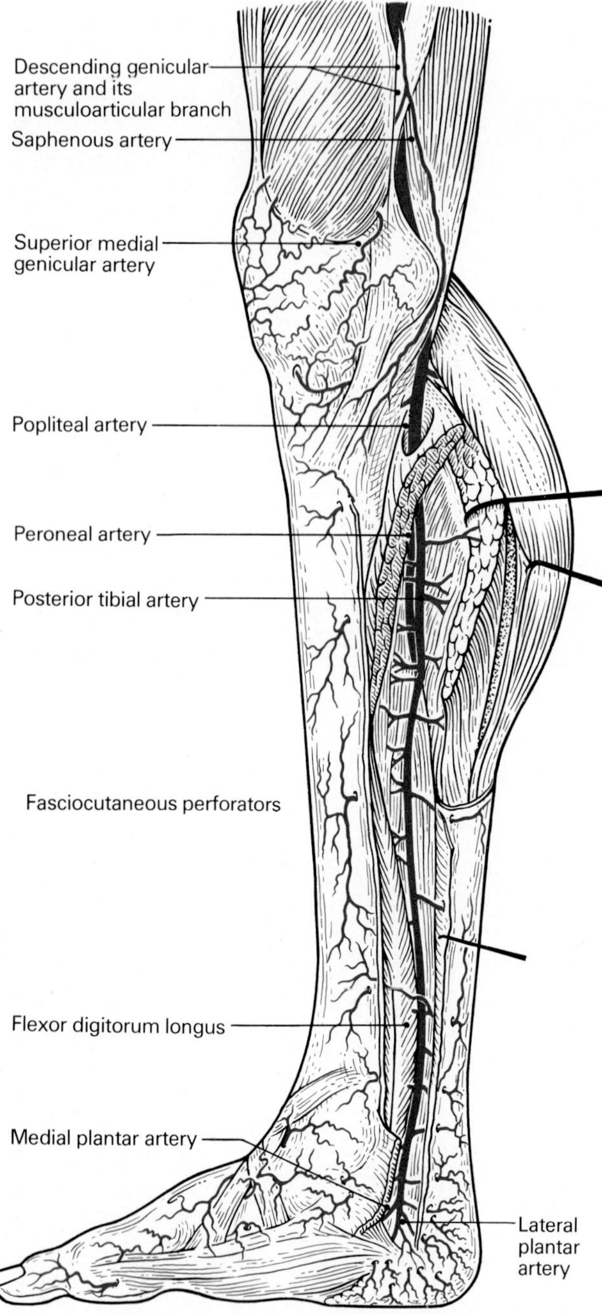

Fig. 6.111 Medial aspect of the lower leg. The deep fascia has been divided overlying the interval between flexor digitorum longus and soleus, and the medial part of soleus arising from the tibia has been divided in order to expose the posterior tibial artery. The diagram does not show that many of the perforators give off, in addition to their branches to skin, a set of vessels to the periosteum on the anterior surface of the tibia.

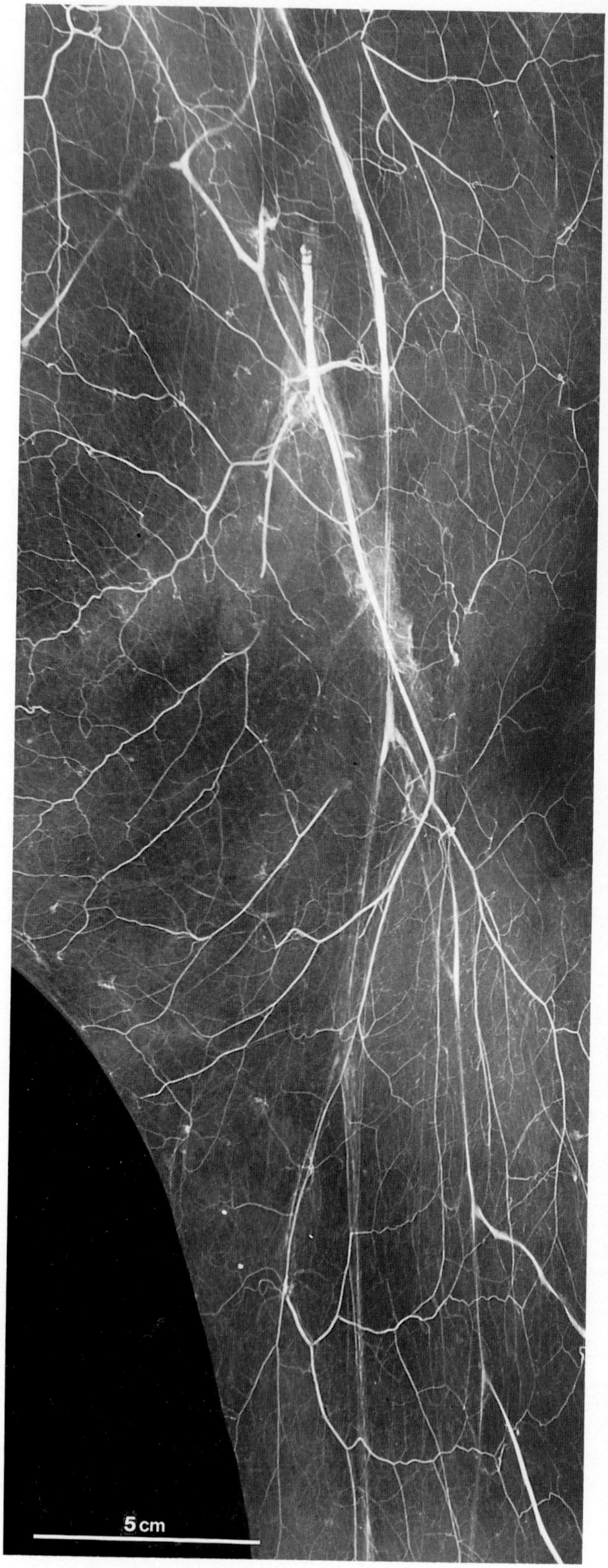

Fig. 6.112 Radiograph of an extremely well-developed saphenous artery which extends onto the medial aspect of the lower leg. A small quantity of contrast medium has entered the long saphenous vein and its close relationship to the artery can be seen.

The sural arteries

The medial head of gastrocnemius is better developed than the lateral head and the medial sural artery is therefore usually slightly greater in diameter than the lateral. Within each head of the muscle, each artery divides into two or three longitudinally running branches, so that each half of the muscle is independent in terms of blood supply. These branches give off multiple small twigs to the muscle and several much larger branches which pierce the surface of the muscle to supply the overlying skin. The lateral sural artery may also give off superficial sural cutaneous branches before it enters the lateral head of gastrocnemius. One always accompanies the medial sural cutaneous nerve, and one may run with the lateral sural cutaneous nerve and its peroneal communicating branch. The cutaneous artery in the midline between the two heads of gastrocnemius initially lies beneath the deep fascia in the company of the medial sural cutaneous nerve. It may carry on with the nerve or pierce the deep fascia to join the short saphenous vein.

The median superficial sural artery

The vessel running in the midline between the heads of gastrocnemius was named by Manchot *arteria suralis superficialis media* and by Adachi and others *arteria saphena parva*. It is currently unrecognised in *Nomina Anatomica* and will be referred to as the median superficial sural artery although another possible name for it might be the small saphenous artery. It arises from the popliteal (48%) from the lateral sural (39%) or from one of the inferior genicular arteries (13%) and pierces the popliteal fascia to accompany the medial sural cutaneous nerve and the short saphenous vein (Figs 6.113 & 6.114). The point at which the artery pierces the deep fascia bridging the groove between the two heads of gastrocnemius is variable but is usually about half-way down the lateral head of gastrocnemius. It follows the lateral edge of the Achilles tendon where it anastomoses with branches of the posterior tibial artery. Rare instances have been recorded in which this vessel was so well developed that it continued all the way down to the foot and communicated with the lateral tarsal artery.

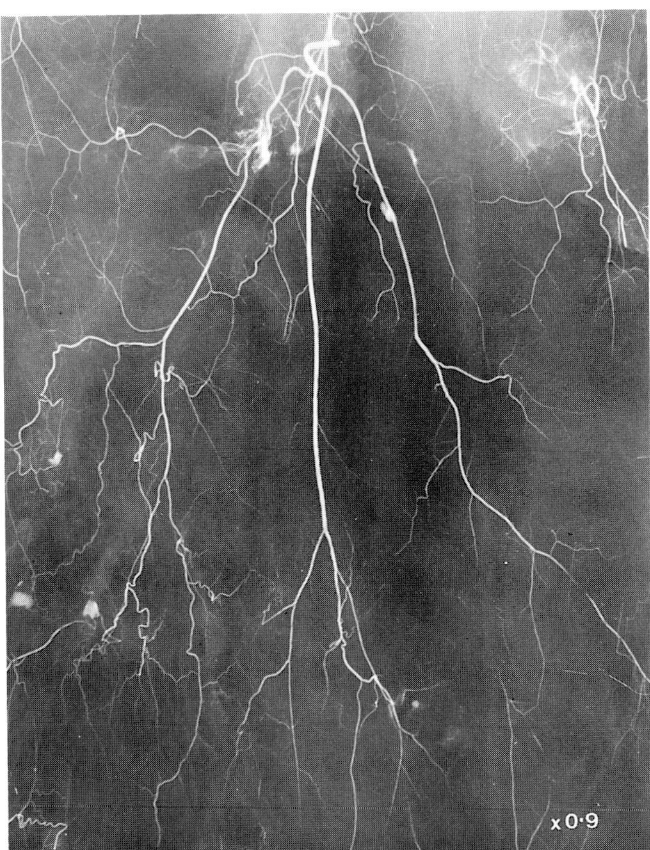

Fig. 6.113 Example of superficial sural artery with medial, median and lateral branches.

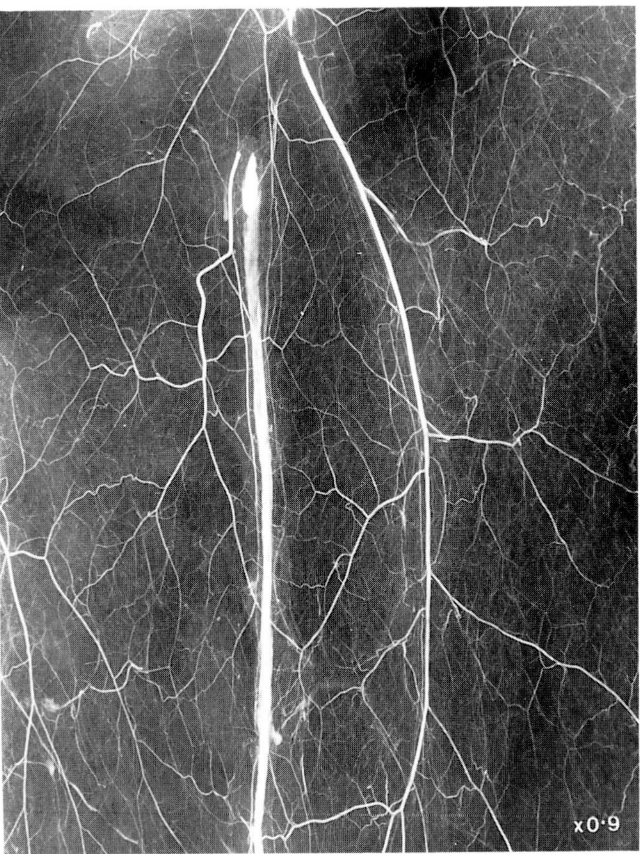

Fig. 6.114 Example of an exceptionally well-developed lateral superficial sural artery and a small median artery. The short saphenous vein has also opacified.

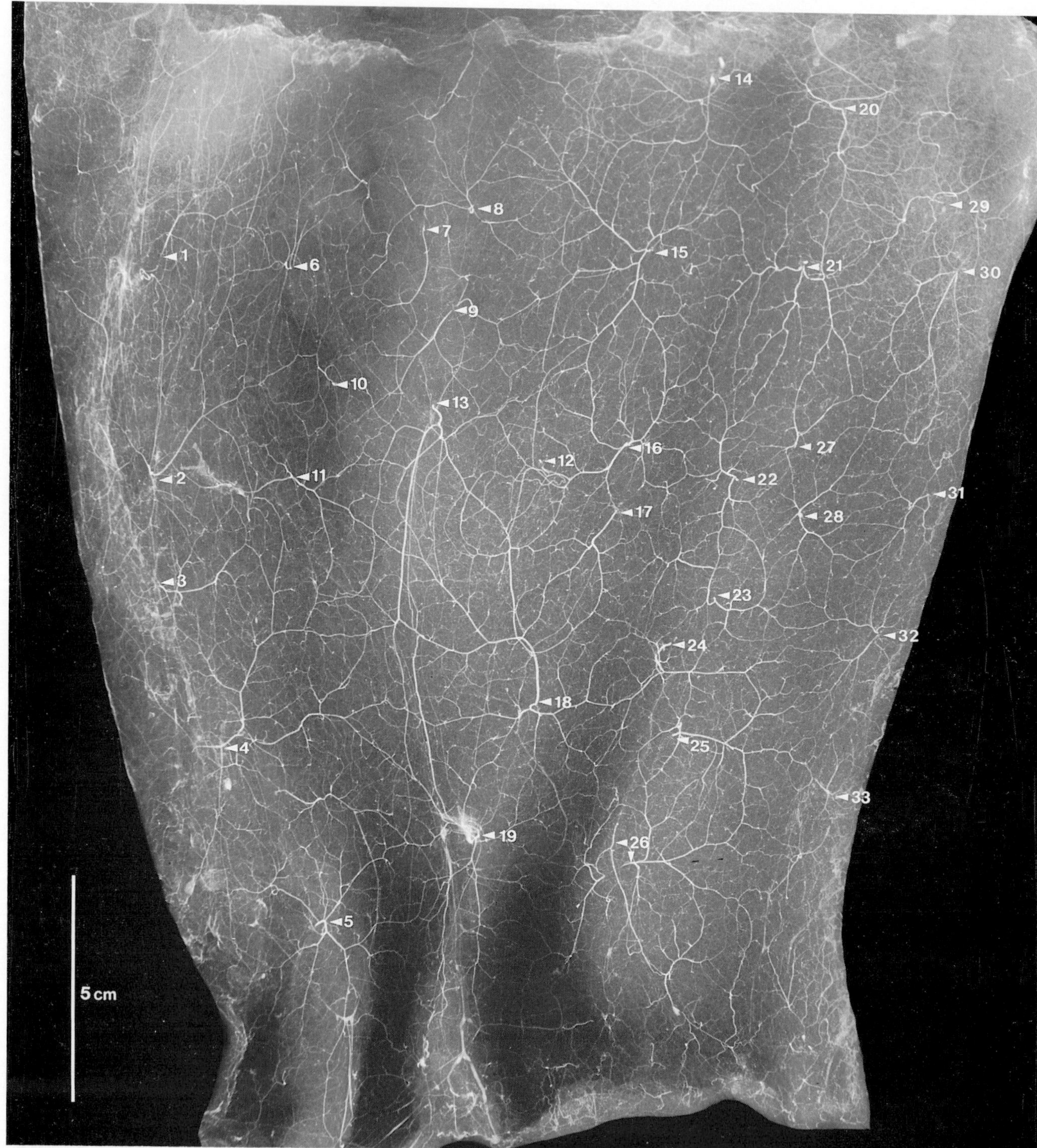

Fig. 6.115 Skin incision over the anterior subcutaneous surface of the tibia, skin and deep fascia removed and laid out flat. Specimen extends from the level of the tibial tuberosity superiorly to the malleoli inferiorly. Origin of perforators:

1–5. Fasciocutaneous perforators from the posterior tibial artery emerging between soleus and flexor digitorum longus,

6–13. Musculocutaneous perforators arising from sural arteries and emerging through the surface of gastrocnemius,

14–19. Fasciocutaneous perforators from the peroneal artery emerging between soleus and peroneus longus, i.e. along the posterior peroneal septum,

20–26. Fasciocutaneous perforators arising from the anterior tibial artery and emerging between peroneus brevis and extensor digitorum longus, i.e. along the anterior peroneal septum,

27 & 28. Fasciocutaneous perforators arising from the anterior tibial artery and emerging between extensor digitorum longus and tibialis anterior,

29–33. Perforators arising from the anterior tibial artery and emerging between tibialis anterior and the anterior edge of the tibia.

The artery accompanying the superficial peroneal nerve

This is similarly unrecognised, but well described in the literature. Sometimes known as the *arteria nervi peronei superficialis*, it arises from the anterior tibial artery and passes with the nerve between extensor digitorum longus and peroneus longus to become superficial. The anterior tibial origin is from the superior branch to the peroneal compartment in 30% of cases, from the inferior branch in 40%, and from both in 30% (Rocha et al, 1987). Occasionally it arises from the peroneal artery and winds superficially round the fibula. Various degrees of development of this vessel have been described, but it is generally very small, and does little more than supply the nerve which it accompanies. Briedenbach has studied its potential for supporting the superficial peroneal nerve as a free vascularised nerve graft (Briedenbach & Terzis, 1983).

SUMMARY OF ANATOMICAL TERRITORIES OF CUTANEOUS SUPPLY

The definition of anatomical territories on the lower leg is a somewhat spurious exercise of limited value since there are such good anastomoses at the level of the deep fascia. The popliteal artery supplies an anatomical territory corresponding to the muscle bellies of gastrocnemius and is often extended downwards in a strip along the dorsal midline to the junction of middle and lower thirds of tibia by the artery accompanying the medial sural cutaneous nerve. The posterior tibial artery covers most of the remaining dorsomedial surface extending almost all the way round to the anterior subcutaneous border of the tibia. This territory is encroached upon superiorly to a variable extent by the saphenous branch of the descending genicular artery. From the anterior subcutaneous surface of the tibia, around the front of the leg to a vertical line about 1.5 cm posterior to the anterior peroneal septum, the skin is supplied by the anterior tibial artery. The peroneal artery covers the remaining posterolateral part of the leg.

As described in Chapter 5, the cutaneous vessels of the lower leg are orientated predominantly along the longitudinal axis of the limb. This applies particularly to the ramifications of the fasciocutaneous perforators, and the direct cutaneous arteries but the musculocutaneous perforators through gastrocnemius tend to fan out more evenly.

BLOOD SUPPLY TO MUSCLES IN THE LOWER LEG

This is summarised in Table 6.13.

Table 6.13 Summary of blood supply to muscles in the lower leg

Muscle	Vascularisation Type	Supplied by branches of
Tibialis anterior	III	Anterior tibial artery
Extensor hallucis	III	Anterior tibial and peroneal arteries
Extensor digitorum longus	III	Anterior tibial and peroneal arteries
Peroneus longus	II	1° Anterior tibial artery (proximally) 2° Anterior tibial or peroneal (distally)
Peroneus brevis	II	1° Anterior tibial or peroneal artery 2° Peroneal artery
Tibialis posterior	III	Posterior tibial and peroneal arteries
Flexor digitorum longus	III	Posterior tibial artery
Flexor hallucis longus	III	Peroneal artery
Gastrocnemius (each head)	I	Sural arteries
Soleus	IV	1° = Popliteal artery 1° = Peroneal artery (posterior tibial in 20%) 2° Lateral sural, peroneal, posterior tibial

FLAPS

Musculocutaneous pedicled flaps may be based on either the lateral or medial head of gastrocnemius and may be extended (if the deep fascia is included) to within 7 or 5 cm of the malleoli respectively. Several purely muscle flaps are possible but not within the scope of this book.

Fasciocutaneous flaps based on branches of the three major vessels may be of Types A, B or C with either a proximally or distally based orientation. In addition the Type C peroneal flaps may incorporate a segment of fibula (p. 389). The most commonly used flaps are:

anterior tibial	Type A proximally based	p. 284
anterior tibial	Type C distally based	p. 284
posterior tibial	Type A prox. or dist. based	p. 410
posterior tibial	Type B distally based	p. 412
peroneal A.	Type B distally based	p. 387
peroneal A.	Type C prox./dist./free	p. 389

Many of the above have also been used as adipofascial flaps without the skin. Neurovascular free flaps based on the medial sural cutaneous nerve are also a possibility (p. 440).

6 ANKLE AND FOOT

THE ANKLE

The region around the ankle joint is supplied by branches of the anterior tibial, peroneal and posterior tibial arteries. These branches anastomose freely and form networks around and below the malleoli (Figs 6.116–6.119).

The anterior tibial artery

This gives off anterior medial and lateral malleolar arteries about two fingers' breadths above the ankle as it passes beneath the tendon of extensor hallucis longus. In addition it gives off one or two small cutaneous twigs directly above the extensor retinaculum. In 24% the anterior malleolar arteries are of equal size, in 69% the lateral is larger, in 7% the medial is larger. Each of the malleolar arteries may be double (10–16%). The anterior lateral malleolar artery crosses the tibia deep to the extensor tendons and in front of the lateral malleolus divides into deep and superficial branches. The deep branches join the plexus on the periosteum and capsule of the ankle joint where they anastomose with branches from the lateral tarsal artery and the perforating branch of the peroneal. (The latter occasionally supplies skin.) The superficial branches pass above, below and sometimes through, the extensor retinaculum to reach the skin. They are very small and fine. The anterior medial malleolar branch runs over the medial malleolus and has deep and superficial branches in the same way as the lateral. In some cases the dorsalis pedis artery sends an ascending branch back to the skin over the ankle joint.

The posterior tibial artery

This contributes to the skin on the posterior and medial aspects of the ankle. The posterior medial malleolar artery sends branches to the malleolar network. Other branches run posteriorly to the skin over the tendo calcaneus and calcaneal branches run postero-inferiorly over the medial surface of the calcaneus. In the midline posteriorly these cutaneous vessels anastomose poorly with branches of the peroneal artery. There is, however, a large anastomosis between posterior tibial and peroneal arteries immediately anterior to the Achilles tendon.

The peroneal artery

This continues dorsally on the posterior surface of the lateral malleolus beneath the peroneal tendons. It sends branches forwards and ends as calcaneal branches directed postero-inferiorly to the skin over the lateral surface of the calcaneus. These are about 5 cm long and about four or five in number. The small saphenous vein overlies the lower part of this artery. The anterior perforating branch of the peroneal in 29% of cases gives origin to the anterior lateral malleolar artery and in some cases to a significantly sized branch to the skin which reaches the surface above the superior part of the extensor retinaculum (see also p. 393).

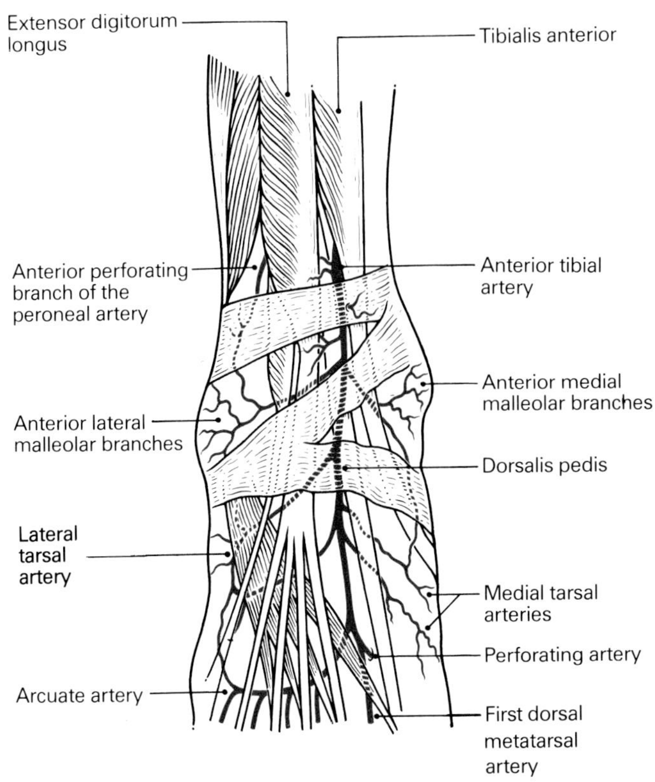

Fig. 6.116 Anterior aspect of the right ankle and tarsus showing the main vessels from which the principal cutaneous vessels arise.

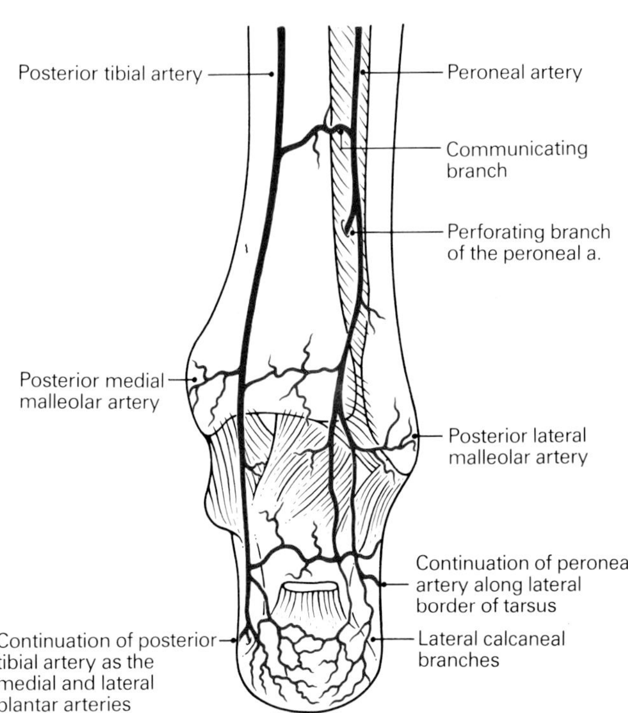

Fig. 6.118 Posterior aspect of right heel and ankle with all tendons removed to show the communications between the peroneal and posterior tibial arteries.

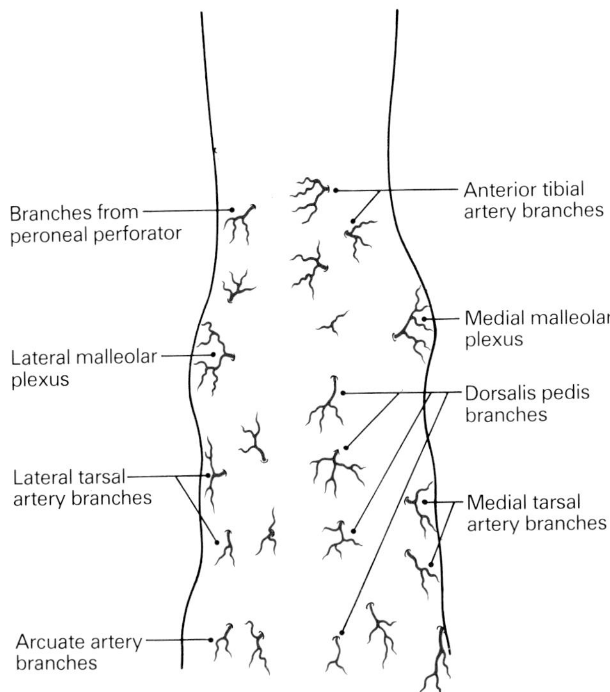

Fig. 6.117 Anterior aspect of the right ankle and tarsus showing the cutaneous branches which one might expect, in principle, to find supplying the skin. In practice multiple very small vessels tend to exist rather than the discrete vessels shown here.

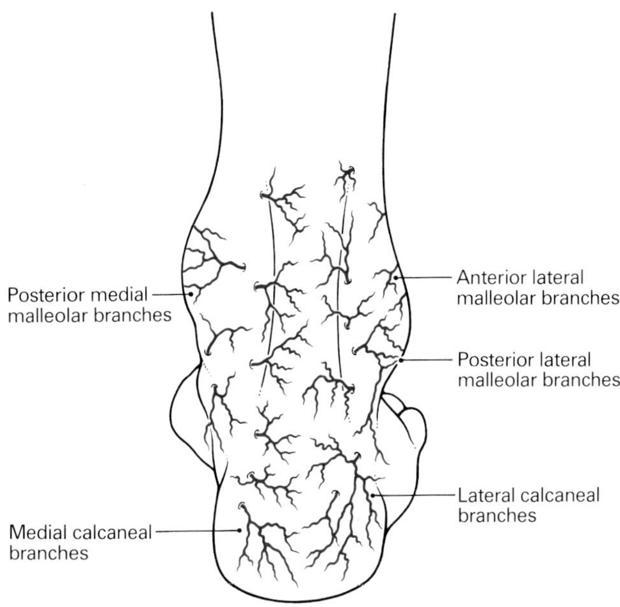

Fig. 6.119 Posterior aspect of right heel and ankle showing cutaneous branches. There is in effect a 'watershed' in the midline posteriorly.

6 THE FOOT

THE DORSUM OF THE FOOT – CLASSICAL DESCRIPTION

This is supplied by the dorsalis pedis artery with a variable contribution from the anterior perforating branch of the peroneal artery. The classical description is that the anterior tibial artery becomes the dorsalis pedis at the level of the ankle joint where it crosses laterally beneath the extensor hallucis longus tendon (for variations see below).

The dorsalis pedis artery

This runs directly along the dorsum of the tarsus to the proximal end of the first intermetatarsal space, where it turns into the sole between the two heads of the first dorsal interosseous muscle to complete the plantar arch (Fig. 6.120). Over the navicular bone it gives off the *lateral tarsal artery* which runs across the tarsus beneath extensor digitorum brevis. This artery is often double (A. tarsea lateralis proximalis et distalis) but the proximal branch is usually the larger. It anastomoses with the lateral malleolar artery above, and the arcuate artery below, and sends some fine twigs to the skin in the region of the cuboid and fifth metatarsal base. Several small *medial tarsal arteries* are given off by the dorsalis pedis. These anastomose on the medial cuneiform with branches of the medial plantar artery and supply bone, ligaments, part of the abductor hallucis and skin. Over the intermediate cuneiform the dorsalis pedis gives off the *arcuate artery* which arches laterally across the bases of the metatarsal bones and anastomoses with the lateral tarsal and lateral plantar arteries. The arcuate artery lies deep to the extensor tendons but gives off small branches between them to the overlying skin, and second, third and fourth dorsal metatarsal arteries which run distally on the corresponding dorsal interosseous muscles to the clefts between the toes where each divides into two dorsal digital branches. The fourth dorsal metatarsal artery gives off a branch to the lateral side of the fifth toe.

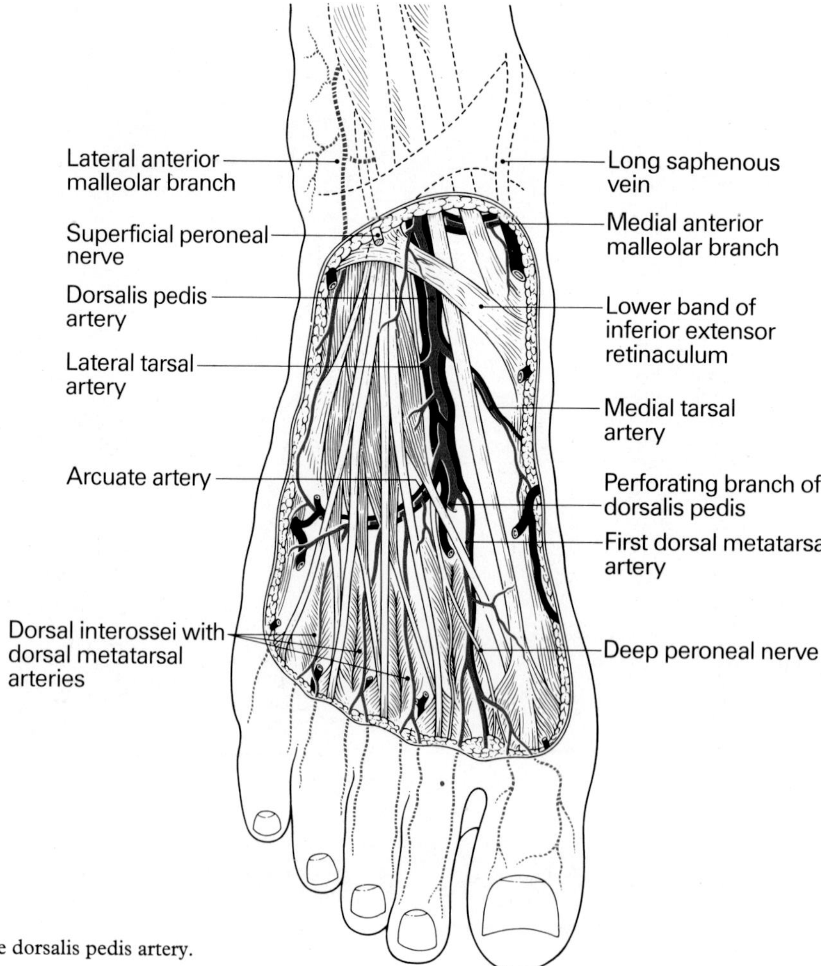

Fig. 6.120 Anatomy of the dorsalis pedis artery.

The dorsal metatarsal arteries

These communicate through the proximal and distal ends of the interosseous spaces with the plantar arch and the plantar metatarsal arteries respectively. The dorsalis pedis artery itself gives off a first dorsal metatarsal artery and then passes through the first interosseous space into the sole. The first dorsal metatarsal artery supplies, via dorsal digital branches, the adjoining surfaces of first and second toes and may also send a separate branch beneath the tendon of extensor hallucis to supply the medial side of the first toe. This may alternatively be supplied by a branch of the medial plantar.

Variations

Variations in this classical pattern are almost the norm, and affect the origin of the dorsalis pedis, its branches, the form of the dorsal arch and the dorsal metatarsal arteries.

Origin of dorsalis pedis. When the anterior tibial fails in the lower leg then the dorsalis pedis artery arises from the anterior perforating branch of the peroneal (37% of cases; Fig. 6.121b). In 1% the dorsalis pedis is formed by the union of two equal roots from the peroneal and the anterior tibial arteries. Rarely the dorsalis pedis may be totally absent or fail to go beyond the navicular (Fig. 6.121c). In the elderly, absence of a dorsalis pedis pulse is common and is due to occlusion of the dorsalis pedis by atherosclerosis or due to more proximal occlusion. Sometimes this results in the dorsalis pedis being fed entirely from the sole through its perforating branch in the first interosseous space.

Branches of the dorsalis pedis. The lateral tarsal artery is usually smaller than the dorsalis pedis (87%), but may be larger than it (5%) or the same size (8%). Clearly when it is larger than the dorsalis pedis it may become the dominant artery to the dorsal arch and feed the dorsal metatarsal arteries from the lateral side (Fig. 6.121d). The medial tarsal arteries do not vary much.

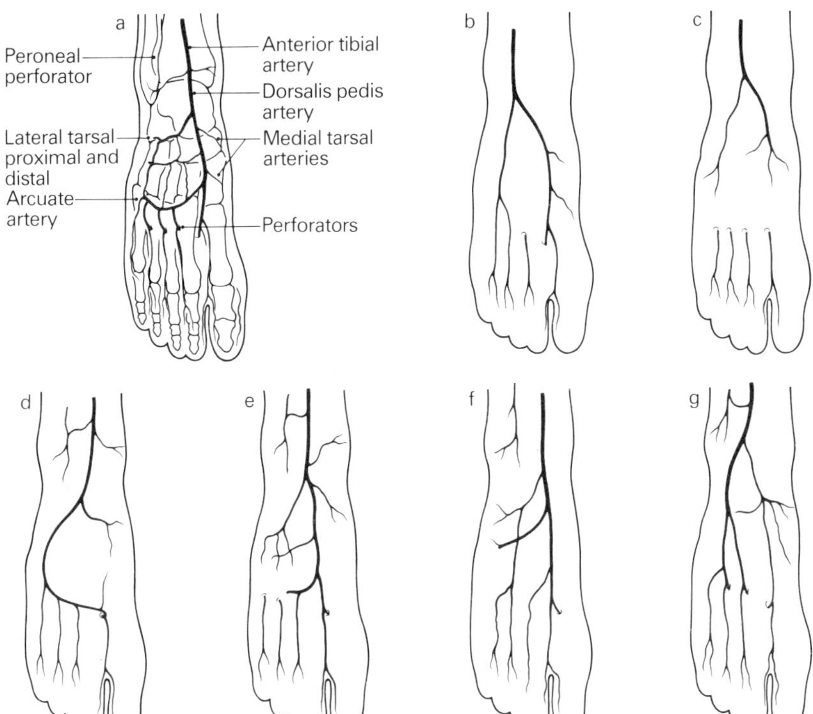

Fig. 6.121 Variations in the dorsal arterial arcades:
a. The 'classical' form,
b. The perforating branch of the peroneal artery takes over the blood supply to the entire dorsum of the foot,
c. The perforating branch of the peroneal artery takes over the supply to the tarsal region while the forefoot is supplied by perforating branches from the plantar metatarsal arteries,
d. The arcuate artery fills from the lateral side via the lateral tarsal artery beyond which the dorsalis pedis is obliterated,
e–g. Various arrangements of the arteries arising from altered patterns of regression and development of the dorsal network.

The dorsal network. A dorsal arch formed by the arcuate artery is far less common than is indicated in classical texts. The arcuate artery is very variable and may be indistinguishable from a strongly developed distal lateral tarsal artery (Fig. 6.121f). Rather than dividing equally between second, third and fourth dorsal metatarsal arteries, the arcuate artery often only supplies the second or the second and third metatarsal arteries (Fig. 6.121e). The other metatarsal arteries are then supplied from the plantar arch via the perforating branches, or from the lateral tarsal arteries, or from both. The various forms may be explained on the basis of a dorsal network (Fig. 6.122), in which only the dorsalis pedis and the proximal tarsal artery are in any way constant while all the other parts may undergo variable interrelated regression or development. If, for example, the second to fourth metatarsal arteries arise from the arcuate then the sagittal communications and the distal lateral tarsal artery regress. When the metatarsal arteries arise from the lateral tarsal then the sagittal communications are well developed (Fig. 6.121g).

Dorsal metatarsal arteries. It appears that in Europeans the second and fourth dorsal metatarsal arteries tend to be fed more from the network on the dorsum of the foot than from the plantar. The first dorsal metatarsal artery has a plantar origin (rather than dorsalis pedis origin) in 9–22% of cases depending on the study (Fig. 6.121c, d). The dorsal metatarsal artery to the lateral side of foot generally arises from the dorsal network but may come from the lateral plantar artery.

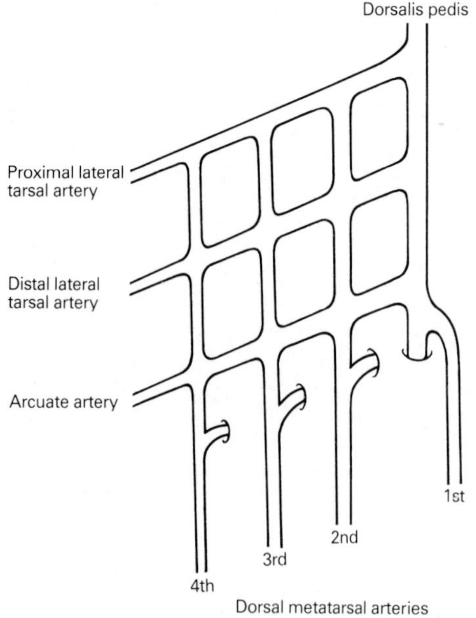

Fig. 6.122 Basic form of the dorsal network.

Cutaneous supply on dorsum of foot

The cutaneous vessels are sparse, short and fine, with a general absence of long or large arteries. The dorsalis pedis gives off a number of small direct branches to the skin between the extensor retinaculum and the first interosseous space. Including the area up to the first web supplied by twigs from the first dorsal metatarsal artery, this area measures only 2–3 cm in width and 7–10 cm in length. Medial to this, over the medial arch but above abductor hallucis, the skin is supplied in turn from the medial malleolar plexus, the cutaneous twigs of the medial tarsal arteries, and the branches to the medial side of the great toe from the medial plantar artery or the first dorsal metatarsal artery. Lateral to the dorsalis pedis territory there are only a few branches arising from the malleolar plexus, the lateral tarsal arteries and the arcuate artery. On the lateral border of the foot there may be cutaneous twigs from an occasional branch of the peroneal (posterior) running forwards beneath the lateral malleolus onto the tarsus where it communicates with the anterior perforating branch of the peroneal and the lateral tarsal artery.

Flaps

The dorsalis pedis artery is the basis for a well-established free flap from the dorsum of the foot. This should be considered only if it is certain that the posterior tibial artery is the dominant source of blood supply to the foot. The largest flap that has been elevated without a delay measured about 9 cm × 8 cm or 10 cm × 12 cm with a delay but such flaps carry a high risk of necrosis in the distal part. This distal segment corresponding to the 3 cm or so lying proximal to the first interdigital cleft is not supplied directly by the dorsalis pedis and constitutes a 'random' area. Delay of the flap, and this portion in particular, in one or more stages improves the chances of survival for the distal part and enable flaps of up to 10 cm × 12 cm to survive on the dorsalis pedis alone. (The medial and lateral tarsal, the arcuate, and the perforating branch are divided: see p. 320 for details.)

Neurovascular free flaps from the first web space may be used. These incorporate the adjacent sides of the first and second toes, the first dorsal metatarsal artery and the deep peroneal nerve.

The second metatarsal and its toe may be used as a free myo-osteo-cutaneous flap.

In certain circumstances, flaps may be created by filleting the toes and turning the flaps back for either plantar or dorsal coverage of small defects. The flaps are supplied by the plantar digital vessels. These are not described further.

Blood supply of muscles on dorsum of foot

Extensor hallucis brevis and extensor digitorum are supplied by several branches of the lateral tarsal artery which enter their deep surfaces. Branches of the arcuate and dorsal metatarsal arteries supply the dorsal interossei.

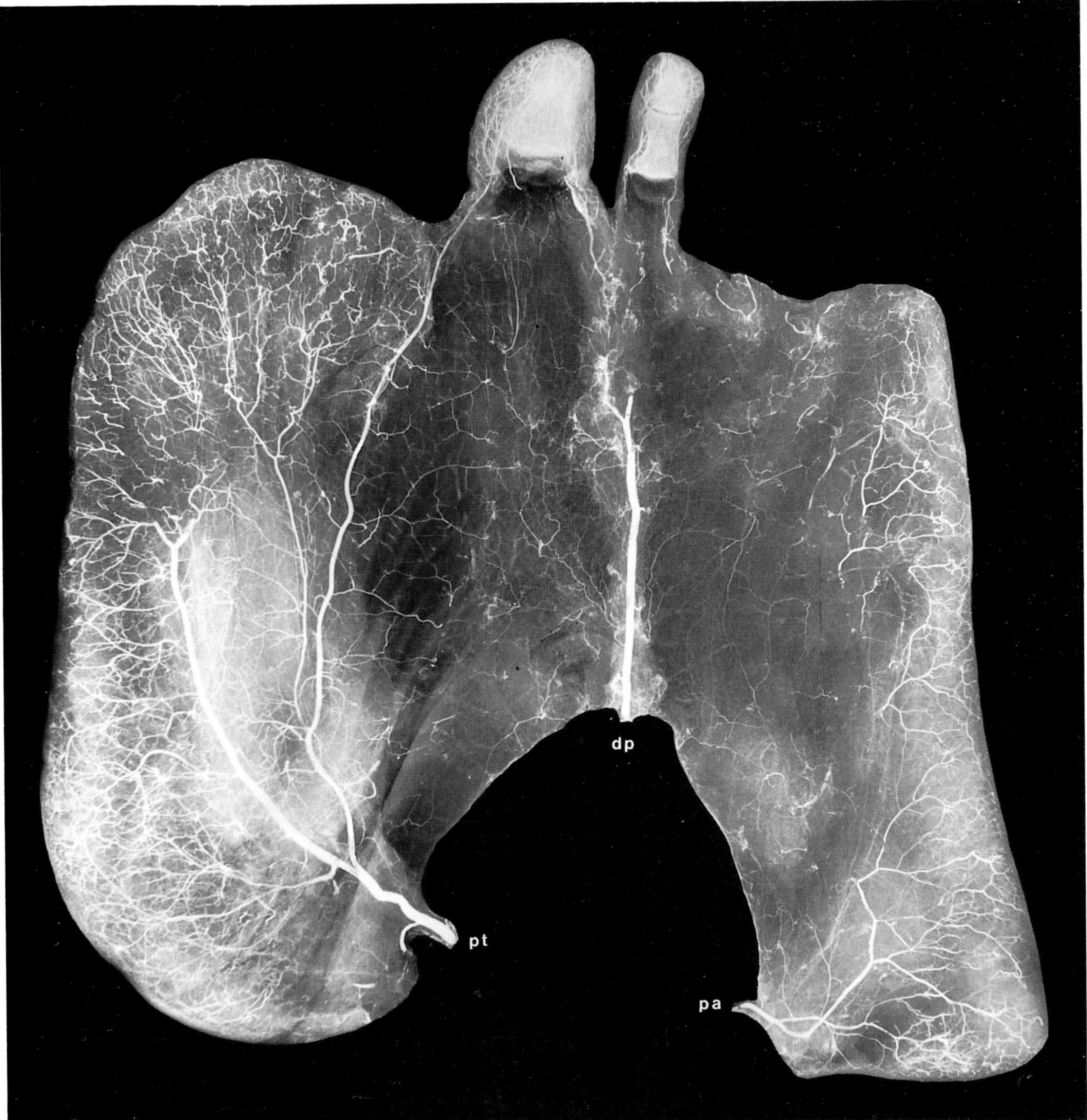

Fig. 6.123 Radiograph of skin of the foot. The specimen was prepared for radiography by an incision which passed down the midline of the heel posteriorly till it reached the weight-bearing surface. Here the incision passed laterally skirting the weight-bearing area and ran along the lateral border of the foot. The incision then passed across the foot distal to the metatarsal heads and ended on the medial side of the metatarsophalangeal joint of the hallux. The hallux and adjacent toe were retained in continuity with the specimen by their dorsal skin attachment only; the other toes were removed. The sole skin was removed in continuity with the plantar aponeurosis and most of flexor digitorum brevis in order to preserve the lateral plantar artery; **pt.** posterior tibial artery, **dp.** dorsalis pedis artery, **pa.** peroneal artery.

THE SOLE OF THE FOOT – CLASSICAL DESCRIPTION

The sole of the foot, together with most of the medial arch, is supplied by the posterior tibial artery. This enters the foot in the company of two veins and the tibial nerve, by passing deep to the flexor retinaculum midway between the medial malleolus and the medial tubercle of calcaneus. It gives off calcaneal branches which pierce the flexor retinaculum to supply fat and skin behind the tendo calcaneus and about the heel. The calcaneal branches also contribute to the supply of abductor hallucis and anastomose with medial malleolar branches. The posterior tibial then divides deep to abductor hallucis into the medial and lateral plantar arteries.

The medial plantar artery

This is the smaller terminal division. It runs forward on the lateral side of the medial plantar nerve between abductor hallucis and flexor digitorum brevis. According to *Nomina Anatomica* it divides into a superficial and a deep branch. However, the deep branch is so inconstant in our cadaver studies and so variously represented in the textbooks that it is better to regard it as a variable sidebranch and think of the superficial ramus as the main stem of the medial plantar artery. This supplies the adjacent flexor and abductor, and gives off cutaneous branches which pass round the sides of abductor hallucis to reach the skin where they augment two or three musculocutaneous perforators leaving the surface of the muscle (Fig. 6.124). It now continues, much reduced in size, along the inferomedial aspect of the first metatarsal, gives off communicating branches to the medial three plantar metatarsal arteries (these arteries are also known as the common plantar digital arteries), and may then end on the medial side of the big toe.

The lateral plantar artery

This lies lateral to the lateral plantar nerve, which it accompanies across the foot towards the base of the fifth metatarsal in the plane between flexor digitorum brevis and flexor accessorius. At the fifth metatarsal it turns medially with the deep branch of the nerve and curves deep in the sole to join the dorsalis pedis artery at the first intermetatarsal space, so forming the plantar arch. The lateral plantar artery gives origin to muscular twigs to abductor digiti minimi and cutaneous twigs which pass round the muscle to reach the skin. Before passing deeply it gives off a plantar digital artery to the lateral side of the little toe.

The plantar arch

This lies on the undersurface of the metatarsals and sends four plantar metatarsal arteries forwards on the interossei, the first perhaps arising from the dorsalis pedis artery. These divide into plantar digital arteries to the adjacent sides of the toes, the first giving a plantar digital artery to the medial side of the big toe. Three perforating arteries link the arch to the dorsal metatarsal arteries through the proximal parts of the intermetatarsal spaces; another four link the plantar and dorsal arteries near their bifurcations. The medial three metatarsal arteries receive communications from the medial plantar artery.

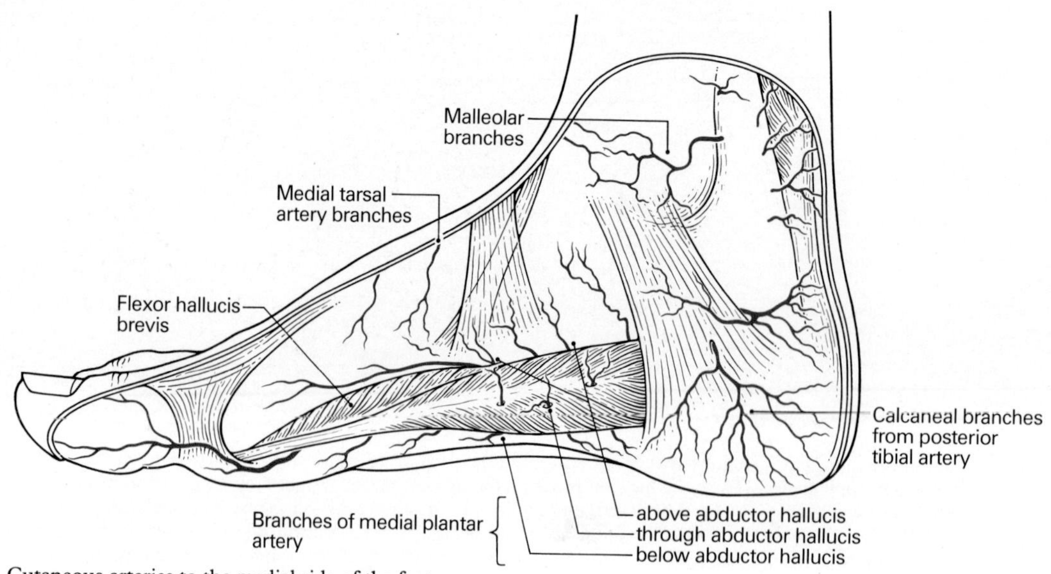

Fig. 6.124 Cutaneous arteries to the medial side of the foot.

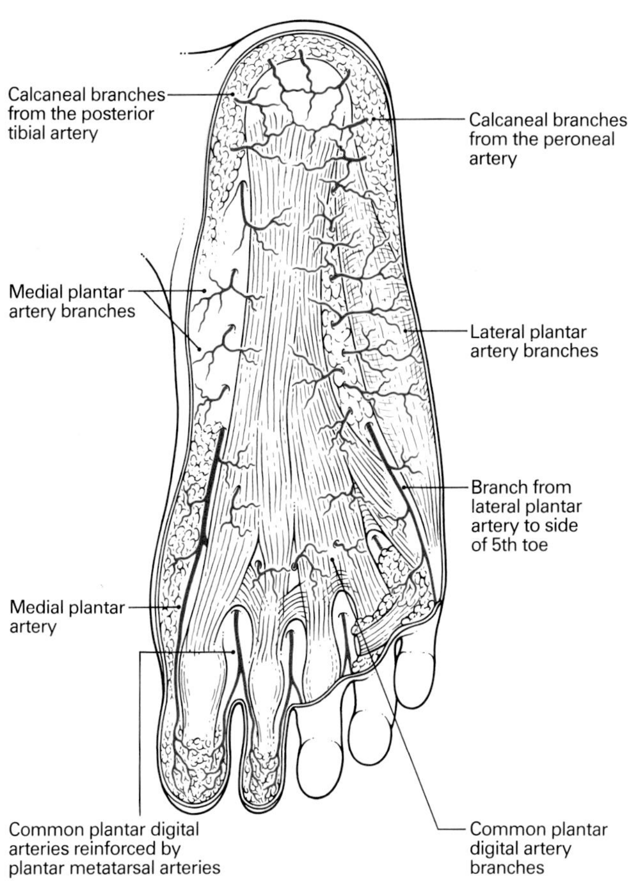

Fig. 6.125 Cutaneous arteries to the sole of the foot. The superficial transverse metatarsal ligament has been divided.

Variations

These concern the relationships of arteries to the tibial and plantar nerves, the relative sizes of medial and lateral plantar arteries, the size of the superficial 'arch', the deep arch and the origins of the plantar metatarsal arteries.

1. The posterior tibial artery usually lies behind the medial malleolus anteromedial to the tibial nerve (87%) but may lie posterolateral to it (13%).

2. The lateral plantar artery is always lateral to the nerve, but the medial plantar artery may lie lateral (83%), medial (9%) or when double, on either side of its nerve (8%) (Fig. 6.126a, b, c).

3. The lateral plantar is generally the larger vessel (80%), but may be smaller (3%) or the same size as the medial (17%).

4. A superficial network lying between the plantar fascia and flexor digitorum brevis is an inconstant finding (probably atavistic). It may contain the following elements: a superficial arch, common plantar digital arteries I to IV, superficial branches to lateral side of fifth toe and is present in approximately 30% of cases but in most of these it is very weak (Fig. 6.126d). The medial plantar artery may supply only the medial side of the great toe and the first cleft (Fig. 6.126e). A well-developed superficial arch may contribute little to the skin of the toes (Fig. 6.126f) or it may give off strong common plantar digital arteries which completely replace the metatarsal arteries as the principal supply to the toes (Fig. 6.126g).

5. The plantar metatarsal arteries I to IV arise from the deep arch. This is formed mainly by the deep perforating branch of the dorsalis pedis (53%) or mainly by the lateral plantar artery (27%) or by both equally.

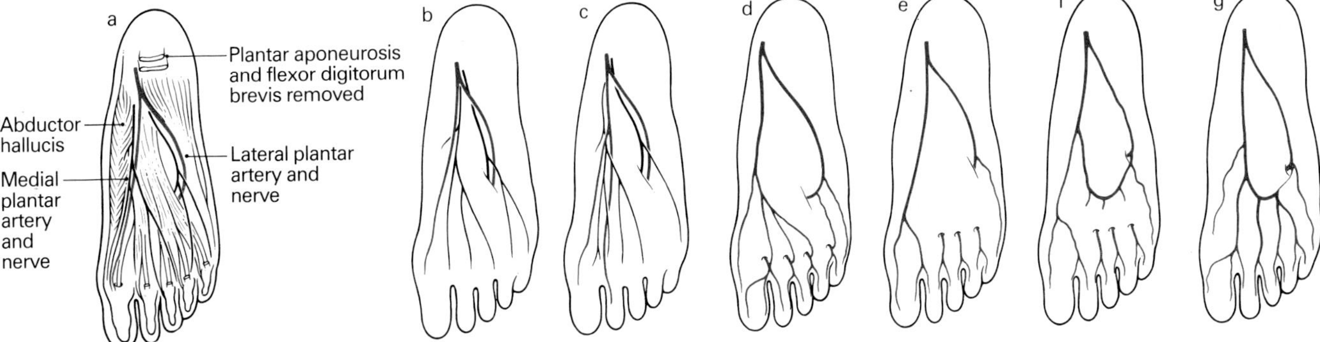

Fig. 6.126 Variations in the plantar arteries:

a. Normal situation, arteries lie lateral to nerves,
b. The medial plantar artery may lie medial to the medial plantar nerve,
c. The medial plantar artery may be double and lie on either side of the medial plantar nerve,
d. There is no superficial plantar arch but the medial plantar artery supplies the toes via common plantar digital arteries which communicate with plantar metatarsal arteries. The arrangement in Fig. 6.123 is probably of this type,
e. No superficial arch; blood supply to toes from plantar metatarsal arteries,
f. Superficial arch present but does not supply toes,
g. Superficial arch forms the principal supply to the sole of the forefoot.

Cutaneous supply of the sole of the foot

The skin is well supplied by numerous small twigs arising out of the vessels described above. These form a dense vascular network in the subcutaneous tissues which can only be visualised by radiography because the tough nature of the fibrous network beneath the skin makes it impossible to dissect out these vessels. Beneath the heel the cutaneous twigs are part of the calcaneal branches of the peroneal and posterior tibial arteries. Further forward the sole is supplied by cutaneous twigs which arise from the plantar arteries and tend to be arranged in two longitudinal rows overlying the edges of flexor digitorum brevis. The medial plantar artery sends a row of small vessels to the skin along the lower margin of the abductor hallucis. Some musculocutaneous vessels also pierce the central two-thirds of the muscle (calcaneal branches of the posterior tibial supply its origin). The skin of the medial arch over the upper border of abductor hallucis also receives several branches from the medial plantar artery (Fig. 6.124). Anteriorly, approaching the ball of the great toe, the superficial branch to the medial side of the hallux lies deeply in the fat and sends several small branches to the skin. Actually in the toe, this vessel lies more superficially. Over the metatarsal heads of the other toes there are cutaneous branches of the common plantar digital arteries, whereas on the toes the digital arteries (generally from the plantar metatarsal arteries) supply the skin. On the lateral side of the sole the vascular plexus is denser, reflecting the greater weight bearing of this side. The lateral plantar artery gives about a dozen branches to the skin which diverge laterally and, for a shorter distance, medially. The posterior branches are longer than the anterior ones and run laterally towards the side of the foot. Over the fifth metatarsal head the superficial branch to the lateral side of the fifth toe appears deep in the fat, gives off branches to the skin, and runs distally coming to lie progressively nearer the surface.

Summary of anatomical territories of cutaneous supply

In general, anastomoses between vessels on the medial side and ones on the lateral side are not well developed except in the region of the heel. This enables medial and lateral anatomical territories to be delineated by an oblique line joining the lateral tubercle of the calcaneus to the second toe. On the lateral side the branches of the lateral plantar anastomose with the vessels on the dorsum of the foot but the edge of the lateral plantar anatomical territory corresponds to the most lateral part of the foot. The medial plantar includes in its territory the medial arch but not the medial part of the heel which is supplied by the posterior tibial artery via its calcaneal branches, and not the plantar surface of the great toe which is usually supplied from the perforating branch of dorsalis pedis via the first plantar metatarsal artery.

Summary of blood supply to muscles in sole

Traditionally, anatomists have described the sole of the foot as being made up of four layers. However, the only muscles of any potential relevance to the blood supply of the skin are abductor hallucis, and abductor digiti minimi in the first layer. Abductor hallucis, arising by a tendon from the medial tubercle of the calcaneus and directly from the flexor retinaculum and the plantar aponeurosis, forms the most superficial muscle along the medial side of the sole. Its vascularisation conforms to the Type II pattern. At its origin it is supplied by small twigs from the calcaneal branches of the posterior tibial and possibly from the lateral plantar, but its main supply is by a branch to the belly of the muscle from the medial plantar artery. Two or three perforators leave the surface of the muscle to supply overlying skin. Abductor digiti minimi arises from both tubercles of the calcaneus and the adjacent plantar aponeurosis, and runs along the lateral border of the sole. It may contribute minimally to the blood supply of the overlying skin but the dominant vessels over the belly of the muscle are the lateral calcaneal branches of the peroneal artery.

Flaps

The anatomy of the sole skin is uniquely adapted for weight bearing. Not only has it a special vascularity but the fibrous septation prevents displacement of subcutaneous fat and confers good sheer resistance. For reconstruction of defects on the sole it is therefore desirable to use similar tissue if at all possible, as this will improve the chances of the graft remaining functional in the long term. The flaps that have been developed on the sole of the foot to meet these aims are of basically 4 types:

Local random transposition flaps
Local transposition flaps are based on a random blood supply, may require a delay and can be used only for closing small defects, largely because the fibrous interconnections between dermis and deeper structures severely limit the mobility and flexibility of the tissues. For this reason also, bilobed flaps have a place in the

sole. Sensation is important on the sole and with time is only poorly recovered in transposition flaps.

Medial plantar flaps from the medial arch

Neurovascular medial plantar flaps from the non-weight-bearing arch region may be either fasciocutaneous or musculocutaneous (when the abductor hallucis brevis is included). The flap may be pedicled, island, or free and is described in detail on page 374.

Lateral calcaneal artery flaps

Lateral calcaneal artery flaps may be pedicled or island flaps; both are supplied by the calcaneal branches of the peroneal artery (p. 395). These may be useful for reconstructing defects over the lower part of the Achilles tendon. The lateral calcaneal flap may also be based distally on the connections that the terminal vessels make deep to the peroneal tendons with lateral tarsal artery branches. This enables a flap to be turned onto the lateral border of the sole posterior to the fifth metatarsal base (p. 397).

Neurovascular toe fillet flaps

Filleted toe flaps are difficult to dissect as neurovascular island flaps based on the lateral plantar artery and the area of skin which they provide is small.

6 EXTERNAL GENITALIA AND PERINEUM

Nomina Anatomica

ARTERIA ILIACA INTERNA
Arteria obturatoria
Ramus pubicus

Arteria pudenda interna
A. rectalis inferior
A. perinealis
Rami scrotales posteriores
Rami labiales posteriores
A. urethralis
A. bulbi penis
A. bulbi vestibuli (vaginae)
A. profunda penis
A. dorsalis penis
A profunda clitoridis
A. dorsalis clitoridis

ARTERIA FEMORALIS
Arteriae pudendae externae
Rami scrotales anteriores
Rami labiales anteriores
Rami inguinales

ARTERIA ILIACA EXTERNA
Arteria epigastrica inferior
Ramus pubicus
Ramus obturatorius
(A. obturatoria accessoria)
A. cremasterica
A. ligamenti teretis uteri

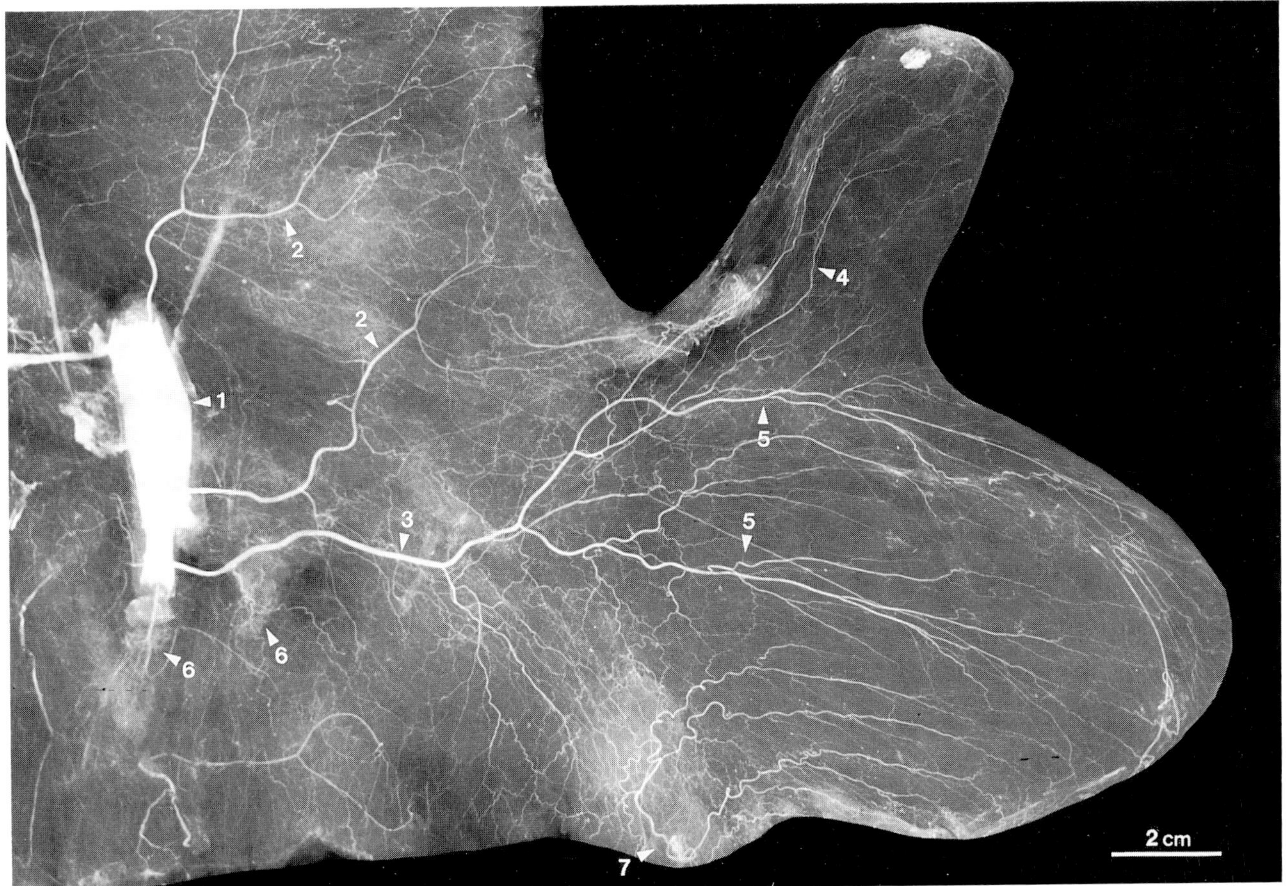

Fig. 6.127 Radiograph of injected skin from groin, suprapubic area, shaft of penis, scrotum, and half of perineum. A segment of the femoral artery has been removed between the inguinal ligament and the point of origin of the profunda femoris artery. Continuity of the cutaneous vessels with the femoral artery has been retained, in the case of the deep external pudendal artery by dividing the long saphenous vein. Veins have not been opacified in this preparation.

1. Femoral artery,
2. Superficial external pudendal arteries (double in this case). The lower of the two sends some small branches onto the shaft of the penis,
3. Deep external pudendal artery. This divides into (4) and (5),
4. Branches to the skin of the penile shaft,
5. Anterior scrotal branches,
6. Branches to lymph nodes,
7. Posterior scrotal branches from the perineal artery.

6

EXTERNAL GENITALIA AND PERINEUM

This region is supplied by branches of the superficial and deep external pudendal arteries and by branches of the internal pudendal artery.

External pudendal arteries

The classic description is that there are two of these arising from the femoral artery. The uppermost passes in front of the femoral vein and is either known as the superior or superficial external pudendal. The lower passes in front of the femoral vein but behind the long saphenous vein and is known as the inferior or deep external pudendal artery. These vessels pass laterally and pierce the deep fascia at the medial and lateral borders of the saphenous opening (located about 1 cm medial and 5 cm distal to the point of emergence of the femoral artery below the inguinal ligament) where they are frequently encountered during a Trendelenburg ligation. Both vessels give off small branches to the inguinal lymph nodes and to the skin over the upper medial part of the femoral triangle. The superior vessel gives off a branch to the skin over the superficial inguinal ring and itself crosses the spermatic cord to supply an area of prepubic and suprapubic skin adjacent to the midline. In the male it sends short branches onto the dorsolateral aspect of the penis (clitoris in the female). The inferior vessel runs horizontally across the upper femoral triangle sending branches to the skin over adductor longus. It gives off two anterior scrotal or labial branches, and in the male ends on the ventrolateral aspect of the penis along which it runs towards the coronal sulcus.

The blood supply of the skin of the shaft of the penis is poorly described in anatomical textbooks. Several claim that the dorsal arteries of the penis vascularise the skin when in fact their main supply is to the glans. The blood supply of the superficial fascia and skin of the shaft of the penis up to the corona, comes from the superficial and deep external pudendal arteries. The deep (inferior) is regularly predominant with the superficial (superior) artery only contributing small short branches to the skin over the base on its dorsal aspect.

The deep external pudendal arteries of the two sides contribute in a variable manner. Three patterns may be

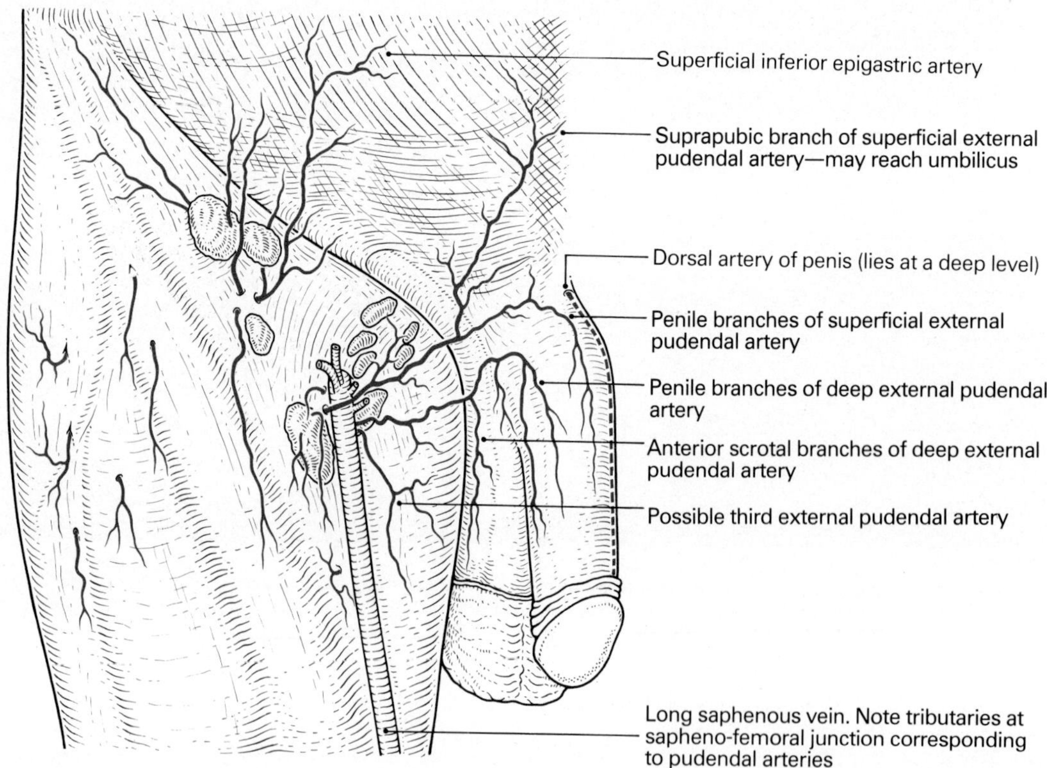

Fig. 6.128 Arrangement of external pudendal arteries. Deep fascia has been left intact. On the shaft of the penis the skin has been removed up to the coronal sulcus.

distinguished which are all equally common (Juskiewenski et al, 1982). In the first type the two arteries participate equally in giving off long branches which run down each side of the shaft from base to coronal sulcus (Fig. 6.129c). In general two branches may be distinguished on each side, a dorso-lateral and a ventro-lateral. In the second type one artery may entirely take over the supply to the shaft skin by giving off a collateral which crosses the midline on the dorsal surface and is distributed to the other side (Fig. 6.129b). In a third type there may be an unequal sharing with the predominating artery giving off a collateral to reinforce the opposite side (Fig. 6.129a).

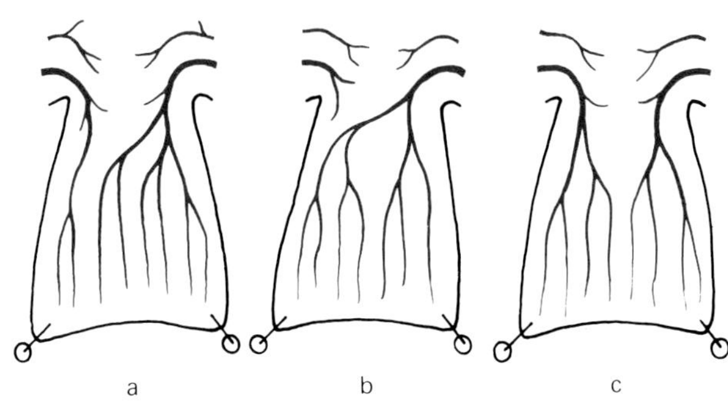

Fig. 6.129 Blood supply to the skin and superficial fascia over the shaft of the penis. The skin has been pinned out flat after longitudinal ventral incision along the raphe. Three types of blood supply may be distinguished which are all equally common: **a.** an asymmetrical distribution of vessels with a strong predominance of one pedicle; **b.** a blood supply entirely dependent on a single deep external pudendal artery; **c.** an approximately equal sharing of the blood supply between the two deep external pudendal arteries. (After Juskiewenski et al, 1982.)

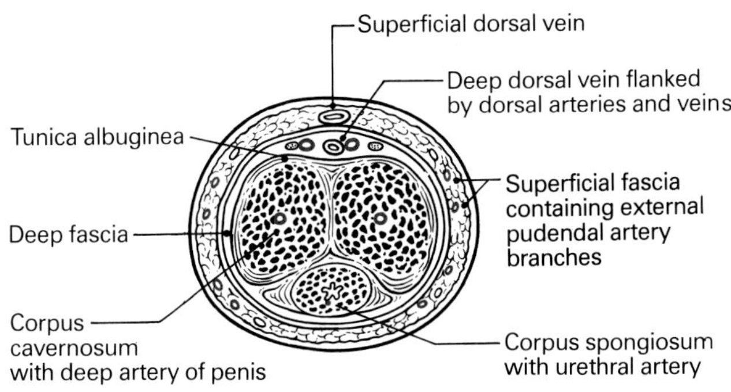

Fig. 6.130 Transverse section through the shaft of the penis showing the superficial and deep arteries. The deep arterial system exists on three planes, superior, middle and inferior. The vessels of the superior system are the dorsal arteries which provide the sole blood supply to the glans. The vessels of the middle plane are the deep arteries of the corpora cavernosa. The vessel of the inferior plane is the urethral artery which is inconstant. The blood supplies to these three planes are complementary – when the arteries in the middle or inferior levels are weak and expire distally then the arterial network lying immediately above it takes over.

Distally fine branches of the deep external pudendal arteries reach the coronal sulcus where they anastomose with branches of the deep arteries (vide infra). The prepuce also derives a blood supply from the deep vessels through small perforators from the corpora cavernosa and corpus spongiosum which are particularly abundant just proximal to the coronal margin on the dorsum of the shaft. This is virtually the only point of anastomosis between the vessels of the skin and those of the deeper structures. Occasionally very fine anastomoses with branches of the dorsal arteries do occur but they are very rare. The artery to the frenulum arises from the dorsal arteries which by this point have come to lie in a ventro-lateral position.

The skin and superficial fascia drain by a network of veins of which the dorsal veins are the most obvious. The deep dorsal veins drain the glans although they may also receive a few veins across the tunica albuginea from the corpora cavernosa (Wagner et al, 1982).

Internal pudendal artery

This arises from the internal iliac artery in a variable manner (p. 223), turns round the back of the ischial spine, and passes along the ischial ramus on the lateral sidewall of the ischiorectal fossa. It gives off *inferior rectal branches* above the ischial tuberosity which cross the ischiorectal fossa to supply anal sphincter musculature and the skin around the anus (Fig. 6.131). A few small branches pass round the lower edge of gluteus maximus to reach the skin of the buttock. At the posterior border of the urogenital diaphragm, the pudendal artery gives origin to the transverse perineal artery and to *posterior scrotal branches*. These often arise in common and both supply skin with the scrotal arteries accompanying, and being distributed with, the posterior scrotal nerves in the cutaneous territory suggested by their name. The pudendal artery continues into the deep perineal pouch below and finally medial to the dorsal nerve, sending the artery of the bulb of the penis and the urethral artery through the perineal membrane to the corpus spongiosum. As it pierces the perineal membrane with the nerve it divides into the deep artery of the penis, which enters and runs forward in the corpus cavernosum, and the smaller *dorsal artery of the penis*, which traverses the layers of the suspensory ligament and descends on the dorsum of the penis medial to the nerve, to supply the deep fascia and the glans.

In the female, the internal pudendal artery is the major source of blood supply to the labia majora and the posterior parts of the labia minora.

Variations

In some studies an inconstant *third external pudendal artery* has been identified which crosses *deep* to the femoral vein. This may replace the inferior external pudendal or be in addition to it. It supplies skin over adductor longus (Chen Er-yu et al, 1982).

The dorsal artery and/or the deep artery of the corpus cavernosum may arise from a vessel termed the *accessory pudendal* which runs entirely within the pelvis. The accessory pudendal takes origin most frequently from the obturator artery but also from the internal iliac or the internal pudendal and runs across the obturator internus muscle to become the dorsal artery of the penis on one side (less commonly the deep artery of the corpus cavernosum). Many examples were recorded by 19th century anatomists with a reported prevalence of 10%.

SUMMARY OF CUTANEOUS BLOOD SUPPLY

The skin of the perianal area, perineum and posterior scrotum is supplied by the internal pudendal; the anterior scrotal skin by the deep external pudendal perhaps aided by cremasteric branches of the inferior epigastric artery; the skin of the shaft of the penis mainly by the deep external pudendal arteries and the glans by the internal pudendal. The veins follow the corresponding arteries.

FLAPS

Flaps have been based on the external pudendal arteries. For the superior external pudendal the axial line suggested runs along a line connecting a point 50 mm distal to the origin of the femoral artery with a point

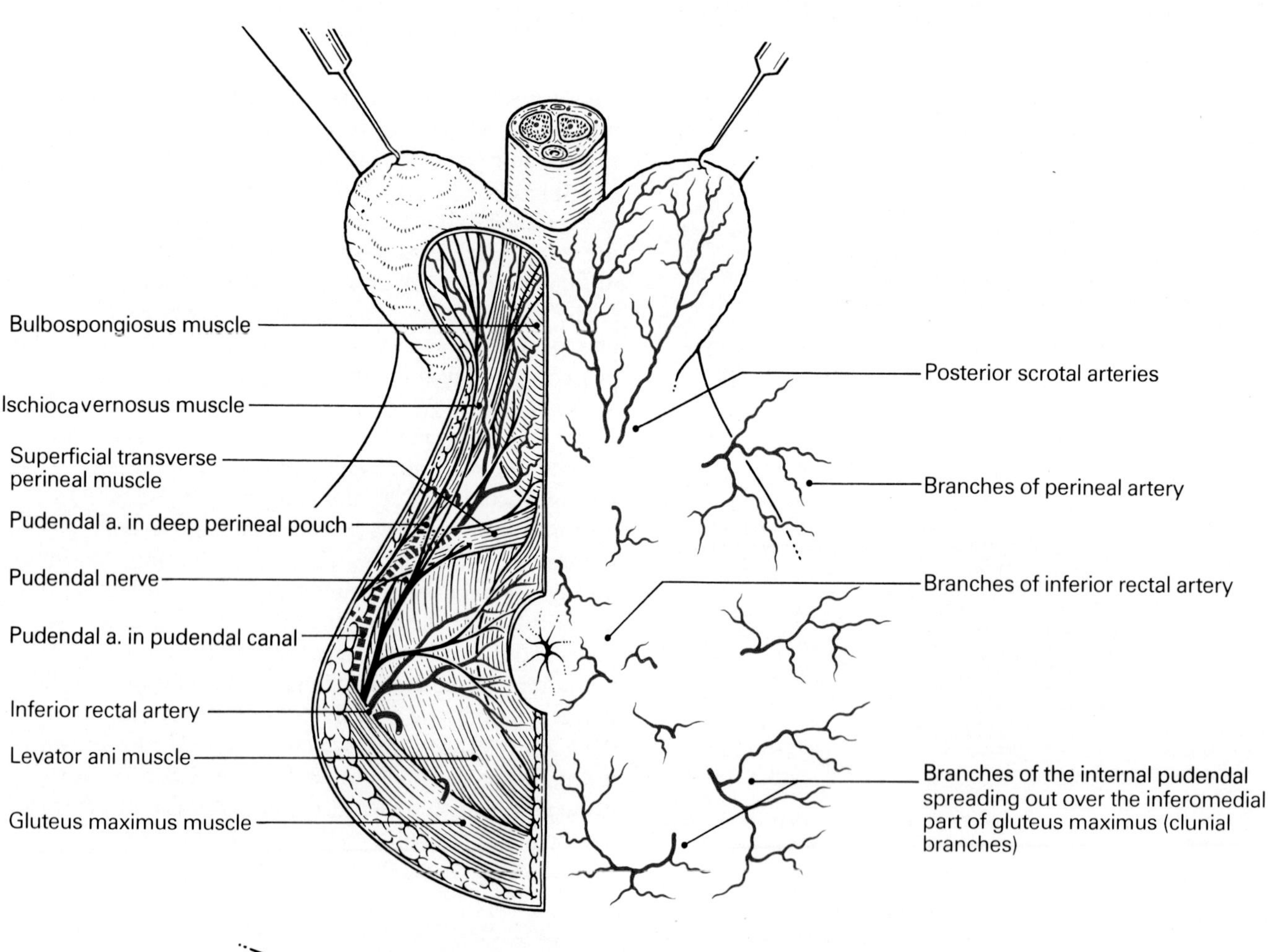

Fig. 6.131 Internal pudendal artery branches to the skin of the perineum and posterior scrotum.

over the pubic tubercle. This may be extended up towards the umbilicus as a unilateral paramedian flap or may be raised as a bilateral flap to a width of about 8 cm (p. 434). For the inferior external pudendal artery flap the axial line runs horizontally, parallel with the pubic crest, from a point 50 mm distal to the origin of the femoral artery. Penile/preputial cutaneous island flaps pedicled on external pudendal vessels have been designed to enable one-stage hypospadias repair or one-stage urethroplasty for strictures anywhere from prostatic urethra to meatus (p. 436).

References

Adachi B 1928 Das Arteriensystem der Japaner. Maruzen, Kyoto

Allen E V 1929 Thromboangiitis obliterans: methods of diagnosis of chronic occlusive arterial lesions distal to the wrist with illustrative cases. American Journal of Medical Sciences 178: 237–244

Allieu Y, Gomis R, Bonnel F, Escare Ph, Hochimora M 1980 The free composed cutaneo-osseous iliac flap (FCCOIF) Anatomia Clinica 2: 83–88

Anson B J, Wright R R, Wolfer J A 1939 Blood supply of the mammary gland. Surgery, Gynaecology and Obstetrics 69: 468–473

Armenta E, Fisher J 1981 Vascular pedicle of the tensor fascia lata myocutaneous flap. Annals of Plastic Surgery 6: 112–119

Badran H A, El-Helaly M S, Safe I 1984 The lateral intercostal neurovascular free flap. Plastic and Reconstructive Surgery 73: 17–25

Bardeen C R 1901 A statistical study of the abdominal and border nerves in man. American Journal of Anatomy 1: 203–228

Barreiro F J J, Valdecasas J G H 1976 Nouvelle conception de la vascularisation artérielle de la main – études anatomique et radiographique. Société Anatomie, Paris

Bean R B 1905 A composite study of the subclavian artery in man. American Journal of Anatomy 4: 303–328

Boyd J B, Taylor G I, Corlett R 1984 The vascular territories of the superior epigastric and the deep inferior epigastric systems. Plastic and Reconstructive Surgery 73: 1–14

Breidenbach W C, Terzis J K 1983 Vascularised nerve grafts. Plastic Surgical Forum 6: 131–133

Brockenbrough E C 1964 Screening for the prevention of stroke. Parks Electronics, Seattle

Budo J, Finucan T, Clarke J 1984 The inner arm fasciocutaneous flap. Plastic and Reconstructive Surgery 73: 629–632

Cabanié H, Garbé J-F, Guimberteau J-C 1980 Anatomical basis of the thoracodorsal axillary flap with respect to its transfer by means of microvascular surgery. Anatomia Clinica 2: 65–73

Carr B W, Bishop W E, Anson B J 1942 Mammary arteries. Quarterly Bulletin of Northwestern University Medical School 16: 150–154

Chen Er-yu et al 1982 Vessels of skin flaps from the groin region: III Macro-microanatomy of the superficial external pudendal vessels. Acta Anatomia Sinica 13: 225

Coleman S S, Anson B J 1961 Arterial patterns in the hand. Surgery, Gynaecology and Obstetrics 113: 409–424

Corso P F 1961 Variations of the arterial, venous and capillary circulation of the soft tissues of the head by decades as demonstrated by the methyl methacrolate injection technique, and their application to the construction of flaps and pedicles. Plastic and Reconstructive Surgery 27: 160–184

Dankmeijer J, Waltman J M 1950 Sur l'innervation de la face dorsale des doigts humains. Acta Anatomica 10: 377–384

Daseler E H, Anson B J 1959 The surgical anatomy of the subclavian artery and its branches. Surgery, Gynaecology and Obstetrics 108: 149–174

Dautel G, Borrelly J, Merle M, Michon J 1989 Dorsal vascular network of the first web space. Surgical and Radiologic Anatomy 11: 109–113

Delaney T A, Gonzales L L 1971 Occlusion of popliteal artery due to muscular entrapment. Surgery 69: 97–101

DesPrez J D, Kiehn C L 1959 Method of reconstruction following resection of anterior oral cavity and mandible for malignancy. Plastic and Reconstructive Surgery 24: 238–249

Dubreuil-Chambardel L 1926 Traité des variations du système artériel. Masson et Cie, Paris

Dufourmentel C, Mouly R 1959 Chirurgie plastique. Flammarion, Paris

Earley M J 1986 The arterial supply of the thumb, first web and index finger and its surgical application. Journal of Hand Surgery 11B: 163–174

Earley M J, Milner R H 1987 Dorsal metacarpal flaps. British Journal of Plastic Surgery 40: 333–341

Eaton R G 1968 The digital neurovascular bundle. Clinical Orthopaedics and Related Research 61: 176–185

Edwards E A 1960 Organization of the small arteries of the hand and digits. American Journal of Surgery 99: 837–846

Elbaz J S, Darcour J C, Ricbourg B 1975 Vascularisation artérielle de la paroi abdominale. Annales de Chirurgie Plastique 20: 19–29

Eustathianos N 1932 Etude anatomique sur les artères temporales superficieles. Annals of Anatomy and Pathology 9: 678–684

Fatah M F, Nancarrow J D, Murray D S 1985 Raising the radial artery forearm flap: the superficial ulnar artery 'trap'. British Journal of Plastic Surgery 38: 394–395

Fisher J 1983 External oblique fasciocutaneous flap for elbow coverage. Presented at ASPRS Meeting, Dallas, November 1983. Abstracted in Plastic Surgical Forum VI, 1983

Fisher J, Bostwick J, Powell R W 1983 Latissimus dorsi blood supply after thoracodorsal vessel division: the serratus collateral. Plastic and Reconstructive Surgery 72: 502–509

Flint M H 1956 Some observations on the vascular supply of the nail bed and terminal segments the fingers. British Journal of Plastic Surgery 8: 186–195

Franchinelli A, Masquelet A, Restrepo Y, Gilbert A 1981 The vascularised sural nerve. International Journal of Microsurgery 3: 57–62

Futrell J W, Johns M E, Edgerton M T, Cantrell R W, Fitz-Hugh G S 1978 Platysma myocutaneous flap for intra-oral reconstruction. American Journal of Surgery 136: 504–507

Gelberman R H, Blasingame J P 1981 The timed Allen test. The Journal of Trauma 21: 477–479

Gillilan L A 1961 The collateral circulation of the human orbita. Archives of Ophthalmology 65: 684–694

Gruber W 1852 Über die neue und constante oberflächliche Ellenbogenbugschlagader des menschen (arteria plicae cubiti superficialis). Zeitschrift der Gesellschaft der Aerzte zu Wein 2: 481–510

Haimovici H 1967 Patterns of arteriosclerotic lesions of the lower extremity. Archives of Surgery 95: 918–933

Harii K 1979 Discussion on Acland's paper 'The Free Iliac Flap'. Plastic and Reconstructive Surgery 64: 257–258

Harii K, Ohmori K, Torii S, Murakami F, Kasai Y, Sekiguchi J, Ohmori S 1975 Free groin skin flaps. British Journal of Plastic Surgery 28: 225–237

Haust S K M D 1979 Variations in the aortic origin of intercostal arteries in man. Anatomical Record 195: 545–552

Hayashi A, Maruyama Y 1990 Anatomical study of the recurrent flaps of the upper arm. British Journal of Plastic Surgery 43: 300–306

Hayashi A, Maruyama Y 1990 The medial genicular artery flap. Annals of Plastic Surgery 25: 174–180

Henry A K 1957 Extensile exposure, 2nd edn. Churchill Livingstone, Edinburgh

Herbert D C 1978 A subcutaneous pedicled cheek flap for reconstruction of alar defects. British Journal of Plastic Surgery 31: 79–92

Hirai M 1980 Digital blood pressure and arteriographic findings under selective compression of the radial and ulnar arteries. Angiology 31: 21–31

Hirai M, Kawai S 1980 False positive and negative results in Allen test. The Journal of Cardiovascular Surgery 21: 353–360

Huber J F 1941 The arterial network supplying the dorsum of the foot. Anatomical Record 80: 373

Huelke D 1958 A study of the transverse cervical and dorsal scapular arteries. The Anatomical Record 132: 233–245

Ikeda A, Ugawa A, Kazihara Y, Hamada N 1988 Arterial patterns in the hand based on a three-dimensional analysis of 220 cadaver hands. The Journal of Hand Surgery 13A: 501–509

Juskiewenski S, Vaysse Ph, Moscovici J, Hammoudi S, Bouissou E 1982 A study of the arterial blood supply to the penis. Anatomia Clinica 4: 101–107

Kaplan E B 1965 Functional and surgical anatomy of the hand. J B Lippincott, Philadelphia

Katai K, Kido M, Numaguchi Y 1979 Angiography of the iliofemoral arteriovenous system supplying free groin flaps and free hypogastric flaps. Plastic and Reconstructive Surgery 63: 671–679

Kirschbaum S 1958 Mentosternal contracture – preferred treatment by acromial ('Charretera') flap. Plastic and Reconstructive Surgery 21: 131–138

Kropp B N 1951 The lateral costal branch of the internal mammary artery. Journal of Thoracic Surgery 21: 421–425

Lai M F, Krishna B V, Pelly A D 1981 The brachioradialis myocutaneous flap. British Journal of Plastic Surgery 34: 431–434

Lamberty B G H, Cormack G C 1982 The forearm angiotomes. British

Journal of Plastic Surgery 35: 420–429
Lamberty B G H, Cormack G C 1983 The antecubital fasciocutaneous flap. British Journal of Plastic Surgery 36: 428–433
Last R J 1984 Anatomy, Regional and Applied, 7th edn. Churchill Livingstone, Edinburgh
Lendrum J 1980 Alternatives to amputation. Annals of the Royal College of Surgeons of England 62: 95–99
Leslie B M, Ruby L K, Madell S J, Wittenstein F 1987 Digital artery diameters: an anatomic and clinical study. The Journal of Hand Surgery 12A: 740–743
Levame J H, Otero C, Berdugo G 1967 Vascularisation arterielle des teguments de la face dorsale de la main et des doigts. Annales de Chirurgie Plastique 12: 316–324
Libersa C, Francke J P, Mauppin J M, Bailleul J P, Gamblin P 1982 The arterial supply to the palm of the hand (arteriae palmae manus). Anatomia Clinica 4: 33–45
Lipschutz B 1916 Studies on the blood vascular tree. I. A composite study of the femoral artery. Anatomical Record 10: 362–370
Lucas G L 1984 The pattern of venous drainage of the digits. The Journal of Hand Surgery 9A: 448–450
Manchot C 1889 Die Hautarterien des Menschlichen Körpers. F C W Vogel, Leipzig
McCormack L J, Cauldwell E W, Anson B J 1953 Brachial and antebrachial arterial patterns. Surgery, Gynaecology and Obstetrics 96: 43–54
McVay C B, Anson B J 1940 Composition of the rectus sheath. The Anatomical Record 77: 213–225
Masquelet A C, Rinaldi S 1985 Anatomical basis of the posterior brachial skin flap. Anatomia Clinica 7: 155–160
Mialhe C, Brice M 1985 A new compound osteo-myocutaneous free flap: the posterior iliac artery flap. British Journal of Plastic Surgery 38: 30–38
Milloy F J, Anson B J, McAfee D K 1960 The rectus abdominus muscle and the epigastric arteries. Surgery, Gynaecology and Obstetrics 110: 293–302
Mitz V, Ricbourg B, Lassau J P 1973 Les branches faciales de l'artère faciale chez l'adulte. Annales de Chirurgie Plastique 18: 339–350
Mütter T D 1842 Case of deformity from burns relieved by operation. American Journal of Medical Sciences 4: 66–80
Nahai F, Brown R G, Vasconez L O 1976 Blood supply to the abdominal wall as related to planning abdominal incisions. American Surgeon 42: 691–695
Nakajima H, Maruyama Y, Koda E 1981 The definition of vascular skin territories with prostaglandin E_1 – the anterior chest, abdomen and thigh-inguinal region. British Journal of Plastic Surgery 34: 258–263
Nathan H, Rubinstein Z, Bogart B 1982 Accessory internal thoracic artery. Anatomia Clinica 3: 333–337
Nicoletis C, Morel-Fatio D 1968 Etranges necroses. Annales de Chirurgie Plastique 14: 56–59
O'Brien B McC, MacLeod A M, Hayhurst J W, Morrison W A 1973 Successful transfer of a large island flap from the groin to the foot by microvascular anastomoses. Plastic and Reconstructive Surgery 52: 271–278
Ohtsuka H 1981 Angiographic analysis of the first dorsal metatarsal arteries and its clinical application. Annals of Plastic Surgery 7: 2–17
Parry S W, Ward J W, Mathes S J 1988 Vascular anatomy of the upper extremity muscles. Plastic and Reconstructive Surgery 81: 358–363
Penteado C V 1983 Anatomosurgical study of the superficial and deep circumflex iliac arteries. Anatomia Clinica 5: 125–127
Penteado C V 1984 Contribution of the superficial and deep circumflex iliac arteries to the blood supply of the anterior third of the iliac crest and adjacent skin. Anatomia Clinica 5: 273–274
Penteado C V, Masquelet A C, Chevrel J P 1986 The anatomic basis of the fascio-cutaneous flap of the posterior interosseous artery. Surgical and Radiologic Anatomy 8: 209–215
Popoff N W 1934 The digital vascular system. Archives of Pathology 18: 295–330
Quain 1844 Anatomy of the arteries of the human body. London
Ramasastry S S, Tucker J B, Swartz W M, Hurwitz D J 1984 The internal oblique muscle flap: an anatomic and clinical study. Plastic and Reconstructive Surgery 73: 721–730
Reid C D, Taylor G I 1984 The vascular territory of the acromiothoracic axis. British Journal of Plastic Surgery 37: 194–212
Revol M P, Lantieri L, Loy S, Guérin-Surville H 1991 Vascular anatomy of the forearm muscles: a study of 50 dissections. Plastic and Reconstructive Surgery 88: 1026–1033
Ricbourg B, Mitz V, Lassau J-P 1975 Artère temporale superficielle. Annales de Chirurgie Plastique 20: 197–213
Rocha R J F, Gilbert A, Masquelet A, Yousif N J, Sanger J R, Matloub H S 1987 The anterior tibial artery flap: anatomic study and clinical application. Plastic and Reconstructive Surgery 79: 396–404
Rowsell A R, Davies D M, Eisenberg N, Taylor G I 1984 The anatomy of the subscapular-thoracodorsal arterial system: study of 100 cadaver dissections. British Journal of Plastic Surgery 37: 574–576
Saijo M 1978 The vascular territories of the dorsal trunk. A reappraisal for potential flap donor sites. British Journal of Plastic Surgery 31: 200–204
Salmon M 1936 Les artères de la peau. Masson et Cie, Paris
Salmon M 1939 Les voies anastomotiques arterielles des membres: Etude anatomique et radiologique. Marseille-Medical 76: 433–476
Senior H A 1919 The interpretation of the arterial anomalies of the human leg and foot. The Journal of Anatomy 53: 142
Smith P J, Foley B, McGregor I, Jackson I T 1972 The anatomical basis of the groin flap. Plastic and Reconstructive Surgery 49: 41–47
Sommerlad B C, Boorman J G 1981 An innervated flap, incorporating supraclavicular nerves, for reconstruction of major hand injuries. The Hand 13: 5–11
Taylor G I, Daniel R K 1975 The anatomy of several free flap donor sites. Plastic and Reconstructive Surgery 56: 243–253
Taylor G I, Ham F J 1976 The free vascularised nerve graft. Plastic and Reconstructive Surgery 57: 413–425
Taylor G I, Townsend P, Corlett R 1979 Superiority of the deep circumflex iliac vessels as the supply for free groin flaps. Experimental and clinical work. Plastic and Reconstructive Surgery 64: 595–604 & 745–759
Taylor G I, Palmer J H 1987 The vascular territories (angiosomes) of the body: Experimental study and clinical applications. British Journal of Plastic Surgery 40: 113–141
Terzis J 1985 Branching of the thoracoacromial axis. Personal communication.
Thoma A, Young J E M 1992 The superficial ulnar artery 'trap' and the free forearm flap. Annals of Plastic Surgery 28: 370–372
Thompson A 1891 Second annual report of the Committee of Collective Investigation of the Anatomical Society of Great Britain and Ireland for the year 1890–1891. Journal of Anatomy and Physiology 26: 77–80
Toldt 1921 Anatomischer Atlas. Hochstetter's Edition. Urban & Schwarzenberg, Berlin
Vasconez L O 1981 Personal communication
Von Mihalik P 1967 The anatomy of the abdominal wall with special reference to the nerves and vessels involved in the incisions for kidney operations. South African Medical Journal 41: 101–103
Wagner G, Willis E A, Bro-Ramussen F, Nielsen M H 1982 New theory on the mechanism of erection involving hitherto undescribed vessels. The Lancet 1: 416–418
Wallace W A, Coupland R E 1975 Variations in the nerves of the thumb and index fingers. Journal of Bone and Joint Surgery 57B: 491–494
Ward G E, Hendrick J W 1950 Diagnosis and treatment of tumours of the head and neck. Williams and Wilkins, Baltimore
Weathersby H T 1954 The volar arterial arches. The Anatomical Record 118: 365–366
Webster J P 1937 Thoraco-epigastric tubed pedicles. Surgical Clinics of North America 17: 145–184
Williams G D, Martin C H, McIntire L R 1934 Origin of the deep and circumflex femoral group of arteries. Anatomical Record 60: 189–196
Zbrodowski A D, Gajisin S, Grodecki J 1981 The anatomy of the digitopalmar arches. Journal of Bone and Joint Surgery 63: 108–113
Zovickian A 1957 Pharyngeal fistulae: repair and prevention using mastoid-occiput based shoulder flap. Plastic and Reconstructive Surgery 19: 355–372

The vascular territories and the clinical application to the planning of flaps

7

Flaps are described under the name of their supplying artery and are listed in alphabetical order. This convention has been adopted because some flaps have several names depending on, for example, their anatomical area of localisation, the person who first described it, or some other feature such as the shape of the flap. The name of the principal supplying vessel provides a constant reference point whilst these other names may come and go in the light of changing fashion. A few flaps (generally musculocutaneous) with more than one supplying vessel are listed under the name of the principal pedicle, e.g. sternomastoid musculocutaneous flap under occipital artery.

However, to aid the search for a specific flap for which perhaps only an eponymous or other 'non-artery' name is known, pages 278–283 list the flaps of each major region of the body and indicate the name of the artery under which further information will be found. The regions listed are head and neck, upper limb, perineum, lower limb and trunk.

7 HEAD AND NECK

UPPER LIMB

7

7 LOWER LIMB

saphenous artery ***see page 428***
sural arteries (gastrocnemius) ***see page 464***
super flap *see posterior tibial artery and peroneal artery*
superficial circumflex iliac artery ***see page 431***
superficial external pudendal artery ***see page 434***
superficial sural arteries ***see page 440***
superior gluteal musculocutaneous flap *see superior gluteal artery*
superior gluteal artery ***see page 336***
superior lateral thigh flap *see profunda femoris lateral perforators*
supramalleolar flap *see peroneal artery – anterior perforating branch*
tensor fasciae latae musculocutaneous flap *see lateral circumflex femoral artery*

PERINEUM

dartos musculocutaneous flap *see deep external pudendal arteries*
superficial external pudendal artery ***see page 434***
deep external pudendal artery ***see page 434***
suprapubic axial pattern flap *see superficial external pudendal arteries*
penile island flaps *see deep external pudendal arteries*

7 TRUNK

7 ANTERIOR TIBIAL ARTERY

Fasciocutaneous flaps
Types A, B and C

Although the broad principles on which the anterior tibial flaps are based are reasonably clear, the details of individual flap sub-types are complex. Figure 7.3 may help in distinguishing the differences between the various subtypes that are in the literature. Theoretically there are more possibilities than this but they are not clinically indicated – for example one would not sacrifice an anterior tibial artery to create a Type C flap for the purpose of filling a proximal defect because there are other ways of dealing with such a problem.

Anatomy (see also p. 231–237)

The anterior tibial artery gives off two major branches to the peroneal compartment which have no formal names in *Nomina Anatomica* but which we will refer to as the superior and inferior lateral peroneal arteries (LPA). The superior artery (~ 1.6 mm D) is always present and arises between 7 and 11 cm below the fibular head; the inferior artery (~ 1.4 mm D) is more variable and may be present in only 70% of cases. Both vessels are destined for the peroneal compartment and on the way give off fasciocutaneous perforators which pass along the anterior peroneal septum to reach the deep fascia in the upper

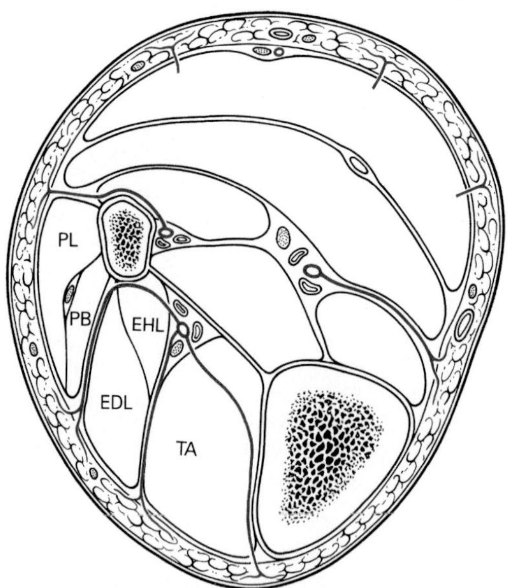

Fig. 7.1 Vascular anatomy. Schematic cross-section through upper third of lower leg to show positions of the branches of the anterior tibial artery to skin. Fig. 7.2 corresponds with this.

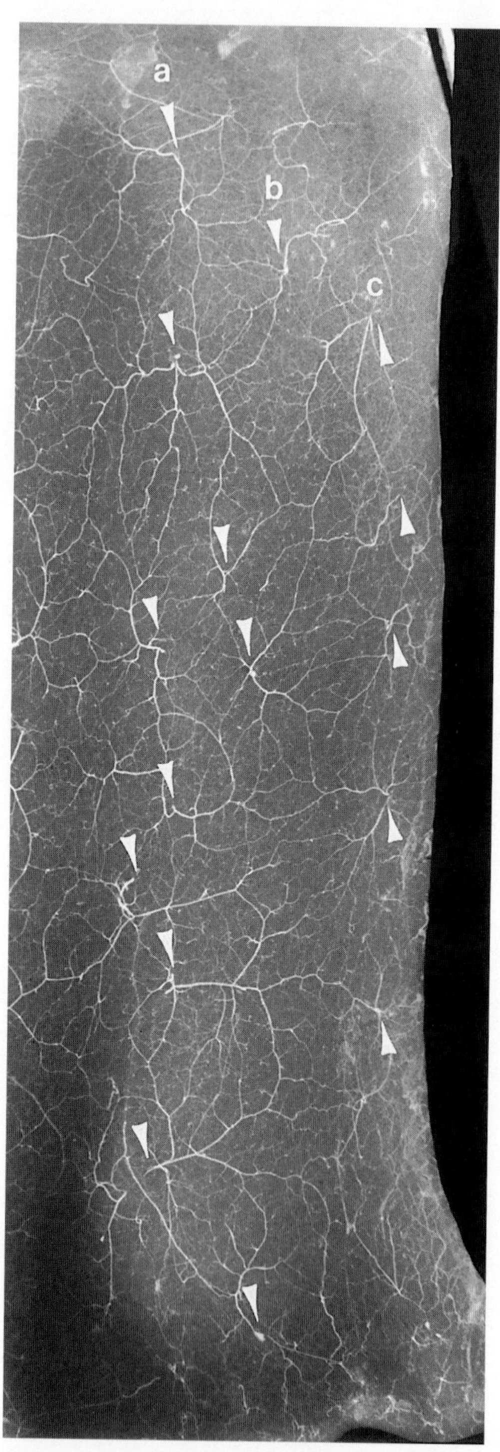

Fig. 7.2 Radiograph of skin and fascia overlying anterior compartment: **a.** perforators along anterior peroneal septum; **b.** perforators between TA and EDL/EDH; **c.** perforators between TA and the edge of the tibia.

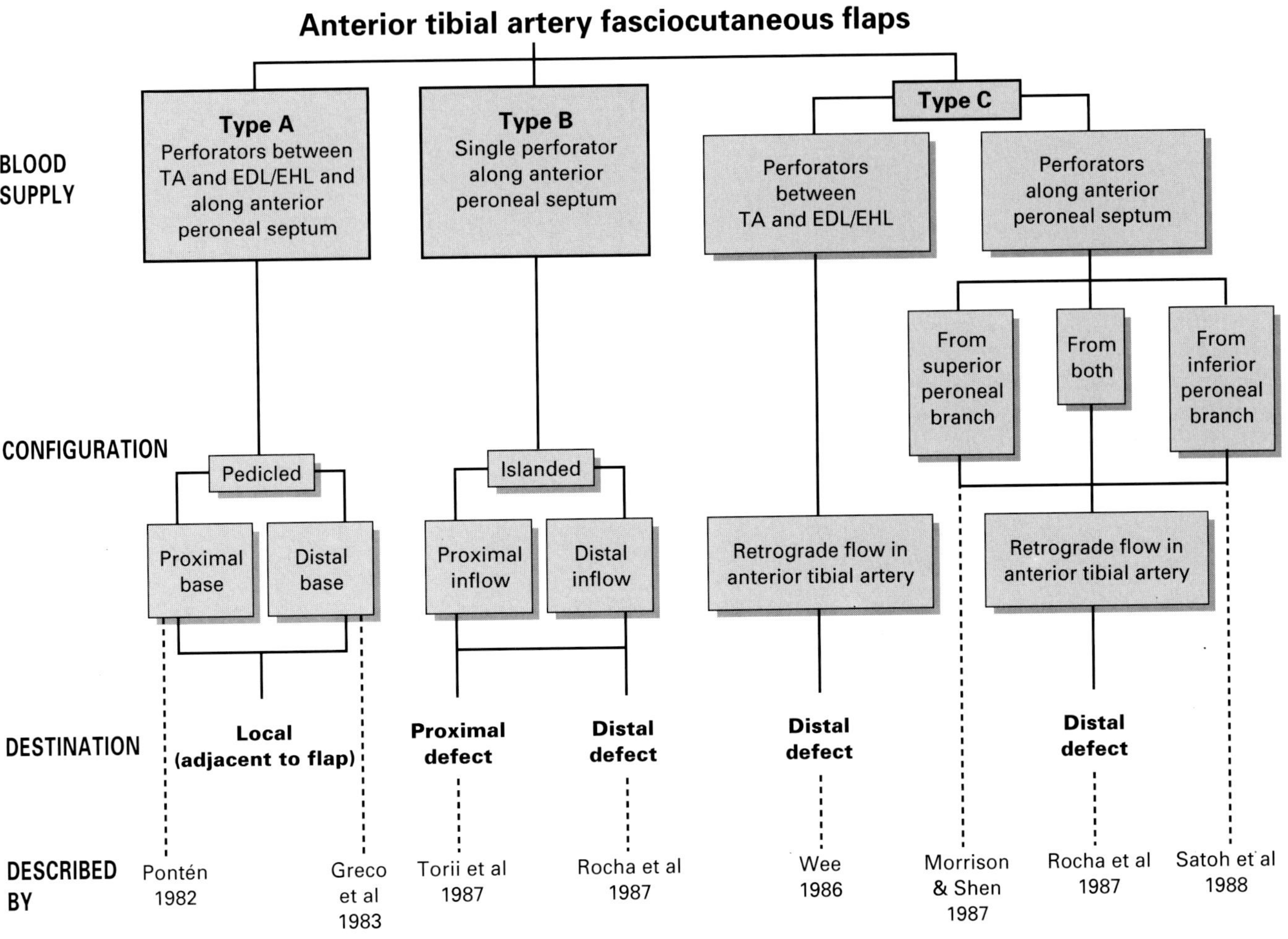

Fig. 7.3 A classification of 'anterior tibial flaps' that combines anatomical and surgical features in order to clarify some of the differences between the various flaps based on fasciocutaneous perforators arising from the anterior tibial artery.

two-thirds of the leg. Branches accompany the superficial peroneal nerve and arise either from the superior lateral peroneal artery (30%) or from the inferior lateral peroneal artery (40%) or from both (30%). The anterior tibial artery itself also gives off further fasciocutaneous perforators along the anterior peroneal septum and also along the fascial septum between tibialis anterior and EDL/EHL. The very small branches that emerge between TA and the edge of the tibia are not used to support flaps.

Flap planning

Choice of flap will depend on the site of the defect to be reconstructed and the need to preserve the anterior tibial artery, although the indications for this are not fully worked out. With the more complex flaps the variations in anatomy are such that it is better to have a thorough familiarity with the anatomy and adapt a flap suited to the individual circumstances, than it is to commence an operation with a fixed plan of raising a particular flap sub-type.

Surgery

With all these flaps it helps to have a tourniquet on the thigh, although the leg is best not exsanguinated as some blood in the perforators greatly aids their identification.

Type A pedicled flaps follow traditional *transposition* and *rotation* flap principles (Fig. 7.4a, b); transposition flaps may be designed with a proximal or a distal base, but rotation flaps always have a superior base because it is necessary to use the slack in the skin below the popliteal fossa to close the defect in the area of the back-cut.[1]

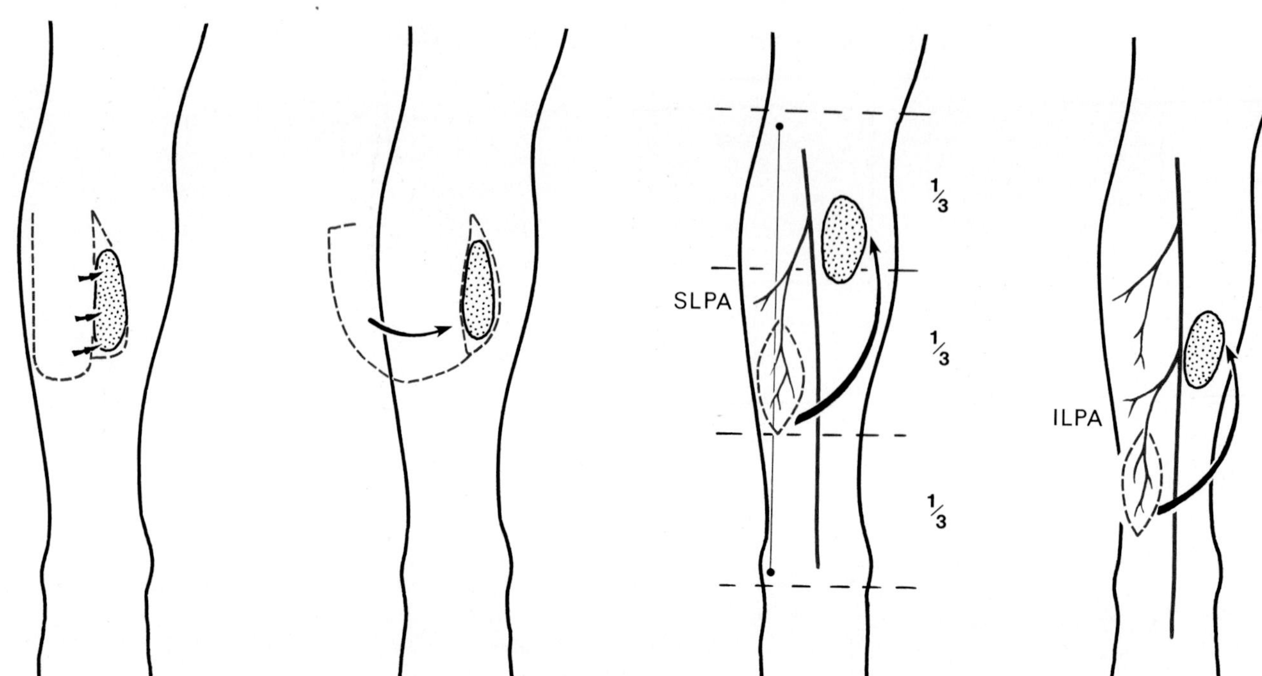

Fig. 7.4 **a.** and **b.** Local transposition and rotation flaps. **c.** Flap based on a perforator arising from the superior lateral peroneal artery branch which may require division distal to the origin of the perforator to mobilise the flap. **d.** Flap based on a perforator arising from the inferior lateral peroneal branch which again may require division for mobilisation.

Type B, proximal inflow (Fig. 7.4c, d). A flap may be carried on a single fasciocutaneous branch of the superior or inferior lateral peroneal artery (LPA).

With the *superior LPA flap*[2] the fasciocutaneous branch is generally given off in the middle third of the leg, so the flap is outlined in this area centered over the anterior peroneal septum which is surface marked by a line drawn between the head of the fibula and the lateral malleolus. Flap elevation, (including the deep fascia), commences at the antero-distal edge of the flap. The aim at this stage is to find the superficial peroneal nerve and the arterial branches that run with it – usually medial to it – and to dissect the nerve free. The vascular pedicle is followed back into the septum between EHL and the peroneal muscles and traced back to the SLPA, taking a strip of the fascial septum adjacent to the vessels. This pedicle will be 5 to 8 cm long so the arc of rotation is limited. Further mobilisation may only be achieved by dividing the main part of the SLPA going to the peroneal muscles in which case the flap may reach the medial side of the knee. Once the flap has been elevated the nerve can be placed in the gap between the muscles which are then sutured together prior to skin grafting the donor site.

With the *inferior LPA flap* (Fig. 7.4d) the skin island is situated more distally as the branch lies approximately at the junction of the middle and the distal thirds. The length of pedicle and arc of rotation may be increased slightly by division of the main part of the artery going to the peroneal muscles.

Type C, distal inflow from ILPA, ATA intact (Rocha et al).[3] In some 30% of cases the inferior and superior LPAs are joined by a large communication along the line of the superficial peroneal nerve allowing the inferior LPA to carry an island skin flap overlying more proximally situated perforators from the superior LPA. This vessel, and the branches which it gives off along the septum to the overlying skin, then has to be dissected out with part of the septum. Figure 7.5a shows how the branch from the superior LPA is divided to allow the flap to be moved to a distal defect. This design enables an 'anterior tibial artery flap' to be moved to a more distal defect *without* sacrifice of the anterior tibial artery but it is only applicable in a limited number of cases and the distance through which the flap can be moved is limited.

More likely to be applicable is the flap in Figure 7.5b in which the skin island is based on the inferior LPA perforators but is extended proximally along the anastomoses that the branches of the perforator make with similar vessels from the superior LPA above the deep fascia. Again the arc of rotation is limited.

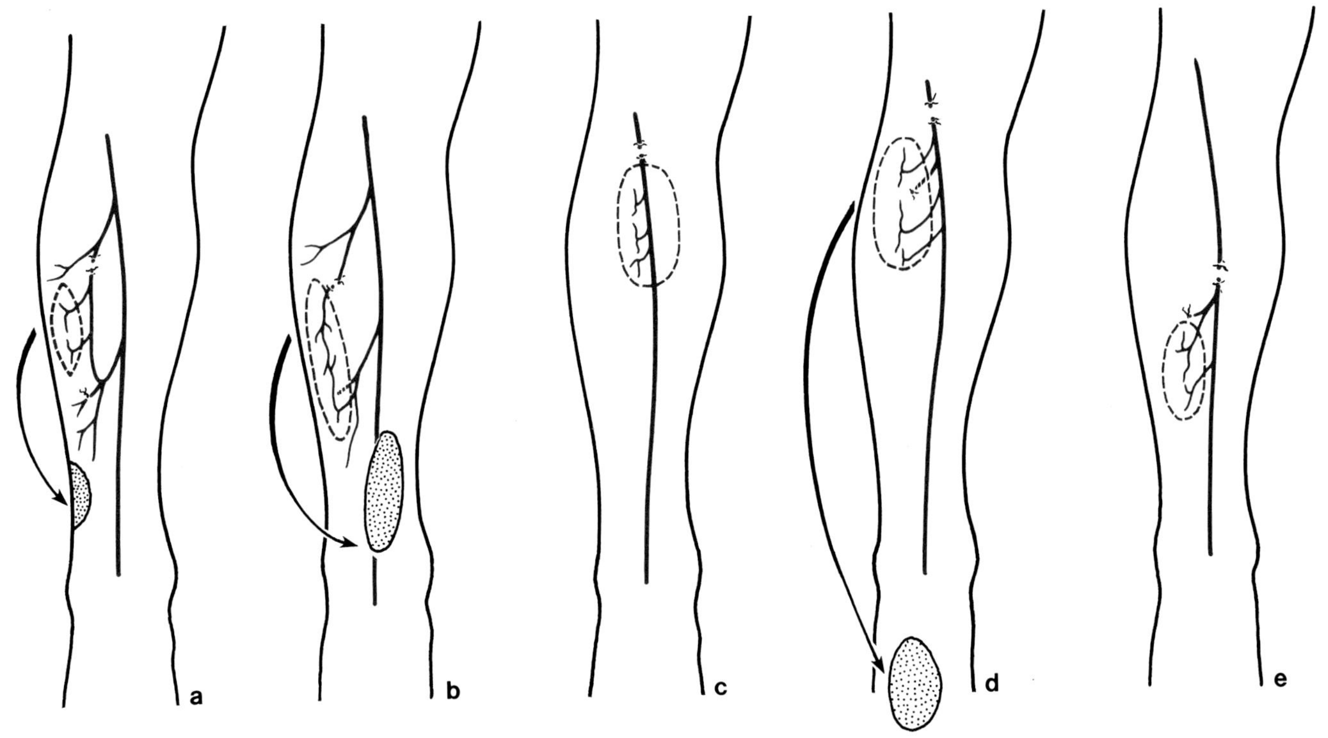

Fig. 7.5 **a.** When there is a good deep lying anastomosis between superior and inferior lateral peroneal arteries (30% of cases), a proximal flap may be moved to a distal defect. **b.** Here the anastomoses are at the level of the deep fascia. **c.** Retrograde flow type C flap with perforators between TA and EDL. **d.** More robust perforators lying along anterior peroneal septum derived from SLPA. **e.** Similar flap but based on perforators from ILPA.

Type C, TA/EDL septum, reverse flow in anterior tibial artery (Fig 7.5c). The perforators along this septum are rather delicate and in raising the septum it is best to include a narrow margin of the lateral edge of TA. The anterior tibial artery and veins are divided and the reach of the flap is therefore considerable (Wee).[4]

Type C, EDL/PB (anterior peroneal septum), reverse flow in anterior tibial artery. The major perforators lie along this septum which is surface marked by a line drawn between the fibular head and the lateral malleolus. Flaps raised in the upper part of the leg depend on fasciocutaneous perforators arising from the anterior tibial artery and from the superior LPA (Fig. 7.5d).[5] Alternatively the flap may be based over inferior LPA branches (Fig 7.5e) which preserves the blood supply to the peroneal compartment from the superior LPA.[6] Alternatively both superior and inferior LPA branches may be used.[3] When raising the flaps the superficial peroneal nerve should be identified and carefully dissected free from the flap – it is then buried in the space between EDL and PB. Venous drainage of these reverse-flow flaps is dependent on a combination of reflux through the valves and bypass of the valves by cross-communications between the venae comitantes and bypass vessels around the valves. Perhaps denervation also has an effect in allowing distension of the veins and incompetence of the valves. Venous anastomosis of one of the venae comitantes to a vein in the recipient site to overcome some of the problems of venous congestion has been recommended by Wee.[4]

References

1. Gréco J M, Simons G, Faugon H 1983 Une arme nouvelle en chirurgie plastique: Le lambeau cutanéo-aponévrotique. Son application dans la réparation des pertes de substance du membre inférieur. Annales de Chirurgie Plastique et Esthétique 28: 211–224
2. Torii S, Namiki Y, Hayashi Y 1987 Anterolateral leg island flap. British Journal of Plastic Surgery 40: 236–240
3. Rocha J F R, Gilbert A, Masquelet A, Yousif N J, Sanger J R, Matloub H S 1987 The anterior tibial artery flap: anatomic study and clinical application. Plastic and Reconstructive Surgery 79: 396–404
4. Wee J T K 1986 Reconstruction of the lower leg and foot with the reverse-pedicled anterior tibial flap: preliminary report of a new fasciocutaneous flap. British Journal of Plastic Surgery 39: 327–337
5. Morrison W A, Shen T Y 1987 Anterior tibial artery flap: anatomy and case report. British Journal of Plastic Surgery 40: 230–235
6. Satoh K, Yoshikawa A, Hayashi M 1988 Reverse-flow anterior tibial flap type III. British Journal of Plastic Surgery 41: 624–627

7 CIRCUMFLEX SCAPULAR ARTERY – horizontal branch

Horizontal scapular flap
Bi-scapular flap
Osteocutaneous composite scapular flap

The vascular anatomy of this fasciocutaneous flap was described by dos Santos[1] and the first published clinical case appears to have been by Gilbert & Test.[2] Numerous publications concerning both anatomical and clinical aspects of this flap appeared during 1982.[3–6] Early reports emphasised that flaps raised on the horizontal branch had limited dimensions, but later experience demonstrated that the midline was not a barrier and that flaps could be reliably raised which crossed the midline and included the territory of the opposite horizontal branch.[7,8]

Vascular anatomy

The subscapular artery arises from the third part of the axillary artery and within 4 cm of its origin gives off the circumflex scapular artery except in a small number of cases (<5%) in which this vessel may arise directly from the axillary artery; renamed, it then continues as the thoracodorsal artery to latissimus dorsi. The circumflex scapular artery grooves the lateral border of the scapula as it passes posteriorly in the triangular space between teres minor above, teres major below and the long head of triceps laterally to divide into cutaneous and muscular branches with the muscular branches given off first. The circumflex scapular artery is accompanied by two veins of which one usually has a large diameter of 2 or 3 mm. Usually the circumflex scapular vein joins the thoracodorsal vein but in about 12% of cases it joins the axillary vein directly.

The cutaneous branches are usually two in number, the horizontal branch which passes laterally parallel to the spine of the scapula, and the parascapular branch which follows the lateral border of the scapula. Often there is a third branch, the ascending scapular, which either arises from the horizontal branch or directly from the circumflex scapular artery (see p. 293). The cutaneous branches spread out at the level of the deep fascia, making this a fasciocutaneous flap. The horizontal branch has been studied by dos Santos in 70 dissections on 70 cadavers.[1] Her findings are summarised in Figure 7.7. The surface marking of the point of emergence of the artery can be estimated by measuring the distance between the scapular spine and the lower pole of the scapula and applying the formula D cm = (L – 2 cm)/2. When checked against dos Santos' figures this is accurate (±0.5 cm) in 68% of cases and in the remainder gives too high or too low a measurement.

The muscular branch ramifies in the infraspinous fossa deep to infraspinatus and supplies the periosteum of the lateral border of the scapula. The scapula also receives a further source of blood supply at its lower pole from a vessel which has been called the angular branch. The origin of this vessel is about evenly divided between firstly a point on the thoracodorsal artery proximal to the serratus collateral take-off, and secondly from the serratus branch itself (Fig. 7.10).

The angular branch has an external diameter of approximately 2 mm and a length between 4 and 5 cm as it passes between latissimus dorsi and teres major to

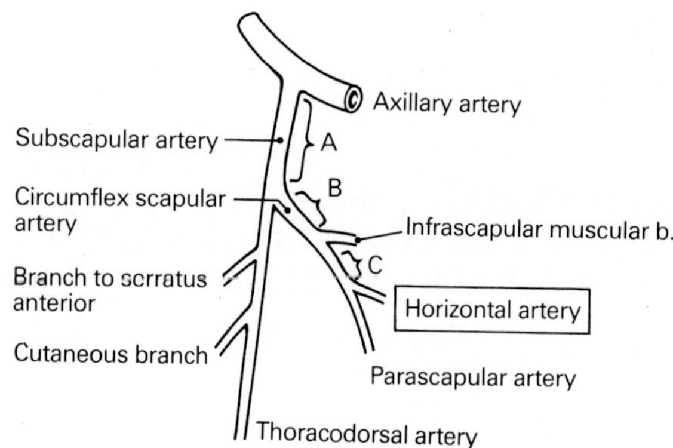

Fig. 7.6 Data on vessel diameters and lengths. (After Nassif et al, 1982)

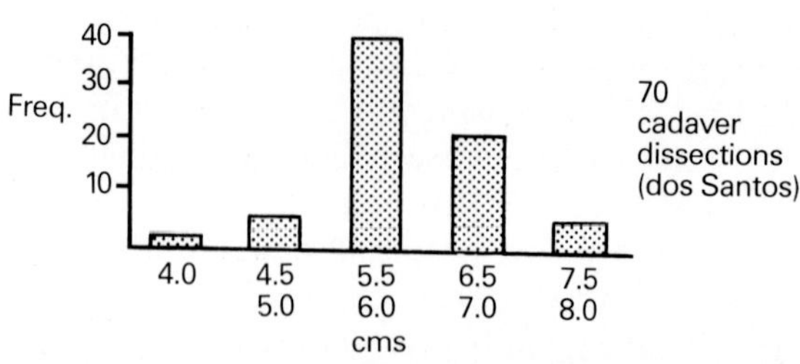

Fig. 7.7 Histogram shows surface marking of point of emergence of the horizontal branch of the circumflex scapular artery in centimetres below the scapular spine (compiled from the figures of dos Santos).

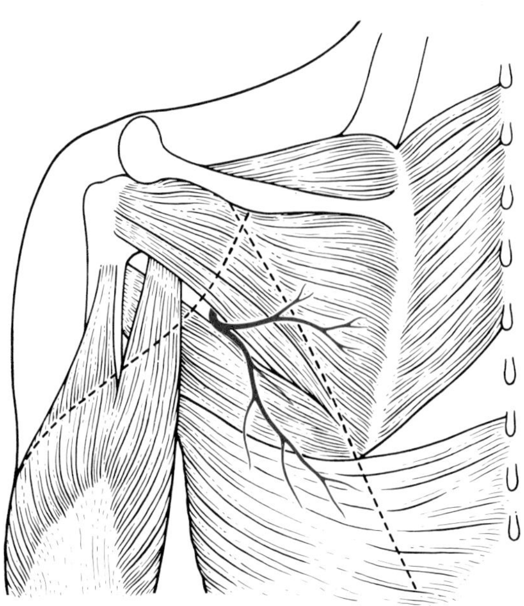

Fig. 7.8 Vascular anatomy. The horizontal and parascapular branches of the circumflex scapular artery are seen emerging between teres minor above and teres major below. Deltoid and trapezius have been omitted for clarity but their margins are indicated by broken lines.

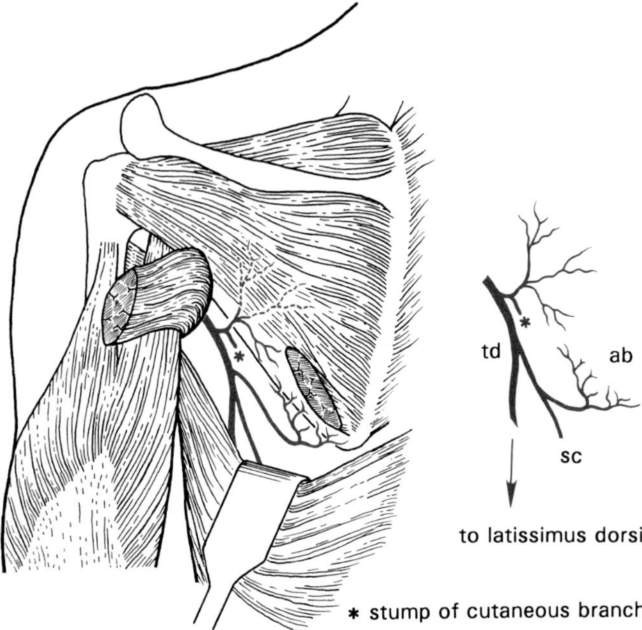

Fig. 7.10 Osteocutaneous flap anatomy. The teres muscle has been divided to display the vessels. The angular branch **ab** arises from the serratus collateral **sc** or the thoracodorsal artery **td**.

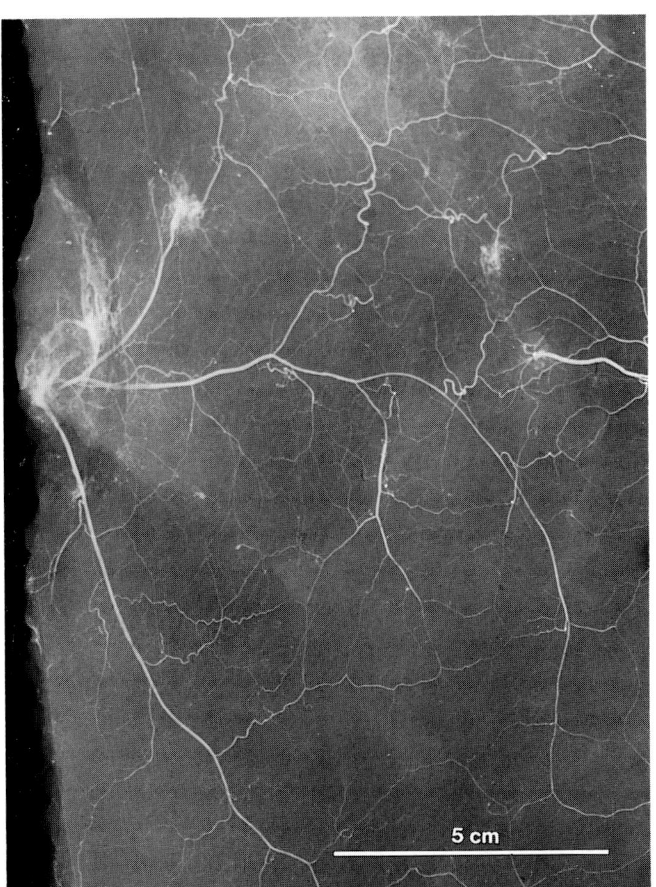

Fig. 7.9 Radiograph of skin and fascia.

reach the lower pole of the scapula approximately 2 to 3 cm above the tip. From this point branches pass both up and down so that this vessel can support an 8 cm length of the lateral scapular border. This vascular anatomy means that bone can be combined with a horizontal scapular flap in three different ways: (a) a lateral scapular strut can be combined on the same pedicle as the flap; (b) a lateral scapular strut can be carried on the angular artery; (c) two separate struts of bone can be carried with independent arterial supplies, although both come together on the single pedicle. In (a) there is limited mobility between bone and flap; in (b) the mobility is greatly enhanced but much more muscle division is required to free the angular artery pedicle; (c) has the advantage that where two bone sites require to be filled or where several osteotomies are required (as in matching the curve of the mandible) the two pedicles maintain blood supply to the separate bone pieces.

Planning

In the method of Urbaniak et al[3] the 'rule of twos' is applied with the subject's arm by his side (Fig. 7.11). This places the medial corner 2 cm from the spinous processes and the lateral corner at a point 2 cm above the posterior axillary crease. The inferior border may extend to a point 2 cm superior to the lower pole of the scapula and the superior border to a point 2 cm inferior to the spine. In an average male these markings create a flap with dimension of approximately 10 cm × 16 cm. However, Urbaniak's method is rather too rigid a schema and later experience has shown that flaps may be extended across the midline. Therefore lengths of up to 40 cm may be achieved although the width is still limited as 10 cm represents the maximum width of defect that may be closed directly at this site.

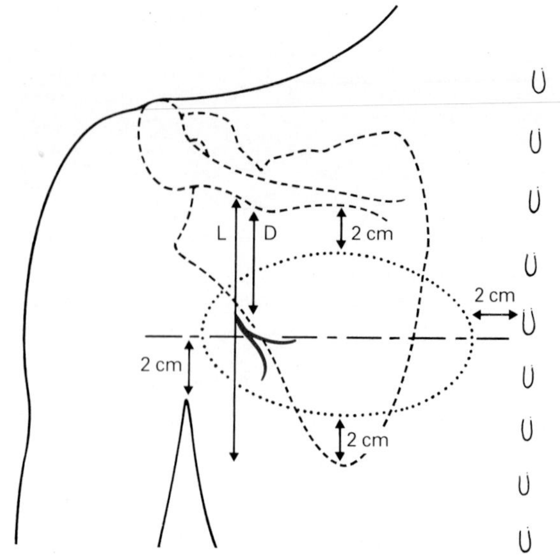

Fig. 7.11 Flap planning. The long axis of the flap lies along the course of the horizontal branch which emerges a distance D cm below the scapular spine where D = 0.5 (L – 2) cm. The boundaries of the flap may be determined by use of 'the rule of 2s'.

Surgery

The elevation of the flap commences with an incision supero-laterally in order to expose the circumflex scapular artery and its paired venae comitantes in the triangular space. This requires retraction of teres minor upwards, triceps laterally, and teres major inferiorly. The dissection proceeds from the medial side in a subfascial plane visualising the vessels and when the flap has been elevated the deeper dissection of the pedicle may be pursued. This requires ligation of muscular branches and becomes more difficult as the plane gets deeper. Removal of most of the circumflex scapular artery will produce a pedicle of 7–10 cm in length with a vessel diameter of 2.5–3.5 mm. There is no potential for an innervated flap.

Elevation of an osteocutaneous flap (Fig. 7.10) involves dissecting out the musculoperiosteal branch which is given off by the CSA 2 to 3 cm further back in the triangular space. An incision is made through the muscles attaching to the scapula in the line of the intended osteotomies and teres major is detached. Following division of the bone, additional exposure is gained for division of subscapularis on the deep surface of the bone, serratus at the lower pole (if appropriate), and additional exposure of the pedicle. The dimensions of the available bone strut vary in length between 10 and 14 cm depending on the size of the individual, and approximately 1.5 cm in width if the intention is to take mainly the sturdy lateral cortico-cancellous edge rather than the thin infraspinous plate of the scapula, although the latter may have application in orbital floor and palate reconstructions. After harvesting the flap the donor defect is reconstructed by reattaching all muscle origins through drill holes in scapular bone with permanent sutures. Suction drains are very important as these wounds tend to develop haematomas.

If bone vascularised by the angular branch is to be harvested then the plane between teres major and latissimus dorsi is opened at an early stage to expose the angular branch and ensure that it is protected before dividing the teres major. Division of the thoracodorsal artery and serratus collateral (if appropriate) will be required depending on the anatomy (Fig. 7.10). The angular branch can support a 6 cm triangle of bone from the lower pole or a 8 cm strut from the lateral edge of the scapula. Closure of the defect again requires extensive suturing of the muscles. As the mobilisation of the teres major is more extensive when raising the angular branch, some devascularisation of the muscle may occur and Coleman & Sultan[10] have pointed out the need to resect any obviously non-viable muscle.

References

1. dos Santos L F 1980 Retalho escapular: um novo retalho livre microcirurgico. Revista Brasileira de Cirurgia 70: 133–144
2. Gilbert A, Teot L 1982 The free scapular flap. Plastic and Reconstructive Surgery 69: 601–604
3. Urbaniak J R, Koman L A, Goldner R D, Armstrong N B, Nunley J A 1982 The vascularized cutaneous scapular flap. Plastic and Reconstructive Surgery 69: 772–777
4. Barwick W J, Goodkind D J, Serafin D 1982 The free scapular flap. Plastic and Reconstructive Surgery 69: 779–785
5. Mayou B J, Whitby D, Jones B M 1982 The scapular flap – an anatomical and clinical study. British Journal of Plastic Surgery 35: 8–13
6. Hamilton S G L, Morrison W A 1982 The free scapular flap. British Journal of Plastic Surgery 35: 2–7
7. Batchelor A G, Bardsley A F 1987 The bi-scapular flap. British Journal of Plastic Surgery 40: 510–512
8. Thoma A, Heddle S 1990 The extended free scapular flap. British Journal of Plastic Surgery 43: 709–712
9. Swartz W M, Banis J C, Newton E D, Ramasastry S S, Jones N F, Acland R 1986 Osteocutaneous scapular flap for mandibular reconstruction. Plastic and Reconstructive Surgery 77: 530–545
10. Coleman J J, Sultan M R 1991 The bipedicled osteocutaneous scapula flap: a new subscapular system free flap. Plastic and Reconstructive Surgery 87: 682–692

CIRCUMFLEX SCAPULAR ARTERY – parascapular branch

Parascapular flap

The parascapular fasciocutaneous free flap was designed and named by Nassif et al[1] after 20 cadaver dissections had demonstrated the constancy of the parascapular branch of the circumflex scapular artery. The parascapular vessel may also be the main source of blood supply to a superiorly based pedicled flap raised from the back for transposition into the axilla.[2]

It shares with the horizontal scapular flap the particular attributes of constant anatomy, large vessels, long pedicle, hairless skin, moderate thickness and minimal donor site morbidity (direct closure possible). There is no potential for an innervated flap.

Anatomy

The salient features of the anatomy of the circumflex scapular artery have already been described in the context of the horizontal scapular flap. It may be questioned whether the parascapular flap is anything other than a scapular flap of a slightly different orientation, since the parascapular artery might be regarded simply as a branch of the horizontal artery. However, the parascapular artery is a vessel in its own right for two reasons. Firstly it is as large, both in diameter and in length, as the horizontal branch. Secondly, although it generally exits through the triangular space in the company of the horizontal branch, it may sometimes reach the surface at an alternative site, specific to it alone, below teres major rather than above it.[3]

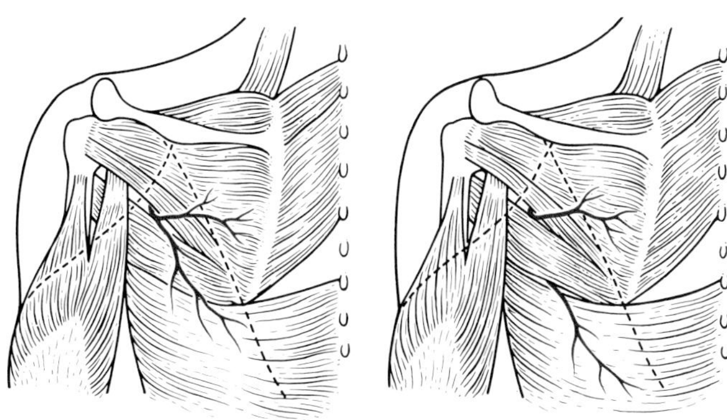

Fig. 7.12 Vascular anatomy. The parascapular branch may emerge in common with the horizontal branch above teres major, or – much less commonly – below teres major.

Flap planning

The upper end of the free flap is located at the level of the emerging branches of the circumflex scapular artery which may be surface marked by the procedure described under the horizontal scapular flap. The lower end of the flap may be situated up to 25–30 cm below this point. The maximum width of flap which still permits direct donor site closure is about 15 cm. The long axis of the flap follows the lateral border of the scapula and extends beyond it. This is different from the vertical scapula flap described by Mayou et al[4] which is centred over the scapula and has the horizontal scapular artery entering its middle rather than its end.

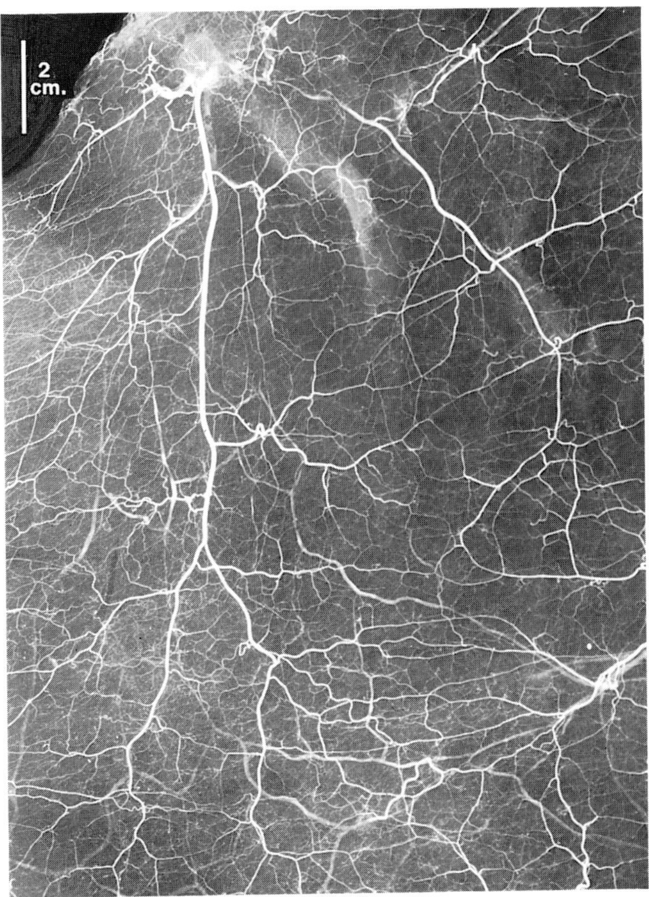

Fig. 7.13 Radiograph of skin and fascia showing a particularly strong parascapular branch.

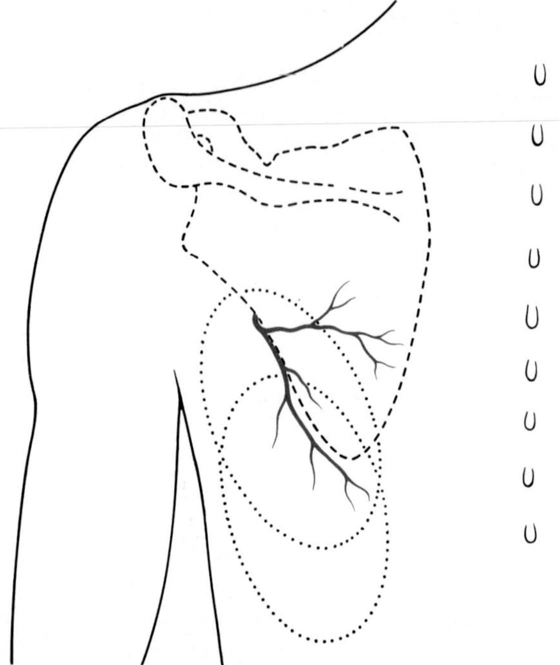

Fig. 7.14 Free flap planning. The orientation of the parascapular flap is indicated by the long axes of the ellipses indicated by dotted outlines. The more distal flap will have a longer pedicle. A larger flap could be raised by incorporating both the horizontal scapular and parascapular branches.

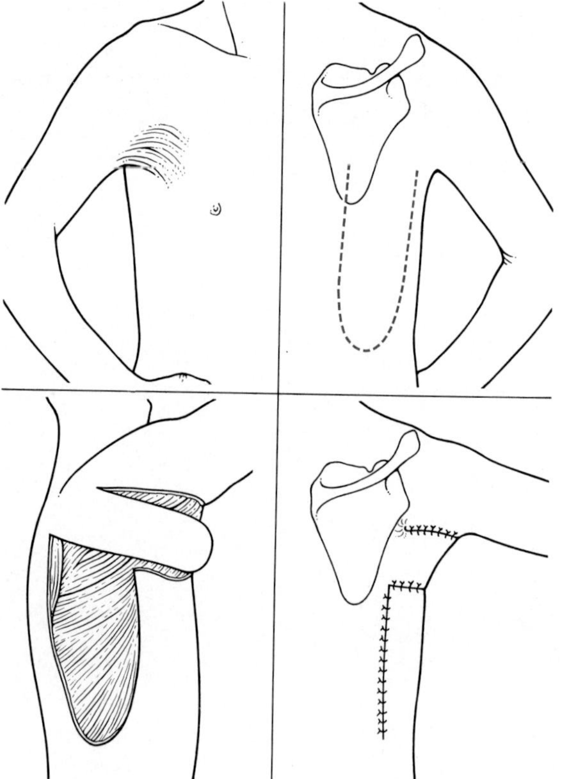

Fig. 7.15 Pedicled flap planning. Design of a pedicled skin flap is shown which incorporates the plexus of fascial vessels arising from the parascapular branch. Flap used in release of post-burn scar contracture of axillary fold.

The pedicled 'axillary' fasciocutaneous (Type A) flap described by Tolhurst & Haeseker[2] for transposition into the axilla after release of post-burn scar contractures owes its marked reliability and safety to this vessel (Fig. 7.15). Tolhurst described a case in which the pedicled flap included a skin grafted area amounting to 10% of the total area of the flap and about 50% of its base. The flap survived in its entirety, presumably because the branches of the parascapular artery escaped the original injury through lying at the level of the fascia and were able to nourish the flap.

A feature of the parascapular flap is that it may be combined with a latissimus dorsi flap to form a large regional unit of transplantable tissue which may be transferred on the one vascular axis, namely the subscapular trunk (except in the minority of cases (<5%) in which thoracodorsal and circumflex scapular arteries arise independently from the axillary artery).

Surgery

The incision starts at the supero-lateral margin of the flap, and may be extended horizontally into the axilla to provide further visualisation of the area between teres major and latissimus dorsi if a long pedicle is required. The location of the pedicle is confirmed, muscular branches are ligated and divided, and the remainder of the flap elevated. Further dissection of the pedicle may be required if more than 5–7 cm of vessel length are required. Widespread undermining, particularly laterally, should permit direct donor site closure.

To remove the parascapular flap in continuity with a latissimus flap the teres major muscle must be divided.

References

1. Nassif T M, Vidal L, Bovet J L, Baudet J 1982 The parascapular flap: A new cutaneous microsurgical free flap. Plastic and Reconstructive Surgery 69: 591–600
2. Tolhurst D E, Haeseker B 1982 Fasciocutaneous flaps in the axillary region. British Journal of Plastic Surgery 35: 430–435
3. Cormack G C, Lamberty B G H 1983 The anatomical vascular basis of the axillary fasciocutaneous pedicled flap. British Journal of Plastic Surgery 36: 425–427
4. Mayou B J, Whitby D, Jones B M 1982 The scapular flap – an anatomical and clinical study. British Journal of Plastic Surgery 35: 8–13
5. Fisette J, Boucq D, Lahaye T, Jacquemin D 1983 Notre expérience du lambeau libre parascapulaire. Annales de Chirurgie Plastique et Esthétique 28: 232–236
6. Fisette J, Lahaye T, Colot G 1983 The use of the free parascapular flap in midpalmar soft tissue defect. Annals of Plastic Surgery 10: 235–238

CIRCUMFLEX SCAPULAR ARTERY – vertical ascending branch

Vertical ascending scapular flap

7

This flap based on the ascending cutaneous branch of the circumflex scapular artery has been developed by Maruyama[1,2] for release of axillary burn scars. The horizontal and parascapular branches of the circumflex scapular artery are larger than the ascending branch so it might be questioned whether this flap actually represents an advance on the two classical flaps. The principal argument that can be put forward for its use is that in general the flap is thinner, particularly at its upper end, than the classical flaps.

Anatomy

No studies of the constancy of the ascending branch appear to have been carried out. Manchot and various German anatomy texts have illustrated this vessel and radiographs of injected specimens confirm its presence (Figs 6.26 & 7.9). The impression from a limited amount of data, is that this vessel tends to branch off the horizontal fasciocutaneous branch, although the origin may be from a trifurcation of the circumflex scapular artery as it emerges from the triangular space.

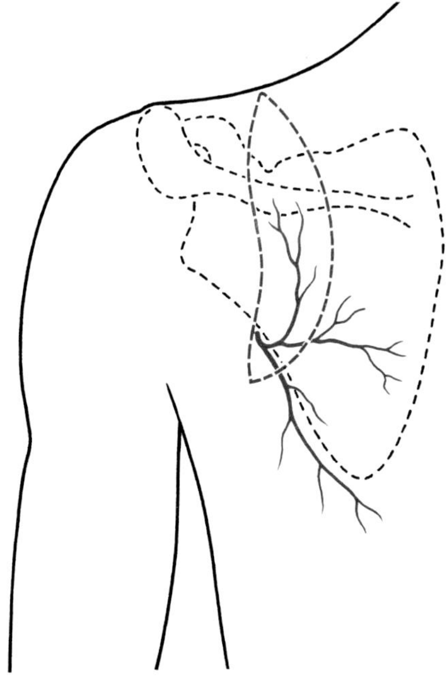

Fig. 7.16 Flap planning. An island flap has been outlined extending upwards from the triangular space.

Flap planning

The flap is outlined extending upwards from the triangular space, with the lateral margin medial to a line from the axilla to the acromion. The width of the flap is limited by the need to obtain direct closure of the donor site and this means that it will be less than 10 cm in width. Maruyama's flaps did not extend beyond the anterior border of the trapezius muscle and therefore 25 cm is about the upper limit for length.

Surgery

Elevation is straightforward and is carried out from medial to lateral including the dorsal thoracic fascia until the branches of the circumflex scapular artery are identified.

References

1. Maruyama Y 1991 Ascending scapular flap and its use for the treatment of axillary burn scar contracture. British Journal of Plastic Surgery 44: 97–101
2. Iwahira Y, Maruyama Y 1992 Free ascending scapular flap. Annals of Plastic Surgery 28: 565–572
3. Ohsaki M, Maruyama Y 1993 Anatomical investigations of the cutaneous branches of the circumflex scapular artery and their communications. British Journal of Plastic Surgery 46: 160–163

7 DEEP CIRCUMFLEX ILIAC ARTERY

DCIA osteocutaneous flap

The first successful transfers of vascularised iliac crest and groin skin were carried out by O'Brien et al in 1976,[1] by Tamai in 1976 and by Taylor et al in 1977,[2] using the superficial circumflex iliac system of vessels. Observations made by Taylor at the time of raising some of these flaps indicated that the deep system was superior in supplying the bone, and this was later confirmed by experimental[3] and clinical[4] studies which also defined more clearly the area of skin which was capable of being perfused by the deep system. Most applications have concentrated on mandibular reconstruction,[5,6] although the flap also has a place in the reconstruction of leg and pelvic defects. Refinements[7] have included reducing the amount of muscle taken with the bone, using only the inner cortex of the ilium, shaping of the bone with osteotomies, and improving the function of reconstructed mandibles by the use of osseo-integrated dental prostheses.

Anatomy

The deep circumflex iliac artery (DCIA) has a diameter of 2 mm (range 1.5–3) at its point of origin from the external iliac artery just above the inguinal ligament. It passes superolaterally towards the anterior superior iliac spine and whilst still medial to it gives off an ascending branch (also known as lateral epigastric) which ascends between transversus abdominis and internal oblique to supply muscle only (see Fig. 6.42). The DCIA then follows the curve of the anterior half of the iliac crest separated from it by the iliacus fascia and the iliacus muscle which it supplies. At about the level of the ASIS the DCIA passes beneath the arch of the transversalis fascia and comes to lie lateral and adjacent to the line of fusion between the iliacus and transversalis fasciae. As it passes back it gives off three to nine musculocutaneous branches to transversus abdominis until some 6 to 9 cm back from the ASIS it penetrates transversus, supplying the muscle and the overlying skin. The area of skin supplied lies behind the ASIS, over the crest and above the crest.

The blood supply to the bone of the iliac crest is via branches of two sorts: (1) musculoperiosteal via the attached muscles – mainly iliacus – and (2) nutrient via the multiple small foramina on the medial aspect of the crest and blade of the ilium.

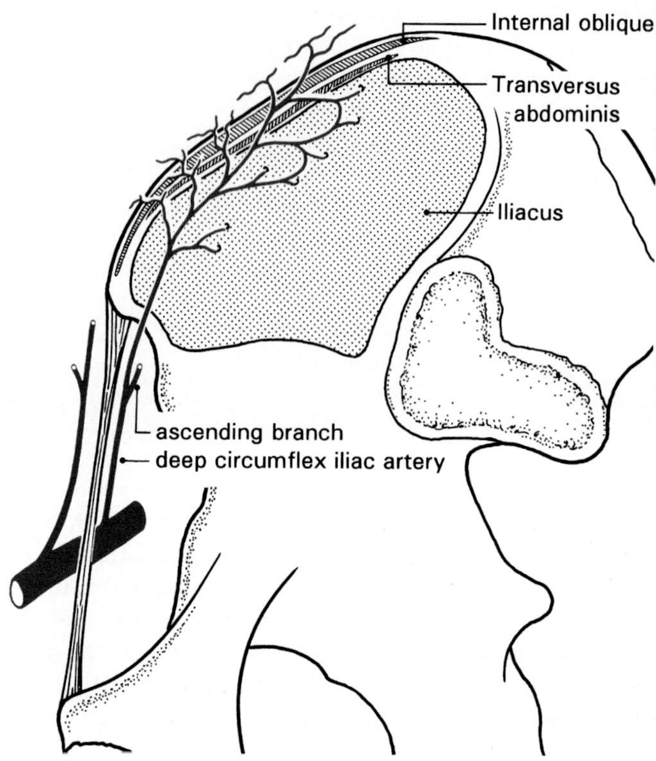

Fig. 7.17 Vascular anatomy. The relationship of deep circumflex iliac artery to inner aspect of ilium is shown.

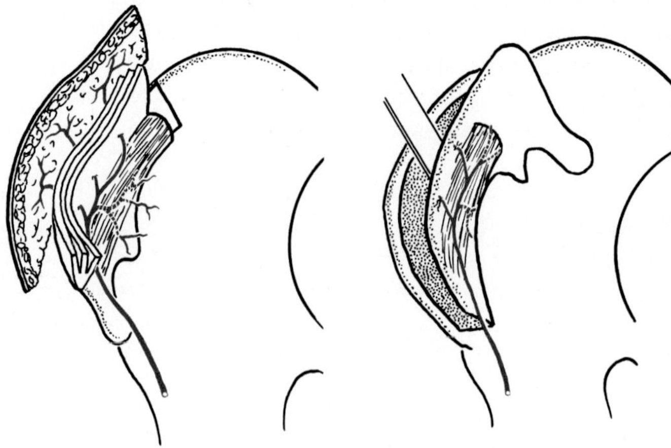

Fig. 7.18 Flap planning: **1.** osteomusculocutaneous; **2.** inner table only.

The paired venae comitantes of the DCIA unite some 2 cm lateral to the external iliac artery to form a single vein 2 to 4 mm in diameter. This vein then diverges from the artery in a superior direction, crossing either in front of or behind the external iliac artery to drain into the external iliac vein.

Significant variations from the normal pattern which may trap the unwary are as follows:

1. The ascending branch may be given off early and may be mistaken for the main trunk of the DCIA.
2. The main trunk of the DCIA may pierce the transversus abdominis muscle medial to the ASIS to lie in a more superficial plane than usual.
3. The DCIA may be duplicated with the medial element supplying iliacus.

Flap planning

There are three flap options: (1) a free osteomusculocutaneous flap; (2) a free musculocutaneous flap; and (3) a free vascularised bone graft, consisting of either the full thickness of the iliac crest or only the inner cortex of the ilium.

The cutaneous portion is designed as a skin ellipse parallel to the iliac crest with two-thirds of the width of the flap above the crest and one-third over/below the crest. The medial end of the ellipse is located overlying or immediately medial to the ASIS. The bone component is designed from the ipsilateral or contralateral ilium depending on the defect and the papers of Taylor[4] and David[7] should be consulted.

Surgery

There are three approaches to exposing the vascular pedicle: (1) by the transinguinal approach as described by Taylor in which the vessels are identified through the posterior wall of the inguinal canal; (2) by an approach through all the muscles above the inguinal canal; or (3) by a sub-inguinal approach in which a small bone block is removed at the lateral attachment of the inguinal ligament and this is then reflected upwards.

Transinguinal approach. The superior border of the skin ellipse is incised, the incision taken through external oblique, and then carried medially parallel to and above the inguinal ligament. The spermatic cord is retracted upwards and the DCIA and vein are approached through the posterior wall of the inguinal canal. To follow the pedicle laterally the transversus abdominis and internal oblique attachments to the inguinal ligament are divided. As the ASIS is approached, the ascending branch of the DCIA and the deep branch to iliacus are identified and care taken not to damage the accompanying vein. Next the internal oblique and transversus muscles are divided 2 cm above and parallel to the crest for a distance of 6 to 8 cm back from the ASIS. Then the transversalis fascia is incised, fat pushed back, the groove between iliacus and transversalis fascia identified, and the iliacus fascia and muscle divided 1 cm medial to this. Access is thereby gained to the medial aspect of the ilium which is further exposed by detaching iliacus whilst leaving periosteum intact. The bone part of the osteocutaneous flap can then be isolated on the medial side and finally the lower border of the skin island is incised, TFL, the glutei, sartorius and the inguinal ligament are detached, and the osteotomies completed levering the bone forward and medially so as to avoid tension on the DCIA pedicle.

Sub-inguinal approach. The medial end of the flap is incised and raised so as to gain access to the ASIS. A pilot hole is drilled in the ASIS at the point of attachment of the inguinal ligament and a malleolar AO screw inserted for 1 cm into this hole. With an osteotome a block of bone carrying the inguinal ligament insertion and this screw are then removed and the whole inguinal ligament and attachments can then be reflected upwards to expose the pedicle. Reconstruction of the donor site is facilitated by fastening the bone block back onto the pelvis by advancing the screw. In other respects the elevation of the flap is similar. Careful closure of the donor site defect is critical and starts with attaching iliacus fascia and muscle to the transversalis fascia and transversus muscle. Internal and external oblique are sutured to the glutei, to TFL and to the fascia lata. With the transinguinal approach the inguinal canal is repaired and the inguinal ligament reattached.

References

1. O'Brien B M, Morrison W A, MacLeod A M, Dooley B J 1979 Microvascular osteocutaneous transfer using the groin flap and iliac crest and the dorsalis pedis flap and second metatarsal. British Journal of Plastic Surgery 32: 188–206
2. Taylor G I, Watson N 1978 One stage repair of compound leg defects with free, revascularized flaps of groin skin and iliac bone. Plastic and Reconstructive Surgery 61: 494–506
3. Taylor G I, Townsend P, Corlett R 1979 Superiority of the deep circumflex iliac vessels as supply for free groin flaps. Experimental work. Plastic and Reconstructive Surgery 64: 595–604
4. Taylor G I, Townsend P, Corlett R 1979 Superiority of the deep circumflex iliac vessels as supply for free groin flaps. Clinical work. Plastic and Reconstructive Surgery 64: 745–759
5. Bitter K, Schlesinger S, Westerman U 1983 The iliac bone or osteocutaneous transplant pedicled to the deep circumflex iliac artery. Journal of Maxillofacial Surgery 11: 241–247
6. Salibian A H, Rappaport I, Allison G 1985 Functional oromandibular reconstruction with the microvascular composite groin flap. Plastic and Reconstructive Surgery 76: 819–825
7. David D J, Tan E, Katsaros J, Sheen R 1988 Mandibular reconstruction with vascularised iliac crest: a 10-year experience. Plastic and Reconstructive Surgery 82: 792–801

7

DEEP INFERIOR EPIGASTRIC ARTERY

Upper rectus abdominis musculocutaneous flap
Extended deep inferior epigastric artery flap
Upper abdominal 'flag flap'
Transverse rectus abdominis musculocutaneous (TRAM) flap

Rectus abdominis musculocutaneous flaps supplied by the deep inferior system may be either pedicled flaps (usually from above the umbilicus) or free flaps (usually from around or below the umbilicus). Pedicled flaps based inferiorly have a wide arc of rotation and may be used for filling defects on the abdomen, flanks, ipsilateral groin, anterior perineum and will reach to the mid-axillary line on the same side or the anterior superior iliac spine on the other side. Flaps may reach defects on the thigh including amputations thereby permitting conservation of bone length. Flaps may also be tunnelled within the pelvis to reach pelvic floor defects or provide vaginal reconstruction. The four variations on inferiorly pedicled flaps described below are only an indication of the many arrangements that are possible.

The lower abdominal transverse ellipse (TRAM flap) is the most common design of free flap because of its application in breast reconstruction. The oblique flap described by Taylor (extended DIEA flap) is a very versatile and reliable free flap and some surgeons have reduced the muscle component of this flap to virtually nil by carefully dissecting the artery and a few selected perforators free from the rectus muscle.

Anatomy

The deep inferior epigastric artery (mean diameter 3.5 mm) arises from the external iliac artery just above the inguinal ligament, and approaches the rectus abdominis from its lateral side. The distance from the insertion of the rectus tendon to the intersection of this artery with the lateral rectus margin – the medial side of Hasselbach's triangle – is around 7 cm although occasionally the artery may pursue a course entirely behind the tendon so that it is hidden from view. This length of the artery is accompanied by two venae comitantes and therefore forms a suitable pedicle for a free microvascular transfer. Milloy et al[2] found that the inferior epigastric artery consisted of a single main stem in 86% of cases and divided into two in 14%. After lying on the posterior aspect of the muscle the vessel(s) usually enters the substance of the muscle in its middle third (78%) but otherwise in the lower third (17%) or upper third (5%).

With all these flaps the blood supply to the skin island is derived from the musculocutaneous perforators through and around the borders of rectus abdominis and depends on the anastomoses which these perforators make with the cutaneous network fed by intercostal arteries, the superficial inferior epigastric artery, the superficial superior epigastric artery and the superficial circumflex iliac arteries.

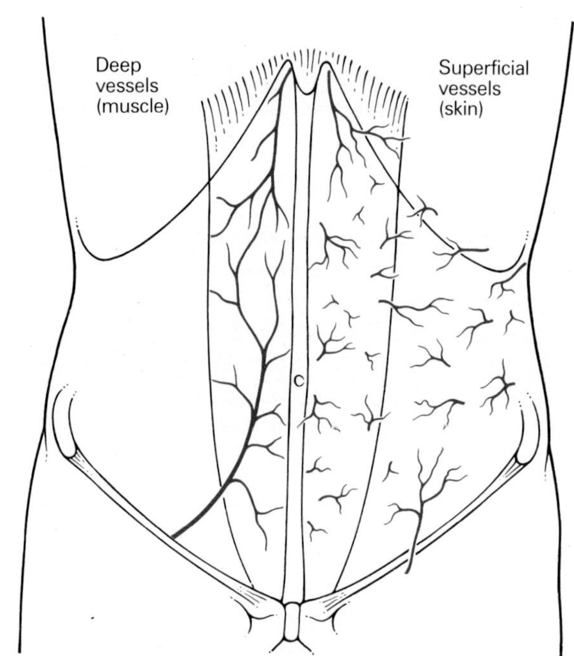

Fig. 7.19 Vascular anatomy. See also radiographs 6.17, 6.36 and 6.38.

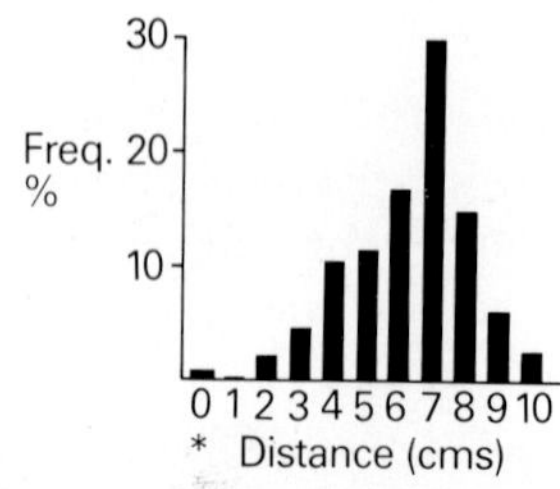

Fig. 7.20 Histogram for point of intersection of the inferior epigastric artery with the lateral border of rectus abdominis in centimetres above the pubic crest (162 muscles). *Epigastric artery entirely behind the tendon of rectus. (After Milloy et al, 1960.)

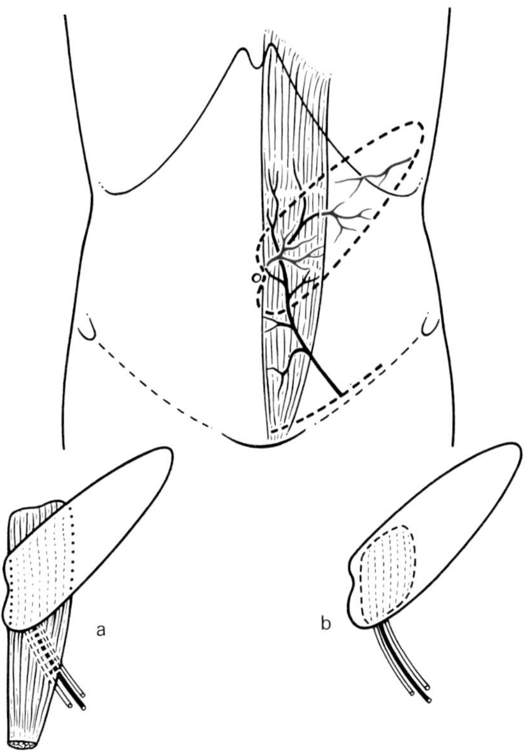

Fig. 7.21 Epigastric free flap after Taylor (1984): **a** and **b** indicate how the muscle component around the vascular pedicle can be reduced to a pad beneath the skin flap.

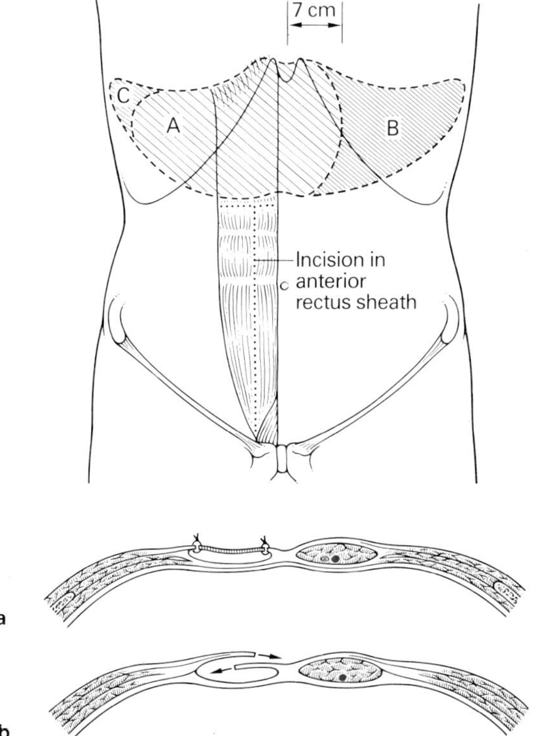

Fig. 7.22 Epigastric 'flag flap' after De La Plaza: **a** indicates method of closure of upper rectus sheath, and **b** the lower rectus sheath.

Surgery

The extended deep inferior epigastric artery flap (DIEA)
The basis of this flap is the fact that the paraumbilical musculocutaneous perforators arising from the inferior epigastric artery tend to fan out away from the umbilicus, and those above the level of the umbilicus are predominantly directed upwards and laterally in the line of the intercostal spaces where they connect with cutaneous branches of the intercostal system. A skin island may therefore be based on these paraumbilical perforators and extended over the costal margin towards the lower pole of the scapula (Fig. 7.21). This may be used as a pedicled flap,[1] or as a free flap.[3] The flap is elevated from lateral to medial so as to include the underlying epimysium. The rectus muscle is mobilised through a longitudinal incision in the anterior wall of the rectus sheath, preserving only the disc of fascia that lies between the skin flap and the rectus muscle, and the superior epigastric artery is ligated cephalad to the flap. The rectus muscle can either be preserved over the vessels, or the vessels can be dissected free of surrounding fibres except beneath the flap where muscle is left surrounding the terminal branches and perforators of the inferior epigastric artery. This can be carried out through a vertical paramedian incision or through a transverse suprapubic incision. The rectus sheath is repaired and the donor site closed directly. Taylor has reported that injection studies suggest the feasibility of combining a segment of the ninth or tenth rib with the flap to create a vascularised osteo-myo-cutaneous graft.

The flag flap
A large transverse ellipse of skin reaching laterally to the anterior-axillary lines is incised on the upper abdomen and inframammary fold area, and is based on one rectus muscle.[4] The lateral parts of the ellipse are in turn lifted towards the midline and the margins of the rectus sheath are incised so that the anterior wall of the sheath remains between the flap and the underlying muscle. At the lower margin of the flap a transverse incision is made through the anterior rectus sheath and the lower sheath is then incised longitudinally all the way down to the pubis along a line lying at the junction of the medial one-third with the lateral two-thirds.

An approximately triangular-shaped piece of the ellipse will serve as the flap (A in Fig. 7.22) based on one rectus muscle. The perforators piercing the uppermost part of the sheath from the superior epigastric artery are small (<0.5 mm D, i.e. smaller than the paraumbilical ones) and are unable to support the ipsilateral tip of the ellipse which is therefore discarded (C). The contralateral half of the ellipse is safely supported up to a point approximately 7 cm across the midline and the skin beyond this (B) is excised but not discarded because it may be de-epithelialised and de-fatted and later used to reconstruct the anterior wall of the upper rectus sheath. The harvested split skin from this same portion may be expanded and used to cover the rectus muscle if an external pedicle is planned. Finally the abdominal skin is advanced upwards and the defect closed with the resulting scar lying in the submammary fold. The umbilicus is relocated.

Upper abdominal ellipse

The principles here are similar except that the skin island is not positioned as high as in the 'flag flap' and the ellipse, which is smaller ($<10 \times 20$ cm), is confined within the costal margins (Fig. 7.23). An island of this size can survive entirely although the contralateral tip may show some vascular stasis.[5] The defect can be closed directly or, in a thin individual, split skin grafted. A better arrangement may be a vertically orientated ellipse sited over the muscle.

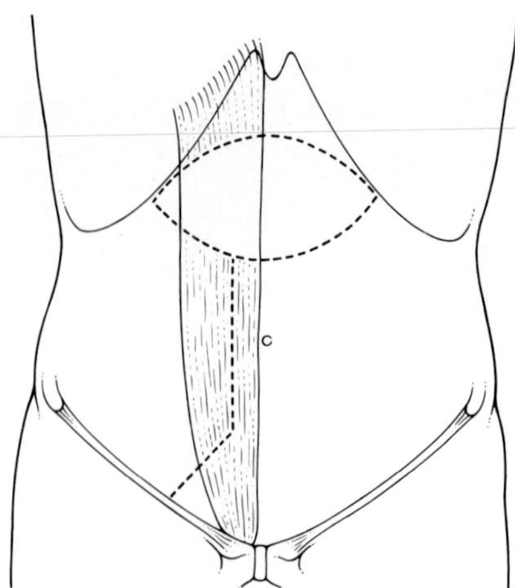

Fig. 7.23 Epigastric pedicled flap after Logan & Mathes (1984). The small skin island is largely confined within the costal margins.

Bilobe modification of extended DIEA flap

This modification may be useful when using a large DIEA flap as a local transposition for closure of upper abdominal wall defects. An inferior lobe of the flap provides a means of achieving direct closure of the defect resulting from transposition of the main part of the flap. The technique is shown in Figure 7.24. To facilitate rotation of the flap without twisting the perforators, the rectus muscle is divided in its lower part whilst preserving the main pedicle intact.

Perineal or vaginal reconstruction

The muscle pedicle may be passed downwards within the pelvic rim either extra- or intraperitoneally for reconstructions in the pelvic floor. For neo-vaginal reconstruction the ipsilateral triangular half of a lower abdominal ellipse may be preferable to a vertical ellipse as this generally allows a greater width of flap and thus diameter of neo-vagina.

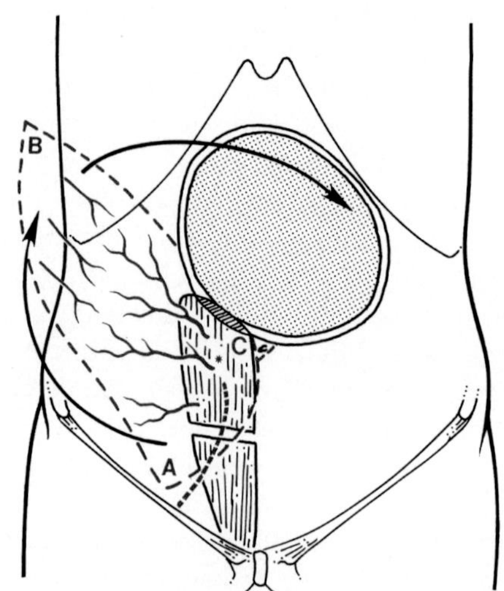

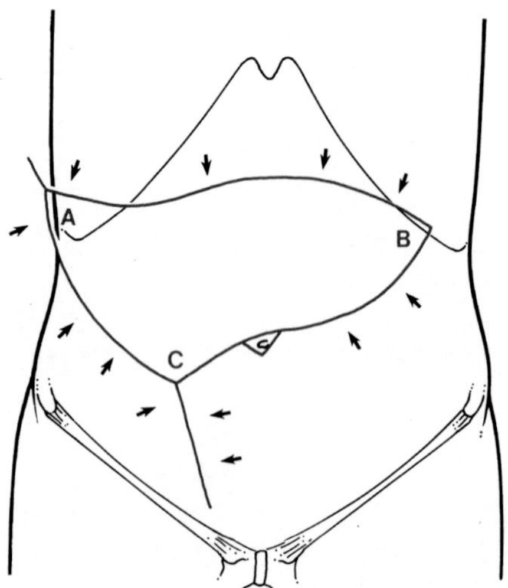

Fig. 7.24 Bilobe flap design and transposition for upper abdominal defect.

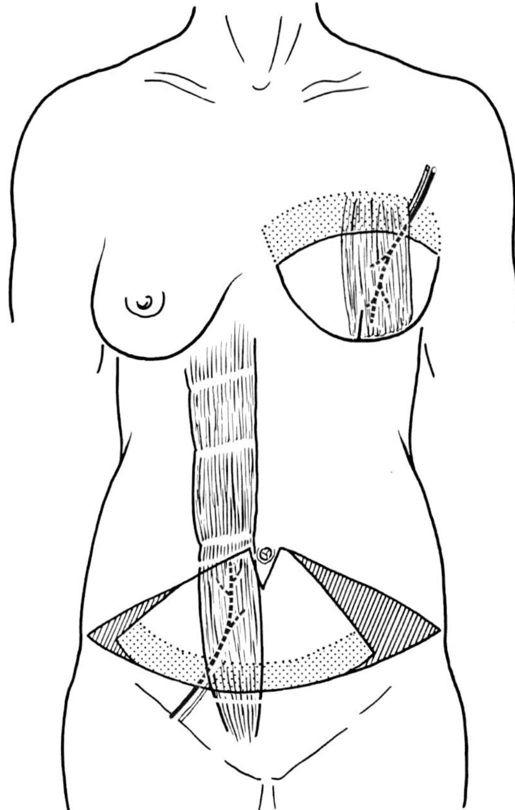

Fig. 7.25 Free TRAM flap with deep inferior epigastric artery and vein anastomosed to vessels in the contralateral axilla. The shaded areas are discarded and the dotted area may be de-epithelialised and inset beneath the upper chest skin.

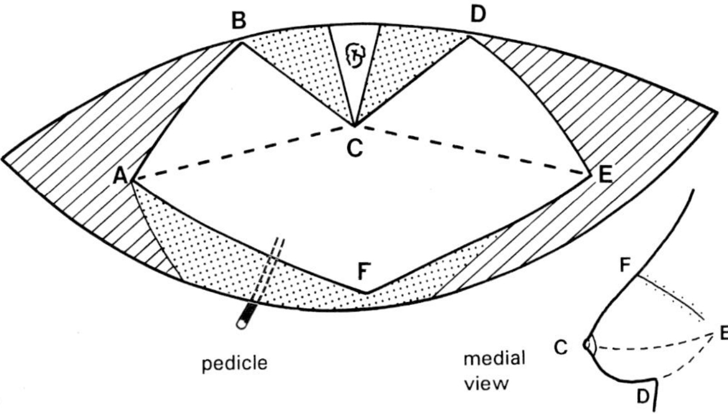

Fig. 7.26 Shaded areas discarded and dotted areas de-epithelialised as required. For a left breast reconstruction the measurements are taken from the right breast and applied as follows:
BC = CD = the normal inframammary fold to nipple distance
ACE = the equator of the normal breast
AB = the length of the inframammary line lateral to the meridian
DE = the length of the inframammary line medial to the meridian
<ABC = <CDE = 90°
FCD = vertical skin defect measured over the curve of the normal breast in the meridian from a projection of the mastectomy scar to the level of the inframammary fold.

The free TRAM flap

The classical transversely-orientated rectus abdominis myocutaneous flap is described under the deep superior epigastric artery. However, since the anastomosis between superior and inferior systems lies above the umbilicus, and since the inferior vessel is by far the larger it makes for a better vascularised and more reliable breast reconstruction if the TRAM flap is transferred as a free flap with anastomosis of the inferior epigastric artery in the axilla.[8] Areas at the ends of the ellipse are discarded and a variable amount may be de-epithelialised to provide bulk beneath the upper chest skin (Fig. 7.25). Alternative designs[9] have been developed to enhance the degree of ptosis obtained in the reconstructed breast (Fig. 7.26).

References

1. Taylor G I, Corlett R, Boyd J B 1983 The extended deep inferior epigastric flap: A clinical technique. Plastic and Reconstructive Surgery 72: 751–764
2. Milloy F J, Anson B J, McAfee D K 1960 The rectus abdominis muscles and the epigastric arteries. Surgery, Gynaecology and Obstetrics 110: 293–302
3. Taylor G I, Corlett R J, Boyd J B 1984 The versatile deep inferior epigastric (inferior rectus abdominis) flap. British Journal of Plastic Surgery 37: 330–350
4. De La Plaze R, Arroyo J M, Vasconez L O 1984 Upper transverse rectus abdominis flap: The flag flap. Annals of Plastic Surgery 12: 410–418
5. Logan S E, Mathes S J 1984 The use of a rectus abdominis myocutaneous flap to reconstruct a groin defect. British Journal of Plastic Surgery 37: 351–353
6. Bostwick J, Hill H L, Nahai F 1979 Repairs in the lower abdomen, groin or perineum with myocutaneous or omental flaps. Plastic and Reconstructive Surgery 63: 186–194
7. Cormack G C, Quaba A A 1991 Case report: Bilobe modification of the deep inferior epigastric artery flap for abdominal wall defect reconstruction. British Journal of Plastic Surgery 44: 541–543
8. Friedman R J, Argenta L C, Anderson R 1985 Case report. Deep inferior epigastric free flap for breast reconstruction after radical mastectomy. Plastic and Reconstructive Surgery 76: 455–458
9. Tobin G R, Day T G 1988 Vaginal and pelvic reconstruction with distally based rectus abdominis myocutaneous flaps. Plastic and Reconstructive Surgery 81: 62–70

7 DEEP SUPERIOR EPIGASTRIC ARTERY

Rectus abdominis musculocutaneous flap

Various pedicled abdominal flaps, based either knowingly or unknowingly on musculocutaneous perforators from the rectus abdominis muscle, had been used for many years prior to 1977 when true island rectus abdominis musculocutaneous (RAM) flaps were introduced.[1] Island RAM flaps pedicled on the superior epigastric artery were initially used for chest and abdominal wall reconstruction[2,3] and later introduced by Robbins[4] for post-mastectomy breast reconstruction as an alternative to the latissimus dorsi flap. He used a longitudinal flap overlying the upper part of the rectus, and others subsequently introduced bipedicle flaps,[5] longitudinal flaps from the central paraumbilical area,[6] supraumbilical horizontal ellipses,[7] infraumbilical horizontal ellipses,[7,8,9] upper abdominal horizontal flaps from one side,[10] and L-shaped flaps[11] (in reality two separate island flaps on one rectus). The major role for all these flaps is in post-mastectomy breast reconstruction when a latissimus flap is considered inappropriate or the patient prefers an abdominal scar. Some of these flaps are intended only for the contralateral breast, some only for the ipsilateral and some for either side. No single flap is suitable for all cases and individual factors, such as the presence of abdominal scars, will preclude flaps in certain positions. Previous radiotherapy to the anterior chest wall, involving the area of the internal thoracic artery, is a relative contraindication.

Anatomy

All these flaps are based on the superior deep epigastric artery which enters the upper part of the rectus sheath between the xiphoid and the seventh costal cartilage where it lies on the posterior surface of the muscle or is occasionally buried in the muscle tissue. The vessel usually enters the sheath as a single trunk behind the medial or the middle third of the muscle (Fig 7.29a & b) and after a short course on the surface enters the muscle where it anastomoses with the inferior epigastric artery approximately half-way between the xiphoid and the umbilicus. Only very rarely is this anastomosis on the posterior surface of the muscle. The superior epigastric artery is therefore the lesser vessel of supply to rectus abdominis and this is reflected by its smaller diameter compared to the inferior epigastric artery (1.6 and 3.4 mm respectively). Branches are given off from the epigastric arcade to rectus abdominis and many of these vessels terminate as perforators to the overlying skin. Several large perforators tend to overlie the lateral edge of the muscle and therefore pierce the anterior rectus sheath just medial to the linea semilunaris. Many smaller perforators emerge round the medial edge of the muscle and lie adjacent to the linea alba with two or three particularly large perforators on each side occurring in the paraumbilical area. All these

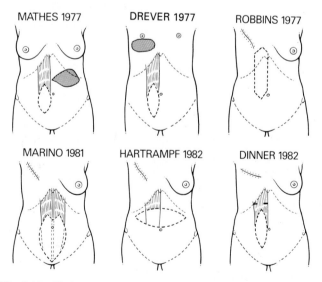

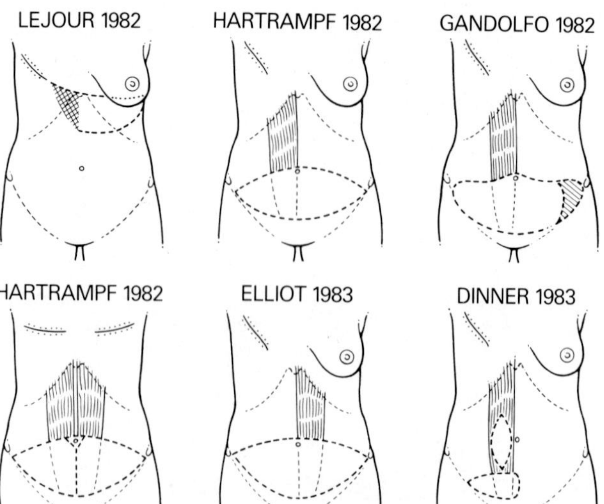

Fig. 7.27 Various designs of superiorly pedicled RAM flaps.

perforators spread out in the subcutis, mainly radiating away from the umbilicus (Fig. 7.31).

In addition, the epigastric arcade gives off several branches on each side which run in the plane between transversus abdominis and internal oblique and either end in the lateral abdominal musculature or anastomose with the deep branches of the intercostal arteries (Figs 6.36. & 6.37 are relevant). Over the lowermost end of rectus abdominis the skin is also supplied by branches of the superficial external pudendal artery.

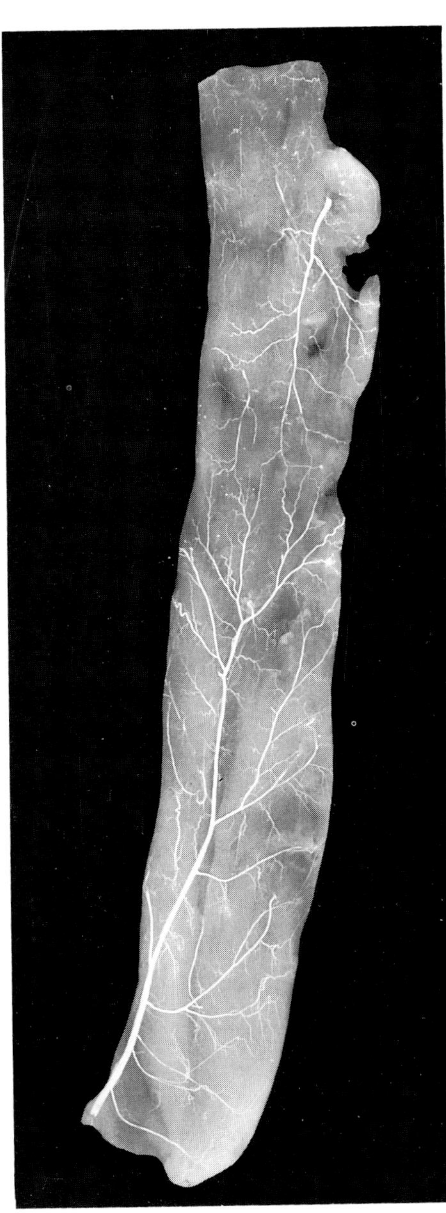

Fig. 7.28 Radiograph of injected rectus abdominis muscle as shown here, reveals a more frequent occurrence of anastomoses.

Surgery

Details of the technique greatly depend on the position of the flap and its intended use. Certain general principles may however be identified.

The *skin island* is positioned as dictated by the requirements of flap size, flap thickness, desired scar position, need for abdominoplasty, presence of previously operated areas, and general patient condition. Paraumbilical perforators are crucial.

The *pedicle* may be situated on the same side as the defect, on the opposite side or may be bilateral. With a lower abdominal ellipse the contralateral pedicle is subjected to less twisting on its course to the defect than an ipsilateral pedicle which may be required to fold on itself if the ellipse is to be positioned with the umbilical area pointing inferiorly. Division of the uppermost of the intercostal nerves supplying the rectus muscle is important to ensure denervation and subsequent atrophy of the muscle, thereby reducing the prominence of the pedicle in the epigastrium. It is not necessary to resect the 7th rib cartilage and dissect the pedicle above the costal margin unless using an upper abdominal horizontal ellipse when resection may be necessary in order to obtain a sufficient arc of rotation. Incisions through the medial and lateral thirds of the muscle sparing the vascular pedicle in the middle will increase the mobility of the pedicle. However, intraoperative flow studies on the

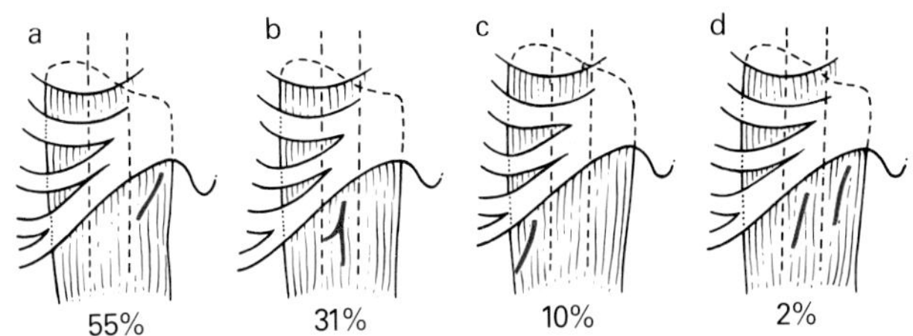

Fig. 7.29 The position of the deep superior epigastric artery on the dorsal aspect of the left rectus muscle after piercing the posterior rectus sheath is shown. The artery frequently appears as two stems but only occasionally do they lie in different thirds (d). (After Milloy et al, 1960.)

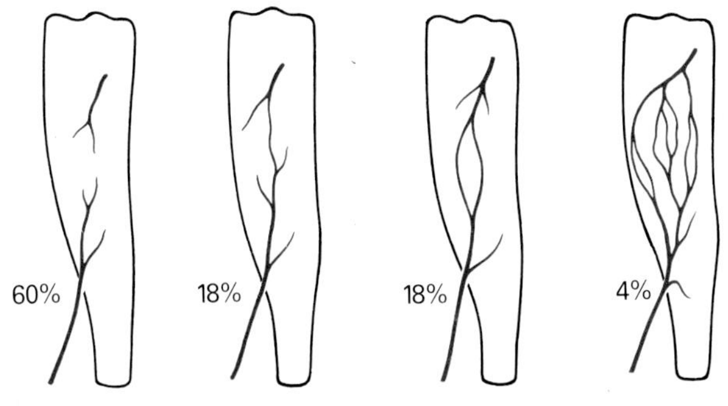

Fig. 7.30 The number of anastomoses between superior and inferior epigastric arteries *demonstrable by dissection* as reported by Milloy et al, 1960.

TRAM flap after division of the DIEA have demonstrated that manual compression of the medial and lateral thirds of the muscle at the cephalic edge of the flap (to simulate division of these parts) reduced the pressure in the DIEA in 80% of cases by an average of 19%.

The *integrity of the abdominal wall* following one of these procedures is an important consideration. Absence of a single rectus muscle does not cause problems but weakness of the rectus sheath consequent on excising parts of it can be problematic. For this reason it is advisable to keep the anterior wall defect above the arcuate line. (This commonly lies half-way between umbilicus and pubis – approximately 8 cm above the pubic crest – but is subject to great variation.) Removal of the anterior sheath below this level requires a synthetic mesh repair. Above this level the anterior sheath can usually be closed directly if a 2 cm strip is preserved medially.

Delays. A prior ligation of the inferior epigastric artery in an endeavour to improve the blood flow to the lower part of the muscle (and thence to skin) from the superior epigastric has been tried with inconsistent results and at the present time the value of such delay remains unproven. However, it is clear from various studies that the deep inferior epigastric vein contains valves which direct blood caudally. When the TRAM flap is isolated on a superior pedicle, flow in these veins is reversed against the direction of the valves. Prior 'delay' directed at ligation of the deep inferior epigastric vein may be effective in improving venous drainage.

'Turbo-TRAM'. To overcome the problems of poor flap perfusion in the area furthest removed from the pedicle when using larger than normal flaps, additional microvascular anastomosis has been carried out of the superficial inferior epigastric artery and vein to vessels in the axilla. In this design the flap is pedicled on the contralateral muscle, inset vertically, and the ipsilateral superficial epigastric a. and v. are anatomosed. This variant has been nick-named the 'turbo-charged TRAM'.

Bipedicled TRAM. To improve the perfusion of the lower abdominal TRAM flap it may be raised with input from both superior epigastric arteries (Fig. 7.32c). As taking both rectus muscles would significantly impair the integrity of the abdominal wall, only partial harvesting of the muscles is carried out. This intramuscular dissection of the pedicle is aided by intraoperative Doppler location of the main vessels. Approximately 30 to 40% of the width of each muscle is preserved laterally where it is innervated by intercostal nerves and supplied by intercostal arteries (see Fig. 6.36). A small strip of <10% of the muscle width is preserved medially and although denervated it is probably vascularised through the connections of the tendinous intersections with the anterior sheath. This allows direct closure of the rectus sheath defects bilaterally with preservation of some rectus function.

A similar intramuscular dissection can be used to raise two flaps for simultaneous bilateral volume replacement following subcutaneous mastectomies (Fig. 7.32d).

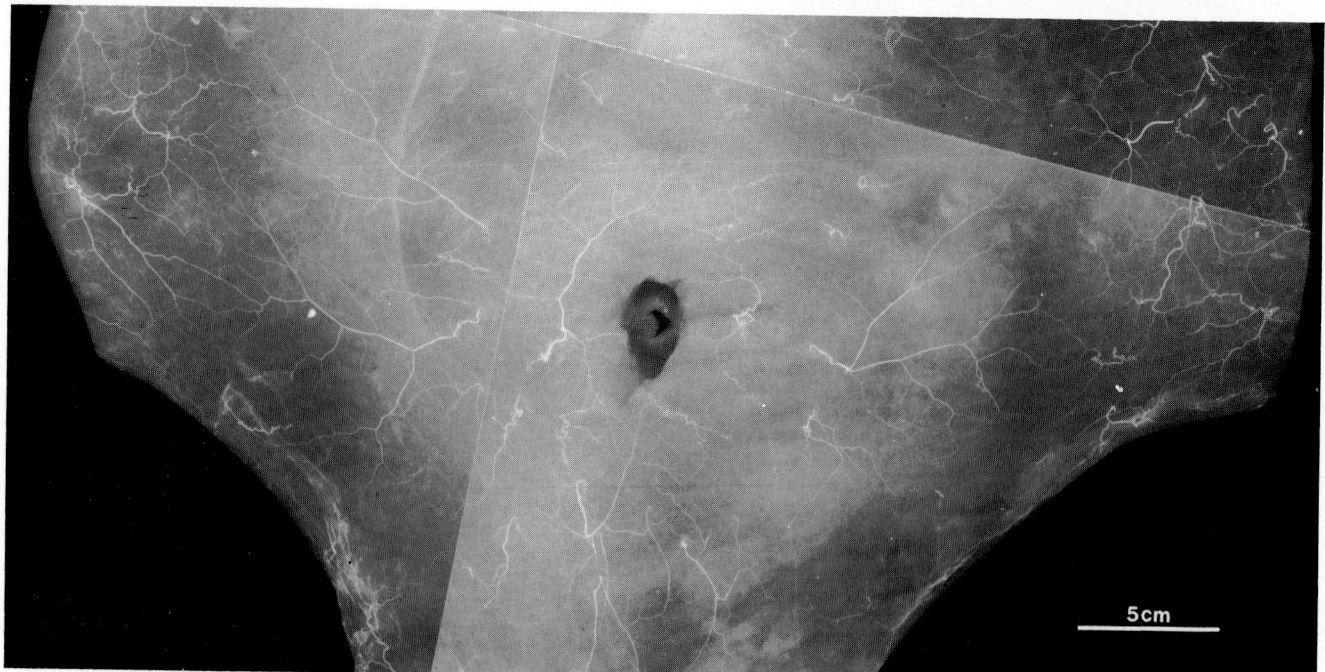

Fig. 7.31 Radiograph of anterior abdominal wall skin and subcutaneous tissues.

References

1. McCraw J B, Dibbell D G, Carraway JH 1977 Clinical definition of independent myocutaneous vascular territories. Plastic and Reconstructive Surgery 60: 341–352
2. Mathes S J, Bostwick J 1977 A rectus abdominis myocutaneous flap to reconstruct abdominal wall defects. British Journal of Plastic Surgery 30: 282–283
3. Drever J M 1970 Total breast reconstruction with either of two abdominal flaps. Plastic and Reconstructive Surgery 59: 185–190
4. Robbins T H 1979 Rectus abdominis myocutaneous flap for breast reconstruction. Australian and New Zealand Journal of Surgery 49: 527–530
5. Marino H Jr, Dogliotti P 1981 Mammary reconstruction with bipedicled abdominal flap: case report. Plastic and Reconstructive Surgery 68: 933–936
6. Dinner M I, Labandter H P, Dowden R V 1982 The role of the rectus abdominis myocutaneous flap in breast reconstruction. Plastic and Reconstructive Surgery 69: 209–214
7. Hartrampf C R, Scheflan M, Black P W 1982 Breast reconstruction with a transverse abdominal island flap. Plastic and Reconstructive Surgery 69: 216–224
8. Gandolfo E A 1982 Breast reconstruction with a lower abdominal myocutaneous flap. British Journal of Plastic Surgery 35: 452–457
9. Scheflan M D, Dinner M I 1983 Transverse abdominal island flap: Indications, contraindications, results, and complications. Annals of Plastic Surgery 10: 24–35
10. Lejour M, De Mey A 1983 Anatomical study and technique of rectus abdominis musculocutaneous flaps (in French). Annales de Chirurgie Plastique et Esthétique 28: 151–158
11. Dinner M I, Dowden R V 1983 The L-shaped combined vertical and transverse abdominal island flap for breast reconstruction. Plastic and Reconstructive Surgery 72: 894–898
12. Harris N R, Webb M S, May J W 1992 Intraoperative physiologic blood flow studies in the TRAM flap. Plastic and Reconstructive Surgery 90: 553–558
13. Carramenha-e-Costa M A, Carriquiry C, Vasconez L O, Grotting J C, Herrera R H, Windle B H 1987 An anatomic study of the venous drainage of the transverse rectus abdominis musculocutaneous flap. Plastic and Reconstructive Surgery 79: 208–213
14. Taylor G I, Corlett R J, Caddy C M, Zelt R G 1992 An anatomic review of the delay phenomenon: II Clinical applications. Plastic and Reconstructive Surgery 89: 408–416
15. Harashina T, Sone K, Inoue T, Fukuzumi S, Enomoto K 1987 Augmentation of circulation of pedicled transverse rectus abdominis musculocutaneous flaps by microvascular surgery. British Journal of Plastic Surgery 40: 367–370

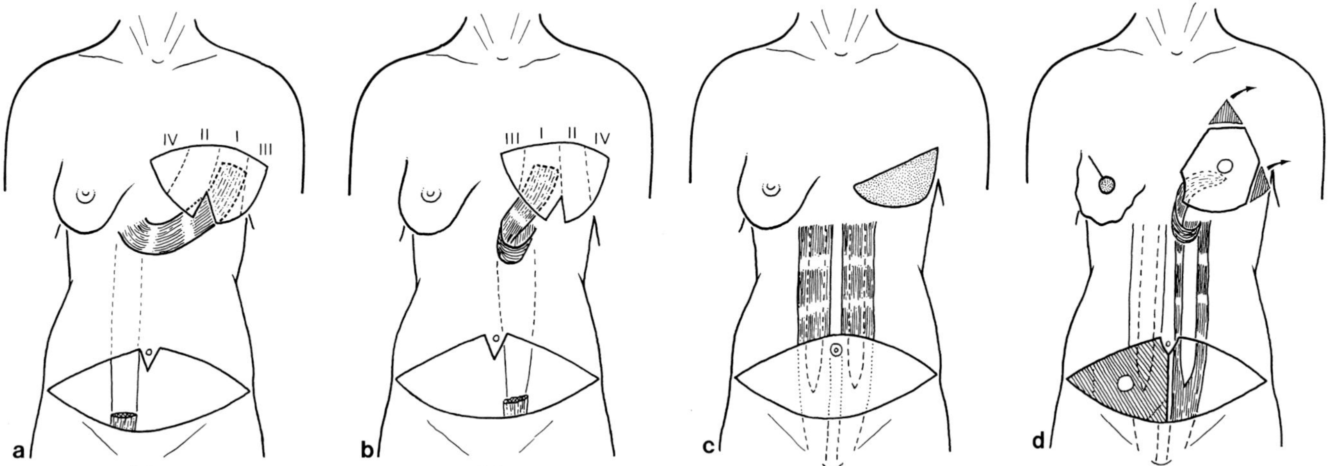

Fig. 7.32 **a.** A contralateral unipedicled flap allows a relatively gentle turning of the muscle but the attachment point on the flap (zone I) may end up fairly lateral on the chest if the ellipse is positioned horizontally. **b.** Ipsilateral unipedicled flap – this requires some folding of the pedicle if the umbilical area is to be inferior but zone I is more medial when the flap reaches the chest. **c.** Bipedicled flap with intramuscular dissection of pedicles. The ellipse may be positioned horizontally, vertically or obliquely on the chest. **d.** Bilateral flaps for simultaneous bilateral volume replacement following subcutaneous mastectomies – tips of the flap are discarded and an excised nipple areolar complex may be replaced with a disc of under-epithelialized skin left on the flap.

7 DIGITAL ARTERIES

Various finger flaps

The anatomy of the digital arteries and nerves has been fully described in Chapter 6 and is not repeated here. Most of the flaps which can be based on these vessels and their branches are summarised below. In addition several random pattern flaps are also described so that the specific flaps may be seen in the more realistic context of other modalities of treatment. It should be self-evident that in any given case it is essential to establish the anatomy of the digital vessels first since the presence of two patent arteries to each finger is not invariable and to use a sole vessel as the support of a flap could seriously compromise the supply of the remainder of the finger.

The principal vascular anomaly to be aware of is that the ulnar digital artery on the little finger and the radial digital artery on the index finger are small in approximately 15% of cases. By contrast the ring and middle fingers conform to the classical concept of two equal-sized digital vessels. It is therefore important to check the perfusion of the digit before isolating a digital artery for a pedicled flap. Many factors need to be taken into consideration when choosing the most appropriate reconstructive method but in a cold climate the sacrifice of a digital artery is a serious matter as cold intolerance may be a problem, particularly in outdoor manual workers.

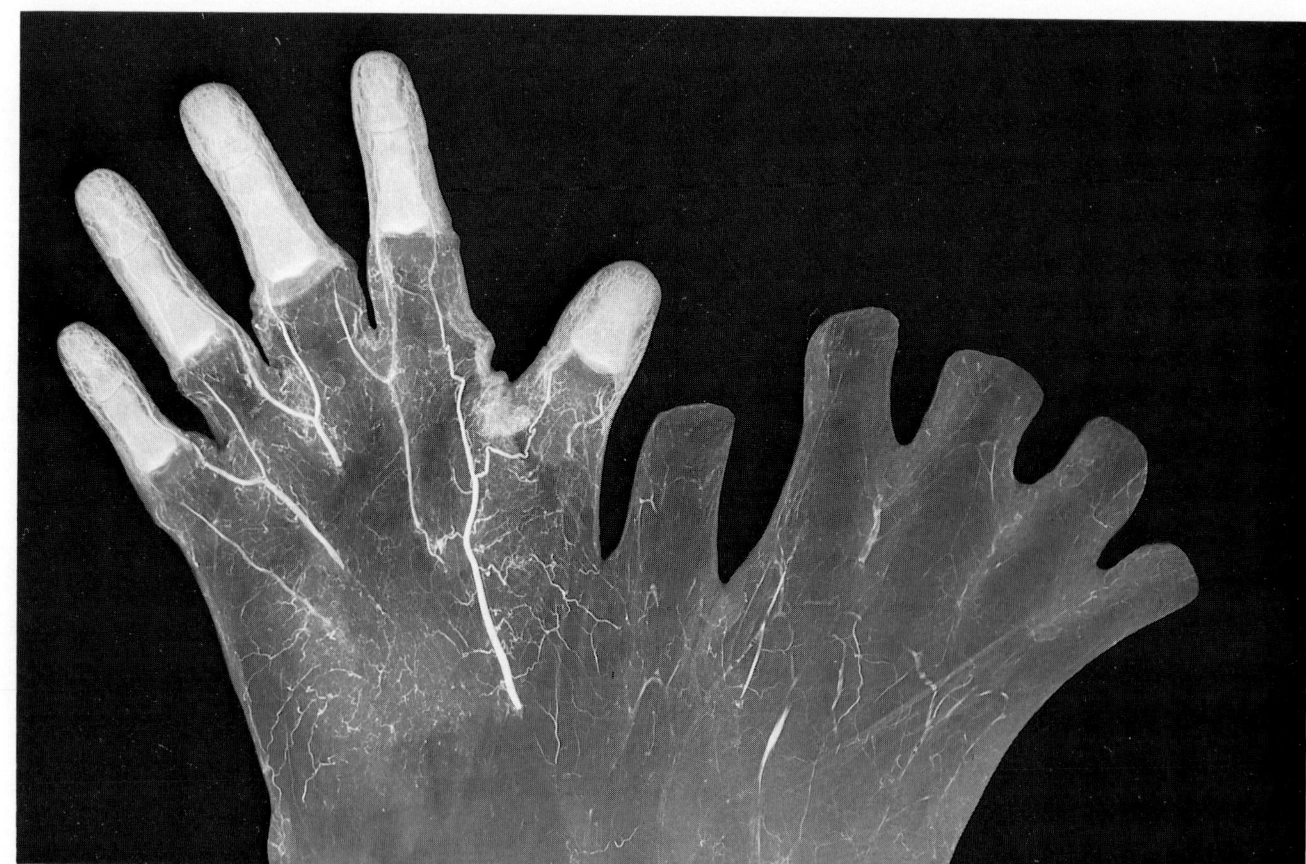

Fig. 7.33 Radiograph of palmar and dorsal skin.

The Atasoy–Kleinert V to Y advancement flap

With amputations through the distal third of the terminal phalanx in a transverse plane, local advancement flaps are very satisfactory. Of these, the triangular volar flap with subcutaneous pedicle and V to Y closure is the most popular and generally associated with the name of Atasoy[1] although previously described by Tranquilli-Leali in 1935.[2] The flap is most appropriate for transverse tip amputations when at least half the length of the nail bed remains. If the bone is longer it can be trimmed to match the nail bed.

The base of the triangle is just less than the overall width of the defect and the two sides of the triangle converge to a point just proximal to the DIP joint crease. With a tourniquet at the base of the exsanguinated finger, skin incisions are made down to the bone near the base of the triangle but through skin only over the remaining parts of the sides of the triangle. The rest of the dissection is carried out with sharp pointed straight scissors while a skin hook is used to put traction on the flap. Dissection is a combination of spreading the points of the scissors and accurately dividing the fibrous septa that are felt to be tethering the flap. Once sufficiently mobile the flap is advanced and sutured first to the nail, and then at the sides of the triangle with direct closure of the apex of the defect. It is acceptable to suture loosely with fat appearing between the skin edges between sutures as this will also prevent a haematoma collecting beneath the flap (no diathermy is used). The tourniquet is removed and the need to readjust any sutures to relieve tension is assessed.

Lateral V to Y advancement (Kutler) flaps

The Kutler method uses two triangular flaps from the sides of the finger which are advanced in a similar fashion to the Atasoy flap to meet in the midline.[3] The dorsal incision is made so as to leave a millimetre of skin at the margin of the nailfold, and extends proximally in the mid-lateral line to the IP joint crease or just proximal to it. The dorsal incision is deepened down to the bone and then moves anteriorly beneath the flap. The volar incision is only carried through skin and takes in approximately one-third of the skin margin of the defect at the end of the finger. Mobilisation is again achieved whilst holding the flap under distal traction with a skin hook, mainly using scissors to divide the fibrous septa. Once the two flaps are mobile they are sutured to each other and in the midline to the remains of the nail otherwise the joined flaps tend to prolapse in a volar direction. In the absence of a nail, a 23 Fg needle inserted into the terminal phalanx in the midline between the two flaps is useful to stabilise the position. The flaps are sutured and the apices closed in a V to Y manner. One of the main criticisms of this method is that the point of convergence of the three scars lies at the point of maximum use of the pulp and annoying sensitivity here can be a problem.

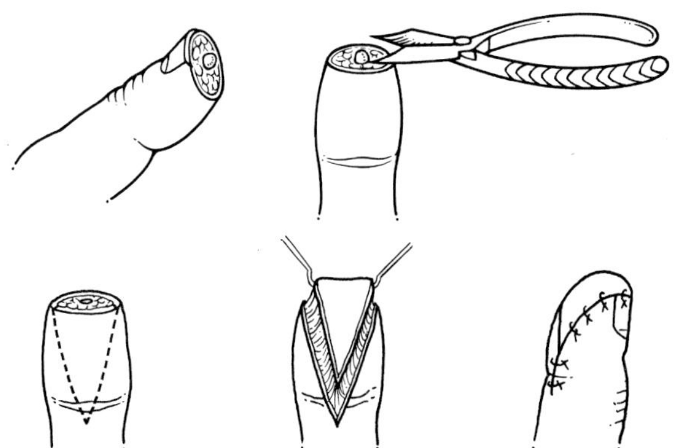

Fig. 7.34 Atasoy–Kleinert V to Y repair.

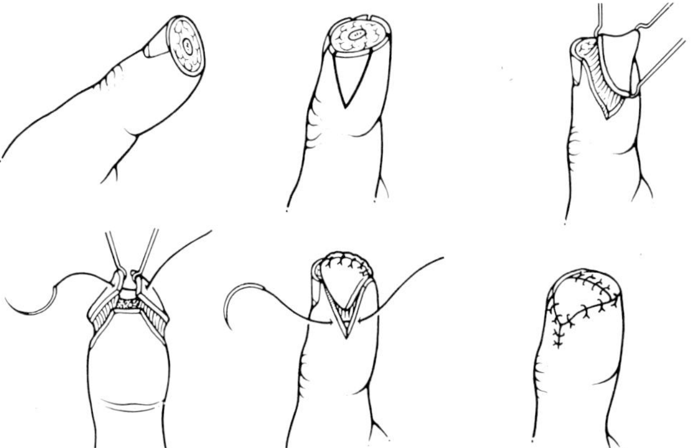

Fig. 7.35 Kutler lateral V to Y repair.

Thenar flaps

These have been widely used for index, middle and some ring fingertip injuries since the technique was described in 1926. This is because a thenar flap provides some of the best tissue for reconstruction, with good colour and texture, and sufficient subcutaneous tissue to restore the bulk of the pad. Sensory recovery is also good as the sensory end-organs are similar to those in the pulp. The original pattern of thenar flap was like a postage stamp with an ulnar attached base.[4] This has been modified by some surgeons to a more rectangular flap with a narrower base attached proximally. Direct cosure of the donor site may be possible when the width of the donor site does not exceed 1.5 cm, otherwise a full thickness graft is the usual method as a split skin graft tends to leave a poor scar. A narrow distally-based flap also works well and the flap is inset with its distal end attached to the proximal part of the recipient defect.[5] When this flap is orientated parallel and slightly over the MCP joint creases, direct closure is easily achieved.[6] Another method of dealing with the donor site involves an initial H-shaped incision to create square proximal and distal flaps.[7] Both are inset on the finger initially so that there are no raw surfaces, and then at division the whole proximal flap is separated from the finger and advanced to close the donor site defect, while the distal flap which is attached on the volar edge of the fingertip defect is detached from the palm and inset over the end of the finger.

With all these flaps care must be taken to avoid damage to the palmar digital nerves of the thumb which lie very superficial at the MCP joint flexion crease. Division is usually carried out on the tenth day.

Palmar, as distinct from thenar, flaps are accompanied by such high complication rates from donor site problems and PIP joint flexion contractures that their use is contraindicated.

Cross fingers flaps

In their standard form these have been in use for over 30 years[8] and are commonly used for volar-oblique amputations through the middle of the distal phalanx. The rectangular flap is raised on the dorsum of a finger middle phalanx with the base of the flap along the medial or lateral side and the flap turned over through 180° (Fig. 7.37). Division of Cleland's ligaments in the base of the flap improves its mobility and if done carefully should not endanger the palmar digital artery branches which support the flap. The flap is situated as follows:

thumb pulp reconstruction	– middle finger, middle phalanx, lateral base
index pulp reconstruction	– middle finger, middle phalanx, lateral base
middle finger pulp	– ring finger, middle phalanx, lateral base
ring finger pulp	– middle finger, middle phalanx, medial base
little finger pulp	– ring finger, middle phalanx, medial base

A variation on the cross finger flap from an adjacent digit is to orientate the flap longitudinally over the dorsum of the middle phalanx with the base of the flap situated distally. The distal basing of the flap does not prejudice its viability as a good blood supply enters it from the superficial arcade over the base of the distal phalanx but it is advisable to restrict the length-to-breadth ratio to 1.5 to 1. Both standard and distally-based cross-over flaps give good skin coverage but it is non-glabrous, may be hairy and does not provide much subcutaneous tissue for reconstructing the bulk of the finger pad. The donor site scar is obvious even when a full thickness graft is used rather than a split skin graft. The recovery of sensibility in the flap can be very good but is unpredictable.

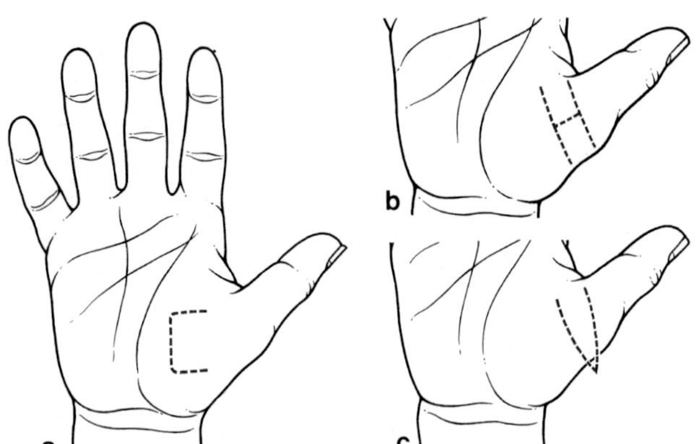

Fig. 7.36 Various thenar flap options.

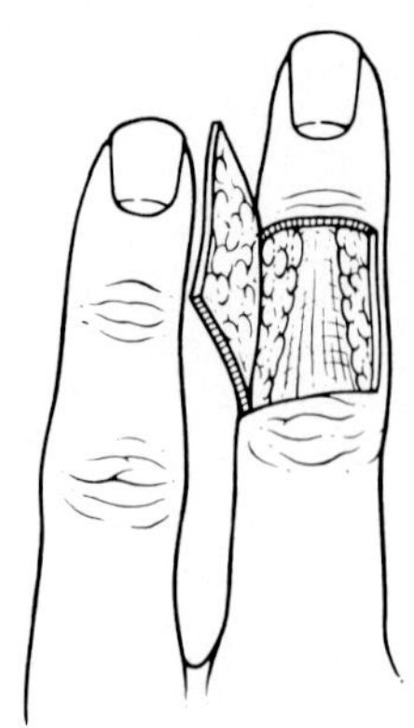

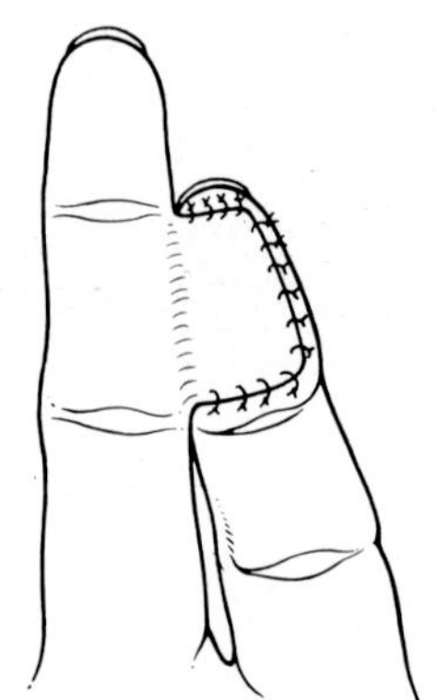

Fig. 7.37 Cross finger flap, dorsum to pulp.

The innervated cross finger flaps

These have been developed in an attempt to improve the sensory result in cross finger flaps.[9,10]

Fingers. After planning the flap in the usual way an incision is made from the proximal corner of the free edge of the flap towards the web space. The dorsal branch of the palmar digital nerve is located and dissected free where it overlies the proximal phalanx, and is then transected about 1.5–2.0 cm proximal to the edge of the flap. The flap is now elevated in the usual way just superficial to the paratenon, so that the ramifications of the isolated nerve are contained in the flap. The recipient finger is prepared by exposing the amputated end of the digital nerve – this requires a proximal mid-lateral line incision on the side of the finger furthest removed from the donor finger – and a neurorrhaphy carried out.

Thumb. For an innervated cross finger flap to the thumb pulp the choice of donor digit is altered from middle finger to index where there are possibilities for innervation using the radial nerve. When incising the margins of the flap the skin incision at the proximal margin is kept superficial and the branches of the superficial radial nerve are located. In the original method[11] these were traced back to the base of the metacarpal from where a further incision was made to the defect on the thumb to allow the radial nerve to be re-routed. This provides a sensate reconstruction, albeit of poor quality, with the added problems of cortical reorientation. More recent elaboration of this concept involves dividing the radial sensory nerve at the time of carrying out the cross finger flap and joining the nerve to the appropriate digital nerve of the thumb.[12] This avoids the problems of orientation. (For a one stage solution to the same problem see under *dorsal metacarpal artery flaps*.)

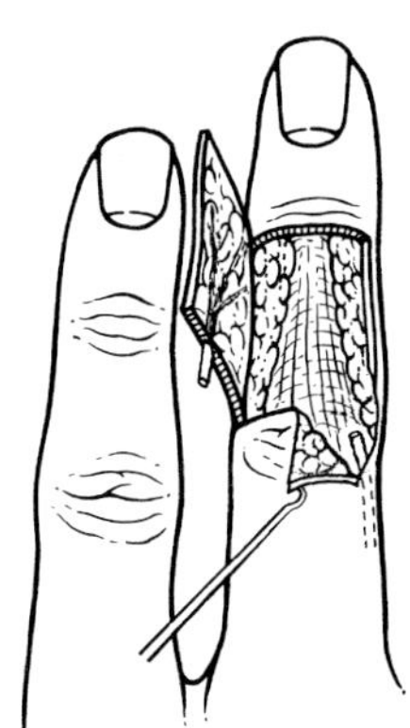

Fig. 7.38 Innervated cross finger flap.

Cross finger flap variations

De-epithelialised cross finger flaps for dorsal defects. Repair of dorsal defects on the fingers should not be carried out with cross finger flaps from the volar surface of an adjoining digit. However a de-epithelialised cross finger flap from the dorsum covered with a split skin graft is an effective method. The skin graft can be laid across both the flap and the donor site defect.[13]

Subcutaneous tissue only. In this modification the skin from the dorsum of the flap is retained on the back of the finger and only the subcutaneous tissue is transferred. This tissue may be applied to a dorsal or a volar defect and needs to be grafted. The skin over the DIP and PIP joints must be avoided when planning the flap as the subcutaneous tissue is too thin. For the rare case requiring an eponychial fold reconstruction, Atasoy[14] has devised an elegant modification in which an appropriately sized and shaped island of skin is preserved along the distal margin of the subcutaneous flap. This skin then comes to lie on the deep surface of the flap when it is turned over into the defect and forms the inner surface of the eponychial fold. A full thickness graft is applied to the dorsum of the subcutaneous tissue flap.

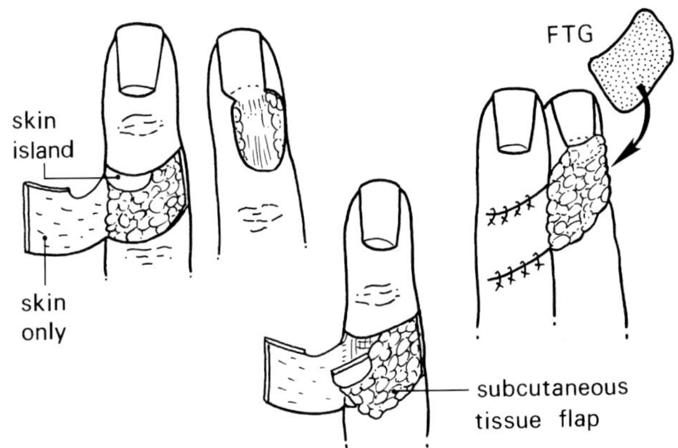

Fig. 7.39 Subcutaneous tissue flap and skin island for eponychial fold reconstruction.

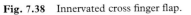

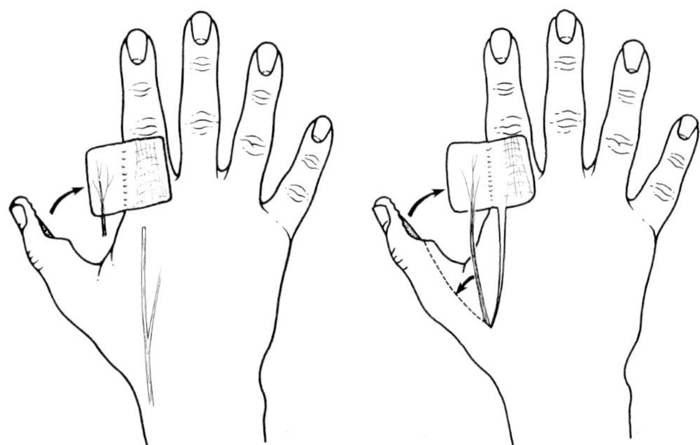

Fig. 7.40 Innervated cross finger flap from index to thumb pulp.

Heterodigital neurovascular island flaps (Littler)

In the original cases the ulnar aspects of the middle and ring fingers were favoured as donor areas since at these sites loss of sensibility is least inconvenient. The island was oval in shape, taking in half the pulp and extending proximally into the middle segment of the finger if necessary[15–18].

The best example of the principle is a flap raised on the medial side of the ring finger and transferred to the thumb or index finger pad. Duparc[19] has listed his indications as follows:

1. thumb pulp destruction
2. thumb reconstruction by pedicle flap and bone grafts
3. isolated pulp anaesthesia caused by destruction of the nerves – only in thumbs
4. median nerve paralysis – only a relative indication
5. anaesthesia of the ulnar border of the little finger.

The skin island is taken from the palmar and medial sides of the terminal phalanx of the ring finger. To preserve the innervation to the adjacent side of the little finger the palmar digital nerve must be split proximal to the web space. Ideally the dorsal digital branch should also be split off the palmar digital nerve in order to preserve sensation on the dorsum of the ring finger, but this is not always done. Where the common palmar digital artery divides in the fourth web space, its little finger digital branch will have to be ligated and divided. The neurovascular pedicle must lie easily in the palm without tension or acute angulation. It has been suggested[20] that when restoring sensation to the thumb the entire territory of the donor digital nerve should be utilised rather than just the small territory over the distal phalanx. In taking the total area supplied by the donor digital neurovascular bundle advantage can also be taken of the dorsal branch of the digital nerve and so an island graft measuring 6 cm × 2–3 cm can be obtained.

Neurovascular exchange island flap

The exchange island is similar to a small Littler flap but is used within the same digit as a means of restoring sensate skin cover to an area of scarred and insensate pulp on the dominant half of a finger. As the digital nerve to the skin island is transferred from one side of the digit to the other, some cortical reorientation is required. Foucher[21] has modified the flap to overcome this problem by dividing the digital nerve on the donor side proximal to the flap and then joining it to the stump of the damaged digital nerve on the recipient side.

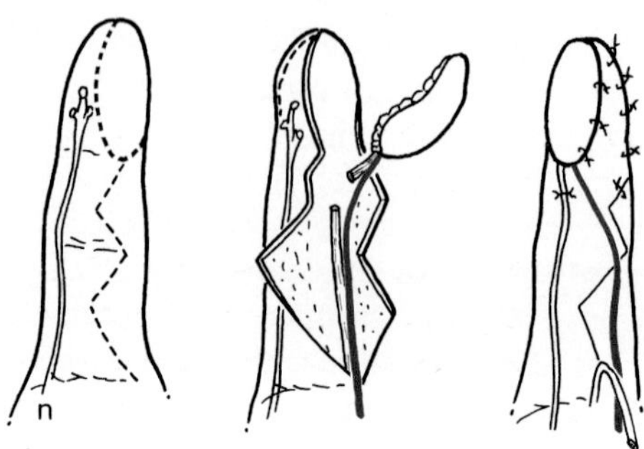

Fig. 7.42 Neurovascular homodigital exchange island flap.

Arterialised island flaps

This arterialised island flap is diamond or elliptical in shape and is taken from the mid-lateral surface of the donor digit, with the exact placement being determined by the desired length of the pedicle. The pedicle includes only the digital artery and some surrounding tissue so as to provide a venous drainage pathway. The digital nerve is not included. A flap of 1.5 cm × 3 cm can be obtained and if the defect is situated over the proximal phalanx it can often be closed without a graft. The flap provides coverage for small defects over critical areas or to release joint and web space scar contractures.[22]

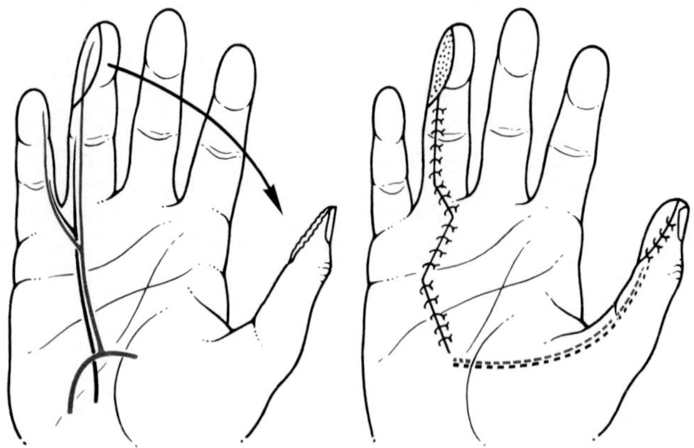

Fig. 7.41 Neurovascular island flap heterodigital transfer.

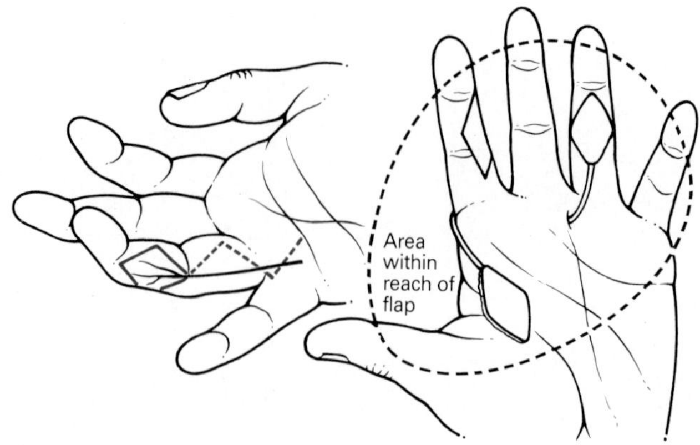

Fig. 7.43 Arterialised island flaps.

Volar advancement flaps on the thumb

For distal pulp amputations of the thumb in which more tissue is lost from the palmar surface than the dorsal surface, various advancement flap options are available.

Moberg flap (Moberg, 1964). The volar skin of the thumb is supplied by the digital arteries while the dorsal skin is supplied by separate vessels – the ulnodorsal vessel being a branch of the first dorsal metacarpal artery and the radiodorsal vessel a branch of the radial artery. This means that on the thumb longitudinal mid-lateral incisions can be made which will not impair the blood supply to the dorsal skin whereas the same incisions on a finger would be likely to produce necrosis of the distal skin because the dorsal digital arteries are short and cannot support the dorsal skin beyond the PIPJ. After making mid-lateral incisions from the defect down to the proximal thumb crease, the volar skin may be elevated on the vascular support of the digital arteries and advanced up to 1 cm to cover a defect at the tip.[23]

Dellon[24] has increased the amount of advancement available from this flap by extending the incisions down to the crease at the base of the thenar eminence and at the same time raising adjoining flaps to still enable primary closure.

Bipedicle island advancement (O'Brien, 1968). A variation on the above for distal thumb defects of about 10–15 mm involves similar mid-lateral incisions which are then joined by a transverse incision at the level of the proximal third of the proximal phalanx taken through skin only. The neurovascular pedicles are then dissected out from beneath the proximal flap to permit mobilisation of the distal skin island. This island is then advanced and the secondary defect filled with a full thickness skin graft.[25] A further option is a V to Y advancement to close the secondary defect.

Unipedicled rotation-advancement flap (Hueston). With smaller defects (~8 mm) it may be possible to avoid bilateral mid-axial incisions and carry out a rotation advancement of the volar thumb skin based only on the vascular pedicle of one side.[26] The base of the flap is classically positioned on the ulnar side of the thumb so as to preserve maximum innervation to the ulnar side of the reconstructed tip. On the free edge of the flap the skin is raised superficial to the neurovascular structures and then incised transversely at the proximal crease. The triangular secondary defect at the base of the thumb requires a full thickness skin graft or alternatively a triangular flap from the side of the thumb can be transposed into the defect as recommended by Foucher.[27] If the base of the flap is positioned on the radial side of the thumb then it may be possible to close the secondary defect by transposing some of the dorsal skin of the first web but the innervation of the tip is likely to be inferior.[28]

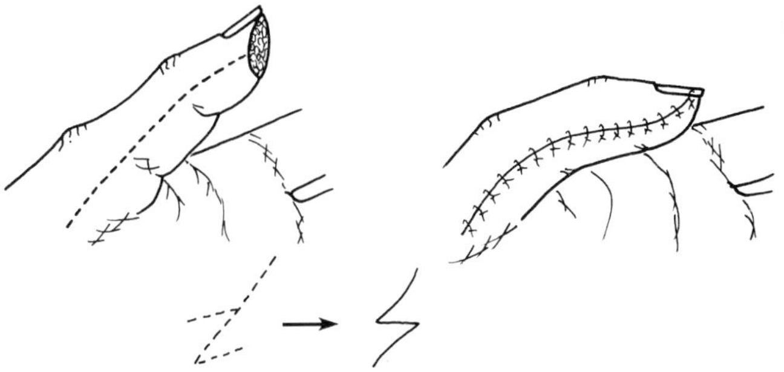

Fig. 7.44 The Moberg advancement flap on the thumb.

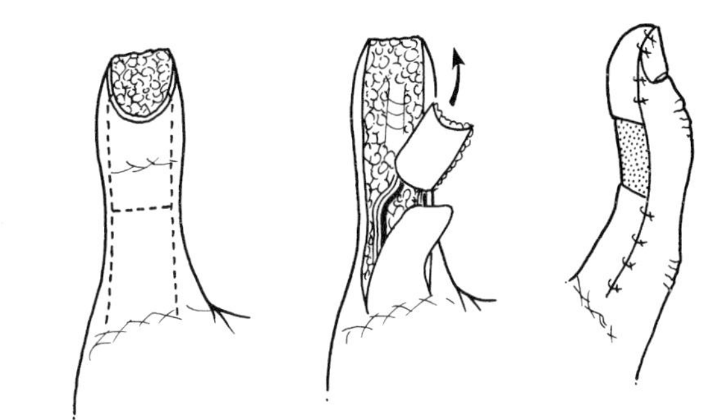

Fig. 7.45 Bipedicle island advancement flap on the thumb.

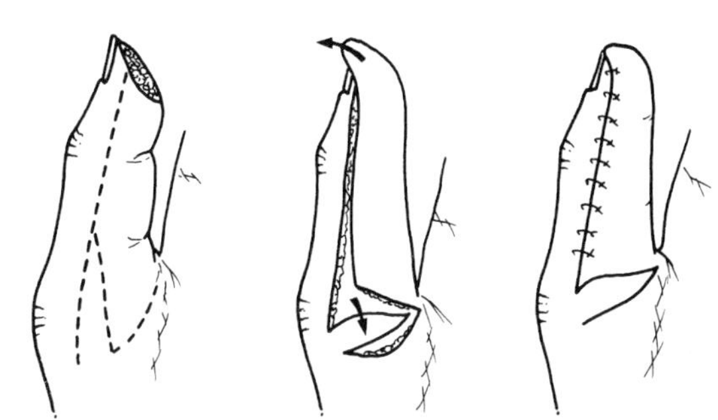

Fig. 7.46 Hueston rotation-advancement flap.

7

Advancement flaps on the digits

Most advancement flaps convert the skin flap into an island because the retention of a skin bridge pedicle, as in the volar advancement flap, does not permit sufficient mobilisation.

Volar advancement flap (Snow, 1967, 1985). This applies the Moberg advancement concept used on the thumb to the fingers[29] but is hazardous because the dorsal skin of a digit does not have independent vascularisation.[30] It has been suggested[31] that the procedure can be applied to a finger if the soft tissues are left attached as a mesentery to the flap. Snow[32] has described dissecting out the dorsal branches of the digital arteries when mobilising the flap, thereby preserving the blood supply to the dorsum.

Unipedicled island advancement flap (Venkataswamy). This reconstructs a lateral or medial oblique tip loss by advancing a triangular island flap from the less damaged side.[33] The base of the flap is as wide as the defect and the other two sides are 2 to $2\frac{1}{2}$ times as long. One side follows the mid-lateral line while the second and longer side crosses the volar side of the digit. The dorsal incision is deepened to a plane beneath the subcutaneous fat so that the neurovascular bundle is raised with the flap. On the volar side the incision is through skin, and fibrous septa are divided with scissors preserving vessels and nerves entering the volar side of the triangle. This should permit adequate mobilisation but if it does not, further separation on the volar side can be carried out to create what is then an island flap based on one neurovascular bundle. After flap advancement the proximal defect is closed in a V to Y manner.

Dorsolateral island advancement flap (Joshi). This flap reconstructs the pulp using a neurovascular island flap from the dorsum and lateral aspect of a finger.[34] The volar margin of the flap borders the defect and then tapers towards the mid-lateral line at the PIP joint crease. The dorsal margin of the flap passes from the defect past the proximal corner of the nail, about 3 mm from it, reaches the midline on the dorsum of the finger and then tapers down to meet the volar incision at the PIP joint crease. From the proximal corner of the flap a mid-lateral incision is made down to the web and the pedicle isolated preserving the dorsal digital branches. The volar margin is incised and the flap elevated in the subcutaneous plane with the neurovascular bundle. The dorsal incision is made and attempts made to retain a dorsolateral vein at this point. The flap is advanced with the MCP joint flexed and the donor site reconstructed with a full-thickness graft.

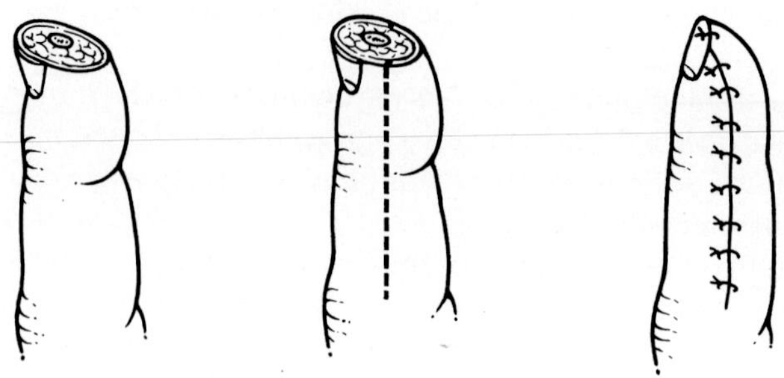

Fig. 7.47 Volar advancement flap on a finger.

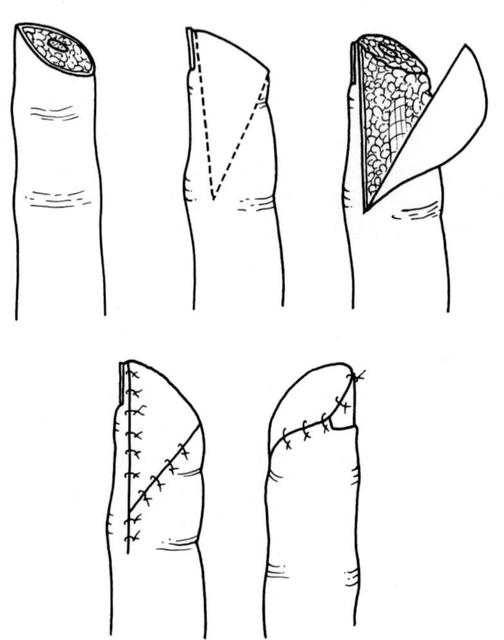

Fig. 7.48 Unipedicled island advancement flap with direct closure of donor site as V to Y.

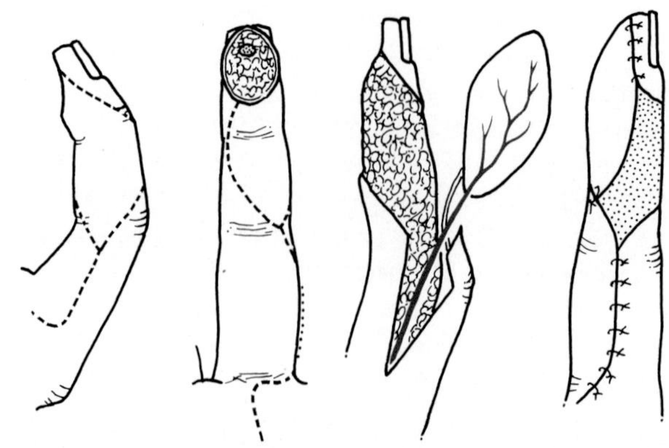

Fig. 7.49 Dorsolateral unipedicled island advancement flap with secondary defect requiring a graft.

Step advancement island flap (Evans, 1988). This flap achieves advancement for tip reconstruction without creating a significant secondary defect.[35] The volar margin of the flap is designed as three triangles, narrow proximally and wide distally, with only the distal flap crossing the midline. In raising the flap these triangles are not separated from the underlying fat whereas the corresponding triangles based on the opposite side of the digit are raised thinly so that a longitudinal midline dissection can be made down to the sheath and then extended beneath the flap so as to raise the neurovascular pedicle with it. The dorsal incision is slightly convex and tapers proximally to meet the volar incision at a point overlying the neurovascular bundle. Mobilisation of the flap takes place deep to the subcutaneous fat and once all the fibrous connections have been divided the incision can be extended proximally over the neurovascular bundle to achieve the necessary degree of mobilisation of the pedicle. The flap is advanced, engaging each triangular flap one step distally, and closing the proximal triangle and the gap over the pedicle directly. Complete apposition of dorsal skin edges is avoided if this would mean putting the flap under tension and any gaps heal secondarily.

Bipedicled island flap (O'Brien). This can be used for reconstructing volar oblique tip amputations on digits in a similar way in which the flap is used on the thumb.[36] Mid-lateral incisions reach from the edges of the defect to the PIP joint. The flap is elevated in the plane beneath the subcutaneous fat with division of Cleland's ligaments. At the proximal ends of the incisons a transverse incision is made through skin only and the neurovascular bundles further mobilised from beneath the proximal skin. After advancing the skin the donor site can generally be closed directly without the aid of grafts. Because there are no incisions dorsal to the arteries at the level of the proximal phalanx, the dorsal branches should have been preserved and the dorsal skin not be at risk. O'Brien has pointed out that one of the advantages of this flap is that when the lateral 'ears' at the end of the flap are joined together in the midline, a very adequately rounded and projecting pulp is obtained.

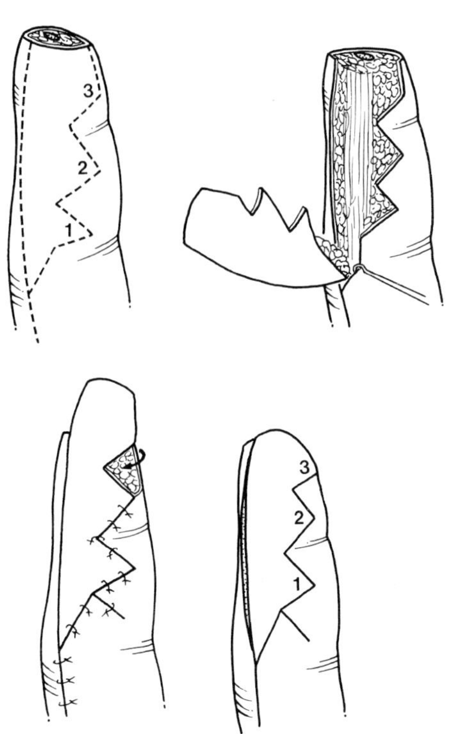

Fig. 7.50 Step-advancement unipedicled island flap with direct closure of donor site.

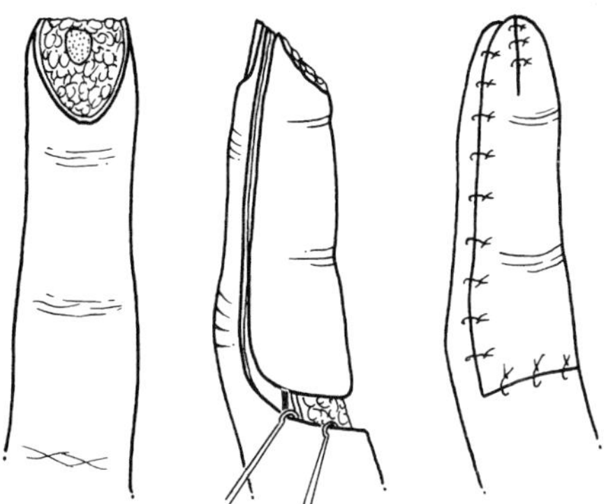

Fig. 7.51 Bipedicled island advancement on a digit.

Other flaps

Retrograde finger dorsum pedicled flap (Ogo). This is a pedicled flap used for pulp reconstruction on the same digit.[37] The territory is that of a standard cross finger flap but moved further distally so as to include the skin over the nail matrix. The pedicle is distally situated, either radial or ulnar based, and the flap is therefore non-sensory. With amputations proximal to the nail matrix the pedicle can be 6 to 8 mm wide. For amputations distal to the nail matrix the pedicle needs to be 8 to 10 mm wide. The flap tends to be white on elevation but pinks up by the following day. This flap has been extensively used by the originators but has been little published in English.

Oblique dorsal flap (Flint & Harrison). This flap for homodigital pulp reconstruction retains good sensation because the palmar digital nerve gives branches of supply to the skin over the dorsum of the DIP joint and these branches are included in the flap together with adjacent branches of the digital artery.[38] The proximal incision runs from the PIP joint crease at the mid-lateral line, obliquely across the dorsum of the finger to the DIP joint crease on the opposite side. The distal incision is placed parallel with this and sufficiently far away to provide enough width of skin to resurface the front of the finger. A back-cut into the base of the flap after locating the vessels, allows transposition into the defect.

Thumb radiodorsal neurovascular flap (Pho). In some respects similar to the Joshi flap but based on the thumb, this flap is supported by the dorsal branches of the radial palmar digital artery given off at the level of the neck of the proximal phalanx of the thumb.[39] The dorsal margin of the flap passes dorsally from the defect some 3 mm away from the nail edge, taking as much as necessary over the dorsum, and then curves down to the mid-lateral line at the proximal third of the proximal phalanx. The volar margin follows the edge of the pulp defect and then approaches the mid-lateral line along which an incision is made to the metacarpal head to expose the pedicle. Flap transposition after mobilising the pedicle is facilitated by flexion at the joints, and the secondary defect is grafted.

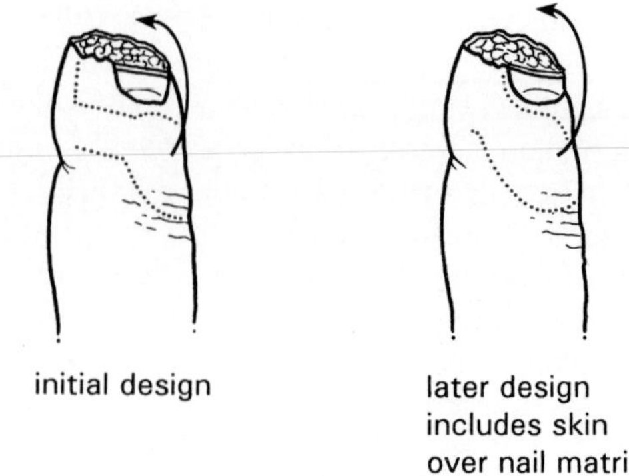

Fig. 7.52 Retrograde finger dorsum pedicled flap.

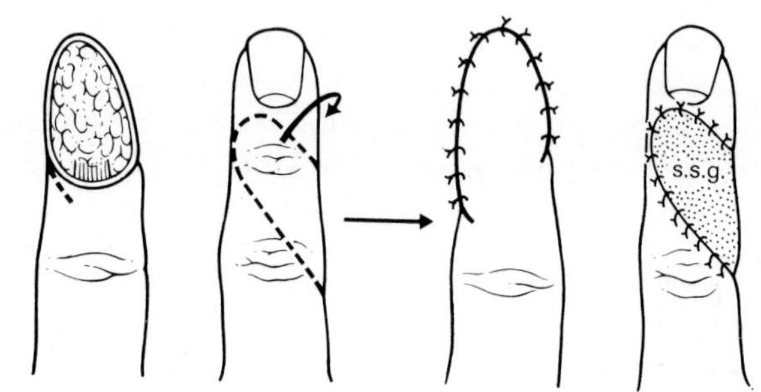

Fig. 7.53 Oblique dorsal neurovascular flap.

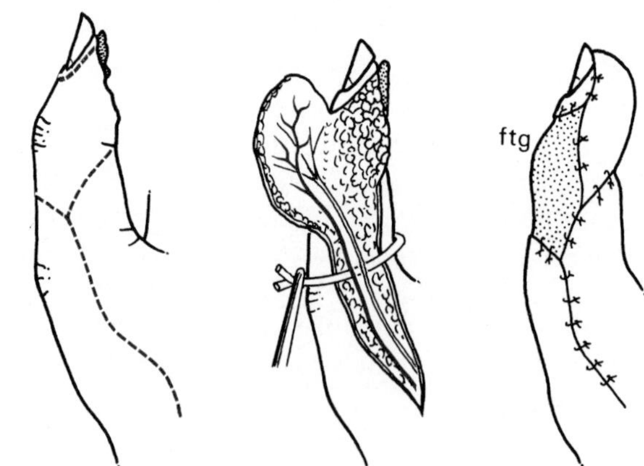

Fig. 7.54 Thumb radiodorsal neurovascular flap.

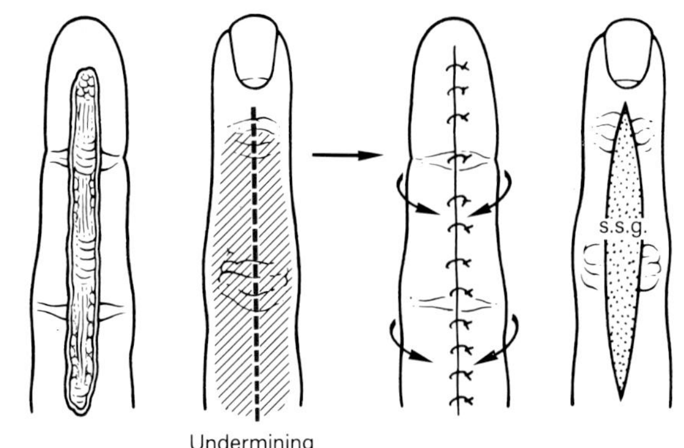

Fig. 7.55 Bilateral bipedicle flaps.

Bilateral bipedicle flaps

For long volar digital skin loss, e.g. grindwheel injuries, it may be useful to elevate longitudinal bipedicle flaps from the sides of the finger for advancement over the exposed flexor tendon. After a dorsal midline incision the flaps are elevated to include the digital neurovascular bundle. The dorsal defect is split skin grafted.

A variety of other dorsal flaps has been designed for a number of specific purposes:

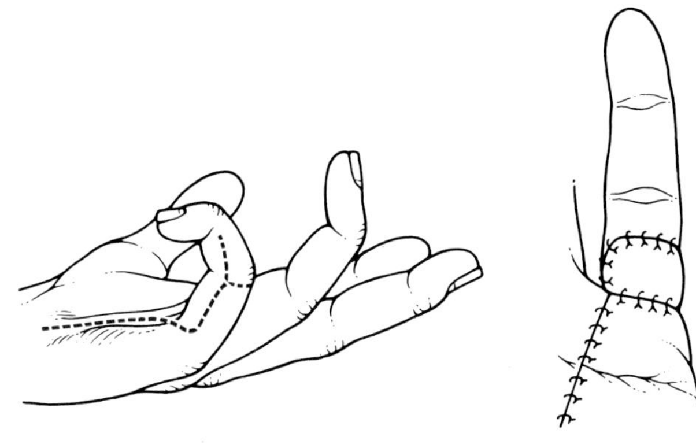

Fig. 7.56 Dorsal fifth finger transposition flap.

Dorsal fifth finger transposition flap

This has been designed specifically for filling the palmar defect over the fifth metacarpal head that results from release of Dupuytren's contracture affecting this finger.[40] The flap lies over the dorso-medial aspect of the proximal phalanx of the fifth finger and extends up to the PIP joint. It is transposed into the space made by an incision that passes transversely across the proximal crease of the finger into the fourth cleft.

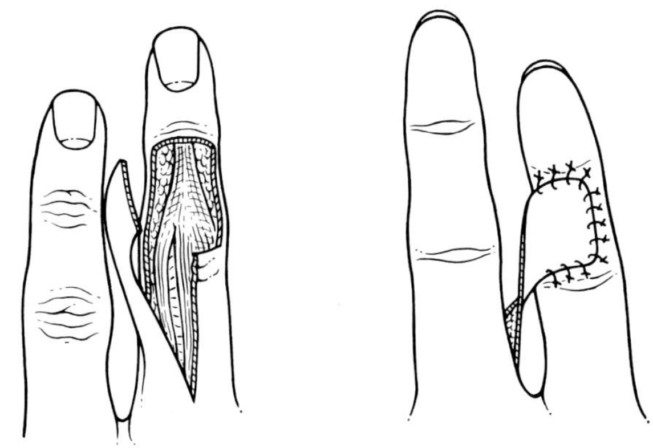

Fig. 7.57 Finger flag flap.

The finger flag flap (Vilain)

This was first described by Vilain in 1952 for providing full thickness skin reconstruction on the palmar or dorsal surface of the middle phalanx of a finger.[41] The name derives from the combined shapes of the square flap and the long narrow pedicle, which resemble a flag and staff respectively. The flap overlies the dorsum of the middle phalanx and the pedicle extends proximally over half the width of the proximal phalanx. The flap transfer may be homodigital for a palmar defect but is certainly heterodigital for a dorsal defect. The flap is not appropriate for homodigital pulp reconstruction, although heterodigital (middle to ring) transfer has been suggested.[42] However, the flap is really of little use, requires two stages, and has been supplanted by more recently developed alternatives described in the foregoing text.

The 'axial flag flap' described by Lister is sited over the dorsum of the proximal phalanx of an index or middle finger and is based on dorsal metacarpal artery branches rather than on digital arteries (see *dorsal metacarpal artery* flaps).

Reverse digital artery flap

This distally based island flap was first described by Weeks & Wray for repair of an exposed PIP joint[43] Development of the flap to reach the fingertip was described by Lai et al, originally in a non-innervated[44] and later in an innervatable form[45] (i.e. with a neurorrhaphy), and by Kojima et al.[46]

The flaps are useful for homodigital reconstruction of skin and pulp loss at the fingertip, or skin loss over a flexor tendon.

The course of the digital arteries and their multiple interconnecting arcades (also termed digitopalmar arches) are described on page 195. These interconnections are important in providing the blood flow into the distal end of the divided digital artery and thereby enabling retrograde perfusion of the flap. An important point is that the digital arteries are not accompanied by venae comitantes and therefore venous drainage of these island flaps is dependent on a cuff of adipose tissue being taken with the artery so as to include enough small vessels to provide a network for drainage.

In the innervated flaps the dorsal branch of the proper digital nerve is taken with the flap. The dorsal branch passes superficial or deep to the digital artery to supply the skin over the side of the proximal phalanx and then joins with the dorsal digital nerve and supplies skin over the dorsum of the middle finger. The anatomy of the dorsal branch is not constant and this has been described on page 196. Lai has defined the configurations of the dorsal branch anatomy as Types I to IV[45]. These correlate with Figure 6.76 as follows I = a, II = c, III = e, IV = b. Type I/a is the most common. The replacement of the dorsal branch by a number of tiny twigs is uncommon (Type IV/b) but precludes the possibility of raising an innervatable flap.

When planning the flap a digital Allen test should be used to confirm that both arteries are adequate. The flaps of Kojima et al were designed to exactly overlie the digital arteries and as a consequence they encroached on volar skin. The flaps of Lai et al are superior in being positioned on the lateral side of the digit so that two-thirds of the flap lies behind the line of the digital artery. This position also facilitates incorporation of the dorsal nerve branch. The standard flap is raised from the side of the proximal phalanx (distal two-thirds), but may be extended proximally to encroach on part of the web skin. From the planned skin island a zig-zag incision is made to the distal defect.

With a tourniquet on the arm the volar and proximal margin of the flap is incised first and the digital artery located and ligated at the proximal margin. It is worth releasing the tourniquet and checking the blood supply to the digit through the contralateral vessel at this point before finally dividing the artery. The remainder of the flap is incised and dissected off the proper digital nerve either dividing the dorsal nerve branch and taking it with the flap or leaving the branch on the finger. If harvesting the flap with the dorsal branch of nerve for an innervated fingertip reconstruction then it is worth dissecting this out proximally so as to have up to 2 cm projecting from the flap for microsurgical attachment to the damaged proper digital nerve.

At the distal end of the flap it is important to leave a cuff of adipose tissue around the digital artery to provide a venous drainage channel.

At the point about which the pedicle turns and between this point and the margin of the distal defect, it may not be possible to close the skin edges of the zig-zag incision, particularly if a neurorrhaphy has been carried out. This distal defect may be closed with a split skin graft and the donor site defect should be reconstructed with a full-thickness graft and tie-over dressing.

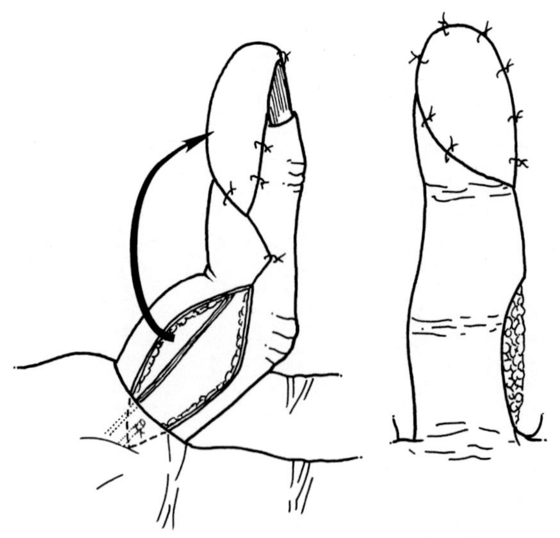

Fig. 7.58 Reverse digital artery flap from side of the proximal phalanx of finger. The palmar digital nerve and its dorsal branch (Type I) are shown in the base of the donor site defect prior to application of a full thickness graft.

References

1. Atasoy E, Iokimidis E, Kasden M L, Kutz J E, Kleinert H E 1970 Reconstruction of the amputated finger tip with a triangular volar flap. Journal of Bone and Joint Surgery 52A: 921
2. Tranquilli-Leali E 1935 Ricostruzione dell'apice delle falangi ungeali mediante autoplastica volare peduncolata per scorrimento. Infort Trauma Lavoro 1: 186–193
3. Kutler W 1947 A new method for finger tip amputation. Journal of the American Medical Association 133: 29–30
4. Gatewood 1926 A plastic repair of finger defects without hospitalisation. Journal of the American Medical Association 87: 1479
5. Barton N J 1975 A modified thenar flap. The Hand 7: 150–151
6. Dellon A L 1983 The proximal inset thenar flap for fingertip reconstruction. Plastic and Reconstructive Surgery 72: 698–702
7. Smith R J, Albin R 1976 Thenar 'H-flap' for fingertip injuries. Journal of Trauma 16: 778–781
8. Gurdin M, Pangman W J 1950 Repair of surface defects of fingers by transdigital flaps. Plastic and Reconstructive Surgery 5: 368–371
9. Berger A, Neissl G 1975 Innervated skin grafts and flaps for restoration of sensation to anaesthetic areas. Chirurgia Plastica 3: 33–38
10. Cohen B E, Cronin E D 1983 An innervated cross-finger flap for fingertip reconstruction. Plastic and Reconstructive Surgery 72: 688–695
11. Bralliar F, Horner R L 1969 Sensory cross-finger pedicle graft. Journal of Bone and Joint Surgery 51A: 1264–1268
12. Gaul J S 1969 Radial-innervated cross-finger flap from index to provide sensory pulp to injured thumb. Journal of Bone and Joint Surgery 51A: 1257–1263
13. Robbins T H 1985 The use of de-epithelialised cross-finger flaps for dorsal finger defects. British Journal of Plastic Surgery 38: 407–409
14. Atasoy E 1982 Reversed cross-finger subcutaneous flap. Journal of Hand Surgery 7: 481–483
15. Moberg E 1955 Discussion on Brooks D. Nerve grafting in orthopaedic surgery. The Journal of Bone and Joint Surgery 37A: 305 & 326
16. Littler J W 1956 Neurovascular pedicle transfer of tissue. Journal of Bone and Joint Surgery 38A: 917
17. Littler W 1960 Neurovascular skin island transfer in reconstructive hand surgery. In: Wallace AB (ed) Transactions of the International Society of Plastic Surgeons. Second Congress, London 1959. E & S Livingstone, Edinburgh, p 175
18. Tubiana R, Duparc M 1961 Restoration of sensibility in the hand by neurovascular skin island transfer. Journal of Bone and Joint Surgery 43B: 474–480
19. Duparc J, Roux F 1973 Restauration de la sensibilité au niveau de la main par transfert d'un transplant cutané heterodigital muni de son pedicule vasculonerveux. Étude critique des resultats. Annales de Chirurgie 27: 497–502
20. Hueston J 1965 The extended neurovascular island flap. British Journal of Plastic Surgery 18: 304–305
21. Foucher G, Braun F M, Merle M, Michon J 1981 La technique du 'débranchement-rebranchement' du lambeau en îlot pédiculé. Annales de Chirurgie 35: 301–303
22. Rose E H 1983 Local arterialised island flap coverage of difficult hand defects preserving donor digit sensibility. Plastic and Reconstructive Surgery 72: 848–857
23. Moberg E 1964 Aspects of sensation in reconstructive surgery of the upper extremity. Journal of Bone and Joint Surgery 46A: 817
24. Dellon A L 1983 The extended palmar advancement flap. Journal of Hand Surgery 8: 190–194
25. O'Brien B M 1968 Neurovascular island pedicled flaps for terminal amputations and digital scars. British Journal of Plastic Surgery 21: 258–261
26. Hueston J T 1966 Local flap repair in fingertip injuries. Plastic and Reconstructive Surgery 37: 349–350
27. Foucher G, Sibilly A, Merle M, Michon J 1985 Le lambeau de Hueston dans les recouverments de pertes de substance distale du pouce. Annales de Chirurgie de la Main 4: 239–241
28. Argamaso R V 1974 Rotation-transposition method for soft tissue replacement on the distal segment of the thumb. Plastic and Reconstructive Surgery 54: 366–368
29. Snow J W 1967 The use of a volar flap for repair of finger tip amputations: a preliminary report. Plastic and Reconstructive Surgery 40: 163–168
30. Shaw M H 1971 Neurovascular island pedicled flaps for terminal digital scars – a hazard. British Journal of Plastic Surgery 24: 161–165
31. Ariyan S 1978 The hand book. Williams & Wilkins, Baltimore
32. Snow J W 1985 Volar advancement skin flap to the fingertip. Hand Clinics 1: 685–688
33. Venkataswamy R, Subramanian N 1980 Oblique triangular flap: a new method of repair for oblique amputations of the finger-tip and thumb. Plastic and Reconstructive Surgery 66: 296–300
34. Joshi B B 1974 A local dorsolateral island flap for restoration of sensation after avulsion injury of fingertip pulp. Plastic and Reconstructive Surgery 54: 175–182
35. Evans D M, Martin D L 1988 Step-advancement island flap for fingertip reconstruction. British Journal of Plastic Surgery 41: 105–111
36. O'Brien B M 1965 Neurovascular pedicle transfers in the hand. Australian and New Zealand Journal of Surgery 35: 2–11
37. Ogo K, Ono N, Tsuchida Y, Takeuchi H, Kagoshima H 1983 Why a cross finger flap? An extended use of the homodigital finger dorsum flap. Proceedings of the International Congress of Plastic Surgery, Montreal 1983: 632–634
38. Flint M H, Harrison S H 1965 A local neurovascular flap to repair loss of the digital pulp. British Journal of Plastic Surgery 18: 156–163
39. Pho R W H 1979 Local composite neurovascular island flap for skin cover in pulp loss of the thumb. Journal of Hand Surgery 4: 11–15
40. Harrison S H, Morris A 1975 Dupuytren's contracture: the dorsal transposition flap. The Hand 7: 145–149
41. Vilain R 1953 Technique élémentaire de réparation des pertes de substance cutanée des doigts. Semaine des Hôpitaux 28: 1223–1229
42. Mitz V, Senly G 1975 A propos de l'utilisation du lambeau en drapeau dans la couverture des perts de substance de la troisième phalange. Annales de Chirurgie Plastique 20: 337–342
43. Weeks P M, Wray R C 1973 Management of acute hand injuries. C V Mosby, St Louis, p 140
44. Lai C S, Lin S D, Yang C C 1989 The reverse digital artery flap for fingertip reconstruction. Annals of Plastic Surgery 22: 495–500
45. Lai C S, Lin S D, Chou C K, Tsai C W 1992 A versatile method for reconstruction of finger defects: reverse digital artery flap. British Journal of Plastic Surgery 45: 443–453
46. Kojima T, Tsuchida Y, Hirase Y, Endo T 1990 Reverse vascular pedicle digital island flap. British Journal of Plastic Surgery 43: 290–295

7 DORSAL METACARPAL ARTERIES

First dorsal metacarpal artery flap
Second dorsal metacarpal artery flap – orthograde flow
Second dorsal metacarpal artery flap – retrograde flow
Distally-based dorsal metacarpal artery flaps

Kuhn[1] and Holevitch[2] were possibly responsible for popularising flaps from the dorsal surface of the index finger proximal phalanx. Foucher & Braun[3] demonstrated that a skin island from the dorsum of the index could be carried on a neurovascular pedicle consisting of the first dorsal metacarpal artery (DMA) and its dorso-radial index branch. This has come to be known as the first dorsal metacarpal flap and its anatomy has been further elucidated by Earley.[4,5]

The second dorsal metacarpal artery has been exploited only more recently. Lister's 'axial flag flap'[6] from the dorsum of the proximal phalanx on a proximal web pedicle included branches of the second DMA but only had a short pedicle. A flap from the contiguous sides of the second web with a second DMA pedicle has been described by Earley,[5] and more fully by Small & Brennen who position the flap more directly over the middle finger proximal phalanx.[8]

Reverse second dorsal metacarpal flaps have been described by Maruyama and Quaba.[9,10]

Anatomy

This is covered fully in Chapter 6.

First dorsal metacarpal artery (FDMA). For the purposes of this discussion this term includes the branch to the dorso-radial aspect of the index proximal phalanx. The FDMA has a course within the fascial layer overlying the first dorsal interosseous muscle in the majority of cases. Here it runs parallel to the index metacarpal, becoming more superficial and branching into smaller vessels as it approaches the metacarpophalangeal joint. In ~ 10% of cases there is no superficial artery available for a flap because the artery has a deep course within the substance of the index head of the first dorsal interosseous muscle. In some cases in which a superficial vessel is present it will be found that at the level of the neck of the second metacarpal the vessel disappears deeply to join vessels in the palm and this situation also precludes the elevation of a flap on the FDMA.

One or two dorsal veins lie more superficially in the same area and the sensory branches of the radial nerve obviously also lie at a superficial level but slightly deeper in the fat than the veins.

Second dorsal metacarpal artery (SDMA). The anatomy of this vessel is more consistent than that of the FDMA and it is also generally larger. Once it has passed beneath the index extensor tendons it has a predictable course lying within the fascia over the second dorsal interosseous muscle. At a point approximately 1 cm proximal to the heads of the metacarpals it gives off a significant branch to the skin. At the web the artery divides into branches which ramify over the dorsal skin of the proximal phalanges of both index and middle fingers. The radial nerve branch to the second space and adjacent dorsal skin of the index and middle fingers runs in approximately the same line as the SDMA but at a level superficial to the index finger extensor tendons.

Third and fourth dorsal metacarpal arteries. The third DMA tends to be small and its branches to skin restricted to the distal part of the area over the third intermetacarpal space. The most significant branch reaches skin about 1 cm proximal to the metacarpal heads. The fourth DMA is larger and as well as the branch in the distal part of the intermetacarpal space it also gives off branches more proximally. Flaps may be based on these branches to the skin.

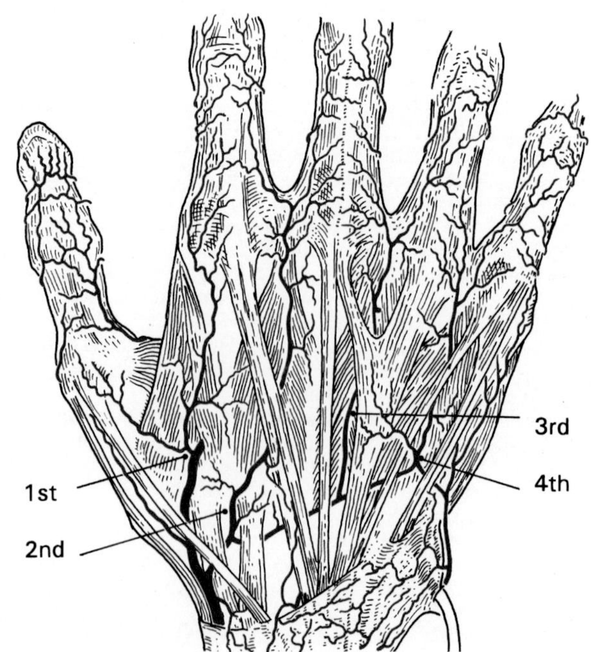

Fig. 7.59 Arterial anatomy on the dorsum of the hand.

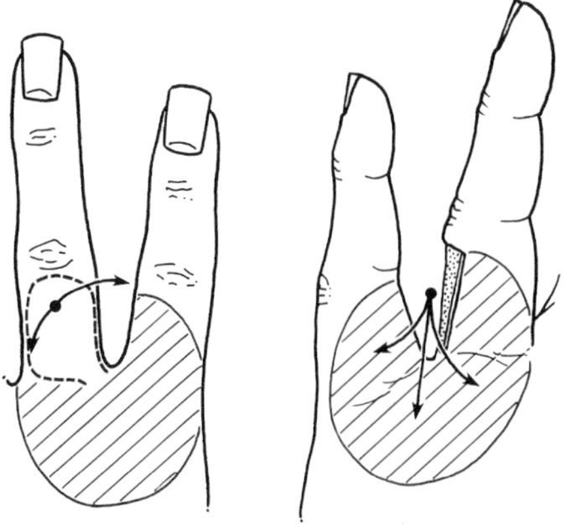

Fig. 7.60 Axial flag flap of Lister based on terminal branches of a second DMA on the middle finger. This can cover a nearby defect on the dorsal or palmar surface. Possible arc of cover indicated by shading.

Surgery

First dorsal metacarpal artery. In order to expose the artery a gently curved incison is made over the dorsum of the first web space. The curve should be convex towards the ulnar side so that the surgeon may have the option of changing to a second DMA dissection without having to make another incision over the dorsum of the hand, in the event that the first DMA does not reach the dorsum of the index finger and therefore cannot support a flap. Through this incision the artery is identified and elevated with a cuff of fascia. Two veins, isolated at a more superficial level, are included as a separate venous pedicle as are branches of the radial nerve if required. The radial edge of the flap is elevated next and then the remainder of the flap is elevated from the paratenon of the extensor tendon.

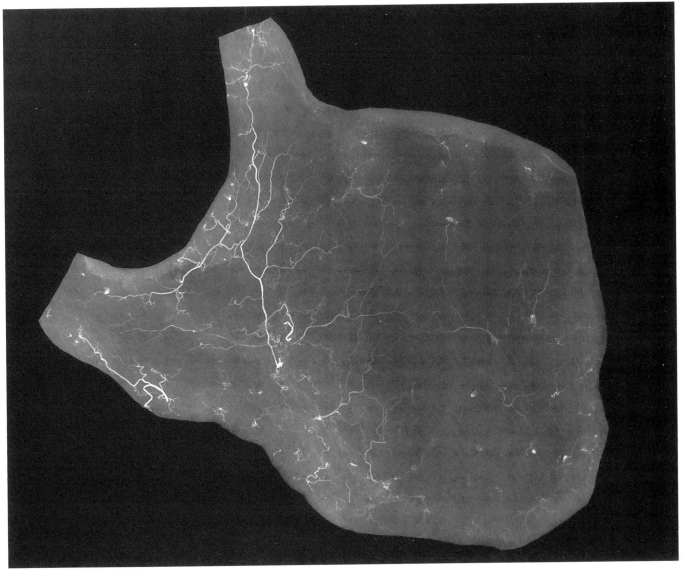

Fig. 7.61 Radiograph of dorsal hand skin shown actual size. The dorso-radial branch of the first dorsal metacarpal artery is clearly seen. Small branches of the other dorsal metacarpal arteries can be seen to anastomose longitudinally.

Second DMA. Either the dorsal skin of the second web is raised with two skin extensions from over the index and middle finger proximal phalanges, or the flap is raised entirely from the skin on the dorsum of the middle or index finger proximal phalanx and adjacent web skin. A proximal skin incision allows the pedicle to be dissected back to the point at which the artery goes deep to the index extensor tendons and if these are retracted even greater mobilisation may be achieved. However, rotation to the thumb is then limited by the radial nerve branches and by superficial veins which lie above the index tendon while the artery lies deep to it. The fascia from over the dorsum of the second dorsal interosseous muscle is included.

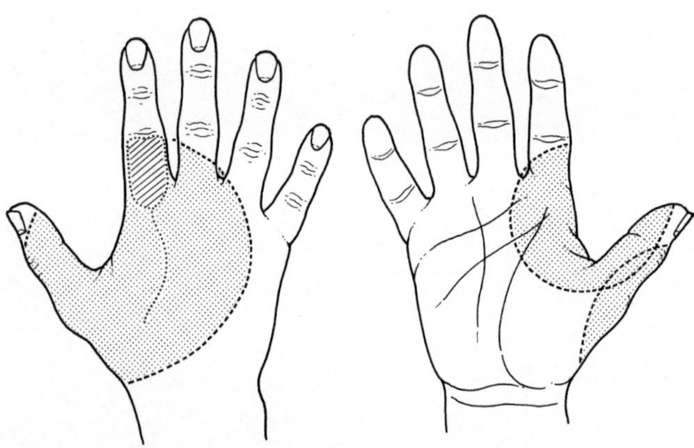

Fig. 7.62 First dorsal metacarpal artery flap planning. The outline of a possible flap is shown in red. Centre of arc of rotation lies at the proximal end of the dorsal incision, and limits of arc of rotation are indicated by shading.

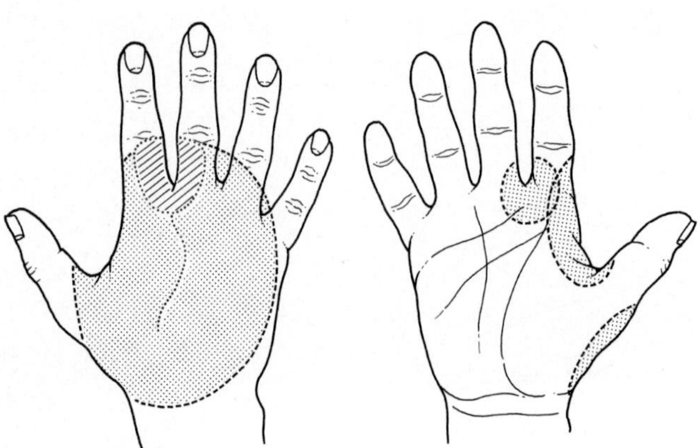

Fig. 7.63 Second dorsal metacarpal artery flap planning. The outline of a possible flap in the second web is shown with the areas that may be covered indicated by shading. The diagram may be a little conservative on the thumb where the flap can just reach to cover an amputation through the interphalangeal joint.

Second DMA with retrograde flow (Maruyama pattern). In this flap the skin island is designed over the intermetacarpal space and is elevated in continuity with the underlying SDMA which is divided at its proximal end beneath the index tendon. Small branches passing between the index and middle finger extensor tendons to reach the overlying skin are preserved. Dissection of the vascular pedicle is continued distally to the web space taking care to preserve the connections between the SDMA and the branches of the palmar digital arteries.

Distally-based dorsal hand flaps. Quaba has shown that it is not necessary to elevate the dorsal metacarpal artery with island flaps from the dorsum of the hand if they are based distally on the branches to skin given off by the second, third and fourth DMAs in the area approximately 1 cm proximal to the metacarpal heads. The skin island is orientated longitudinally so as to incorporate the longitudinal vascular network formed by anastomoses between successive branches of individual dorsal metacarpal arteries. Venous drainage is ensured by the

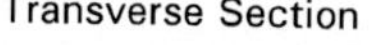

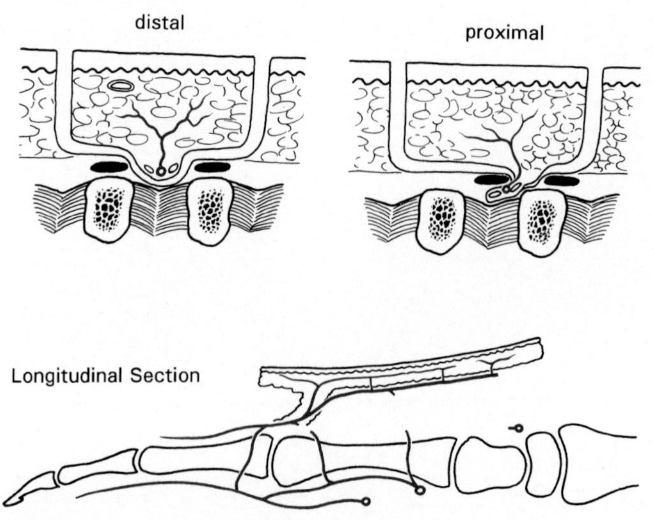

Fig. 7.64 Second DMA reverse-flow flap anatomy (Maruyama pattern).

preservation of a substantial cuff of tissue around the arterial pedicle and some subcutaneous veins may also be preserved at the (anatomically) distal end of the flap. Flow in these veins is reversed from normal. The proximal limit of these flaps is determined by the wrist joint and this enables the arc of rotation to include the dorsal aspects of the fingers to just beyond the PIP joints. The donor site on the dorsum of the hand is often amenable to direct closure.

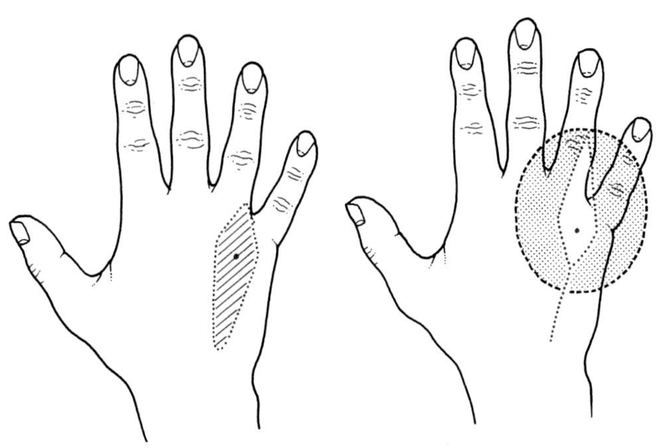

Fig. 7.67 Fourth DMA distally-based flap planning. A similar scheme may be applied to the second or third DMA where the flap can be made longer. Note that recipient site for the flap will have to be in continuity with donor site of flap.

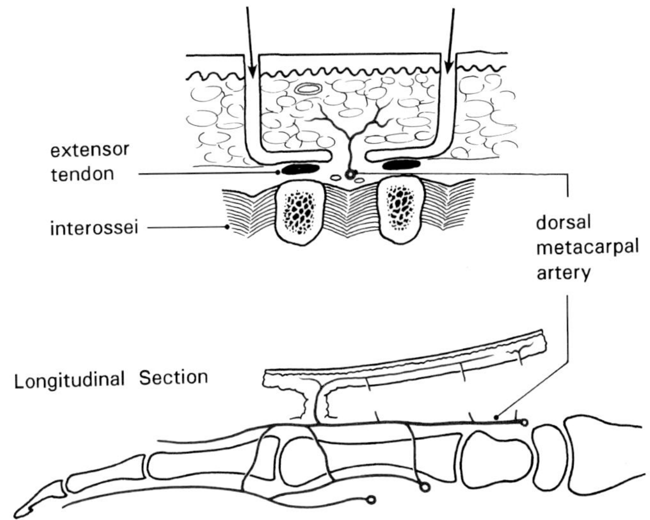

Fig. 7.65 Second DMA distally-based flap anatomy (Quaba pattern).

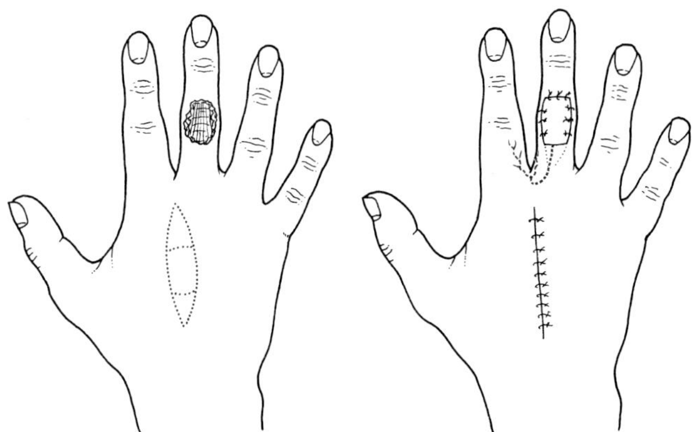

Fig. 7.66 Second DMA reverse-flow example to cover defect on middle finger. Note that recipient site for the flap and the donor site are separate from each other.

References

1. Kuhn H 1961 Reconstruction du pouce par 'Lambeau de Hilgenfeldt'. Annales de Chirurgie Plastique 6: 260–268
2. Holevitch J 1963 A new method of restoring sensibility to the thumb. Journal of Bone and Joint Surgery 45B: 496–502
3. Foucher G and Braun J-B 1979 A new island flap transfer from the dorsum of the index to the thumb. Plastic and Reconstructive Surgery 63: 344–349
4. Earley M J 1986 The arterial supply of the thumb, first web and index finger and its surgical application. Journal of Hand Surgery 11: 163–174
5. Earley M J, Milner R H 1987 Dorsal metacarpal flaps. British Journal of Plastic Surgery 40: 333–341
6. Lister G D 1985 Local flaps to the hand. Hand Clinics 1: 621–640
7. Small J O and Brennen M D 1988 The first dorsal metacarpal artery neurovascular island flap. The Journal of Hand Surgery 13B: 136–145
8. Small J O, Brennen M D 1990 The second dorsal metacarpal artery neurovascular island flap. British journal of Plastic Surgery 43: 17–23
9. Maruyama Y 1990 The reverse dorsal metacarpal flap. British Journal of Plastic Surgery 43: 24–27
10. Quaba A A, Davison P M 1990 The distally-based dorsal hand flap. British Journal of Plastic Surgery 43: 28–39

7 DORSALIS PEDIS ARTERY

Dorsalis pedis flap
Dorsal metatarsal flap

The possibility of raising a free flap based on the dorsalis pedis artery was suggested by O'Brien & Shanmugan in 1973[1] and described by McCraw & Furlow in 1975.[2] A thorough understanding of the underlying anatomical vascular basis of this flap, and the indications for its use, has been slowly established since then. Its principal advantage is thinness, even in the obese individual, and it has the possibility of providing crude sensory innervation by the superficial peroneal nerve.

Dorsalis pedis compound osteocutaneous flaps incorporating the second metatarsal have been described but are not considered here, nor are toe transplants based on this vessel system.

Anatomy

Variations in the so-called normal pattern of distribution of the arterial network on the dorsum of the foot have been described on page 261, but it should be noted that atherosclerotic occlusion of the dorsalis pedis artery at the ankle is relatively common in the elderly and furthermore the presence of a palpable pulse on the dorsum of the foot must not be taken as evidence of a normal supply since the dorsalis pedis may be filled via its lateral tarsal branch anastomosing with the perforating branch of the peroneal or the lateral plantar artery, or it may be filled from the plantar arch via its perforator in the first interosseous space. These conditions may be established by arteriography or with the aid of a directional Doppler probe.

The cutaneous branches of the dorsalis pedis artery enter the skin in a fairly small strip only 2 or 3 cm wide extending from the extensor retinaculum to a point approximately half-way along the first interosseous space. Beyond this point the skin is supplied by the first dorsal metatarsal artery (FDMA) which lies beneath the tendon of extensor hallucis brevis. The disposition of the FDMA is variable and is crucial to the supply of the distal part of the flap. In a variety of studies the FDMA has been found to have a plantar origin, rather than a dorsalis pedis origin, in between 9 and 22% of cases. When it has a deep origin it passes up through the interosseous muscles of the first space and reaches the skin just distal to the extensor hallucis brevis tendon. When it arises from the dorsalis pedis it lies on the fascia of the first dorsal interosseous muscle. Irrespective of origin it usually divides into branches for the adjacent sides of the toes of the first web and may also give off branches to the medial side of the great toe.

The skin lateral to the area fed directly by the dorsalis pedis is supplied by multiple branches from the

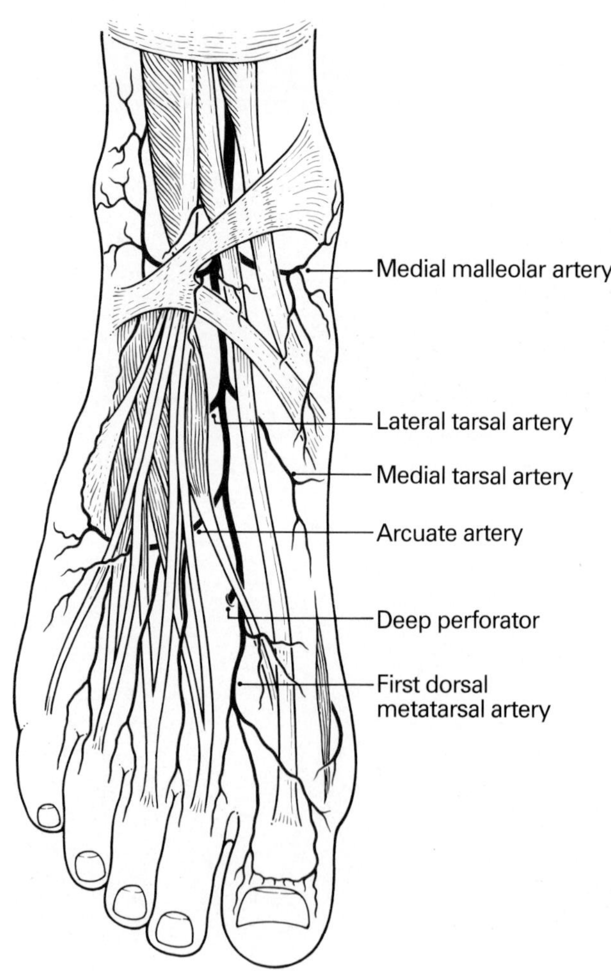

Fig. 7.68 Vascular anatomy. The superior extensor retinaculum and the Y-shaped inferior extensor retinaculum are shown. The lateral tarsal artery and the arcuate artery pass deep to extensor digitorum brevis and the long extensor tendons. In the case illustrated the first dorsal metatarsal artery arises from the dorsalis pedis. The tendon of the short extensor passing to the great toe lies between this artery and the flap and must be divided.

lateral tarsal and acuate arteries although these vessels cannot be included in the flap since they lie deep to extensor digitorum brevis and the long extensor tendons. When elevated as part of a flap this skin is therefore dependent for its blood supply on subcutaneous anastomoses between cutaneous branches of these vessels and branches directly off the dorsalis pedis artery.

There are numerous veins in the flap which drain to the long and short saphenous veins as well as to the paired venae comitantes of the dorsalis pedis artery. The latter often communicate with the dorsal venous arch over the distal part of the first interosseous space.

The superficial peroneal nerve supplies sensation to all of the dorsum of the foot except for the first web space which is supplied by the deep peroneal nerve. Two-point discrimination is poor and averages about 15 mm.

Planning – dorsalis pedis flap

The proximal margin of the flap overlies, or is just proximal to, the lower band of the bifurcate inferior extensor retinaculum which passes from the upper surface of the calcaneus to the medial border of the foot where it attaches to the navicular and blends with the plantar aponeurosis. The flap extends across the width of the dorsum of the foot but does not pass round the borders of the foot. Distally the incision is made proximal to the web spaces of the toes. This distal portion of the flap is the part most prone to necrosis and therefore several experienced surgeons have advocated a conservative policy of performing a delay procedure on this distal portion in all cases. Such a delay involves elevation of the distal part of the flap with ligation of the perforating branches through the interosseous spaces, especially the first. Much of the

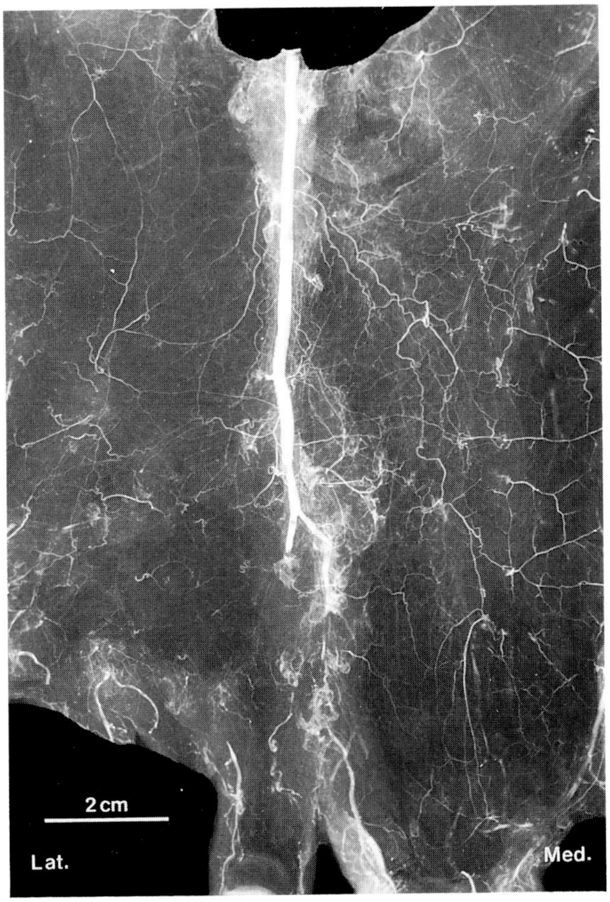

Fig. 7.69 The radiograph shows skin from the dorsum of the foot in continuity with the first two toes only. The first dorsal metatarsal artery was inadvertently divided in elevating the skin, hence the discontinuity in the vessel on the radiograph. All the branches to the skin are very fine indeed.

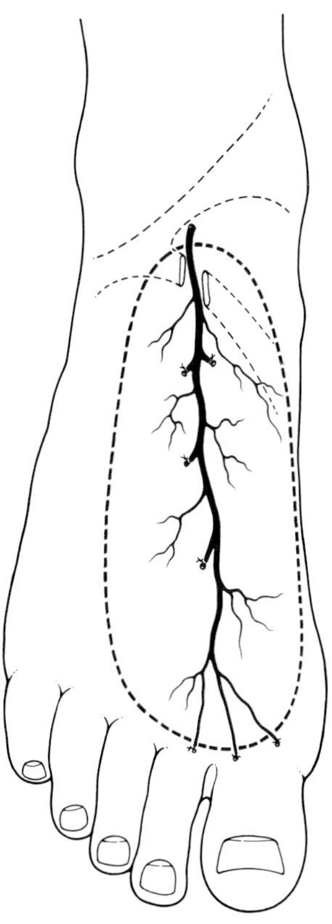

Fig. 7.70 Planning the dorsalis pedis flap elevation. The lower band of the inferior extensor retinaculum has been divided and the major branches of the dorsalis pedis artery ligated and divided.

blood supply to the distal part of the flap comes from the first dorsal metatarsal artery and the variable arrangement of this vessel may determine the tendency for necrosis. May[3] has suggested that a delay is necessary only in those cases where the first dorsal metatarsal artery arises deeply and cannot be incorporated in the flap. It is suggested that the distal end of the flap should be elevated and if this reveals a deep FDMA then the deep perforating branch of the dorsalis pedis artery and the FDMA should be divided, and the flap should be sutured back in its bed. In this minority of cases such a delay manoeuvre will encourage the blood supply to the tip of the flap to come from the more proximal superficial dorsalis pedis artery territory. In most cases it will be possible to elevate the whole flap primarily because the FDMA is superficial and is included within the flap.[4–7]

The flap is elevated under tourniquet in a plane which leaves sufficient paratenon behind for 'take' of the split skin graft. The dissection is carried from the medial side over the tendon of extensor hallucis longus and then on the lateral side of this tendon it passes deeply onto the bone so as to include the dorsalis pedis artery and its venae comitantes with the flap. The lower band of the inferior extensor retinaculum can be divided vertically so that the dorsalis pedis artery can be identified and dissected more easily, and a longer pedicle obtained. If the flap includes the skin overlying the area between the upper and lower bands of the inferior extensor retinaculum then care must be taken to preserve the cutaneous branches of the dorsalis pedis in that region. The dissection proceeds laterally initially above the periosteum of the tarsal bones and then over the long extensor tendons. The tendon of the extensor hallucis brevis muscle passes between the vessel system and the skin and must be divided.

A frequently stated objection to this flap is that it is difficult to get the donor site to heal with a split skin graft. If difficulties in achieving successful graft take are anticipated, particularly in the crevice between the first and second metatarsals, then delayed application of the graft until after granulation tissue has filled the hole has been recommended.

Planning – dorsal metatarsal flap

The small branches to skin from the first dorsal metatarsal artery in the distal part of the foot may be used to support small longitudinally orientated skin flaps from over the dorsum of the first inter-metatarsal space (Fig. 7.71). After transposition through 90° these flaps are useful for filling the defect resulting from release of scar contractures on the dorsum of the foot.[8] If correction of toe hyperextension has required capsulotomy and tendon lengthening these flaps can be particularly helpful. The skin flap may be designed with a distal skin pedicle or may be isolated on a pedicle of subcutaneous tissue; no attempt is made to skeletonise the pedicle down to vessels as they are only 0.7 mm in size at the very largest. The donor site can often be closed directly.

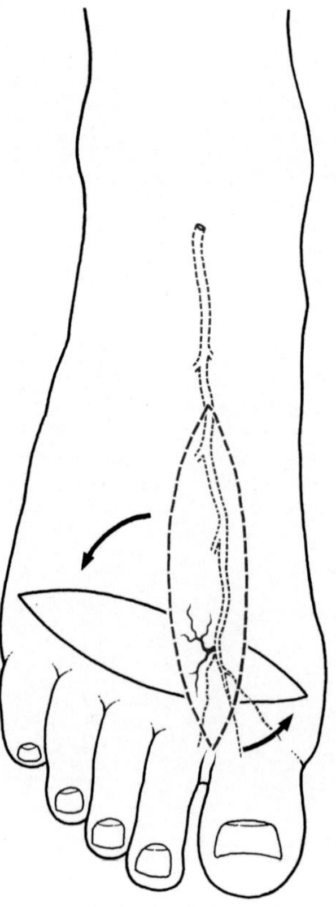

Fig. 7.71 Planning of dorsal metatarsal flap. The outline of an elliptical flap is shown based on the distal cutaneous branch over the first inter-metatarsal space. Transposition is possible into the transverse defect resulting from scar release.

Planning – reverse-flow dorsalis pedis flap

This flap may be useful for covering exposed metatarsal heads in traumatic amputations of the toes or distal forefoot.[9] The dorsalis pedis artery is ligated proximally at the level of the inferior limb of the extensor retinaculum as there are no direct branches to skin through this. Blood flow into the flap is dependent on the deep connections of the dorsalis pedis with the plantar arch and on distal anastomoses of the FDMA.[10] Superficial saphenous system veins and venae comitantes of the dorsalis pedis artery are also ligated at the proximal margin of the flap. Venous drainage of the flap depends on connections that the superficial system makes with the deep system around the dorsalis pedis and in turn connections that these venae comitantes make with the plantar system through the first inter-metatarsal space. Provided that the flap has a reasonably large attachment to the dorsalis pedis artery below the extensor retinaculum, it is possible to extend the proximal limit of the flap some 3 cm above the inferior limb of the extensor retinaculum.

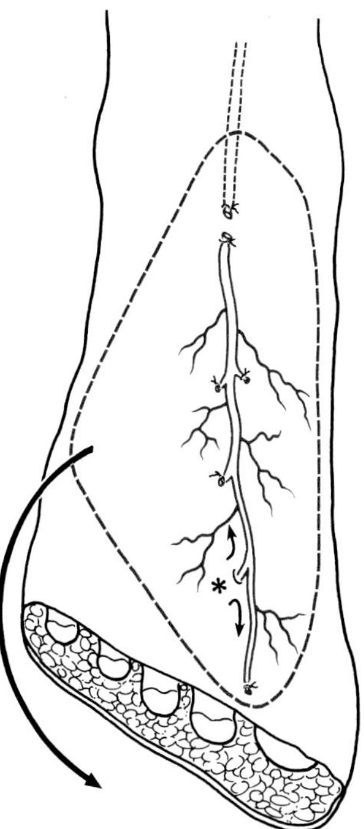

Fig. 7.72 Reverse-flow dorsalis pedis flap planning. Outline of a possible flap for cover of the end of the foot is shown. The area of the flap taken from above the inferior limb of the extensor retinaculum does not receive branches directly from the dorsalis pedis artery but is supported on the rest of the flap.

References

1. O'Brien B McC, Shanmugan M 1973 Experimental transfer of composite free flaps with microvascular anastomoses. Australian and New Zealand Journal of Surgery 43: 285–288
2. McCraw J B, Furlow L T Jr 1975 The dorsalis pedis arterialized flap: A clinical study. Plastic and Reconstructive Surgery 55: 177–185
3. May J W 1977 Letter to the Editor, Plastic and Reconstructive Surgery 59: 909
4. Franklin J D 1979 Use of the free dorsalis pedis flap in head and neck repairs. Plastic and Reconstructive Surgery 63: 195–204
5. Man D, Acland R D 1980 The microarterial supply of the dorsalis pedis flap and its clinical applications. Plastic and Reconstructive Surgery 65: 419–423
6. Chem R C, Franciosi L F N 1983 Dorsalis pedis free flap to close extensive palatal fistulae. Microsurgery 4: 35–39
7. Leeb D, Ben-Hur N, Mazzarella 1977 Reconstruction of the floor of the mouth with a free dorsalis pedis flap. Plastic and Reconstructive Surgery 59: 379–381
8. Earley M J, Milner R H 1989 A distally based first web flap in the foot. British Journal of Plastic Surgery 42: 507–511
9. Ishikawa K, Isshiki N, Suzuki S, Shimamura S 1987 Distally based dorsalis pedis island flap for coverage of the distal portion of the foot. British Journal of Plastic Surgery 40: 521–525
10. Valenti P, Masquelet A C, Bégné T 1990 Anatomic basis of a dorso-commissural flap from the 2nd, 3rd and 4th intermetacarpal spaces. Surgical and Radiological Anatomy 12: 235–239

DORSAL SCAPULAR ARTERY

Lower trapezius musculocutaneous flap

The possibility of carrying skin on the lower part of the trapezius muscle supplied by the dorsal scapular artery/deep branch of the transverse cervical artery was demonstrated by Mathes & Nahai.[1] The cutaneous component may take the form of an island of skin[2,3] or a superiorly-based pedicled flap.[1,4]

Anatomy

The lower part of the trapezius arises from the spinous processes and supraspinous ligaments of the lower thoracic vertebrae. The lowermost fibres ascend almost vertically to insert into a tubercle at the medial end of the lower lip of the spine of the scapula. The middle part of the muscle arises from the lower part of the ligamentum nuchae and upper thoracic spinous processes and runs laterally to be inserted into the medial border of the acromion and the upper border of the crest of the scapular spine. This part of the muscle overlies the rhomboid muscles which are also relevant structures to the elevation of the flap. The rhomboideus minor and rhomboideus major arise from the lower part of the ligamentum nuchae, the seventh cervical spine and the spines and supraspinous ligaments of the first five thoracic vertebrae; they insert into the medial border of the scapula. The rhomboids often form one quadrilateral muscle crossing erector spinae, but the division between them is taken to be at the second thoracic spine.

The lower part of trapezius is supplied by the dorsal scapular artery or deep branch of the transverse cervical artery: (see p. 142 for an explanation of this confusing terminology and details concerning the origin of the dorsal scapular artery and its relationship to trunks of the brachial plexus). The dorsal scapular artery passes downwards lying medial to the vertebral border of the scapula, initially deep to the rhomboids, and in approximately 90% of cases gives off a branch to trapezius as it lies level with the base of the scapular spine. This branch pierces one of the rhomboids or

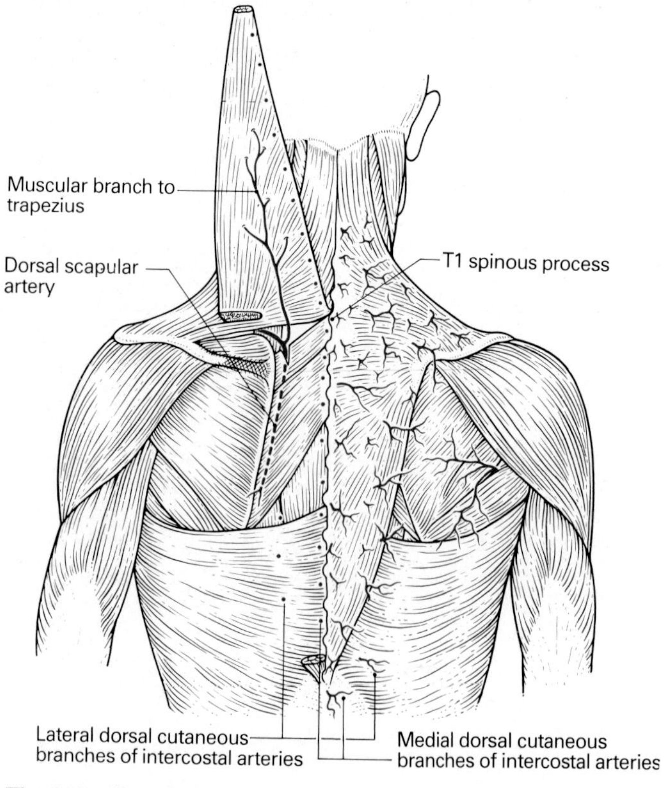

Fig. 7.73 Vascular anatomy. The principal vessels involved are shown.

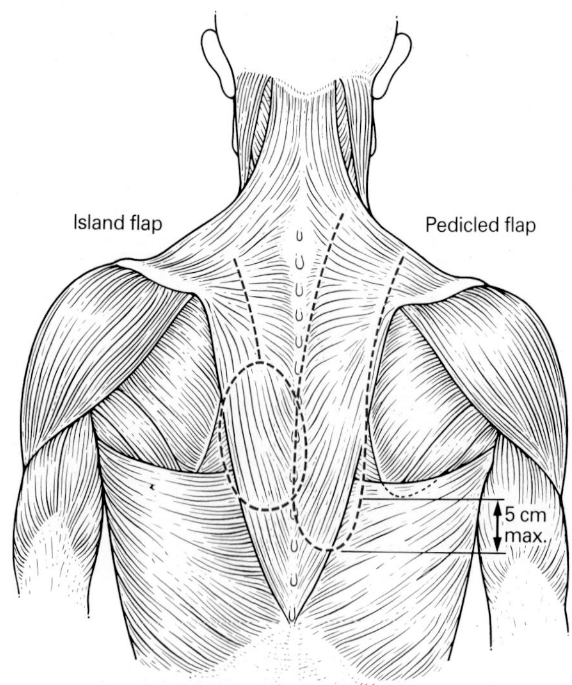

Fig. 7.74 Flap planning. The end of the flap may overlap the lateral edge of trapezius to overlie latissimus dorsi. The flap should not extend more than 5 cm below the lower pole of the scapula.

passes between rhomboideus major and minor to reach the deep surface of trapezius where it supplies the lower third of the muscle. Within the muscle it anastomoses with medial and lateral dorsal cutaneous branches of the posterior intercostal arteries. These vessels are on their way through trapezius to reach the overlying skin and it is via the intramuscular anastomoses with these cutaneous arteries that the dorsal scapular artery is able to supply skin.

Flap elevation

The patient should be positioned lying on the opposite side to that of the intended flap with the scapula brought into a position of protraction by flexion and adduction of the arm at the shoulder. This opens the space between the medial margin of the scapula and the vertebral spines. The cutaneous element of the flap is designed either as an island or a pedicled flap. With a skin island a proximal incision is also required towards the lower neck (Fig. 7.74). The skin incisions are made and the skin adjoining the lateral side of the flap is elevated off the scapula so as to expose the lateral edge of the trapezius musle. Beneath the lowermost part of the muscle lies latissimus dorsi (arising from the lower six thoracic spines) and it is here that blunt dissection commences in order to elevate trapezius. This proceeds upwards raising the muscle from the underlying rhomboid muscles. Perforating lateral dorsal cutaneous rami are ligated and divided, and the origin of the lower part of trapezius from the midline is detached. The dorsal scapular artery branch with its accompanying veins will be seen passing into the undersurface of the muscle and this vascular pedicle is mobilised – this may involve dividing some of the upper fibres of rhomboideus minor. The musculocutaneous island may now be transferred into the recipient site; either (i) by tunnelling it under the lower fibres of the upper part of the trapezius muscle, or (ii) by dividing the muscle and passing the pedicle through a subcutaneous tunnel if the accessory nerve has already been sacrificed, or (iii) by exteriorising the muscle pedicle and covering it with a split skin graft. The donor site may be closed directly.

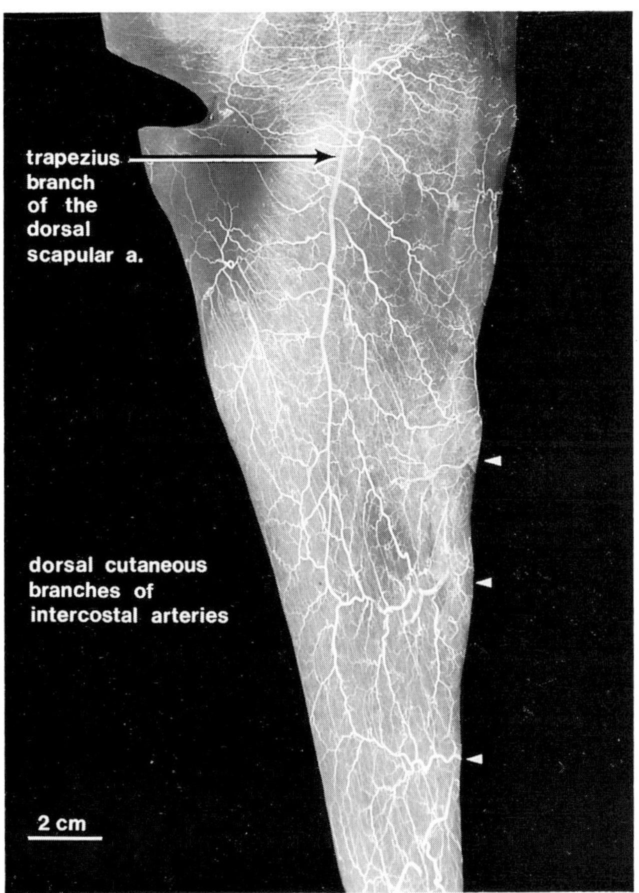

Fig. 7.75 Radiograph of injected lower part of trapezius muscle.

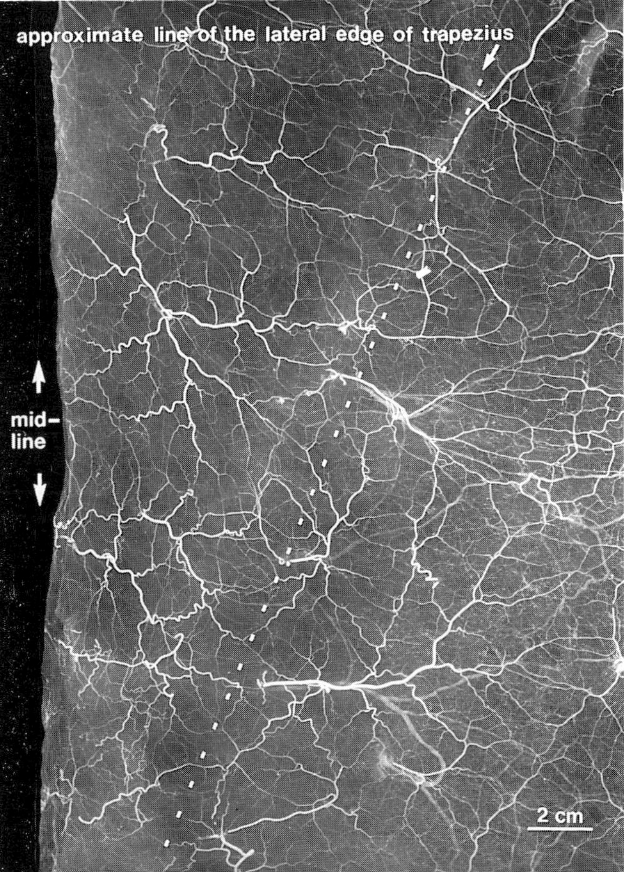

Fig. 7.76 Radiograph of skin and subcutaneous tissues from region overlying the lower part of trapezius.

References

1. Mathes S J, Nahai F 1979 Clinical atlas of muscle and musculocutaneous flaps. C V Mosby Company, St Louis
2. Baek S M, Biller H F, Krespi Y P, Lawson W 1980 The lower trapezius island myocutaneous flap. Annals of Plastic Surgery 5: 108–114
3. Yoshimura Y, Maruyama Y, Takeuchi S 1981 The use of lower trapezius myocutaneous island flaps in head and neck reconstruction. British Journal of Plastic Surgery 34: 334–337
4. Maruyama Y, Nakajima H, Fujino T, Koda E 1981 The definition of cutaneous vascular territories over the back using selective angiography and the intra-arterial injection of prostaglandin E_1: some observations on the use of the lower trapezius myocutaneous flap. British Journal of Plastic Surgery 34: 157–161
5. Seyfer A E 1988 The lower trapezius flap for recalcitrant wounds of the posterior skull and spine. Annals of Plastic Surgery 20: 414–418

FACIAL ARTERY

Nasolabial pedicled flaps
Subcutaneously-pedicled sliding island flaps
Facial artery island flaps

7

Flaps raised from the 'spare' skin of the nasolabial fold fall into three categories – conventional pedicled flaps (superiorly or inferiorly based), subcutaneously-pedicled sliding island flaps, and facial artery island flaps.

Conventionally-pedicled nasolabial flaps may be used either for intraoral reconstructions such as closure of large palatal fistulae or may be used for external cover in local reconstructions, usually of an ala or side of nose. The former tend to be inferiorly-based flaps and the latter superiorly-based, although in terms of the historical development of the nasolabial flap concept this is not the case. For example the first use of a nasolabial flap to repair a palatal fistula occurred in 1868 when Thiersch dissected a superiorly-based nasolabial flap consisting of the whole thickness of the cheek and folded it into the mouth skin-side downwards to close a palatal fistula of traumatic origin. Despite Thiersch's precedence the nasolabial flap repair of the palate is more commonly associated with the name of Esser who in 1917 described his use of inferiorly-based nasolabial flaps of skin only[1] (Fig. 7.77e). The flap was tucked into the mouth through a short incision passing through the cheek deep to the base of the flap while the flap itself was twisted through nearly 180° to bring its raw surface upwards. Since then the operation has been modified by several surgeons[2,3] sometimes by the addition of a split skin graft to the undersurface of the flap to provide lining. Wallace[4] has described the operation and outlined the indications for its use in palatal reconstruction.

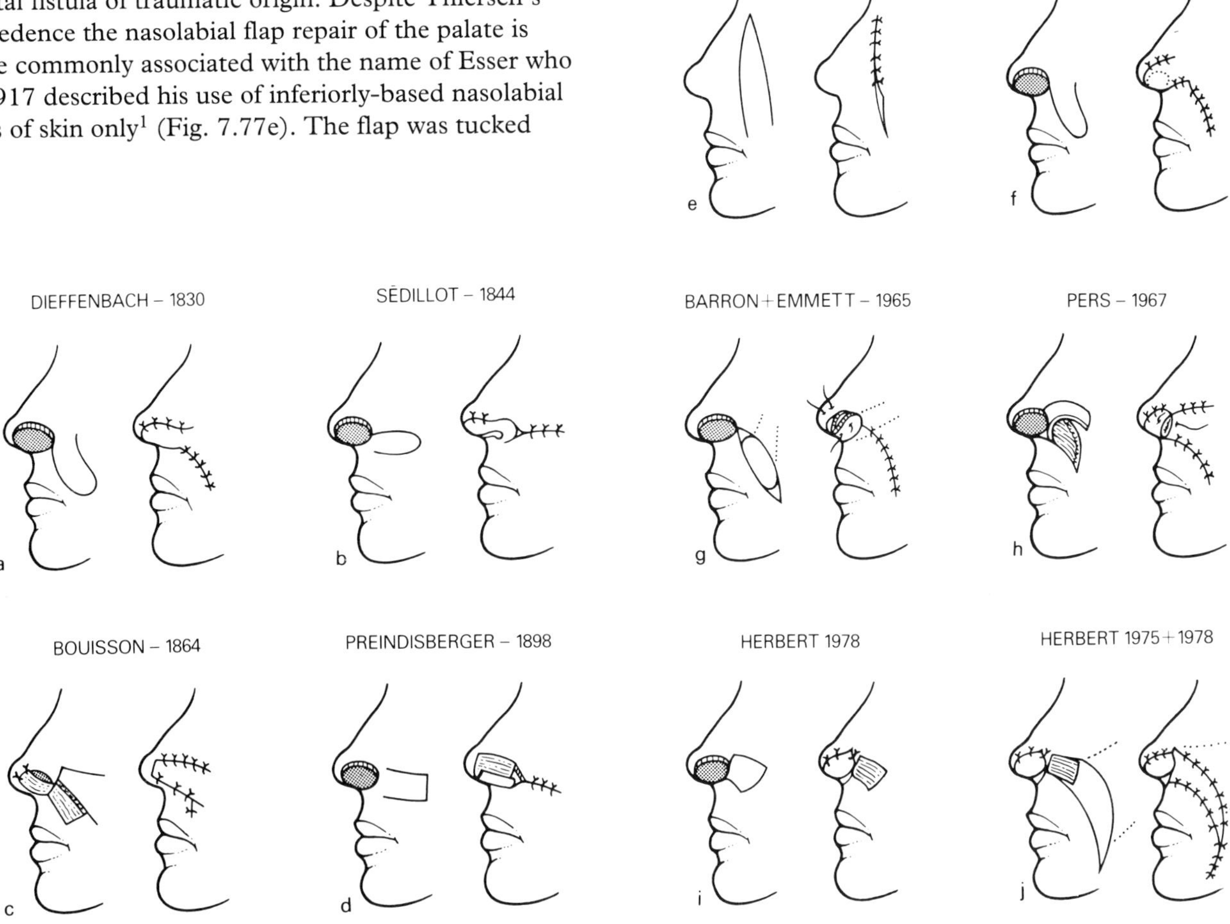

Fig. 7.77 Historical evolution of the nasolabial flap concept (see text).

The use of nasolabial flaps as traditional transposition flaps for repair of defects of the nose and cheek also has a long history which can be traced through several phases of evolution (excluding any possible use by ancient Indian rhinoplasty practitioners).

In the first phase, corresponding to the 19th century, the results of attempts to use these flaps in reconstruction of full thickness defects were compromised by failure to line the flaps with epithelium (Fig. 7.77a, b), or by failure to provide adequate external cover when the flaps were used for vestibular lining (Fig. 7.77c, d) Then in the early part of this century better methods of covering the reversed cheek flap were developed so that it could be used as a reliable source of vestibular lining in combination with either a cheek rotation or a forehead flap. More recently the innovative method of folding the flap has developed so that the flap provides both internal and external cover. Early versions utilised a long pedicled flap extended down into the cheek and folded on itself (Fig. 7.77f) while the most modern techniques depend on subcutaneously-pedicled island flaps.

Subcutaneously-pedicled nasolabial flaps specifically for the purpose of reconstructing full thickness alar and nose defects were developed by Pers[5] (Fig. 7.77h). This flap was based on a 1 cm wide pedicle of subcutaneous tissue situated at the nostril margin. Pers' flaps were about 7 cm long with the shorter lower border following the nasolabial sulcus. The flaps were mobilised up to a point about 1 cm from the base so that the flap could be hinged over to provide internal lining. This left the apex hanging downwards and it could then be brought up to the uppermost corner of the defect, the resulting fold creating a soft alar margin. The reliability of this flap was greater than might reasonably have been expected in the light of the available knowledge at that time. This led Herbert to investigate the detailed blood supply to this region of the face in cadavers.[6] He demonstrated that the medially-based nasolabial flap could have its pedicle reduced to 0.5 cm without endangering the blood supply.[7] This manoeuvre enhanced the mobility of the flap and was combined with a further innovation whereby the secondary defect was closed with a subcutaneously-pedicled nasolabial island flap rather than by the cheek rotation flap used by Pers. This secondary flap was based on a lateral pedicle and therefore was dependent on a different set of vessels from those supplying the medially-based flap.

Nasolabial island flaps pedicled on the facial artery and anterior facial vein have also been described. This modification of the classical nasolabial flap may be useful for the repair of defects of the floor of the mouth as by skeletonising the pedicle the flap achieves greater mobility and reach. Also advantageous is the lack of bulk passing over the alveolus that is associated with the classical flap. As first reported,[8] the flap was passed directly into the floor of the mouth over the mandible but Piggot et al[9] have demonstrated the possibility of passing the flap under the mandible. The flap is elevated from superior to inferior and is raised at a level just deep to the vessels. Of necessity this means that parts of levator labii superioris, zygomaticus major and zygomaticus minor must be removed where they lie between the vessels and the skin.

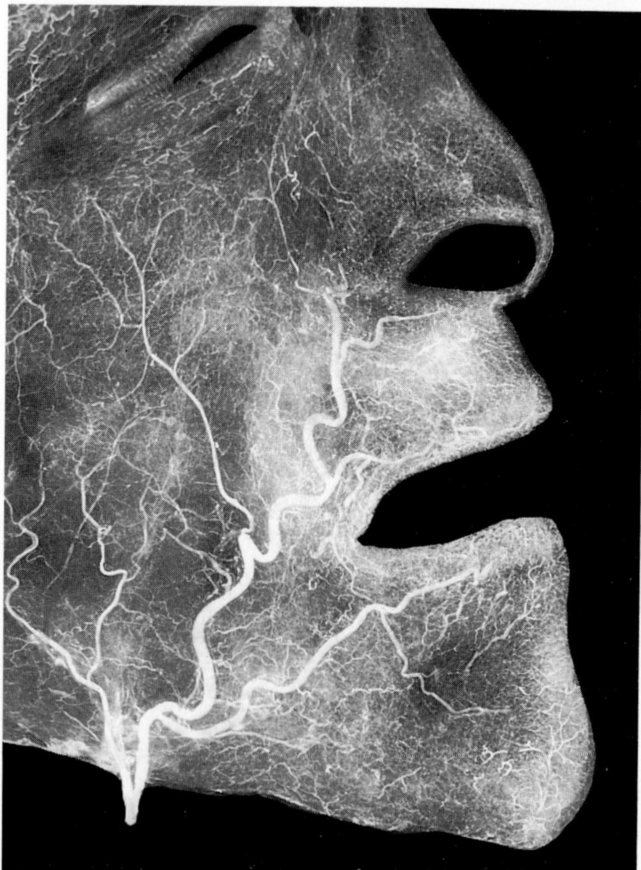

Fig. 7.78 Radiograph of injected skin with facial artery in continuity.

Anatomy

The region of the cheek lying lateral to the alar base is involved in all these flaps and receives its blood supply by multiple small branches from the alar branch given off by the superior labial as it passes into the upper lip. It turns round the lateral side of the alar base lying deep in the groove between the alar and the cheek, buried in the fibres of orbicularis oris and the levator labii superioris alaequi nasi. It runs parallel to the margin of the nostril and ends on the dorsum of the nasal tip by anastomosing with the alar branch of the superior labial artery of the other side. The facial artery, now the angular artery, also gives off a couple of branches to the subcutaneous tissues at this point. Other areas of the face where the tissues are particularly well served by arterial branches are also illustrated in Figure 7.79, namely at the medial canthus of the eye, below the modiolus, and over the maxilla beneath the lateral canthus of the eye, just anterior to masseter.

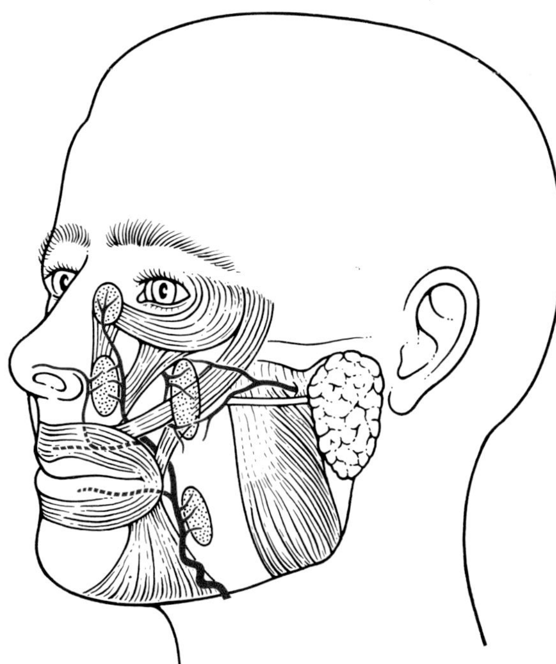

Fig. 7.79 Areas of subcutaneous tissue particularly well served by branches from the facial, infraorbital and transverse facial arteries are indicated by shading. (Modified after Herbert)

Surgery

The Pers and Herbert medially-based flaps undoubtedly depend on the numerous branches in the nasolabial fold lateral to the alar base. The Herbert sliding nasolabial flap[10] which is advanced upwards with a V to Y closure in the lower end of the nasolabial fold (Fig. 7.77j) is based on a lateral pedicle. These flaps may also be used to fill defects of the inner canthus and side of the nose. In order to achieve sufficient mobility it has been found necessary to divide the perforators entering above the zygomaticus major but the posterolateral and inferior perforating groups of vessels are preserved. Where much migration of the flap is required it should be planned to reach as far as the lower border of the mandible otherwise the level of the angle of the mouth represents the minimum length. When advancement above the level of the alar base is planned the flap should generally not be advanced more than 2 cm since advancement more than this was found by Herbert to impair the perfusion of the flap in the majority of cases.[10]

References

1. Esser J F S 1918 Deckung von Gaumendefekten mittels gestielter Naso-Labial-Hautlappen. Deutsche Zeitschrift für Chirurgie 147: 128–135
2. Georgiade N G, Mladick R A, Thorne F L 1969 The nasolabial tunnel flap. Plastic and Reconstructive Surgery 43: 463
3. Zarem H A 1971 Current concepts in reconstructive surgery in patients with cancer of the head and neck. Surgical Clinics of North America 51: 149–173
4. Wallace A F 1966 Esser's skin flap for closing large palatal fistulae. British Journal of Plastic Surgery 19: 322–326
5. Pers M 1967 Cheek flaps in partial rhinoplasty: A new variation: the in and out flap. Scandinavian Journal of Plastic and Reconstructive Surgery 1: 37
6. Herbert D C, Harrison R G 1975 Nasolabial subcutaneous pedicle flaps. I. Observations on their blood supply. British Journal of Plastic Surgery 28: 85–89
7. Herbert D C 1978 A subcutaneous pedicled cheek flap for reconstruction of alar defects. British Journal of Plastic Surgery 31: 79–92
8. Rose E H 1981 One-stage arterialized nasolabial island flap for floor of mouth reconstruction. Annals of Plastic Surgery 6: 71–75
9. Piggot T A, Logan A M, Knight S L, Milner R H 1987 The facial artery island flap. Annals of Plastic Surgery 19: 260–265
10. Herbert D C, DeGeus J 1975 Nasolabial subcutaneous pedicle flaps. II. Clinical experience. British Journal of Plastic Surgery 28: 90–96
11. Gewirtz H S, Eilber F R, Zarem H A 1978 Use of the nasolabial flap for reconstruction of the floor of the mouth. American Journal of Surgery 136: 508–511

7 FACIAL ARTERY – submental branch

Platysma musculocutaneous flaps

The combination of platysma and overlying skin as an 'apron flap' was described by Ward & Hendrick in 1950. This was later modified by DesPrez & Kiehn[1] who de-epithelialised the proximal segment (Fig. 7.82) in order to be able to introduce the skin paddle into the floor of the mouth. In 1978 this was recognised to be a musculocutaneous flap[2] and several variations on this principle have since evolved. In these, the cutaneous paddle is usually designed as an ellipse over the lower or upper part of the muscle.

Anatomy

The platysma muscle extends as a thin broad sheet over almost the whole of the ventral and lateral sides of the neck. Distally it covers the clavicle and extends to the second rib. Superiorly it is attached to the lower border of the mandible but the posterior superficial fibres carry on into the superficial parotid fascia and angle of the mouth. The fibres lie in thin parallel bundles and approach the midline superiorly (Fig. 7.81). Frequently some of the medial fibres do not reach the chin but end in the superficial fascia.

It is important to appreciate the variability of the muscle. It may be unilaterally or bilaterally absent; it is rarely foreshortened but may be lengthened and extend down to the fourth rib. Rarely the two anterior edges may blend together in the midline throughout their length (Fig. 7.81d). Fibre bundles crossing the midline are more often found above the level of the laryngeal prominence (Fig. 7.81c). Occasionally fibres reach high up on the face – up to the zygomatic arch and orbicularis oculi has been recorded. It may be joined by slips of muscle from the mastoid process, the occipital bone or from the fascia over the upper part of trapezius (Occipitalis minor).

Platysma is innervated by the cervical branch of the facial nerve which enters the muscle along two lines; the upper runs parallel and close to the edge of the mandible, the lower lies slightly caudal to the middle of the muscle. Occasionally additional motor fibres from C3 and 4 run with the transverse nerve of the neck and either communicate with the facial nerve branches to be distributed with them, or run to the muscle direct. The sensory innervation of the skin over platysma comes from the transverse nerve of the neck (C2,3), and over the lower part from the supraclavicular nerves (C3,4).

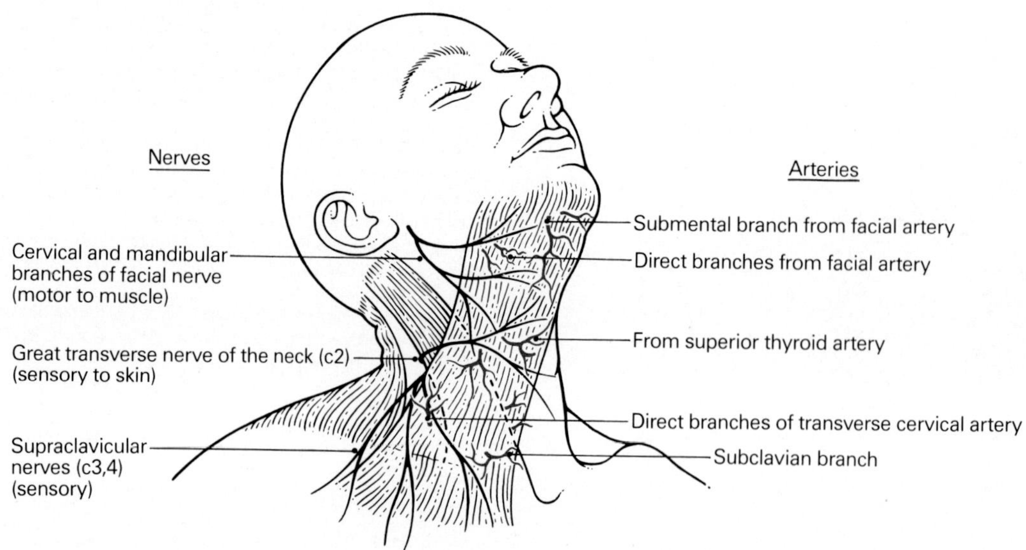

Fig. 7.80 Anatomy of blood supply and nerve supply to platysma and skin.

The muscle is vascularised by branches of the facial artery, the superior thyroid artery, the transverse cervical artery and the subclavian artery. (Contributions from the hyoid branch of the lingual artery have also been described but not confirmed.) These branches form a plexus in and beneath the muscle from which the skin is supplied (Fig. 7.80). These arteries are described in greater detail on page 135, but the principal ones are the submental branch of the facial superiorly, and the superior thyroid and transverse cervical inferiorly.

The venous drainage is by veins lying deep to platysma. Anteriorly these are the anterior jugular vein (one each side) arising from the submental venous plexus, and laterally the external jugular vein receiving blood from the retromandibular vein and draining downwards across the sternomastoid towards the middle of the clavicle. Just above the clavicle anterior and external jugular are connected by a horizontal vein which may lie either superficial or deep to sternomastoid.

Planning

The cutaneous paddle is usually designed as an ellipse to permit direct closure of the donor site or perhaps as a 60° rhomboid to permit Limberg flap closure. The maximum dimensions are about 10 cm × 6 cm.

Figure 7.83 shows the usual arrangement with the skin paddle situated over the lower part of the muscle, but above the clavicle. From this position an arc of rotation based on facial and submental vessels takes the flap up to the malar region and upper lip. A skin paddle extending lower than the clavicle would require an extensive attachment to the underlying platysma

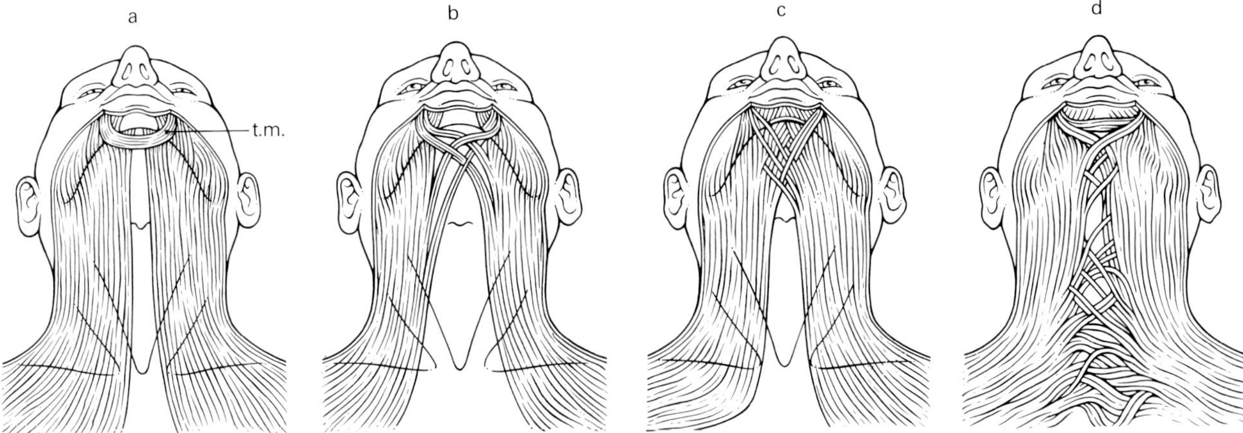

Fig. 7.81 Variations in development of platysma (it may be absent). **tm.** transversus menti. (**a, b & c.** after Schmidt D 1894. Arch. f. Anat 269–291, No. 2, 19 & 24; **d.** after v. Lanz 1922 Z. f. Morph. Anthrop. 22: 373)

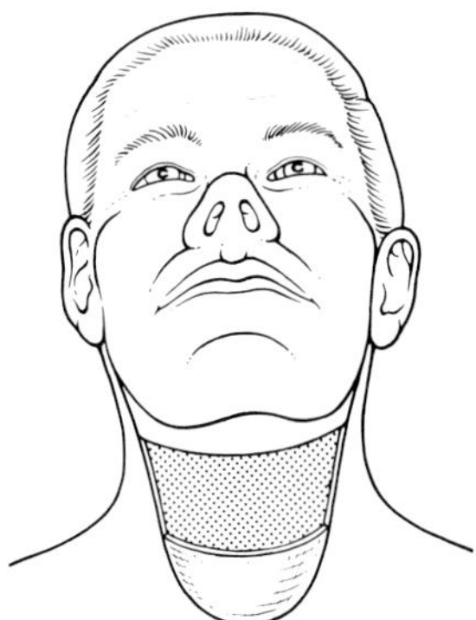

Fig. 7.82 'Apron flap' (c. 1959). The proximal shaded part is de-epithelialised and supports the distally situated skin paddle.

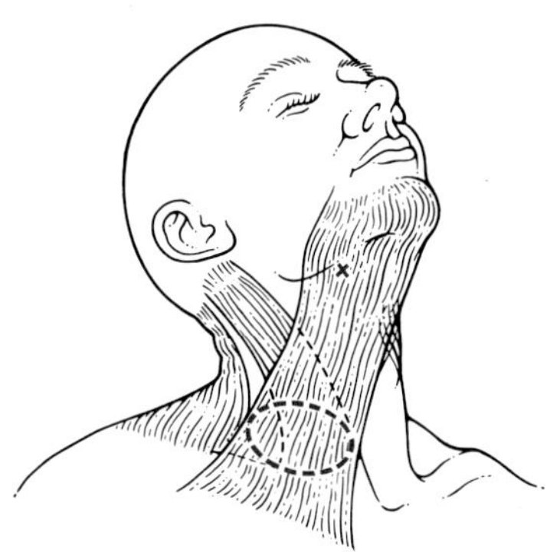

Fig. 7.83 Inferiorly situated skin paddle is indicated. **X** marks the point of rotation.

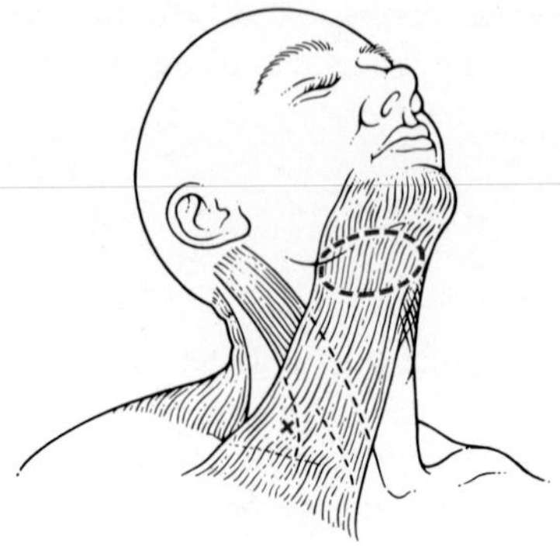

Fig. 7.84 Superiorly situated skin paddle. **X** marks the point of rotation.

(minimum skin island diameter of 6 cm) to be sure that blood could reach the skin, and an intact superior thyroid pedicle, which would restrict the arc of rotation. Cases have been reported[3] in which the flap was used in the presence of a previously divided facial artery but nevertheless survived. This was no doubt due to the extensive anastomoses of the submental artery above the mandible and across the midline which enable it to still pass on blood to the flap in the absence of facial artery input. Other surgeons[4] have stated that the flap cannot be used with a block dissection of the neck because the facial artery is divided proximal to its submental branch. In theory the sensory branches to the flap could be preserved and reattached to a suitable nerve in the recipient area and indeed an instance has been described in which the transverse nerve of the neck was joined to the mental nerve in order to provide sensibility to a lip reconstruction.[5]

Figure 7.84 shows the superiorly-situated skin paddle pedicled on the branch of the transverse cervical artery. A requirement for this design is less frequent but it may, for example, be appropriate in closing a tracheostomy.

Surgery

The flap requires meticulous dissection and even then there are likely to be minor post-operative complications in many cases (42% of 24 patients in one reported series[4]). The dissection is well escribed by Hurwitz et al[3] who make the important point that fascia over sternomastoid must be included with the flap, as also must its continuation over the posterior triangle. Apart from protecting the vasculature on platysma this also helps one to include the external and anterior jugular veins which are necessary for venous drainage of the flap.

With an inferiorly-situated flap the procedure commences with a skin incision around the flap and undermining of the proximal skin between the facial defect and the flap. A small incision beneath the mandible may aid this. The distal part of the muscle is then elevated until branches of the superior thyroid artery are encountered at the anterior border of sternomastoid. Once the cutaneous branch of the superior thyroid is identified, other branches may be ligated and divided to reduce the tethering effect of the vessel on the arc of rotation of the flap. The supraclavicular and transverse cervical nerves are divided, but the motor innervation from the facial nerve is preserved.

References

1. DesPrez J D, Kiehn C L 1959 Method of reconstruction following resection of anterior oral cavity and mandible for malignancy. Plastic and Reconstructive Surgery 24: 238–249
2. Futrell J W, Johns M E, Edgerton M T, Cantrell R W, Fitz-Hugh G S 1978 Platysma myo-cutaneous flap for intraoral reconstruction. American Journal of Surgery 136: 504–507
3. Hurwitz D J, Rabson J A, Futrell J W 1983 The anatomic basis for the platysma skin flap. Plastic and Reconstructive Surgery 72: 302–312
4. Coleman J J, Jurkiewicz M J, Nahai F, Mathes S J 1983 The platysma musculocutaneous flap: Experience with 24 cases. Plastic and Reconstructive Surgery 72: 315–321
5. Hurwitz D J, Kerber C W 1981 Haemodynamic considerations in the treatment of arteriovenous malformations of the face and scalp. Plastic and Reconstructive Surgery 67: 421–432
6. Suárez Nieto C, Lorenzo Gallego L, Galán Cortes J C 1983 Reconstruction of the posterior wall of the pharynx using a myocutaneous platysma flap. British Journal of Plastic Surgery 36: 36–39

FEMORAL ARTERY – fasciocutaneous branches

Medial thigh flap

The possibility of raising fasciocutaneous flaps from the anteromedial thigh based on fasciocutaneous perforators from the femoral artery was first reported by Baek[1] who described the anatomy and a single demonstrative clinical case.[2] Further cases based on similar principles, although not on precisely the same vessels, have been developed by Song.[3] The authors have described the relevant anatomical findings in 50 preserved cadavers and injection studies of fresh cadavers;[4] those findings are summarised here.

Anatomy

The course of the femoral artery along the length of the thigh may be roughly divided into three equal parts. In the first third it lies in the femoral triangle, in the remaining two-thirds it lies in the sub-sartorial canal with the third part under cover of the fascia between vastus medialis and the abductors. In the lower two-thirds of its course it gives off branches to muscles and fasciocutaneous branches which pass in the fascia around the sides of sartorius to reach the skin overlying the muscle. Here the perforators divide into mainly ascending and descending branches which form a plexus at the level of the deep fascia with an axiality aligned parallel with the long axis of sartorius (Figs 7.85 & 7.86). Perforators pass round both borders of sartorius and range in size between 0.5 and 1.0 mm in internal diameter excluding the descending genicular artery and its saphenous branch which forms the basis for another specific flap.[5]

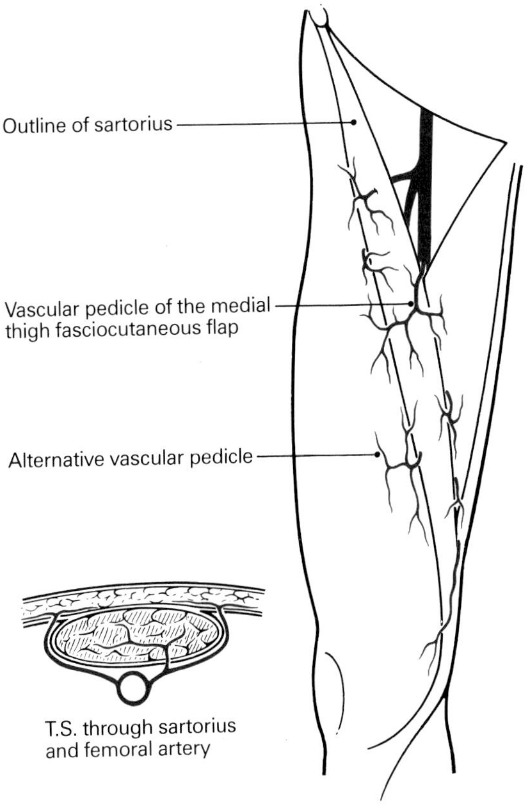

Outline of sartorius

Vascular pedicle of the medial thigh fasciocutaneous flap

Alternative vascular pedicle

T.S. through sartorius and femoral artery

Fig. 7.85 Vascular anatomy. Branches of the femoral artery are shown emerging along the borders of sartorius to supply the skin. The smaller diagram shows the relationship of these branches to the muscular branches of supply to sartorius.

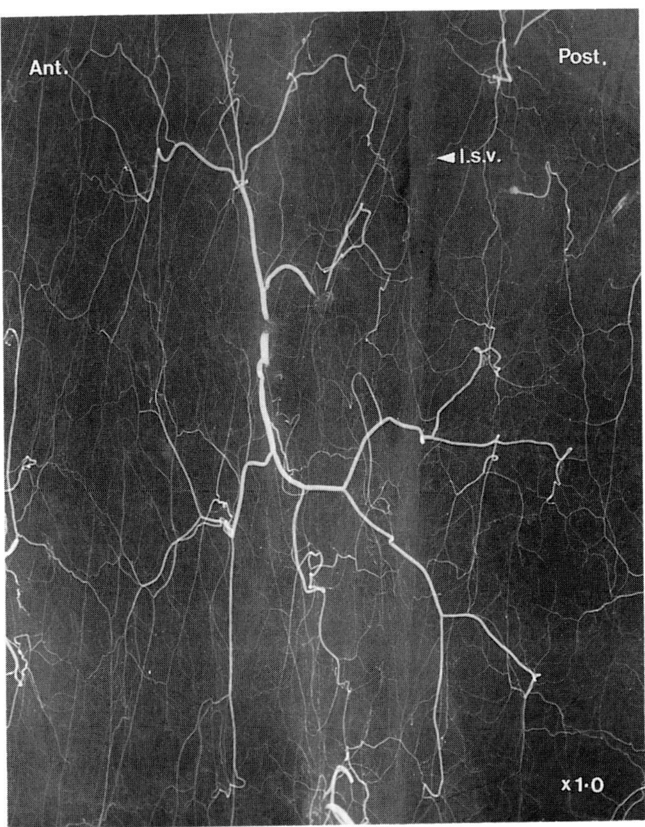

Fig. 7.86 The radiograph of skin shows a single perforator from the lowermost part of the femoral triangle. The shadow of the long saphenous vein may be vaguely discerned (it is not filled with contrast medium).

In approximately 78% of cases there is a perforator, generally the largest of all the perforators (excluding the saphenous artery), passing round the superior/medial border of sartorius in the apex of the femoral triangle. This is the vessel described by Baek on which he based the medial thigh flap. In addition to supplying skin this vessel always supplies muscle so that at its point of origin from the femoral artery it is larger in diameter than the cutaneous branch alone. The cutaneous branch measures 0.5–1.2 mm in internal diameter and at its origin measures up to 1.5 mm ID. It is accompanied by a vein which provides venous drainage of the area supplied by the artery. Injection of this artery stains an elliptical area of skin approximately 7 cm × 12 cm in size over the anteromedial part of the thigh. The ellipse is orientated with the long axis vertically and the upper part of the ellipse overlies the apex of the femoral triangle.

Song et al[3] have described an anteromedial thigh flap based on a cutaneous branch of the lateral circumflex femoral artery which emerges in the narrow triangular interval between sartorius, rectus femoris and vastus medialis and supplies skin. The authors have found this to be an uncommon vessel. Song states that in those cases in which the artery is 'too slender or non-existent' a branch of the femoral which arises at the junction of the middle and lower thirds of the thigh and supplies sartorius, can be found. He suggests the use of the cutaneous branch of this vessel which provides a pedicle of up to 5 cm in length with an external diameter of 2 mm. This vessel emerges around the inferior border of sartorius and, although not the same as the vessel on which Baek based his flap, the principle is obviously the same. Indeed there are always several perforators emerging around the borders of sartorius whose pattern is not absolutely constant and it is somewhat artificial to place too heavy an emphasis on attempting to surface-mark any one of these with any degree of exactness. Exploration of the area is certain to reveal at least one vessel with sufficient size and area of distribution to support a flap.

Koshima et al[6] have also described flaps based on these perforators and have stressed the variable position of the main perforator which they, like Song, found lateral to sartorius.

The area of the anteromedial thigh is innervated by the medial anterior cutaneous nerve of the thigh (Fig. 7.87). This is one of the three cutaneous divisions of the femoral nerve and crosses medially in front of the artery at the apex of the femoral triangle. It sends a proximal branch to the skin near the great saphenous vein and a middle branch over sartorius to the skin over the medial side of the thigh before finally ending as a distal branch over the medial side of the knee.

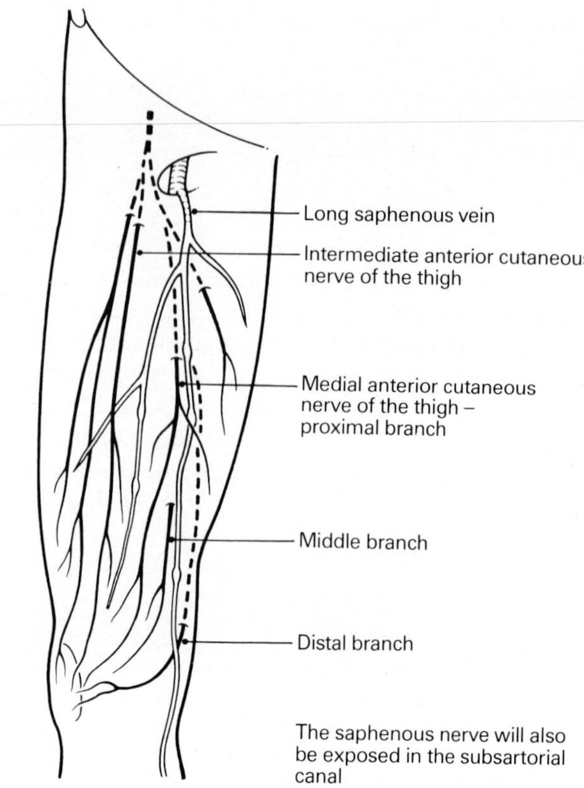

Fig. 7.87 Cutaneous nerves and veins in the area of the flap.

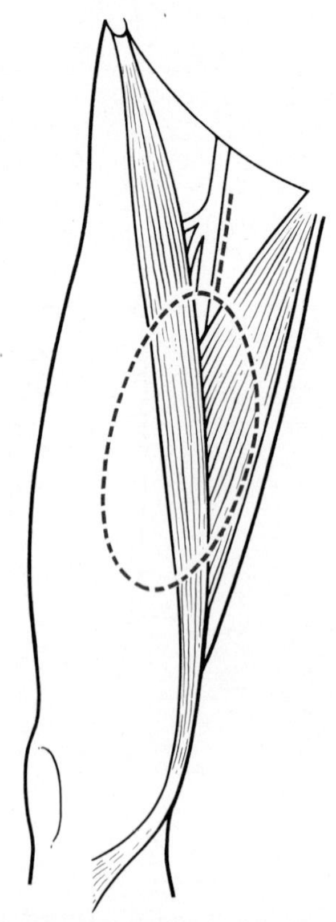

Fig. 7.88 Flap planning. Since most of the perforators incline distally an initial proximal incision will reveal any potential pedicle and will allow the precise location of the flap to be adjusted accordingly.

Flap elevation

The exact location of the vascular pedicle is first identified and the position of the flap is then adjusted so as to be centred over its branches. A vertical incision over the lower part of the femoral triangle is deepened through the fascia to expose the femoral artery which is then followed down towards the subsartorial canal where the arterial pedicle will be found arising from its medial side. If an innervated flap is required damage to the medial cutaneous nerve of the thigh must be avoided as it crosses the femoral triangle; it can later be dissected out once the flap has been prepared. The pedicle is dissected and the muscular branch to sartorius ligated. The anterior and posterior margins of the flap are then incised and the flap is elevated from anterosuperior to posteroinferior. The deep fascia must be elevated with the flap since the arterial plexus largely lies at this level. The long saphenous vein passes through the posterior part of this flap and Baek recommends that this should be dissected free from the undersurface of the flap so as to leave the vein intact on the thigh; depending on the position of the vein, however, this may involve dividing vital vessels in the fascial plexus and may compromise the circulation to parts of the flap.

The donor site may be closed directly.

References

1. Baek S M 1982 Two new neurovascular free flaps: medial and lateral thigh flaps. 51st Annual Meeting of the American Society of Plastic and Reconstructive Surgeons. Honolulu, Hawaii. Abstracted in Plastic Surgical Forum 5: 27
2. Baek S M 1983 Two new cutaneous free flaps: the medial and lateral thigh flaps. Plastic and Reconstructive Surgery 71: 354–363
3. Song Y G, Chen G Z, Song Y L 1984 The free thigh flap: a new free flap concept based on the septocutaneous artery. British Journal of Plastic Surgery 37: 149–159
4. Cormack G C, Lamberty B G H 1985 The blood supply of thigh skin. Plastic and Reconstructive Surgery 75: 342–354
5. Acland R D, Schusterman M, Godina M, Eder E, Taylor G I, Carlisle I 1981 The saphenous neurovascular free flap. Plastic and Reconstructive Surgery 67: 763–774
6. Koshima I, Soeda S, Yamasaki M, Kyou J 1988 The free or pedicled anteromedial thigh flap. Annals of Plastic Surgery 21: 480–485

7

GLUTEAL ARTERIES – superior and inferior

Gluteal musculocutaneous flaps

Anatomy

Gluteus maximus is made up of large coarse fibre bundles which have an extensive origin from the ilium between the posterior gluteal line and the crest, from the aponeurosis of erector spinae, and from the sacrotuberous ligament and the back of the sacrum and coccyx. The parallel bundles are directed downwards and laterally with the greater part of the muscle inserting into the posterior border of the iliotibial tract and only the lower deep fibres inserting into the gluteal tuberosity of the femur.

Although gluteus maximus is usually classified as a Type III muscle on account of its two dominant vascular pedicles, an additional contribution from the first profunda perforator which enters the lower insertion of the muscle is of practical significance. Usually the inferior gluteal artery is dominant over the superior, and supplies approximately two-thirds of the muscle, but this pattern may be reversed. Small branches of supply also reach the muscle from the medial and lateral circumflex femoral, the lateral sacral and the internal pudendal arteries – but flaps cannot be based on these vessels alone. The surface markings of the gluteal arteries are summarised in Figure 7.89. For further details concerning the distribution of these arteries and the inferior gluteal nerve, see page 220.

Territory

It is necessary to be able to define the edges of the

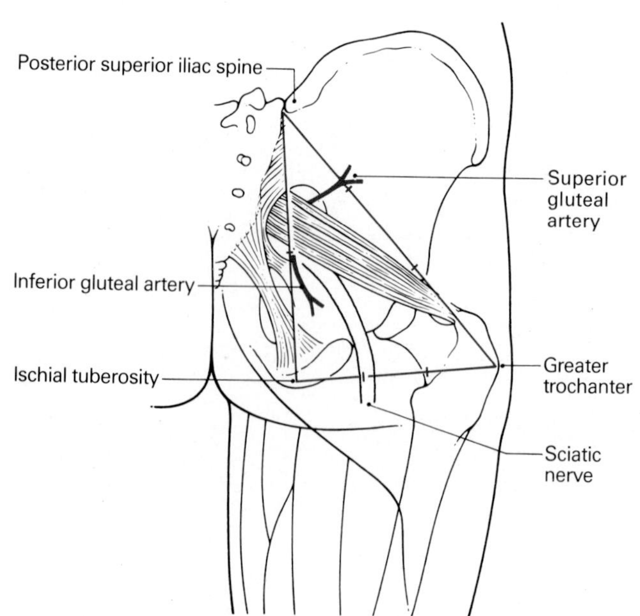

Fig. 7.89 Surface markings of the approximate points of emergence into the buttock of the superior and inferior gluteal arteries related to palpable bony landmarks.

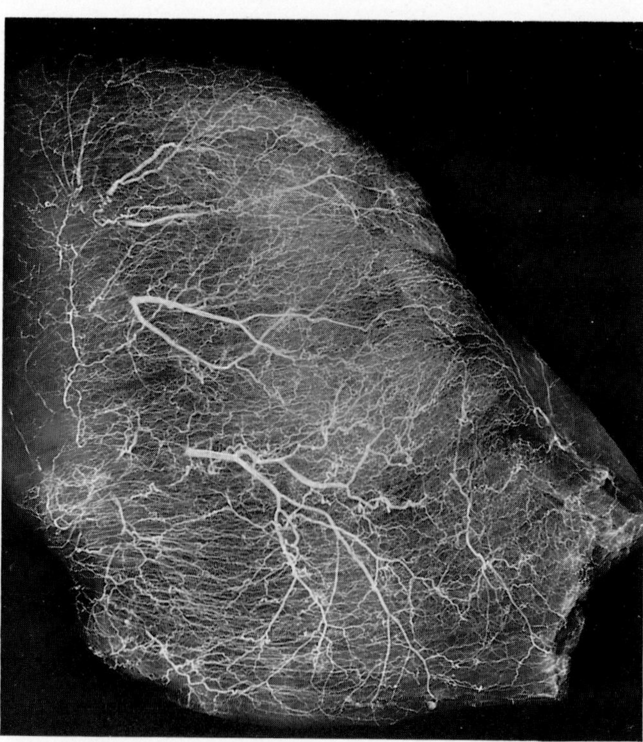

Fig. 7.90 Radiograph of injected gluteus maximus muscle. See Fig. 6.77 for a radiograph of buttock skin, and Fig. 6.97 for the branches of the inferior gluteal artery which extend down the posterior thigh to support the gluteal thigh flap.

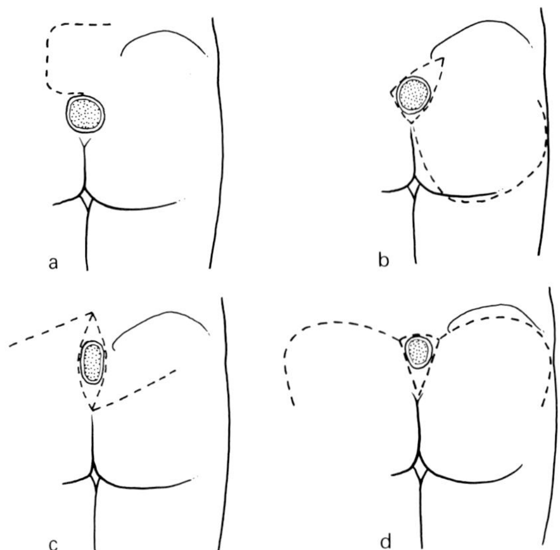

Fig. 7.91 Various local skin flaps.

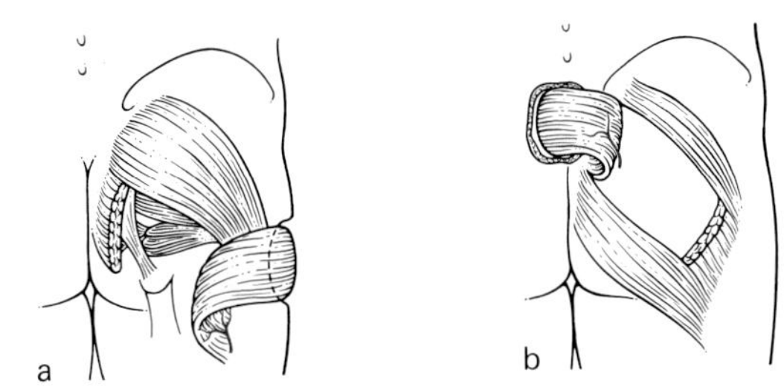

Fig. 7.92 Various local muscle flaps.

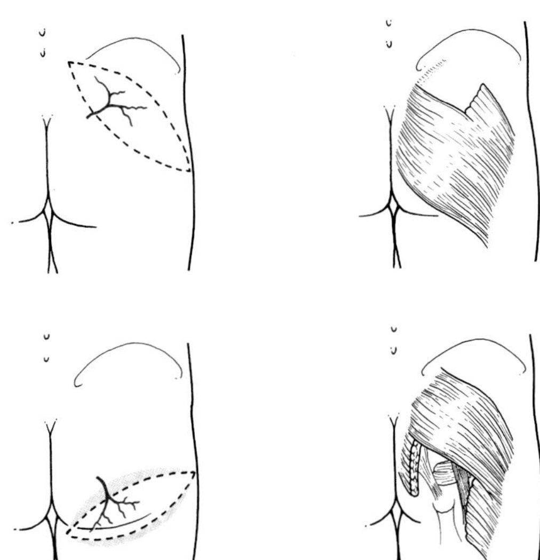

Fig. 7.93 Superior and inferior gluteal free flaps.

gluteus maximus and a guide to the upper border is provided by marking a point on the iliac crest approximately four fingers' breadths along from the posterior superior iliac spine. Although the skin area anterior to this may receive contributions from the superior gluteal artery, it is through its deep branch and not by musculocutaneous perforators from gluteus maximus. The bony attachments to the sacrum, and the greater trochanter of the femur are palpable. Inferiorly the edge of gluteus maximus does not coincide with the fold of the buttock. In this region the territory of the inferior gluteal artery extends downwards onto the posterior thigh because it gives off branches at the level of the deep fascia which accompany the posterior cutaneous nerve of the thigh. The principal of these branches may measure up to 1 mm in diameter and run for up to 10 cm down the posterior thigh although this is not an invariable finding. Cut ends of these vessels are seen at the inferior border of the muscle in the radiograph of gluteus maximus shown in Figure 7.90.

Flaps

Local rotation and transposition skin flaps (Fig. 7.91). These were the traditional means of obtaining sacral cover prior to the development of musculocutaneous flaps. These are of limited mobility if direct skin closure is to be obtained either by means of direct advancement/rotation or by means of a Bürow's triangle. Larger advancements require that the secondary defect be split skin grafted.

Muscle flaps (Fig. 7.92). These were an established reconstructive technique for bringing additional 'padding' into the area of a pressure sore before the advent of the musculocutaneous flap. Part of the gluteus maximus is mobilised on its vascular pedicle and rotated or turned over into the defect with a local skin flap being transposed over the muscle. Muscle is based on the superior gluteal artery for sacral pressure sores and on the first profunda perforator for trochanteric defects. Ger & Samuel[1] reviewed ten years' experience of these in 1975.

Gluteal free flaps (Fig. 7.93). Three types of free flap are possible: (1) musculocutaneous free flaps based on the superior gluteal artery in which a part of the upper gluteus maximus is taken with an ellipse of overlying skin extending from upper sacrum to greater trochanter (Shaw[2]); (2) inferior gluteal flaps in which the skin island is orientated obliquely along the gluteal crease (Paletta et al[3]); (3) the gluteal thigh flap (vide infra) may be used as a neurovascular free flap (Hurwitz et al[4]).

Vertical sliding gluteus maximus musculocutaneous flap (Fig. 7.94a). The whole of the muscle with the overlying skin and attached posterior thigh can be advanced vertically based only on the inferior gluteal pedicle.

Horizontal sliding gluteus maximus musculocutaneous flap (Fig. 7.94b, c). A triangular flap can be advanced medially and the secondary defect closed in a V-Y manner.[5] The origin of the muscle from sacrum, ilium and sacrotuberous ligament must be detached, the insertion into the greater trochanter divided, and the vascular pedicle of the relevant part of the muscle preserved. Movement is limited by the vessels to a maximum of about 6 cm.

Inferolateral flaps (Fig. 7.94d). These are based on the branches of the first profunda perforator and musculocutaneous perforators through the distal part of the muscle.[6] The flap includes the insertion of gluteus maximus (which is detached from the iliotibial tract), and the skin of the posterior thigh lateral to the midline. It is advanced supero-laterally over the greater trochanter with V-Y closure of the secondary defect.

Inferior gluteal flap (Fig. 7.94e). This is another sliding or island transposition musculocutaneous flap. It may be used for ischial defects when the skin island is placed superolateral to the defect and is based on the inferior gluteal artery. The inferior part of the muscle is split from the superior, the inferior part of the gluteal insertion is divided, and the musculocutaneous unit is swung around the sacral origin. The secondary defect is closed in a V-Y manner.[5] With the island transposition flaps a modification is to have the skin island separated from the defect by an intact intervening skin bridge. The flap is transferred into the defect via a subcutaneous tunnel.

The gluteal thigh flap (Fig. 7.94f). This is an inferior gluteal musculocutaneous flap based on the inferior gluteal artery with a fasciocutaneous extension of up to 15 cm down the midline of the posterior thigh.[4,6] The extension is based on the branches of the inferior gluteal artery which extend down the posterior thigh at the level of the deep fascia in the company of the posterior cutaneous nerve of the thigh. The lower part of gluteus maximus is mobilised as required by detaching origin and insertion, and splitting the muscle between fibre bundles up to the level of the lower border of piriformis. The posterior cutaneous nerve of the thigh and the deep fascia have to be included in the flap. The flap may be used in various ways: for local skin cover by rotation around the inferior gluteal pedicle; for filling deep pelvic cavities by inserting the de-epithelialised distal portion; or as a neurosensory free flap. If the width of the flap is restricted to a maximum of 10 cm primary closure of the donor site may be possible.

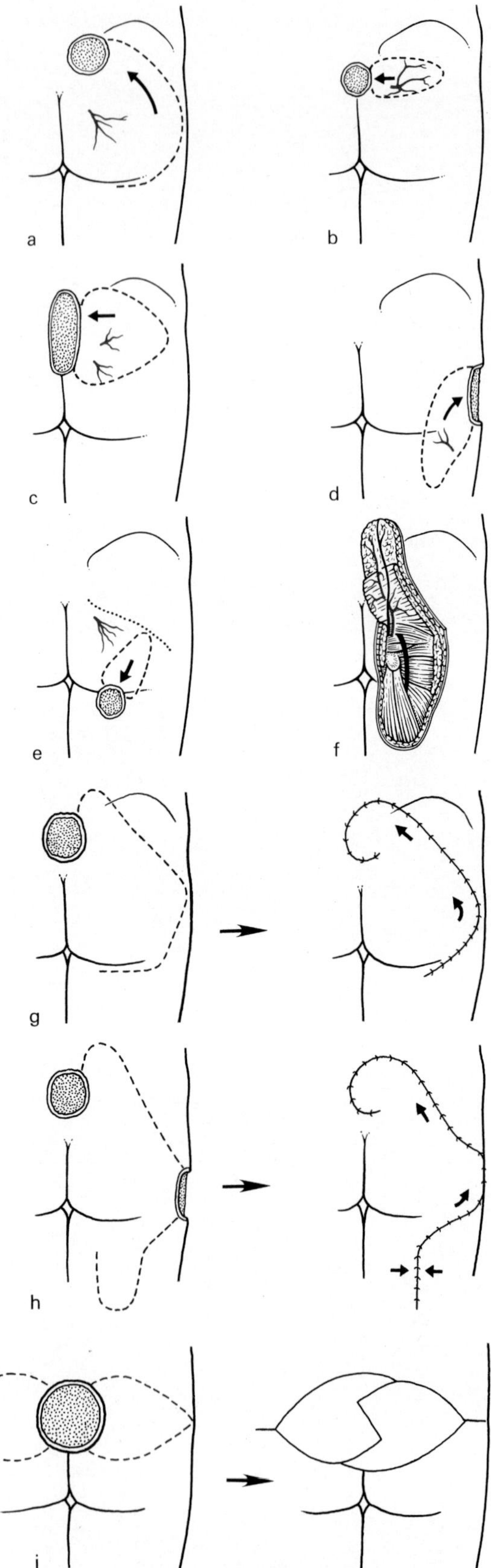

Fig. 7.94 Various designs of musculocutaneous flaps (see text).

Total gluteus maximus rotation flap for sacral defect (Fig. 7.94g). An incision is made at the midpoint of the greater trochanter and deepened to reach the plane deep to the gluteal fascia. The separation is continued medially to the iliac crest where the muscle is detached from bone and the plane of separation extended inferiorly to below the level of the defect. The incision is then extended from the trochanter inferiorly along the gluteal fold. The superior gluteal vessels often need division but inferior gluteal vessels must be preserved. The entire skin muscle unit is then rotated to cover the sacral defect.

Total rotation flap plus inferior gluteal thigh extension (Fig. 7.94h). The elevation of this flap is similar to the forgoing with the addition of the inferior gluteal flap extension. This modification is designed to permit simultaneous closure of sacral and trochanteric pressure sores.

Bilateral V to Y advancement flaps (Fig. 7.94i). In this modification of the V–Y advancement principle the flaps are raised with extra skin in the form of 'horns' at the corners of the advancing edges. The flaps are also undermined and only left attached to gluteus maximus in their central third so that some rotation can also be carried out thereby bringing one corner of each flap into the centre of the defect. This manoeuvre helps to reduce the tension across the central area that would otherwise result from apposing the bases of the two triangular flaps. It also places a Z-shaped scar across the centre of the wound.

Posterior iliac osteo-myocutaneous free flap. A free flap based on the superior gluteal artery and its intermediate branch has been described by Mialhe & Brice.[9] This branch runs on the periosteum of the posterior iliac crest and enables a mono-cortical bone block (8 cm × 13 cm) with a thick cancellous component to be removed with an overlying island of gluteus maximus and skin measuring up to 10 × 14 cm.

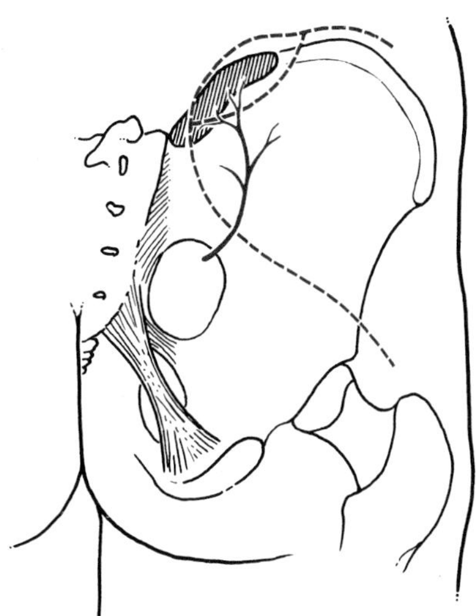

Fig. 7.95 Markings of skin incision for harvesting skin island and bone component of the posterior iliac free flap.

Sliding musculocutaneous flaps are technically straightforward because the intermuscular planes are fairly obvious, and healing is rapid because of the good vascularity. In general, these flaps work well for pressure sores given the limitations of any method that does not provide protective sensation. The subcutaneous connective tissue network linking the muscle with the dermis is preserved and confers good sheer resistance, and the added bulk of the muscle provides a layer of padding between the skin and the underlying bone.

Although the intention here is not to enter into a discussion of the relative merits of these different procedures but simply to present their anatomy, it is appropriate to point out that although there are many gluteal flaps, there may be preferable methods for reconstruction in the buttock area. For example, other techniques of bringing skin into the sacral area include sensory island flaps based on an intercostal neurovascular pedicle, lumbosacral flaps based on lateral dorsal cutaneous branches of the lumbar arteries, and extended tensor fasciae latae flaps. Nor has any description been given of hamstring musculocutaneous flaps, of posterior thigh advancement flaps for ischial pressure sores, or of vastus lateralis muscle flaps and gluteus medius/proximal TFL flaps for trochanteric sores. Consideration must also be given to the functional deficit that will result in the non-paraplegic from interfering with a muscle of locomotion.

References

1. Ger R, Samuel L 1976 The surgical management of decubitus ulcers by muscle transplantation. Plastic and Reconstructive Surgery 58: 419–428
2. Shaw W W 1983 Breast reconstruction by superior gluteal microvascular free flaps without silicone implants. Plastic and Reconstructive Surgery 72: 490–499
3. Paletta C E, Bostwick J, Nahai F 1989 The inferior gluteal free flap in breast reconstruction. Plastic and Reconstructive Surgery 84: 875–883
4. Hurwitz D J, Swartz W M, Mathes S J 1980 The gluteal thigh flap: a reliable sensate flap for the closure of buttock and perineal wounds. Plastic and Reconstructive Surgery 68: 521–530
5. Scheflan M, Nahai F, Bostwick J 1981 Gluteus maximus island musculocutaneous flap for the closure of sacral and ischial ulcers. Plastic and Reconstructive Surgery 68: 533–538
6. Ramirez O M, Hurwitz D J, Futrell J W 1983 The expansive gluteus maximus flap. Plastic and Reconstructive Surgery 74: 757–770
7. Parkash S, Banerjee S 1986 The total gluteus maximus rotation and other gluteus maximus musculocutaneous flaps in the treatment of pressure ulcers. British Journal of Plastic Surgery 39: 66–71
8. Heywood A J, Quaba A A 1989 Modified gluteus maximus V–Y advancement flaps. British Journal of Plastic Surgery 42: 263–265
9. Mialhe C, Brice M 1985 A new compound osteomyocutaneous free flap: the posterior iliac artery flap. British Journal of Plastic Surgery 38: 30–38

7 INFERIOR CUBITAL ARTERY

Antecubital fasciocutaneous flap

This flap is based on a fasciocutaneous perforator which emerges in the lower part of the antecubital fossa. The anatomy was described by the authors[1] in 1982 and clinical cases reported in 1983[2] which demonstrated the use of both pedicled and free flaps based on this vessel.

Anatomy

The radial artery, in its course down the forearm, gives off a succession of fasciocutaneous perforators to the skin. The most proximal of these arises in the antecubital fossa and reaches the surface by passing up in the fascia between brachioradialis and pronator teres. This perforator measures from 0.5–1.0 mm in internal diameter and has been named the inferior cubital artery. In 16 out of 37 dissected cadaver arms it was found[1] that the perforator arose from the radial recurrent artery rather than the radial itself (Fig. 7.100). The surface marking of the origin of the vessel varies from 2 to 5 cm (average 4 cm) below the mid-point of the inter-epicondylar line on the anterior aspect of the forearm (Fig. 7.96). The cephalic vein, as it gives off its median cubital branch, also gives off a deep branch which communicates with the deep venae communicantes of the radial artery. It is in the fork of this inverted V that the inferior cubital perforator reaches the skin (Fig. 7.97) and this provides a further indication of the position of the vessel when raising the flap. From this point the vessel tends to run distally along the line of the cephalic vein, i.e. directed towards the radial styloid process, but it may fan out widely over the muscle bellies of the forearm muscles.

The venous drainage of the forearm skin is mainly through the superficial venous system although small vessels pass along the fascial septa and communicate with the deep venae comitantes.

The area of skin lying along the line of the cephalic vein is supplied by the lateral cutaneous nerve of the arm (which is the cutaneous termination of the musculocutaneous nerve).

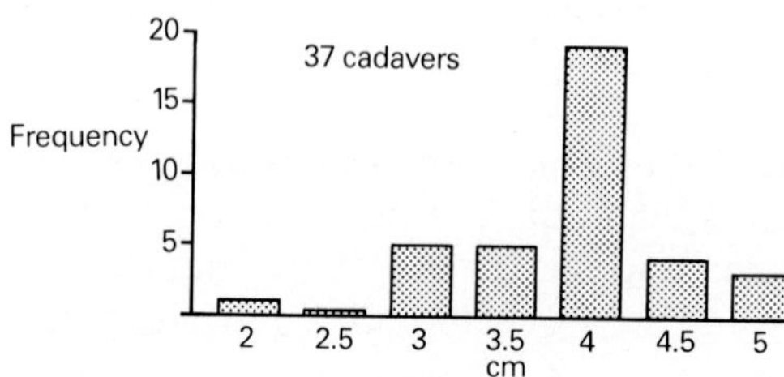

Fig. 7.96 Histogram for the surface marking of the inferior cubital artery in centimetres below the midpoint of the inter-epicondylar line.

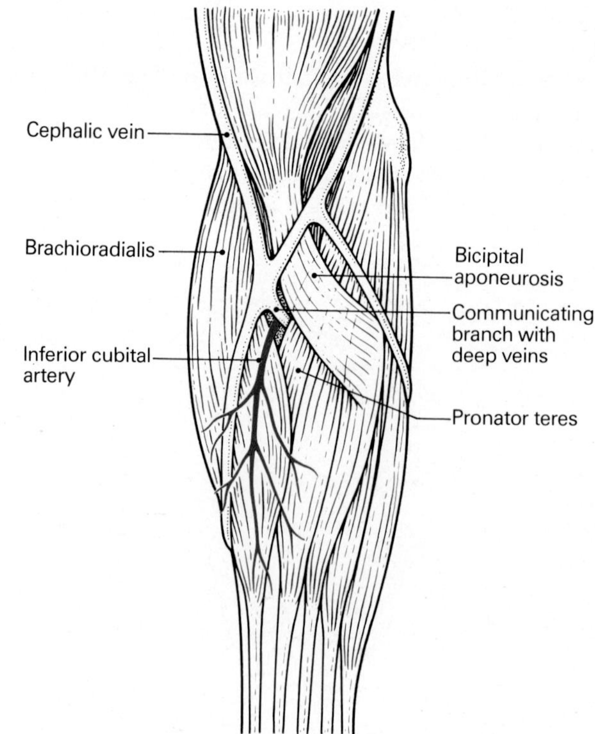

Fig. 7.97 Vascular anatomy. The point of emergence and the course of the inferior cubital artery are indicated. This is the first and largest perforator arising from the radial artery or from its first branch, the radial recurrent artery.

Surgery

The flap may be raised either as a pedicled flap or as a free flap. As a pedicled flap the base lies 4 cm below the inter-epicondylar line and the axial line extends distally along the forearm. The deep fascia is elevated with the flap and an extensive cuff of fascial septum preserved in the lower part of the antecubital fossa to enclose and protect the inferior cubital artery. The forearm skin is thin, with little subcutaneous fat, and transillumination may be useful in seeing the vessel. The maximum length-to-breadth proportions attained without complications have been about 4:1 (17 cm × 4 cm). This gives the end of the flap a wide arc of rotation so that it may be useful for covering exposed elbow joints or prostheses and is capable of reaching (with a back-cut) the olecranon region. It may be preferable to the brachioradialis musculocutaneous flap which has been recommended for elbow coverage but is considerably more bulky.

Free flaps of the same territory are based on the inferior cubital and radial arteries. The inferior cubital artery supplying the flap is rather too small and short for direct anastomosis and therefore a length of the radial artery is taken in continuity with it. This has three significant advantages. Firstly, the arterial pedicle may be made any length up to 20 cm and by proximal dissection of the cephalic vein a similarly long venous pedicle may be obtained. Secondly, anastomosis of both ends of the radial artery in the recipient site creates a 'through-flow' situation which may create more physiological flow in the inferior cubital artery than is the case with an 'end artery' flap, and through the haemodynamic improvement reduce circulatory complications in the flap. Thirdly, the combination of a long flap with a long pedicle allows greater versatility in flap positioning in the recipient site.

There are two situations in which this flap would not be feasible. Firstly, in the absence of a significantly sized inferior cubital artery, and secondly, in the

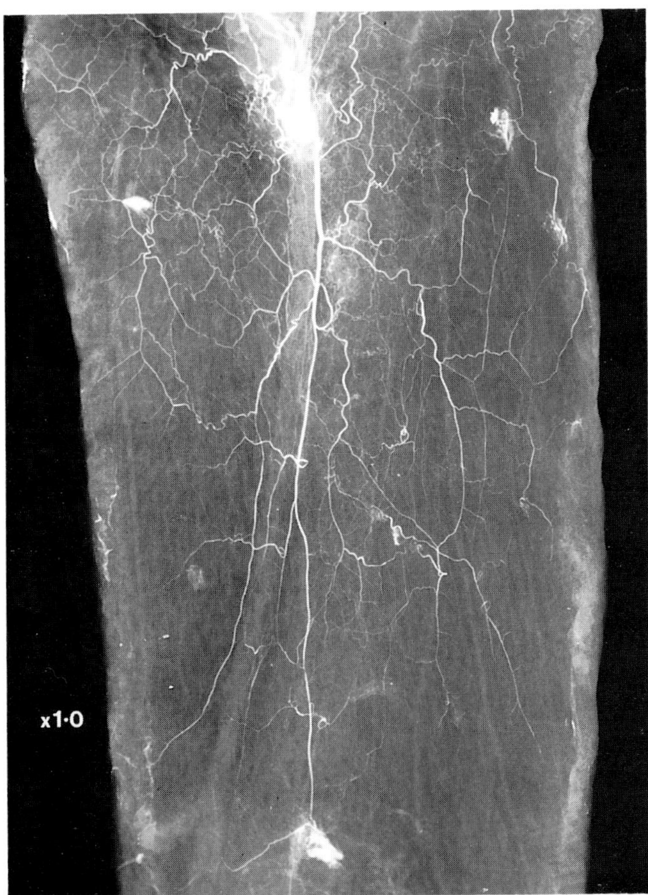

Fig. 7.98 Radiograph of skin showing inferior cubital artery lying alongside cephalic vein.

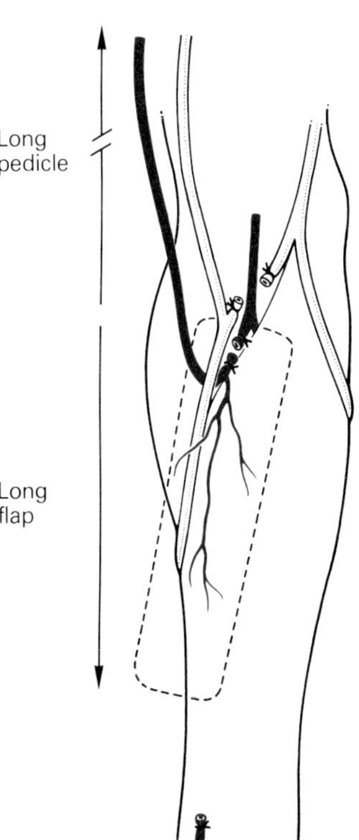

Fig. 7.99 Flap planning. With a free flap long segments of the cephalic vein and radial artery may be removed. Here the radial artery is shown after it has been divided distally and turned upwards so that an equivalent length of vein may be removed.

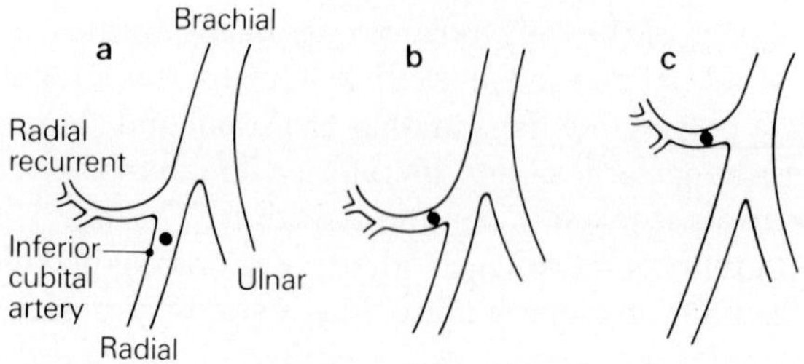

Fig. 7.100 Variations in the site of origin of the inferior cubital artery. Type c precludes the possibility of raising a free flap of the type shown in Fig. 7.99.

presence of such an artery when it arises from a radial recurrent which had its point of origin from the brachial artery rather than the radial artery. This is rare (Fig. 7.100)

After marking out the course of the arteries and veins the flap is elevated in the manner of the Chinese radial forearm flap by removing the skin and deep fascia in continuity with the radial artery and the fascial septum between brachioradialis and flexor carpi radialis. Perforators in the septum may then be divided, except for the inferior cubital artery which is left entering the proximal end of the flap. Division of the radial artery both proximal to this vessel and 5 cm or more above the wrist isolates the arterial input. The venous drainage is through the cephalic vein which is dissected out proximally from the upper arm to the required length of the pedicle.

References

1. Lamberty B G H, Cormack G C 1982 The forearm angiotomes. British Journal of Plastic Surgery 35: 420–429
2. Lamberty B G H, Cormack G C 1983 The antecubital fascio-cutaneous flap. British Journal of Plastic Surgery 36: 428–433
3. Dickinson J C, Roberts A H N 1986 Fasciocutaneous cross-arm flaps in hand reconstruction. The Journal of Hand Surgery 11B: 394–398

INTERCOSTAL AND LUMBAR ARTERIES – dorsal cutaneous branches

'Reverse' latissimus dorsi musculocutaneous flap

The conventional latissimus dorsi musculocutaneous flap is based on the main thoracodorsal artery pedicle which enters the muscle approximately 5 cm below its humeral insertion. By a 'reverse' flap is meant one based on the segmental perforators entering the posterior origin of the muscle. The posterior skin and muscle may be advanced medially, based on these perforators,[1] or various designs of musculocutaneous flap may be based on them. The application of these flaps lies in the reconstruction of midline defects, and some posterior chest wall defects. A particular feature of some of these flaps is that they may be designed so as to retain cutaneous sensation.

Anatomy

Latissimus dorsi arises from the lumbar and lower six thoracic spines and supraspinous ligaments by means of the posterior layer of the thoracolumbar fascia which also gives it an origin from sacral spines and posterior iliac crest. In addition, it arises by muscular fibres from the posterior part of the outer lip of the iliac crest lateral to erector spinae, and also by muscle fibres from the three or four lower ribs: the latter slips of origin interdigitate with the lower slips of the external oblique. (Descriptions exist in the anatomical literature of cases where the muscle was underdeveloped to varying degrees, muscle fibres on occasions only arising from the ribs and none from points inferior or medial to the ribs.)

The supplementary vascular pedicles come from the lateral of the two dorsal cutaneous branches given off by each of the lower five intercostal arteries, the subcostal and the upper lumbar arteries. Of these various vessels, three or four are usually particularly well developed while the others are much smaller. Often it is the lateral dorsal cutaneous branches of the lower intercostal arteries which are the largest. These arteries, accompanied by veins and cutaneous nerves, pass through erector spinae (lying between longissimus and iliocostalis) with a distal inclination. They pass through the extensive origin of latissimus dorsi between 4 and 8 cm from the midline. On their way through latissimus dorsi the lateral perforators give off branches which run between the muscle fibre bundles and anastomose within the muscle with terminal branches of the thoracodorsal system. From these two sets of vessels, musculocutaneous perforators reach the skin over the muscle. It follows that a pedicled musculocutaneous flap may be designed with a medially situated base and a skin island overlying the lower dorsal part of the

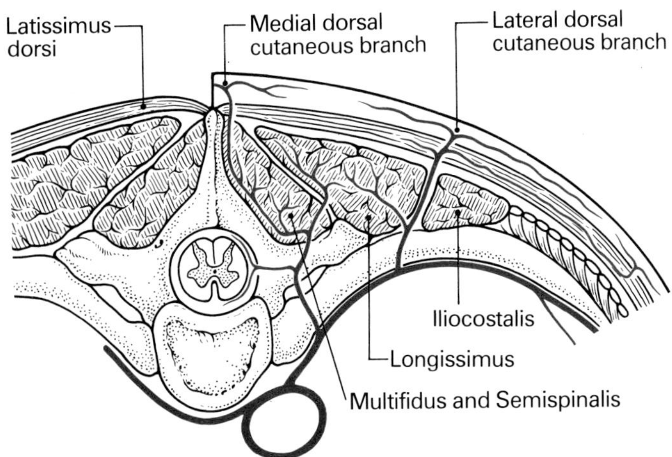

Fig. 7.101 Schematic transverse section to illustrate the disposition of medial and lateral dorsal cutaneous branches of an intercostal artery. A similar arrangement applies to the segmental lumbar arteries.

muscle. Such a flap may carry sensation since the dorsal (posterior primary) rami of the lower six thoracic nerves turn backwards into the deep muscles and divide into medial and lateral branches on each side of longissimus. The lateral branches wind downwards and laterally, becoming successively longer and more vertical. Both medial and lateral branches supply the deep muscles, but the medial branches of the upper six thoracic nerves and the lateral branches of the lower six are also cutaneous (Fig. 7.102). The dorsal rami of the first, second and third lumbar nerves are similar but follow a much more vertical course such that the cutaneous nerves cross the iliac crest and are distributed to the superolateral part of the buttock (as superior clunial or gluteal branches). The dorsal rami of the fourth and fifth lumbar nerves are wholly muscular but the first sacral dorsal ramus again reaches skin over the superomedial part of the buttock by piercing gluteus maximus (middle clunial branches). Depending on the position of the flap, some of the thoracic nerves may be incorporated. Other flaps may be designed with skin islands over the anterolateral part of the latissimus dorsi muscle, and rely on the intramuscular anastomoses between the thoracodorsal and intercostal systems.

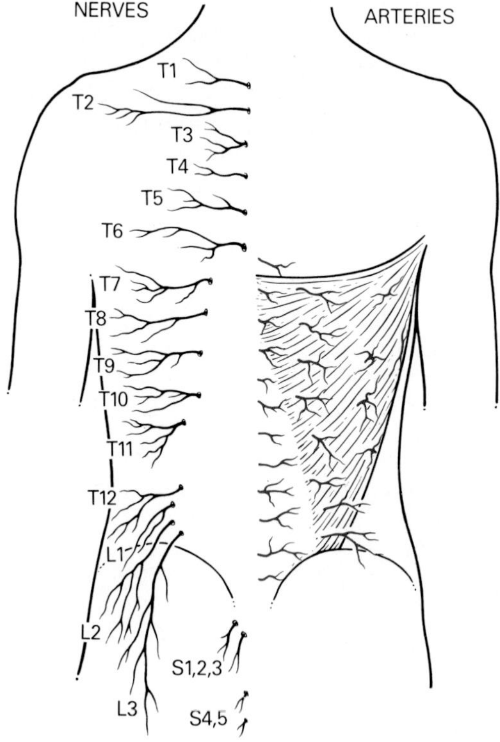

Fig. 7.102 Cutaneous nerves are illustrated on the left side and cutaneous arteries are superimposed on the outline of latissimus dorsi on the right. Medial dorsal cutaneous branches do not exist bilaterally at each level and occasional lateral dorsal branches fail.

Planning

The flap can be designed transversely of any width, although clearly it must not be so narrow that it fails to include sufficient perforators, and must incorporate muscle, or lower down, aponeurosis. It may be extended

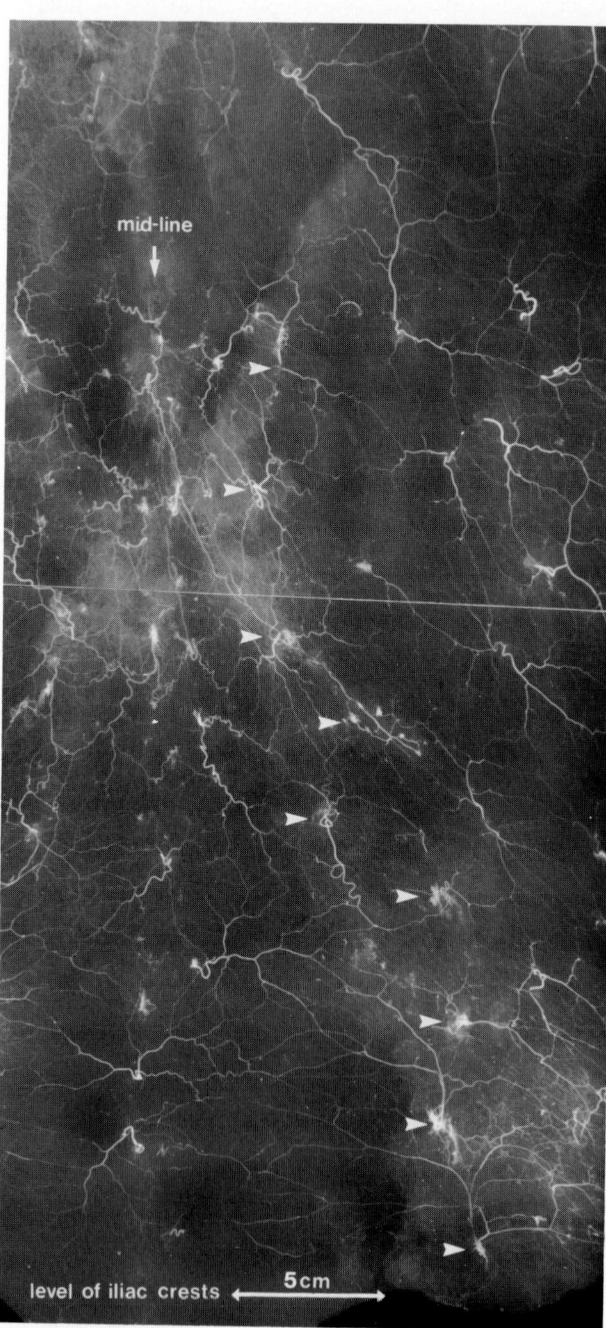

Fig. 7.103 On this radiograph of dorsal skin the lateral dorsal cutaneous branches have been indicated with arrows. See Fig. 7.298 to see the anastomoses which branches of these vessels make with branches of the thoracodorsal system within the muscle.

as far forwards as the anterior edge of the muscle. The flap may be designed either as an island of skin on a subcutaneous muscle pedicle,[2,5] or as a pedicled flap of skin and muscle.[4] In the latter case the donor site must be in continuity with the defect (Fig. 7.104). The advantage of this flap when repairing skin defects over the spine, especially in spina bifida, is that there is a good pad of muscle between the skin and underlying bone.

Surgery

The actual surgery is straightforward but care needs to be taken when separating latissimus from the posterior abdominal/chest wall to preserve the perforating vessels emerging between iliocostalis and longissimus, and their accompanying cutaneous nerves.

An alternative to elevating a circumscribed flap is to carry out a posterior advancement of skin and muscle by dissecting beneath latissimus dorsi and incising the thoracolumbar fascia lateral to sacrospinalis whilst leaving the posterior perforators intact. The skin is left intact anteriorly but the fascia at the anterior margin of latissimus is divided (blindly) to enable one to gain 5 cm of posterior advancement of the skin and muscle.[1]

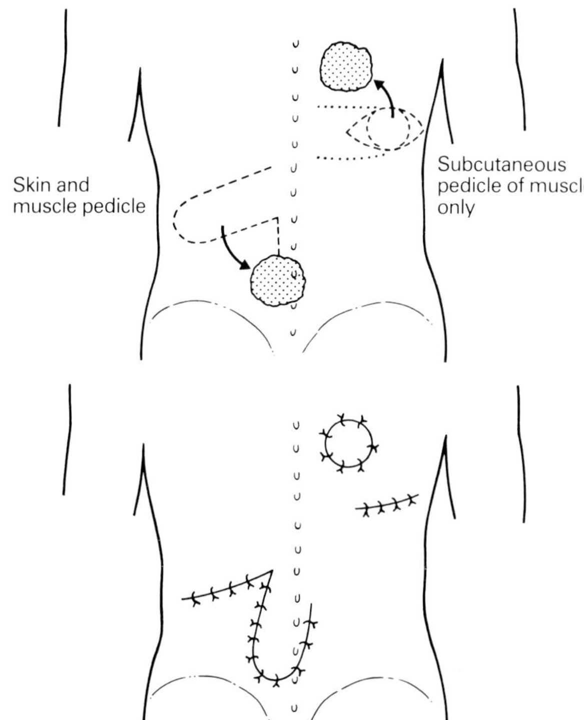

Fig. 7.104 Examples of two forms of the 'reverse' latissimus flap.

In 1971 a case was reported[6] in which longitudinal bipedicle compound musculocutaneous flaps from each side of the spine had been advanced medially to close a large meningomyelocoele defect[6]. The authors did not consider the blood supply of the flaps in detail but clearly the dorsal perforators were important. An interesting addition to this procedure was the manoeuvre of splitting sacrospinalis longitudinally to its medial margin where the bifid spinous processes were encountered. These were transected with an osteotome and the whole skin/muscle/bone flap advanced to the midline. More commonly, however, the muscle alone is turned over medially to close a spina bifida defect and the muscle is then split skin grafted.

References

1. McCraw J B, Penix J O, Baker J W 1978 Repair of major defects of the chest wall and spine with the latissimus dorsi myocutaneous flap. Plastic and Reconstructive Surgery 62: 197–206
2. Bostwick J, Scheflan M, Nahai F, Jurkiewicz M J 1980 The 'reverse' latissimus dorsi muscle and musculocutaneous flap: anatomical and clinical considerations. Plastic and Reconstructive Surgery 65: 395–399
3. Muldowney J B, Magi E, Hein K, Birdsell D 1981 The reverse latissimus dorsi myocutaneous flap with functional preservation — report of a case. Annals of Plastic Surgery 7: 150–151
4. McGregor J C 1983 The 'reverse' latissimus dorsi musculocutaneous flap. Case report. Journal of the Royal College of Surgeons of Edinburgh 28: 154–156
5. Stevenson T R, Rohrich R J, Pollock R A, Dingman R O, Bostwick J 1984 More experience with the 'reverse' latissimus dorsi musculocutaneous flap: precise location of blood supply. Plastic and Reconstructive Surgery 74: 237–243
6. DesPrez J D, Kiehn C L, Eckstein W 1971 Closure of large meningomyelocoele defects by composite skin muscle flaps. Plastic and Reconstructive Surgery 47: 234–238

7 INTERCOSTAL ARTERIES – lateral cutaneous branches

Intercostal flaps
Upper quadrant flap
Lower quadrant flap
Free flap

The possibility of using the intercostal vessels as the basis of free flaps was discussed by Daniel & Williams in 1973.[1] Dibbell in 1974[2] described a case in which an island of abdominal skin was transferred in four stages on its T10 neurovascular pedicle to the site of a sacral decubitus ulcer in a 3-year-old patient.[2] Improvements followed in the technical aspects of raising the pedicle and the method was elaborated and extended to include double vascular pedicles for large flaps raised without a delay. Indications for the use of the intercostal flap have been listed as the provision of stable sensate skin over kyphosis ulcers in young meningomyelocoele patients, and cover of sacral pressure sores in selected recurrent cases and paraplegics.[3]

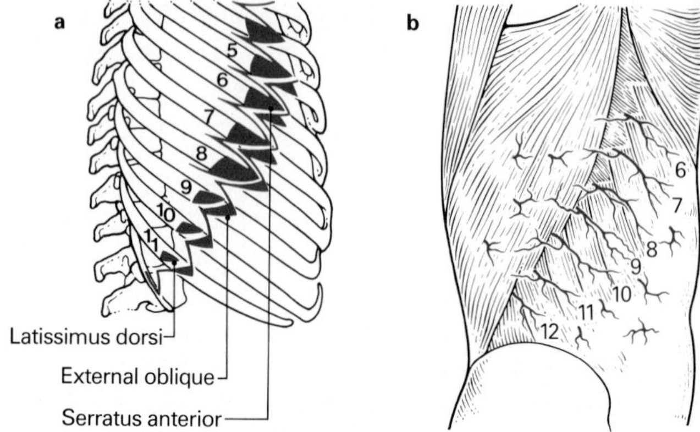

Fig. 7.105 Vascular anatomy of lateral cutaneous branches: **a.** shows the origins of the external oblique muscle from ribs; **b.** shows lateral cutaneous branches and musculocutaneous perforators through external oblique.

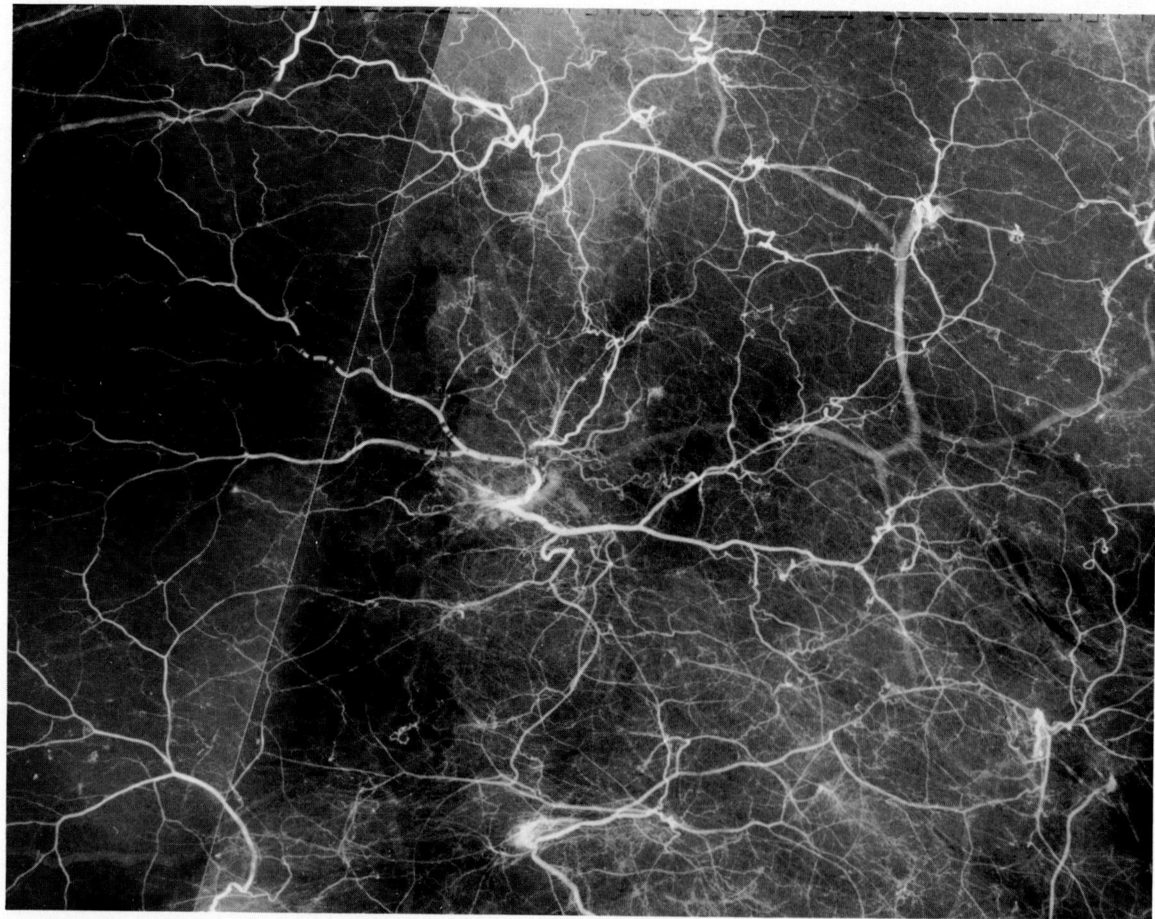

Fig. 7.106 Radiograph of skin specimen showing typical lateral cutaneous branches of the intercostal arteries. See also Figs 6.27–6.31.

The problem of raising a reliable, large flap without a delay has been overcome by incorporating a large amount of abdominal musculature in the flap. This method was developed by Little et al[4] and termed the *upper quadrant flap* but it is in principle an extended intercostal flap. The indications for such a tissue transfer are limited to large difficult trunk wounds of impaired vascularity where more conventional flaps are either inadequate or unavailable.

A *lower quadrant* external oblique musculocutaneous flap pedicled on the mid-lateral line to carry skin from the lower abdomen to the site of a post-mastectomy breast reconstruction has been based on branches of the intercostal arteries.[5]

Recently a purely cutaneous *neurovascular free flap* has been described based on the lateral cutaneous branches of the intercostal vessels and nerves.[6]

Anatomy

The anatomy of the vessels has been fully described on pages 153–165. In summary, in the course of its travel along the costal groove segment of an intercostal space, the intercostal artery gives off a number of musculocutaneous perforators which pass through the overlying internal and external intercostal muscles to reach the skin. The lateral cutaneous branch is a particularly large perforator which consistently arises in the distal part of the costal groove and is accompanied by a lateral cutaneous nerve, and by venae comitantes. These structures reach the surface where the respective slip of external oblique takes origin from its rib. The lower posterior intercostal arteries continue on into the anterior abdominal wall running between transversus abdominis and internal oblique and terminate by anastomosing in its plane with branches from the epigastric arcade. The posterior intercostal vessels also give off branches which run in a more superficial plane on the deep surface of external oblique where they supply the muscle and, via perforators, the overlying skin.

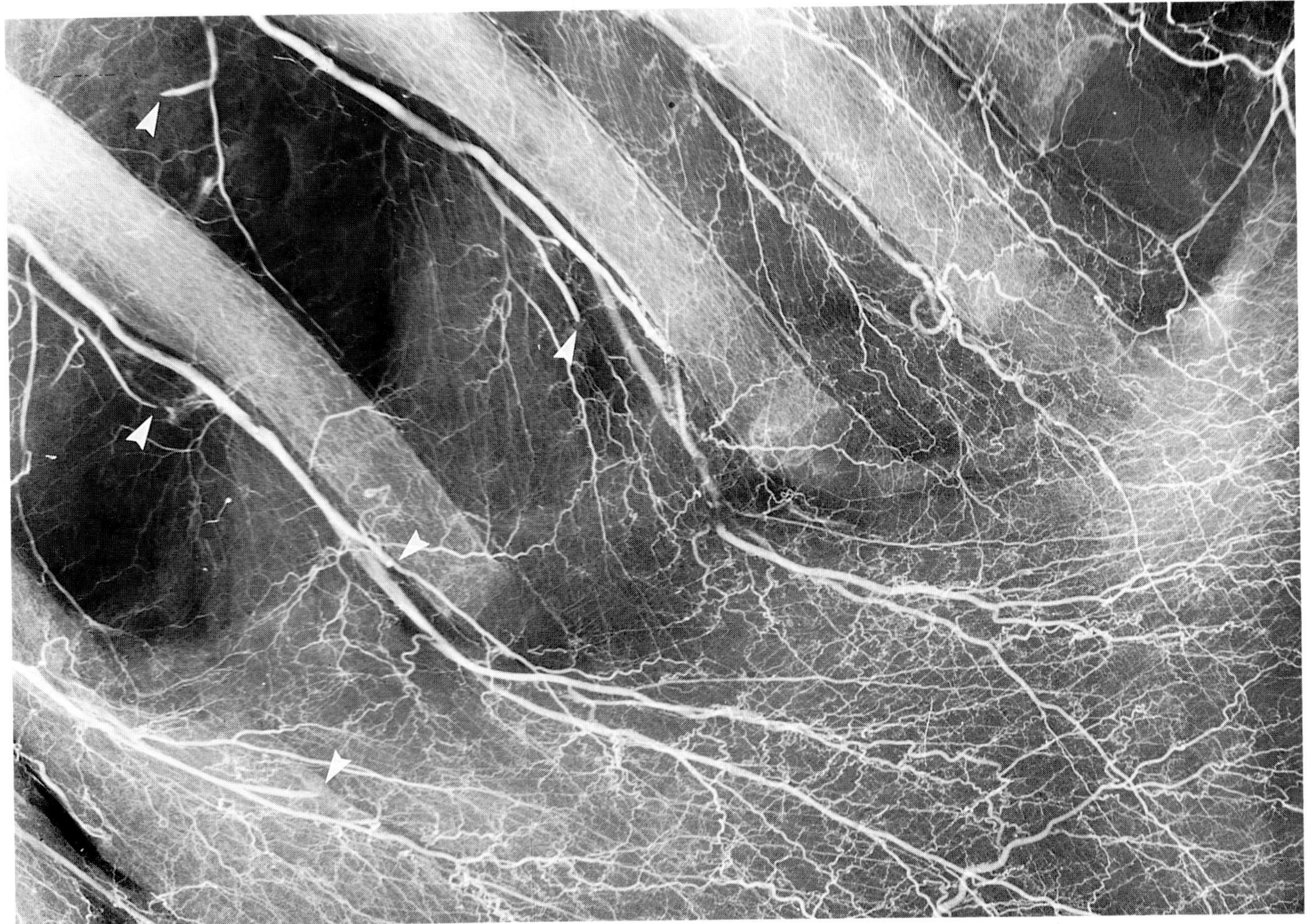

Fig. 7.107 Musculature of the right hypochondrium. Arrows show where branches of the intercostal arteries become cutaneous.

Flap planning and surgery

Posterior intercostal artery flap

The position of the flap is determined by the location of the recipient defect but it will generally be planned so as to overlie the ninth or tenth intercostal space and have dimensions of up to 18 cm × 12 cm. The flap is positioned as far forwards as necessary with the proviso that flaps which reach the anterior midline and do not incorporate rectus muscle are probably best either delayed or based on a double intercostal pedicle. The maximum width of defect that can be closed primarily is ~12 cm. In elevating the flap, the outline is first incised and the pedicle then elevated from distal to proximal. The thoracic musculature is preserved beneath the posterior skin incision but anteriorly the incision goes through muscle and divides the neurovascular bundle as it passes into the abdominal wall. The skin overlying the chosen intercostal space is carefully incised so as to avoid damaging the lateral cutaneous branch which is followed into the flap. Rather than dissecting the intercostal vessels out from their groove as suggested in the Preliminary Report of Daniel et al,[7] the pedicle is exposed by subperiosteal excision of the rib of the donor space. The entire contents of the intercostal space, including a portion of rib periosteum, are then incorporated into the pedicle.

Extended intercostal flap

In this flap the abdominal paddle extends to the midline and is centred on the umbilicus for T10 or a little higher for T9. The pedicle includes skin and subcutaneous fat as well as the entire contents of the chosen intercostal space up to the posterior axillary line, thereby removing the need for careful avoidance of the lateral cutaneous branch and speeding the dissection of the pedicle. Ribs still need to be removed from their periosteal beds. The abdominal paddle is removed with underlying rectus muscle, anterior sheath and lateral half of posterior sheath. The paddle is then joined to the pedicle by dissection at the level of the intact peritoneum, taking the overlying muscle from the upper quadrant between the two. The muscle component therefore contains the intercostal vessels between the muscle layers without them having to be visualised. However the donor defect is clearly very extensive.

External oblique musculocutaneous flap

This consists of a paddle of skin and fat which is triangular in shape with the base of the skin island lying along the midline between umbilicus and pubis, and two sides which converge on the anterior superior iliac spine. The external oblique aponeurosis and anterior rectus sheath on the undersurface of the skin island are also incised and elevated. A 10 cm wide strip of external oblique is separated along its lower margin from the iliac crest and is elevated from the underlying internal oblique. Small branches of the intercostal vessels which lie in this plane are protected and two lateral perforating vessels are conserved as the muscle is partly detached from the ribs. In breast reconstruction the abdominal skin is elevated in the usual manner for a lipectomy and

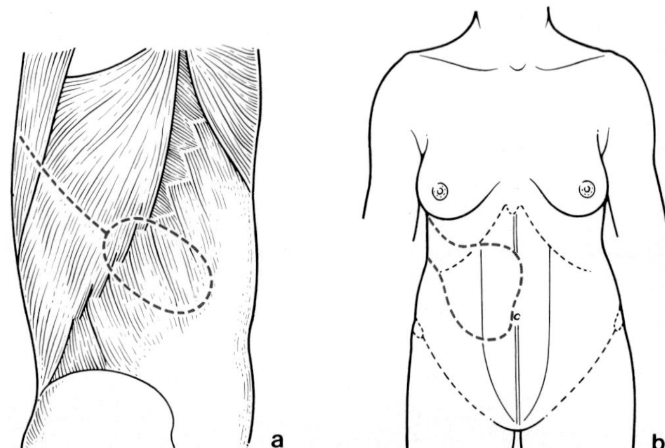

Fig. 7.108 Flap planning. **a.** Posterior intercostal artery island flap. Diagram shows incision for dissection of the pedicle and the outline of the skin paddle. Muscle is preserved between the skin paddle and the underlying intercostal neurovascular bundle. **b.** Extended intercostal/upper quadrant flap. Flap extends to midline and includes muscle. Pedicle includes skin and muscle in addition to the intercostal neurovascular bundle(s).

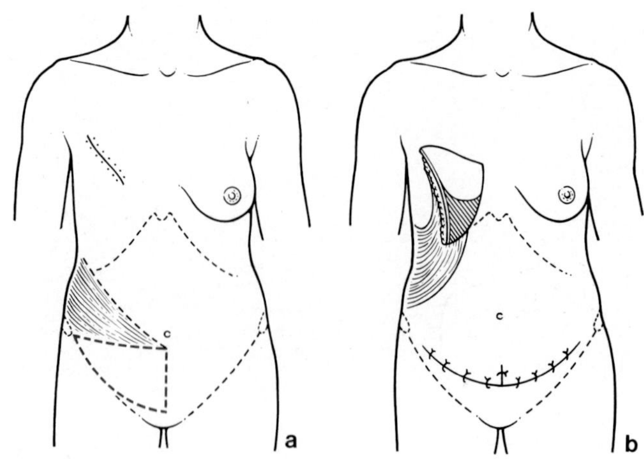

Fig. 7.109 Lower quadrant external oblique musculocutaneous flap: **a.** shows the outline of the flap and the external oblique pedicle. **b.** A variable amount of the flap may be de-epithelialised (shaded area) and tucked up to provide bulk. Direct skin closure after excising some contralateral skin, and relocation of umbilicus.

the flap tunnelled beneath this to reach the breast defect where portions of the flap are de-epithelialised and buried as required. The abdominal lipectomy is completed by excising the excess skin of the opposite side and closing in the usual way. At a second stage operation the muscle pedicle may be divided and turned upwards to further augment the breast volume.

Lateral cutaneous flap
In this flap the lateral cutaneous neurovascular bundle is removed in continuity with as much of the posterior intercostal artery as is required for the vascular pedicle. Figure 7.105 shows how the line along which these vessels emerge slopes postero-inferiorly. Therefore, to ensure that the lowermost branches are included in the flap, its posterior margin must lie three fingers' breadths behind the mid-axillary line (Fig. 7.110). The posterior and inferior incisions are made, then elevation of the flap commences at the posterior margin and proceeds forwards over latissimus dorsi at a sub-epimysial level so as to incorporate the posterior branches in the flap. When the anterolateral edge of latissimus appears in the dissection, this is an indication that the neurovascular bundles are about to be encountered. These are visualised and the largest selected as the basis of the flap. This bundle is traced back into its intercostal space and the overlying fibres of external oblique, latissimus and the intercostals are divided to gain access to the main intercostal neurovascular bundle. This is freed from the costal groove by incising the periosteum at the lower border of the rib and peeling it down from the roof of the costal groove. The anterior continuation of the intercostal artery is ligated and the remainder of the flap is elevated. Flaps up to 24 cm × 17 cm have been used successfully, with pedicle lengths of 8–15 cm.

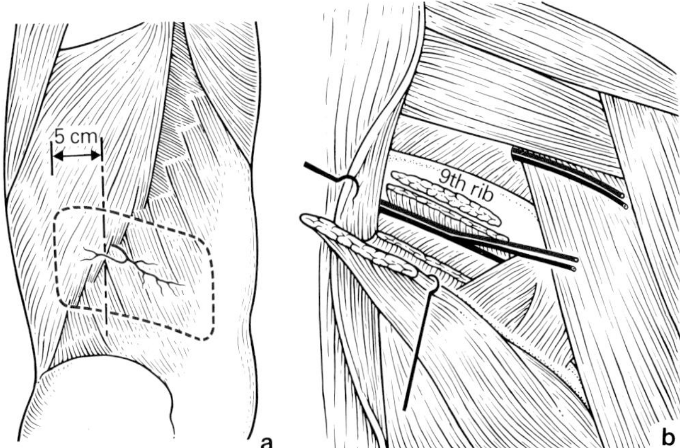

Fig. 7.110 Lateral cutaneous branch free flap. **a.** Posterior edge of flap lies 5 cm posterior to the mid-axillary line. **b.** Exposure of the pedicle in the ninth intercostal space is shown.

The same vessels may also be used to support a horizontally orientated pedicled flap for local transposition, e.g. breast reconstruction or transfer to the arm.[9]

References

1. Daniel R K, Williams H B 1973 The free transfer of skin flaps by microvascular anastomoses. Plastic and Reconstructive Surgery 52: 16–31
2. Dibbell D G 1974 Use of a long island flap to bring sensation to the sacral area in young paraplegics. Plastic and Reconstructive Surgery 54: 220–223
3. Daniel R K, Kerrigan C L, Gard D A 1978 The great potential of the intercostal flap for torso reconstruction. Plastic and Reconstructive Surgery 61: 653–665
4. Little J W, Fontana D J, McCulloch D T 1981 The upper quadrant flap. Plastic and Reconstructive Surgery 68: 175–184
5. Marshall D R, Anstee E J, Stapleton M J 1982 Soft tissue reconstruction of the breast using an external oblique myocutaneous abdominal flap. British Journal of Plastic Surgery 35: 443–451
6. Badran H A, El-Helaly M S, Safe I 1984 The lateral intercostal neurovascular free flap. Plastic and Reconstructive Surgery 73: 17–25
7. Daniel R K, Terzis J K, Cunningham D M 1976 Sensory skin flaps for coverage of pressure sores in paraplegic patients: A preliminary report. Plastic and Reconstructive Surgery 58: 317–328
8. Kerrigan C L, Daniel R K 1979 The intercostal flap: An anatomical and hemodynamic approach. Annals of Plastic Surgery 2: 411–421
9. Fisher T 1985 External oblique fasciocutaneous flap for elbow coverage. Plastic and Reconstructive Surgery 75: 51–59

7 INTERNAL THORACIC ARTERY

Deltopectoral flap

The great potential in head and neck reconstruction of a medially-based pedicled flap from the anterior chest was first demonstrated by Bakamjian in 1965[1] who used a deltopectoral flap to reconstruct the upper oesophagus. He reported further refinements in 1967, 1968, 1971 and 1973. The basic flap may be modified in numerous ways: for example, the end may be split either longitudinally or tangentially;[2] a double-sided 'sandwich' may be performed on the end of the flap; or the pedicle may be de-epithelialised so as to leave only a terminal 'island' of skin.

Harii[4] has described the deltopectoral free flap transferred only on the second perforating branch and its venae comitantes.

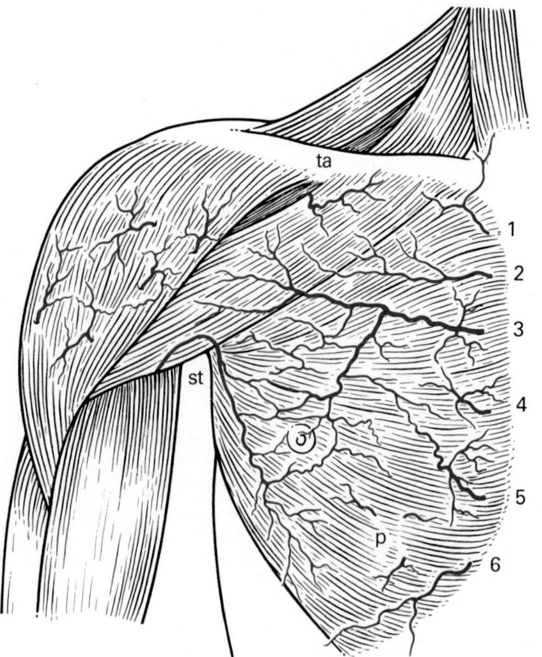

Fig. 7.111 Vascular anatomy. A particularly large perforator is shown emerging through the third intercostal space. A superficial thoracic artery lies over the lateral part of pectoralis major. (After Manchot, 1889.)

Anatomy

The conventional pedicled flap is based on the first, second and third perforating branches of the internal thoracic artery although the flap may survive on only a single one of these if the vessel is large. Commonly the flap is based on only the second and third perforators. The primary deltopectoral flap raised without a prior delay extends up to the deltoid area and includes the territory of the cutaneous branches of the thoraco-acromial axis. The area over deltoid is supplied by musculocutaneous perforators through the muscle from the deltoid branch of the thoraco-acromial axis and also from the anterior circumflex humeral artery. The ability of the internal thoracic artery perforators to 'take over' the territory overlying the anterior deltoid is unpredictable and a flap raised to extend over deltoid as a one-stage procedure will suffer distal necrosis in approximately 10% of cases. Reliability can be greatly enhanced by carrying out a delay on this part of the flap about one week before raising the flap. The delay consists of incising the margins of this distal part of the flap, elevating the end by sharp dissection in the sub-fascial plane, and ligating the cutaneous branch of the thoraco-acromial axis. A delay is particularly indicated with long flaps, especially when modified, with elderly patients, and where there may previously have been damage to the vessels. In general, the perforator emerging through the medial end of the second intercostal space is the largest with the gradation in size of the vessels in the other spaces following the pattern $2 > 3 > 4 > 1$ but this is not invariably the case and $4 > 2 > 1 > 3$ has been observed. The external diameter of these arteries ranges up to 1.2 mm with the second perforator nearly always larger than 0.8 mm. The perforators pierce the intercostal spaces between 10 and 20 mm out from the lateral edge of the sternum.

Venae comitantes accompany the arteries and constitute the principal routes for venous drainage of the flap since subcutaneous veins on the anterior chest tend to run towards the axilla. The venae comitantes measure from 1.2 to 1.5 mm in external diameter.

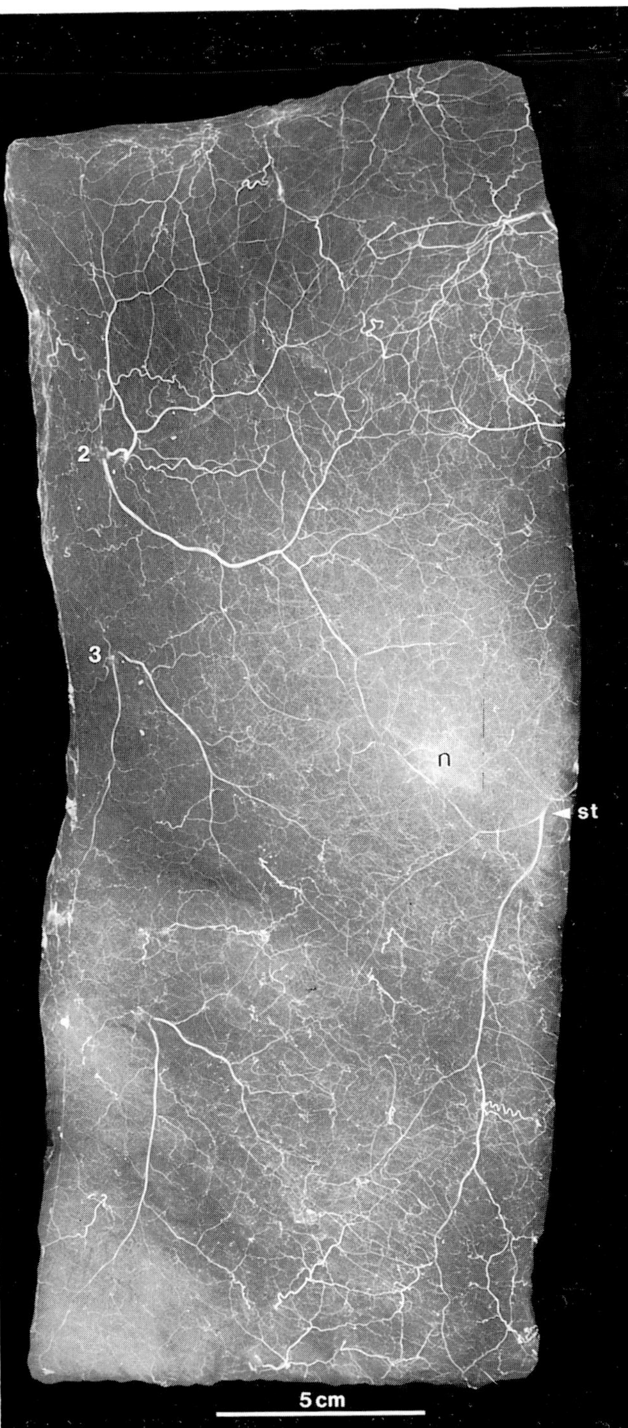

Fig. 7.112 Radiograph of a paramedian strip of left anterior chest skin. The superior margin of the specimen resulted from an incision which passed along the line of the clavicle. The left-hand edge corresponds to the midline over the sternum. A large perforator can be seen (2) which has passed through the second intercostal space and immediately divided into ascending and descending branches. The latter branch is inclining downwards and anastomosing with branches of the superficial thoracic artery (**st**); **n** denotes nipple shadow. See also the upper part of Fig. 6.17 which has two good examples of large perforators through the second intercostal spaces passing laterally towards the shoulders.

Flap planning

The boundaries of the flap are not rigidly defined but the following outline is representative. The base of the flap is situated 2 cm from the sternal edge, with the upper margin following the infraclavicular line, and the lower margin following a line parallel with this lying 2 fingers' breadths above the male nipple. To be of a useful length the flap must extend beyond the deltopectoral groove onto the anterior deltoid. With a preliminary delay it is possible to extend the flap beyond the lateral profile of the shoulder or down onto the anterior aspect of the upper arm. The arc of rotation of the flap takes in the neck, head and face below the zygoma on the side of the flap, or the neck and shoulder on the contralateral side (depending on the breadth of the patient's shoulders and length of neck).

The free flap is raised within the same territory as the pedicled flap with the axis overlying the second intercostal space.

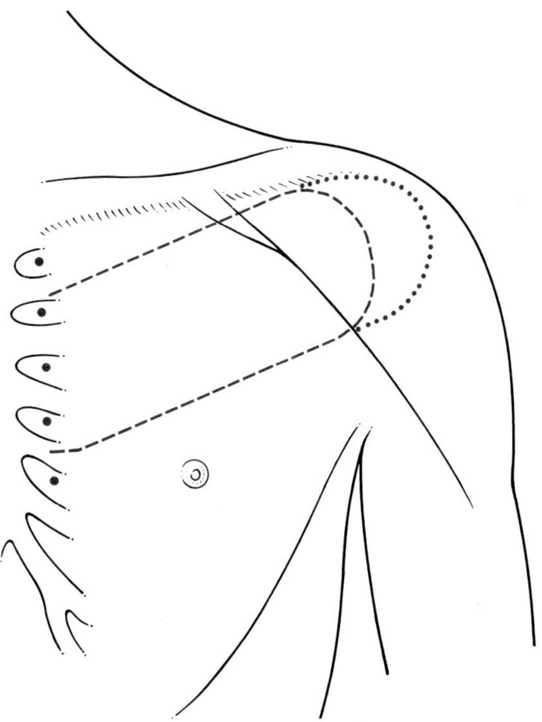

Fig. 7.113 Flap planning. A possible outline for a pedicled deltopectoral flap based mainly on the third perforator is indicated (broken line). An extension onto the anterior part of deltoid constitutes a random element on the end of the axial part and is less reliable (dotted line). A free flap would be raised within the same outlines.

7

Flap elevation

The flap is elevated from lateral to medial by sharp dissection in the subfascial plane which is straightforward with little bleeding because the only large perforator comes from the thoraco-acromial axis through the clavipectoral fascia of the infraclavicular triangle. Elevation proceeds medially right up to the emerging perforators. It will be found that the lower edge of the flap is longer than initially apparent and is longer than the upper edge due to the excess skin that lies in the lower anterior axillary fold. As a result, when the flap is swung upwards into the region of the head and neck the axis point of rotation lies at the upper attachment of the base of the flap, i.e. the part nearest to the defect. Also when the flap is swung upwards it will be seen that the pedicle tubes very readily.

The donor site may be split skin grafted in whole or in part, or – less commonly – the chest skin is extensively undermined and the defect closed directly.

References

1. Bakamjian V Y 1965 A two stage method of pharyngo-oesophageal reconstruction with a primary pectoral skin flap. Plastic and Reconstructive Surgery 36: 173–184
2. Krizek T J, Robson M C 1973 Split flap in head and neck reconstruction. American Journal of Surgery 126: 488–491
3. Bakamjian V Y, Holbrook L A 1973 Prefabrication techniques in cervical pharyngo-oesophageal reconstruction. British Journal of Plastic Surgery 26: 214–221
4. Harii K, Ohmori K, Ohmori S 1974 Successful clinical transfers of ten free flaps by microvascular anastomoses. Plastic and Reconstructive Surgery 53: 259–270
5. McGregor I A, Jackson I T 1970 The extended role of the deltopectoral flap. British Journal of Plastic Surgery 23: 173–185
6. Gingrass R P, Culf N K, Garrot W S, Mladick R A 1972 Complications with the deltopectoral flap. Plastic and Reconstructive Surgery 49: 501–507

INTEROSSEOUS RECURRENT ARTERY (a branch of the posterior interosseous artery)

Anconeus musculocutaneous flap Interosseous recurrent fasciocutaneous flap

An inferiorly pedicled musculocutaneous flap incorporating the anconeus muscle has been utilised based on the interosseous recurrent artery.[1, 2, 3] The anatomy and flap outlines are indicated in Figures 7.114–7.117.

Chang et al[4] have described an interosseous recurrent flap designed along the lateral intermuscular septum posterior to the epicondyle which may be interpreted as an extended anconeus flap. However, communications between the interosseous recurrent artery and the middle collateral artery are sparse (as outlined on p. 183) and extension of the flap above the level of the lateral epicondyle is therefore limited.

References

1. Cardany C R 1985 Anconeus Flap. Personal communication.
2. Vasconez L O 1981 Personal communication.
3. Cohen B Unpublished work.
4. Chang C C, Maruyama Y, Onishi K, Iwahira Y, Fujita R, Shimizu K 1987 Fasciocutaneous flaps of the upper arm (abstract). Journal of Japan Society of Plastic and Reconstructive Surgery 6: 550

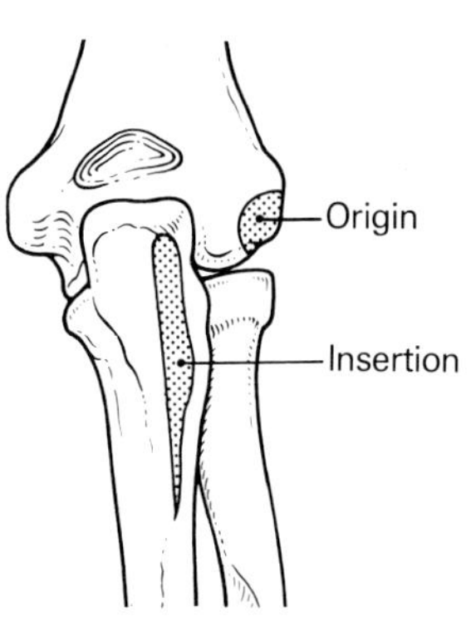

Fig. 7.115 Bony attachments of anconeus.

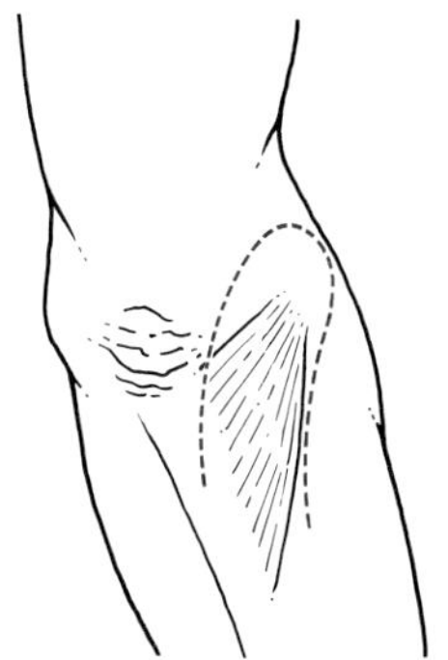

Fig. 7.116 Flap planning.

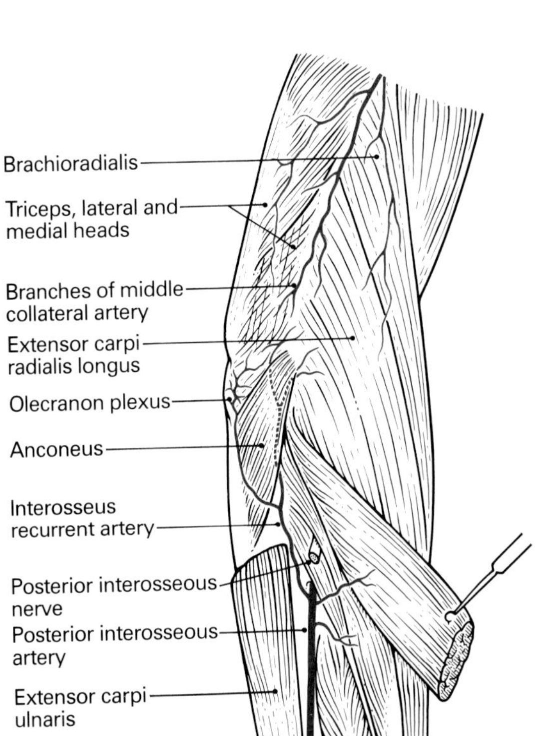

Fig. 7.114 Vascular anatomy. Posterolateral view of the right elbow showing blood supply to anconeus. Extensor carpi ulnaris has been partially excised; extensor digitorum has been divided and retracted; the posterior interosseous nerve has been excised (for clarity).

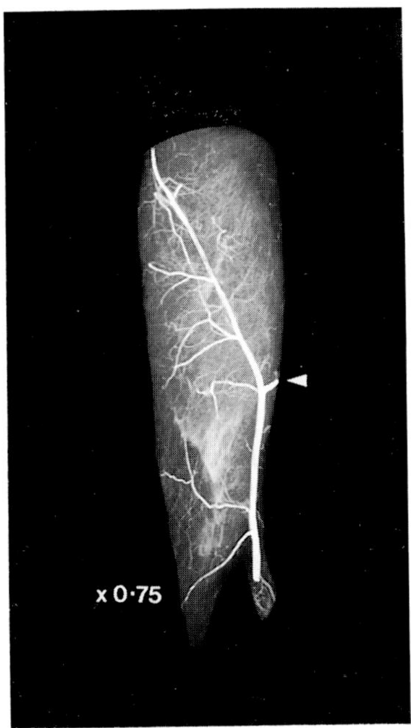

Fig. 7.117 Radiograph of anconeus. An arrow indicates a cutaneous branch of the interosseous recurrent artery.

7 LABIAL ARTERY

Abbe flap
Estlander flap
Gillies fan flap
Karapandžić flap

Many different varieties of local flaps have been described for the repair of lip defects. The four described here have been chosen to illustrate different principles but all depend on labial arteries for their survival.

Anatomy

The facial artery gives off the inferior labial artery near the angle of the mouth. This passes deep to depressor anguli oris and penetrates orbicularis oris to run a tortuous course in the lower lip between this muscle and the mucous membrane. There is some variation in the size and number of inferior labial vessels and a single inferior labial artery on each side is not invariable. It anastomoses with the inferior labial of the other side at almost full diameter and, by branches, anastomoses with the mental branch of the inferior alveolar artery. The superior labial artery also arises from the facial artery but sometimes from the transverse facial artery. It follows a similar course along the edge of the upper lip between orbicularis oris and the mucous membrane, giving off an alar branch and a nasal septal branch. It anastomoses at full diameter with its opposite number.

Abbe flap

The Abbe flap is a full-thickness lower lip flap with a vermilion-based pedicle containing the inferior labial artery. The flap is used for repairing or augmenting the upper lip – a lip-switch procedure (Fig. 7.118 a–c). The flap is named after Robert Abbe who, in 1897, swung such a flap from a full lower lip into an upper lip which was tight and scarred as the result of a previous bilateral cleft lip repair. Prior to Abbe, however, vermilion-based flaps had been used by several people and were first reported by the Italian Sabattini in 1837. Abbe flap designs over the years have included triangular, W, split apex, rectangular and shield shapes (Fig. 7.118d). The shape of the defect will be determined by the objective of the procedure, and the flap will be fashioned so as to correspond in shape. The design of the pedicle is important and affects the accuracy with which the flap may be inset into the recipient defect. Early flaps included all of the red margin of the lip, thereby creating a bulky pedicle which interfered with positioning of the flap. More accurate knowledge of the anatomical localisation of the inferior labial vessels enables the pedicle to be positioned behind the orbicularis oris with little reduction of its vascular input.

On the side of the pedicle, the skin is incised from the apex of the V (assuming a triangular-shaped flap) up to a point 2 mm proximal to the mucocutaneous junction. The incision is then deepened until most of the muscle has been divided, and then the pedicle containing the inferior labial artery is dissected. Once this has been safely done the free margin of the flap may be incised. When insetting the flap, a small Z plasty on the red margin may be routinely incorporated in order to counteract the slight notching of the red margin which tends to follow straight suturing over the lip. The pedicle may be divided 10–14 days later. It is worth noting that histological and histochemical studies of muscle biopsies taken from Abbe flaps and from the normal lateral lip elements of six patients, showed that motor reinnervation occurred in these flaps.[2]

A one-stage modification of the Abbe flap has also been described in which the lower lip island is raised on a skeletonised inferior labial artery pedicle which is dissected back to the oral commissure (Hu et al, 1993).[3]

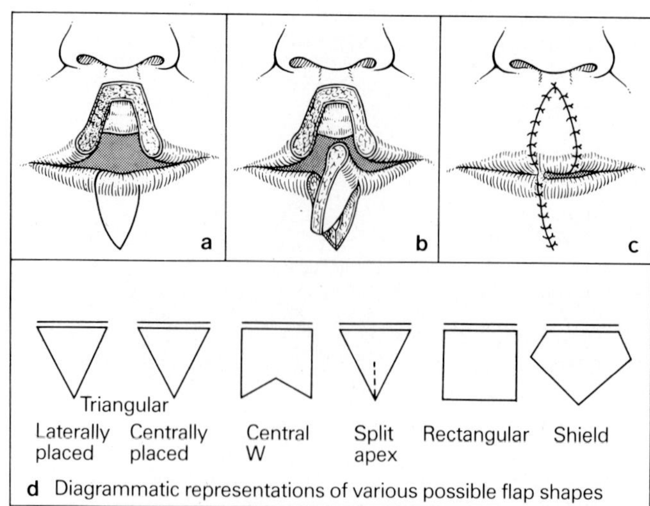

Fig. 7.118 Abbe flap for central defect of upper lip (**a–c**).
d. Diagrammatic representations of various possible flap shapes.

Estlander flap

In 1872 Estlander[4] described an operation for the repair of lateral defects of the lower lip using a flap from the corner of the mouth based on a narrow superior labial artery pedicle (Fig. 7.119 a–c). This operation produces a new, medially displaced commissure at the point of rotation but the resulting rounded corner has an unnatural appearance and requires correction by a secondary procedure which reconstructs the commissure. A further problem is that the closure of the donor site may produce a scar which transgresses the nasolabial fold.

With a median defect of the lower lip an Estlander type of flap may be used if the median defect is first closed by swinging a flap from the lateral half of the lower lip; an Estlander flap is raised and rotated into the lateral secondary defect (Fig. 7.119 d–f). Again the lateral commissure will require reconstruction.

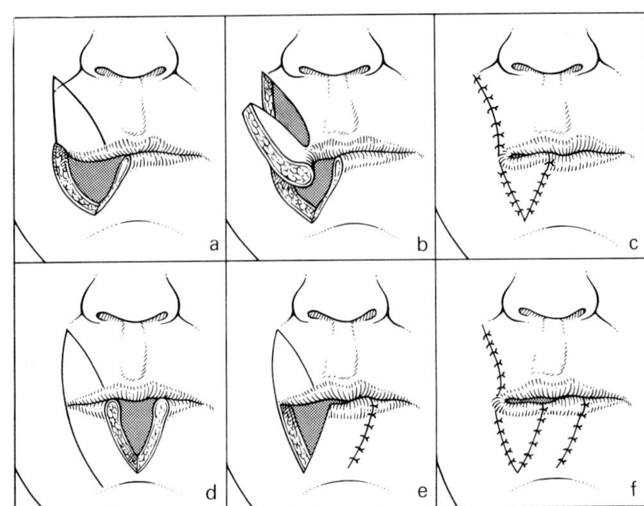

Fig. 7.119 Estlander flaps for lateral (**a–c**) and central defects (**d–f**).

Abbe–Estlander flap

Most authors apply this term to an upper-to-lower lip-switch which does not involve the corner of the mouth. The flap may be basically triangular as in the classic Estlander or modified in various ways. Figure 7.120 shows how the excisional defect may be designed in the form of 'W' with the infero-lateral corner forming a 30° angle. In placing the inferior margin, use is made of any natural crease that may be present between the lower lip and the chin. The donor flap is outlined on the upper lip between two vertical lines, the first parallel to and just lateral to the philtral margin, while the position of the second is determined by the desired width of the flap. The flap width should not exceed 2 cm and should be half that of the defect and therefore a 4 cm defect can be repaired. The pedicle containing the superior labial artery is preserved on the medial side and therefore supplies the flap through its anastomoses with the vessel of the opposite side. A Bürow's triangle situated lateral to the alar base forms an eccentric apex to the defect and allows advancement of the remaining lateral lip so that the final scar will lie along the alar base and philtral margin.

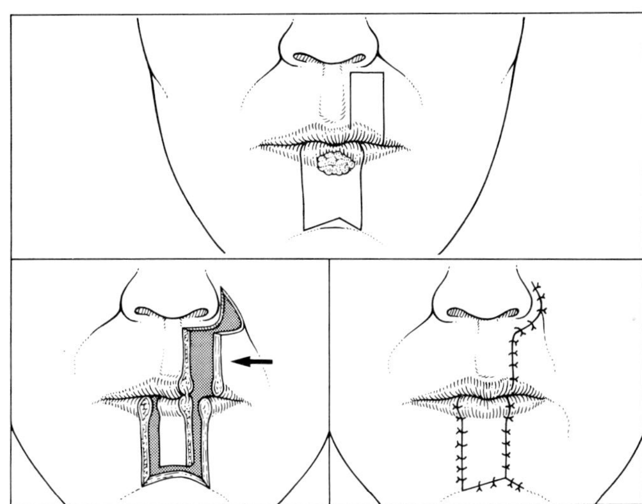

Fig. 7.120 Abbe–Estlander flap (one of several possible versions).

Gillies fan flap

The fan flap principle[5] was developed to deal with excisions of more than half the lower lip, or rectangular defects, for which lip-switch flaps were less appropriate. A fan-shaped flap based on the superior labial vessels of the normal lip and of a depth to match the defect is constructed and rotated into the lower lip until flap red margin meets lip red margin (Fig. 7.121). The secondary defect is closed by using the slack skin of the cheek. This classic fan-flap tends to reduce the size of the mouth considerably and an alternative approach is to

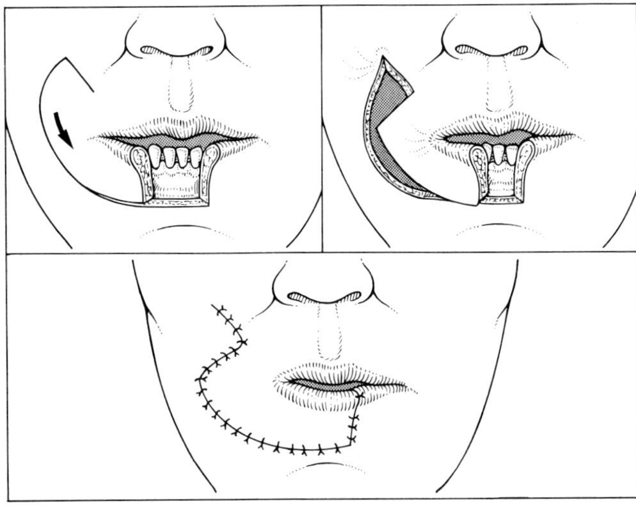

Fig. 7.121 Classical Gillies fan flap.

use a vertical rectangular-shaped flap which rotates around the corner of the mouth without altering the position of this point, and brings an incised side up into the position of the lower lip (Fig. 7.122). Here the skin and mucosa may be sutured together to produce a red margin or the vermilion may be reconstructed more effectively with a tongue flap. The width of the rectangular flap is made equal to the vertical height of the lip defect and the flap length to the horizontal width of the defect plus the width of the flap. The secondary defect is closed by bringing the skin of the cheek downwards and medially, and may be aided by rounding off the corners of the 'rectangle' when it is first elevated.

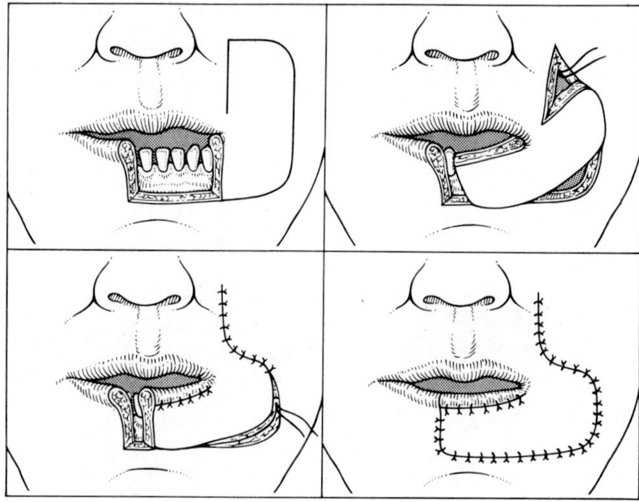

Fig. 7.122 McGregor modification of Gillies fan flap.

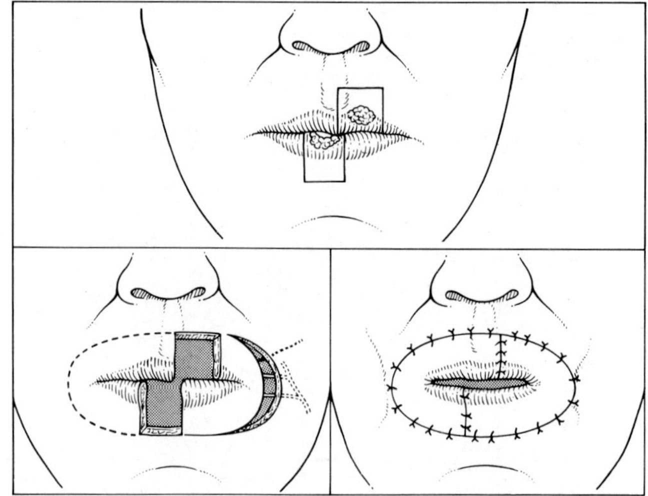

Fig. 7.123 Karapandžić neurovascular musculocutaneous flaps.

Karapandžić neurovascular fan flaps

It will be apparent that both the classic and the modified fan flaps are devoid of motor and sensory innervation, perhaps most significantly with bilateral flaps, although some recovery does slowly take place in most cases.

To deal with this, and the problem of coincident defects of both the upper and the lower lips when a fan flap would not survive, Karapandžić has raised bilateral flaps of orbicularis oris, lips and skin based on the superior and inferior labial vessels and with as many sensory and motor nerve fibres preserved as possible (Fig. 7.123). The skin incisions parallel the lip margins at a distance equal to the depth of the defects, the flaps are then mobilised and rotated into the defects until they meet. This restores the anatomical continuity of the orbicularis oris muscle and retains maximum function. Occasionally, correct flap function in the region of the commissure may need to be restored by attaching a bundle of fibres from the anterior part of masseter. The technique is not suitable for all defects, but works best with central excisions, and works least with defects at the angle because of difficulty in regaining symmetry of the lips.

References

1. Abbe R 1898 A new plastic operation for the relief of deformity due to double hare lip. Medical Record 53: 477–478
2. Thompson N, Pollard A C 1961 Motor function in Abbe flaps. British Journal of Plastic Surgery 14: 66–75
3. Hu H, Song R, Sun G 1993 One-stage inferior labial flap and its pertinent anatomic study. Plastic and Reconstructive Surgery 91: 618–623
4. Estlander J A 1872 Eine Methode aus der einen Lippe Substanzverluste der anderen zu ersetzen. Translated by: Sundell B 1968 Plastic and Reconstructive Surgery 42: 361–366
5. Gillies H D, Millard D R 1957 The Principles and Art of Plastic Surgery. Butterworth, London
6. McGregor I A 1983 Reconstruction of the lower lip. British Journal of Plastic Surgery 36: 40–47
7. Karapandžić M 1974 Reconstruction of lip defects by local arterial flaps. British Journal of Plastic Surgery 27: 93–97
8. Jabaley M E, Orcutt T W, Clement R L 1976 Applications of the Karapandžić principle of lip reconstruction after excision of lip cancer. American Journal of Surgery 132: 529–532

LATERAL CIRCUMFLEX FEMORAL ARTERY – ascending branch

Tensor fasciae latae musculocutaneous flap

The tensor fasciae latae flap is a reliable musculocutaneous unit with a constant vascular pedicle of relatively large size, but limited length, which can be equally readily used as a transposition, island or free flap.[1, 2] Several variations and refinements have been described, e.g. combination with gluteus medius as a rotation advancement flap,[3] as a mainly fascial flap for abdominal wall reconstruction,[4] as a bilobed flap,[5] or as a bipedicle flap.

Anatomy

The tensor fasciae latae (note this is often misspelt as tensor fascia lata – the muscle is the tensor *of* the fascia *of* the thigh) arises from a narrow strip of the ilium between the origin of gluteus minimus and the anterior part of the iliac crest. An important point is that the muscle lies *between* the laminae of the iliotibial tract and is inserted into the tract just below the level of the greater trochanter. This is a Type I muscle with a single vascular pedicle entering on its deep surface consisting of an artery of 2–3 mm in diameter and paired venae comitantes. This artery comes from the ascending branch of the lateral circumflex femoral artery and enters the muscle approximately 9 cm below the anterior superior iliac spine (variations in the origin of this vessel have been described in Chapter 6).

The ascending and transverse branches are generally given off together and then divide with the ascending branch supplying parts of the minor gluteal muscles and the upper part of vastus lateralis as well as TFL. The transverse branch supplies vastus lateralis and participates in the cruciate anastomosis. The branch to gluteus minimus is significant and must be divided when freeing the vascular pedicle. Branches may also be

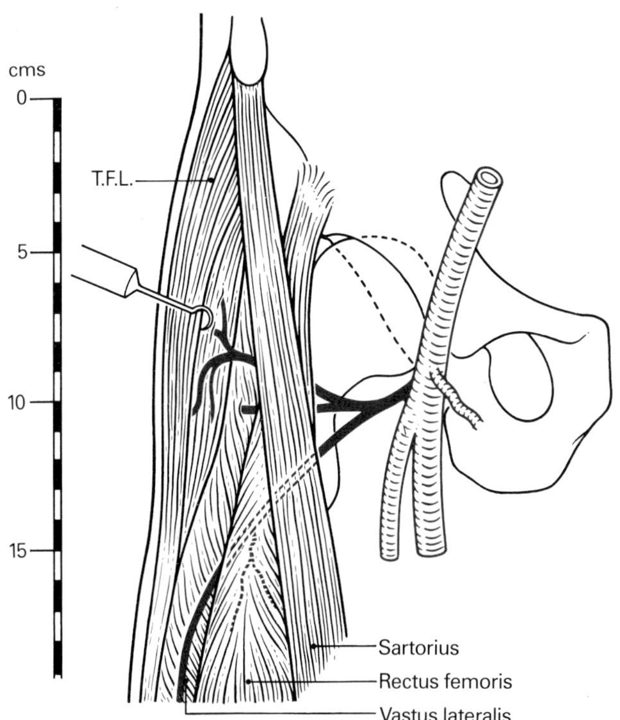

Fig. 7.124 Vascular anatomy. Ascending, transverse and descending branches of the lateral circumflex femoral artery showing the ascending branch piercing the deep surface of TFL 8–10 cm below the anterior superior iliac spine.

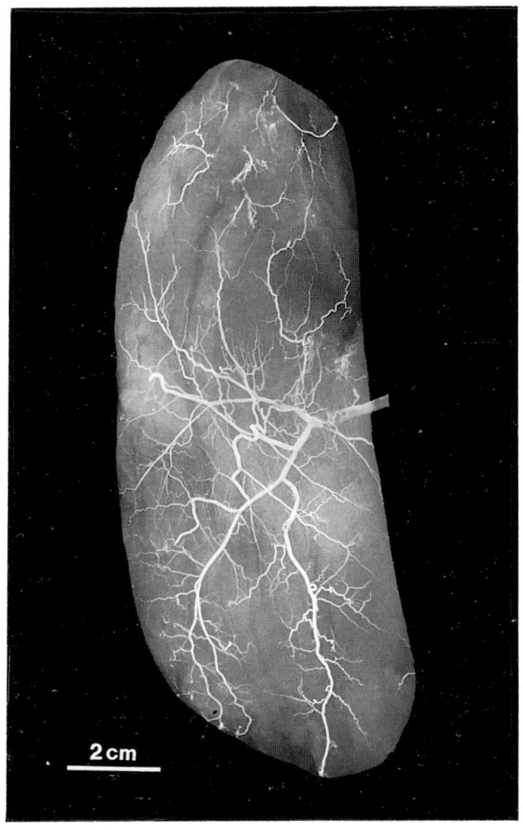

Fig. 7.125 Radiograph of tensor fasciae latae muscle.

given off to sartorius and rectus femoris from the ascending branch or the combined trunk of ascending and transverse branches.

On entering the muscle, the arterial pedicle divides into several branches which run superiorly and inferiorly between the muscle fibre bundles and give off, or themselves terminate as, musculocutaneous perforators to the overlying skin. There are about seven of these comparatively large perforators which is generous for a muscle of this small size. These perforators anastomose inferiorly through large channels with branches of the first profunda perforator and anastomose posteriorly with branches of the superior gluteal artery. Anastomoses with the superior gluteal system also occur in the fascia behind TFL, between it and gluteus medius. Within the superior part of the muscle, branches supply the periosteum of the iliac crest and penetrate the bone – the flap therefore has the capability of transferring a vascularised bone graft.

The area of the flap is innervated by the lateral cutaneous branch of T12, the lateral cutaneous branch of the iliohypogastric nerve and the lateral cutaneous nerve of the thigh. The muscle is innervated by the superior gluteal nerve.

Flap planning

The flap usually measures 10–12 cm in width and is centred over the muscle with the upper border along the iliac crest. The flap may be raised in a short form approximately 20 cm long or in a long form some 30 cm in length although it has been stated that it may be raised (when delayed) to within 8 cm of the knee joint. The short flap can easily be transposed over the trochanteric area while the longer flap will cover trochanteric and ischial areas at the same time. The anatomical vascular basis of the long flap is the excellent longitudinal network of vessels overlying the tract formed by large-bore anastomoses between individual branches of profunda perforators which emerge along the lateral intermuscular septum and fan out over the

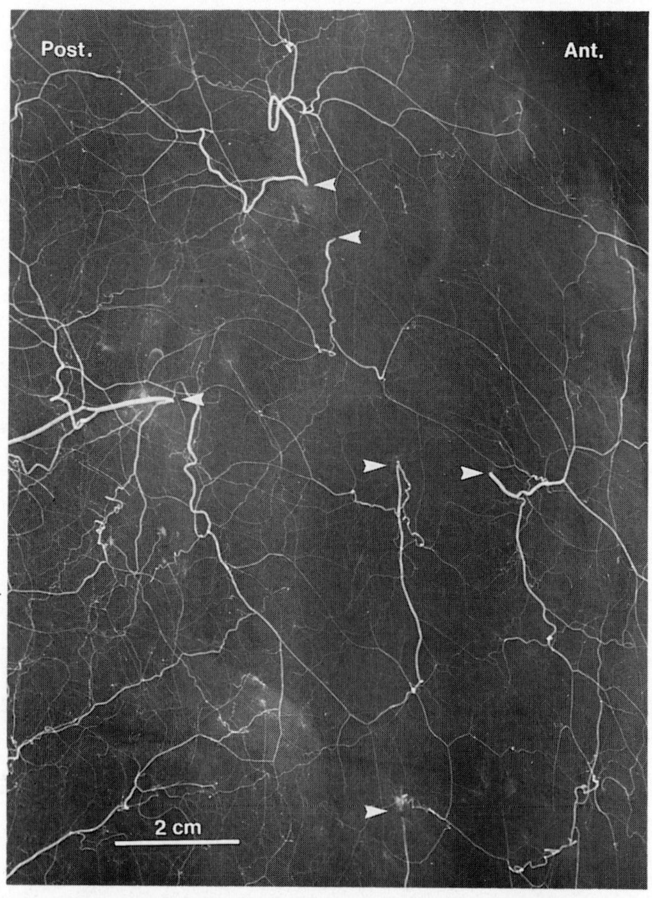

Fig. 7.126 Radiograph of skin from area overlying TFL showing several musculocutaneous perforators.

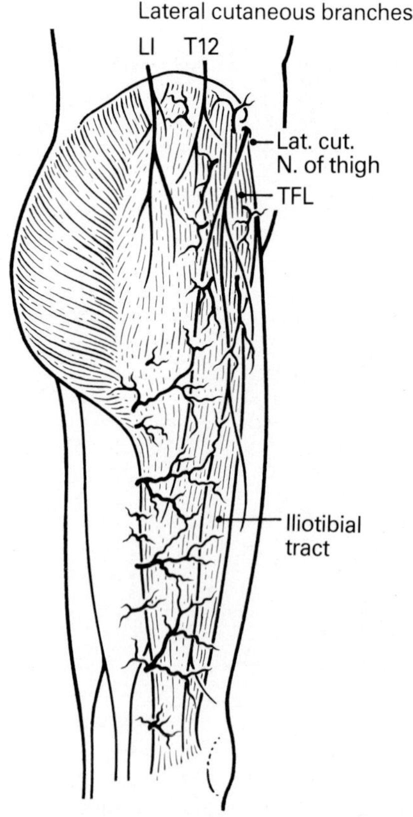

Fig. 7.127 Flap planning.

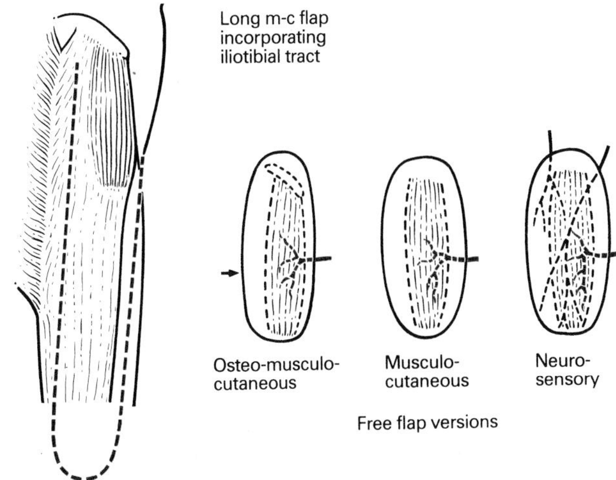

Fig. 7.128 Various flap options are available.

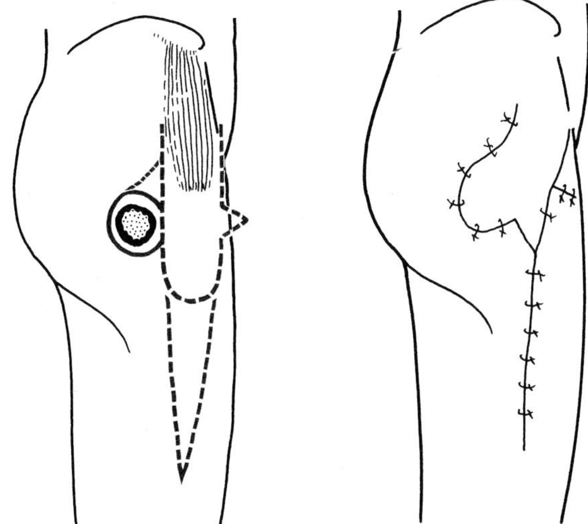

Fig. 7.129 TFL flap for trochanteric pressure sore. Note bilobed arrangement to facilitate closure of the upper end of the donor site wound where it is under most tension.

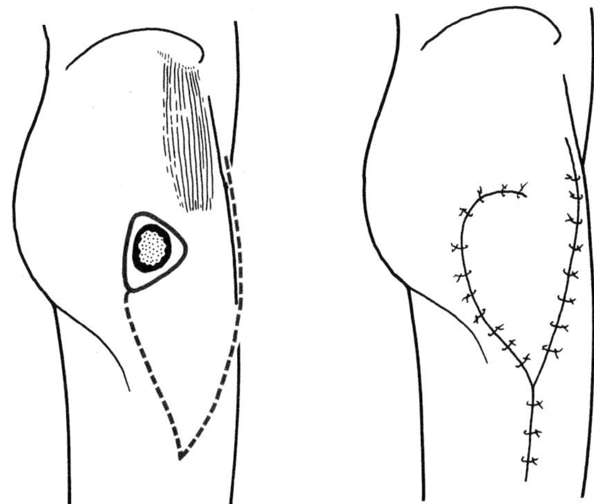

Fig. 7.130 V to Y advancement of the TFL flap for closure of trochanteric pressure sore.

iliotibial tract. The tract is raised with the flap and its inextensibility prevents the flap being stretched and thereby prevents the anastomotic channels being narrowed. The ability to create long flaps is not a function of the vascularity of the tract itself which is relatively poorly vascularised and has no perforators piercing it from the underlying vastus lateralis. This also implies that the tract cannot be expected to act as a vascularised carrier for a more distally situated island of skin raised on the inferior part of the tract.

The frequently illustrated artery which is reputed to run down the tract (above it in some reports, beneath it in others) is something that the authors have never seen. The source of this confusion has probably been the descending branch of the lateral circumflex femoral artery which descends within the anterior part of vastus lateralis but may lie deep or superficially in the interval between vastus lateralis and rectus femoris. Here it is a short distance from the anterior edge of the tract but this vessel is generally not elevated with the flap.

Flap elevation

The distal margin of the flap is incised first and the incision carried down through skin and fascia onto vastus lateralis. The anterior and posterior margins are incised, and the flap elevated from distal to proximal with anchoring sutures inserted between skin and tract. As the muscle lies between the laminae of the tract, continued upward elevation of the tract ensures that the muscle is incorporated in the flap. Used as a local transposition flap visualisation of the pedicle may not be necessary, but for island and free flap versions the pedicle is dissected out at this stage. The position of this pedicle 7–9 cm below the anterior superior iliac spine in the interval between rectus femoris and vastus lateralis and the need to divide gluteal branches have already been mentioned.

References

1. Hill H L, Nahai F, Vasconez L O 1978 The tensor fascia lata myocutaneous free flap. Plastic and Reconstructive Surgery 61: 517–521
2. Nahai F, Hill H L, Hester T R 1979 Experiences with the tensor fascia lata flap. Plastic and Reconstructive Surgery 63: 788–799
3. Little J W, Lyons J R 1983 The gluteus medius – tensor fasciae latae flap. Plastic and Reconstructive Surgery 71: 366–370
4. Lynch S M 1981 The bilobed tensor fascia lata myocutaneous flap. Plastic and Reconstructive Surgery 67: 796–798
5. Caffee H H 1983 Reconstruction of the abdominal wall by variations of the tensor fasciae latae flap. Plastic and Reconstructive Surgery 71: 348–351
6. Scheflan M 1981 The tensor fascia lata: variations on a theme. Plastic and Reconstructive Surgery 68: 59–68
7. Paletta C E, Freedman B, Shehadi S I 1989 The V Y tensor fasciae latae musculocutaneous flap. Plastic and Reconstructive Surgery 83: 852–857

7

LATERAL CIRCUMFLEX FEMORAL ARTERY – descending branch

Rectus femoris musculocutaneous flap

The rectus femoris muscle was used as a transposition flap for several years[1, 2] before it evolved as a musculocutaneous flap early on in the period of musculocutaneous flap development.[3, 4] It has a reliable vascular pedicle and considerable length (7 cm × 40 cm) which gives it an arc of rotation about a point 7 cm below the inguinal ligament which takes in the anterior groin, perineum and abdominal wall up to the umbilicus and also the trochanter and ischium posteriorly. However, because this muscle is necessary for fully functional knee extension and thigh flexion in the non-paraplegic patient it is not really expendable and defects in the area which can be covered by this flap can be reconstructed with alternative less essential musculocutaneous units (e.g. TFL, gracilis).

Anatomy

Rectus femoris arises by a short strong tendon which is made up of a superficial part attached to the anterior inferior iliac spine and a deeper part attached above the brim of the acetabulum, the so-called straight and reflected heads. The muscle fibres arise in bipennate fashion from the deep aspect of the tendon and its prolongation in the substance of the muscle, and are inserted into an aponeurosis on the deep surface of the lower two-thirds of the muscle. The tendon, separated from the femur by the suprapatellar bursa, inserts into the upper pole of the patella. It is a Type II muscle supplied by a single dominant vascular pedicle derived from the lateral circumflex femoral artery and a number of smaller secondary pedicles.

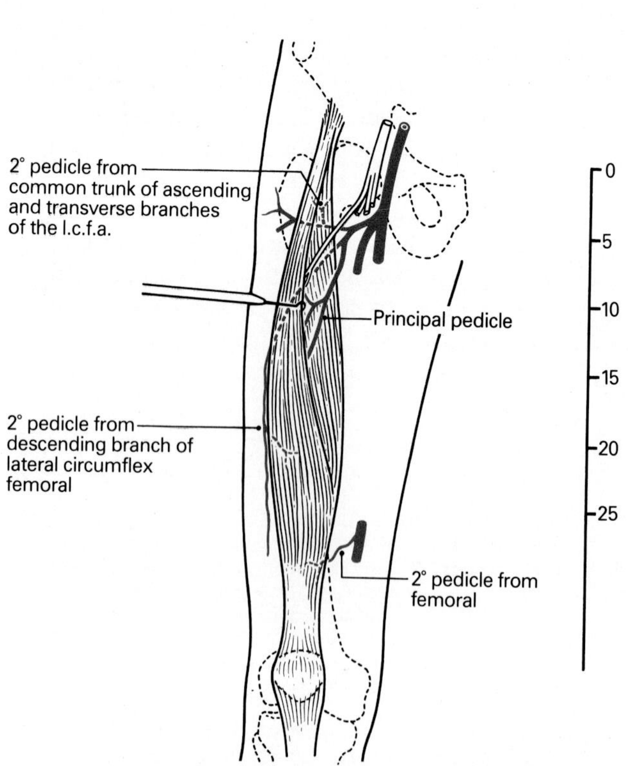

Fig. 7.131 Vascular anatomy. The primary pedicle is constant, the secondary pedicles more variable.

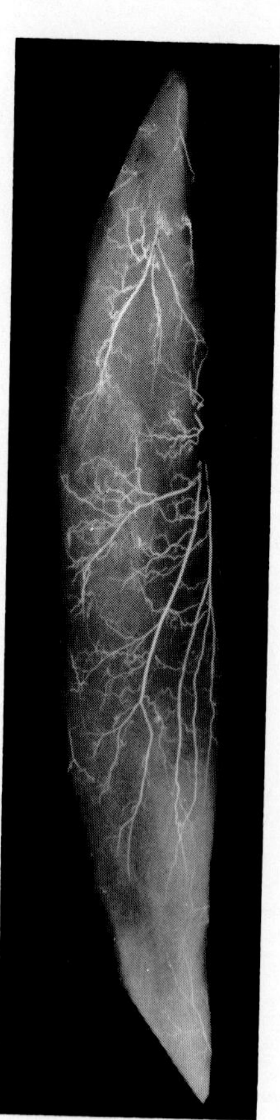

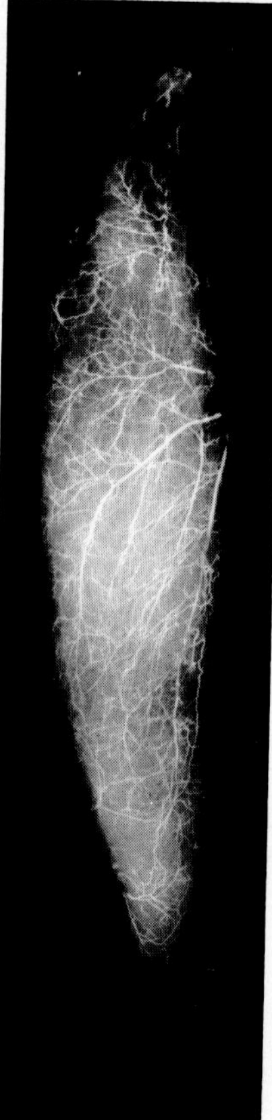

Fig. 7.132 Radiographs of two injected rectus femoris muscles.

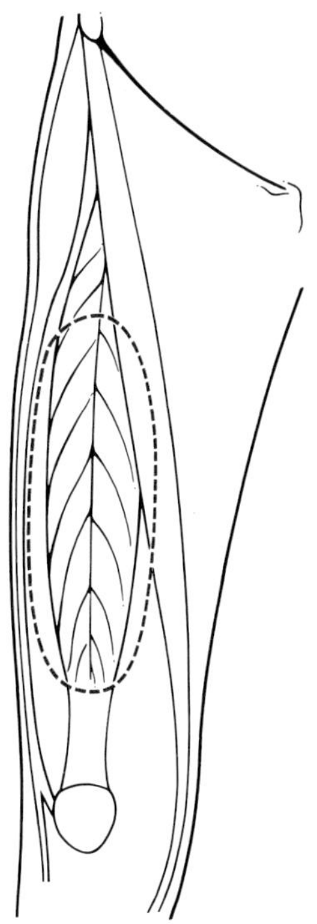

Fig. 7.133 Flap planning. The flap overlies the lower two-thirds of the muscular part of rectus femoris.

The main pedicle comes from the descending branch of the lateral circumflex femoral artery and enters the muscle at the junction of its proximal and middle thirds. The variations in the manner of origin of this vessel have been described on page 236 but it generally arises some 5 cm below the top of the symphysis pubis and runs downwards for 5–8 cm to enter the muscle on its posterior surface deep to the medial border (the medial border has been turned forwards in Fig. 7.131). At this point therefore the vascular pedicle, which is usually accompanied by a motor branch from the femoral nerve, lies approximately 10–13 cm beneath the inguinal ligament. It divides into a superior branch and an inferior branch; the superior divides into ascending and descending parts which lie within the muscle nearer its posterior surface; the inferior branch runs axially downwards in the muscle nearer its anterior surface and gives off musculocutaneous perforators to the overlying skin. Sometimes this vessel may lie on the posteromedial surface of the muscle rather than within it, in which case it will give off vessels which pass round the medial side of the muscle.

Secondary pedicles are found entering the muscle superiorly from the ascending branch of the lateral circumflex femoral artery, and inferiorly from branches of the femoral artery directly or via its branches to vastus medialis.

The descending branch of the lateral circumflex femoral artery lies in the interval between rectus femoris and vastus lateralis supplying the latter, but may also give off very small branches to the lower part of rectus femoris and may send fasciocutaneous perforators to the skin in the interval between rectus femoris and vastus lateralis.

The territory of skin supportable by perforators from the muscle takes in superiorly the area between sartorius and tensor fasciae latae. The distal part of the territory is less reliable, largely because in some individuals the rectus femoris becomes entirely tendinous from a point approximately 20 cm above the upper pole of the patella.

The sensory innervation of the territory of the flap comes from the intermediate anterior cutaneous nerve of the thigh (Fig. 7.134).

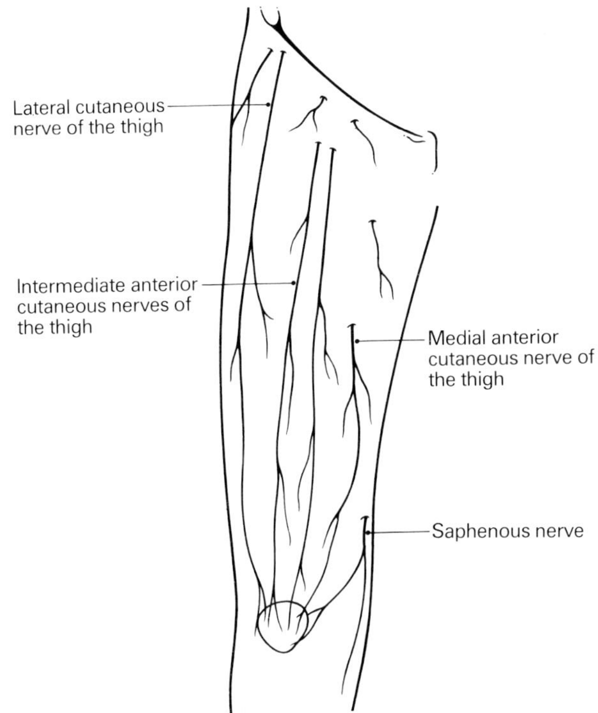

Fig. 7.134 Cutaneous innervation in the area of the flap is illustrated.

Flap elevation

The flap may be constructed with a skin pedicle or with an island centred over the proximal two-thirds of the muscle. The elevation commences distally with division of the tendon of insertion (preserving the integrity of the suprapatellar bursa) and continues upwards deep to the muscle until the pedicle is reached. With narrow flaps the donor defect may be closed directly.

References

1. Ger R, 1971 The surgical management of decubitus ulcers by muscle transposition. Surgery 69: 106–110
2. Ger R, Levine S A 1976 The management of decubitus ulcers by muscle transposition. Plastic and Reconstructive Surgery 58: 419–428
3. McCraw J B, Dibbell D G, Carraway J H 1977 Clinical definition of independent myocutaneous vascular territories. Plastic and Reconstructive Surgery 60: 341–352
4. Bhagwat B M, Pearl R M, Laub D R 1978 Use of the rectus femoris myocutaneous flap. Plastic and Reconstructive Surgery 62: 698–701
5. Larson D L, Liang M D 1983 Quadriceps musculocutaneous flap: a reliable sensate flap for the hemipelvectomy defect. Plastic and Reconstructive Surgery 72: 347–353
6. Ger R, Duboys E 1983 Prevention and repair of large abdominal wall defects by muscle transposition: a preliminary communication. Plastic and Reconstructive Surgery 72: 170–175

LATERAL CIRCUMFLEX FEMORAL ARTERY – transverse and descending branches

Vastus lateralis musculocutaneous flap

The use of a vastus lateralis muscle flap to repair trochanteric pressure sores was first reported in the 1940s[1] and 'rediscovered' in the 1970s.[2, 3, 4] At that time it was not appreciated that there were vascular connections between the anterior part of the muscle and the overlying skin. Subsequently it was recognised that a skin island could be carried on the distal part of the muscle that lay anterior to the iliotibial tract because although no perforators pass through the tract itself, there are musculocutaneous perforators anterior to it, particularly in the lower half of the thigh.[5, 6]

More recently it has been appreciated that it is not always necessary to include the muscle with the skin and such a flap may be used as a free flap. This is, in effect, a fasciocutaneous flap with some additional supply by one or two musculocutaneous perforators which are dissected free from the anterior part of the muscle.

Anatomy

Vastus lateralis is a Type II muscle with a dominant proximal pedicle from the lateral circumflex femoral artery augmented by multiple perforators from the posterior compartment which pierce the lateral intermuscular septum close to the femur and end in the muscle. The lateral circumflex pedicle is in two parts:

The transverse branch of the LCFA runs into the proximal part of vastus lateralis. In a few cases (~6%) musculocutaneous perforators may pass through the upper anterior part of the muscle to reach skin.

The descending branch of the LCFA runs down behind the anterior edge of vastus lateralis in the company of the nerve of supply to the muscle and terminates either in skin (10%) or by entering the muscle (90%). Near its origin it also gives branches to rectus femoris and vastus intermedius. The surface marking of the descending branch is represented by the lower two-thirds of a line drawn between the mid-point of the inguinal ligament, and the mid-point of a line between the anterior superior iliac spine and the superolateral corner of the patella.

The way in which the nerve of supply and the descending branch run together along the antero-medial border of the vastus lateralis is characteristic. As their branches enter the muscle multiple neurovascular hila are formed, with one of these in the proximal third and three in the proximal and middle thirds, sometimes creating a plane splitting the muscle into anterior and posterior parts.

In approximately 60% of cases several of these muscle branches exit from the surface of the muscle to pierce the deep fascia over the anterior part of the muscle (not the part beneath the iliotibial tract) and supply the skin.

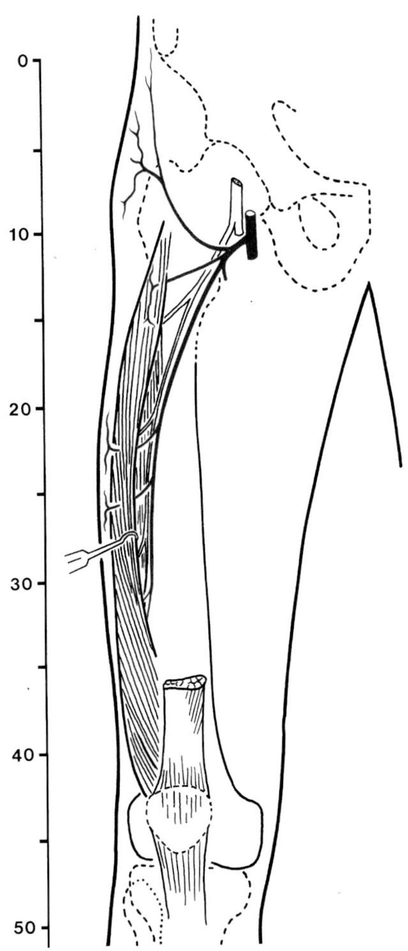

Fig. 7.135 The lateral circumflex femoral artery and its ascending, transverse and descending branches are shown. The supply to vastus lateralis entering on the medial aspect of the muscle is displayed and the approximate distance below the anterior superior iliac spine is indicated in centimetres.

In approximately 40% of cases one or two septocutaneous perforators are also given off in the intermuscular septum and reach the deep fascia at a point approximately 2 cm inferolateral to the mid-point of the previously mentioned line between the anterior superior iliac spine and the superolateral corner of the patella.

Flap planning

The application for this flap lies in the repair of trochanteric pressure sores and the salvage of the open wounds following removal of infected hip arthroplasties and bone destroyed by osteomyelitis. The shape of the skin island as dictated by the defect is outlined over the distal part of the muscle anterior to the iliotibial tract. Maximum dimensions will not exceed 12 cm × 8 cm, with the most distal part of the flap at least 4 cm above the proximal end of the patella.

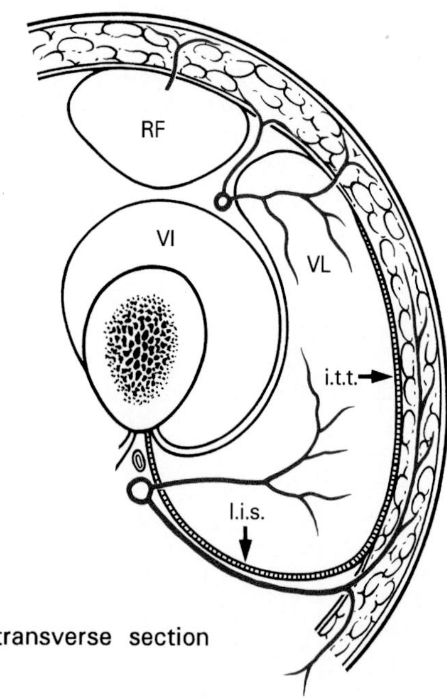

Fig. 7.136 Vascular anatomy. Medial and posterior vascular pedicles of vastus lateralis are indicated schematically. Perforators to skin lie anterior to the iliotibial tract and do not perforate it. The numbers of perforators reaching the skin via the septum and through the anterior part of the muscle are inversely related to each other.

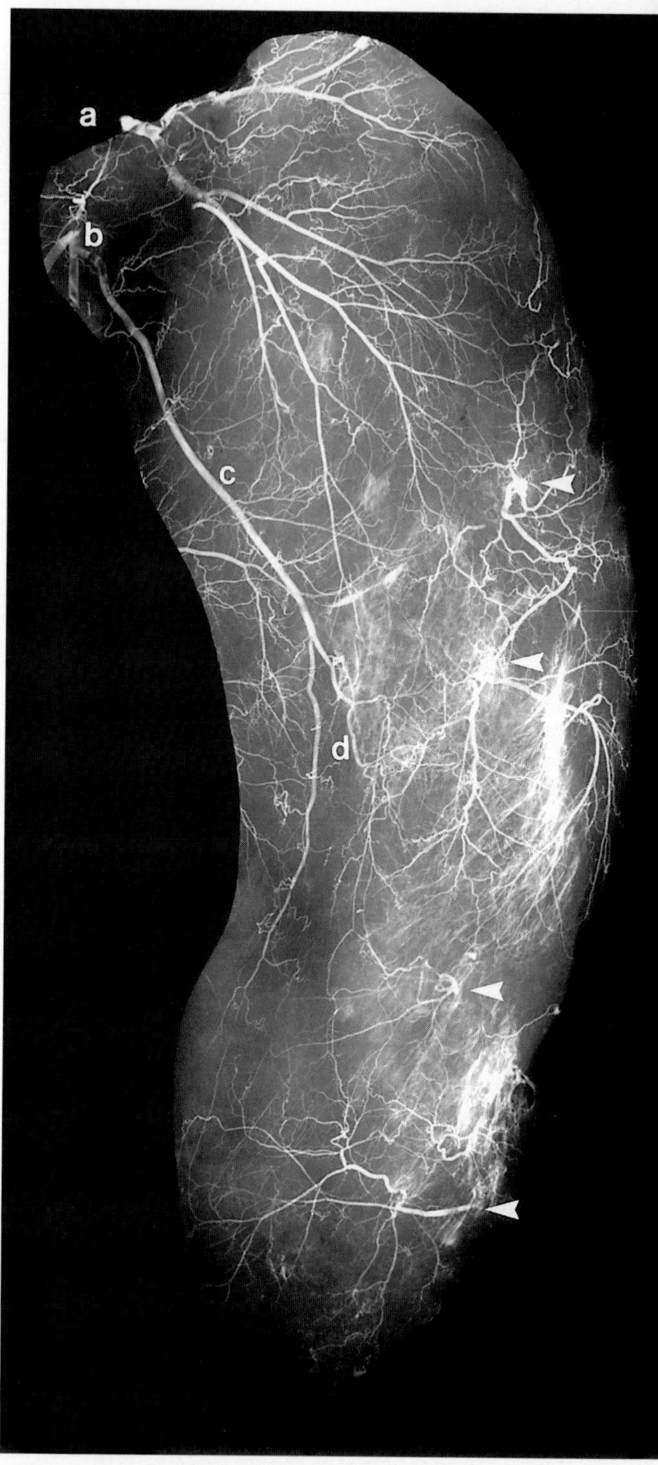

Fig. 7.137 Radiograph of injected vastus lateralis and vastus intermedius which have been raised together. Vessels are indicated as follows: **a.** transverse branch of lateral circumflex femoral artery; **b.** quadriceps group of arteries (branches to rectus femoris and vastus intermedius cut short) with **c.** the descending branch giving off **d.** a branch to vastus lateralis. Arrows indicate several branches of the profunda perforators entering the posterior part of the vastus lateralis.

Flap elevation

In elevating the flap wide exposure of the vastus lateralis is required and this is done through an incision over the anterior part of the muscle which splits the fascia lata. The surface marking for this incision is a little lateral to the previously described line between the ASIS and patella and will join the defect and the flap. Vastus lateralis is separated from rectus femoris and vastus intermedius, with branches of the descending artery to these latter muscles requiring division. Proximally, the pedicle to the muscle is preserved and vastus lateralis is separated from intermedius by sharp dissection, turning to blunt dissection as the plane between the deep surface of lateralis and the superficial surface of intermedius is developed distally. Vastus lateralis is divided distally when sufficient length has been obtained. The muscle must be mobilised from the femur to allow rotation in a posterior arc but it should be noted that the vastus lateralis muscle also receives a blood supply on its posteromedial aspect from terminal branches of the profunda femoris perforators, and therefore mobilisation of this muscle off the femur can be a bloody procedure.

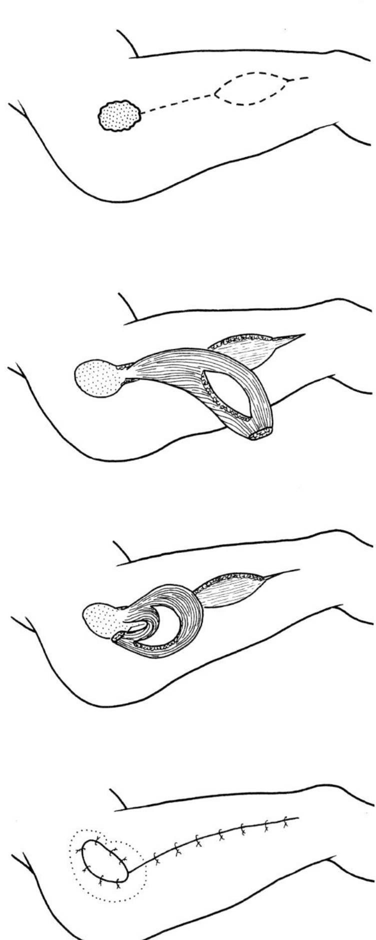

Fig. 7.138 Vastus lateralis musculocutaneous flap with skin island used to fill defect resulting from excision of trochanteric pressure sore.

References

1. Conway H, Kraissl C J, Clifford R H, Gelb J, Joseph J M, Leveridge L L, 1947 The plastic surgical closure of decubitus ulcers in patients with paraplegia. Surgery, Gynaecology and Obstetrics 85: 321–332
2. Mathes S J, Nahai F 1979 Clinical atlas of muscle and musculocutaneous flaps. Mosby, St. Louis, p 51
3. Minami R T, Hentz V R, Vistnes L M 1977 Use of vastus lateralis muscle flap for repair of trochanteric pressure sores. Plastic and Reconstructive Surgery 60: 364–368
4. Dowden R V, McCraw J B 1980 The vastus lateralis muscle flap: technique and applications. Annals of Plastic Surgery 4: 396–404
5. Bovet J L, Nassif T M, Guimberteau J C, Baudet J 1982 The vastus lateralis musculocutaneous flap in the repair of trochanteric pressure sores: technique and indications. Plastic and Reconstructive Surgery 69: 830–834
6. Hauben D J, Smith A R, Sonneveld G J, Van der Meulen J C 1983 The use of the vastus lateralis musculocutaneous flap for the repair of trochanteric pressure sores. Annals of Plastic Surgery 10: 359–363
7. Wolff K-D, Grundmann A 1992 The free vastus lateralis flap: an anatomic study with case reports. Plastic and Reconstructive Surgery 89: 469–475

7

LATERAL CIRCUMFLEX FEMORAL ARTERY – descending branch

Anterolateral thigh fasciocutaneous flap

This flap is based on the perforators to skin arising from the descending branch of the lateral circumflex femoral artery with the descending branch forming a very adequate pedicle for a free flap. In a pedicled form the length of the pedicle (maximum ~12 cm) will permit an arc of rotation which takes in the groin and suprapubic areas.

Anatomy

The descending branch gives off perforators to skin in the intermuscular septum between vastus lateralis and rectus femoris. The largest of these generally reaches the deep fascia at a point approximately 2 cm inferolateral to the mid-point of a line between the anterior superior iliac spine and the superolateral corner of the patella. If a fasciocutaneous perforator is not present in this area then it is likely that a musculocutaneous one will be. In either situation a blood supply from the descending branch of the LCFA to anterolateral thigh skin is assured, and even if the descending branch arises not from the LCFA, but directly from the profunda femoris or the femoral artery (a rare variation that is described on pages 236 and 237), then this vessel is still likely to give off a perforator. However, the occasional absence of a vessel has been

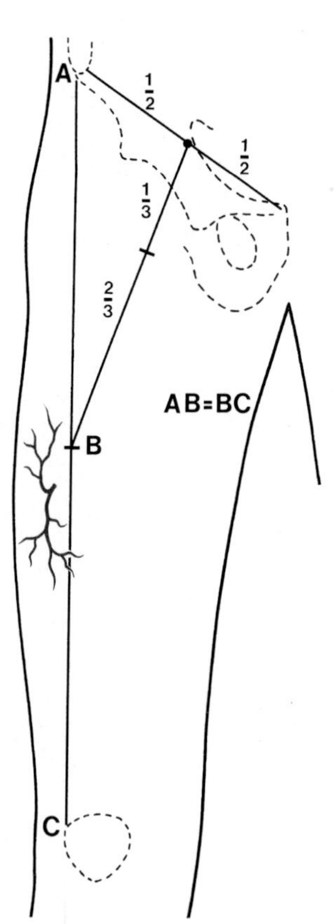

Fig. 7.139 Vascular anatomy. The surface marking of the usual position of the largest perforator is shown together with the surface marking of the descending branch pedicle.

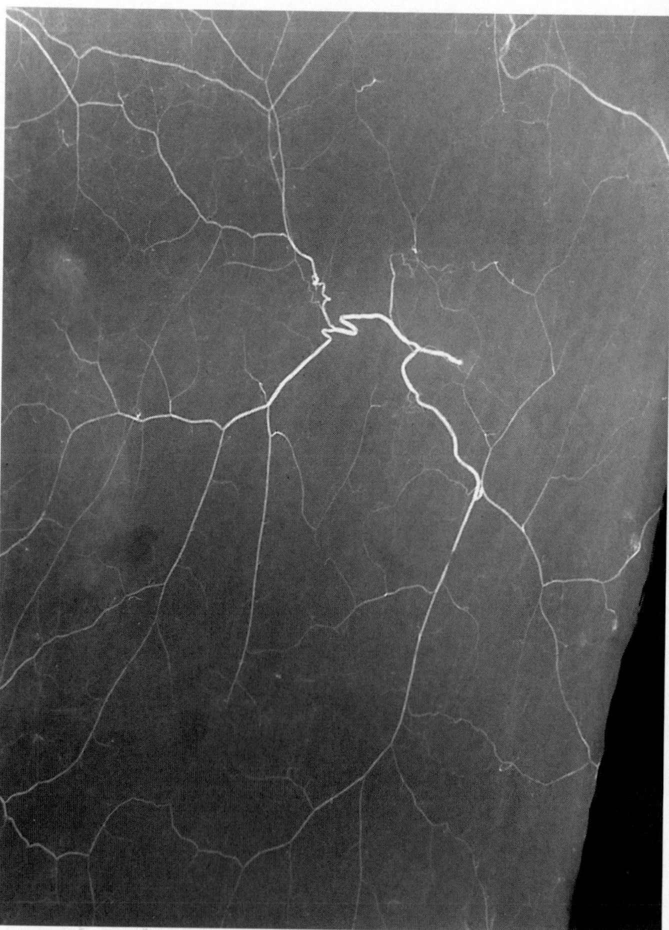

Fig. 7.140 Radiograph of perforator.

reported, although when this happened the surgeon was able to convert to an anteromedial flap without difficulty. Occasionally the descending branch may be in two parts running in parallel in the intermuscular septum. The branch lying in the superficial part of the septum is small and contributes little to the overlying skin and on seeing this the surgeon may be discouraged from further exploration, but in a deeper position than normal in the septum there will be a large branch with perforators through the anterior part of the muscle to the overlying skin.

Flap planning

A flap of maximum dimensions 15 cm × 30 cm may be planned centred on the point described above. The pedicle has a length of between 8 and 12 cm and a diameter of 2.1 ± 0.1 mm. Veins accompany the perforators but an additional large vein of 3 to 4 mm diameter will be encountered in the subcutaneous tissues draining the anterolateral thigh into the long saphenous vein over the femoral triangle. It is not recommended that this vessel be used as the sole means of draining a free flap. Survival is reliable when the venae comitantes of the descending branch are used.

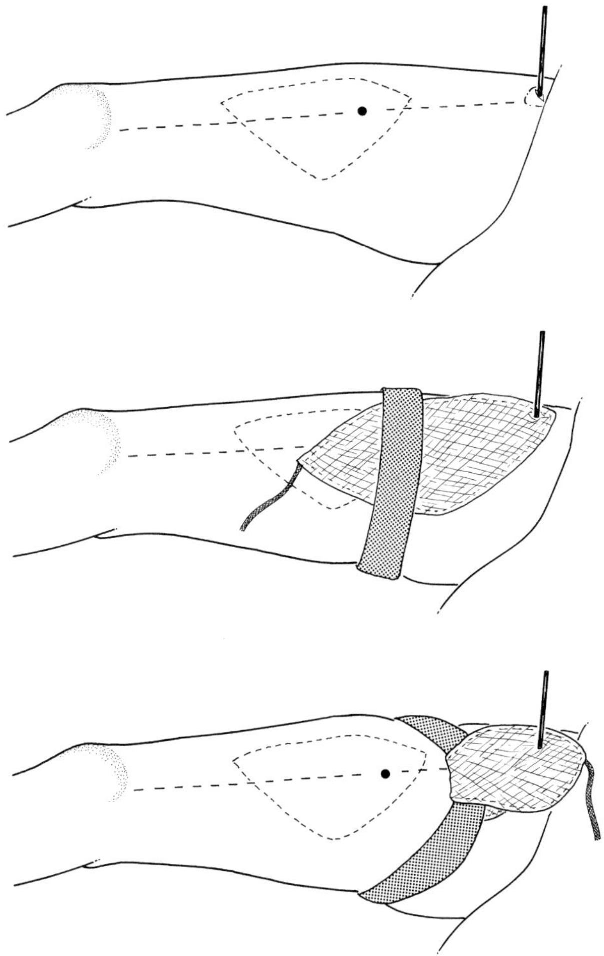

Fig. 7.141 Method of applying tourniquet for free flap elevation illustrated on lateral aspect of left thigh.

Flap elevation

The medial edge of the flap and deep fascia are incised first. The lateral cutaneous nerve of the thigh will be encountered and may be dissected free of the anterior margin of the flap (depending on the size of flap). Elevation is continued to expose the intermuscular septum between rectus femoris and vastus lateralis which is explored for the descending branch. The disposition of peforators is determined at this point and branches to muscle that are not passing through to supply the skin are ligated and divided. In the absence of septocutaneous perforators it will be necessary to preserve and dissect out perforators from the anterior 2 cm of vastus lateralis which pass through on their way to the skin. This requires division of intervening muscle fibres which will be found easier if a sterile Esmarch tourniquet has previously been applied to the thigh as shown in Figure 7.141. The posterior part of the flap can then be incised once the vascular supply to the flap is assured. The Esmarch tourniquet is then removed and the pedicle pursued proximally – this will require a vertical incision from the cephalic edge of the flap. Although the blood supply to vastus lateralis is not compromised by removal of the descending branch, it is important not to dissect out the descending branch above the point at which the blood supply to rectus femoris is given off. It is at about this level that the venae comitantes of the descending branch unite to form a single vein before joining with veins from rectus femoris. After repair of the muscle the donor site will almost certainly need to be grafted.

References

1. Xu Da-Chuan, Zhong Shi-zhen, Kong Ji-ming, Wang Guo-ying, Lui Mu-zhi, Luo Li-sheng, Gao Jian-hua 1988 Applied anatomy of the anterolateral femoral flap. Plastic and Reconstructive Surgery 82: 305–310
2. Song Y G, Chen G Z, Song Y L 1984 The free thigh flap: a new free flap concept based on the septocutaneous artery. British Journal of Plastic Surgery 37: 149–159
3. Koshima I, Fukuda H, Utunomiya R, Soeda S 1989 The anterolateral thigh flap; variations in its vascular pedicle. British Journal of Plastic Surgery 42: 260–262
4. Zhou G, Qiao Q, Chen G Y, Ling Y C, Swift R 1991 Clinical experience and surgical anatomy of 32 free anterolateral thigh flap transplantations. British Journal of Plastic Surgery 44: 91–96
5. Bégué T, Masquelet A C, Nordin J Y 1990 Anatomical basis of the anterolateral thigh flap. Surgical and Radiologic Anatomy 12: 311–313

7 LATERAL PLANTAR ARTERY

Calcaneal advancement flap
Flexor digitorum brevis musculocutaneous flap

The calcanceal branches of the lateral plantar artery have been used to support a local pedicled suprafascial flap for reconstructing ulcers on the heel. The lateral plantar artery itself may support both pedicled[1, 2] and island subfascial[3, 4] flaps from the sole – the latter include the flexor digitorum brevis muscle.

Anatomy

The posterior tibial artery consistently divides into its medial and lateral plantar branches at the posterior edge of the sustentaculum tali. The point of division may lie up to 1 cm proximal to this point, but rarely lies distal to it, and if so only by a couple of millimetres. The lateral plantar artery, at or just after its origin, gives off one or more calcaneal arteries which pierce flexor digitorum brevis and the plantar aponeurosis near their attachment to the medial tubercle of the calcaneus. These calcaneal branches then pass posteriorly and laterally over the inferior surface of the heel supplying the skin (Fig. 7.142). The lateral plantar artery continues in a distal direction at the same time passing across the foot lying in the plane between flexor digitorium brevis and flexor accessorius (supplying them both) until it reaches the lateral border of the plantar aponeurosis. Here it runs for a short distance parallel to the lateral border of the foot, gives off a branch to the lateral side of the fifth toe and then curves medially across the foot beneath the metatarsal shafts to form the deep plantar arch and anastomoses with the perforating branch of the dorsalis pedis artery in the first interosseous space.

Sensory innervation over the sole is provided by branches of the lateral plantar nerve in the lateral third and by branches of the medial plantar nerve over the medial two-thirds.

Flap elevation

Calcaneal flap

A defect over the posterior part of the heel may be covered by a rotation advancement flap based on the calcaneal branches of the lateral plantar artery.[1] The flap is outlined with the base centred on a point just distal to the medial tubercle of the calcaneus (Fig. 7.144). In order to gain additional mobility of a large flap for covering larger defects it may be necessary to enlarge the flap in a distal direction away from the heel. The flap is elevated by dissection directly on the surface of the bone up to the anterior border of the calcaneus where the calcaneal vessels are carefully preserved. With

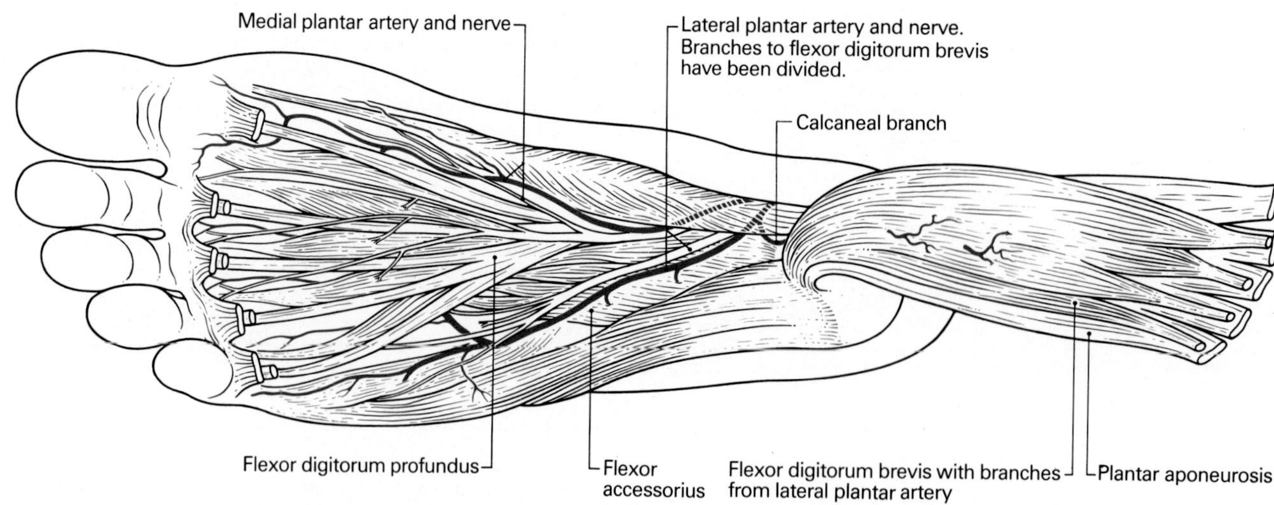

Fig. 7.142 Vascular anatomy. Flexor digitorum brevis has been reflected with the plantar aponeurosis in this schematic illustration to show the deep-lying position of the lateral plantar artery. Branches passing from the artery to FDB and the skin of the lateral and posterior parts of the sole have been divided.

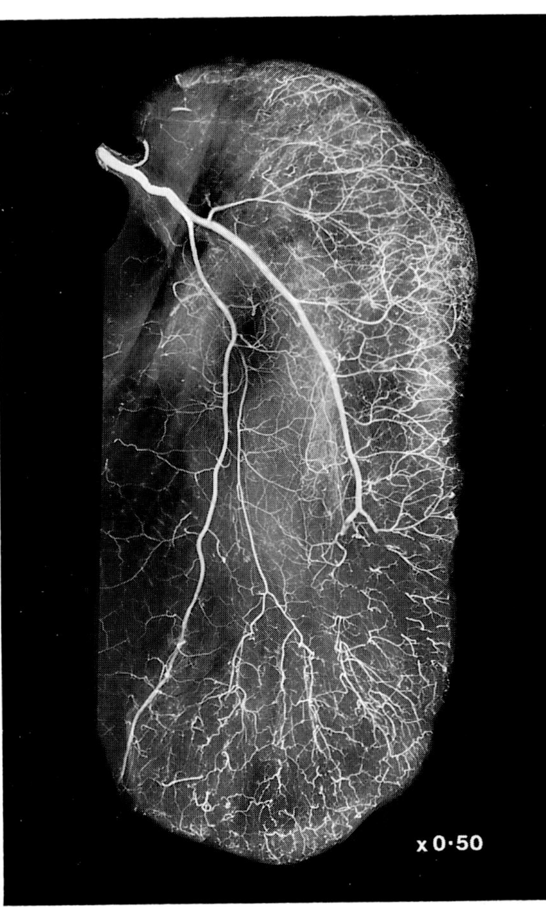

Fig. 7.143 Radiograph of sole skin including FDB and the plantar aponeurosis. (In creating this specimen the skin incision passed down the dorsal midline of the heel and then passed along the lateral margin of the weight-bearing surface of the heel and along the lateral border of the sole.)

an enlarged flap the dissection may proceed either superficial or deep to the plantar aponeurosis preserving the vessels – dissection deep to the plantar fascia after dividing its proximal attachment is easier. With rotation advancement, direct closure of small defects is possible.

Lateral plantar flap

For larger defects a larger flap with a smaller pedicle may be raised from the heel, lateral side of sole and non-weight-bearing midsole on the lateral plantar artery. An incision along the lateral side of the foot allows the plantar aponeurosis and flexor digitorum brevis to be divided proximally. Alternatively this may be carried out from the medial side.[3] Dissection beneath these structures in a medial direction will reveal perforating branches from the lateral plantar artery to the skin and these are followed down to their parent vessels. Deep muscular branches of the vessels are divided. The innervation of the toes may be preserved by longitudinally splitting off those branches which are going to the flap. The distal part of the lateral plantar artery, the plantar aponeurosis and flexor digitorum brevis are all divided at the distal skin incision which lies proximal to the weight-bearing area beneath the metatarsal heads. All these structures are removed with the flap. This incision then curves across the non-weight-bearing underside of the arch of the foot to the medial side of the heel leaving the medial plantar artery and nerve intact. Once sufficient mobility has been achieved, by division of fibrous connections to deeper structures, the flap may be rotated posteriorly. Split skin grafting of the midsole area will be necessary.

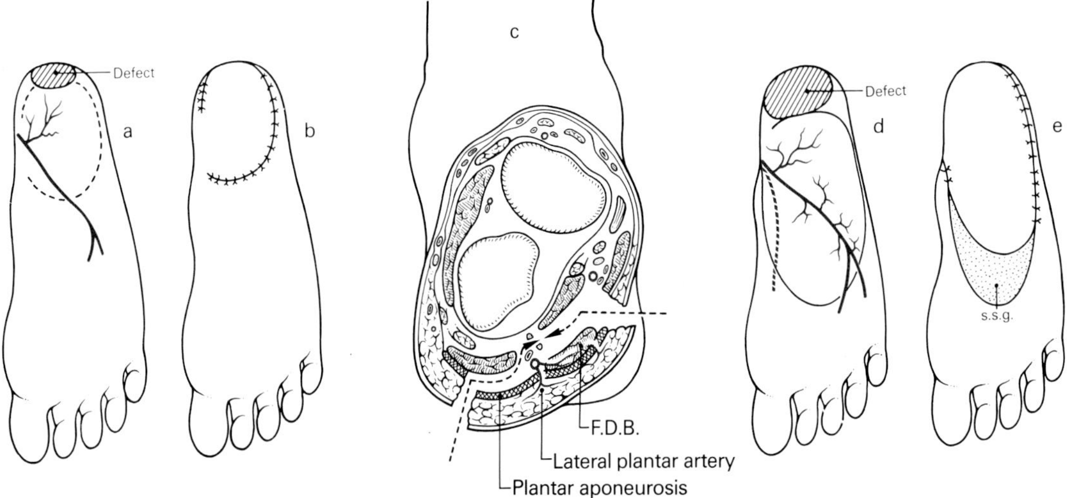

Fig. 7.144 Flap planning: **a–b** calcaneal flap; **c–e** flexor digitorum brevis musculocutaneous flap (**c.** is a vertical section through the plane of the talo-navicular and calcaneo-cuboid joints).

Combined medial and lateral plantar arteries

The flexor digitorum brevis musculocutaneous flap has also been used based on both of these vessels together.[4] Clearly it is essential to be certain of the patency and ability of the dorsalis pedis artery to supply the deep plantar arch through its perforating branch in the first interosseous space. The long-term effects on the blood supply to the distal foot are uncertain.

Retrograde lateral plantar flap

Reiffel et al[1] have described a retrograde lateral plantar flap which allowed distal advancement of a flap to cover an ulcer over the fourth and fifth metatarsal heads. The lateral plantar artery was divided proximally and received its blood supply through anastomoses of the deep arch.

References

1. Reiffel R S, McCarthy J G 1980 Coverage of heel and sole defects: A new subfascial arterialized flap. Plastic and Reconstructive Surgery 66: 250–260
2. McCarthy J G 1984 Subfascial arterialized sole of the foot flap. Plastic and Reconstructive Surgery 73: 691
3. Hartrampf C R, Scheflan M, Bostwick J 1980 The flexor digitorum brevis muscle island pedicle flap: a new dimension in heel reconstruction. Plastic and Reconstructive Surgery 66: 246–270
4. Ikuta Y, Murakami T, Yoshioka K, Tsuge K 1984 Reconstruction of the heel pad by flexor digitorum brevis musculocutaneous flap transfer. Plastic and Reconstructive Surgery 74: 86–94
5. Hidalgo D A, Shaw W W 1986 Anatomic basis of plantar flap design. Plastic and Reconstructive Surgery 78: 627–636
6. Shaw W W, Hidalgo D A 1986 Anatomic basis of plantar flap design: clinical applications. Plastic and Reconstructive Surgery 78: 637–649
7. Sakai S, Terayama I 1991 Modification of the island subcutaneous pedicle flap for the reconstruction of defects of the sole of the foot. British Journal of Plastic Surgery 44: 179–182

LATERAL THORACIC ARTERY
SUPERFICIAL THORACIC ARTERY

Lateral thoracic flap
External mammary flap

Several flaps have been described from the region of the lateral chest wall and axilla and have been variously called lateral thoracic, external mammary, thoracodorsal, axillary or thoracodorsal axillary flaps. They are broadly divisible into two groups. Firstly, there are those which are based on the lateral thoracic and superficial thoracic arteries – they are described here. Secondly there are those which are based on a cutaneous branch of the thoracodorsal artery – they are described on page 478. It is obviously also possible to have flaps which include both vessels, and flaps which include varying quantities of latissimus dorsi and its overlying skin based on the main stem of the thoracodorsal artery.

Anatomy

The variations in the origins of the superficial thoracic and lateral thoracic arteries have been described on page 162. The lateral thoracic artery arises from the axillary artery or one of its branches and follows the lateral border of pectoralis minor beneath the lateral edge of pectoralis major. Taylor & Daniel[1] were unable to identify this vessel in 3 out of 20 cadaver dissections and Harii et al[2] failed to find the vessel in 2 out of 11 clinical cases. When present, the artery descends no further than the fifth interspace and supplies pectoralis minor, pectoralis major and serratus anterior and gives off branches in the female which pass round the lateral border of pectoralis major to supply the breast. The artery may itself pierce the deep fascia to become cutaneous at about the level of the fourth interspace, or may give off cutaneous branches. These may communicate with the cutaneous branch of the thoracodorsal artery.

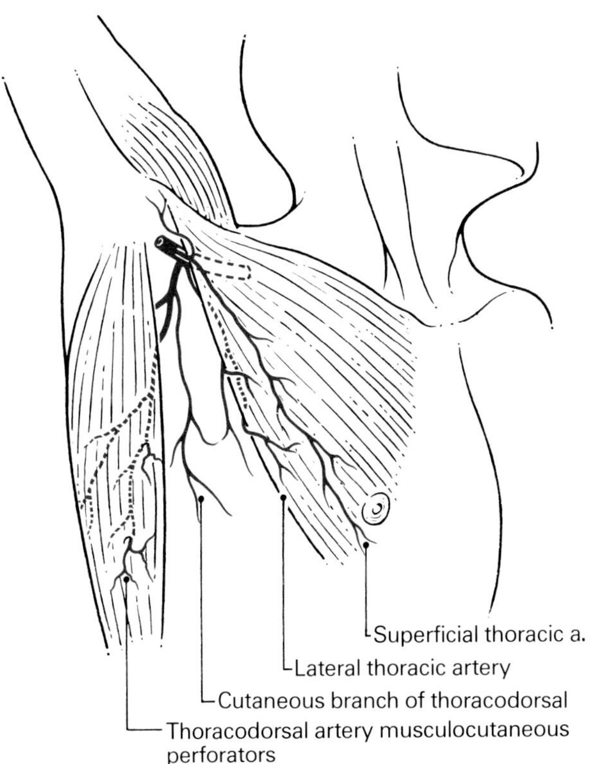

Fig. 7.145 Vascular anatomy. A schematic diagram in which all the possible vessels contributing to the lateral thoracic area are shown.

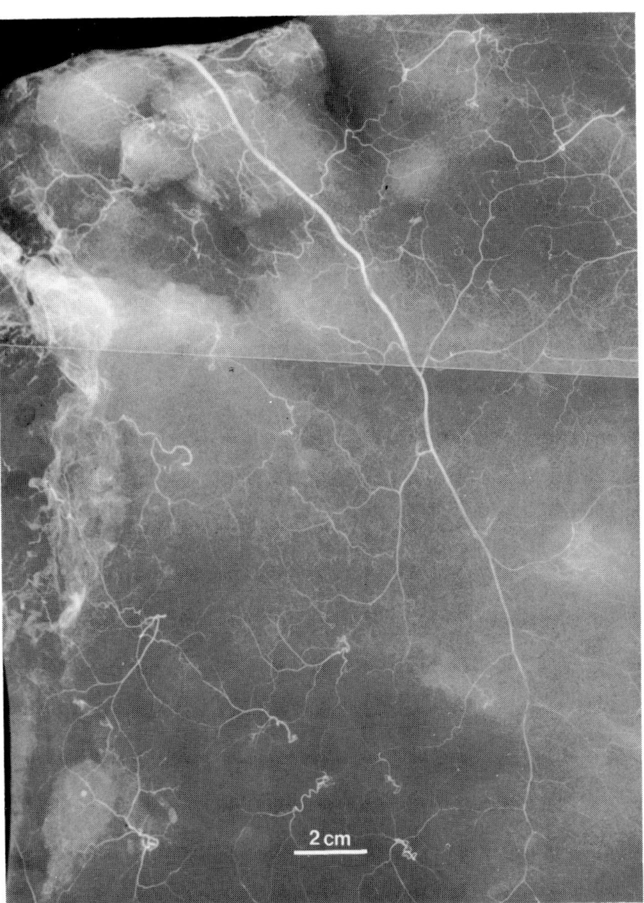

Fig. 7.146 Radiograph of skin showing a superficial thoracic artery.

The superficial thoracic artery is neglected in contemporary anatomy texts and is omitted from *Nomina Anatomica*. Adachi and Manchot both illustrated it and said it was commonly present but its prevalence has not been accurately documented. It has also been named the accessory lateral thoracic artery[3] but its course is different from that of the lateral thoracic in that it is a direct cutaneous artery exclusively supplying the superficial tissues and lies on top of the lateral part of pectoralis major. It often extends down to the fifth and sixth interspace. It originates directly from the anterior surface of the axillary or the brachial artery within 4 cm of the lower border of the tendon of insertion of pectoralis major and, according to Harii, has a diameter of 1.2–1.5 mm but we have come across examples with internal diameters in excess of 1.5 mm in male subjects (e.g. Fig. 7.146). Harii also described this artery as giving off a branch to the inner aspect of the upper arm and found that dye injected into the vessel stained an area centred on the axillary hair region which included the upper lateral quadrant of the breast and part of the inner side of the upper arm (Fig. 7.145). The vein accompanying the artery flows into the axillary vein.

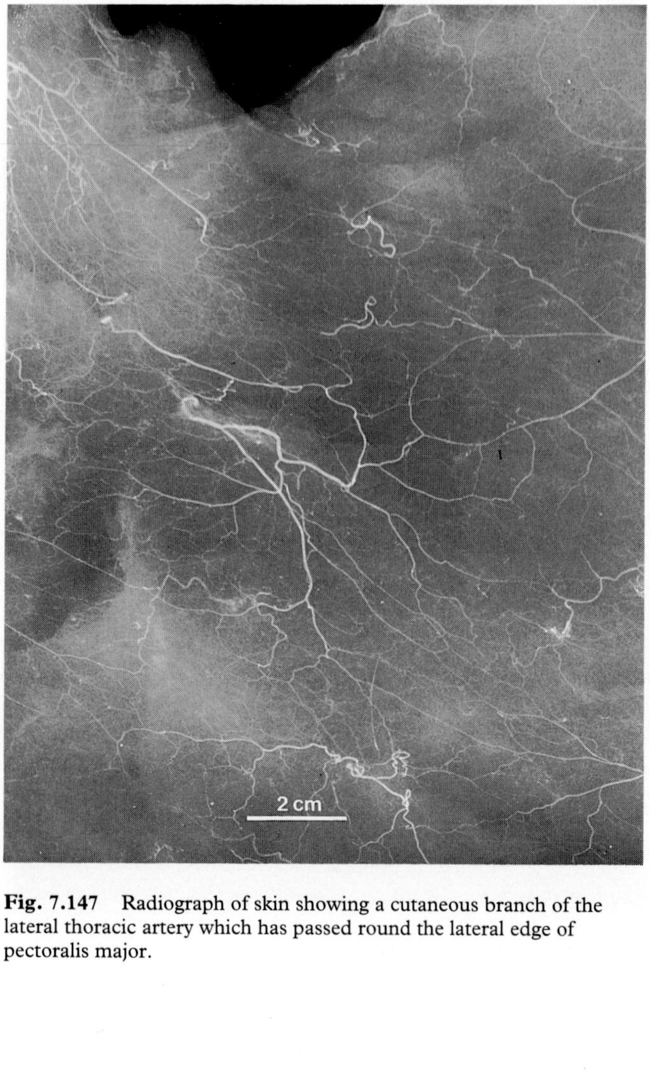

Fig. 7.147 Radiograph of skin showing a cutaneous branch of the lateral thoracic artery which has passed round the lateral edge of pectoralis major.

Free flap elevation

The vessels have been used to support free flaps.[2, 4, 5, 6] Since the arrangement of the arteries in the trapezoidal area bounded by the axillary artery, the lateral borders of latissimus dorsi and pectoralis major, and the seventh rib is so variable the exact outlines of a flap cannot be planned in advance. The first stage therefore is to abduct the arm and incise the skin overlying the pulsating path of the axillary artery. The axillary artery is dissected out and the various branches which could possibly support a flap are exposed. The flap is then developed so as to take advantage of the largest of those supplying an adequate area of skin.

If the lateral thoracic artery is chosen, the pedicle will have to be dissected from beneath pectoralis major and muscle branches ligated. No such problems accompany dissection of the superficial thoracic artery. The epimysium is dissected off the muscle and retained on the undersurface of the flap.

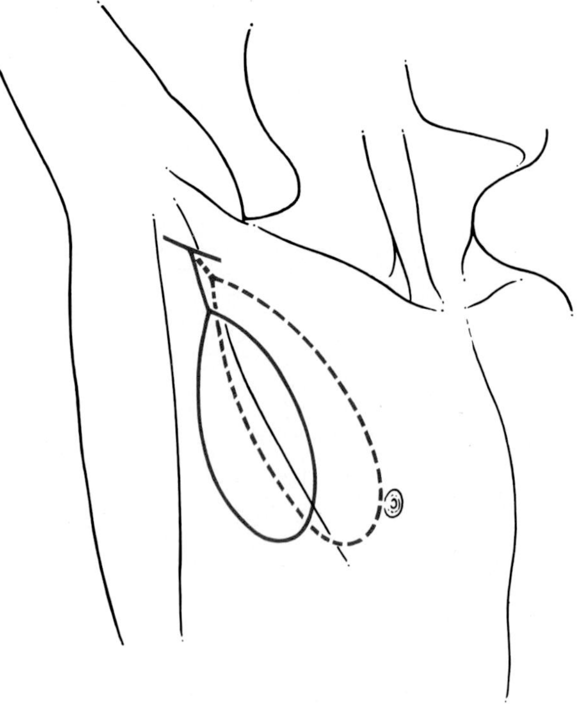

Fig. 7.148 Flap planning. Approximate outlines are shown for flaps based on cutaneous branches of the lateral thoracic artery (continuous line), and on the superficial thoracic artery (broken line).

Pedicled flap elevation

A pedicled flap from the lateral chest wall has been described and termed the lateral thoracic region flap.[7] The incorporation of the word 'region' indicates that this flap is based on more than just the lateral thoracic artery. Branches of any of the vessels shown in Figure 7.145 may be included but due to variability of these vessels not all will be present at the same time. There may also be a supply from the acromio-thoracic axis via its pectoral branch which sends terminal branches around the lateral border of pectoralis major to the skin and which also anastomoses with the lateral thoracic artery. The outlines of such a flap are shown in Figure 7.149.

The surface marking of the anterior border of the flap commences at the 3rd intercostal space and follows a line dropped vertically downwards from the coracoid process, crossing the infero-lateral border of the pectoralis major and running over the serratus anterior and external oblique muscles to a point not more than 3 cm below the costal margin. The posterior incision starts at the same level, i.e. 3rd interspace, at a point 2 cm medial to the lateral border of latissimus dorsi and passes vertically downwards crossing the infero-lateral border of the muscle and extends to not more than 3 cm below the costal margin. The anterior and posterior margins may be joined by a curve such that the end of the flap lies 4–6 cm below the costal margin in the mid-axillary line.

In elevating the flap particular attention is paid to taking the fascia and vessels for up to 1 cm from beneath the infero-lateral border of pectoralis major. Perforators from the intercostal vessels require ligation but otherwise the elevation is straightforward.

Extensive undermining of the skin over the anterior and posterior chest walls will enable direct closure of the donor site defect in some cases (e.g. pedicled transfer to upper limb). The deforming effect on the female breast is likely to make this unacceptable in some cases however.

A smaller pedicled flap, termed the subaxillary flap, has also been standardised by these authors[8] for pedicled reconstruction of the opposite hand. This is based on a single vessel and measures up to 7 cm × 20 cm.

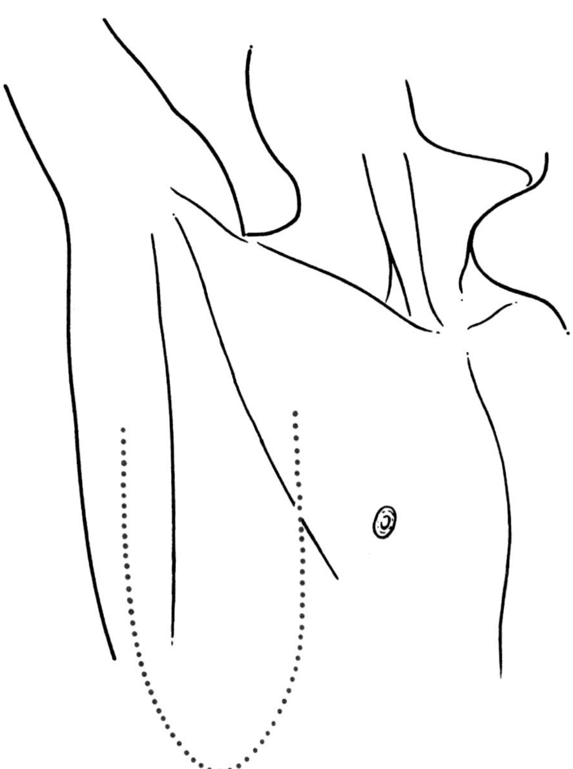

Fig. 7.149 Pedicled flap planning. The outlines of a possible flap are shown. The surface markings are described in the text.

References

1. Taylor G I, Daniel R K 1975 The anatomy of several free flap donor sites. Plastic and Reconstructive Surgery 56: 243–253
2. Harii I, Torii S, Sekiguchi J 1978 The free lateral thoracic flap. Plastic and Reconstructive Surgery 62: 212–222
3. Anson B J, Wright R R, Wolfer J A 1939 Blood supply of the mammary gland. Surgery, Gynaecology and Obstetrics 69: 468–473
4. Ricbourg B, Lassau J P, Violette A-M, Merland J J 1975 A propos de l'artère mammaire externe. Origine, territoire et intérêt pour les transplants cutanés libres. Archives d'Anatomie Pathologique 23: 317–322
5. Ricbourg B 1975 Un nouveau site donneur pour transplant cutané: le territoire mammaire externe. Lettre d'information du Groupe d'Advancement pour la Microchirurgie 2: 1–9
6. Coninck A de, Vanderlinden E, Boeckx W 1976 The thoracodorsal skin flap: A possible donor site in distant transfer of island flaps by microvascular anastomosis. Chirurgia Plastica 3: 283–291
7. Bhattacharya S, Bhagia S P, Bhatnagar S K, Chandra R 1990 The lateral thoracic region flap. British Journal of Plastic Surgery 43: 162–168
8. Chandra R, Kumar P, Abdi S H M 1988 The subaxillary pedicled flap. British Journal of Plastic Surgery 41: 169–173

7

MEDIAL PLANTAR ARTERY

Medial plantar flap – proximally based
– distally based
– free flap
– cutaneous branch variant

As originally described,[1,2] this flap included the abductor hallucis muscle because this was thought to be the principal source of blood supply to the skin over the midsole. In fact cutaneous branches of the medial plantar artery pass in the fascia round the muscle to appear at its superior and inferior borders. This has enabled the same area of midsole skin to be raised as a fasciocutaneous flap without the muscle, based only on the cutaneous branches emerging between abductor hallucis and flexor digitorum brevis.[3,4] This modification confers two advantages: firstly, it lessens the functional and cosmetic deformity at the donor site; and secondly, it removes a wad of tissue from beneath the flap which can otherwise result in mobility of the skin and a feeling of instability when it is transferred to a weight-bearing area.

Anatomy

Irrespective of whether the flap is raised with or without abductor hallucis, it is this muscle which provides the key to the anatomy. Abductor hallucis arises from the medial tubercle of the calcaneus, the adjacent plantar aponeurosis and the distal part of the flexor retinaculum. Between calcaneal and retinacular origins it forms a tendinous arch through which the plantar neurovascular bundles run. It lies on flexor hallucis brevis, becomes tendinous about half-way along the foot and gains insertion into the medial sesamoid and medial tubercle on the base of the proximal phalanx. The calcaneal branches of the posterior tibial artery supply its origin, and the medial plantar artery which comes to lie between it and flexor digitorum brevis supplies its belly. The medial plantar artery sends branches to the skin both above and below abductor hallucis, principally the latter.

The second important anatomical point concerns the location of the spot where the posterior tibial artery and the tibial nerve divide into their plantar branches. Several anatomical studies have found this point to be consistently related to the posterior edge of the sustentaculum tali with little variation. The point of division may lie up to 1 cm proximal to this point, but rarely lies distal to it, and if so only by a couple of millimetres. The division of the tibial nerve into its medial and lateral branches lies proximal to the division

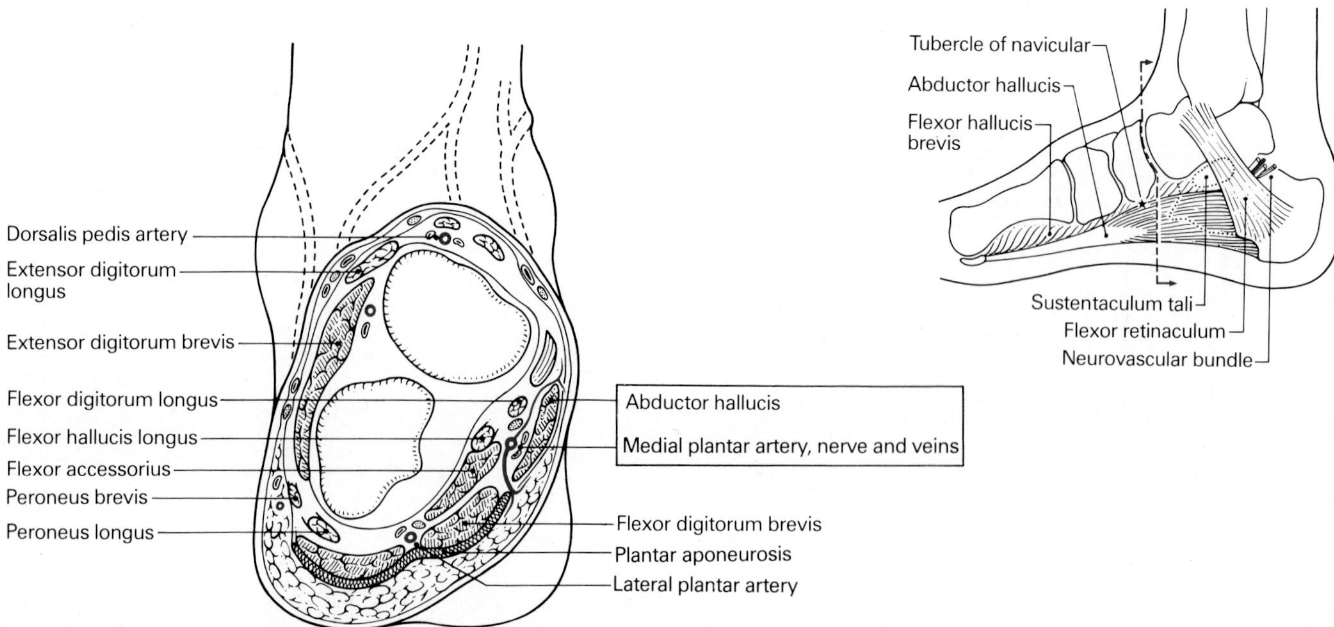

Fig. 7.150 Vascular anatomy. Diagram shows section through the tarsus along Chopart's line (see inset top right). The relationship of the medial plantar neurovascular bundle to abductor hallucis and the medial edge of the plantar aponeurosis can be seen.

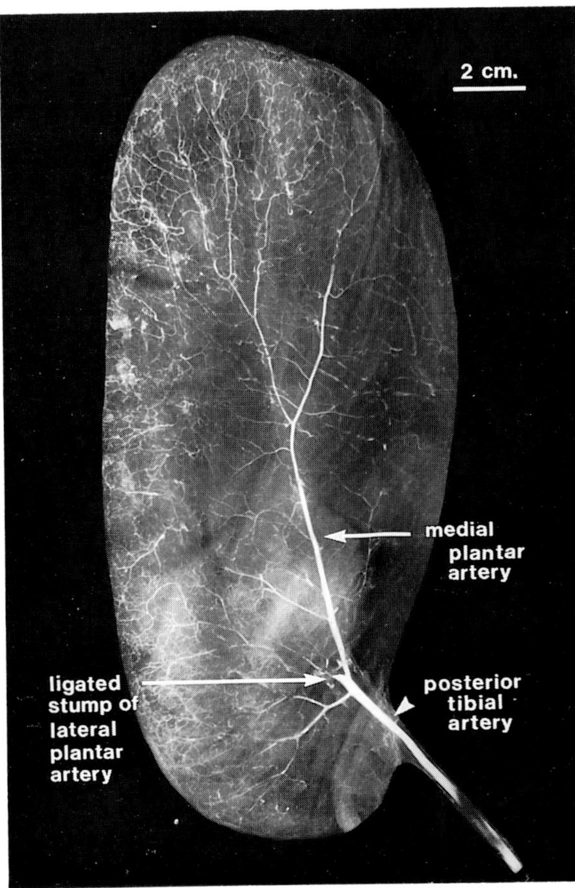

Fig. 7.151 Radiograph of sole skin.

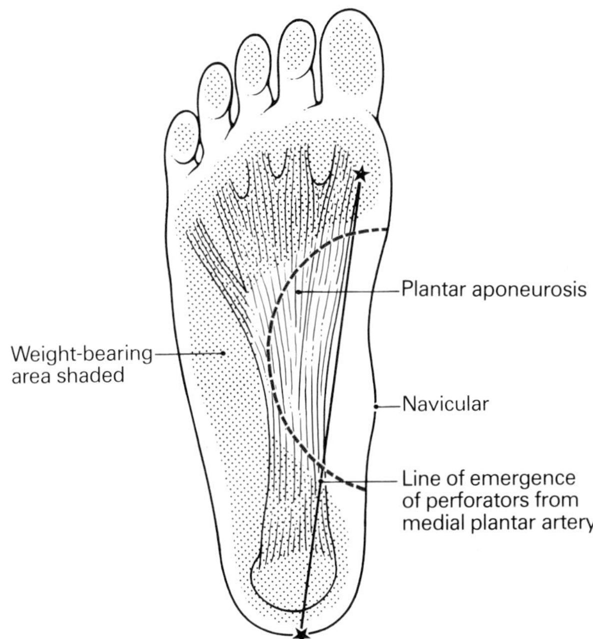

Fig. 7.152 Flap planning. The flap is raised from the non-weight-bearing area of the underside of the medial longitudinal arch. The medial edge of the plantar aponeurosis – corresponding to a line between the head of the first metatarsal and the centre of the heel – indicates the area where the perforators emerge.

of the artery in 90% of cases. The medial plantar artery lies lateral to its accompanying nerve in ~80% of cases.

Venous drainage of the area is by two communicating sets of veins; a superficial network visible through the skin which drains into the great saphenous vein and a deeper system which drains via venae comitantes of the medial plantar artery. Venous drainage through the deep system alone is sufficient to allow the flap to be made into an island or used as a free flap with anastomosis of the venae comitantes.

Sensory innervation of the medial two-thirds of the sole is from the medial plantar nerve and innervation of the lateral third from the lateral plantar nerve.

Flap planning

In planning the flap, the weight-bearing areas are avoided and the flap should not extend above the tuberosity of the navicular. A proximal incision up to the posterior edge of the sustentaculum tali is required for dissection of the pedicle. The lateral edge of abductor hallucis marks the line along which the perforators emerge and over which the flap is centred. It can be approximately marked out on the surface by a line drawn between the centre of the heel posteriorly and the medial sesamoid of the great toe (Fig. 7.152). This also corresponds to the medial edge of the plantar aponeurosis which can be brought into prominence by passively dorsiflexing the great toe and thereby putting the medial part of the plantar aponeurosis under tension. With this manoeuvre the edge can be palpated and often springs into view. Flaps may be raised with dimensions of up to 10 cm length × 7 cm width.

Flap elevation – proximally based

The flap is elevated from distal to proximal in a plane superficial to abductor hallucis so as to include the plantar fascia. The septum between abductor hallucis and flexor digitorum brevis containing the medial plantar artery and its fasciocutaneous perforators is removed in continuity with the flap. The distal branches of the medial plantar artery are divided. Using magnification, the cutaneous branches innervating the flap can be dissected from the main stem of the medial plantar nerve and stripped proximally. Alternatively, if one of the plantar digital nerves is the predominant source of cutaneous nerve filaments to the flap then the digital nerve may be divided distally and elevated with the flap (this saves the difficulty of splitting off nerve fibres, ensures the integrity of the cutaneous filaments, and allows easier neurorrhaphy at the recipient site).

As the neurovascular structures are followed proximally they pass beneath abductor hallucis and it is necessary to divide the origin of the muscle in order to mobilise the pedicle all the way up to the point where the posterior tibial artery divides. This gives an arc of rotation which allows the flap to be brought over the weight-bearing surface of the heel. Although not primarily intended for reconstructing the area on the back of the heel over the insertion of the Achilles tendon this has been achieved through further increasing the mobility of the flap by dividing the lateral plantar artery (having established that the perforating dorsalis pedis is able to send blood through into the sole of the foot). Mobilisation of the distal posterior tibial artery enables the flap to reach the Achilles tendon or the lower anterior tibia. When this more extensive mobilisation is carried out,[4] no attempt should be made to retain cutaneous innervation to the flap from the medial plantar nerve since an interfascicular dissection over this distance is impractical.

When it is intended to use this flap as a free flap then the neurovascular bundle is divided just distal to the point of division of the tibial artery. A modification of this flap is one raised on both the medial and lateral plantar arteries – see lateral plantar artery (p. 368).

Miyamoto et al have made a study of the sensory disturbances in the forefoot resulting from elevation of this flap.[5]

Flap elevation – distally based

The same medial plantar flap can also be raised on a distal pedicle for forefoot defect reconstruction.[6, 7] In this design the flap will clearly be without innervation and the flap is dependent for its blood supply on the distal anastomoses of the medial plantar artery branches with the distal plantar arch branches supplied by the lateral plantar artery and also by the penetrating branch through the first interosseous space from the dorsalis pedis artery. The skin island is placed proximally in the donor area and flap elevation commences at the posterior margin of the skin island. The medial and lateral borders of the flap are then incised and elevated with the medial plantar artery. The presence of retrograde flow into the medial plantar artery is checked before this is finally divided and the elevation of the anterior margin of the flap completed.

Flap variant on cutaneous branch

All of the foregoing flaps are based on the branches of the medial plantar artery which emerge around the lateral and inferior border of abductor hallucis. However, as shown in Fig. 7.150, there are also branches of the medial plantar artery emerging above the supero-medial border of the muscle. A small number of surgeons have demonstrated that these branches alone may also support a flap, albeit rather smaller in size than the classical flap.[8] Terminology for these branches has not been formalised but the usual arrangement is that shortly after its origin the medial plantar artery gives off a deep branch that passes deeply close to the navicular to join the deep arch. This deep vessel is not available for a flap but in approximately two-thirds of cases it gives off a 'cutaneous' branch that runs more superficially beneath the upper edge of abductor hallucis giving off branches to skin. Alternatively this vessel may arise directly from the medial plantar artery rather than from its deep branch (approximately one-third of cases). Irrespective of origin this vessel appears to have a constant course crossing the terminal part of the tibialis posterior tendon to lie on the navicular and medial cuneiform. It generally extends as far as the mid-shaft of the first metatarsal but may be a large vessel going on to replace the first plantar metatarsal artery. Mobilising a flap on this vessel requires division of the deep branch of the medial plantar artery, and division of the main part of the medial plantar artery – either distal to the origin of the cutaneous branch for a proximally-based flap, or proximal to the origin of the cutaneous branch for a distally-based flap. The principal advantage of this flap is that the abductor hallucis muscle does not have to be divided but there is no potential for making this a sensate flap.

References

1. Shanahan R E, Gingrass R P 1979 Medial plantar sensory flap for coverage of heel defects. Plastic and Reconstructive Surgery 64: 295–298
2. Harrison D H, Morgan B D G 1981 The instep island flap to resurface plantar defects. British Journal of Plastic Surgery 34: 315–318
3. Morrison W A, Crabb D McK, O'Brien B McC, Jenkins A 1983 The instep of the foot as a fasciocutaneous island and as a free flap for heel defects. Plastic and Reconstructive Surgery 72: 56–63
4. Baker G L, Newton E D, Franklin J D 1990 Fasciocutaneous island flap based on the medial plantar artery: clinical applications for leg, ankle and forefoot. Plastic and Reconstructive Surgery 85: 47–58
5. Miyamoto Y, Ikuta Y, Shigeki S, Yamura M 1987 Current concepts of instep island flap. Annals of Plastic Surgery 19: 97–102
6. Amarante J, Martins A, Reis J 1988 A distally based medial plantar flap. Annals of Plastic Surgery 20: 468–470
7. Masquelet A C, Penteado C V, Romana M C, Chevrel 1988 The distal anastomoses of the medial plantar artery: surgical aspects. Surgical and Radiologic Anatomy 10: 247–252
8. Romana M C, Masquelet A C 1989 Vascularization of the inner border of the foot: surgical applications. Surgical and Radiologic Anatomy 11: 177–178

MIDDLE COLLATERAL ARTERY

Lateral arm flap

A Type C fasciocutaneous flap based on the middle collateral artery, similar in principle to the radial artery (Chinese) forearm flap, may be raised from the outer aspect of the upper arm. This has been described by the authors[1, 2] and by Katsaros et al.[3] A similar flap has been based on the radial collateral artery and has been described by Song.[4] This is not described here because we have studied the middle collateral artery and found it to be the more consistent of the two. By contrast, the anatomy of the radial collateral artery is less well documented and the artery is in any case more complex in its relations.

Anatomy

The middle collateral artery is one of the two terminal divisions of the profunda brachii. It passes down on the lateral intermuscular septum posterior to brachioradialis. (Note that there is confusion in the plastic surgery literature concerning the nomenclature of this vessel.) The other terminal branch is the radial collateral artery which accompanies the radial nerve in the septum anterior to brachioradialis. The exact point of division of the profunda brachii artery varies but the surgically accessible length does not extend more than 6 or 7 cm above the level of the deltoid insertion. The vessel supplies skin by four or five fasciocutaneous perforators along the lateral intermuscular septum from the lower edge of the deltoid downwards with the uppermost of these branches generally being the largest.

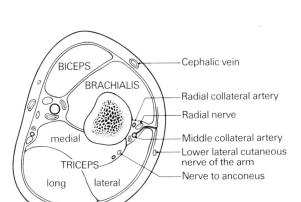

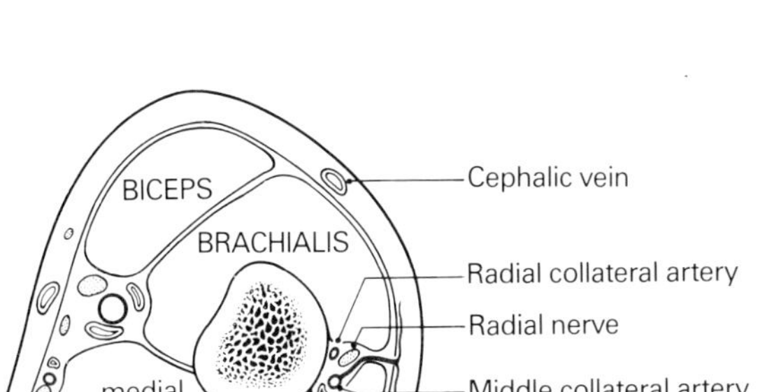

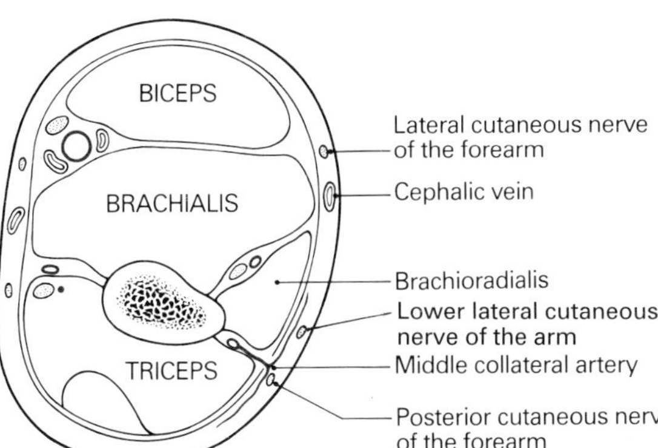

Fig. 7.153 Schematic transverse sections through the upper arm at mid-shaft and lower third levels showing the location of the vessel in the lateral intermuscular septum.

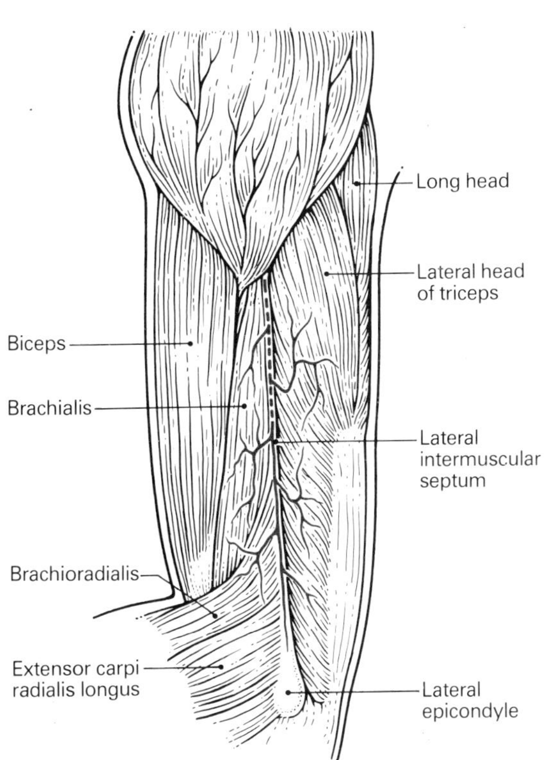

Fig. 7.154 View of lateral aspect of the upper arm showing the branches of the middle collateral artery. The flap directly overlies this area.

From this level the middle collateral artery travels downwards on the septum for between 7 and 13 cm before penetrating the deep fascia. If the deep fascia is reached at an early stage then the artery continues on downwards lying on it although it usually lies deeply on the septum and may extend distally beyond the lateral epicondyle. The fasciocutaneous perforators fan out at the level of the deep fascia in anterior and posterior directions with a distal inclination. At its upper end the middle collateral artery measures ~1.5 mm ID (range 0.9–2.4).

The artery is accompanied by a vena comitans and the cephalic vein passes through the anterior part of the artery's territory. The flap is innervated by the lower lateral cutaneous nerve of the arm which passes round the humerus in the radial groove, pierces the lateral head of triceps and runs near the cephalic vein to the skin of the lower lateral part of the upper arm. The flap therefore has the capability for enabling a neurosensory reconstruction to be carried out. The posterior cutaneous nerve of the forearm passes through the lower part of the lateral intermuscular septum and can complicate the dissection. It supplies skin down to the wrist but its territory is partly overlapped by other nerves so that its division leaves a permanently anaesthetic area confined to the posterolateral upper third of the forearm.

Territory

The axis of the flap lies on the lateral intermuscular septum and extends from the deltoid insertion downwards for 10–12 cm. The nearer the flap approaches the lateral epicondyle the greater will be the likelihood of the posterior cutaneous nerve of the forearm running into the flap. The flap may extend both anteriorly and posteriorly for up to 6 cm. It may incorporate in its anterior part the cephalic vein which generally lies 4 to 5 cm anterior to the lateral intermuscular septum. However, if direct closure of the donor site is required then the maximum width of the flap measures 6 cm.

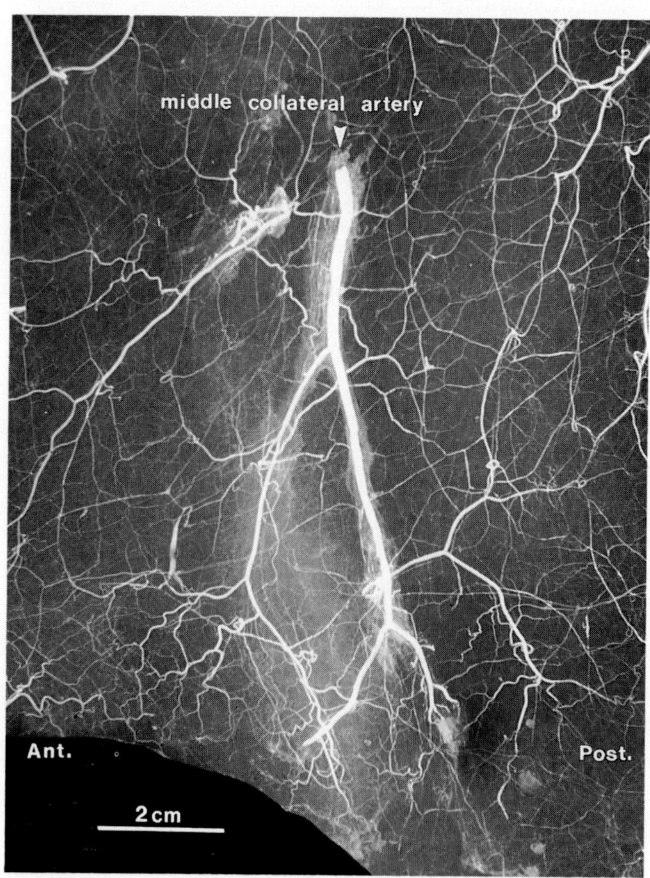

Fig. 7.155 Radiograph of skin and deep fascia including the fascial septum containing the middle collateral artery which has *not* been dissected out from above the level of the deltoid insertion.

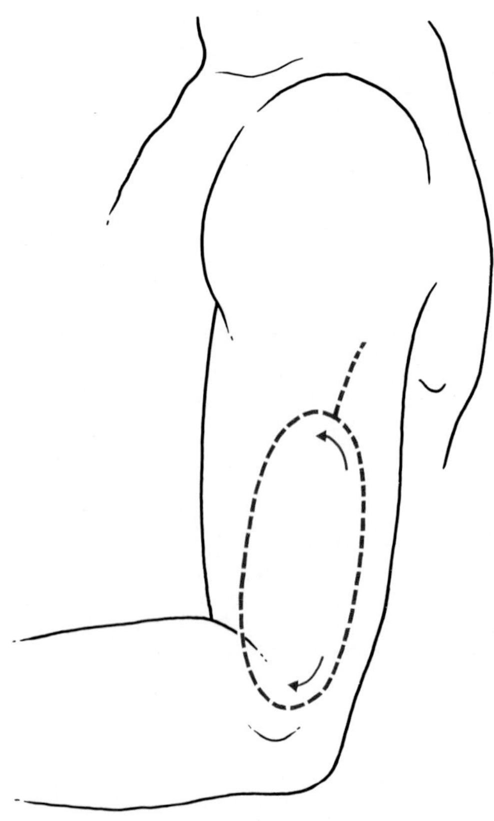

Fig. 7.156 Flap planning. Approximate outline of a possible flap is shown.

Flap elevation

The essential point is that the flap is raised to include the deep fascia over biceps and triceps, in addition to the lateral intermuscular septum which must be freed where brachioradialis arises from it. All borders of the flap can be marked out prior to elevation and a short incision extending upwards along the posterior edge of deltoid facilitates dissection of the pedicle. The margins are incised and the elevation off biceps and triceps proceeds from the posterior margin and then the anterior margin up to the lateral intermuscular septum. The cephalic vein, if lying within the territory of the flap, is divided during this stage. At the proximal end of the flap the pedicle is then developed by opening the plane between the deltoid insertion and triceps to find the middle collateral artery and veins. To do this, fibres of the medial head of triceps are separated from the posterior aspect of the lateral intermuscular septum and small vessels running to the muscle are divided. Once ligated as high and deep as possible or desirable the pedicle is drawn laterally and freed from its medial attachments by dividing the lateral intermuscular septum medial to the vessel. A 2 or 3 mm cuff of muscle may be preserved on the lateral intermuscular septum to protect the vessels and small muscular branches require ligation. The artery will be found to be approaching the deep fascia until finally it may pierce it. From this point to the inferior end of the flap the dissection is simpler although the posterior cutaneous nerve of the forearm may have to be dissected out by division of the deep fascia.

If dissection of the pedicle from beneath a large deltoid with a tight posterior margin is difficult and is preventing an adequate length from being mobilised, then a posterior approach to the profunda brachii artery may be useful. The incision is carried round to the posterior midline, where it is deepened by splitting the lateral and long heads of triceps to reveal the radial nerve crossing the deep head of the triceps. The profunda artery lies lateral and deep to the nerve and by this approach the pedicle may be pursued up to the lower border of teres major.

In many cases the donor site can be closed directly.

Flap variants

Katsaros et al[3] have shown that an osteo-myo-fasciocutaneous composite tissue transfer may be created by incorporating with the skin element a segment of the lateral supracondylar ridge and shaft of the humerus measuring up to 10 cm × 1 cm. For the bone segment to receive a blood supply from the middle collateral artery it is necessary to include a portion of the brachioradialis in front of the septum and a portion of the medial head of triceps from behind the septum. (The radial nerve must be retracted well away during the osteotomy to prevent injury.)[5]

Katsaros et al have also shown that a strip of the triceps tendon may be removed with the flap. There is potential application for this modification in the reconstruction of defects of the dorsum of the hand where skin and extensor tendons have been lost.

Yousif et al[6] have demonstrated the use of the fascia only flap which may be particularly applicable to the reconstruction of defects on the dorsum of the hand where a split skin graft onto the fascia provides acceptable durability without the bulk of a skin flap.

Matloub et al[7] have described the innervated flap which incorporates the lower lateral cutaneous nerve of the arm.

A distally pedicled version of the flap based on the interosseous recurrent artery has been described (p. 353) but is not as reliable as the reverse pedicled lateral arm flap based on the radial recurrent artery which is larger and has better anastomoses with the radial collateral artery (p. 201).

References

1. Lamberty B G H, Cormack G C Fasciocutaneous vessels. Winning essay in 1983 Scholarship Awards of the Plastic Surgery Educational Foundation. Presented at ASPRS, Dallas, Nov. 1983
2. Cormack G C, Lamberty B G H 1984 Fasciocutaneous vessels in the upper arm – application to the design of new fasciocutaneous flaps. Plastic and Reconstructive Surgery 74: 244–249
3. Katsaros J, Schusterman M, Beppu M, Banis J C, Acland R D 1984 The lateral upper arm flap: Anatomy and clinical applications. Annals of Plastic Surgery 12: 489–500
4. Song R, Song Y, Yu Y, Song Y 1982 The upper arm free flap. Clinics in Plastic Surgery 9: 27–35
5. Scheker L R, Kleinert H E, Hanel D P 1987 Lateral arm composite tissue transfer to ipsilateral hand defects. The Journal of Hand Surgery 12A: 665–672
6. Yousif N J, Warren R, Matloub H S, Sanger J R 1990 The lateral arm fascial free flap: its anatomy and use in reconstruction. Plastic and Reconstructive Surgery 86: 1138–1145
7. Matloub H S, Sanger J R, Godina M 1983 The lateral arm flap. A neurosensory free flap. In: Transactions of the 8th International Congress of Plastic Surgery, p 126
8. Katsaros J, Tan E, Zoltie N, Barton M, Venugopalsrinivasan, Venkataramakrishnan 1991 Further experience with the lateral arm free flap. Plastic and Reconstructive Surgery 87: 902–910

7 **OCCIPITAL ARTERY**

Sternocleidomastoid musculocutaneous flap

In 1955 Owens[1] described the use of the sternomastoid muscle to carry neck skin for the repair of cheek defects, and Bakamjian[2] later suggested this flap for the repair of palatal defects. These, and an extensive series reported by Littlewood,[3] were similar in that the flaps were really pedicled skin flaps augmented by muscle.

O'Brien[4] described a single case in which he had carried a 'paddle' of skin situated over the lower end of the muscle and pedicled about the superior attachment, and Ariyan did much to publicise this method.[5, 6]

Anatomy

The sternocleidomastoid muscle has three principal arterial pedicles and a number of minor ones (Fig. 7.157).

The *superior pedicle* is a branch given off in about 70% of cases by the occipital artery within 1 cm of its point of origin from the external carotid (in 20% this branch arises directly from the external carotid). It measures about 2.5 mm in diameter and varies between 3 and 4 cm in length; the hypoglossal nerve hooks round it. It inclines posteriorly, laterally and downwards giving off branches to lymph nodes and enters sternocleidomastoid about 1.5–2 cm back from the anterior edge of the muscle. It generally runs with or just below the accessory nerve, and is accompanied by two veins, thereby constituting the principal neurovascular pedicle of the muscle. As a rough guide the surface marking of the point of entry into the muscle lies some two fingers' breadths below the mastoid process. In the muscle it divides into two or three branches with the upper branch being short and the lower extending some way distally.

The *middle pedicle* is formed by a branch of the superior thyroid artery and measures 0.3–1.5 mm in diameter with a length of 4–6 cm. It passes vertically downwards and then curves laterally across the anterior surface of the common carotid artery and the internal jugular vein. Before entering the muscle it usually divides into two or more branches which form into ascending and descending groups. The ascending group enters the middle third of the muscle; the descending group enters at the junction of middle and lower thirds. Small branches are given off to lymph nodes and to some of the infrahyoid strap muscles. An accompanying vein may drain into the internal jugular.

The *inferior pedicle* arises from the suprascapular artery or from the transverse cervical but it is very inconstant. It crosses the deep surface of the clavicular head of sternocleidomastoid giving it two or three branches, and reaches the sternal head where it divides into terminal twigs. It often gives off a cutaneous branch through the clavicular head of the muscle which supplies skin over and below the medial end of the clavicle.

There is obviously a reciprocal relationship between these three pedicles so that all three are never well developed in the same individual, but in general the superior and middle pedicles share the supply of most of the muscle, with the inferior pedicle serving only a small part at the lower end. Figure 7.158 demonstrates the degree of intramuscular anastomosis between the separate pedicles.

Accessory pedicles arise from the posterior auricular artery (two or three branches to superficial and deep surfaces), from the occipital (note that the occipital

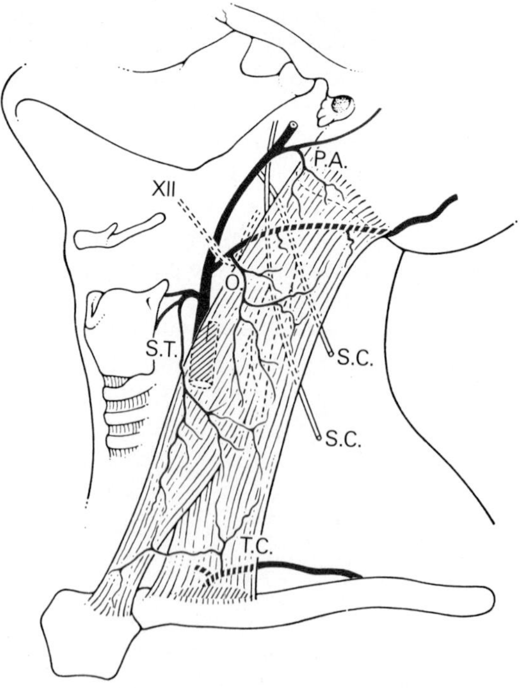

Fig. 7.157 Vascular pedicles of sternomastoid: **P.A.** branch of the posterior auricular artery; **O.** branch of occipital artery; **S.T.** branch of superior thyroid artery; **T.C.** branch from thyrocervical trunk (suprascapular artery or transverse cervical artery); **S.C.** supraclavicular nerves.

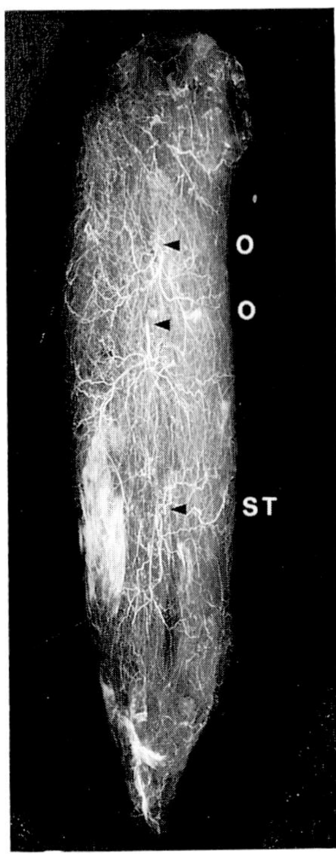

Fig. 7.158 Radiograph of sternomastoid muscle: **O.** branches of occipital artery; **S.T.** branch from superior thyroid artery. There is some extravasation of barium within the muscle.

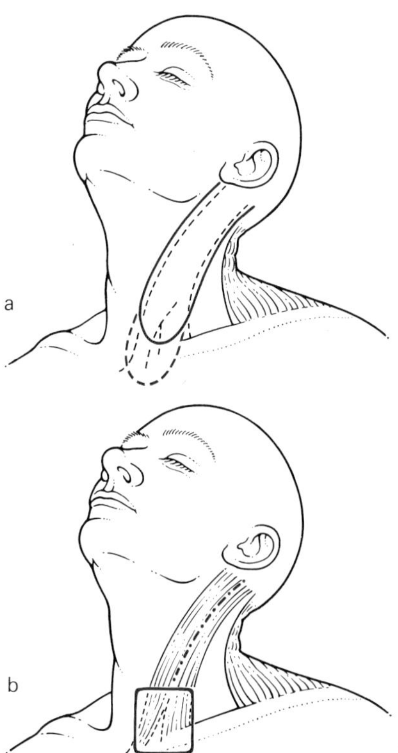

Fig. 7.159 Flap planning: **a.** a pedicled musculocutaneous flap may extend down to the sternoclavicular joint; **b.** a skin island may be carried on the lower end of the muscle.

artery may occasionally pass superficial to sternomastoid) and from the inferior thyroid (in 8%).

Surgery

Pedicled flap

When the donor defect is to be closed directly, the width of the flap is limited to 6 cm and the flap is centred over the muscle. When the donor defect is to be skin grafted, the flap may be broadened to 12–14 cm. The standard flap is 6 cm × 24 cm and extends up to 4 cm below the clavicle. Any extension distally beyond the clavicle requires a delay procedure.

Island flap

The investing layer of the deep cervical fascia splits to enclose sternocleidomastoid. Consequently when elevating the muscle it is possible to include the anterior layer but to leave the posterior layer intact and in continuity with the fascia over the cervical triangles thereby leaving the underlying neck structures undisturbed. The lower end of the flap is raised first together with the deep fascia and the dissection is then carried upwards ligating and dividing the branches from the thyrocervical trunk and from the superior thyroid artery (plus any small accessory pedicles that may be present). The occipital artery branches are preserved.

The flap can reach defects inferior to a line extending from the top of the ear to the lateral part of the nose and the midline of the upper and lower lips. Intraorally the flap will reach the hard and soft palate superiorly, and it will reach past the midline anteriorly and posteriorly. On the whole, however, this is not a very reliable flap with a reported 20% failure rate and a minor flap loss in an additional 15% of one series and partial epithelial loss in 50% of another series.[5]

References

1. Owens N 1955 A compound neck pedicle designed for the repair of massive facial defects: formation, development, and application. Plastic and Reconstructive Surgery 15: 369–389
2. Bakamjian V 1963 A technique for primary reconstruction of the palate after radical maxillectomy for cancer. Plastic and Reconstructive Surgery 31: 103–117
3. Littlewood A H M 1967 Compound skin and sternomastoid flaps for repair in extensive carcinoma of the head and neck. British Journal of Plastic Surgery 20: 403–419
4. O'Brien B 1970 A muscle-skin pedicle for total reconstruction of the lower lip. Plastic and Reconstructive Surgery 45: 395–399
5. Ariyan S 1979 One stage reconstruction for defects of the mouth using a sternomastoid myocutaneous flap. Plastic and Reconstructive Surgery 63: 618–625
6. Ariyan S 1980 The sternocleidomastoid myocutaneous flap. The Laryngoscope 90: 676–679

OCCIPITAL ARTERY

Upper trapezius musculocutaneous flap

Since 1842 when Mutter[1] devised a flap of skin and subcutaneous tissue from the neck and shoulder region for release of post-burn scar contractures, there have been many variations on this theme. Several people have described the epaulette flap, whose base 'includes the lateral and upper part of the neck, inclined a little towards the nape; it spreads over the entire shoulder'[2] (Fig. 7.160). Chretien et al[3] developed an 'extended shoulder flap' which extended from the midline to the deltoid region, measured 12–18 cm in width at the base and 7–13 cm over the shoulder, but required three delay procedures before it was safe to use. It was, however, McCraw[4] who realised the possibility of raising virtually the same flap in one stage by the expedient of including the underlying fibres of the upper part of trapezius so that the occipital artery supply to the muscle would, via perforators, enhance the vascularity of the skin flap. With short flaps the need for a prior delay procedure is thereby removed but with longer flaps a bipedicle delay with undermining is recommended.[5]

Anatomy

The occipital artery gives off a number of branches (p. 136) but in the context of this flap its trapezius branch and its direct cutaneous descending branches are important. The trapezius branch is given off to the uppermost part of the muscle at the level of the mastoid process as the artery emerges from beneath longissimus capitis. This vessel gives off perforators which can be seen on the radiograph of skin overlying trapezius (Fig. 7.162). Within the muscle the trapezius branch anastomoses with the transverse cervical artery which supplies the lateral part of the muscle. The direct cutaneous branches are given off by the horizontal part of the occipital artery which lies on semispinalis in the interval between trapezius and sternomastoid. These branches descend to supply upper posterior neck skin. The branch to trapezius is not seen during the elevation of the flap as the superior/lateral incised margin of the flap does not extend as high on the neck as the inferior/medial margin.

Surgery

The principal landmark is the anterior border of trapezius. The anterior edge of the flap follows this line from a point about 5 cm below the superior nuchal line to the lateral edge of the acromion. The posterior boundary lies parallel to the anterior and extends from the dorsal midline to the spine of the scapula with a flap width of 7–10 cm. The flap can measure approximately 7 cm × 30 cm without a delay and 7 cm × 35 cm with one delay. The delay procedure involves making parallel incisions and undermining only the distal part of the

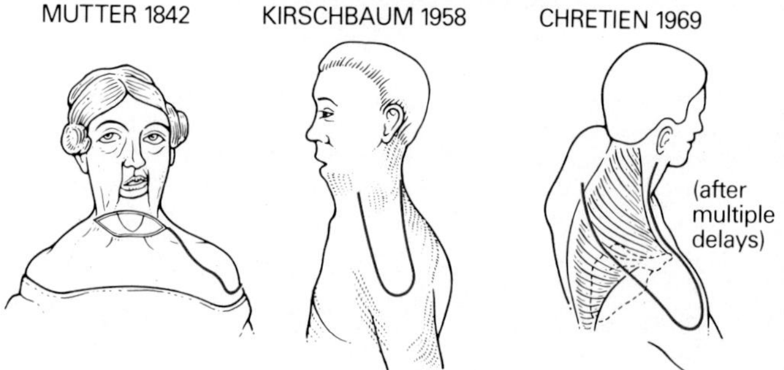

Fig. 7.160 Early designs of neck/shoulder flaps which did not include muscle.

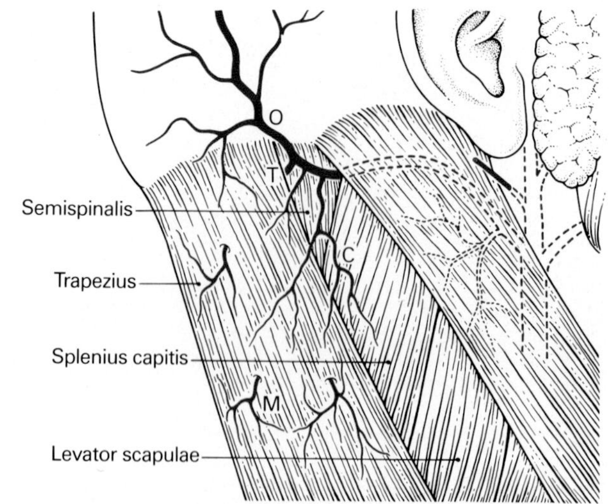

Fig. 7.161 Vascular anatomy. The occipital artery (**O**) lies on semispinalis and gives off direct cutaneous branches (**C**) and a trapezius branch (**T**) which gives rise to musculocutaneous perforators (**M**).

bipedicle flap some 8–10 days prior to elevation of the entire flap (Fig. 7.163).

In elevating the flap, the trapezius muscle is only included in the upper part of the flap and not in the lower lateral part where the muscle receives its blood supply from the transverse cervical artery. However, in the distal part, the deep fascia overlying trapezius is included in the flap, thereby leaving the muscle bare. Therefore the musculocutaneous component of the flap has a 2:1 length-to-breadth ratio whereas viewed overall the skin element has proportions of 3:1. The site for dividing the antero-superior part of the muscle lies just above the junction of the upper two-thirds with the lower one-third (Fig. 7.164). This preserves the nerve supply to the remainder of the muscle where it enters at or just below this point. The muscle fibres are then split to the midline and dissected free from underlying structures. Further mobility may be gained by dividing the midline attachment of trapezius to nuchal fascia. The arc of rotation of the longer version of this flap takes in the anterior floor of mouth, tonsil, cheek and temporal fossa. The flap does not carry sensory innervation. The loss of function is generally unimportant but the cosmetic defect resulting from inequality of shoulder and neck contour between the two sides may be significant. Closure of the donor site requires the use of split skin grafts.

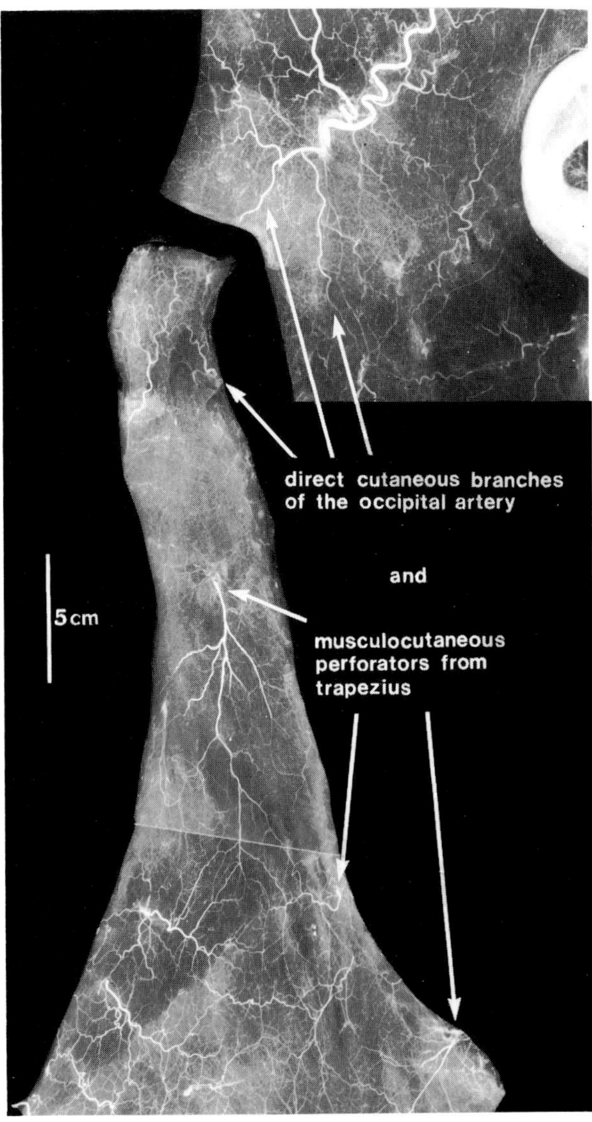

Fig. 7.162 Radiograph of skin overlying the upper part of trapezius.

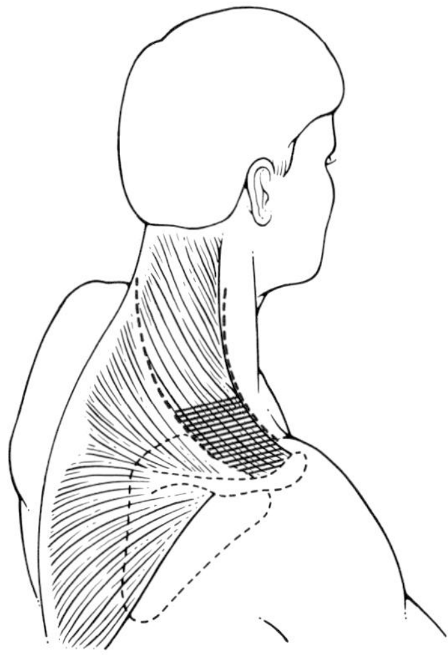

Fig. 7.163 Flap planning and execution of the preliminary delay. Broken lines show the position of the parallel incisions and the shaded area indicates the distal portion of the skin flap which is undermined.

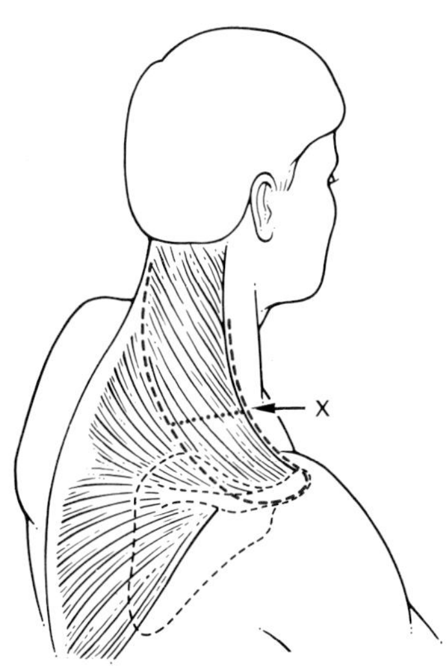

Fig. 7.164 Outline of incision for elevation of flap – note superior extension in midline. **X** marks the level for division of trapezius.

References

1. Mutter T D 1842 Cases of deformity from burns relieved by operation. American Journal of Medical Science 4: 66
2. Kirschbaum S 1958 Mentosternal Contracture. Preferred treatment by Acromial ('Charretera') flap. Plastic and Reconstructive Surgery 21: 131–138
3. Chretien P B, Ketcham A S, Hoye R C, Gertner H R 1969 Extended shoulder flap and its use in reconstruction of defects of the head and neck. American Journal of Surgery 118: 752–755
4. McCraw J, Dibbell D, Carraway J 1977 Clinical definition of independent myocutaneous vascular territories. Plastic and Reconstructive Surgery 60: 341–352
5. McCraw J, Magee W P, Kalwaic H 1979 Uses of the trapezius and sternomastoid myocutaneous flaps in head and neck reconstruction. Plastic and Reconstructive Surgery 63: 49–57
6. Kazanjian V H, Converse J M 1949 The surgical treatment of facial injuries. Williams & Wilkins, Baltimore

PERONEAL ARTERY

Fasciocutaneous postero-lateral leg flaps
— proximally based
— distally based

Pontén[1] first described the use of proximally based flaps consisting of skin, fat and deep fascia on the lower leg. The vascular anatomy of these flaps was investigated by Haertsch,[2] and further clinical examples reported by Barclay et al.[3] Distally based flaps supplied by one specific perforator from the peroneal artery have been described by Donski & Fogdestam[4] and others.[5–8] Initially these flaps were raised with a pedicle that included skin but further experience showed that this was not always necessary and skin islands may be carried satisfactorily on pedicles consisting of deep fascia and subcutaneous tissues. A further variation is the islanded skin flap overlying a perforator which is turned through 180° to fill an adjacent defect.

Anatomy

The peroneal artery is a constant major vessel in the posterior compartment of the lower leg but is not always dispensable since it may take over the distal territory of an underdeveloped or absent posterior tibial artery. It is on average 4.2 mm in diameter at its origin (normal diameter in 85%, hypertrophied in 11%, decreased in 4%). It lies between tibialis posterior, the interosseous membrane and flexor hallucis longus and gives off seven main sets of branches:

Medial branches are given off to muscles, interosseous membrane and periosteum of fibula. There are up to ten of these small short vessels.

Lateral branches are given off to peroneal muscles, periosteum of fibula, and skin via fasciocutaneous perforators. There are five to twelve of these branches with an average diameter of 1.2 mm (range 0.5–2 mm) and several smaller branches. These vessels branch off the peroneal artery at various angles between 20° and 95° (average 40°).

A nutrient vessel to the fibula is given off about 7 cm from the origin of the artery and penetrates the shaft of the bone on its posterior or medial surface posterior to the interosseous membrane. The nutrient foramen lies in the middle third of the bone on average 17 cm from the styloid process of the fibula (range 14–19 cm).

A transverse communicating branch is given off approximately 6 cm above the tip of the lateral malleolus. This communicates with the posterior tibial artery.

A perforating branch pierces the interosseous membrane above the lateral malleolus and communicates with the lateral anterior malleolar branch of the anterior tibial artery.

Lateral malleolar branches may communicate with the lateral tarsal branches of the dorsalis pedis artery.

Calcaneal branches communicate with calcaneal branches of the posterior tibial artery.

Fasciocutaneous flaps situated over the posterolateral aspect of the leg are dependent for their blood supply on the lateral branches. Only about five perforators reach the deep fascia along the posterior peroneal septum lying at 3–5 cm intervals down the length of the leg. These vessels have an internal diameter of 0.1–0.4 mm and tend to be smaller in the lower third of the leg. The largest perforators, and the highest concentration of perforators, have been found by the authors to lie within a 10 cm long rectangle whose upper edge lies 10 cm below the fibular styloid (Fig. 7.167).

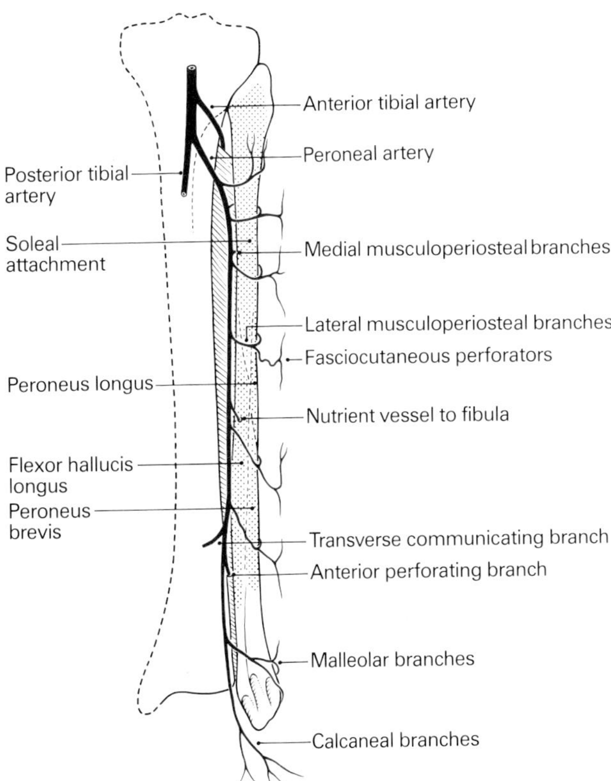

Fig. 7.165 Schematic diagram of peroneal artery branches and of the muscle attachments to the posterior surface of the fibula.

7

Flap planning

These fasciocutaneous flaps may be designed in a pedicled form with either a proximal or distal pedicle, or they may be designed as skin islands located over a single perforator. Pedicled flaps may be further subdivided on the basis of whether or not the pedicle includes skin. Pedicled and islanded forms will be described in turn:

Proximally pedicled fasciocutaneous flaps
The proximally pedicled flaps are best reserved for defects on the anterior and anterolateral aspects of the upper half of the leg. There is the disadvantage that if the flap is placed in the lower third of the leg where the fibula is subcutaneous, then bone will be exposed on transposition of the flap, and although this will accept a graft it makes for an unsatisfactory donor site.

The position of the base of the flap is largely determined by the location of the defect requiring reconstruction combined with Doppler probe aided identification of a larger perforator, but it will generally be sited in the area about 10 or 20 cm below the head of the fibula. The flap is orientated longitudinally overlying the posterior peroneal septum which is surface marked by a line drawn between the fibular styloid and the posterior edge of the lateral malleolus. The greater the proportion of the flap lying in front of the septum, the greater are the chances of including perforators from the anterior tibial artery emerging along the anterior peroneal septum whereas if the flap is sited more behind the posterior peroneal septum musculocutaneous perforators through the lateral head of gastrocnemius and branches from the sural arteries will tend to be included. Flaps of 8 cm × 20 cm are reliable and longer ones may occasionally be successful.

The pedicles of these flaps need not necessarily contain skin.

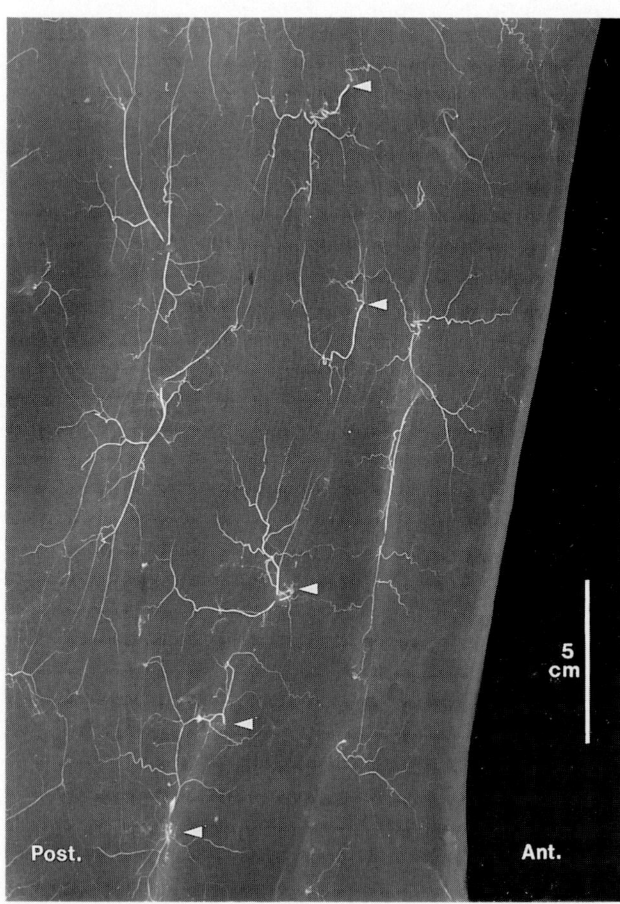

Fig. 7.166 Radiograph of skin overlying posterior peroneal septum showing a series of fasciocutaneous perforators.

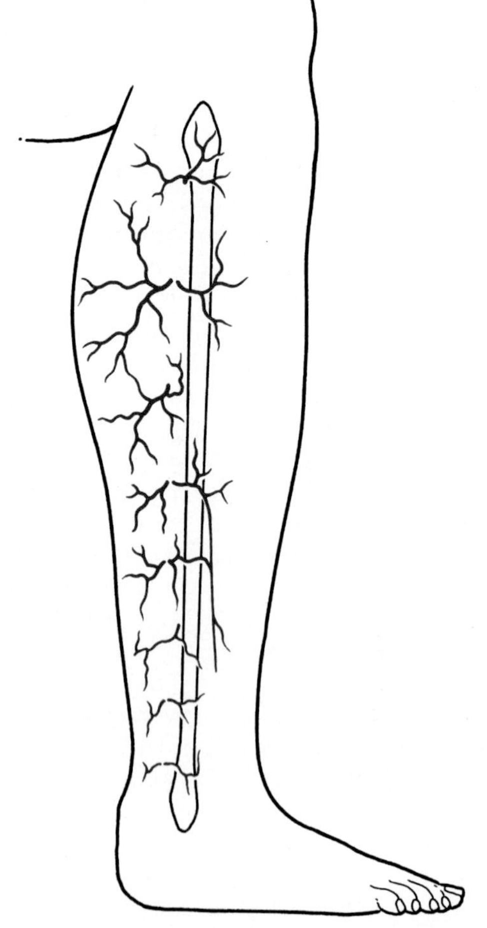

Fig. 7.167 Disposition of perforators in the area of the posterior peroneal septum. Note that the most superior perforator does not arise from the peroneal artery, the others do.

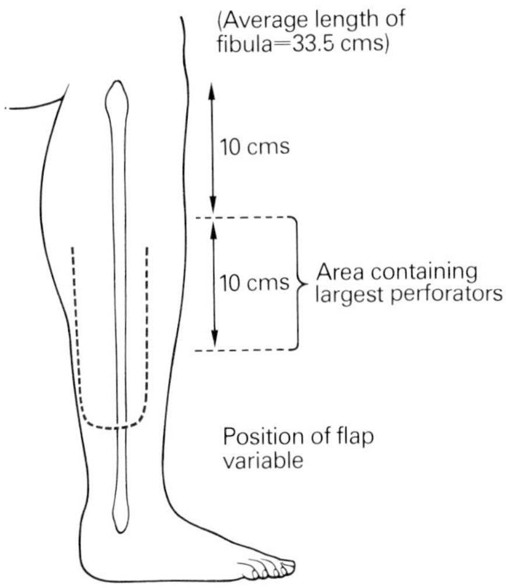

Fig. 7.168 Conventional proximally-based pedicled flap.

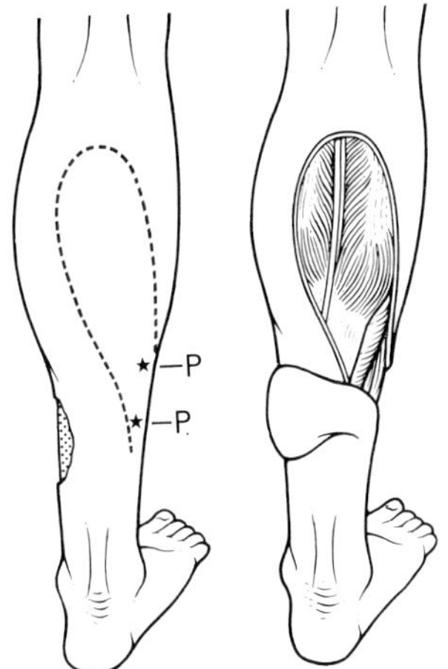

Fig. 7.169 Distally-based pedicled flap based on one or two perforators and inclined medially so as to take skin from over the calf.

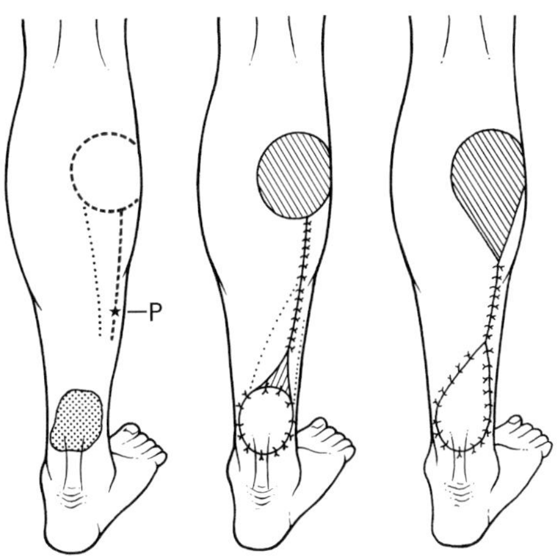

Fig. 7.170 Distally-based pedicled flap with a pedicle consisting of deep fascia and skin only. The pear-shaped flap for a circular defect avoids tight closure of the skin over the pedicle.

Distally pedicled fasciocutaneous flaps
These flaps have a base overlying a single-peroneal artery perforator located in the posterior peroneal septum generally in the lower third of the leg. The flap is directed upwards but the end of the flap should not overlie the area of the neck of the fibula otherwise the common peroneal nerve will be exposed in the base of the secondary defect. Instead the axis of the flap inclines upwards and medially so as to take skin from over the calf muscles. This part of the flap may be much wider than the pedicle. The upper limit of the territory is bounded by the lower border of the popliteal fossa, the lateral border by the subcutaneous crest of the fibula, and the medial border by a line approximately 2–3 cm behind the medial edge of the tibia. The perforator about which the flap is usually pedicled lies approximately 10–12 cm above the tip of the lateral malleolus. Various authors in studying the arrangement of the peroneal perforators have given different measurements but the use of a Doppler probe will greatly help in the planning of the flap. In planning the length of the flap it should always be 1 cm longer than seems to be necessary as this avoids any traction on the perforator once the flap has been transposed and inset into the recipient site.

Skin island overlying a perforator
This technique is possible on a large peroneal perforator but in general it is better reserved for the medial side of the leg where the posterior tibial artery perforators are larger and the accompanying veins are also of greater diameter.

Flap elevation

Flap elevation commences laterally elevating skin and fascia towards the posterior peroneal septum where the perforators become visible. The locations of the perforators may then lead to modification of the design of the flap and positioning of its base. The attachment of the deep fascia to the posterior peroneal septum is divided and perforators more proximal than the one chosen to act as the axis of the flap are divided. The remainder of the flap is then raised starting below the popliteal fossa and sparing the sural nerve if possible.

If a fascio-subcutaneous pedicle is planned then an incision is made between the perforator at the base of the pedicle and the planned skin island, and skin flaps with a thin layer of fat are reflected on both sides for 2 to 3 cm. A 4 to 6 cm wide fascio-subcutaneous pedicle is then raised. Otherwise flap elevation is similar.

References

1. Pontén B 1981 The fasciocutaneous flap: its use in soft tissue defects of the lower leg. British Journal of Plastic Surgery 34: 215–220
2. Haertsch P 1981 The blood supply to the skin of the leg: a post mortem investigation. British Journal of Plastic Surgery 34: 470–477
3. Barclay T L, Cardoso E, Sharpe D T, Crockett D J 1982 Repair of lower leg injuries with fasciocutaneous flaps. British Journal of Plastic Surgery 35: 127–132
4. Donski P K, Fogdestam I 1983 Distally based fasciocutaneous flap from the sural region. Scandinavian Journal of Plastic and Reconstructive Surgery 17: 191–196
5. Greco J M, Simons G, Faugon H 1983 Une arme nouvelle en chirurgie plastique: le lambeau cutanéo-aponévrotique. Son application dans la réparation des pertes de substance du membre inférieur. Annales de Chirurgie Plastique et Esthétique 28: 211–224
6. Le Huec J C, Midy D, Chauveaux D, Calteux N, Colombet P, Bovet J L 1988 Anatomic basis of the sural fasiocutaneous flap: surgical applications. Surgical and Radiologic Anatomy 10: 5–13
7. Carriquiry C, Costa A, Vasconez L O 1985 An anatomic study of the septocutaneous vessels of the leg. Plastic and Reconstructive Surgery 76: 354–361
8. Ferreira M C, Gabbianelli G, Alonso N, Fontana C 1986 The distal pedicle fascia flap of the leg. Scandinavian Journal of Plastic and Reconstructive Surgery 20: 133–136

PERONEAL ARTERY – nutrient artery to fibula and cutaneous branches

Type C fasciocutaneous flaps – pedicled
– free flaps
Type C osteofasciocutaneous flaps
Vascularised fibular graft – free
– pedicled

Free vascularised fibular grafts were described by Taylor[1] in 1975 and by Gilbert[2] in 1979, with the incorporation of the fibular epiphysis and growth plate being a subsequent development.[3, 4] Complex defects which required soft tissue cover of the vascularised bone graft were handled either by harvesting part of the soleus muscle with the bone and grafting onto the muscle (Baudet, 1982)[5] or by using such a piece of muscle as a carrier for an island of skin (Zhong-Wei, 1980).[6] Yoshimura (1983, 1984)[7, 8] and Chen (1983)[9] popularised the combination of a fibular graft with a skin island based on the posterior peroneal septum perforators, both as a means of reconstructing a complex defect and as a means of monitoring the perfusion of the bone graft. Many studies have reported on the anatomy and clinical application of these flaps.[10–13] Initially the concept was of a fascio- or septo-cutaneous flap based on the posterior peroneal septum but then in 1986 Harrison stressed the importance of raising muscle with the flap,[14] and only since then have the details of the anatomy become fully understood.

Anatomy

The broad principles on which these flaps are raised are (i) that perforators pass along the posterior peroneal septum to reach skin, (ii) the largest perforators from the peroneal artery lie between 10 and 20 cm below the head of the fibula, and (iii) if the septum and perforators are retained between the skin island and the peroneal vascular pedicle then the skin island should survive. In clinical practice flaps have not been as reliable as expected and this is attributable to variation in the detailed anatomy of exactly where the perforators lie in relation to the septum. Many of the earlier studies were in conflict but the present understanding of the situation is best summarised by Figure 7.171 in which it can be seen that the perforators to skin lie either (i) on the anterior surface of the septum, (ii) on the posterior surface of the septum but closely attached to muscle, or (iii) they pass through the substance of soleus to reach skin. For descriptive purposes these have been designated as septal, septomuscular and musculocutaneous perforators.[15] Since the disposition of muscle around the posterior surface of the fibula changes throughout the length of the bone it is also to be expected that at different levels the predominating perforator type will also vary. The musculocutaneous and septomuscular perforators are encountered mainly in the proximal part of the leg where the bulk of soleus lies, and septocutaneous are encountered mainly distally. Pure septocutaneous perforators lying on the anterior aspect of the lateral septum were not found in 20% of cases in one study,[15] while no musculocutaneous or septomuscular perforators were found in 6%.

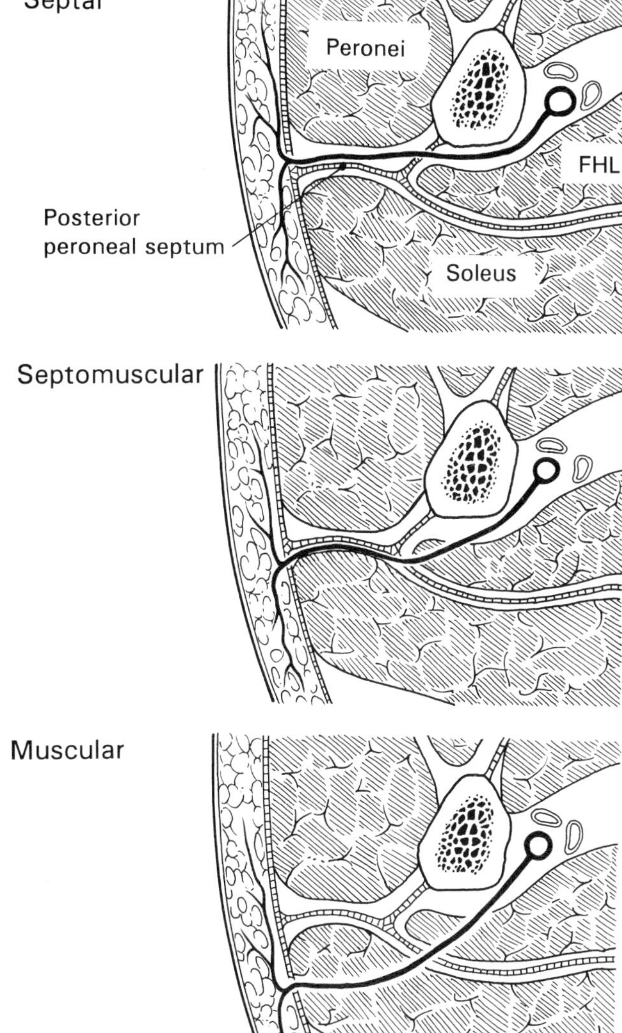

Fig. 7.171 Vascular anatomy. Variations in the positions of the perforators 'along' the posterior peroneal. These have been described as septal, septomuscular and musculocutaneous.

Flap planning

The usual arrangement is to design the skin island as a longitudinally orientated ellipse overlying the posterior peroneal septum, the location of the septum being surface marked by a line drawn between the head of the fibula and the posterior edge of the lateral malleolus. Even if the required shape of flap is not elliptical it may still be worth raising a long ellipse with a corresponding long length of septum so as to obtain as many perforators as possible to the deep fascia. The cutaneous ends of the flap that are in excess of requirements can later be excised. The skin ellipse is positioned so that one-third of it lies anterior to the line of the septum and two-thirds posterior to it. Maximum dimensions are 5 cm anterior and 10 cm posterior to the line, or alternatively the boundaries of the territory can be taken as the subcutaneous border of the tibia anteriorly and the midline posteriorly. The maximum concentration of large perforators from the peroneal artery is located between 10 and 20 cm below the head of the fibula and therefore the skin ellipse is centred on this area. That at 10 cm is usually the largest perforator. Around the upper end of the fibula there are contributions from the popliteal, anterior and posterior tibial arteries which give origin to the first perforator. The positioning of the skin island will obviously be modified if the flap is intended not as a free flap but as a proximally or distally pedicled flap.

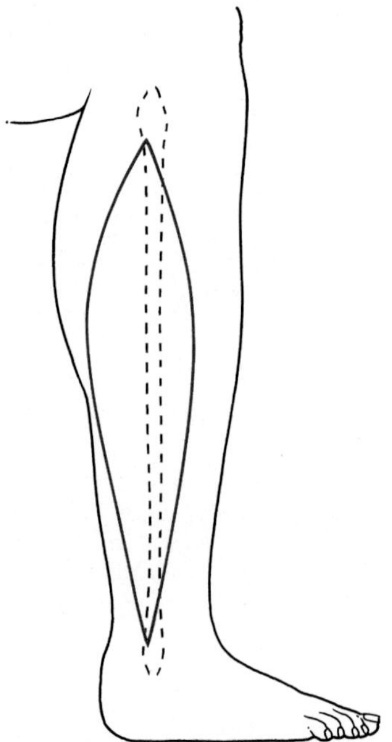

Fig. 7.172 Flap planning. Surface marking of the posterior peroneal septum is shown with the elliptical flap overlying this with two-thirds of the flap posterior to the line.

Flap elevation

Type C fasciocutaneous flaps. Lack of appreciation of the variations in perforator anatomy and failure to account for this in raising the flaps probably underlie most of the difficulties that have been encountered with flap failures. The key point is to ensure that enough muscle cuff is taken posterior to the septum to ensure incorporation of septomuscular and musculocutaneous perforators lying within soleus and flexor hallucis longus.

Elevation commences at the anterior margin of the flap which is raised with the fascia from over the peroneal compartment up to the posterior peroneal septum. Depending on how wide the flap is, peforators along the anterior peroneal septum may require division. The posterior peroneal septum is divided where it attaches to the fibula and the dissection then keeps close to the bone. The posterior skin incision is then made and the flap elevated with fascia. The short saphenous vein and lateral sural nerve will need to be dealt with. When the edge of soleus is approached the incision is deepened through the muscle so as to leave a 1 cm portion on the septum. The septum between the superficial and deep posterior compartments is then incised and part of flexor hallucis is also taken to protect the perforators. The peroneal artery and veins are then dissected free and divided.

There are three versions of this flap: the proximally-pedicled flap, the distally-pedicled flap and the free flap.

Distally pedicled flap. In this version the flap is situated over the upper third of the fibula. It should be noted that the first perforator, which lies at the neck of the fibula, arises either from the popliteal, posterior or anterior tibial artery and not from the peroneal. The peroneal artery is

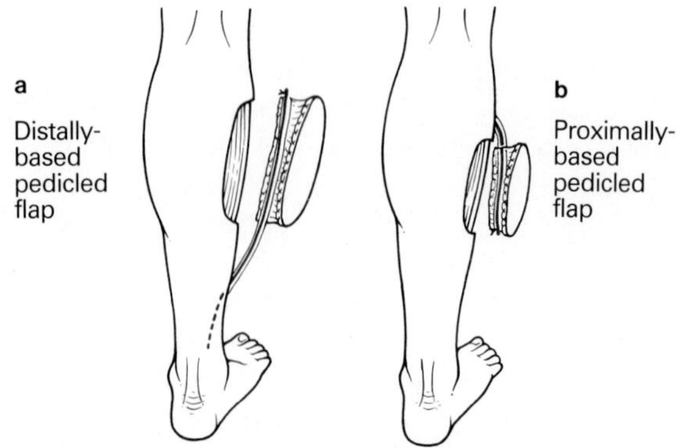

Fig. 7.173 Proximally and distally pedicled flaps.

ligated and divided proximal to the flap, and the skin island is then swung downwards to fill a defect in the distal leg. The flap is supported by retrograde flow in the peroneal artery which is fed by its distal anastomoses with the anterior and posterior tibial arteries. The point of rotation is the transverse communicating branch of the peroneal artery which lies approximately 6 cm above the tip of the lateral malleolus, and this takes the flap down to the region of the ankle joint. A microsurgical anastomosis of a vena comitans of the peroneal artery or of the short saphenous vein to a superficial vein at the recipient site is desirable.[11]

Proximally pedicled flap. With orthograde flow in the peroneal artery and its venae comitantes this is a reliable flap but there are many other possible flap options for reconstructing defects around the region of the knee which do not sacrifice a major leg vessel so the applications for this pedicled flap are few.

Free flap. The skin island is taken with an appropriate length of the peroneal artery and venae comitantes so that orthograde flow in the vessels can be achieved after anastomosis in the recipient site.

Osteofasciocutaneous free flap (Type C skin island with fibula shaft). These composite flaps are unlikely to be used in the pedicled form (i.e. on the same leg) but are frequently used to reconstruct defects of tibia and skin on the opposite leg where trauma has resulted in a bone defect of over 10 cm, or on another long bone after tumour ablation or destruction by osteomyelitis.

The same principles of flap planning are used as when planning the skin island of the Type C flap. The probable location of the nutrient foramen is 17 cm from the styloid process of the fibula (range 14.2–19 cm).[16]

In raising the composite flap the order of elevation is different because early mobilisation of the fibula facilitates exposure of the peroneal pedicle. The skin and fascia are incised posteriorly and reflected forwards to the edge of soleus where the incision passes deeply through soleus some 5 to 10 mm posterior to the line of the emerging perforators. (Some authors[12] have reported successful transfers without incorporating the muscle cuff but in general it seems safer to do so.) The upper and lower ends of the fibula are divided with a Gigli saw which allows the fibula to be turned forwards. Flexor hallucis longus is divided longitudinally to expose the peroneal artery and veins which are then ligated and divided at their lower ends. The anterior incision is now made and skin and fascia reflected back to the posterior peroneal septum where the incision is deepened through peroneus longus 2 or 3 mm in front of the septum. Some 3 or 4 mm from the fibula the incision passes anteriorly to separate the extensors from the bone while leaving a small cuff of muscle on the periosteum to protect the periosteal vessels. Retraction exposes the interosseous membrane which is divided and the sole remaining attachment of the fibula is now the tibialis posterior muscle. This is separated by pulling the lower end of the fibula laterally away from the leg and dividing the muscle from below upwards whilst preserving a 1 cm cuff on the bone to protect the circular and nutrient arteries.

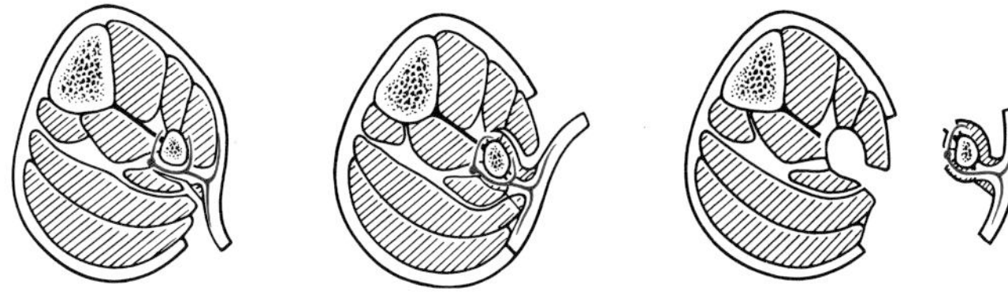

Fig. 7.174 Stages in raising the composite flap; posterior dissection first, then anterior, then bone mobilisation and completion of anterior dissection, then final freeing of pedicle working from both sides.

It is advisable to leave intact the lower 5 cm of fibula to maintain the ankle mortise and in children a screw passed across the lower end of the fibula segment into the tibia may help to prevent valgus deformity.

Free vascularised fibular diaphysis graft. The specific indications for this technique are few and include replacement of tibial bone defects in excess of 10 cm where there is no loss of skin cover, certain cases of congenital pseudoarthrosis of the tibia, long bone defects secondary to tumour ablation, and some deformities of the forearm bones such as radial club hand where it is also desirable to transfer the fibular epiphysis. It should be noted that in the skeletally immature the epiphysis has a separate blood supply from the diaphysis. Up to six arteries arising from the popliteal and anterior tibial arteries contribute to the epiphysis with the major contribution being from the inferior lateral genicular artery.[16] Although separate anatomosis of one of these vessels to maintain epiphyseal circulation would be theoretically ideal, in practice in children these vessels are too small for anastomosis, and blood supply to the epiphysis is maintained by harvesting a cuff of soft tissue around the vascularised bone graft and its epiphysis so as to provide a route of communication between the metaphyseal and epiphyseal blood supplies because there are no vessels crossing the growth plate.

The fibular shaft is harvested by a slightly different technique from that used to raise the fibular with an accompanying skin flap. This is because it is not necessary to see the soleus when harvesting bone only. Several techniques have been described but we favour the following. An incision is made over the peroneal compartment down to the muscle. The posterior deep fascial edge is raised off the peronei, the muscles are

7

retracted by the assistant and the anterior aspect of the posterior peroneal septum is exposed. Through this septum perforators can be seen passing along its posterior surface to the skin. The posterior peroneal septum is divided close to the fibula and the perforators coagulated and divided. At this stage it is not necessary to proceed any further round the back of the fibula. The peroneal muscles are now separated from the fibula, dividing muscle fibres some 5 mm from the bone. Care is taken over the peroneal nerve. This dissection is continued through the anterior peroneal septum and round the anterior aspect of the fibula releasing extensor hallucis until the interosseous membrane is exposed – this is carefully divided. At the distal end, between 5 and 10 cm from the malleolus, the peroneal vascular bundle diverges slightly medially from the fibula. With division of the interosseous membrane the artery can be identified at this level from the anterior aspect which is much easier than trying to dissect it out from behind the fibula. A space between the vascular pedicle and the fibula is then created at the desired level of bone section and a Gigli saw passed. The bone is divided and with lateral traction of the end of the bone graft the distal end of the peroneal vascular pedicle is exposed, ligated and divided. The graft is retracted laterally and it is then easier to divide the remaining muscle attachments of tibialis posterior and flexor hallucis starting distally and working both from medial and postero-lateral approaches around the fibula. The upper osteotomy is made and the peroneal artery then traced up to its origin from the posterior tibial artery where artery and venae comitantes are ligated and divided. The tourniquet should be released and the leg bandaged for a while before returning to it to secure haemostasis, suture the muscles and close the wound over a suction drain.

Pedicled vascularized fibular graft. This may occasionally be indicated for a congenital pseudoarthrosis or tibial defect. A segment of the middle of the fibula is mobilised on a distal pedicle and transposed into the defect in the distal tibia.[17] A cross leg pedicled transfer may very occasionally be indicated. Note that there is a cross anastomosis by a large vessel between the posterior tibial artery and the peroneal artery above the level of the ankle.

References

1. Taylor G I, Miller G D H, Ham F J 1975 The free vascularised bone graft. Plastic and Reconstructive Surgery 54: 274–285
2. Gilbert A 1979 Surgical technique – vascularized transfer of the fibula shaft. International Journal of Microsurgery 1: 100–102
3. Weiland A J, Kleinert H E, Kutz J E, Daniel R K 1979 Free vascularized bone grafts in surgery of the upper extremity. Journal of Hand Surgery 4: 129–144
4. Pho R W H, Patterson M H, Kour A K, Kumar V P 1987 Free vascularised epiphyseal transplantation in upper extremity reconstruction. The Journal of Hand Surgery 13B: 440–447
5. Baudet J, Panconi P, Cox M, Schoofs V 1982 The composite fibula and soleus free transfer. International Journal of Microsurgery 4: 11–16
6. Zhong-Wei C, Yueh-Se 1980 Microsurgery in China. Clinics in Plastic Surgery 7: 437–473
7. Yoshimura M, Shimamura K, Iwai Y, Yamauchi S, Ueno T 1983 Free vascularised fibular transplant. A new method for monitoring circulation of the grafted fibula. Journal of Bone and Joint Surgery 65A: 1295–1301
8. Yoshimura M, Imura S, Shimamura K, Yamauchi S, Nomura S 1984 Peroneal flap for reconstruction in the extremity: preliminary communication. Plastic and Reconstructive Surgery 74: 402–409
9. Chen Z, Yan W 1983 The study and clinical application of the osteocutaneous flap of fibula. Microsurgery 4: 11–16
10. Chen Y, Zheng B, Zhu J, Zheng B, Gu Y, Wu M, Li H 1985 Microsurgical anatomy of the lateral skin flap of the leg. Annals of Plastic Surgery 15: 313–318
11. Gu Y, Wu M, Li H 1985 Lateral lower leg skin flap. 1985 Annals of Plastic Surgery 15: 319–324
12. Wei F, Chen H, Chuang C, Noordhoff M S 1986 Fibular osteocutaneous flap: anatomic study and clinical application. Plastic and Reconstructive Surgery 78: 191–199
13. Yoshimura M, Shimada T, Hosokawa M 1990 The vasculature of the peroneal tissue transfer. Plastic and Reconstructive Surgery 85: 917–921
14. Harrison D H 1986 The osteocutaneous free fibular graft. Journal of Bone and Joint Surgery 68B: 804–807
15. Schusterman M A, Reece G P, Miller M J, Harris S 1992 The osteocutaneous free fibula flap: is the skin paddle reliable? Plastic and Reconstructive Surgery 90: 787–793
16. Bonnel F, Lesire M, Gomis R, Allieu Y, Rabischong P 1981 Arterial vascularization of the fibula. Microsurgical transplantation techniques. Anatomia Clinica 3: 13–22
17. Townsend P L G 1990 Vascularised fibular graft using reverse peroneal flow in the treatment of congenital pseudoarthrosis of the tibia. British Journal of Plastic Surgery 43: 261–265

PERONEAL ARTERY – Supramalledar anterior perforating branch

Supramalleolar flap

This island fasciocutaneous flap was developed by Masquelet, Beveridge et al.[1, 2] Because the vascular inflow (and therefore the pivot point) is located under the distal part of the flap, it may be useful for defects over the malleoli, dorsum of foot and heel although the donor site on the front of the lower leg, which always has to be skin grafted, may be cosmetically unacceptable.

Anatomy

The flap is based on the anterior perforating branch of the peroneal artery which pierces the intermuscular septum and appears on the front of the leg approximately 5 cm above the lateral malleolus. Here it divides into two branches; one is a *deep branch* which runs distally in the loose areolar tissue under the deep fascia, running over the bones of the tarsus and anastomosing widely with other vessels – principally branches of the anterior tibial and dorsalis pedis arteries, but also with the terminal part of the peroneal artery as it lies on the calcaneus deep to the peroneal tendons. The other branch is a *superfical cutaneous branch.*

The superficial cutaneous branch emerges between extensor digitorum longus and peroneus brevis muscles and is largely expended in proximally-directed branches. These proximally-directed branches run superficially and supply a potential territory of up to 8 cm × 16 cm.

Variations. The size of the cutaneous branch of the peroneal anterior perforating artery may be inversely related to the size of the anterior malleolar artery given off by the anterior tibial artery. Variations in the relative contributions of the peroneal and anterior tibial arteries to the dorsum of the foot are covered on page 261. Anomalies such as the dorsalis pedis artery being the distal continuation of the peroneal anterior perforating branch may make this flap impractical since ligation of the artery might render the forefoot ischaemic.

Flap planning

The planning starts by placing the inferior end of the flap over the anterior perforating artery in the groove that can be palpated above and medial to the lateral malleolus. The margins of the flap are outlined above this point with dimensions of up to 8 cm × 16 cm although Masquelet et al state that the superior end of the flap may be sited as far as half-way up the fibula. The lateral border must not extend posterior to the line of the fibula and the anterior/medial edge will overlie the superficial peroneal nerve. Depending on the length of pedicle required, a further incision will be necessary extending downwards for 5 cm from the end of the flap along a line directed towards the fifth toe.

Flap elevation

This commences at the anteromedial border of the flap. In deepening the skin incision down to the deep fascia care must be taken to identify the superficial peroneal nerve to protect it from injury, and to dissect it free from the flap. The deep fascia is elevated with the flap and as the medial half of the flap is raised the perforating branch will come into view. If the flap is to be used as a local

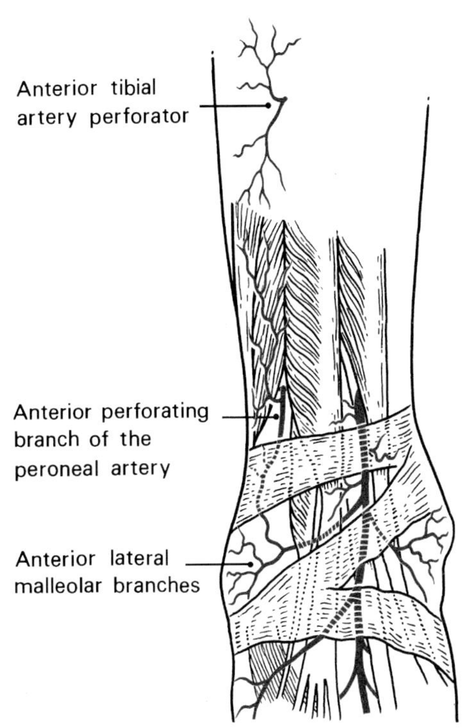

Fig. 7.175 Vascular anatomy. Cutaneous and deep branches of the peroneal anterior perforating artery are shown.

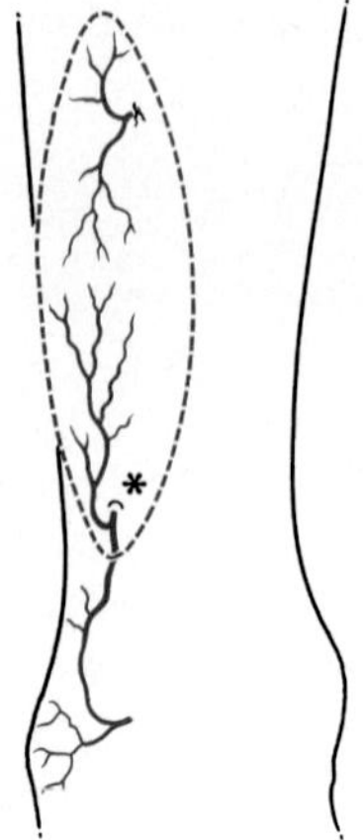

Fig. 7.176 Version of the flap for local transposition.

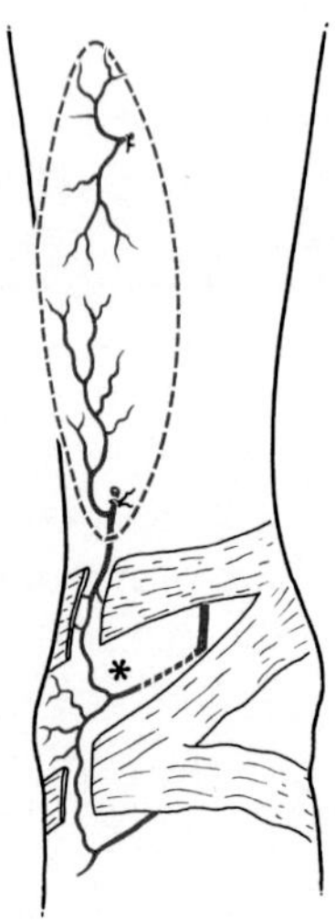

Fig. 7.177 Original version of the flap pedicled on the deep branch.

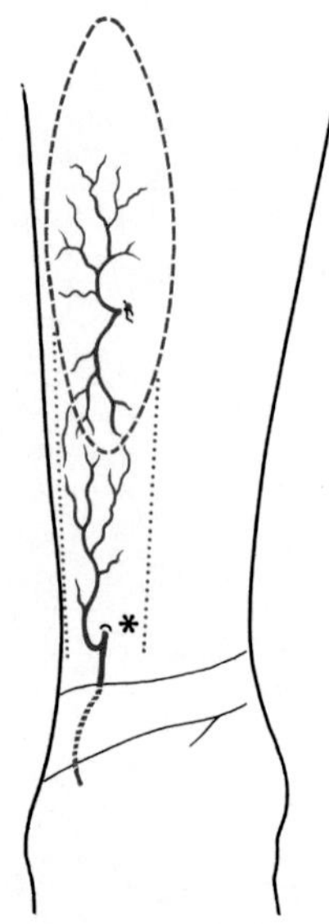

Fig. 7.178 Modified version of the flap positioned more proximally and pedicled on a fascio-subcutaneous tissue pedicle.

transposition flap for adjacent defects over the malleoli or the anterior aspect of the ankle, then this identification of the perforating branch will pinpoint the centre of the arc of rotation and will permit adjustment of the previously planned superior and inferior flap margins before they are incised. The remainder of the flap is then elevated and the perforator and its accompanying venae comitantes freed sufficiently to permit rotation of the flap about this point.

If the flap is intended for a more distal defect in the foot then a longer pedicle and a point of rotation located more distally on the foot are required. This can be achieved by division of the anterior perforating artery deep to the point at which it divides into superficial and deep branches. Inflow into the flap is then not from the peroneal artery but by reversed flow in the deep branch which receives blood via its numerous connections over the dorsum of the foot. This deep branch is on average 6.5 cm long (range 4.4–9 cm) and 1.0 mm in diameter. It is dissected out by dividing the overlying superior part of the extensor retinaculum. By this means a pedicle length of up to 8 cm may be achieved. However, in two out of 40 dissections Masquelet et al found that instead of a single identifiable deep branch (with venae comitantes) there was instead a network of finer vessels. If this should be the case then some vascular insufficiency of the flap might be expected.

In a subsequent report Masquelet et al presented a modification in the design of the flap to overcome the problem of an inadequate deep branch.[3] They suggested that the skin island should be placed, not over the perforating branch, but proximal to it. A long pedicle to reach defects on the foot can then be achieved by dissecting out a pedicle of subcutaneous tissue and deep fascia 2 to 3 cm wide between the flap and the peroneal perforating artery. The point of rotation of the flap is then the perforating artery but in the presence of a strong deep branch the fascio-subcutaneous pedicle can be lengthened further by division of the peroneal perforator and distal dissection of the descending branch in the originally described manner. The authors caution that the longer the pedicle is made, the smaller should be the skin island and the mid-point of the leg represents the proximal limit of the territory.

References

1. Masquelet A C, Beveridge J, Romana C, Gerber C 1988 The lateral supramalleolar flap. Plastic and Reconstructive Surgery 81: 74–81
2. Beveridge J, Masquelet A C, Romana M C, Vinh T S 1988 Anatomic basis of a fasciocutaneous flap supplied by the perforating branch of the peroneal artery. Surgical and Radiologic Anatomy 10: 195–199
3. Valenti P, Masquelet A C, Romana C, Nordin J Y 1991 Technical refinement of the lateral supramalleolar flap. British Journal of Plastic Surgery 44: 459–462

PERONEAL ARTERY – calcaneal branches

Lateral calcaneal flap
Distally-based retrograde-flow calcaneal flap

This pedicled neurovascular flap was introduced by Grabb & Argenta[1] in 1981 as a means of reconstructing a skin defect over the lower 3–5 cm of the Achilles tendon or over the calcaneus on its posterior and/or plantar surface. There are two versions of the pedicled flap, a long and a short, depending on whether the plantar surface of the heel is also going to be repaired. Holmes & Rayner[2] have modified the flap to an island form with a subcutaneous pedicle.

Anatomy

The 'lateral calcaneal artery' described by Grabb & Argenta is not recognised by this name by anatomists. The vessel concerned is the terminal part of the peroneal artery and its calcaneal branches, of which there are usually four or five.

At the level of the ankle the peroneal artery lies deeply in the fat between the Achilles tendon and the peroneal tendons. It follows the curve of the peroneus longus tendon round the lateral malleolus lying about 1 cm posterior to it (Fig. 7.179). Palpable landmarks are the lateral edge of the Achilles tendon and the tip of the lateral malleolus. At the level of the ankle the peroneal artery lies 5–8 mm in front of the Achilles tendon, and then curves downwards to a point 30 mm inferior to the tip of the fibula. From here the artery continues towards the tuberosity of the fifth metatarsal where it anastomoses with branches of the lateral plantar artery deep to abductor digiti minimi and with the lateral tarsal artery deep to the tendon of peroneus brevis. Throughout the curved part of its course the peroneal artery gives off calcaneal branches which run posteriorly and inferiorly to form a network beneath the skin, overlying the lateral, posterior and inferior surfaces of the calcaneus (rete calcaneum of *Nomina Anatomica*). There are usually four or five of these calcaneal branches and always at least two.

Venous drainage of the area is through the small saphenous vein which lies immediately anterior to the peroneal artery but at a more superficial level. It has an extensive network of comparatively large veins draining into it but, as in other regions, the venous anatomy is variable.

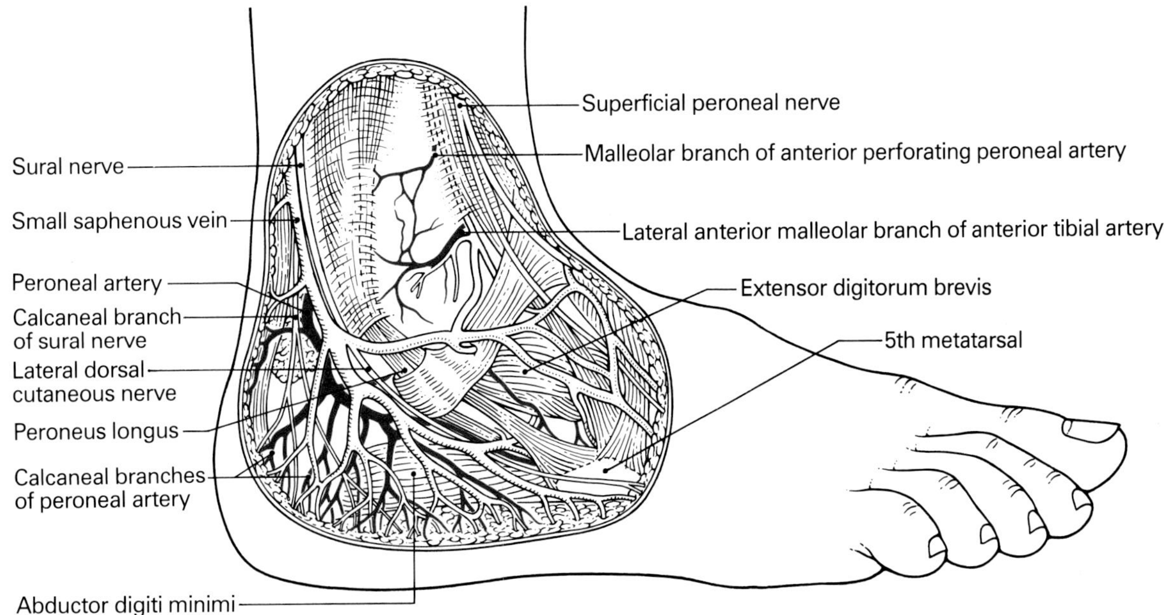

Fig. 7.179 Vascular anatomy. Note also the nerves related to this flap; the calcaneal branch of the sural nerve and, more anteriorly but still between the arterial supply to the flap and the overlying skin, the lateral dorsal cutaneous nerve of the foot. (Margins of area displayed bear no relation to shape of flap.)

7

The nerve supply comes from the sural nerve (S1) which lies just in front of the small saphenous vein. It gives off calcaneal branches to the heel and then, renamed the lateral dorsal cutaneous nerve, curves beneath the lateral malleolus and supplies the lateral side of the foot and the fifth toe.

Planning

The peroneal artery is always present although it may be reduced in size; furthermore it is usually unaffected by arteriosclerosis. Nevertheless it is wise to check the state of the vessel pre-operatively with a Doppler probe, especially if a long flap is planned. The pedicled flap may be designed in a short or a long version.

Short type (Fig. 7.181). The base lies approximately 1 cm above the point of maximum lateral convexity of the malleolus and extends from the lateral edge of the Achilles tendon to the back of the lateral malleolus. This distance measures 3–4 cm. The flap extends vertically downwards with a slight anterior inclination to take it away from the posterior surface of the heel. It reaches the lateral edge of the plantar surface of the heel but does not encroach on the weight-bearing area. This distance measures about 8 cm. The flap can be made slightly wider at its tip than at its base if required.

Long type (Fig. 7.182). The base is the same but the flap curves anteriorly towards the tuberosity at the base of the fifth metatarsal, running parallel to the tendon of peroneus longus. The anterior edge of the flap crosses the retinaculum of the peroneal muscles and the posterior edge crosses abductor digiti minimi.

Island type (Fig. 7.183). The island may lie within the territory of the long or short flap. A proximal incision for dissection of the pedicle can be extended to 4 cm

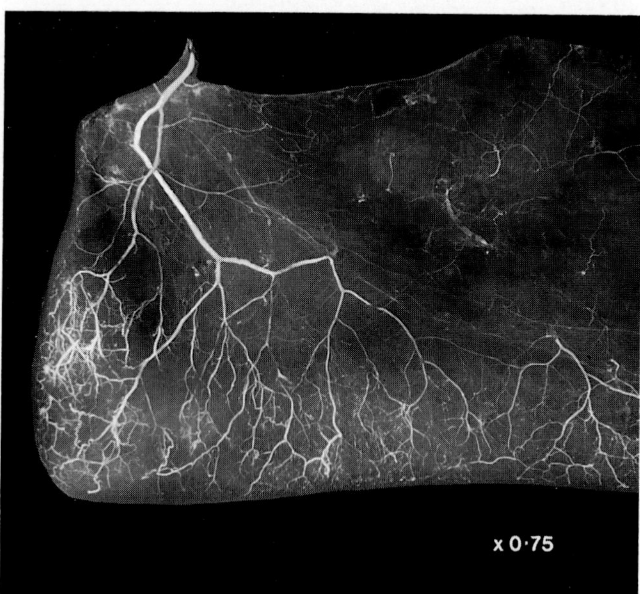

Fig. 7.180 Radiograph of skin over lateral aspect of calcaneum. In preparing this specimen for radiography the skin was incised in the dorsal midline downwards as far as the weight-bearing area of the heel. The incision then passed laterally along the lateral edge of the weight-bearing skin. The specimen included all the tissues between the periosteum of the calcaneum and the overlying skin in the area of the flap but preserved the peroneal tendons and covering retinaculum. This accounts for the abrupt termination of the main stem of the artery which at that point passed deeply beneath the tendon of peroneus brevis but branches to skin re-emerged further distally.

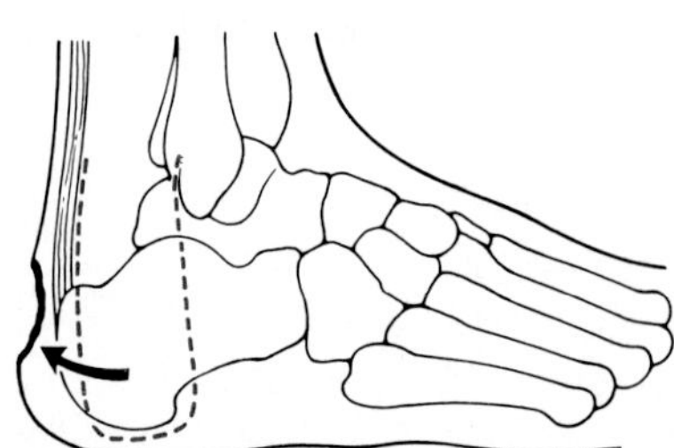

Fig. 7.181 Short type.

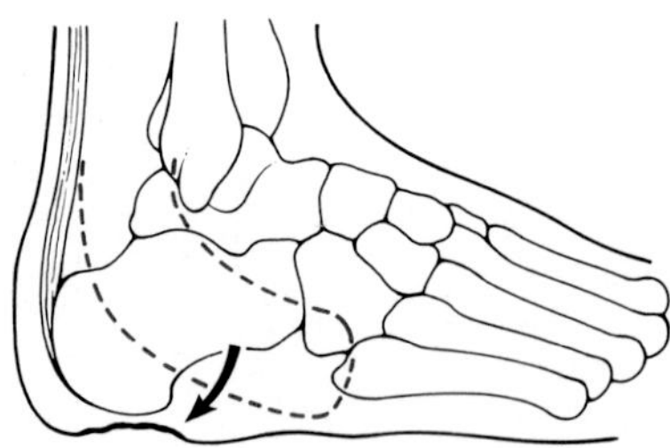

Fig. 7.182 Long type.

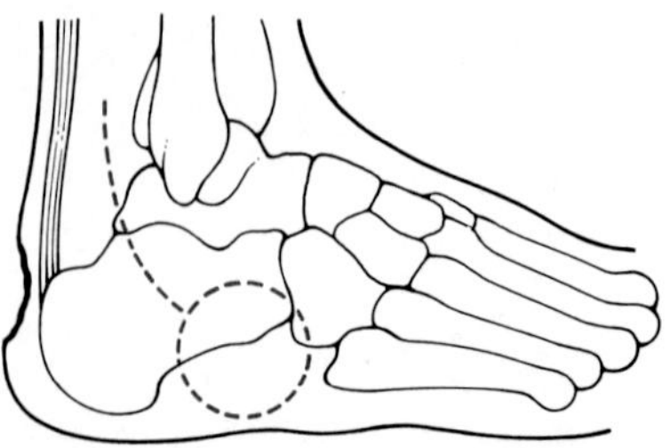

Fig. 7.183 Island type.

above the tip of the fibula. Note that in planning the flap, an increase in the arc of rotation is gained by moving the flap distally and not by moving the pivot point proximally.

Reverse type (Fig. 7.184). The base of the flap lies parallel to the peroneus brevis tendon but some 10 mm posterior to it, with a variable width between points 1 cm and 5 cm from the 5th metatarsal tuberosity. The flap extends posteriorly up to the edge of the Achilles tendon and may extend superiorly to a horizontal level corresponding to the point of maximum convexity of the fibular malleolus.

Surgery

Short type. The posterior incision is made and the correct plane is found by dissecting down to the periosteum over the calcaneus and undermining at this level. The neurovascular structures lie on the deep surface of the subcutaneous tissues. The anterior incision will require division of large veins.

Long type. The posterior incision follows the lateral edge of the Achilles tendon down to the calcaneus and then curves forwards towards the fifth metatarsal. The key to finding the right plane is again to start the undermining over the calcaneus and then to take it forwards over abductor digiti minimi. The anterior incision curves round the lateral malleolus and runs parallel to the posterior. Grabb & Argenta recommended that the distal end of the flap should not be incised at this stage. They applied a clamp across the distal end of the flap and carried out a fluorescein test. The flap was only divided if the full length of the flap fluoresced. If it did not then they divided the distal end of the flap in stages commencing one week after the first operation.

Island type. The proximal skin incision is made through the dermis and the margins elevated at the subdermal level so as to preserve the venous network on the pedicle. The dissection of the pedicle is carried out from distal to proximal, preserving paratenon over the tendons.

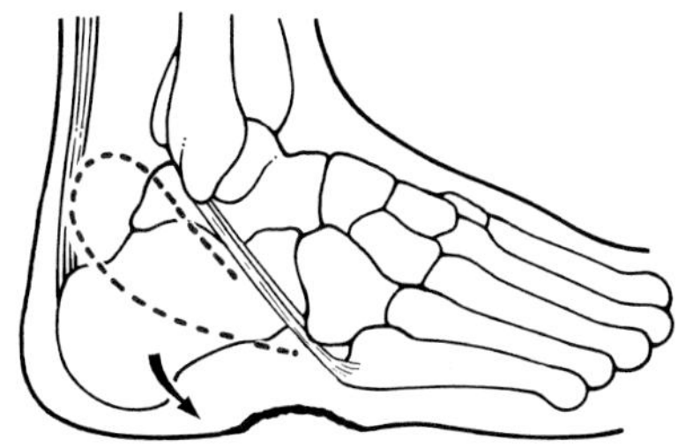

Fig. 7.184 Distally-based retrograde-flow flap.

The donor site is split skin grafted, and sufficient soft tissue should therefore be left on the os calcis so as to ensure 'take' of the graft.

The principal advantage of the island type of flap is that the pedicle is more flexible and thereby permits easier rotation of the flap with less likelihood of kinking the pedicle. With the island flap it may be possible to cover defects on the medial side of the foot just below and behind the medial malleolus. In this application excessive tension on the pedicle and necrosis of skin that has been undermined to create a tunnel for the pedicle are recognised hazards.

Reverse type. The elevation of the flap commences at the proximal end of the flap behind the lateral malleolus with the intention of exposing the terminal part of the peroneal artery (lateral calcaneal artery). This can then be clamped and pulsation distal to the clamp will reveal whether there is retrograde flow into the vessel. The flap is then elevated in a distal direction just above the periosteum of the calcaneus. Rather than try to dissect the very small vessels off the inferior peroneal retinaculum, Ishikawa et al advise detaching the lowermost calcaneal attachment of the inferior peroneal retinaculum off the calcaneum and elevating it with the flap. However, the distal anastomoses of the artery may lie around the peroneus brevis tendon where it emerges beyond the retinaculum. The flap may be islanded but a good subcutaneous pedicle must be preserved to include enough subcutaneous veins to provide an adequate venous drainage system for the flap.

References

1. Grabb W C, Argenta L C 1981 The lateral calcaneal artery skin flap. Plastic and Reconstructive Surgery 68: 723–730
2. Holmes J, Rayner C W R 1984 Lateral calcaneal artery island flaps. British Journal of Plastic Surgery 37: 402–405
3. Yanai A, Park S, Iwao T, Nakamura N 1985 Reconstruction of a skin defect of the posterior heel by a lateral calcaneal flap. Plastic and Reconstructive Surgery 75: 642–646
4. Gang R K 1987 Reconstruction of soft tissue defect of the posterior heel with a lateral calcaneal artery island flap. Plastic and Reconstructive Surgery 79: 415–419
5. Hovius S E R, Hofman A, Van der Meulen J C 1988 Experiences with the lateral calcaneal flap. Annals of Plastic Surgery 21: 532–535
6. Ishikawa K, Isshiki N, Hoshino K, Mori C 1990 Distally based lateral calcaneal flap. Annals of Plastic Surgery 24: 10–16

POPLITEAL ARTERY
– ascending branch
– inferior anastomotic artery
– superior lateral genicular artery

Popliteo-posterior thigh flap
Lateral genicular flap }
Genus lateralis flap }
Lower lateral thigh flap

Reconstruction of defects about the knee joint may be achieved with a variety of local flaps. Three of these are based on branches of the popliteal artery and have been termed the popliteo-thigh flap,[1] the lateral genicular flap (= genus lateralis flap),[2, 3, 4] and the lower postero-lateral thigh flap.[5] All are fasciocutaneous flaps.

Anatomy

The branches of the popliteal artery are described in detail on pages 244 to 246 but the key facts relating to these flaps will be summarised here.

1. The popliteal artery may give off an ascending branch from its proximal part, which reaches the deep fascia in the midline between biceps femoris and semimembranosus some 10 cm above the plane of the knee joint.
2. At a point between 3 and 5 cm below the adductor hiatus the popliteal gives off on its lateral side a vessel which supplies branches to vastus lateralis and biceps femoris before passing along the lateral intermuscular septum and emerging on the lateral aspect of the lower thigh to supply skin. It reaches skin approximately 9 cm above the plane of the knee joint. Masquelet,[4] in describing this vessel, uses the term Bourgery's artery or the inferior anastomotic artery.
3. Further on, the popliteal artery gives off the well-recognised superior lateral genicular artery which also reaches skin over the lateral inter-muscular septum approximately 5 cm above the plane of the knee joint.
4. The lateral branches to skin from the inferior anastomotic artery and from the superior lateral genicular artery are to some extent inversely related in size.
5. The lowermost (probably 4th) perforating branch of the profunda femoris may terminate by passing along the lateral intermuscular septum to reach skin approximately 13 cm above the knee joint.

The approximate points at which the various arteries reach the skin are indicated in centimetres above the plane of the knee joint in the following table:

Vascular pedicle	Mean	Range
Lower profunda perforator	13	Inconstant
Inferior anastomotic artery	9	8–10
Superior lateral genicular A	5	3–8

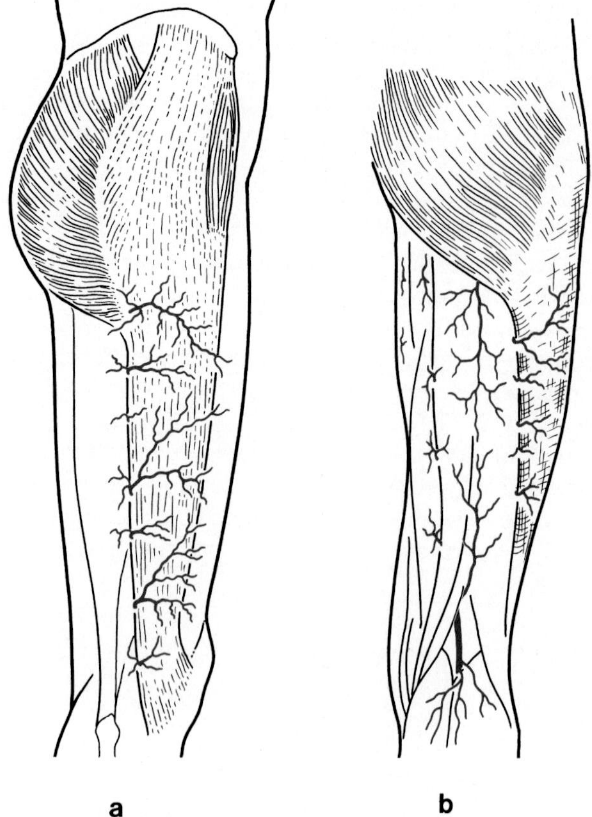

Fig. 7.185 Vascular anatomy: **a.** on the lateral aspect of the thigh perforators reach skin along the lateral intermuscular septum and fan out over the iliotibial tract; **b.** on the posterior thigh there is an ascending branch of the popliteal artery.

Popliteo-thigh flap (Fig. 7.187)

The vessel of the flap is not constant and Doppler flowmeter assessment may be helpful. It generally reaches the deep fascia some 8 to 10 cm above the plane of the knee joint in the company of venae comitantes and ascends in the midline. Here it may anastomose with the branch of the inferior gluteal artery that runs downwards in the company of the posterior cutaneous nerve of the thigh. This means that the flap may be extended upwards certainly to the level of the midthigh and on occasion as far as the gluteal crease. Maximum limits for the width of the flap have not been established but if the donor site is to be closed directly, then the width will be limited to a maximum of 10 cm. The arc of rotation takes in the area over the patella, the

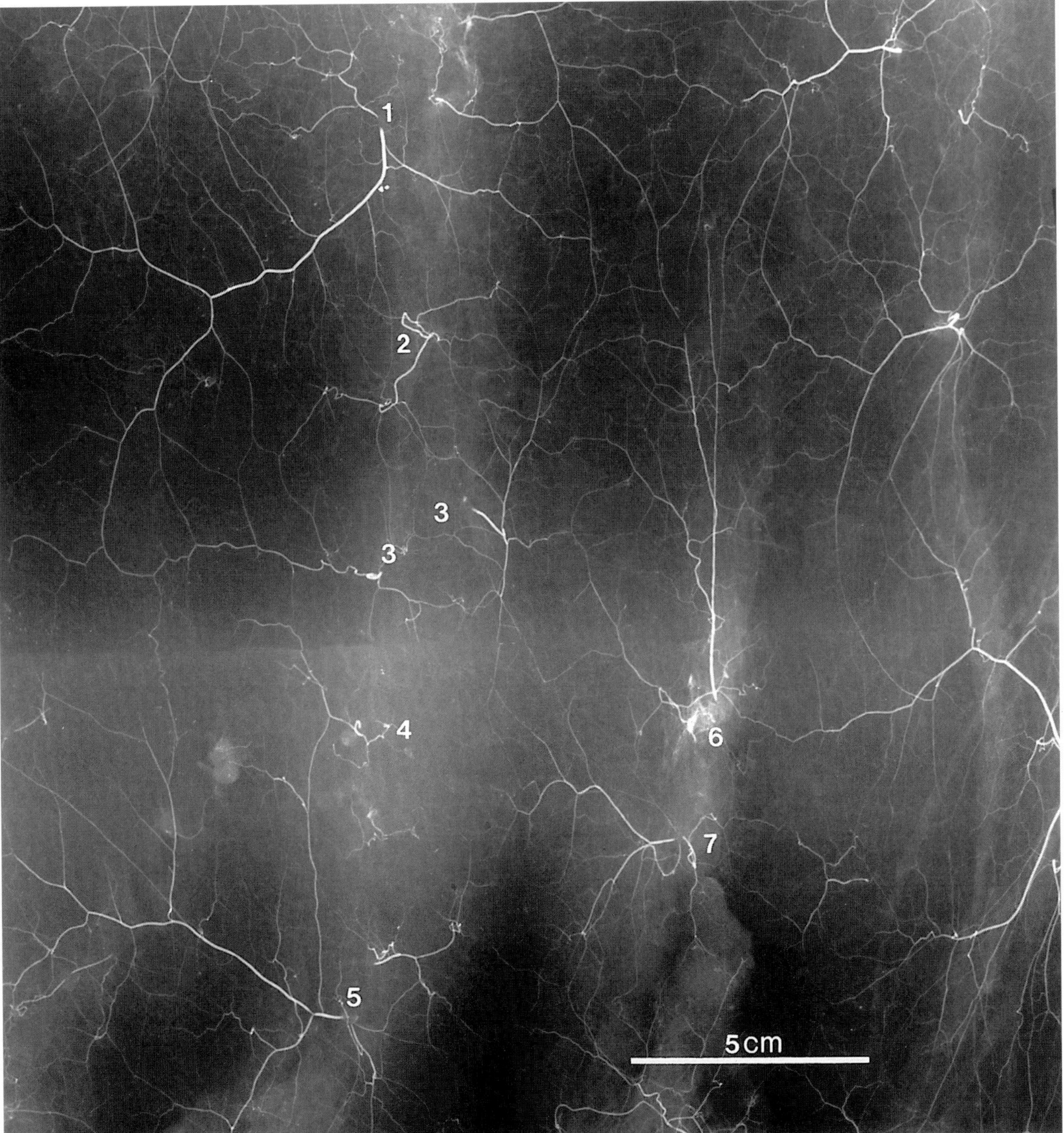

Fig. 7.186 Radiograph of the lower half of posterior and lateral thigh skin. The line of the lateral intermuscular septum occupies the centre of the picture and the skin to the left of this overlies the iliotibial tract (compare with Fig. 6.84). **1.** is from the third profunda femoris perforator, **2.** and **3.** are probably from the fourth profunda perforator, **4.** from the inferior anastomotic artery, in this case much smaller than **5.** from the superior lateral genicular artery. **6.** the ascending branch of the popliteal and **7.** another branch of the popliteal.

calf, and the sides though not the front, of the upper quarter of the leg.

In elevating the flap it is best to start at its lower end, taking the skin in continuity with the deep fascia and the septum between the biceps femoris and the semimembranosus. This will enable the vascular axis of the flap to be established. The remainder of the flap can then be elevated together with the intermuscular septum.

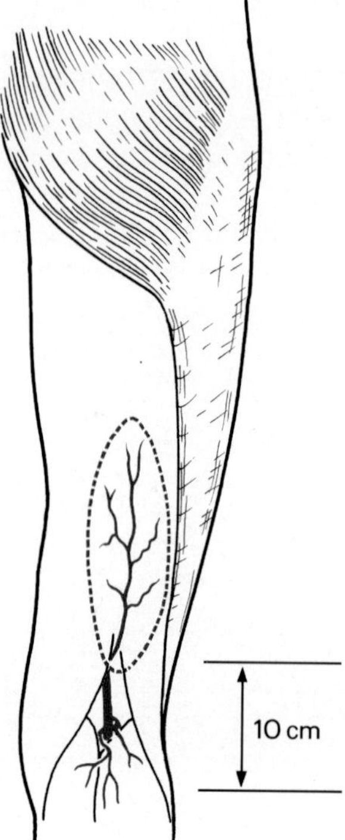

Fig. 7.187 Popliteo-posterior thigh flap.

Lateral genicular flap (Fig. 7.188)

An islanded flap based specifically on the cutaneous termination of the superior lateral genicular artery may be called the genus lateralis or lateral genicular flap. If the flap is based on the inferior anastomotic artery (Bourgery's A.) then it may be hard to know what to call it. However, unless the pedicle is dissected back, it will be hard to differentiate between these two vessels, indeed, both may be included in the flap. They both emerge along the fascial septum in the manner of septocutaneous perforators and then fan out above, rather than on, the iliotibial tract. This is probably because the tract is aponeurosis (of TFL) rather than deep fascia and it follows that the tract does not contribute significantly to the vascularity of the flap. In our experience, supported by others,[2] it is not necessary to raise the tract with the flap unless this is required as part of the reconstruction, e.g. for knee joint capsule or quadriceps mechanism.

Lower lateral thigh flap (Fig. 7.189)

It may be difficult to distinguish an artery emerging on the lateral thigh between 8 and 10 cm from the plane of the knee joint as being derived from the popliteal as opposed to the lowermost profunda femoris perforator. Such a vessel may be incorporated in the lateral genicular flap when it is created with a broad pedicle situated vertically so as to overlie the lateral intermuscular septum. This might best be termed a lower lateral thigh flap thereby maintaining a logical scheme to the naming of flaps on the lateral thigh as suggested by Laitung, viz:

Thigh flap	*Cutaneous vessel*
superior	1st profunda femoris perforating A.
middle	3rd profunda femoris perforating A.
lower	4th PFPA, inferior anastomotic A., and superior lateral genicular A.

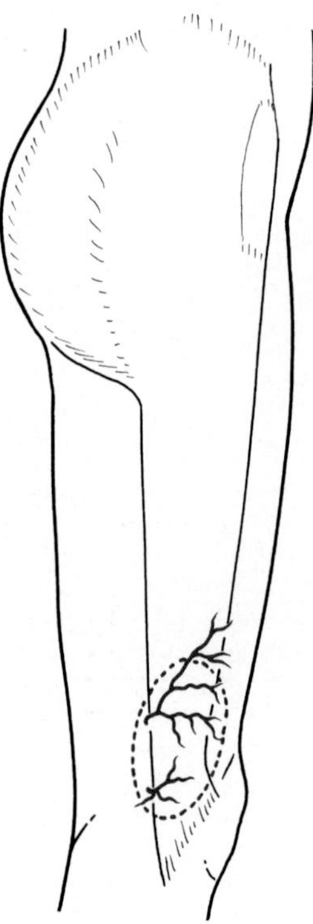

Fig. 7.188 Lateral genicular flap.

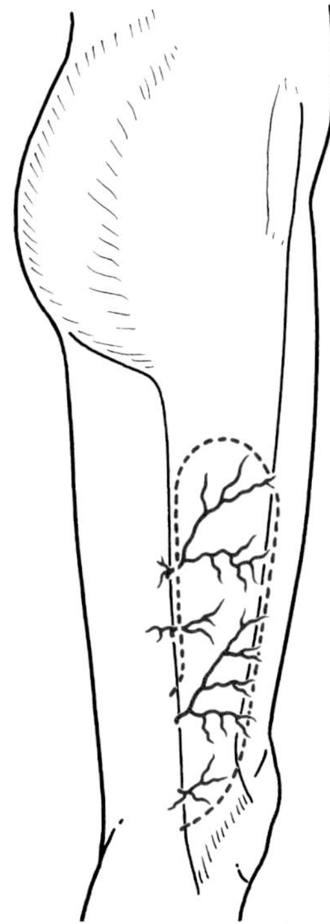

Fig. 7.189 Lower lateral thigh flap.

The longest flap successfully raised by the authors measured 25 cm and was based on two vessels as in Fig. 7.189. Generally 20 cm vertically by 10 cm horizontally will be the safe limits of the flap which is raised so as to leave a thin layer of loose areolar tissue over the iliotibial tract to ensure a successful take of a skin graft. Exposure and mobilisation of the pedicle, if required, will necessitate some division of the vastus lateralis and short head of biceps femoris.

Posterolateral thigh flap (Fig. 7.190)

When the lower lateral flap is designed with a broad horizontal base situated so as to include the vertical midline branch of the popliteal artery then this may become a posterolateral thigh flap.

References

1. Maruyama Y, Iwahira Y 1989 Popliteo-posterior thigh fasciocutaneous island flap for closure around the knee. British Journal of Plastic Surgery 42: 140–143
2. Hayashi A, Maruyama Y 1990 The lateral genicular artery flap. Annals of Plastic Surgery 24: 310–317
3. Oberlin C, Alnot J Y, Duparc J 1988 La couverture par lambeau des pertes de substance cutanée de la jambe et du pied, à propos de 76 cas. Revue de Chirurgie Orthopedique et Reparatrice de l'Appareil Moteur 74: 526–538
4. Masquelet A C, Bessa J, Romana M C 1989 Bourgery's artery: anatomic basis for a new cutaneous skin flap. Surgical and Radiologic Anatomy 11: 249–253
5. Laitung J K G 1989 The lower postero-lateral thigh flap. British Journal of Plastic Surgery 42: 133–139
6. Satoh K, Gyoutoku H, Usami Y 1990 Suprapopliteal flap. Annals of Plastic Surgery 24: 459–466

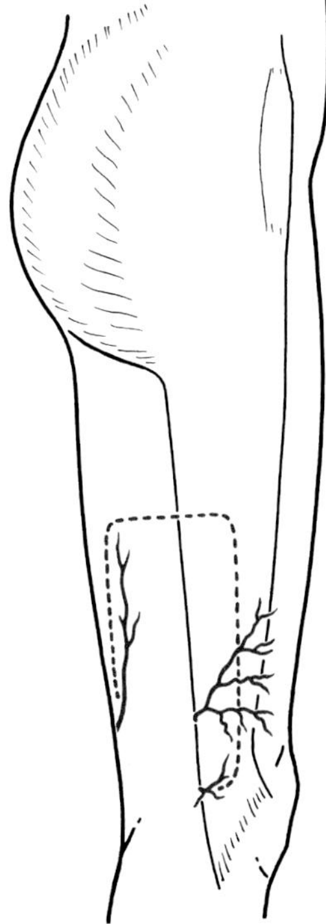

Fig. 7.190 Lower posterolateral thigh flap.

POSTERIOR AURICULAR ARTERY

Fasciocutaneous free flap

The possibility of raising a free flap of skin from behind the ear based on the posterior auricular artery was first demonstrated by Fujino et al.[1, 2] His flap measured 4 cm × 5 cm × 6 cm and was used for nasal reconstruction.

A pedicled flap of postauricular skin, combined with a postero-superior extension consisting of fascia from beneath the hair-bearing parietal scalp has also been described. This was designed by Song[3] for use in ear reconstruction and the purpose of the fascial component was to act as a well-vascularised layer which would cover a fabricated cartilagenous auricle and/or the defect resulting from moving the postauricular skin, and would readily accept a split skin graft. Chul Park et al[4] have described pedicled flaps based on branches of the artery used for reconstructing small ear defects.

Kohle and Leonard have also described free flaps.[5, 6]

Anatomy

The posterior auricular artery arises from the external carotid (85%) or the occipital artery (15%) and passes up between the mastoid process and the ear to reach the deep fascia at a variable level but usually at about the level of the external auditory meatus where it divides into two terminal branches. These posterior auricular vessels are small and somewhat unreliable. In the case reported by Fujino the artery measured 0.7 mm in diameter, and of the four veins present, the largest measured 1.0 mm and the next largest only 0.5 mm in diameter. The auricular branch of the artery passes up deep to the auricularis posterior muscle, gives off three or four branches to the cranial surface of the auricle and anastomoses with parietal branches of the superficial temporal artery. One or two of its branches pierce the concha to supply skin on the external surface of the auricle. The occipital branch runs back over the insertion of sternomastoid, supplies skin and the occipital belly of occipito-frontalis and anastomoses with the occipital artery.

A significant feature of the skin behind the ear is that it has an extensive small vessel plexus. As a result, in the Europid the characteristic colour which the plexus gives to a vascularised flap may mean that the skin is too red for a good match on parts of the face whereas in the Oriental the skin appears to be a better colour match to that of the nose, cheek or eyelid.

Surgery

Due to the variability of the vessel no firm guidelines can be given to developing the free flap; note, however, that the auricular branch will need to be freed from beneath auricularis posterior.

The use of a skin and fascial flap for otoplasty is illustrated in Figures 7.193A–D. In Figure 7.193A the superficial temporal artery and the posterior auricular artery have been marked, and the intended shape and position of the ear reconstruction outlined using a reversed pattern prepared from the normal ear. In Figure 7.193B the incisions are shown by which an antero-inferiorly pedicled flap of retroauricular skin and fascia are created. The incisions labelled 'a' delineate the sides of the flap and pass through the full thickness of skin and deep fascia; branches of the superficial temporal and occipital arteries will need to be ligated and divided. The line labelled 'c' indicates an incision

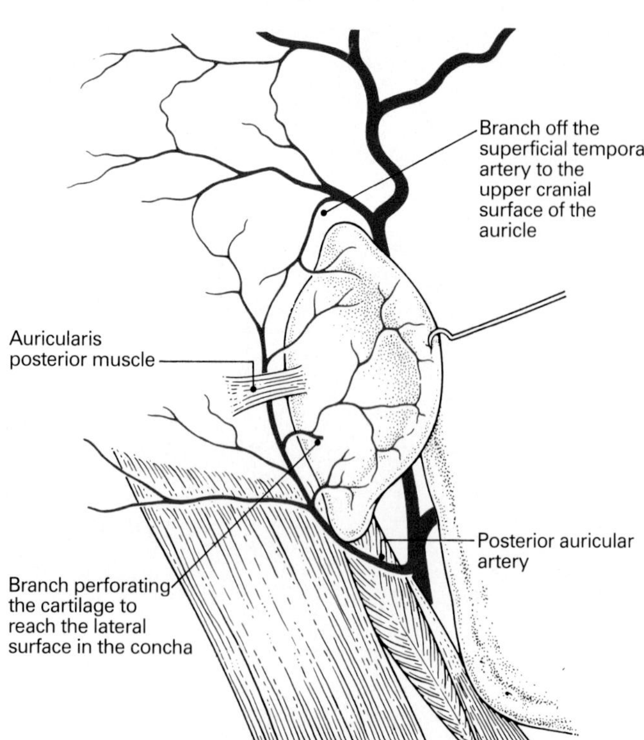

Fig. 7.191 Vascular anatomy. Schematic situation – the branch from the superficial temporal artery is not always present.

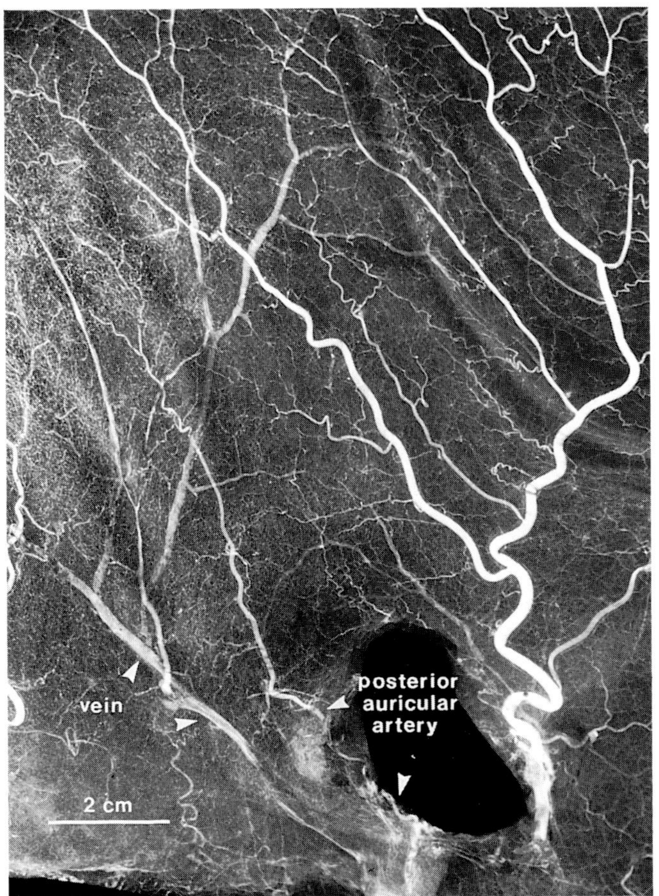

Fig. 7.192 Radiograph of postauricular skin. The auricle has been removed from the specimen. The branch from the superficial temporal artery shown in Fig. 7.191 is not present.

which passes through dermis only; the hair-bearing scalp between 'b' and 'c' is then elevated off the underlying fascia so that the vessels supplying the fascia are preserved. The fascia is then divided along 'b' and can be elevated in an anterior direction until the whole skin and fascial flap is attached only by its pedicle. The cartilage framework for the reconstruction is sculptured from the sixth and seventh costal cartilages in the usual way and is placed beneath the elevated flap. A wedge of cartilage is fixed in position so as to hold the carved auricle out from the side of the skull at an angle of about 30°. The skin and fascial flap is tucked round behind the ear to cover its cranial surface and the fascial flap also extends onto the temporal bone. The incisions are closed and a split skin graft sutured over the bare fascia (Fig. 7.193C). Rudimentary auricular remnants 'd' around the external auditory means may be used to fashion a tragus and ear lobule.

References

1. Fujino T 1975 Third International Symposium on Microsurgery, East Grinstead
2. Fujino T, Harashina T, Nakajima T 1976 Free skin flap from the retroauricular region to the nose. Plastic and Reconstructive Surgery 57: 338–341
3. Song R, Chen Z, Yang P, Yue J 1982 Reconstruction of the external ear. Clinics in Plastic Surgery 9: 49–52
4. Chul Park, Keuk Shun Shin, Ho Suck Kang, Young Ho Lee, Jae Duk Lew 1988 A new arterial flap from the postauricular surface: its anatomic basis and clinical application. Plastic and Reconstructive Surgery 82: 498–504
5. Kolhe P S, Leonard A G 1987 The posterior auricular flap: anatomical studies. British Journal of Plastic Surgery 40: 562–569
6. Leonard A G, Kolhe P S 1987 The posterior auricular flap: intra-oral reconstruction. British Journal of Plastic Surgery 40: 570–581

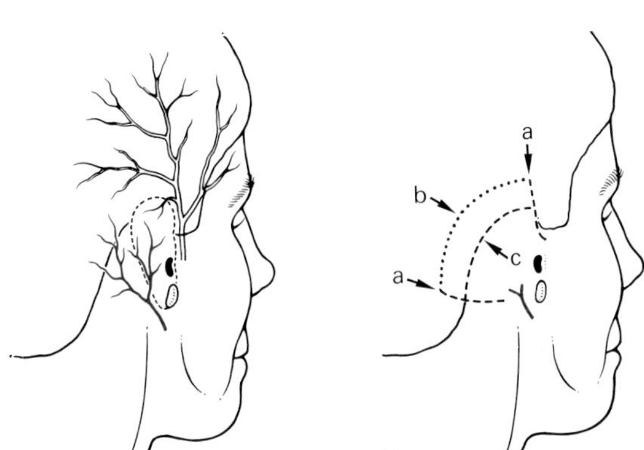

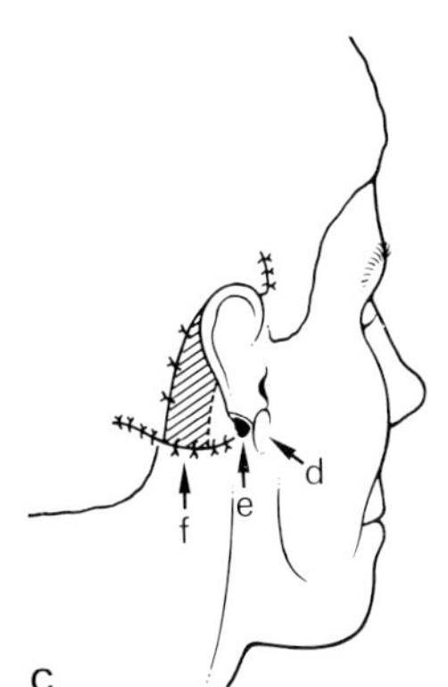

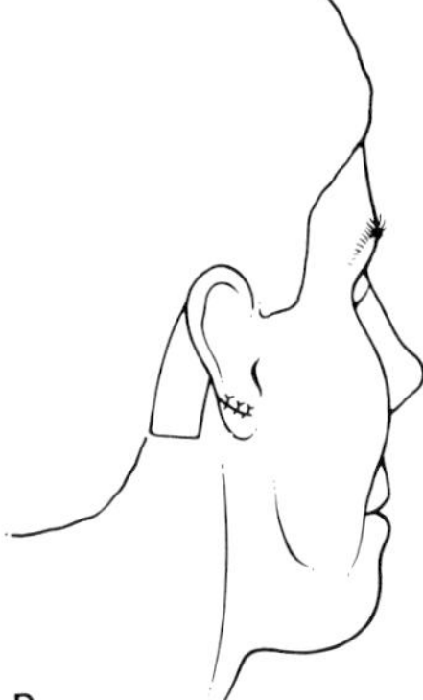

Fig. 7.193 Ear reconstruction using a flap based on the posterior auricular artery. **A.** Principal landmarks, **B.** Planning of incisions and creation of flap, **C.** Covering the cartilage model, **D.** Final stage.

7 POSTERIOR CIRCUMFLEX HUMERAL ARTERY – cutaneous branch

Deltoid flap

The deltoid flap was designed by Franklin[1] and is based on a branch of the posterior circumflex humeral artery which pierces the posterior edge of deltoid and runs vertically upwards towards the acromion. This vessel was known to 19th-century anatomists and was termed the arteria deltoidea subcutanea posterior by Manchot but it is not currently recognised in *Nomina Anatomica*. The deltoid flap is a recent development and is invariably used as a free flap.

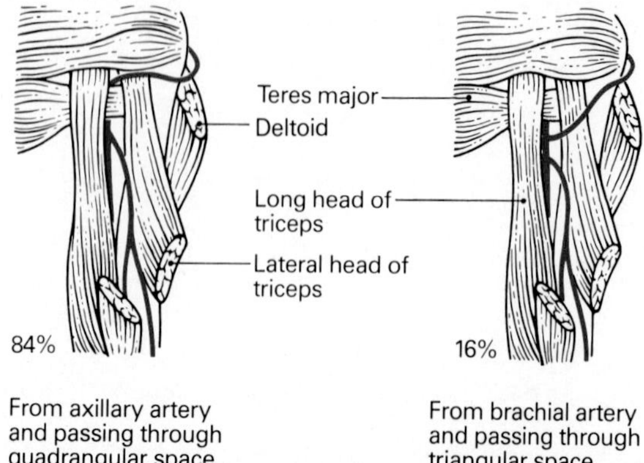

Fig. 7.194 Origin and course of the posterior circumflex humeral artery.

Anatomy

The posterior circumflex humeral artery (for variations see p. 182) passes posteriorly round the humerus either above or below teres major to anastomose beneath deltoid with the anterior circumflex humeral artery (Fig. 7.194). It gives off multiple branches of supply to the muscle, and some of these vessels then pierce the surface of the muscle to supply skin and anastomose in the subcutis with adjacent perforators. The arteria deltoidea subcutanea is a particularly large and constant branch to the skin. It measures 0.75–1.5 mm in internal diameter at its point of origin from the posterior circumflex humeral artery close to where that vessel approaches teres minor. It either passes round the posterior border of deltoid or pierces the muscle near its edge to then run vertically upwards in the subcutaneous fat towards the acromion giving off multiple branches which fan out mainly anterosuperiorly but also posterosuperiorly (Figs 7.195 & 7.196). It anastomoses anteriorly with musculocutaneous perforators from the anterior circumflex humeral artery, posteromedially with small branches from the circumflex scapular artery, and superiorly with the supraclavicular artery and the rete acromiale branches of the thoracoacromial axis.

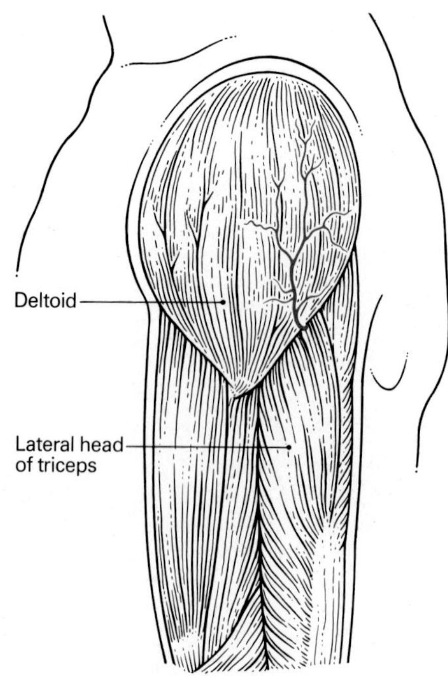

Fig. 7.195 Vascular anatomy. Emergence and course of the posterior deltoid subcutaneous artery.

Planning

The point of emergence of the cutaneous artery around the edge of deltoid is established by drawing a line on the back of the arm between the acromion and the medial epicondyle of the humerus. The vessel lies at or immediately posterior to the point where this line crosses the posterior border of deltoid. From this point the vessel passes vertically upwards and such a line marks the axis of a long ellipse which constitutes the territory of the flap (Fig. 7.197). The upper limit of this flap can be taken to the acromion but it is best not to go onto it. The upper lateral cutaneous nerve of the arm may accompany the artery around the posterior part of deltoid and is distributed to the lower part of the flap. The vessel is accompanied by venae comitantes in the manner of a direct cutaneous artery.

Surgery

After marking the outlines of the flap, the postero-inferior margin is incised over 5–8 cm to confirm the location of the vessel supporting the proposed flap. Care must be taken to ensure that this initial incision lies posterior to the fascial 'septum' between the posterior margin of deltoid and the lateral head of triceps. Dissection proceeds down the posterior aspect of this fascial septum – deep to deltoid towards the neck of the humerus – in a relatively bloodless plane except for one large branch from the PCHA which pierces the lateral head of triceps. If the vessel of the flap runs around the posterior edge of deltoid in the expected position then the posterior margin incision is extended superiorly over the posterior part of deltoid. The anterior margin of the ellipse is then incised and the remainder of the flap is then elevated from anterior to posterior in a plane immediately on deltoid with division of several musculocutaneous perforators (i.e. incision of the margin proceeds anticlockwise on the left side or clockwise on the right side). This leads onto the anterior aspect of the inferior part of the fascial 'septum' whose posterior border has already been freed from triceps. The arterial and venous pedicles lie within this septum. If the artery supplying the flap actually pierces the posterior part of deltoid then this will be seen when the elevation of the flap off deltoid is nearly completed and the muscle fibres between the vessel and the free posterior margin of the muscle must then be divided in

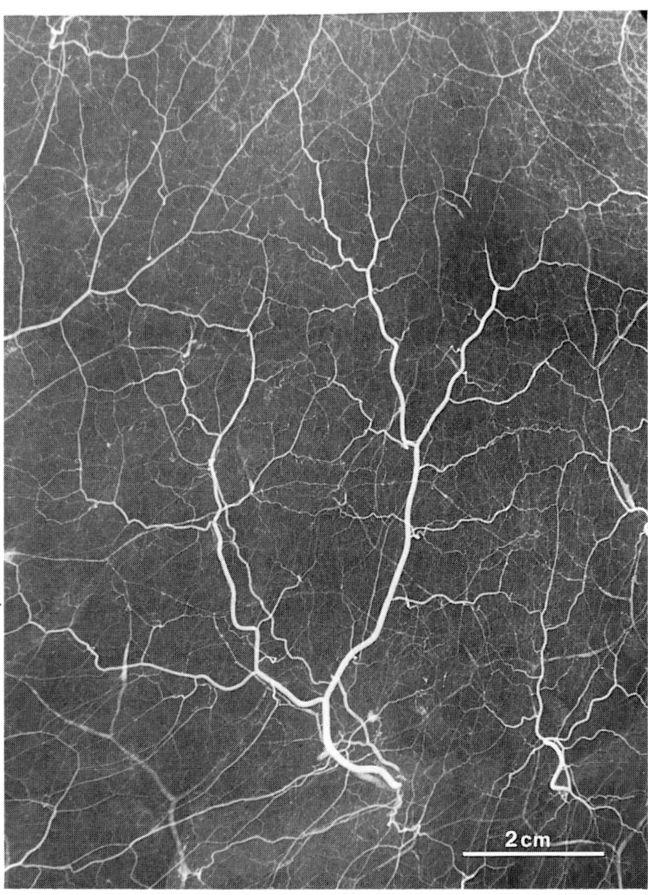

Fig. 7.196 Radiograph of the cutaneous part of the posterior deltoid subcutaneous artery. The segment of the pedicle which lies deep to deltoid has not been removed with the specimen.

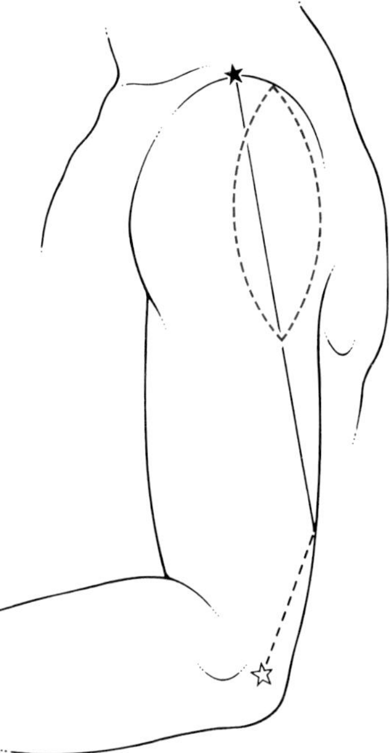

Fig. 7.197 Flap planning. The artery turns round the posterior border of deltoid where this is crossed by a line between the medial epicondyle of the humerus and the tip of the acromion. The long axis of the elliptical flap ascends vertically from this point.

order to free the pedicle. The pedicle is then mobilised and this requires strong upward retraction of the posterior border of deltoid by an assistant. The pedicle can be traced up to the PCHA and a portion of this may be removed in order to provide a pedicle of sufficient length and adequate diameter for microvascular anastomosis. Venae comitantes of the cutaneous artery supplying the flap provide venous drainage – these drain into veins accompanying the PCHA. The deep dissection of this pedicle is made difficult by the limited exposure and the presence of the axillary nerve.

References

1. Franklin J D 1984 The deltoid flap: anatomy and clinical applications. In: Bunke H J, Furnas D W (eds) Symposium on clinical frontiers in reconstructive microsurgery. Vol 24. C V Mosby, St Louis, p 63–70
2. Cormack G C, Lamberty B G H 1984 Fasciocutaneous vessels in the upper arm – application to the design of new fasciocutaneous flaps. Plastic and Reconstructive Surgery 74: 244–249
3. Rijavec M C, Ruiz S 1983 The deltoid flap (Spanish). Cirurgia Plastica Argentina 7: 8
4. Murray R A, Rabt M T, Singh G B, Russell R C 1985 The deltoid free flap; anatomical studies and clinical experiences. British Journal of Plastic Surgery 38: 437
5. Russell R C, Guy R J, Zook E G, Merrell J C 1985 Extremity reconstruction using the free deltoid flap. Plastic and Reconstructive Surgery 76: 586–595
6. Harashina T, Inoue T, Tanaka I, Imai K, Hatoko M 1990 Reconstruction of penis with free deltoid flap. British Journal of Plastic Surgery 43: 217–222

POSTERIOR INTEROSSEOUS ARTERY

Posterior interosseous artery flap
Fasciocutaneous posterior forearm flap
Osteocutaneous flap

A septocutaneous island flap based on the posterior interosseous artery (PIA) was first presented by Zancolli at a meeting in Sweden in 1985 and published in English by Zancolli and Angrigiani in 1988.[1] Other reports[2, 3, 4] have further confirmed the feasibility of raising a skin island in the proximal forearm supplied by the PIA and isolating this on a distal pedicle with retrograde flow in the artery. In this design the flap has application in reconstruction around the first web space, the wrist area, and the dorsum of the hand. Its combination with a segment of the ulna for thumb reconstruction has been described.[5] A distally situated skin island on a proximal pedicle is a possible method of transferring a skin island into the area in front of the elbow or over the olecranon but would not be a flap of first choice.

Flaps based on the interosseous recurrent artery (with or without the anconeus muscle) are described under the interosseous recurrent artery.

Anatomy

The posterior interosseous artery (PIA) enters the posterior compartment of the forearm at the lower border of supinator where it joins the deep radial nerve. At this point its external diameter averages 1.7 mm (range 1.2–2.6 mm). Here the PIA gives off the interosseous recurrent artery which passes back beneath anconeus to the elbow, giving off two or three perforators which pass round the lateral border of that muscle. The PIA, accompanied by venae comitantes, then passes down the forearm deep to the interval between the extensor digiti minimi (the most ulnar part of extensor digitorum) and the extensor carpi ulnaris, crossing in turn the origins of the abductor pollicis longus, extensor pollicis longus and extensor indicis. It ends by anastomosing over the distal radius with the terminal branches of the anterior interosseous artery and with the dorsal carpal arch (Fig. 7.199b). In its course it gives off up to six significantly sized perforators and several minute ones which pass up along the fascial septum between extensor digiti minimi and extensor carpi ulnaris (Fig. 7.199a). Other important relationships in its course are that it gives off up to 20 branches which cross superficially over the deep radial nerve to reach the extensor muscles while it is itself crossed by the branch of the radial nerve that innervates extensor carpi ulnaris.

Of the perforators the most proximal is generally the largest and the remainder are distributed either at regular intervals down the forearm or in proximal and distal groupings. The width of the skin territory supplied by the PIA is of the order of 5 cm.

Venae comitantes are variable with either one or two present.

It has been found that in a small number of cases the PIA may be rapidly dissipated in the proximal part of the posterior compartment and that the distal part is taken over by a large perforator from the anterior interosseous artery which perforates the interosseous membrane in the middle part of the forearm.

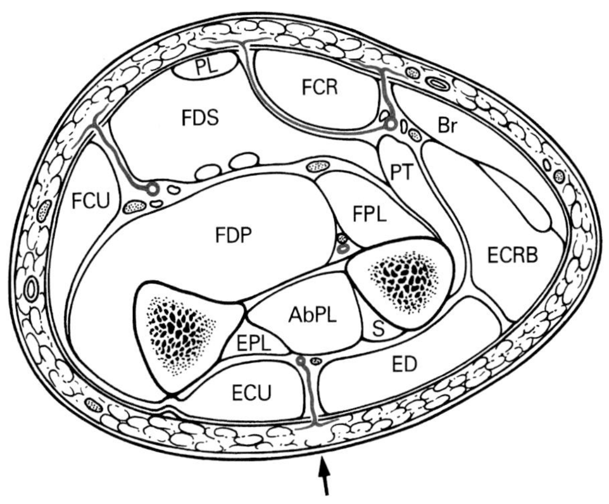

Fig. 7.198 Vascular anatomy. Transverse section of forearm in middle third showing location of posterior interosseous artery, perforators to skin and the part of the ulna that may be harvested in the composite flap.

Flap planning

The surface marking of the intermuscular septum between EDM and ECU is made with the elbow flexed and the forearm in the neutral position mid-way between full supination and full pronation. A line is drawn between the lateral epicondyle and the distal radio-ulna joint with a slight ulnar convexity. The point of entry of the PIA into the posterior compartment is surface marked on this line at the junction of its proximal third with its distal two-thirds. The location of the anastomosis between the terminal PIA and the terminal AIA is marked some 2 cm proximal to the radio-carpal joint. This marking determines the most distal point about which the arc of rotation may be taken although the centre of rotation may of course be more proximally located if desired. The flap is then outlined so that the distance from the rotation point to the proximal end of the defect to be reconstructed on the hand is not more than the distance from the distal edge of the flap to the rotation point. The outline of the flap is then dictated by the defect and will generally be located with its centre just distal to the point where the PIA enters the posterior compartment at the junction of the upper one-third with the lower two-thirds.

Surgery

The incision starts distally at the rotation point and passes proximally along the marked line and then around the radial margin of the proposed flap. Starting at this radial edge the flap is elevated off the extensor digitorum communis and the fascial septum between EDM and ECU identified. The septum is traced deeply to reveal the PIA and the continuation of the deep radial nerve. At the proximal end of the PIA it will be possible to see whether or not the flap is supplied by a large

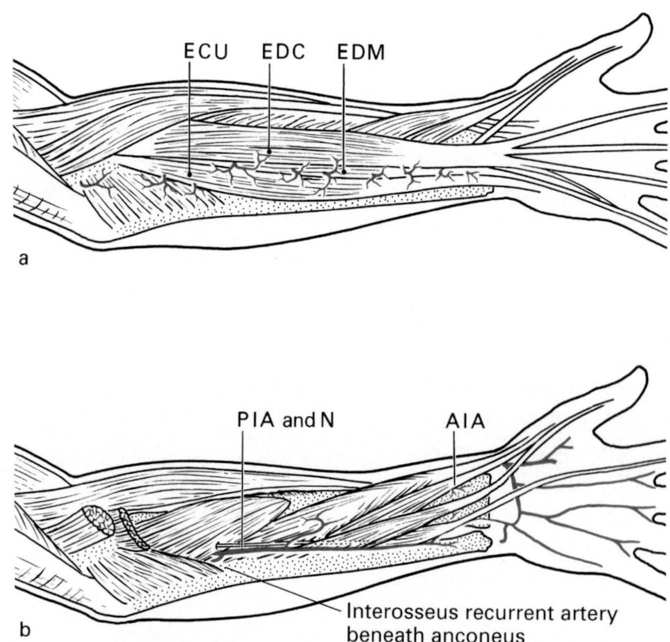

Fig. 7.199 Vascular anatomy: **a.** disposition of perforators; **b.** superficial muscles removed to show deep pedicle and relationship to deep part of radial nerve.

perforator arising from the interosseous recurrent artery. If so the proximal arterial division will have to be through the PIA before it branches and through its interosseous recurrent branch above the point where it gives off its perforator; otherwise the PIA is ligated distal to the origin of the recurrent branch and proximal to its first perforator. Having established the presence of perforators to the marked outline of the intended flap, the ulnar border may then be incised, the flap elevated off the muscles up to the septum, and the flap then raised with its vascular pedicle whilst preserving the deep radial nerve. The numerous branches of the artery to the muscles will need to be divided. The maximum width of the flap that is supported by perforators probably does not exceed 8 cm at the maximum (the anatomical territory of supply is approximately 5 cm in width). If the flap is less than 4 cm in width then it will usually be possible to close the donor site directly.

If bone is required with the flap this is raised from the proximal third of the ulna. Vascularisation of the bone is through an attached cuff of the extensor pollicis longus muscle with preservation of the branches from the PIA to this piece of muscle. In the descriptions of this method by Costa et al[4, 8] an 8 cm long segment of ulna was raised from the radial side of the ulna by separating it from the interosseous membrane (Fig. 7.198). In the reported cases in which a bone segment was used it was for lengthening a thumb amputation stump. In this situation the damage to the extensor pollicis longus will be of no consequence as there will be no interphalangeal joint for the tendon to extend. Use of such a vascularised bone segment for other reconstructions would probably not be acceptable because of the interference with EPL.

Technical aspects are crucial to the success of the flap. The nutrient vascular pedicle is working at a low pressure and external compression must be avoided. A volar slab holding the wrist at 40° of extension should be used for one week to decrease dorsal skin tension over the pedicle.

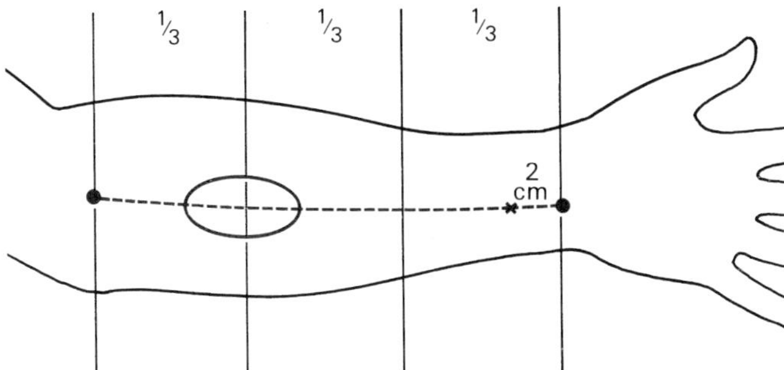

Fig. 7.200 Flap planning. See text for explanation.

References

1. Zancolli E A, Angrigiani C 1986 Posterior interosseous island forearm flap. The Journal of Hand Surgery 138: 130–135
2. Penteado C V, Masquelet A C, Chevrel J P 1986 The anatomic basis of the fascio-cutaneous flap of the posterior interosseous artery. Surgical and Radiologic Anatomy 8: 209–215
3. Costa H, Soutar D S 1988 The distally based island posterior interosseous flap. The British Journal of Plastic Surgery 41: 221–227
4. Costa H, Smith R, McGrouther D A 1988 Thumb reconstruction by the posterior interosseous osteocutaneous flap. British Journal of Plastic Surgery 41: 228–233
5. Ding Y, Sun G, Lu Y, Ly S 1989 The vascular microanatomy of skin territory of posterior forearm and its clinical application. Annals of Plastic Surgery 22: 126–134
6. Nakajima H, Fujino T, Adachi S 1986 A new concept of vascular supply to the skin and classification of skin flaps according to their vascularization. Annals of Plastic Surgery 16: 1–17;
7. Landi A, Luchetti R, Soragni O, De Santis G, Sacchetti G L 1991 The distally based posterior interosseous island flap for the coverage of skin loss of the hand. Annals of Plastic Surgery 27: 527–536
8. Costa H, Comba S, Martins A, Rodrigues J, Reis J, Amarante J 1991 Further experience with the posterior interosseous flap. British Journal of Plastic Surgery 44: 449–455
9. Arnež Z M 1992 Letter to Editor: Posterior interosseous flap. British Journal of Plastic Surgery 45: 181–184

7 POSTERIOR TIBIAL ARTERY

Lower leg fasciocutaneous flap
— proximal base
— distal base
— islanded on single perforator

The development of the fasciocutaneous concept was largely initiated by Pontén's demonstration of the safety and reliability of lower leg flaps which had been raised so as to include the deep fascia.[1] Some of these flaps were situated on the medial aspect of the leg and depended for their survival on the anastomoses at the level of the deep fascia between fasciocutaneous perforators from the posterior tibial artery. The early flaps of this design were all proximally-based. In 1986 Amarante et al[2] demonstrated that distally-based flaps were just as reliable and much more useful for reconstructing defects in the lower third of the leg and around the heel and ankle. Further development of this concept has led to flaps being islanded on a single perforator with its accompanying venae comitantes and rotated through up to 180° on such a pedicle.[3, 4]

Anatomy

The first cutaneous vessel on the medial side of the lower leg usually arises from the inferior medial genicular artery but the saphenous branch of the descending genicular artery may occasionally extend below the level of the knee joint. Below this the posterior tibial artery gives off a series of five or six perforators. These vessels emerge between soleus and flexor digitorum longus and frequently perforate the deep fascia at circumscribed openings which also serve as the routes by which perforating veins connect the superficial venous network to the deep veins. The perforators tend to be largest proximally with an internal diameter of 0.3–0.77 mm. On reaching the deep fascia they divide into two or three branches which diverge anteriorly and posteriorly in a slightly descending direction. These vessels then give off multiple finer branches which ascend and descend so as to interconnect adjacent perforators. This plexus lies at the level of the deep fascia and supplies the skin.

Posteriorly in the calf region these vessels meet the medial superficial sural artery and musculocutaneous perforators through gastrocnemius from the medial sural artery; lower down over the Achilles tendon these branches of the posterior tibial anastomose with branches from the peroneal artery. Anteriorly these perforators anastomose with the plexus around the knee, especially the branches of the medial inferior genicular and saphenous arteries. Lower down, over the anterior border of the tibia the perforators anastomose with branches of the anterior tibial artery and with the artery that accompanies the superficial peroneal nerve.

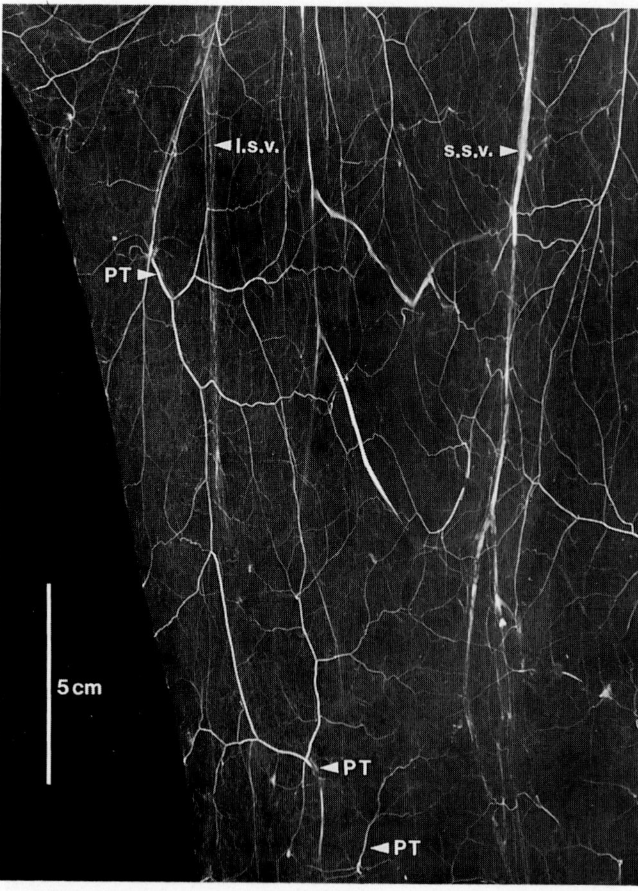

Fig. 7.201 The radiograph of skin shows two large perforators labelled **PT**. A small amount of contrast has penetrated through into the venous side of the circulation and delineates the long and short saphenous veins. The left-hand edge of the specimen was created by a longitudinal incision over the middle of the subcutaneous surface of the tibia. The arterial branches coming into the specimen in its superior part are terminal branches of the saphenous artery which may extend for a variable distance onto the medial aspect of the lower leg.

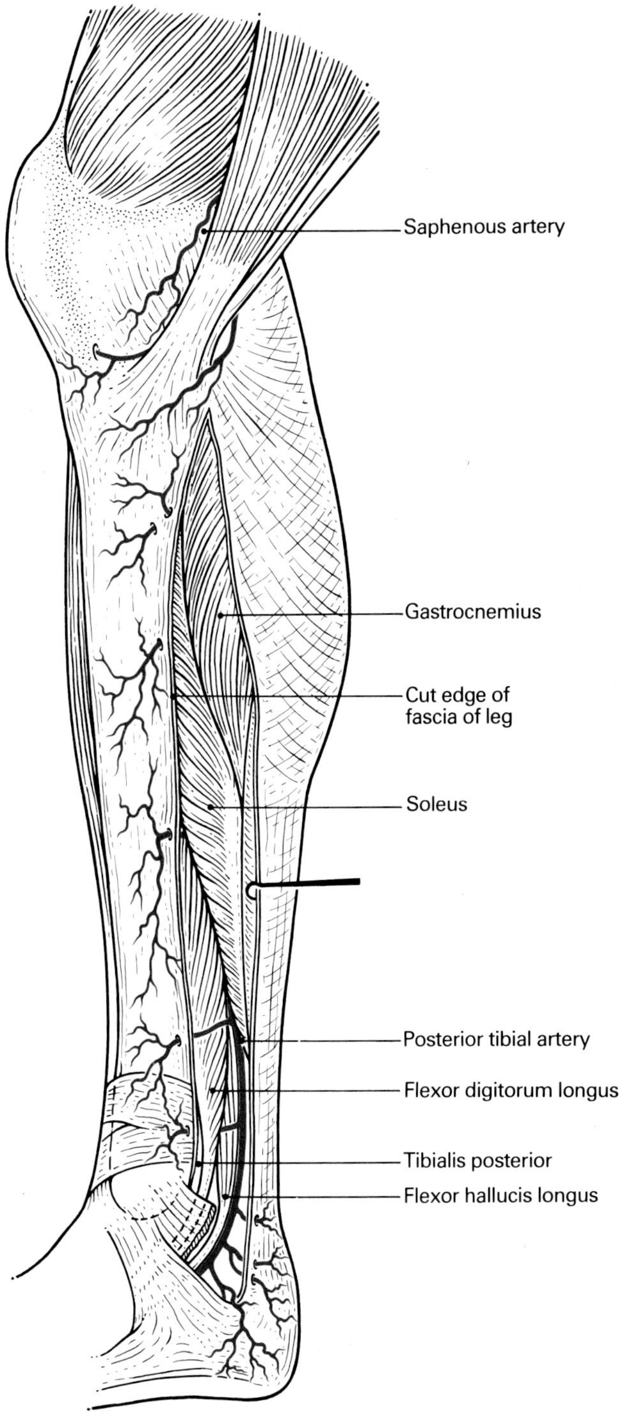

7

Flap planning

Proximally-based flaps (Fig. 7.203)
The flap design is obviously determined by the defect and whether the flap is intended for the opposite or the same leg, but in general terms the medial leg fasciocutaneous flap is designed with the base situated proximally and with proportions of up to 3:1. Flaps of even greater length than this up to 5:1 have survived. Inclusion of the saphenous vein is beneficial to the venous drainage of the flap. The flap is often used to procure skin cover over exposed tibia and therefore tends to be situated with more of the flap lying behind rather than in front of the line of the emerging perforators. The incisions are carried through skin, subcutaneous fat and fascia and the dissection is then carried out from one of the long incisions. A thin layer of loose areolar tissue exists beneath the fascia and should as far as possible be left undisturbed on the underlying structures so as to provide a good base for split skin grafting the donor site. As the base of the flap is approached care must be taken to conserve a suitable major perforator to supply the flap. Pontén has stated that a limited back-cut through the deep fascia may be required at this point to enable the flap to be more easily rotated into the defect, but this must clearly spare any major perforators and fascial vessels.

Fig. 7.202 Vascular anatomy. Branches of the posterior tibial artery are shown reaching the medial side of the leg by passing between soleus and flexor digitorum longus where they then fan out superiorly and inferiorly on the superficial surface of the deep fascia. The emerging perforators also give off branches to the periosteum of the subcutaneous surface of the tibia but these have *not* been shown on the diagram.

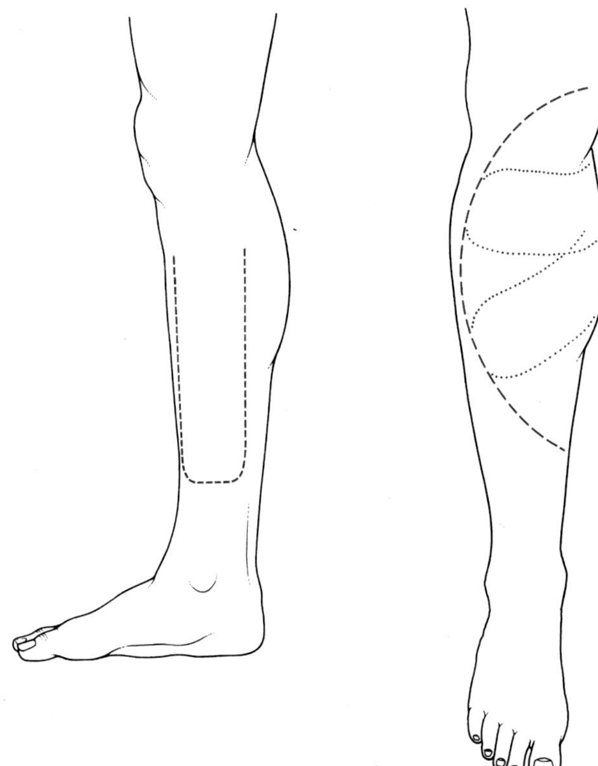

Fig. 7.203 Flap planning. A typical flap outline is shown on the left but position and dimension vary. Arc of rotation shown on right.

Distally-based flaps (Fig. 7.204a)

This flap is the medial equivalent of the distally-based flap on the lateral aspect supplied by peroneal artery perforators (see Fig. 7.169). In the example shown in Figure 7.204a the flap is used for reconstructing a distal defect as a two stage procedure but a more common application is for cover of a contiguous pre-tibial defect. The flap is usually based on a single perforator from the posterior tibial artery which reaches the deep fascia at a level approximately 8 cm above the tip of the medial malleolus. The next most distal perforator lying approximately 4 cm above the malleolus also contributes to the vascular input to the base of the flap. The locations of the perforators should be confirmed preoperatively with a Doppler probe. The flap extends proximally from the 8 cm perforator to overlie the medial head of gastrocnemius and is supported by the fascial plexus. The proximal limit of the flap lies approximately 10 cm below the plane of the knee joint. Flap elevation commences at the posterior margin over the muscle where the plane is easy to find – it is more difficult to elevate the flap from the anterior border as the plane is less clear at the medial margin of the tibia. Perforators above the level of the base of the flap pedicle must be divided. The pedicle may be made much narrower than the skin paddle at the end of the flap and this aids the rotation of the pedicle. The donor site always needs to be skin grafted.

Islanded flaps (Fig. 7.204b)

In this form of the distally-based flap the skin is islanded on a single distal perforator and inverted through 180° to achieve closure of a defect around the ankle or lower third of the leg. Flap and defect must be in continuity. In this application the flap is designed somewhat smaller than it would have been with a skin and fascia pedicle. Venous drainage problems may occur with this design and small areas of marginal skin in the distal part of the flap may necrose but the flap has the advantage of being a single-stage procedure without the need for a second stage division and insetting of the pedicle.

Bipedicle flap design

This may occasionally be useful for a long narrow area of skin loss over the front of the tibia.

Other flap variants

With all these flap options available the need to dissect out and divide a posterior tibial artery to create a Type C posterior tibial flap seems unnecessary although this has been done to create a free flap,[5] a regional pedicled flap,[6] and a cross leg flap.[7]

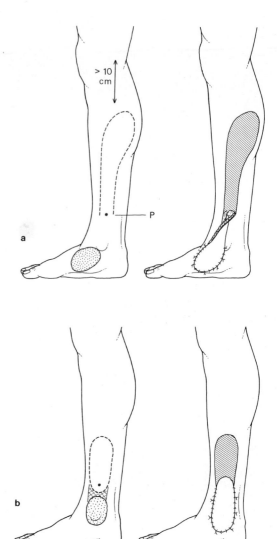

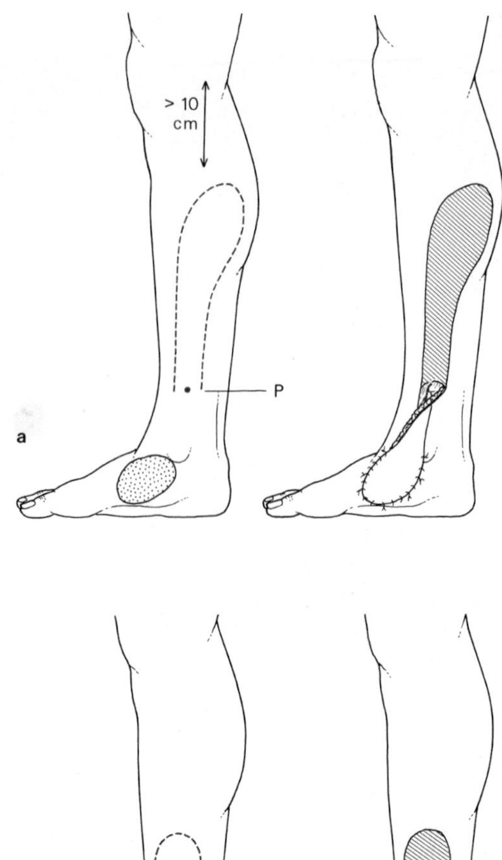

Fig. 7.204 **a.** Distally-based pedicled flap (P marks perforator). **b.** Islanded flap based on a single distal perforator.

References

1. Pontén B 1981 The fasciocutaneous flap: its use in soft tissue defects of the lower leg. British Journal of Plastic Surgery 34: 215–220
2. Amarante J, Costa H, Reis J, Soares R 1986 A new distally based fasciocutaneous flap of the leg. British Journal of Plastic Surgery 39: 338–340
3. Shalaby H A, Higazi M, Mandour S, El-Khalifa M A, Ayad H 1991 Distally based medial island septocutaneous flap for repair of soft-tissue defects of the lower leg. British Journal of Plastic Surgery 44: 175–178
4. El-Saadi M M, Khashaba A A 1990 Three anteromedial fasciocutaneous leg island flaps for covering defects of the lower two-thirds of the leg. British Journal of Plastic Surgery 43: 536–540
5. Okada T, Yasuda Y, Kitamaya Y, Tsukada S 1984 Salvage of an arm by means of a free cutaneous flap based on the posterior tibial artery. Journal of Reconstructive Microsurgery 1: 25–75
6. Hong G, Steffens K, Wang F B 1989 Reconstruction of the lower leg and foot with the reverse pedicled posterior tibial fasciocutaneous flap. British Journal of Plastic Surgery 42: 512–516
7. Sharma R K, Kola G 1992 Cross leg posterior tibial artery fasciocutaneous island flap for reconstruction of lower leg defects. British Journal of Plastic Surgery 45: 62–65

Gracilis musculocutaneous flap

The possibility of elevating the gracilis muscle on its proximal vascular pedicle with a flap of overlying skin supported by the muscle was first demonstrated by Orticochea[1] although the use of the muscle alone for anal sphincter reconstruction had been described by Pickrell much earlier.[2] As one of the 'early' musculocutaneous flaps it was initially used extensively for groin, ischial and perineal repairs[3, 4] but has been largely superseded by more reliable flaps (such as the tensor fasciae latae) except for certain specific indications such as reconstruction of the male external genitalia, vaginal reconstruction[5] and closure of vesico-vaginal fistulae where it is still a flap of first choice. This is partly due to its proximity and also to the fact that cutaneous sensory innervation through the obturator nerve can be maintained in the pedicled flap. It has also been used as a free flap.[6, 7]

Anatomy

Gracilis arises by a thin aponeurosis from the medial margin of the ischiopubic ramus and the adjacent body of the pubis. It is widest and thickest superiorly (approximately 6 cm × 2 cm) and narrows as it descends, to end as a rounded tendon which crosses the medial side of the knee between sartorius and semitendinosus to be inserted into the upper medial tibia. Its nerve supply comes from the anterior division of the obturator nerve. Its vascular supply conforms to the Type II pattern with a primary dominant pedicle arising from the profunda femoris artery and entering the muscle on its deep surface at the junction of the upper one-third with the lower two-thirds. The vessel measures between 1 and 2 mm in diameter and is accompanied by paired venae comitantes. A secondary pedicle arises from the superficial femoral artery, passes between adductors longus and brevis, gives off a branch to adductor magnus and finally enters gracilis in its lower third. A further, but usually very minor, vascular input occurs at the origin of the muscle from the medial circumflex femoral artery. These vessels and the degree of development of the intramuscular anastomoses can be seen in the radiographs of the muscle (Fig. 7.206).

The branch from the profunda femoris does not come directly off the main stem of the vessel but is usually a branch of what may be called the adductor artery. This vessel arises from the profunda at approximately the same level as the first perforator and passes medially between adductor longus and adductor brevis supplying them and ending in gracilis. This vessel has often been confused with the medial circumflex femoral artery which passes round the femur at a much higher level between psoas and pectineus although it often has a branch which follows the same course between the adductors as the 'adductor artery'. This branch is unnamed in current *Nomina Anatomica* although previously it was known as the ramus superficialis of the medial circumflex femoral artery. The adductor artery is shown in Figure 7.205 entering the muscle approximately 8 cm beneath the pubic crest.

Musculocutaneous perforators from the surface of the muscle supply the immediately overlying skin and an additional area extending beyond this. Studies have shown that in the superior third of the muscle there are on average two or three large calibre musculocutaneous perforators augmented by three small calibre perforators,

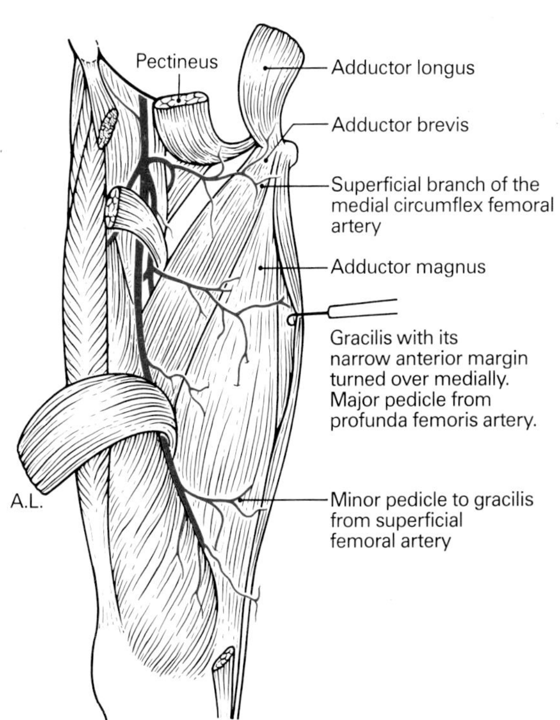

Fig. 7.205 Vascular anatomy. The principal vascular pedicles of gracilis are shown.

7

while in the middle third there are only two small calibre perforators, and in the lower third effectively no perforators. This lower part of the thigh is preferentially supplied by two fasciocutaneous perforators arising from the superficial femoral artery either as part of the sartorius system or emerging between gracilis and semimembranosus approximately 8 and 15 cm above the plane of the knee joint. Sometimes the lower pedicle of gracilis divides before entering the muscle with the side branch reaching skin as a fasciocutaneous perforator.

Flap planning

The cutaneous territory which can be reliably carried on the major pedicle is elliptical in shape with maximum dimensions of 8 cm × 20 cm and lies entirely posterior to a line drawn between the pubic tubercle

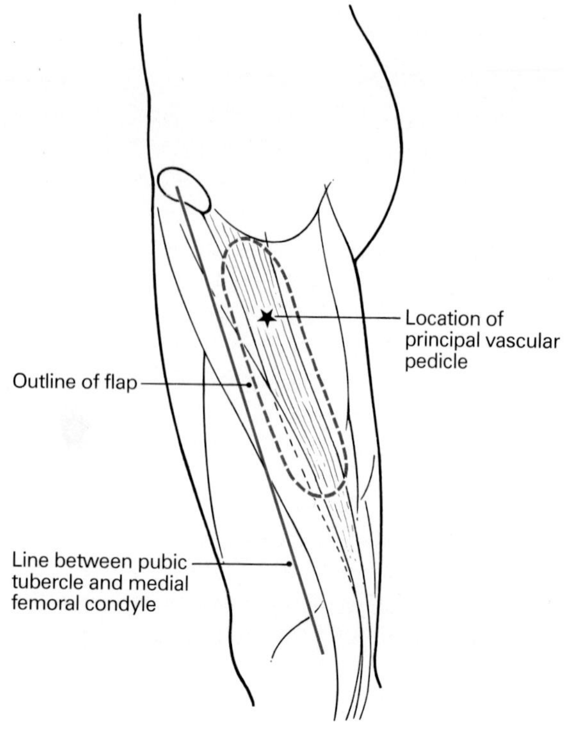

Fig. 7.207 Flap planning. The territory of the gracilis musculocutaneous flap based on its major vascular pedicle is shown. The area of the flap lies posterior to a line between the pubic tubercle and the medial femoral condyle.

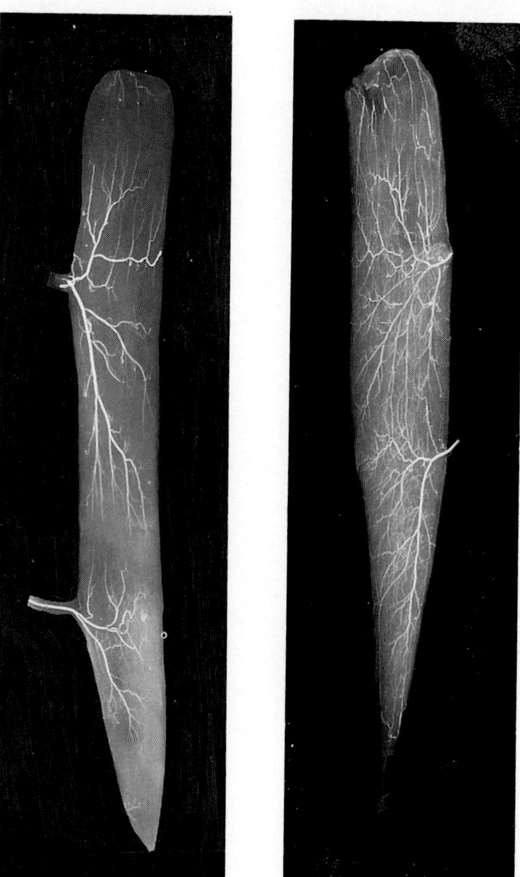

Fig. 7.206 Radiographs of injected gracilis muscles.

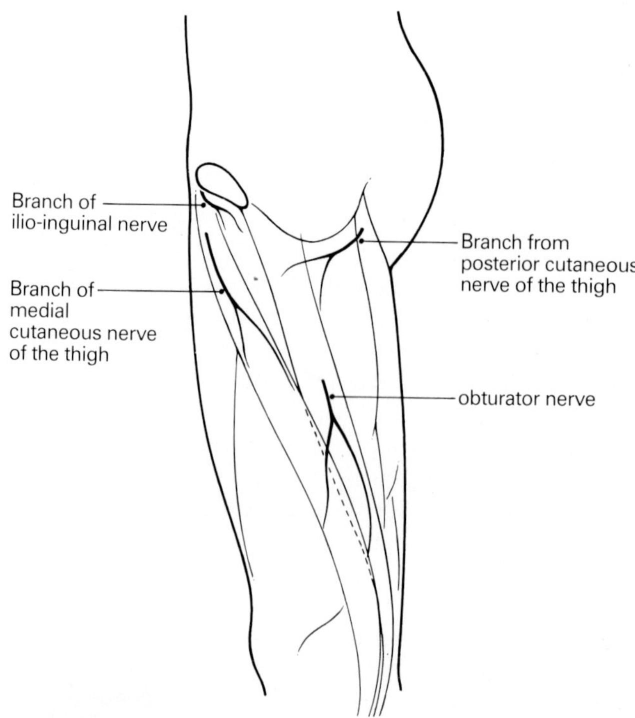

Fig. 7.208 Cutaneous innervation in the area of the flap.

and the semitendinosus tendon at the knee. The reach of the flap lies within an arc of rotation approximately 20 cm in radius centred on the site of the dominant vascular pedicle between 7 and 9 cm beneath the public crest.

An alternative design of the flap for perineal reconstruction is as a triangle with base superiorly and apex over the middle third of the muscle.[9] The skin triangle can then be advanced after mobilisation of the muscle and division of the muscle at the proximal and distal margins of the flap. The donor site is closed in a V to Y manner.

Flap elevation

The elevation commences with an incision along the anterior margin of the flap and exposure of the main vascular pedicle. This is found by dividing the fascia over adductor longus and peeling it back with the flap. The vessels will then be revealed lying between adductor magnus posteriorly and adductor longus anteriorly. The distal end of the muscle is now transected, the pedicle from the superficial femoral artery ligated and divided, and the posterior margin of the flap incised so that only the main vascular pedicle and the proximal attachment of the muscle to bone tether the flap. The sensory innervation from the obturator nerve is preserved but the other proximal attachments may be divided if this limits the mobility of the flap. The flap may be transferred into the perineum by undermining the skin between the donor site and the perineum with the flap being passed through this tunnel pivoted on the neurovascular pedicle. The donor site can be closed directly.

References

1. Orticochea M 1972 The musculocutaneous flap method: an immediate and heroic substitute for the method of delay. British Journal of Plastic Surgery 25: 106–110
2. Pickrell K, Georgiade N, Maguire C, Crawford H 1956 Gracilis muscle transplant for rectal incontinence. Surgery 40: 349–363
3. Labandter H P 1980 The gracilis muscle flap and musculocutaneous flap in the repair of perineal and ischial defects. British Journal of Plastic Surgery 33: 95–98
4. Wingate G B 1978 Repair of ischial pressure ulcers with gracilis myocutaneous island flaps. Plastic and Reconstructive Surgery 62: 245–248
5. McCraw J B, Massey F M, Shanklin K D, Horton C E 1976 Vaginal reconstruction with gracilis myocutaneous flaps. Plastic and Reconstructive Surgery 58: 176–183
6. Harii K, Ohmori K, Sekiguchi J 1976 The free musculocutaneous flap. Plastic and Reconstructive Surgery 57: 294–303
7. Mathes S J, Nahai F, Vasconez L O 1978 Myocutaneous free-flap transfer – anatomical and experimental considerations. Plastic and Reconstructive Surgery 62: 162–166
8. Giordano P A, Abbes M, Pequignot J P 1990 Gracilis blood supply: anatomical and clinical re-evaluation. British Journal of Plastic Surgery 43: 266–272
9. Peled I J 1990 Reconstruction of the vulva with V-to-Y advancement myocutaneous gracilis flap. Plastic and Reconstructive Surgery 86: 1014–1016

7 PROFUNDA FEMORIS POSTERIOR PERFORATORS

Hamstring musculocutaneous flaps

The biceps femoris muscle transposition was developed in the 1940s for the treatment of ischial pressure sores in paraplegics[1] and the transposition of biceps femoris and semitendinosus muscles into the patella was advocated for the relief of quadriceps paralysis caused by femoral nerve injury or residual poliomyelitis.[2] Since then a greater understanding of the principles of the musculocutaneous system of perforators to skin has resulted in the use of the hamstring muscles as carriers for islands of skin from the posterior thigh.[3–5]

Musculocutaneous flaps may be based on semitendinosus or biceps femoris or both. In the latter, the muscles are divided proximally and distally and are raised with an overlying triangle of skin – the whole unit may then be transferred upwards by V–Y advancement to cover ischial defects.[4, 5] One major advantage of using a large musculocutaneous triangular island flap and advancing it to cover ischial defects is that the flap may be re-elevated and advanced on subsequent occasions should the pressure sore recur.[6]

Biceps femoris may be transferred with a skin flap to the anterolateral thigh and inserted into the patella to reconstruct traumatic injuries in which a skin defect coexists with damage to the quadriceps muscle.[7]

Muscle anatomy

Biceps femoris. The long head of the muscle arises in common with semitendinosus from the ischial tuberosity and inclines laterally to form, in the lower part of the thigh, a long flattened tendon which is joined on its deep aspect by the fibres of the short head and inserts into the lateral side of the head of the fibula. The short head arises from the lateral lip of the linea aspera, the upper part of the lateral supracondylar line and the lateral intermuscular septum, and extends proximally as far as gluteus maximus.

Semitendinosus arises by a short tendon from the lower medial part of the ischial tuberosity in common with biceps femoris, forms a muscular belly, and then narrows progressively to a large rounded tendon which is inserted into the medial surface of the tibia below the insertion of gracilis. It is not uncommon to find a tendinous intersection running obliquely across the middle of the muscle belly.

The nerve supply to semitendinosus and to the long head of biceps comes from the 'nerve to the hamstrings' branch of the sciatic (tibial component). The nerve supply to the short head is from a separate branch (peroneal component). The nerve branches enter biceps along an elongated transfascicular hilum with the lower branch entering the muscle in the company of an arterial pedicle in two-thirds of cases. (Brash recorded the positions of nerve entry as proximal third of belly in 41%, proximal/middle junction 21%, middle third 38%.)

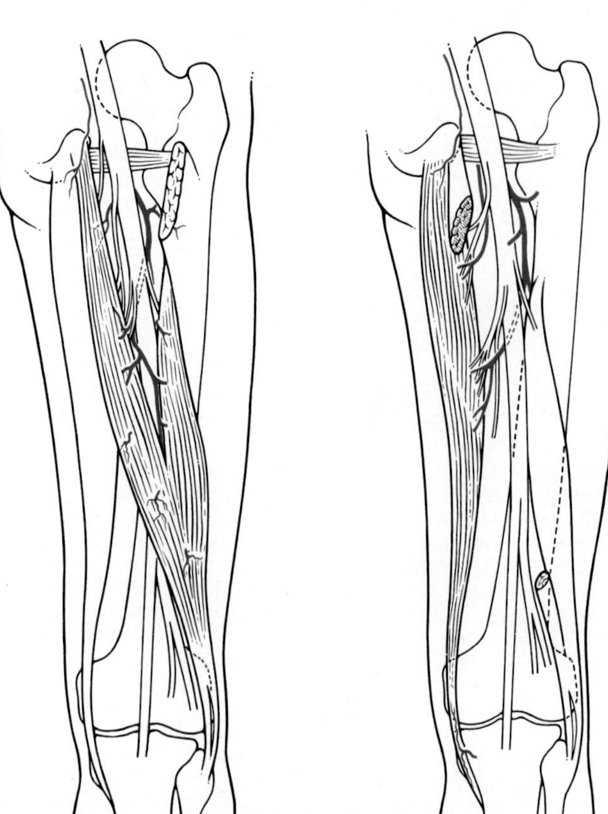

Fig. 7.209 Vascular anatomy. Branches of profunda perforators to semitendinosus on right and biceps femoris on left.

Vascular anatomy

The vascularisation of *biceps* has been classified as Type II but this is a little misleading since there may be up to four separate major vascular pedicles and several accessory pedicles entering the muscle (Fig. 7.209). However three of the major pedicles usually arise from the first profunda perforator and one of these tends to be predominant. This primary pedicle enters the muscle at the junction of its upper and middle thirds but the distal half of the muscle also receives major pedicles; these facts combine to limit the arc of rotation of the muscle.

The first profunda perforator descends in the posterior compartment for 6–10 cm, gives off two or three variously sized branches to the deep surface of the upper third of biceps, and divides into medial and lateral branches (often beneath the sciatic nerve). The lateral terminal branch disappears into the middle part of the long head of biceps – often dividing into two secondary branches in the company of the nerve of supply. If the second perforator is underdeveloped this lateral terminal division also sends a long branch obliquely inferiorly and laterally to the lower part of the long head. The medial terminal branch may give off a branch in about a third of cases which passes round the medial edge of the sciatic nerve, crosses its posterior surface and returns towards the long head of biceps – clearly this may tether transposition of the muscle.

The second perforator supplies the short head and the lower part of the long head. The third perforator supplies the short head. Within the muscle there are no anastomoses between vessels supplying the long and short heads.

Biceps receives additional vascular pedicles at its superior end from the inferior gluteal artery (on its superficial surface) and the medial circumflex femoral (on its deep surface) and at the lower end from the

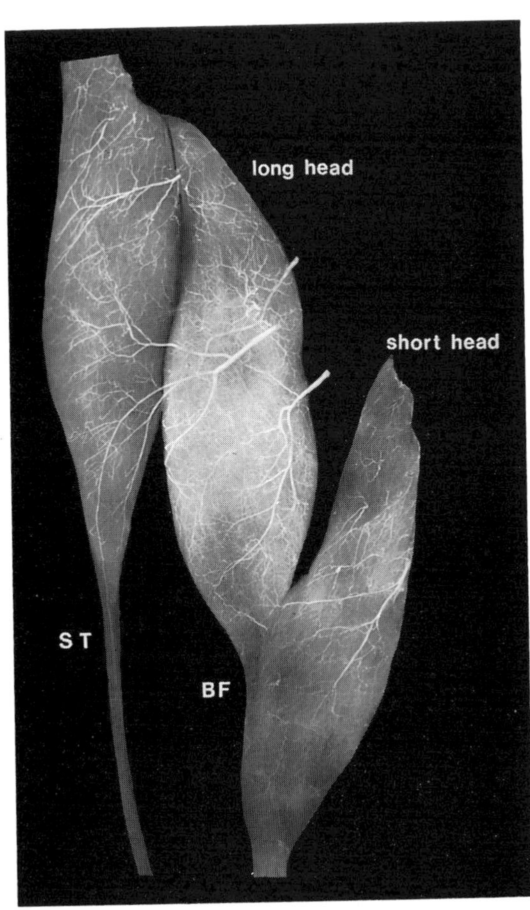

Fig. 7.210 Radiograph of hamstring muscles.

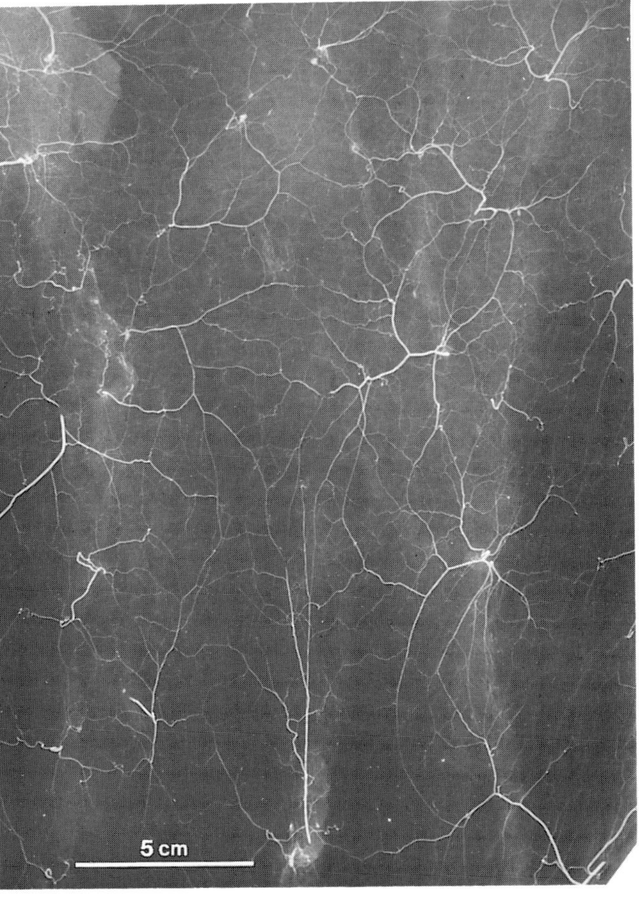

Fig. 7.211 Radiograph of posterior thigh skin showing emerging perforators.

superior lateral genicular artery. The artery accompanying the sciatic nerve (arteria comitans nervi ischiadici) has been described as important in supplying biceps but this is only exceptionally rarely the case.

Semitendinosus has a Type II pattern of vascularisation with a primary dominant pedicle entering the muscle belly from the first profunda perforator and a smaller pedicle above this from the medial circumflex femoral artery. In addition, small branches of the inferior gluteal and inferior medial genicular supply the tendons of origin and insertion respectively.

Flap planning

Musculocutaneous perforators reach the skin from the surface of biceps. In addition, one or two fasciocutaneous perforators consistently emerge between semitendinosus and biceps within the 12 cm above the plane of the knee joint but above this level fasciocutaneous perforators are far less consistently present. A large island of skin (12 cm × 35 cm) may be raised over the muscle extending beyond its margins.[3] Smaller islands may be carried over the lower third of the muscle belly and rotated about a point 10 cm below the ischial tuberosity (Fig. 7.212). Note that the flap may be constructed so as to preserve the innervation from the posterior cutaneous nerve of the thigh. Semitendinosus supplies musculocutaneous perforators to the medial posterior thigh skin which generally emerge close to the edges of the muscle. Flaps tend not to be raised on this muscle alone but rather over biceps and semitendinosus in conjunction (Fig. 7.213).

For functional reconstruction of composite defects on the anterolateral thigh, the biceps femoris musculocutaneous flap may be designed using the long head as shown in Figure 7.214 and transferred round to the front of the thigh with insertion of the biceps tendon into the patella. Quaba et al have used flaps up to 12 cm × 35 cm in size centred on the long head of biceps with a rotation point between 10 and 14 cm below the ischium. The inferior limit of the flap may be extended down to the popliteal skin crease if necessary.

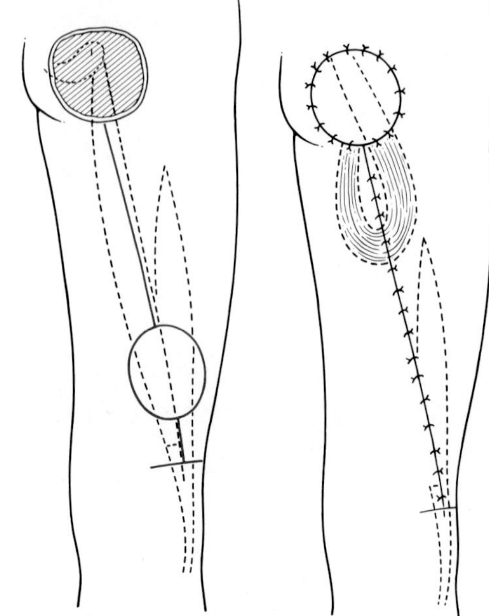

Fig. 7.212 Flap planning. Biceps femoris musculocutaneous island flap used to fill an ischial defect.

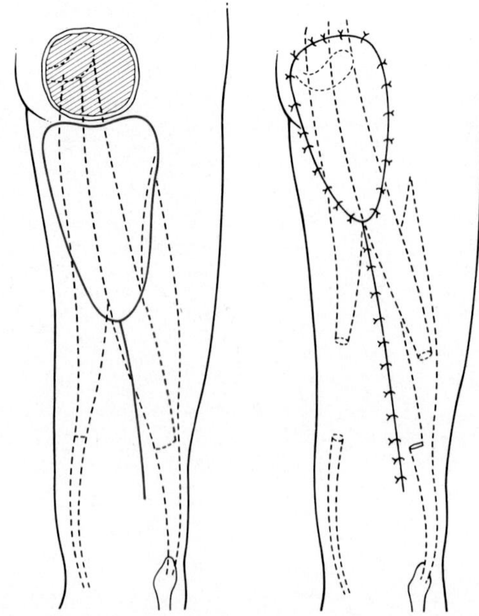

Fig. 7.213 Flap planning. V–Y advancement of a skin island based over the proximal parts of semitendinosus and the long head of biceps femoris.

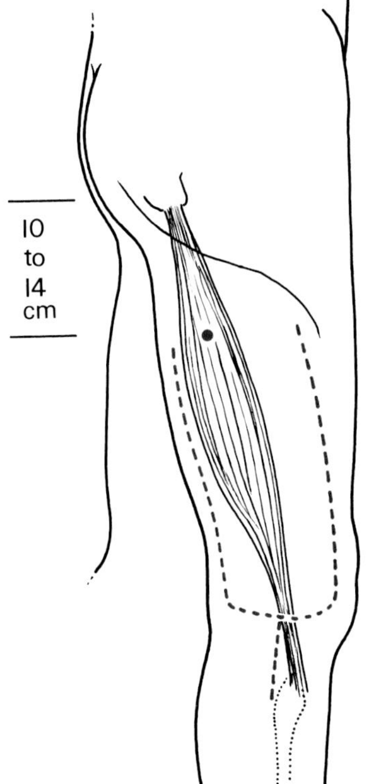

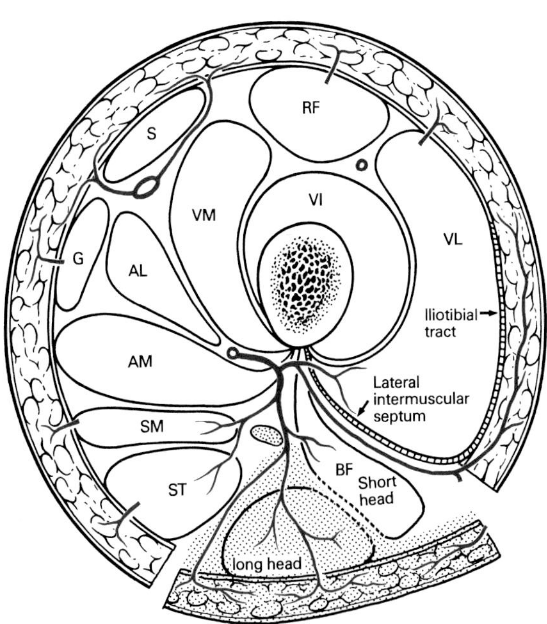

Fig. 7.214 Planning and elevation of the musculocutaneous biceps femoris transfer to replace damaged quadriceps muscle and overlying skin.

Surgery

V-Y advancement flap

An incision is made distally from the lower end of the proposed triangular flap towards the fibula to identify the biceps femoris. Dissection then proceeds proximally up the lateral and then the medial side of the flap. The muscles are then divided distal to the flap, lifted up, and the undersurface of the hamstrings mobilised whilst preserving the vascular pedicles. The proximal ends of the muscles are detached from the ischium and the flap advanced. As an alternative with small ischial defects, it may be sufficient to only incise the distal half of the medial side of the flap, thereby creating a hatchet flap with a pedicle rather than a true skin island.

Biceps transfer to patella

In elevating the pedicled flap the tendon is first separated from the fibula taking care to preserve the fibular collateral ligament. The long head is freed on its medial side from semitendinosus and the vascular pedicles identified. The lateral side is then elevated and the two heads of biceps separated. This starts at a point just below where the vessels have already been identified entering the long head and proceeds by sharp dissection freeing the oblique fibres of the short head from those of the long.

References

1. Conway H, Kraisel L J, Clifford R H, Gelb J, Joseph J M, Leveridge L L 1947 Plastic surgical closure of decubitus ulcers in patients with paraplegia. Surgery, Gynaecology and Obstetrics 85: 321–332
2. Schwartzman J R, Crego C H 1948 Hamstring-tendon transplantation for the relief of quadriceps femoris paralysis in residual poliomyelitis. A follow-up study of 134 cases. Journal of Bone and Joint Surgery 30A: 541–548
3. McCraw J B, Dibbell D G, Carraway J H 1977 Clinical definition of independent myocutaneous vascular territories. Plastic and Reconstructive Surgery 60: 341–352
4. Hurteau J E, Bostwick J, Nahai F, Hester R, Jurkiewicz M J 1981 V-Y advancement of hamstring musculocutaneous flap for coverage of ischial pressure sores. Plastic and Reconstructive Surgery 68: 539–542
5. Hagerty R F, Hagerty R C, Hagerty H F 1980 The hamstring myocutaneous flap in repair of ischial decubiti. Annals of Plastic Surgery 5: 227–231
6. Kroll S S, Hamilton S 1989 Multiple and repetitive uses of the extended hamstring V to Y myocutaneous flap. Plastic and Reconstructive Surgery 84: 296–302
7. Quaba A A, Chapman R, Hackett M E J 1983 Extended application of the biceps femoris musculocutaneous flap. Plastic and Reconstructive Surgery 81: 94–105

7 PROFUNDA FEMORIS LATERAL PERFORATORS

Superior lateral thigh pedicled island flap
Middle lateral thigh free flap

The possibility of raising a free flap from the lateral aspect of the thigh based on a single emerging branch of one of the lateral branches of a profunda femoris perforator was first demonstrated by Baek in 1983.[1] Baek used the lateral branch of the third perforator to support a free flap. Maruyama et al[2] have based a local pedicled island flap on the lateral branches of the first perforator. Further aspects of the anatomy of the vessels concerned have also been reported by the authors.[3]

Nomenclature for flaps based on the various lateral thigh flaps varies in the literature. Standardisation along the lines indicated on page 401 is to be recommended, with division of the flaps into superior, middle and lower categories as suggested by Laitung. Particularly in the middle of the thigh it is impossible to be certain precisely which profunda perforator the vessels of the flap arise from.

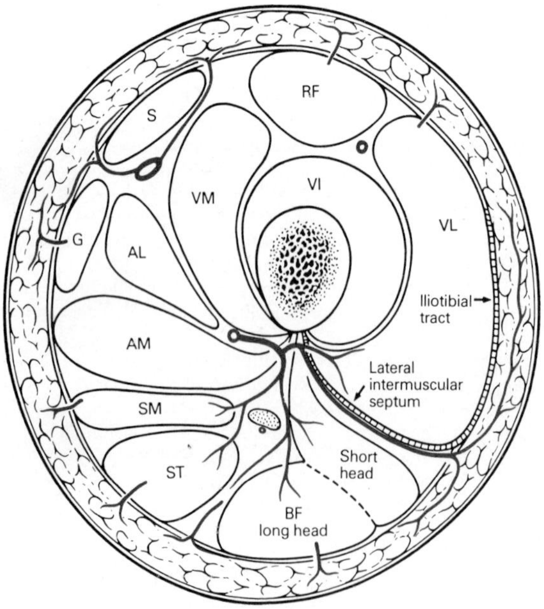

Fig. 7.215 Schematic transverse section through the mid-thigh showing the posterior and lateral branches of the profunda perforators.

Anatomy

The profunda femoris artery usually gives off four branches which pierce the insertion of adductor magnus to enter the posterior compartment (range 2–6). Here the profunda perforators give off branches to the hamstring muscles and each then ends by dividing into two branches at the point where the lateral intermuscular septum meets the shaft of the femur. (This point lies deep to the origin of the short head of

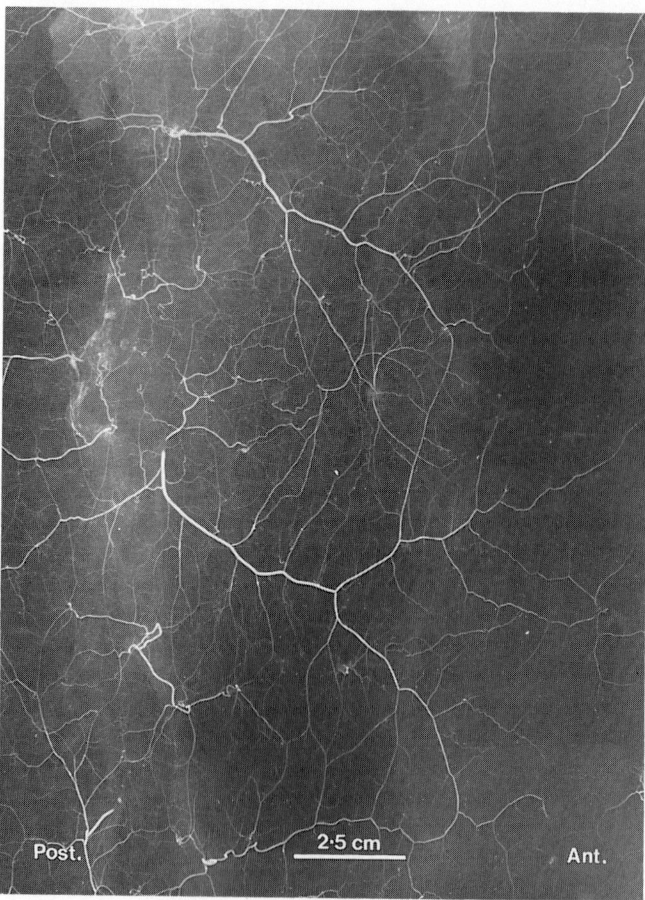

Fig. 7.216 The radiograph shows a specimen of thigh skin supplied by two perforators which have emerged along the posterior edge of the lateral intermuscular septum which lies towards the left side of the radiograph. Only the subcutaneous portions of these perforators are included in the specimen, the deep-lying sections on the posterior aspect of the septum have not been dissected out. (See also Fig. 6.93.)

biceps femoris from the lateral lip of the linea aspera of the femur.) One branch pierces the lateral intermuscular septum to enter and supply the posterior parts of vastus lateralis. The other branch passes horizontally in a lateral direction towards the iliotibial tract, closely applied to the posterior aspect of the lateral intermuscular septum (Fig. 7.215). The first perforator is a little different in that it sends a large branch to the lowermost part of the insertion of gluteus maximus which gives off branches which run between the muscle fibre bundles and emerge at the posterior edge of the iliotibial tract.

Baek has drawn attention to the lateral branch of the third profunda perforator as being a significantly sized vessel of 1.0–1.5 mm in external diameter and lying midway between the greater trochanter and the lateral condyle of the femur. The authors have found in a study of 50 preserved cadaver specimens that there was also a large perforator consistently emerging within 3 cm of the lower border of gluteus maximus or actually piercing the very lowermost part of the muscle insertion into the iliotibial tract and lateral intermuscular septum (Fig. 7.217). Furthermore in 60% of cases this vessel, which was a branch of the first profunda perforator, was the largest of all the perforators emerging along the length of the lateral thigh. This perforator is the basis of the island flap described by Maruyama et al.[2]

In both cases the branches of the perforator fan out over the iliotibial tract in an anterior direction giving off branches which pass superiorly and inferiorly where they anastomose with the branches of adjacent perforators. These anastomoses tend to be of a considerable diameter (for anastomoses). As a consequence, dye injected into a single perforator tends to stain an elliptical area of skin which has its long axis orientated longitudinally. It is expected that when these connections with neighbouring perforators are interrupted then blood flow will be channelled into the more anteriorly directed branches and therefore the potential territory of the flap is not necessarily elliptical in the long axis of the limb. The true anterior limits of the territories of these flaps have not yet been established.

In addition to these two principal perforators there are several other smaller branches emerging along the lateral intermuscular septum so that from the four profunda perforators a total of up to nine vessels may emerge along the length of the posterior border of the iliotibial tract. Of these, three tend to be large and the rest much smaller in size (Fig. 7.216). All these perforators anastomose longitudinally and this is the explanation for the unexpectedly great distance for which these flaps may be extended down the lateral thigh.

Venous drainage of the flap is by paired venae comitantes of the cutaneous perforators. These tend to join together to form a single vein when they approach the femur.

The nerve supply of the area is by the lateral cutaneous nerve of the thigh which emerges beneath the lateral end of the inguinal ligament, divides into two branches and runs down over the iliotibial tract. Over the insertion of gluteus maximus inferior clunial branches of the posterior cutaneous nerve of the thigh supply the skin.

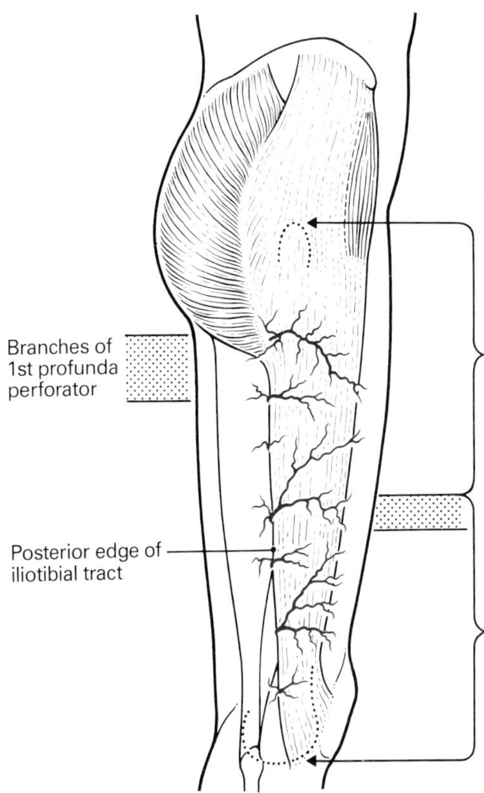

Fig. 7.217 Vascular anatomy. The locations of the principal perforators in relation to the tract and to the greater trochanter and knee joint are shown.

Flap elevation

First perforator. Due to the relationship of the insertion of gluteus maximus to the vessels it is difficult to get a good length of pedicle when flaps are based on the lateral branch of the first perforator and therefore these flaps are probably best used as local island flaps for transposition into ischial or trochanteric defects. The skin island is elliptical and is orientated with the long axis extending down the leg. Maruyama has reported flaps of 8 cm × 25 cm and 7 cm × 23 cm based on the first perforator. It may be important to elevate the underlying deep fascia and iliotibial tract with these flaps as this will protect the anastomoses between successive perforators and prevent them coming under tension. The outline for this flap indicated in Figure 7.218 is not intended to be precise.

Second or third perforator. A flap based on these perforators is rather different from the one described above. It is not adjacent to any commonly occurring defect and is designed for use as a free flap since a useful length of pedicle can be dissected out from along the lateral intermuscular septum. The flap is raised without the deep fascia and is therefore largely confined to the territory of a single perforator and is of limited size but has advantages of thinness and the possibility of innervation through the lateral cutaneous nerve of the thigh. Since the majority of the perforator branches run in an anterior direction it is best to plan the flap with one-third to one-quarter of it lying behind the lateral intermuscular septum and the rest in front. The elevation commences posteriorly at a level immediately above the deep fascia. The emerging cutaneous branches are visualised and the position of the largest determines the further elevation of the major part of the flap. The vascular pedicle is traced down the posterior aspect of the lateral intermuscular septum by strong retraction of vastus lateralis and biceps femoris. The remainder of the flap is then elevated off the iliotibial tract and if all is well the pedicle can then be divided.

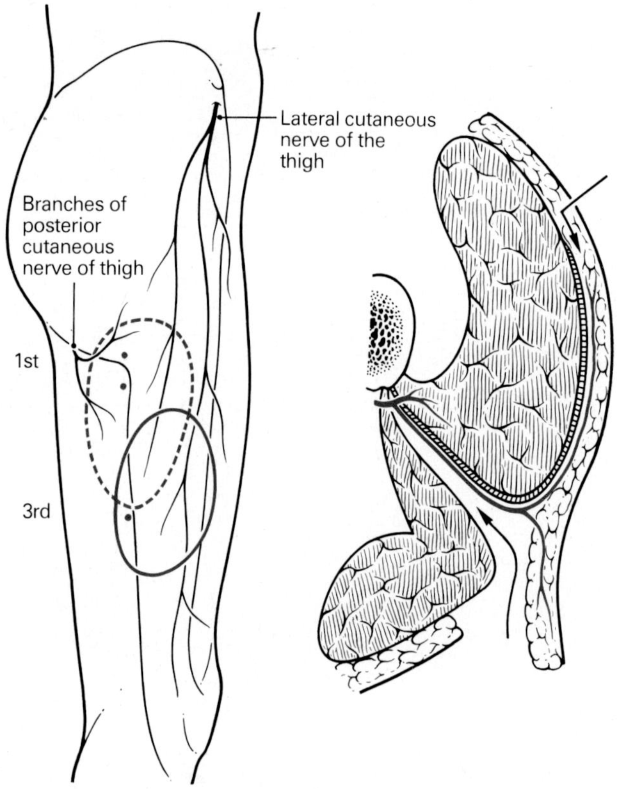

Fig. 7.218 Flap elevation. The approximate territories of branches of the first and third profunda perforators are shown on the left. Plane of flap elevation shown on right.

References

1. Baek S-M 1983 Two new cutaneous free flaps: The medial and lateral thigh flaps. Plastic and Reconstructive Surgery 71: 354–363
2. Maruyama Y, Ohnishi K, Takeuchi S 1984 The lateral thigh fasciocutaneous flap in the repair of ischial and trochanteric defects. British Journal of Plastic Surgery 37: 103–107
3. Cormack G C, Lamberty B G H 1985 The blood supply of thigh skin. Plastic and Reconstructive Surgery 75: 342–354

RADIAL ARTERY

Radial artery fasciocutaneous flap
'Chinese' forearm flap
Osteo-fasciocutaneous flap

This free flap was first described by Yang Guofan et al in 1981 in Chinese,[1] hence the alternative designation of the flap as the Chinese forearm flap. In 1981 the use of neurovascular free forearm flaps was reported by Stock in the German literature, while the first reports in English were an abstract of Yang Guofan's original report of 60 cases, an article by Song[2] reporting 31 such forearm flaps and a report by Mühlbauer et al.[3]

Whilst the commonest application of the flap is in intraoral lining reconstruction,[4] the possibilities are exceedingly diverse and range from thumb reconstruction[5] to one-stage penile reconstruction.[6]

Anatomy

The radial artery sends a series of perforators along the fascial septum between brachioradialis and flexor carpi radialis. Distally one or two of these perforators may be displaced to lie between the tendons of flexor carpi radialis and flexor digitorum superficialis. These perforators fan out at the level of the deep fascia, forming a plexus from which the skin is supplied with blood. In the proximal third of the forearm these perforators, including the so-called 'inferior cubital artery', tend to spread out in a predominantly

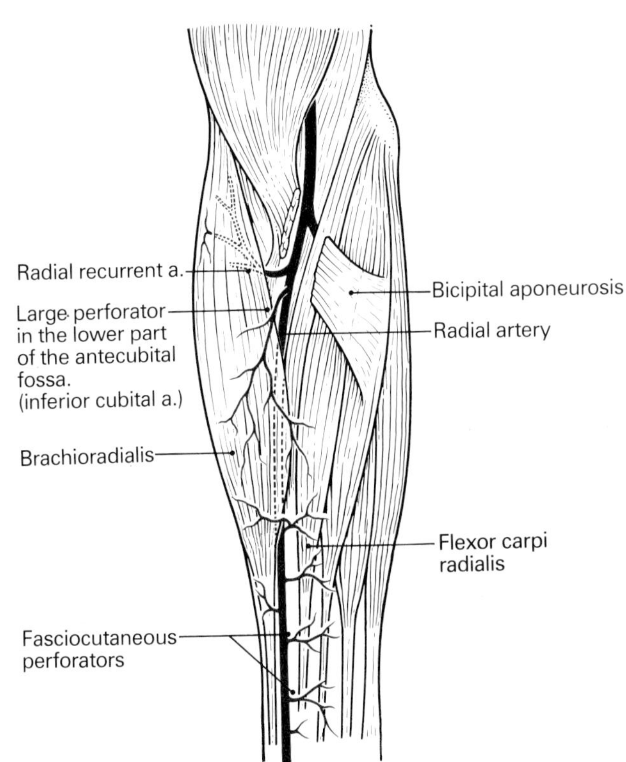

Fig. 7.219 Vascular anatomy. Fasciocutaneous branches of the radial artery are shown. Musculocutaneous perforators through brachioradialis are sparse.

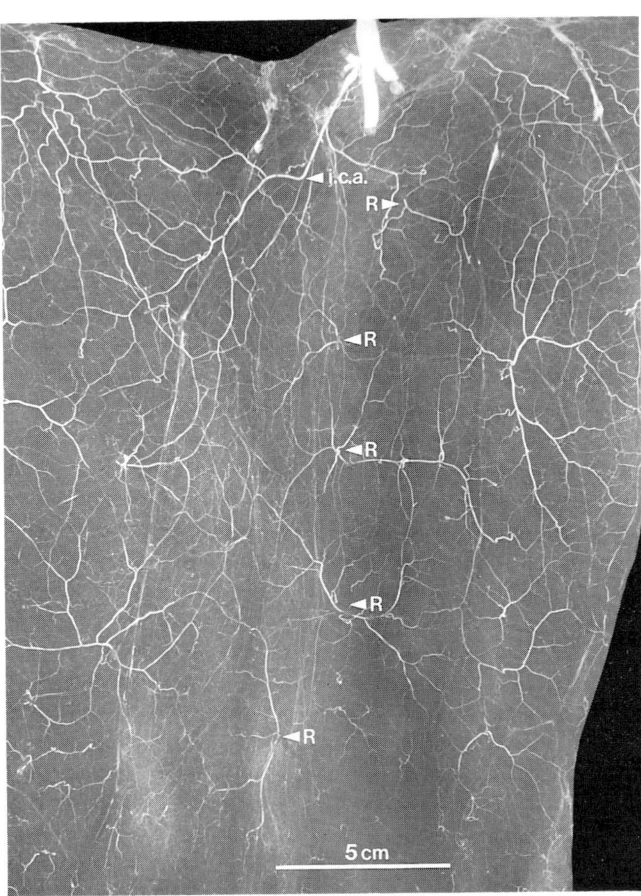

Fig. 7.220 The radiograph shows the part of the forearm skin supplied from the radial artery; arrows indicate perforators. (Proximal end at top of picture)

longitudinal direction. By contrast, in the distal third of the forearm the fasciocutaneous perforators tend to be orientated more transversely. These perforators supply most of the anterior forearm skin but are no more significant than the perforators from the ulnar artery which number between three and five and lie mainly in the proximal forearm between flexor carpi ulnaris and flexor digitorum superficialis. The description of a flap based on the inferior cubital artery should also be noted (p. 340).

The deep fascia is particularly thick proximally where it covers the bulk of the forearm flexors but thins out distally until it reaches the distal wrist crease where it starts to thicken as it joins with the flexor retinaculum.

The venous drainage of the skin is through both the superficial system of veins and also through the deep venae comitantes of the radial artery. The superficial veins contain obviously effective valves but the findings concerning the deep veins have been conflicting. Although valves are definitely present in freshly examined material, their functional effectiveness is in doubt. The undoubted ability of blood to flow in a reversed direction along these veins may be due to the presence of cross communications between venae comitantes allowing blood to bypass the valves (see p. 123). It is recommended that drainage of the flap be arranged through the superficial system.

Anomalies of the radial artery are listed on page 178.

Flap planning

The vascular supply to the hand is assessed by various methods in the light of the known variability of the vasculature. The location of the flap is determined by the best compromise between the various dictates of skin thickness, hairiness, flap size, length of arterial pedicle, requirements for innervation and inconstant anatomical features such as location of superficial veins.

Flap elevation

Standard free flap

The skin is incised and the incision deepened through the deep fascia. A suitable superficial vein is preserved at the proximal end of the flap during this incision and is dissected out up to the antecubital fossa or further proximally (cephalic vein) if a longer venous pedicle is required. The venae comitantes of the radial artery are an alternative drainage system for the flap but they are smaller in size and generally not the first choice for a free flap unless it is a small and distally situated flap. Elevating the deep fascia is easiest proximally over the fleshy parts of the muscle and more difficult distally over the tendons where care must be taken to preserve a layer of paratenon for protection and to enable a split skin graft to take. The superficial branches of the radial nerve often lie at the lateral margin of the flap and injury to these should be avoided. The medial edge of brachioradialis muscle and its tendon are retracted with skin hooks and the fascial septum containing the perforators connecting with the radial artery and venae comitantes is dissected free. Numerous branches to muscles require to be divided before the flap and its pedicle are finally free. It is not usually necessary to replace the radial artery with a reversed vein graft.

Osteo-fasciocutaneous free flap

The skin flap may be combined with bone by raising the radial artery in continuity with the fascia containing branches which run down onto the radius. These branches are shown in Figure 7.222a and consist of branches to flexor pollicis longus and two or three fascioperiosteal branches to the lateral aspect of the bone

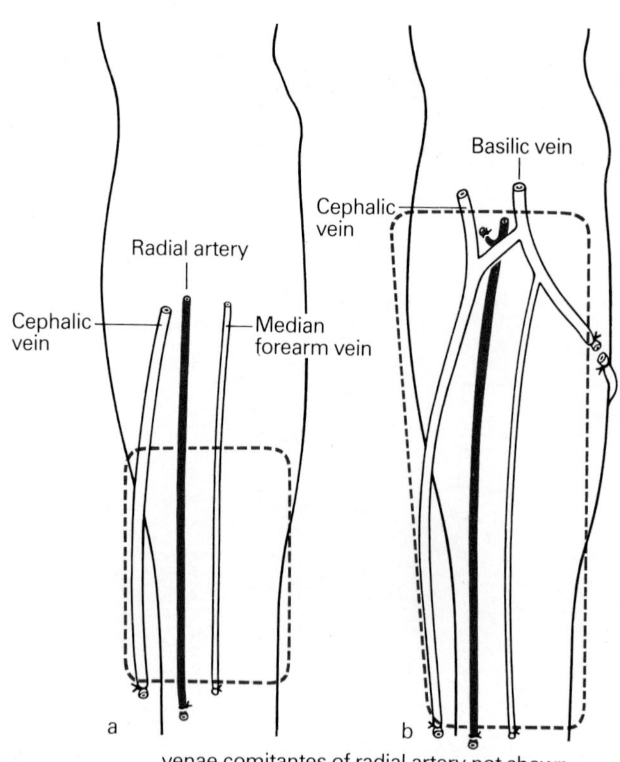

Fig. 7.221 Flap planning. **a.** Free flaps may be small and confined mainly to the distal part of the forearm, or **b.** may incorporate most of the volar forearm skin and even extend onto the lowermost part of the upper arm.

between the pronator teres insertion and the brachioradialis insertion. Up to half the cross-sectional area of the bone may be safely removed. The average length of this segment of lateral cortex is 10 to 12 cm.[7] Because of the segmental blood supply to the harvested segment, osteotomies to change the shape of the bone strut are possible without impairing its viability.

Double and triple paddle flaps

The reconstruction of complex defects may require two or sometimes even three paddles of skin, e.g. large buccal carcinoma excisions requiring one paddle for intra-oral lining and one for overlying skin. The radial forearm flap is particularly adaptable in this regard and several paddles, with intervening de-epithelialised areas, may be carried on the one pedicle. This principle is also applied when the flap is used for penile reconstruction with one tubed paddle forming neo-urethra and the other the covering skin.

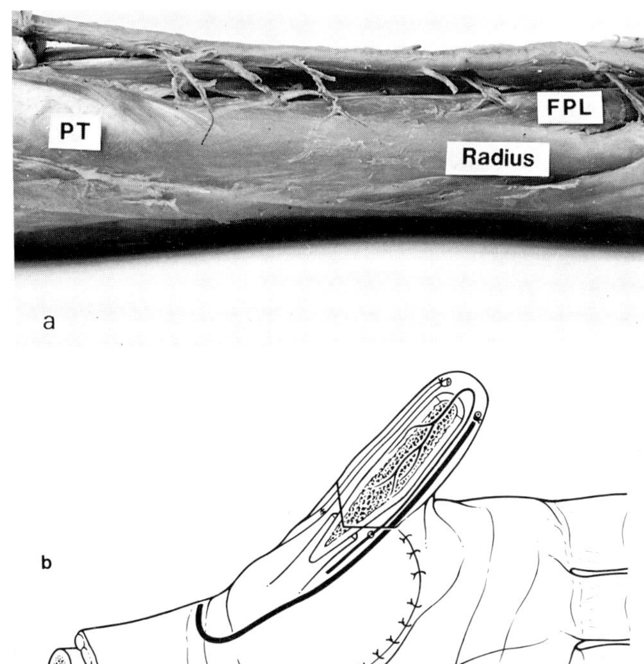

Fig. 7.222 Myo-osteo-fasciocutaneous tissue transfer. **a.** Photograph shows fascioperiosteal branches of the radial artery and branches to flexor pollicis longus (**FPL**) through which vessels reach the bone (**PT.** insertion of pronator teres). **b.** Diagram shows method of thumb reconstruction using a composite flap supported by a distally pedicled radial artery. The cephalic vein has been used for venous drainage and a segment of the lateral cutaneous nerve of the forearm which innervates the flap has been joined to a digital nerve.

Distally pedicled (reverse flow) flaps

In the presence of intact palmar arches and a good inflow from the ulnar artery, a forearm flap can be raised for transfer to the hand with the radial artery and venae comitantes dissected down to the level of the anatomical snuff box. A damaged palm with disruption of the palmar arches is not necessarily a contraindication to the use of the reverse flow flap because the radial artery also has anastomoses around the wrist, but in these circumstances it is recommended that the distal part of the flap pedicle should be left undisturbed and the pivot point should be at least 1 inch, and preferably 2 inches, proximal to the wrist crease.[8]

The composite flap may be pedicled distally and used to reconstruct hand defects needing bone[9] or may be used to replace an amputated thumb by creating an opposition post with a segment of radius enveloped by the flap (Fig. 7.222b).[4]

Other flap variants

The flap may be variously combined with palmaris longus or brachioradialis tendons, with cutaneous nerves, or may be used as a fascia only flap. The radial artery may be used to bridge a gap in another major vessel by anastomosing both ends whilst at the same time supporting a flap to reconstruct a soft tissue defect.

References

1. Yang Guofan et al 1981 Forearm free skin flap transplantation (in Chinese). National Medical Journal of China 61: 139. Abstracted in Plastic and Reconstructive Surgery 69: 1041
2. Song R, Gao Y, Song Y, Yu Y, Song Y 1982 The forearm flap. Clinics in Plastic Surgery 9: 21–26
3. Mühlbauer W, Herndl E, Stock W 1982 The forearm flap. Plastic and Reconstructive Surgery 70: 336–344
4. Soutar D S, Scheker L R, Tanner N S B, McGregor I A 1983 The radial forearm flap: a versatile method of intra-oral reconstruction. British Journal of Plastic Surgery 36: 1–8
5. Biemer E, Stock W 1983 Total thumb reconstruction: a one-stage reconstruction using an osteo-cutaneous forearm flap. British Journal of Plastic Surgery 36: 52–55
6. Chang T-S, Hwang W-Y 1984 Forearm flap in one-stage reconstruction of the penis. Plastic and Reconstructive Surgery 74: 251–258
7. Cormack G C, Duncan M J, Lamberty B G H 1986 The blood supply of the bone component of the compound osteocutaneous radial artery forearm flap: an anatomical study. British Journal of Plastic Surgery 39: 173–175
8. Naasan A, Quaba A A 1990 Successful transfer of two reverse forearm flaps despite disruption of both palmar arches. British Journal of Plastic Surgery 43: 476–479
9. Foucher G, van Genechten F, Merle N, Michon J 1984 A compound radial artery forearm flap in hand surgery: an original modification of the Chinese forearm flap. British Journal of Plastic Surgery 37: 139–148

7 RADIAL RECURRENT ARTERY

Brachioradialis musculocutaneous flap
Radial recurrent fasciocutaneous flap (reverse lateral upper arm flap)

The use of the muscle alone as a local rotation flap was described in 1980,[1,2] followed by the use of the musculocutaneous flap in 1981.[3] The muscle alone has also been transferred distally on a reverse-flow radial artery pedicle (with venae comitantes) for use in reconstructing defects on the dorsum of the hand.[4]

It was subsequently demonstrated that muscle was not essential for the viability of the flap.[5] A flap may be raised in a septocutaneous manner based on the fasciocutaneous perforators from the radial recurrent artery and its anastomoses with the radial collateral artery.[6] This may be termed the radial recurrent fasciocutaneous flap or the reverse lateral upper arm flap.

N.B. The term 'lateral arm flap' is usually applied to the flap based on the middle collateral artery. The 'reverse lateral arm flap' being described here is not a distally based version of the lateral arm flap based on the middle collateral artery because that vessel anastomoses (poorly) behind the lateral epicondyle with the interosseous recurrent artery. 'Lateral arm flap' and 'reverse lateral arm flap' are therefore not opposite versions of the same flap although this impression is sometimes given in the literature.

Anatomy

The blood supply to brachioradialis comes from the radial recurrent artery, which is given off by the radial artery in the cubital fossa. This vessel ascends on the medial surface of brachioradialis and above the lateral epicondyle anastomoses with the radial collateral branch of the profunda brachii artery. The radial recurrent artery gives off several branches to the muscle, the usual arrangement being that the first branch is large and enters the muscle distal to the elbow joint, while subsequent branches are smaller. Some of the smaller vessels accompany the muscular branches of the radial nerve which nearly always enter the muscle well above the lateral epicondyle forming distinct neurovascular hila in about 50% of cases. A nerve branch may also run down to enter about the level of the epicondyle and may be associated with the nerve of supply to extensor carpi radialis longus. The radial recurrent artery also supplies extensor carpi radialis longus and brevis.

In addition to these muscle branches the radial recurrent artery gives off branches to skin along the fascial septum between brachialis and brachioradialis. In two-thirds of cases it anastomoses at a point approximately 3.5 cm above the lateral epicondyle (range 1.5–6.5 cm) with the radial collateral artery by a vessel approximately 0.3 mm in calibre. In the remaining third of cases the anastomosis is by multiple very fine vessels not visible with the naked eye. The anastomosis lies deep in the fascial septum between the muscles and needs to be included in the reverse fasciocutaneous flap.

Territory

The territory of the musculocutaneous flap overlies the proximal part of the muscle and therefore includes the lower third of the lateral upper arm and the proximal lateral forearm. The fasciocutaneous flap is generally raised as an elliptical island over the septum between brachialis and brachioradialis. The donor site can be closed directly in most cases.

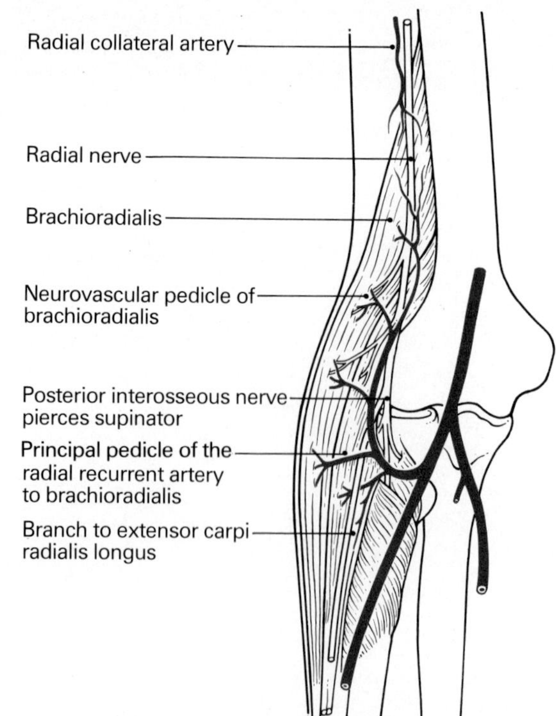

Fig. 7.223 Vascular anatomy. Brachioradialis and extensor carpi radialis longus have been turned laterally to expose the radial recurrent artery and the muscular branches of the radial nerve.

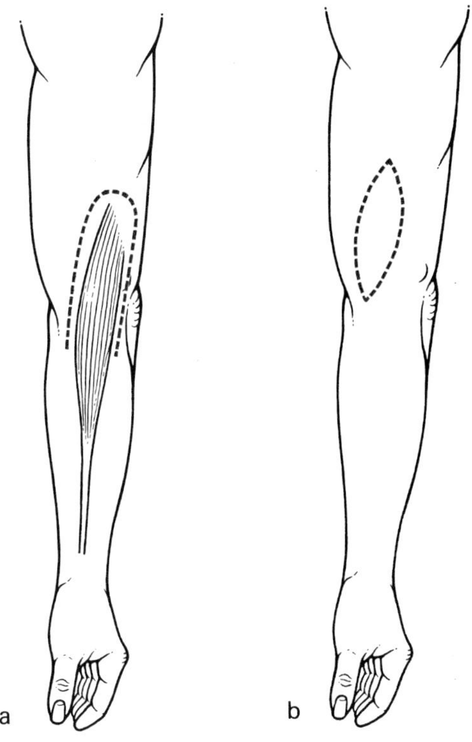

Fig. 7.224 Flap planning.

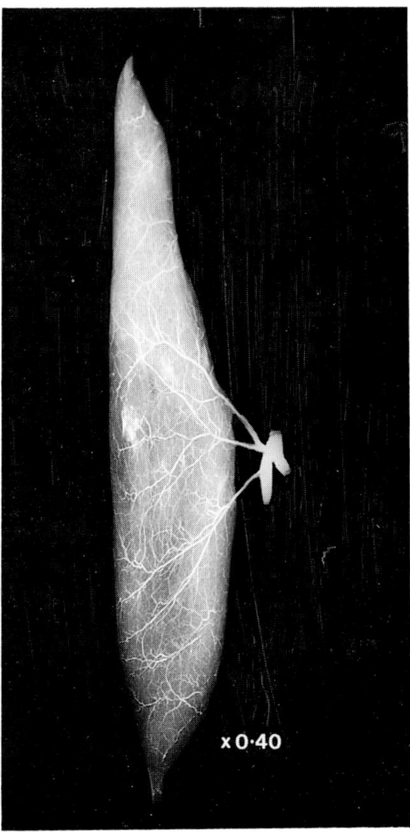

Fig. 7.225 Radiograph of brachioradialis. The radial recurrent artery was not identifiable in this case and branches to the muscle came directly off the radial artery just after the brachial bifurcation.

Surgery

Musculocutaneous flap (Fig. 7.224a)
The base of the flap is situated about 5 cm below the lateral epicondyle and the flap extends proximally over brachioradialis. The proximal limit of the flap, including a random-pattern cutaneous extension, has been reported to be the mid-humeral level. The incision for the medial margin of the flap provides access to the vascular pedicle and exposure of the nerve to brachioradialis which will need to be divided to allow transposition of the end of the flap. The arc of rotation takes in the olecranon region and the flap may be useful for providing cover of an exposed elbow joint open on its postero-lateral surface, although an antecubital forearm flap might be a less bulky alternative. Disadvantages of the flap include the donor defect and the fact that the radial nerve will then be left in a superficial position without muscular cover.

Fasciocutaneous flap (Fig. 7.224b)
The incision is commenced on the anterior or posterior border of the skin island near the epicondyle and deepened through the fascia to expose the radial recurrent vessels lying deep in the fascial septum. The incision is extended away from the lateral epicondyle and the radial collateral vessels divided at the upper end of the flap. The radial nerve should be avoidable by virtue of its deeper position in the septum. The flap is useful for reconstruction of defects over the antecubital fossa, e.g. from release of scar contractures, when the flap can be transposed into the defect and the donor site closed directly in most cases.

References

1. Gilbert A, Restrepo J 1980 Le long supinateur: anatomie et utilisation comme lambeau de rotation musculaire. Annales de Chirurgie Plastique 25: 72–75
2. Lendrum J 1980 Alternatives to amputation. Annals of the Royal College of Surgeons of England 62: 95–99
3. Lai M F, Krishna B V, Pelly A D 1981 The brachioradialis myocutaneous flap. British Journal of Plastic Surgery 34: 431–434
4. McGeorge D D, Arnstein P M, Stilwell J H 1991 The distally-based brachioradialis muscle flap. British Journal of Plastic Surgery 44: 30–32
5. Maruyama Y, Takeuchi S 1986 The radial recurrent fasciocutaneous flap: reverse upper arm flap. British Journal of Plastic Surgery 39: 458–461
6. Hayashi A, Maruyama Y 1990 Anatomical study of the recurrent flaps of the upper arm. British Journal of Plastic Surgery 43: 300–306
7. Culbertson J H, Mutimer K 1987 The reverse lateral arm flap for elbow coverage. Annals of Plastic Surgery 18: 62–68

7

SAPHENOUS ARTERY

Saphenous artery flap
Reverse saphenous artery flap
(Medial condylar bone flap – see p. 504)

This fasciocutaneous free flap was described by Acland et al[1] in 1981. The flap has a reliable supporting artery and a distinct nerve supply, and is useful because of the long pedicle and the thinness of the flap. However, the flap requires careful dissection and details of the vascular anatomy are crucial if the flap is to be developed correctly as the dissection proceeds.

Anatomy

The saphenous artery which supplies the flap is a branch of the descending genicular artery. This arises from the medial side of the femoral artery immediately before the femoral artery passes through the hiatus in adductor magnus (Fig. 7.226). The descending genicular artery and saphenous nerve pierce the fascia over the femoral artery (membrana vastoadductoria) and run distally under cover of sartorius. The artery divides within 3 cm of its origin into musculo-articular, periosteal and saphenous branches. The musculo-articular branch supplies vastus medialis and the capsule of the knee joint and anastomoses with the superior medial genicular artery. The saphenous branch is 1.5–2.0 mm in diameter.[2] It is accompanied by two venae comitantes and the saphenous nerve and descends under sartorius for about a hand's breadth. Here it gives off branches of supply to sartorius and several fasciocutaneous perforators which pass round the edges of the muscle of reach the skin. These perforators emerge both anterior and posterior to the muscle with the more proximal perforators tending to run anterior. There may be up to four of these and in about 50% of cases they constitute the dominant source of supply to the area of skin immediately in front of sartorius, which is otherwise fed by musculocutaneous perforators from vastus medialis. At the level of the femoral condyle the muscular fibres of sartorius are replaced by a thin flattened tendon which curves obliquely forward to expand into a broad aponeurosis which gains attachment to the upper part of the medial surface of the tibia immediately in front of gracilis and semitendinosus. The saphenous artery and nerve continue their straight course and emerge from behind the tendon as it curves forward. They continue onto the leg lying first in the deep fascia and then branching out into the

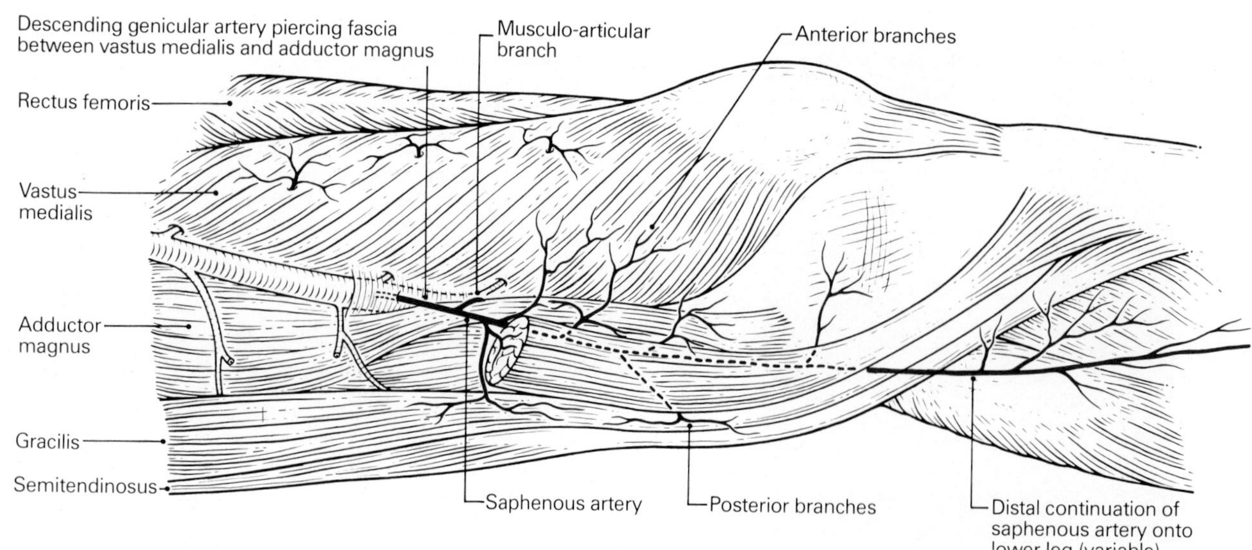

Fig. 7.226 Vascular anatomy of saphenous artery. Venae comitantes, the saphenous nerve, and the great saphenous vein have been omitted for clarity.

subcutaneous tissue over the medial side of the knee and the proximal part of the lower leg. There are instances recorded in the anatomical literature where a well-developed saphenous artery reached the foot, but usually the cutaneous branches do not extend for more than 12 cm below the knee joint. Very small vascular filaments may continue to run with the saphenous nerve thereby enabling a substantial length of this nerve to be used as a vascularised free nerve graft.[2]

The nerve supply to the skin on the medial side of the knee is from three nerves. In the proximal part of the saphenous territory the middle and distal branches of the medial femoral cutaneous nerve approach the knee (Fig. 7.228). Fine terminal obturator branches may also encroach. In the distal part of the saphenous territory the nerve supply is by direct branches of the saphenous nerve and by twigs which accompany the arteries. The infrapatellar branch turns forwards round the tendon of sartorius.

The venous drainage is by venae comitantes of the saphenous artery and also by the great saphenous vein which tends to run with the saphenous nerve in front of the artery.

Surgery

The final decision as to the location of the flap is delayed until the dissection has revealed whether or not the main strength of the saphenous artery is expended early on in anterior branches. If these are well developed the flap is sited over their territory (Fig. 7.228a); alternatively, if there are no anterior branches then the cutaneous distribution of the saphenous artery will fall within a more postero-inferior territory (Fig. 7.228b).

In order to establish the vascular topography the elevation must proceed from proximal to distal and

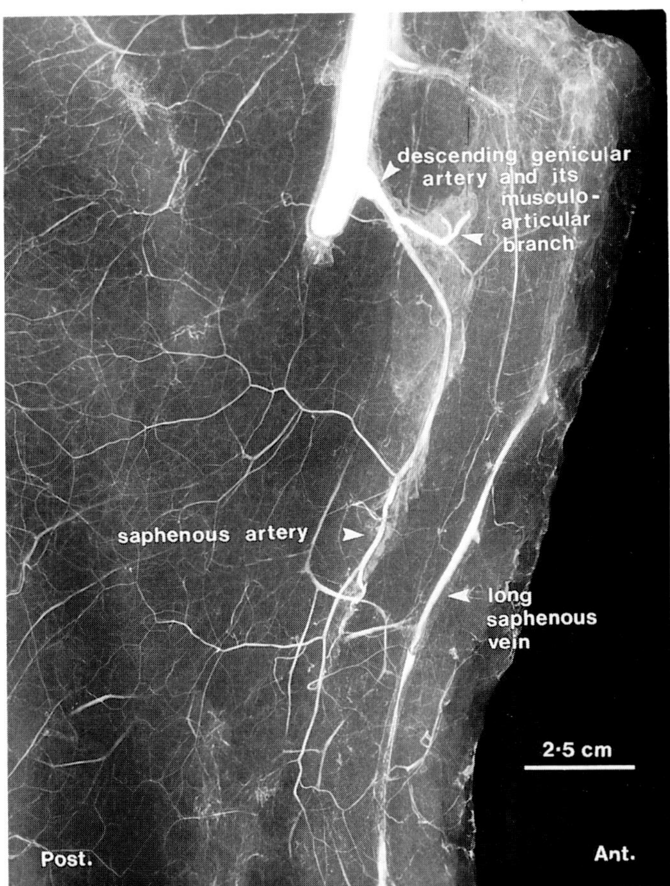

Fig. 7.227 Radiograph of skin showing saphenous artery (a segment of the femoral artery has been removed in continuity with the descending genicular artery). See also Fig. 6.112 for a further example of the saphenous artery.

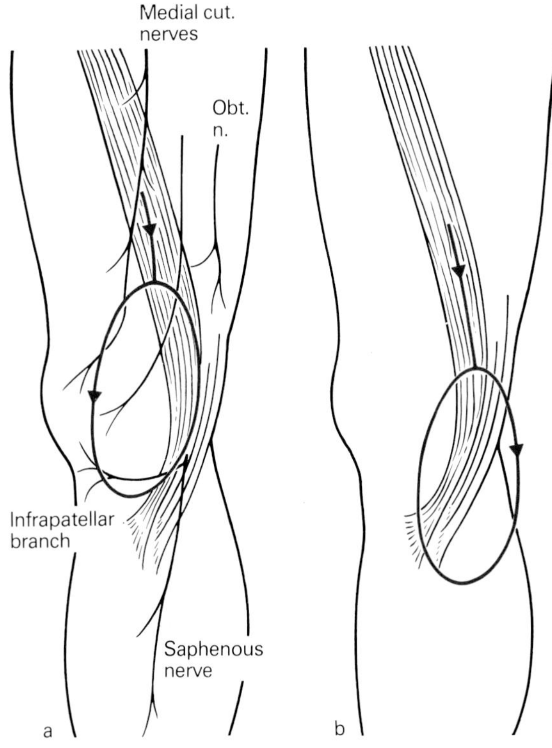

Fig. 7.228 Flap outlines for **a.** predominantly anteriorly emerging branches (cutaneous nerves also shown on this diagram), and **b.** posteriorly emerging branches.

commence with an incision over sartorius with its distal end some 12 cm above the knee. The incision is carried through the deep fascia over sartorius with preservation of overlying branches of the medial cutaneous nerve of the thigh. The deep fascia is elevated off the anterior part of sartorius which is displaced posteriorly, thereby revealing the saphenous artery in the space beneath. The state of its branches is ascertained, and the skin and subcutaneous tissue retracted away from the limb inferiorly in order to reveal the situation beyond the end of the skin incision. Some blunt dissection is required to free the vessels and the incision may be cautiously extended.

If strong anterior branches are present the skin incision is extended anteriorly to include these branches. The flap is then raised from anterior to posterior with division of sartorius (Fig. 7.228a).

If strong posterior branches are present in combination with the artery and its cutaneous branches below the sartorius tendon, then the incision is extended posteriorly and the flap is placed more posteriorly and distally. Elevation proceeds from posterior to anterior (Fig. 7.228b).

If both anterior and posterior branches are present then the flap needs to be placed over both and the sartorius muscle divided or a segment of it incorporated in the flap. Saphenous vein and cutaneous nerves are dissected out with an adequate proximal length as required.

The donor defect may be closed directly if less than 6 cm across. The largest successful reported flap has measured 8 cm × 29 cm.[1]

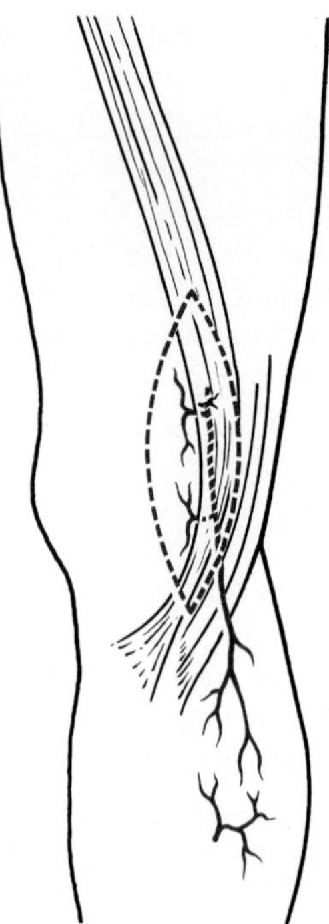

Fig. 7.229 Flap outline for a distally pedicled flap to be transferred to below the knee. In the situation shown where most of the vessels to skin lie anterior to the muscle it will be necessary to pass the flap under the sartorius.

Reverse saphenous artery flap

This development of the saphenous artery flap was described by Torii et al in 1988. By dividing the descending genicular artery and isolating the skin island on a distal pedicle, transposition to a more distal defect becomes possible. In the cases reported by Torii all the flaps were used to resurface areas of ulceration on amputation stumps and the largest flap measured 23 cm × 7 cm. With a flap of this width the flap will include the long saphenous vein as well as the saphenous artery and its venae comitantes. Generally the pivot point determining the arc of rotation will be no further distally than 5 cm below the plane of the knee joint although in theory the anastomosis between the distal end of the saphenous artery and the first perforator from the posterior tibial artery could form the axis point for distal rotation of the flap. If the flap is supplied by perforators reaching skin around the anterior edge of sartorius then the flap will either have to be tunnelled under the muscle to deliver it distally or sartorius will need to be divided.

References

1. Acland R D, Schusterman M, Godina M, Eder E, Taylor G I, Carlisle I 1981 The saphenous neurovascular free flap. Plastic and Reconstructive Surgery. 67: 763–774
2. Briedenbach W C, Terzis J K 1984 The anatomy of free vascularised nerve grafts. Clinics in Plastic Surgery 11: 65–71
3. Koshima I, Endou T, Soeda S, Yamasaki M 1988 The free or pedicled saphenous flap. Annals of Plastic Surgery 21: 369–374
4. Torii S, Hayashi Y, Hasegawa M, Sugiura S 1989 Reverse flow saphenous island flap in the patient with below-knee amputation. British Journal of Plastic Surgery 42: 517–520
5. Bertelli J A 1992 The saphenous posteromedial cutaneous island thigh flap and the saphenous superomedial cutaneous island leg flap. Surgical and Radiologic Anatomy 14: 187–189

SUPERFICIAL CIRCUMFLEX ILIAC ARTERY

Groin flap
Extended groin flap
Sartorius-cutaneous groin flap

7

An axial pattern flap based on the superficial circumflex iliac artery and the superficial venous network of the groin area was first reported as a pedicled skin flap by McGregor & Jackson in 1972.[1] The anatomy was further described by Smith et al.[2] O'Brien reported the use of the groin flap as a free flap in 1973[3] and since then several series have been reported. Acland[4] has modified the free flap so as to lengthen the vascular pedicle by displacing the skin island laterally and has termed this the free iliac flap. Several other reports have detailed the vascular anatomy and served to emphasise the variable nature of the vessels involved.[5] These aspects of the anatomy are dealt with in detail in Chapter 6 where further papers concerned exclusively with the vascular variability are referenced.

Used as a pedicled flap the groin flap has advantages: it can reliably be raised with a good length-to-breadth ratio; it can be readily tubed; and direct closure of the donor site is possible with the resultant scar in a cosmetically advantageous position.

The development of many alternative free flaps during the 1980s decreased the attractiveness of the groin free flap which had acquired a reputation for having a higher than average complication rate, largely arising from problems associated with the small size and variability of the vessels. Several authors have advised against use of the flap and quoted failure rates of up to 20%. However, advances in technology, allied with special techniques to overcome the vessel size problem, still make this flap a realistic option in skilled hands. A series of 73 free groin flaps carried out by a very experienced team between 1985 and 1990 showed 3 complete failures (4%) and 3 partial failures (Chuang et al, 1992).[6] Exploitation of the side branches, either the superficial inferior epigastric or the branch to sartorius, as shown in Figure 7.235, can make anastomosis significantly easier by increasing the diameter at the end of the artery.

Anatomy

The superficial circumflex iliac artery (SCIA) commonly arises from the femoral artery and in 50% of cases this will be by a common trunk with the superficial inferior epigastric artery. The point of origin lies approximately 3 cm below the mid-inguinal point (range 0.5–8 cm). The vessel measures between 1.3 and 2 mm in diameter but will be smaller than this (and therefore unsuitable for anastomosis) if the vessel is double or if it gives off a sizeable descending branch which is present in some degree in half the cases (Fig. 7.230). The SCIA lies beneath the deep fascia but always pierces it before it reaches a point 2.5 cm medial to the anterior superior iliac spine (ASIS), and commonly pierces it 2.5 cm medial to the lateral edge of sartorius (range 0.5–5.0 cm). The main stem of the SCIA (or its branches) follows a course towards the ASIS running approximately parallel to the inguinal ligament. As it passes laterally the quantity of overlying subcutaneous fat reduces and the vessel therefore comes to lie nearer to the skin.

In approximately 80% of cases the SCIA divides at a point between 2 and 3.5 cm from its origin into deep and superficial branches. The superficial branch is

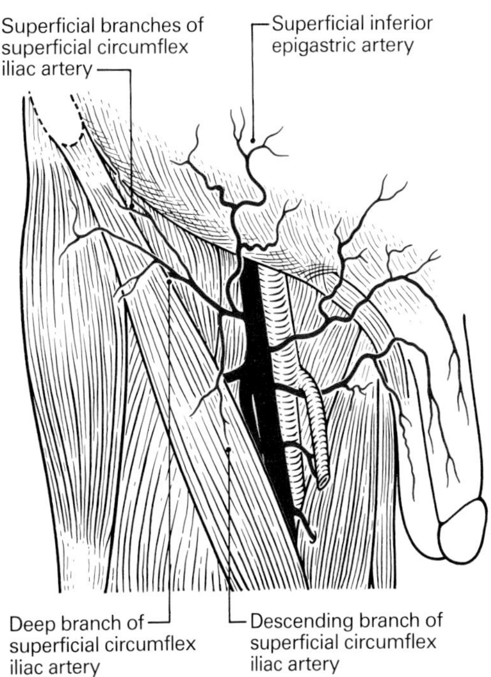

Fig. 7.230 Vascular anatomy. The superficial circumflex iliac artery runs below and parallel to the inguinal ligament. It gives off a deep branch at the medial edge of sartorius while superficial branches continue on to the region below and overlying the anterior superior iliac spine. A descending branch is generally also present but has been little described.

tortuous and supplies lymph nodes, fat and skin. The deep branch is straighter, supplies muscles, but eventually penetrates the deep fascia also. Both may supply the flap equally or alternatively the vessels are inversely proportional to each other in size. Distally the vessels anastomose with the periosteal vessels over the ASIS, and with the superior gluteal, deep circumflex iliac and lateral circumflex femoral arteries.

The veins of the area comprise a superficial set and a deeper set of venae comitantes. The superficial vein lies superficial to the artery and is often joined by the superficial inferior epigastric vein to form a moderate sized vessel of about 3 mm in diameter which drains into the saphenous bulb. The venae comitantes are a less important route of drainage and may also join the sapheno-femoral junction or may pass deeply beneath the femoral artery to enter the femoral vein.

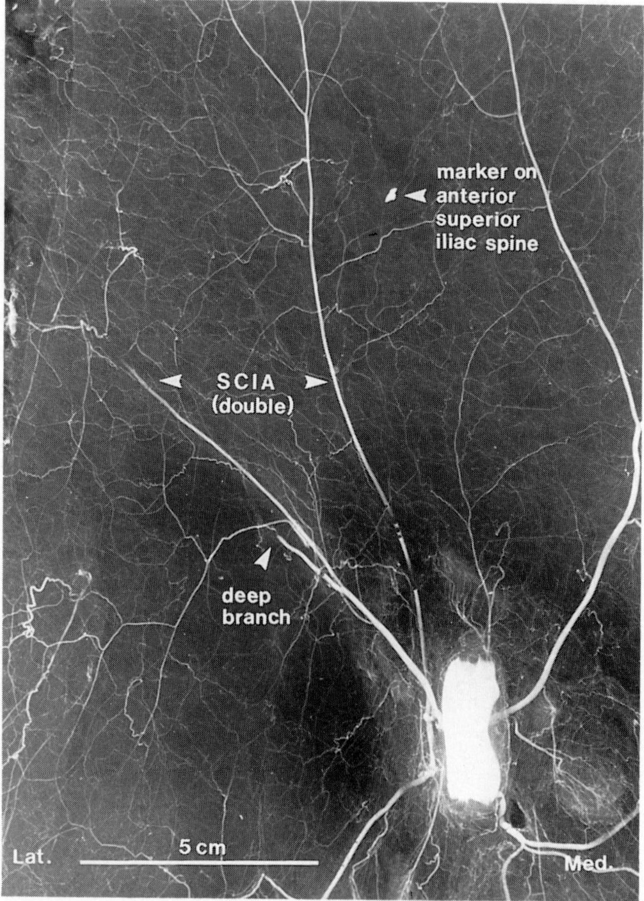

Fig. 7.231 The radiograph shows a slight departure from the classical description. (A short segment of the femoral artery has been removed in continuity with the skin specimen.)

The principal nerve of the area which is likely to complicate the elevation of the flap is the lateral cutaneous nerve of the thigh which divides into anterior and posterior branches and supplies the skin over the lower lateral part of the buttock and the anterolateral aspect of the thigh as far as the knee. These branches emerge into the thigh from beneath the lateral end of the inguinal ligament and run in front of, or through, sartorius to pierce the deep fascia and become superficial at varying distances below the inguinal ligament.

Surgery

Pedicled flaps. The approximate outlines of the pedicled flap are shown in Figure 7.232. This is based on a presumed course of the SCIA parallel to, and 3 cm below, the inguinal ligament but pre-operative determination of the course of the artery with a Doppler probe may lead to modification of the position of the flap. The upper and lower margins of the flap lie 5 cm on either side of this line since a width of 10 cm represents the upper limit with which direct closure may still be achieved. Flaps have been raised up to 27 cm × 17 cm but required skin grafting of the donor site. The flap may extend 5 cm beyond the ASIS. Elevation of the flap commences laterally and since the vessels lie superficially at this point the elevation may be above the fascia lata. At the lateral border of sartorius, if not before this point, the fascia is incised and medial to this line it is included in the flap. The fascia is also incised along the lower edge of the inguinal ligament since above this line the elevation proceeds in a plane superficial to the external oblique aponeurosis. The elevation may cease at the medial border of sartorius or be carried further in which case the deep muscular branch of the SCIA is divided. Various aspects of tubing the flap so as to avoid compression at the base where the flap is thicker, and so as to induce a spiral rotation to the tube, have been well described by Schlenker.[7]

Free flaps. The skin island is orientated over the presumed course of the vessels (Fig. 7.234) with the medial margin overlying the femoral artery. In contrast to the pedicled flap, the first stage is to explore the vessels and establish the vascular anatomy. The flap may then be elevated, once again including the deep fascia, but now visualising the deep branch of the SCIA, and dividing its muscular branches. In the lateral modification of the groin flap (the 'free iliac flap')[4] a long horizontal T-shaped incision is made over the course of the vessels (Fig. 7.234), the SCIV is mobilised and retracted and the SCIA sought by incising the

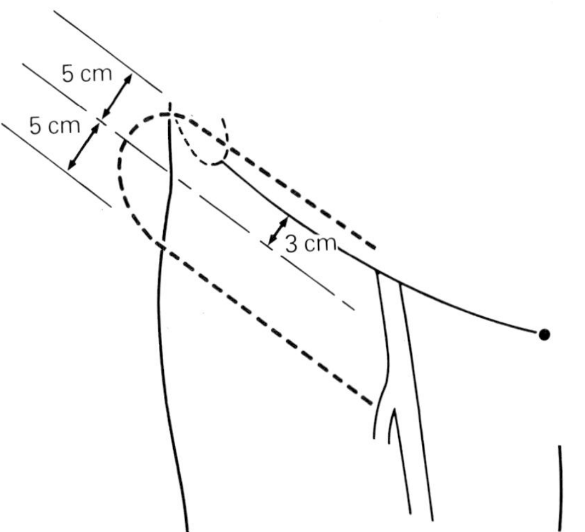

Fig. 7.232 Pedicled flap planning. The axial line of the flap lies 3 cm below the inguinal ligament. The margins of the flap lie above and below this line, parallel to it, and up to 5 cm from it.

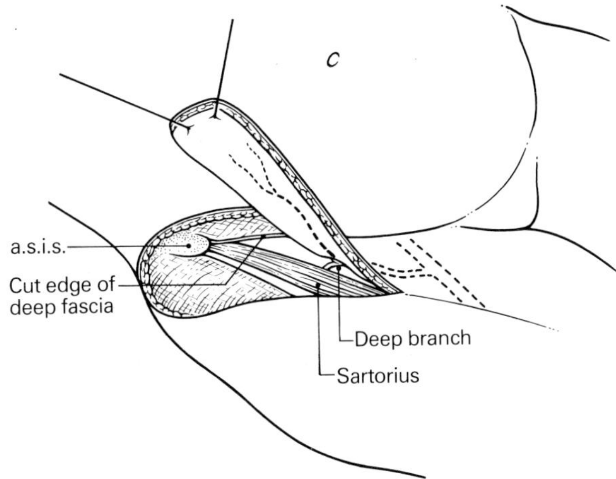

Fig. 7.233 Elevation of the pedicled form of the flap. Elevation commences laterally and includes the deep fascia over sartorius and medial to it – note the cut edge of the deep fascia at the lower border of the inguinal ligament.

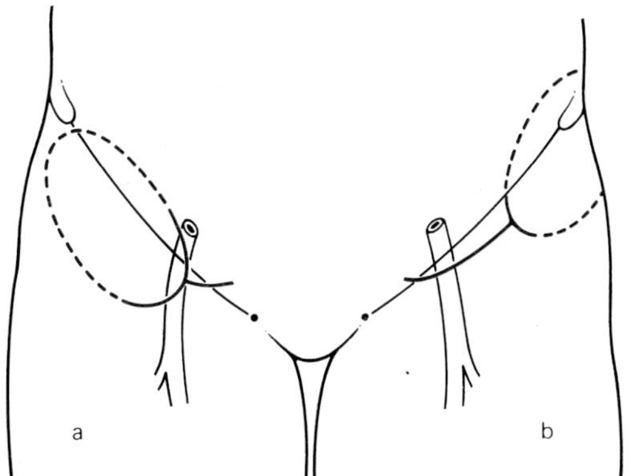

Fig. 7.234 Free flap planning: **a.** 'conventional' flap; **b.** 'extended' groin flap (see text). Initial incision shown by continuous line, remainder of flap then developed in a variable manner depending on vascular anatomy (dotted line).

femoral sheath and exposing the origin of the vessel. The superficial and deep branches are traced laterally, their relative contributions to the supply of the flap assessed, and the larger of the two preserved with the flap. In a modified technique described by Chuang[8] (who also orientates the flap more obliquely with the axial line drawn between SCIA origin and ASIS), a segment of sartorius is raised with the flap (the *sartorius-cutaneous groin flap*). In carrying out the lateral to medial flap elevation the fascia is divided at the lateral edge of sartorius as described above. The muscle is then elevated from its posterior fascia, divided superiorly and inferiorly, and then the fascia is divided at the medial edge of the muscle from below once the pedicle has been visualised. The flap then incorporates both the deep and superficial branches of the SCIA and no direct exploration of the deep branch is required.

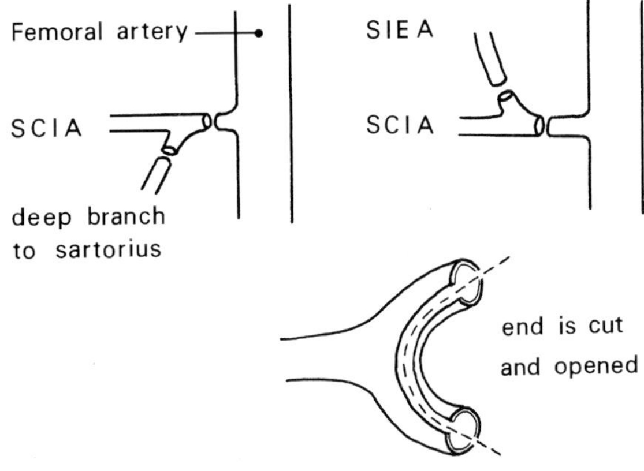

Fig. 7.235 Method of increasing the available end diameter for anastomosis of the free flap by utilising either the superficial inferior epigastric or the deep branch to sartorius.

References

1. McGregor I A, Jackson I T 1972 The groin flap. British Journal of Plastic Surgery 25: 3–16
2. Smith P J, Foley B, McGregor I A, Jackson I T 1972 The anatomical basis of the groin flap. Plastic and Reconstructive Surgery 49: 41–47
3. O'Brien B McC, MacLeod A M, Hayhurst J W, Morrison W A 1973 Successful transfer of a large island flap from the groin to the foot by microvascular anastomoses. Plastic and Reconstructive Surgery 52: 271–278
4. Acland R D 1979 The free iliac flap. A lateral modification of the free groin flap. Plastic and Reconstructive Surgery 64: 30–36
5. Ohmori K, Harii K 1975 Free groin flaps: their vascular basis. British Journal of Plastic Surgery 28: 238–243
6. Chuang D C C, Jeng S F, Chen H T, Chen H C, Wei F C 1992 Experience of 73 free groin flaps. British Journal of Plastic Surgery 45: 81–85.
7. Schlenker J D 1980 Important considerations in the design and construction of groin flaps. Annals of Plastic Surgery 5: 353–357
8. Chuang D C C, Colony L H, Chen H C, Wei F C 1989 Groin flap design and versatility. Plastic and Reconstructive Surgery 84: 100–107.

7 SUPERFICIAL EXTERNAL PUDENDAL ARTERY DEEP EXTERNAL PUDENDAL ARTERY

Paramedian axial-pattern flap
Penile island flaps
Dartos musculocutaneous flap

The superficial external pudendal artery supplies mainly a paramedian zone of suprapubic skin extending up towards the umbilicus, but may also send a branch onto the dorsum of the penis. The artery is the basis of an axial-pattern flap as described by Dias.[1,2,3]

The deep external pudendal artery supplies mainly penile and scrotal skin in the male, or labial skin in the female. It is the basis for several penile island flaps used in urethral reconstruction and in hypospadias repair.[4–7]

The skin of the scrotum is closely applied to the dartos muscle with no intervening subcutaneous fat. Composite skin/dartos flaps may be raised with either a skin and muscle pedicle or with the skin component reduced to an island carried on the deep external pudendal artery and dartos muscle pedicle.[8,9]

Anatomy

The origin of the superficial and deep external pudendal arteries from the femoral artery at the level of the sapheno-femoral junction has been described in Chapter 6 (p. 270). Note that both vessels supply superficial fascia and skin, the designation 'deep' merely indicating that in passing medially from the femoral artery one of the vessels passes under the saphenous vein, i.e. between it and the femoral vein. The superficial artery by contrast crosses superficial to the femoral vein. An alternative arrangement is that the femoral artery gives off a single trunk about 2 mm in diameter which then divides into two vessels which follow the same course as the arteries would have taken if they had arisen separately.

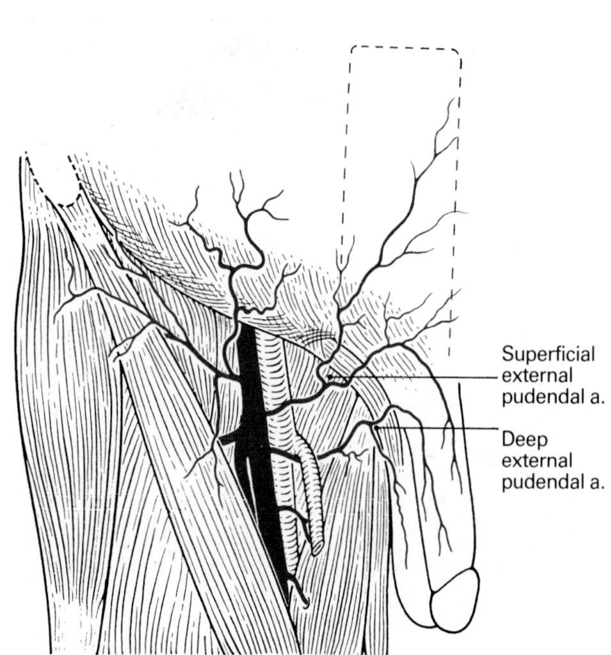

Fig. 7.236 Vascular anatomy. This also shows the outline of a paramedian flap based on the superficial external pudendal artery. The medial incision may reach the level of the crest of the pubic symphysis but the lateral margin must stop at least 2.5 cm above the pubic tubercle. Anastomoses exist across the midline and a flap of twice the width may be raised on the vessels of both sides.

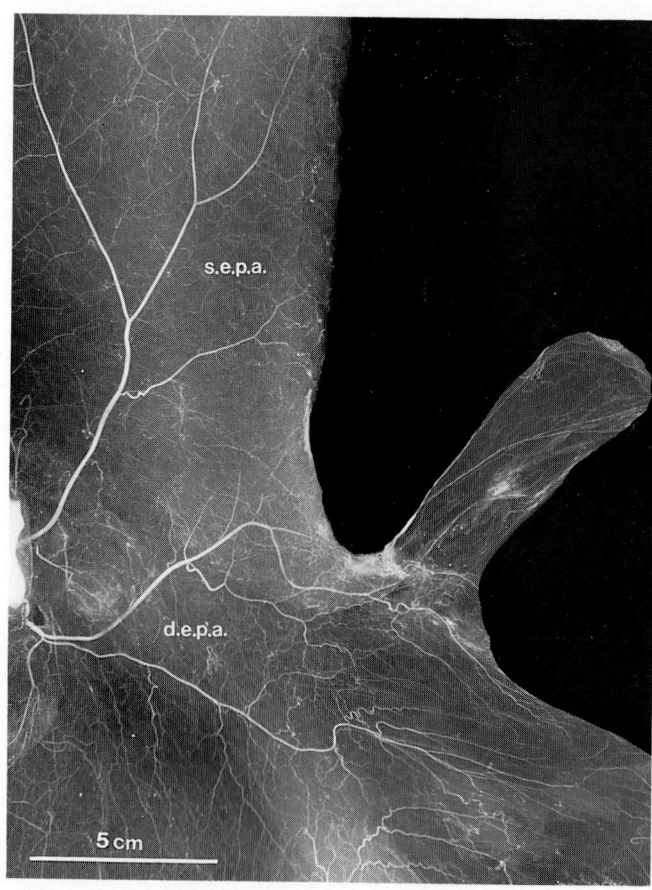

Fig. 7.237 Radiograph of skin from right side of midline.

The *superficial* or superior vessel passes up towards the pubic tubercle giving off a few small branches to the skin and a branch which supplies the region of the superficial inguinal ring and may enter the inguinal canal. It crosses over the spermatic cord and at this point is just superficial to Scarpa's fascia. It then continues up towards the umbilicus gradually becoming more superficial. Vessels of each side communicate across the midline and approximately half-way between the symphysis and the umbilicus the superficial external pudendal artery branches out into three or four longitudinal vessels. The vessels anastomose with musculocutaneous perforators through rectus abdominis and with the superficial inferior epigastric artery.

The *deep* artery has a more horizontal course and runs over the upper part of the thigh, gives off branches to the scrotum, and runs onto the shaft of the penis where it spreads out to supply the superficial fascia and skin up to the coronal sulcus. Branches from the deep artery tend to lie in a more lateral position on the shaft than branches of the superficial artery. Veins accompany the arteries.

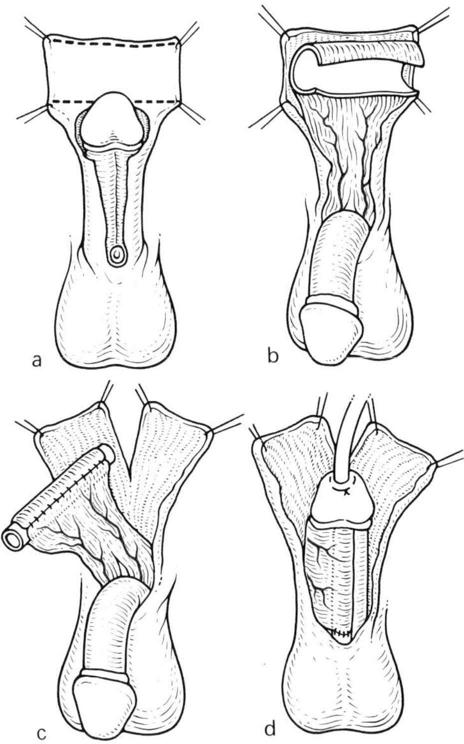

Fig. 7.238 Duckett repair of hypospadias – method of repair after release of chordee: **a.** ventral preputial skin displayed; **b.** development of island flap on a fascial pedicle; **c.** formation of neourethral skin tube; **d.** anastomosis of skin tube and passage through glans. Byars flaps will be brought round for ventral closure and their tips excised. (Redrawn after Duckett, 1980.)

The glans is supplied by the dorsal arteries of the penis (derived from the internal pudendal artery) and drains through the deep dorsal veins which also receive a few veins across the tunica albuginea from the corpora cavernosa. The prepuce also receives blood from the deep vessels through small perforators from the corpus spongiosum and corpora cavernosa which are particularly abundant just proximal to the coronal margin on the dorsum of the penis.

Surgery

Suprapubic abdominal flaps. A long narrow flap some 4 cm wide may be constructed on one side of the midline based on one vessel, or if greater width is required a bilateral flap of up to 9 cm width may be raised. It may be raised to just below the umbilicus and is elevated in a plane just deep to Scarpa's fascia. The lateral incision may be taken down to the level of the pubis but must stay at least 2.5 cm lateral to the pubic tubercle to ensure incorporation of the vessels.

Penile island flaps. The following two operations out of some of the 150 different ones reported for hypospadias repair, indicate the way in which these vessels may be used to support an island flap on a vascularised subcutaneous pedicle.

For the one-stage hypospadias repair in the child, Duckett[4] has developed a transverse preputial island flap as a modification of the Asopa procedure.[5] A circumferential incision is made just proximal to the corona down to the tunica albuginea, and on the ventral surface is brought proximally to include the meatus (Fig. 7.238a). The dorsal skin and prepuce are then dissected free from the shaft working in the avascular plane above the tunica but beneath the pudendal vessels. A rectangle of skin is outlined on the ventral shiny undersurface of the prepuce some 12–15 mm in width and 30–40 mm long. The distal and lateral sides of this rectangle are incised but the proximal margin, which coincides with the edge resulting from the circumferential incision, carries the blood supply to the flap in a subcutaneous tissue pedicle and only the skin is incised. The subcutaneous vascular pedicle is developed by dissecting it off the dorsal skin and the island, fashioned into a tube, is swung round onto the ventral surface of the penis.

A similar technique in principle is one which uses instead a vascularised flap of dorsal preputial skin.[6]

For the circumcised adult with a stricture anywhere between meatus and prostate, Quartey[7] has developed a transverse island flap from the penile shaft. The skin incision commences at the frenum and passes circularly on one side just proximal to the corona. The length of

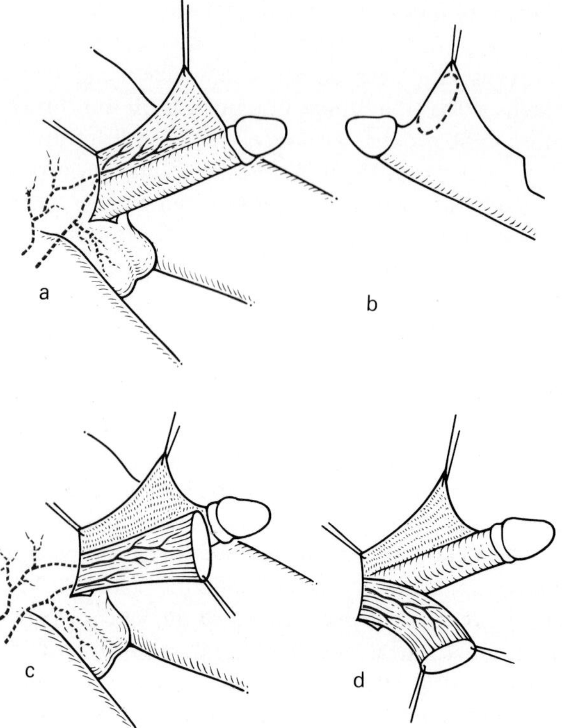

Fig. 7.239 Quartey technique for fashioning an island of skin on the penile shaft just proximal to the coronal sulcus; **c.** shows the subcutaneous pedicle being dissected off the undersurface of the dorsal skin.

this incision is equal to the length of urethra requiring repair and is deepened down to the tunica albuginea. A ventral midline incision is then made from the frenum to the peno-scrotal junction and deepened down to the corpus spongiosum. The penile skin together with the subcutaneous tissue containing the pudendal vessels is then dissected off the tunica albuginea as a flap (Fig. 7.239a). Next the transverse skin island for the urethroplasty is outlined transversely at the coronal margin of the flap. The proximal side is only incised skin-deep preserving the vessels in the subcutaneous tissue which is then dissected off the dorsal skin. The largest flap reported measured 6 cm × 3 cm and there was no difficulty in recovering the shaft with skin.

Dartos musculocutaneous flaps. These have been used for ischioperineal pressure areas, groin defects and penile skin defects.[8] The flap is raised from the unilateral anterior scrotum, since the posterior part of the scrotum has a separate blood supply from the branches of the internal pudendal artery. Bilateral flaps can be used if required, but a flap pedicled on one side should probably not be extended across the midline. These flaps can be sensate since branches of the ilioinguinal nerve are included. Tiwari et al[9] described the elevation of a skin island, pedicled on dartos only. They recommended injecting saline beneath the skin in the area of the pedicle to facilitate dissection of the skin off the underlying muscle; this skin is then discarded and the island flap passed through a subcutaneous tunnel to reach the recipient site. Flaps with dimensions of up to 5 cm × 4 cm may be raised and the donor sites closed directly.

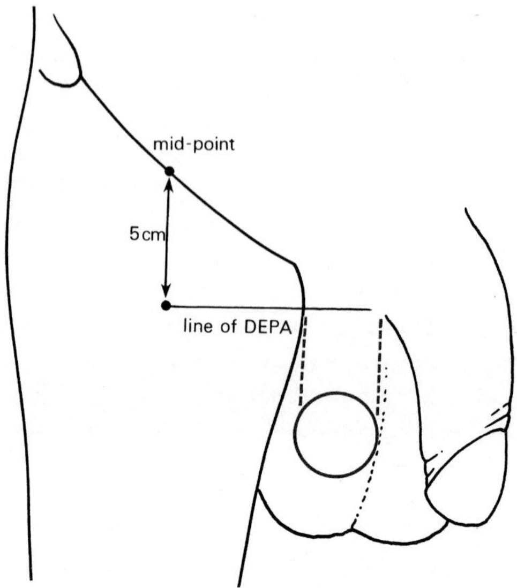

Fig. 7.240 Dartos musculocutaneous island flap. The flap is positioned adjacent to the midline raphe. The muscle pedicle is the same width as the skin island, and the base of the pedicle is located over the anterior scrotal neck. The base of the pedicle is on the same horizontal level as the junction between the undersurface of the penile shaft and the scrotum.

References

1. Dias A D 1984 The superficial external pudendal artery (SEPA) axial-pattern flap. British Journal of Plastic Surgery 37: 256–261
2. Patil U A, Dias A D, Thatte R L 1987 The anatomical basis of the SEPA flap. British Journal of Plastic Surgery 40: 342–347
3. Dias A D, Thatte R L, Patil U A, Dhami L D, Prasad S 1987 The uses of the SEPA flap in the repair of defects in the hands and fingers. British Journal of Plastic Surgery 40: 348–359
4. Duckett J W 1980 Transverse preputial island flap technique for repair of severe hypospadias. Urological Clinics of North America 7: 432–439
5. Asopa H S, Elhence E P, Atria S P, Bansal N K 1971 One-stage correction of penile hypospadias using a foreskin tube. A preliminary report. International Surgery 55: 435–440
6. Carmignani G, Belgrano E, Gaboardi F, Farina F P 1982 Microsurgical one-stage repair of hypospadias with a rectangular transverse dorsal preputial vascularised skin flap. Journal of Microsurgery 3: 222–227
7. Quartey J K M 1983 One stage penile/preputial cutaneous island urethroplasty for urethral stricture: a preliminary report. Journal of Urology 129: 284–287
8. Mendez-Fernandez M A, Hollan C, Frank D H, Fisher J C 1986 The scrotal myocutaneous flap. Plastic and Reconstructive Surgery 78: 676–678
9. Tiwari V K, Kumar P, Sharma R K 1991 The dartos musculocutaneous flap. British Journal of Plastic Surgery 44: 33–35

SUPERFICIAL INFERIOR EPIGASTRIC ARTERY

Hypogastric flap

The possibility of raising a long flap from the anterior abdominal wall without the need for several preliminary delays was demonstrated by Shaw in 1944[1,2] when he reported the hypogastric flap based on the superficial inferior epigastric artery although French surgeons had probably been doing this since 1930. The flap has been superseded by others and is now rarely used in the original form although Barfred[3] has reported the use of the flap is 28 instances on 26 patients with major necrosis in four cases. However, the development of the groin flap revived interest in this vessel since the superficial inferior epigastric artery anastomoses with the superficial circumflex iliac artery. It may on occasions be the larger of the two vessels and may arise from the superficial circumflex iliac in approximately 50%. Such a situation allows a large island flap to be created which incorporates parts of the territories of both vessels but is based on only one dominant artery.[4] Recently the SIEA has been used to support a horizontal ellipse of lower abdominal skin which is used as a pedicled flap for coverage of hand and forearm defects.[5]

Anatomy

The superficial inferior epigastric artery arises from the femoral artery either directly or via a common trunk with the superficial circumflex iliac in the 5 cm segment beneath the inguinal ligament (Fig. 7.241) and measures up to 2.5 mm in diameter. It pierces the cribriform fascia and ascends in the subcutaneous tissues for up to 15 cm lying within the area shown in Figure 7.241 which indicates the region containing the commonest locations of the artery. Its course tends to be vertical or slightly laterally inclined; its medial branches anastomose with musculocutaneous perforators from the epigastric arcade, and its lateral branches anastomose with intercostal arteries. The venous drainage of this area is mainly through the superficial inferior epigastric vein which lies superficially and may be seen through the skin, but when it is small the venae comitantes of the SIEA may substitute. The superficial inferior epigastric vein often unites with the superficial circumflex iliac vein to form a common trunk which joins the great saphenous vein, but in some cases they flow separately into the great saphenous vein.

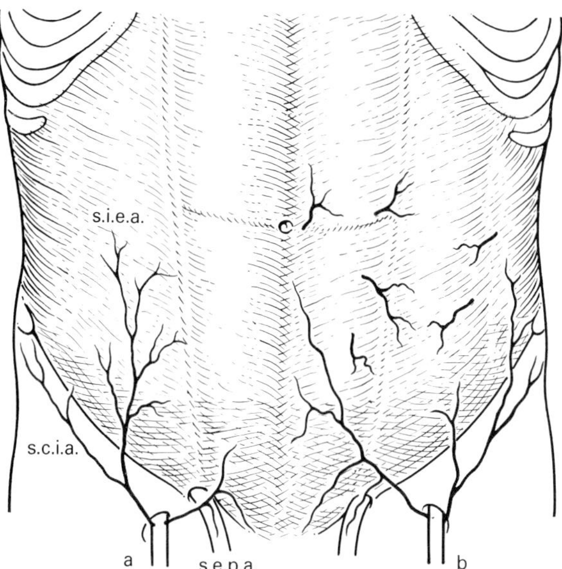

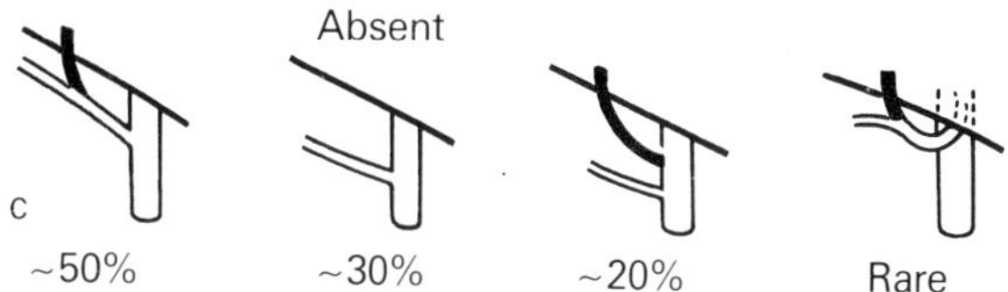

Fig. 7.241 Vascular anatomy: **a.** well-developed superficial inferior epigastric artery; **b.** poorly developed SIEA, supply of lower abdominal area taken over by well-developed SEPA and musculocutaneous perforators; **c.** variability in the origin of the SIEA from the SCIA or the femoral artery.

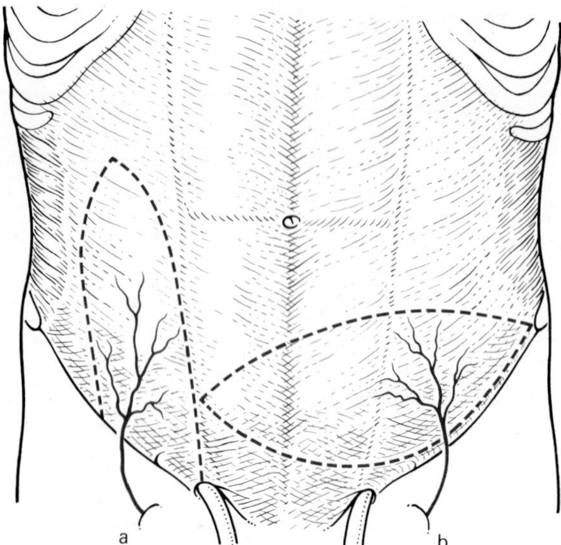

Fig. 7.242 Flap planning. **a.** Conventionally pedicled vertical hypogastric flap. Base consists of skin and subcutaneous fat containing the pedicle. **b.** Modified horizontal paddle with subcutaneous pedicle containing vessels. Ability to support the end of the ellipse which lies on the other side of the midline is variable.

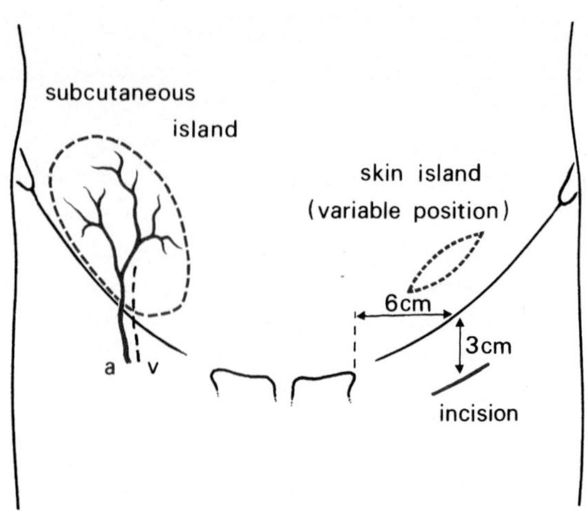

Fig. 7.244 Flap planning. Incisions for elevating the flap of subcutaneous tissue only. The upper incison can be made into a small skin ellipse for flap monitoring.

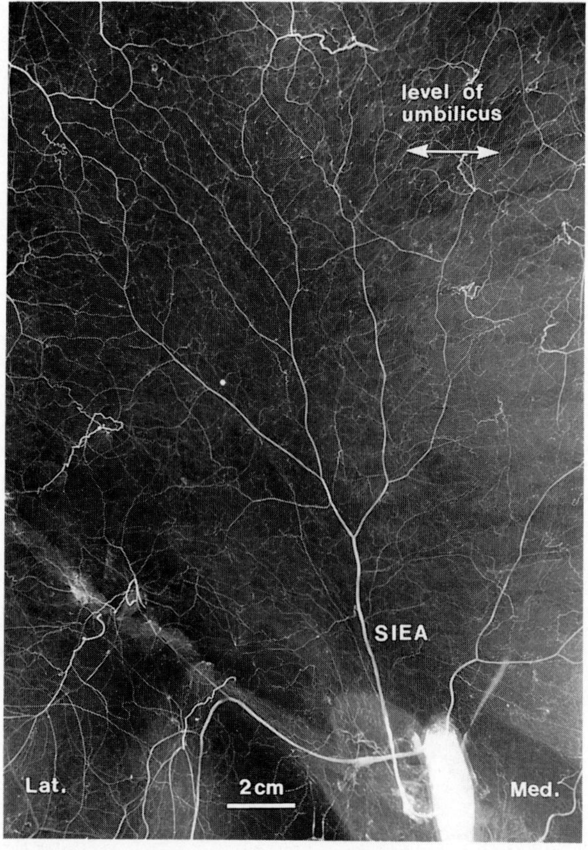

Fig. 7.243 Radiograph illustrating a particularly well-developed example of the SIEA.

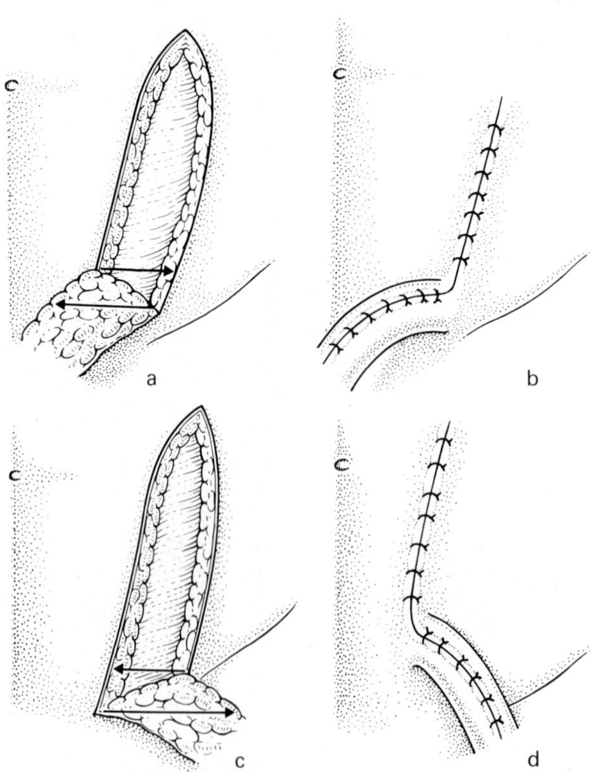

Fig. 7.245 This illustrates the method of tubing the base of the flap in such a way as to turn the raw surface at the end of the flap in either a lateral (**a & b**) or medial (**c & d**) facing direction.

Flap planning

The classical flap. The superficial inferior epigastric vein is used as a guide in planning the flap which is outlined between two parallel incisions tapering to a blunt point 2 cm above the level of the umbilicus. Shaw quoted various dimensions for the flap ranging in length from 5 to 18 cm and in width from 3 to 7 cm. The flap is raised just superficial to Scarpa's fascia or may include the fascia, and the margins of the donor defect are then undermined for closure in the fatty areolar layer beneath the fascia. Additional relaxation may be obtained by incising the fascia parallel with the skin margins. By staggering the inferior ends of the incisions and undermining to achieve mobility for closure of the angles, it is possible to rotate the base through an arc of up to 180°. If the medial incision is shorter then the open surface of the flap will rotate laterally (Fig. 7.245a, b), whereas if the lateral incision is shorter then the flap will be rotated medially (Fig. 7.245c, d). The final amount of rotation depends on the amount of staggering of the original incisions and the width of the flap. Formation of the flap into a tube can be easily achieved.

The horizontal ellipse. A lenticular-shaped horizontally-located skin island with maximum dimensions of approximately 25 cm length × 15 cm width may be based on one superficial inferior epigastric artery.[5] The flap can be designed to cross the midline for a couple of centimetres but survival beyond this is unlikely (Fig. 7.242b). The inferior incision is made first and the vascular pedicle identified and preserved. The inferior and superior incisions are completed to the level of the external oblique aponeurosis from which the entire flap can be elevated. The flap can be thinned by reducing the fat beneath Scarpa's fascia. The advantages of this flap are that the donor site is closed at the time of the initial flap elevation except for a 2 cm gap to allow passage of the vascular pedicle and the narrow pedicle allows considerable mobility of the flap when compared to the standard groin flap. Stevenson et al[5] have successfully rotated the flap through an arc of 120° without vascular compromise.

Kelleher et al[6] have described a related, but much broader-based, lower abdominal flap supplied by both superficial inferior epigastric arteries for extensive injuries of the distal upper limb.

The subcutaneous tissue only flap. This is a good donor site when a flap of fatty tissue is required for subcutaneous tissue augmentation, and the flap can include a small skin island as a monitor if required. Two skin incisions are made parallel to the line of the groin skin crease and are used to expose the pedicle and dissect out the flap. It is best to position the lower incision inferolateral to the probable site of origin of the SIEA. This avoids accidental damage to the pedicle when deepening the approach and a dissection in a superior and medial direction is convenient for the surgeon seated on the side of the flap. An incision is made centred on the mid-point of the inguinal ligament and approximately 4 cm below it for exposure of the pedicle and a second parallel incision is made above the inguinal ligament in a position dictated by the size of the required flap. The presence of the SIEA is confirmed first by dissecting the pedicle and its size assessed. If suitable, the superior incision is made (± monitoring flap) and a subcutaneous undermining carried out which allows the margins of the skin wounds to be retracted to the limits of the proposed flap. These limits are incised and the fat flap dissected off the external oblique muscle commencing superiorly and working inferiorly towards the pedicle which is skeletonised last. The monitoring island tends to be very pale and hard to assess.

References

1. Shaw D T 1944 Open abdominal flaps for repair of surface defects of the upper extremity. Surgical Clinics of North America 24: 293–308
2. Shaw D T, Payne R L 1946 One stage tubed abdominal flaps. Surgery, Gynaecology and Obstetrics 83: 205–209
3. Barfred T 1976 The Shaw abdominal flap. Scandinavian Journal of Plastic and Reconstructive Surgery 10: 56–58
4. Harii K, Ohmori K, Torii S, Sekiguchi J 1978 Microvascular free skin flap transfer. Clinics in Plastic Surgery 5: 239–263
5. Stevenson T R, Hester T R, Duus E C, Dingman R O 1984 Superficial inferior epigastric artery flap for coverage of hand and forearm defects. Annals of Plastic Surgery 12: 333–339
6. Kelleher J C, Sullivan J G, Baibak G J et al 1982 Large combined axial vessel pattern abdominal pedicle flap: Indications for its use in surgery of the hand. Orthopaedic Review 11: 33–48
7. Hester T R Jr, Nahai F, Beegle P E, Bostwick J 1984 Blood supply of the abdomen revisited, with emphasis on the superficial inferior epigastric artery. Plastic and Reconstructive Surgery 74: 657–666
8. Stern H S, Nahai F 1992 The versatile superficial inferior epigastric artery free flap. British Journal of Plastic Surgery 95: 270–274

7 SUPERFICIAL SURAL ARTERY

Calf fasciocutaneous free flap
Calf island pedicled flap
Lateral sural artery pedicled flap

Taylor & Daniel[1] described a free flap from the posterior calf region in 1975. Their flap required that a branch of one of the sural arteries should be dissected out of its bed within one of the bellies of gastrocnemius whilst preserving its musculocutaneous branches to an overlying island of calf skin. Incorporation of the terminal branches of the posterior cutaneous nerve of the thigh would permit this flap to carry sensation.

More recently an easier way of elevating a fasciocutaneous flap from the same region has been described by Walton & Bunkis[2] who have reported its use in 14 cases (with two failures).[3] This flap is based on a branch of the popliteal or of a sural artery which runs beneath the deep fascia between the two heads of gastrocnemius. It may also carry sensation through any of the cutaneous nerves of the region.

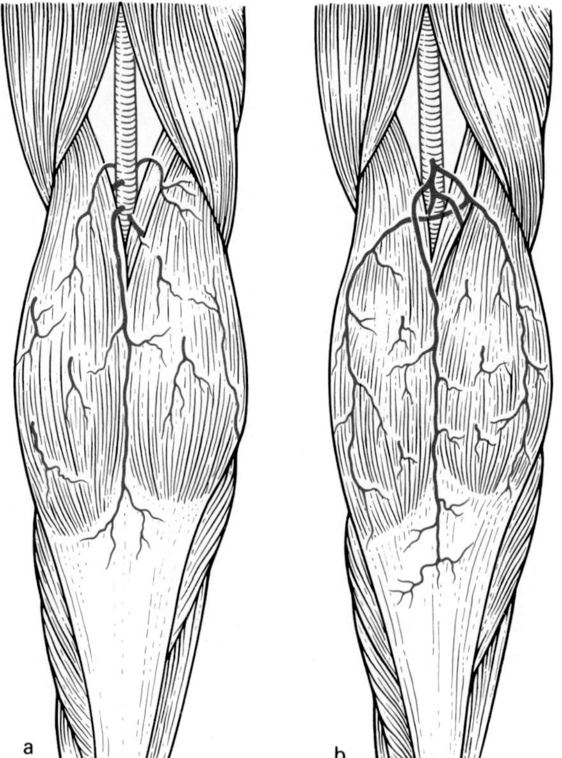

Fig. 7.246 Vascular anatomy. Varying degrees of development of the median, medial, and lateral superficial sural arteries are shown. These vessels arise either directly from the popliteal artery or from sural arteries.

Anatomy

There are up to three vessels arising from the popliteal artery and running down over gastrocnemius. The best description of these arteries has been given by Manchot (1889) who used the Latin terms Arteriae suralis superficialis medialis, lateralis et mediana. The English equivalents seem suitable terms to use in describing these vessels in the absence of any official designation in *Nomina Anatomica*. The median superficial sural artery has been described by Haertsch[4] and has also been described in the context of the vascularised sural nerve graft by Briedenbach & Terzis,[5] and by Frachinelli et al.[6]

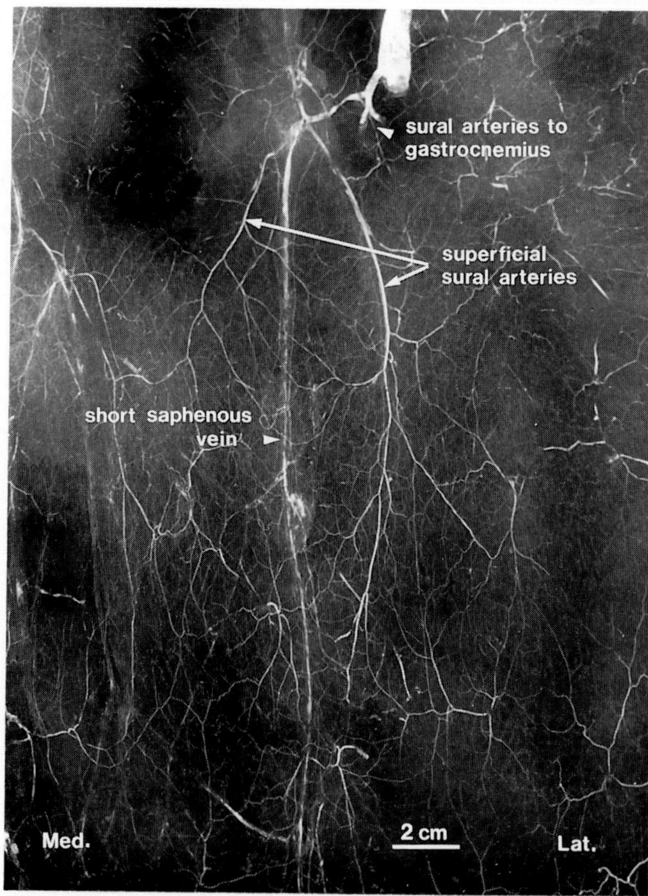

Fig. 7.247 Radiograph of skin showing medial and lateral superficial sural arteries, the lateral being larger than the medial. A segment of the popliteal artery has been removed in continuity with the vessels.

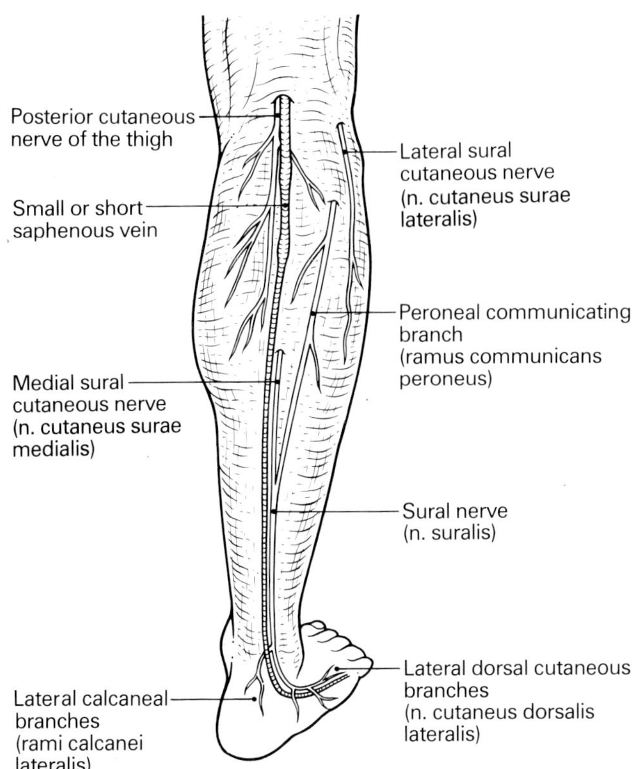

Fig. 7.248 Cutaneous innervation in the area of the flap. Note that the short saphenous vein may alternatively lie with the medial sural cutaneous nerve beneath the surface of the deep fascia between its two layers.

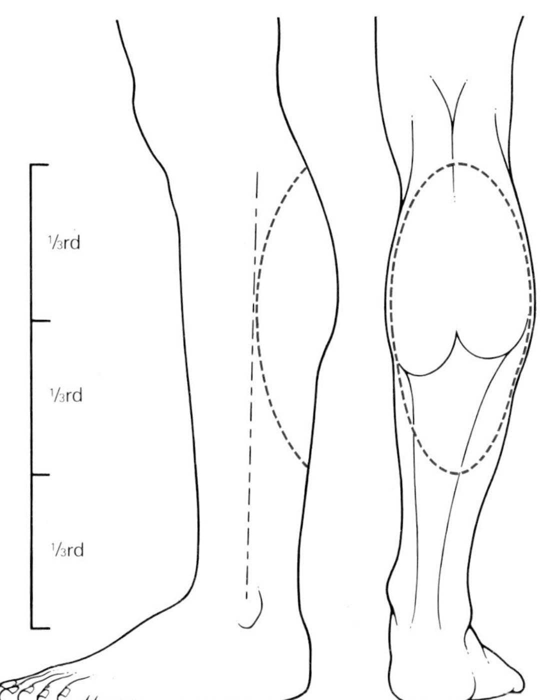

Fig. 7.249 Flap planning. The flap lies in the upper two-thirds of the lower leg and does not extend forwards beyond the mid-lateral axial lines.

The median superficial sural artery is present in ~95% of cases and arises from the popliteal artery (~65%) or from either the medial (~20%) or lateral (~8%) sural arteries or sometimes the common stem of origin of the two. At its point of origin at the level of the tibial condyles it measures approximately 1.2 mm in external diameter (range 1.0–2.0 mm). The vessel runs between the two heads of gastrocnemius and after 2 or 3 cm reaches the midline beneath the deep fascia where it lies in the company of the medial sural cutaneous nerve. (This nerve becomes the sural nerve once joined by the peroneal communicating branch: see Fig. 7.248 for an indication of the somewhat confusing terminology for nerves in this area.) At approximately the point where it joins the nerve it may give off a branch to the skin. The median superficial sural artery is accompanied by one or two small veins approximately 1.3 mm in diameter while the much larger short saphenous vein generally lies above the deep fascia and penetrates it only in the popliteal fossa. The artery descends in the groove between the two gastrocnemius muscles down to the commencement of the Achilles tendon and very occasionally beyond this point.

The medial and lateral superficial sural arteries arise from the popliteal artery and vary inversely in size with the median superficial sural artery. Usually these vessels are short and fine, and only reach small areas over the heads of the gastrocnemius, but when the median superficial sural artery is underdeveloped they may extend down to the Achilles tendon. Manchot described cases in which all three vessels were equally developed and anastomosed with each other in the middle third of the leg (Fig. 7.246b).

The venous anatomy parallels the arterial anatomy in approximately 80% of cases with the venae comitantes draining into the popliteal or sural vessels either separately or after forming a common trunk.

Flap planning

Dye injection of the isolated median superficial sural artery discolours the skin of the upper half of the calf with lesser mottled discoloration evident in the lower half of the leg. This is in accordance with our own and Haertsch's radiographs. The clinical experience of Walton et al[3] indicates that the territory of the flap may extend round to the medial and lateral mid-axial lines with the length of the flap extending from the popliteal crease to the junction of the middle and lower thirds of the leg. The largest reported clinical case[2] used a flap measuring 11 cm × 19 cm.

Li et al have used the lateral sural artery based posterolateral calf flaps in 17 patients to reconstruct defects around the knee. They orientated their flaps on the posterolateral aspect of the leg between the plane of the knee joint superiorly and the lower end of the gastrocnemius inferiorly. In cadavers they found that the lateral sural artery was fairly constant and had an outside diameter of 0.4 to 0.6 mm at its origin. In their clinical series the largest flap measured 25 cm × 15 cm which is surprisingly large for such a small vessel. However, the distribution can be extensive as shown in the radiograph in Figure 7.247.

Flap elevation

Walton & Bunkis recommend prior delineation of the vessel with a Doppler probe. The flap is then centred over this vessel and elevated from distal to proximal in the subfascial plane. The sural nerve lies above or below the deep fascia depending on whether one is at the lower or upper end of the flap respectively (Fig. 7.248) and should be included in the flap irrespective of whether or not an innervated flap is required since the superficial sural artery lies in close relationship to the nerve and might be damaged by its dissection. Other cutaneous nerves impinging on the territory of the flap are shown in Figure 7.248. The posterior cutaneous nerve of the thigh is the primary choice for a small innervated flap and is located above the fascia when the superior margin of the flap is incised. Also in this region it is probably worth isolating a superficial vein as a reserve in the event of the venae comitantes of the artery being too small for anastomosis. However, the main use of this flap is not as a free flap but as a local pedicled flap for reconstructions around the knee as described by Moscona et al.[8]

When raising the posterolateral calf/lateral sural flap key points are protection of the common peroneal nerve when incising the lateral border of the flap, and dividing all veins and nerves down to the muscle at the distal end of the flap, including the lateral sural nerve and the peroneal communicating branch which are raised with the flap. This makes the flap sensate and is an advantage of this flap over the reverse pedicled flaps available in the area for reconstructions around the knee. The axis point of rotation is located at the lower part of the popliteal fossa. Flaps less than 4 cm wide enable direct closure of the donor site.

References

1. Taylor G I, Daniel R K 1975 The anatomy of several free-flap donor sites. Plastic and Reconstructive Surgery 56: 243–253
2. Walton R L, Bunkis J 1984 The posterior calf fasciocutaneous free flap. Plastic and Reconstructive Surgery 74: 76–85
3. Walton R L, Logan S E, Bunkis J, Asko S 1983 Experience with two fasciocutaneous free flap models. Plastic Surgical Forum 6: 158–160
4. Haertsch P A 1981 The blood supply to the skin of the leg: a post-mortem investigation. British Journal of Plastic Surgery 34: 470–477
5. Breidenbach W C, Terzis J K 1983 Vascularised nerve grafts. Plastic Surgical Forum 6: 131–133
6. Frachinelli A, Masquelet A, Restrepo J, Gilbert A 1981 The vascularised sural nerve. International Journal of Microsurgery 3: 57–62
7. Satoh K, Fukuya F, Matsui A, Onizuka T 1989 Lower leg reconstruction using a sural fasciocutaneous flap. Annals of Plastic Surgery 23: 97–103
8. Moscona A R, Govrin-Yehudain J, Hirshowitz B 1985 The island fasciocutaneous flap; a new type of flap for defects of the knee. British Journal of Plastic Surgery 38: 512–514
9. Li Z, Liu K, Lin Y, Li L 1990 Lateral sural cutaneous artery island flap in the treatment of soft tissue defects at the knee. British Journal of Plastic Surgery 43: 546–550

SUPERFICIAL TEMPORAL ARTERY

Laterally based forehead flaps

In 1893 Dunham described a laterally based forehead flap which 'was so cut as to contain, traversing its pedicle and ramifying in it, the anterior temporal artery. It had rather a long pedicle, about an inch wide, attached in front of the ear, and the mass of the flap was from the upper forehead where it slightly crossed the median line'.[1] The end of the flap was inset into a defect of the left side of the nose and cheek and in the second stage of this operation Dunham dissected the anterior temporal artery and veins free from the pedicle, returned the proximal part of the skin flap to the forehead and buried the vessels beneath the skin of the cheek.

The ability of a narrow pedicle containing the superficial temporal artery to support a forehead flap was further demonstrated clinically by Monks (lower eyelid reconstruction 1898),[2] Horsley (cheek defect reconstruction 1916),[3] Esser (1917, 1931), Gillies (1949) and many others. Despite this early history of the forehead flap being characterised by fairly narrow pedicles and despite Wilson's advocacy of the 2 cm wide pedicle,[4] in common practice the base of the flap tended to be wider. Indeed Cramer & Culf[5] suggested that the base should be kept wide and the posterior incision inclined posteriorly at its lower end so as to obtain some additional inflow into the base of the flap from the posterior auricular artery. In general, however, the base has tended to be located entirely in front of the ear at the level of the tragus.

It must be said that the development of alternative flaps for intra-oral reconstruction, particularly the free Chinese forearm flap, combined with a feeling that the cosmetic disfigurement resulting from having a split skin graft on the forehead is unacceptable, has meant that this flap no longer enjoys the popularity that it once did.

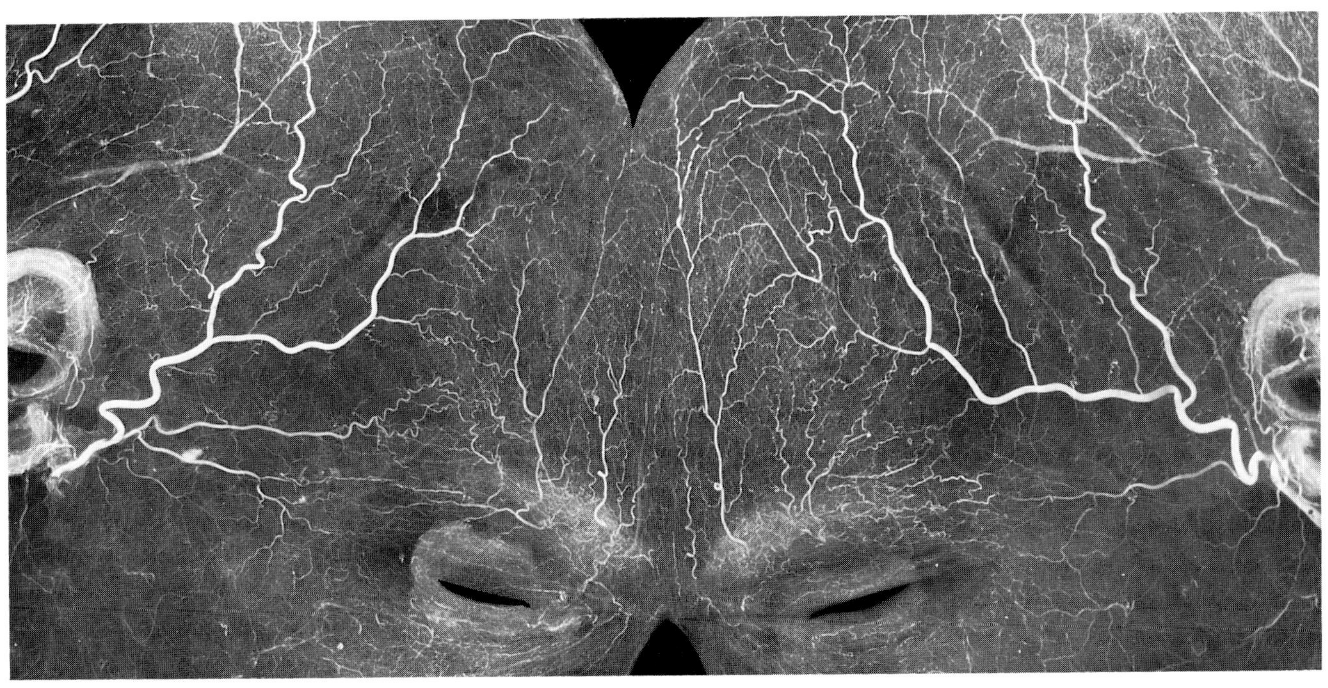

Fig. 7.250 Radiograph of forehead skin.

Anatomy

A thorough understanding of the vascular anatomy underlying forehead flaps has been provided by the cadaver injection studies of Conway et al[6], Corso[7] and Behan & Wilson.[8] These studies have shown that the dynamic territory of the forehead flap is made up of four anatomical territories, namely that of the feeding frontal branch of the superficial temporal, the two supratrochlear arteries and the contralateral frontal branch of the superficial temporal. When the flap is situated over the vertex only the two parietal branches of the superficial temporal are involved. All these vessels anastomose extensively through large diameter vessels, which readily allow the separate anatomical territories to link up and form an axial territory. The anatomy of the superficial temporal artery has been described on page 138, but the following points are worthy of note:

1. The zygomatico-orbital artery may arise directly from the STA or from its frontal branch. This affects the course of the frontal branch and in the latter situation confusion as to which is truly the frontal branch can occur.
2. The STA pierces the fascia at a variable level.
3. The avascular plane lies deep to the galea.

The flap that can be raised primarily on a broad pedicle containing one STA and its accompanying veins, extends across the width of the forehead and reaches from the eyebrows to the normal position of the frontal hairline. The flap may therefore be up to about 30 cm long and this sort of length can generally be achieved without a delay.

Surgery

The laterally based forehead flap is usually elevated so as to include the hairless skin of the forehead and part of the temporal hair-bearing sideburn area. In the bald individual it may be preferable for cosmetic reasons to take the flap from the top of the head, basing it on the parietal branch of the superficial temporal artery rather than its frontal branch. A third possibility which is suitable when only a small area of forehead skin is required for the reconstruction, is to create a sickle-shaped pedicle based on the parietal branch and to curve this forwards so that the tip of the flap lies on the forehead immediately anterior to the hairline. These three basic types are illustrated in Figure 7.251. A fourth possibility is a double flap which can be passed down like a visor over the face to reconstruct the chin.[9]

Islanded versions of the flap are possible but are probably best restricted to islands based on the posterior branch in bald individuals since the anterior branch does not appear to be constantly accompanied by such a reliable venous drainage system.

Elevation of the flap is straightforward except at the base where the blood vessels must be protected. The plane of dissection lies beneath the galea and the pedicle is elevated down to the level of the middle of the tragus; below this level the artery lies deep to the fascia.

Use of the flap for intra-oral lining was described by Blair in 1941.[10] When used for intra-oral lining the flap may be led into the mouth in essentially four different ways.

1. As described by McGregor (1963)[11] the flap was turned downwards with its raw surface facing laterally and was then passed through an incision in the cheek approximately 1.5 cm below the zygomatic arch and along a tunnel in the cheek created by blunt dissection (Fig. 7.252a). The precise course taken by the flap depends on whether or not the ramus of the mandible has been resected and on the position of the defect but the flap usually takes the most direct course to the defect.

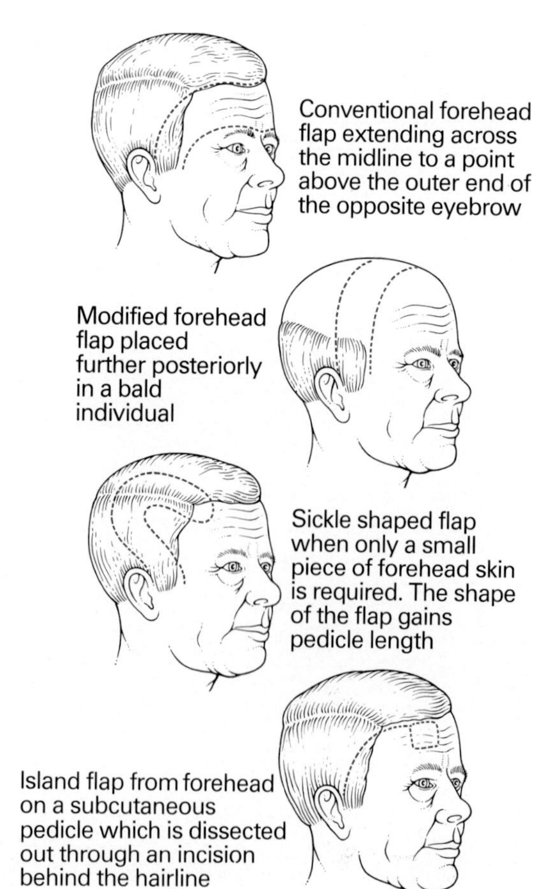

Conventional forehead flap extending across the midline to a point above the outer end of the opposite eyebrow
Modified forehead flap placed further posteriorly in a bald individual
Sickle shaped flap when only a small piece of forehead skin is required. The shape of the flap gains pedicle length
Island flap from forehead on a subcutaneous pedicle which is dissected out through an incision behind the hairline

Fig. 7.251 Flap planning. Various possible designs are shown.

2. Millard[12] described passing the flap through a much lower route, in fact a submandibular incision created for removal of an inferior alveolar carcinoma.

3. Hoopes & Edgerton[13] created a tunnel by elevating the skin and subcutaneous tissues at the base of the pedicle and folding the flap inward so that it passed down between the zygomatic arch and the overlying skin (Fig. 7.252b).

4. Subsequently Davis & Hoopes[14] suggested passing the flap deep to the zygomatic arch although there seems to be little space for it in this location (Fig. 7.252c).

On balance the method least likely to compromise the circulation in the flap is the first of those cited above.

Full thickness cheek defects may be reconstructed by either lining the end of the flap with a split skin graft[15] or folding the end over to form a sandwich with skin on both surfaces,[16] or by constructing a bipolar flap with the anterior part of forehead skin based on the frontal branch for internal lining, and the posterior part based on the parietal branch for external cover.[17]

Finally the forehead is covered with a thick split skin graft. Excision of an extra amount of skin so that the margins of the defect coincide with the eyebrows and the hairline may lessen the cosmetic disability and bevelling the margins of the defect aids the achievement of a smooth contour between graft and surrounding skin.

Islanded flaps based on the posterior branch can achieve a long pedicle if the anterior branch is divided and the superficial temporal artery dissected free down to the level of the tragus.

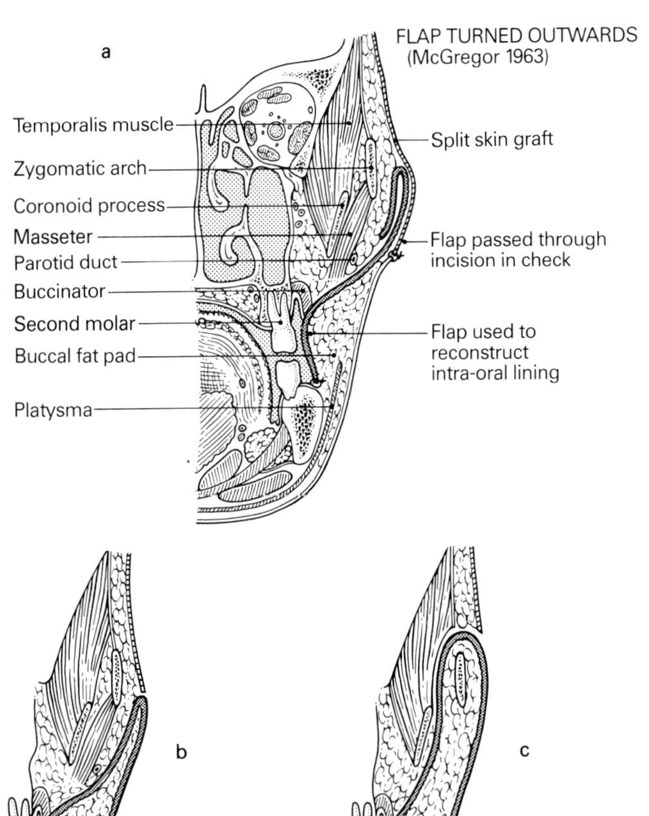

Fig. 7.252 Routes for tunnelling a forehead flap into the mouth for intra-oral reconstructions, shown on a coronal section at the level of the second molar tooth.

References

1. Dunham M T 1893 A method for obtaining a skin flap from the scalp and a permanent buried vascular pedicle for covering defects of the face. Annals of Surgery 17: 677–679
2. Monks G H 1898 The restoration of a lower eyelid by a new method. Boston Medical and Surgical Journal 139: 385–387
3. Horsley J S 1916 Transplantation of the anterior temporal artery. Clinical Journal, London 45: 193–196
4. Wilson J S 1967 The application of the 2–centimetre pedicle flap in plastic surgery. British Journal of Plastic Surgery 20: 278–296
5. Cramer L R, Culf N K 1969 Use of pedicle flap tissues in conjunction with a neck dissection. In: Gaisford J C (ed) Symposium on Cancer of the Head and Neck. C B Mosby Company, St Louis
6. Conway H, Stark B, Kavanagh J D 1952 Variations of the temporal flap. Plastic and Reconstructive Surgery 9: 410–423
7. Corso P F 1961 Variations of the arterial, venous and capillary circulation of the soft tissues of the head by decades as demonstrated by the methyl methacrolate injection technique, and their application to the construction of flaps and pedicles. Plastic and Reconstructive Surgery 27: 160–184
8. Behan F C, Wilson J S P 1973 The vascular basis of laterally based forehead island flaps, and their clinical application. Presented at the Second Congress of the European Section of the International Confederation of Plastic and Reconstructive Surgery, Madrid. Royal College of Surgeons of England, London
9. Rawat S S 1977 Bipedicled (vascular) forehead flap. British Journal of Plastic Surgery 30: 42–43
10. Blair V P, Moore S, Byars L T 1941 Cancer of the face and mouth. C V Mosby, St Louis
11. McGregor I A 1963 The temporal flap in intra-oral cancer: its use in repairing the post-excisional defect. British Journal of Plastic Surgery 16: 318–335
12. Millard D R 1964 A new approach to immediate mandibular repair. Annals of Surgery 160: 306–313
13. Hoopes J E, Edgerton M T 1966 Immediate forehead flap repair in resection for oro-pharyngeal cancer. American Journal of Surgery 112: 527–533
14. Davis G N, Hoopes J E 1971 New route for passage of forehead flap to inside of mouth. Plastic and Reconstructive Surgery 47: 390–392
15. Gillies L D, Millard D R Jr 1957 Principles and Art of Plastic Surgery. Little Brown, Boston
16. Champion R 1960 Closure of full-thickness cheek loss by forehead flap. British Journal of Plastic Surgery 13: 76–78
17. Narayanan M 1970 Immediate reconstruction with bipolar scalp flap after excisions of huge cheek cancers. Plastic and Reconstructive Surgery 46: 548–553

7 SUPERFICIAL TEMPORAL ARTERY

Scalp flaps

A number of pedicled hair-bearing scalp flaps have been designed based on the parietal branches of the superficial temporal artery. The temporo-parieto-occipital flaps associated with the name of Juri,[1] and the lateral scalp flap associated with Elliot,[2] are designed for transposition into the frontal region to reconstruct the anterior hairline. For reconstruction of frontal and occipital defects Orticochea has developed a triple scalp flap technique and one or two of these flaps are based on the superficial temporal vessels.[3] Free hair-bearing flaps have also been described by several authors.[1,4]

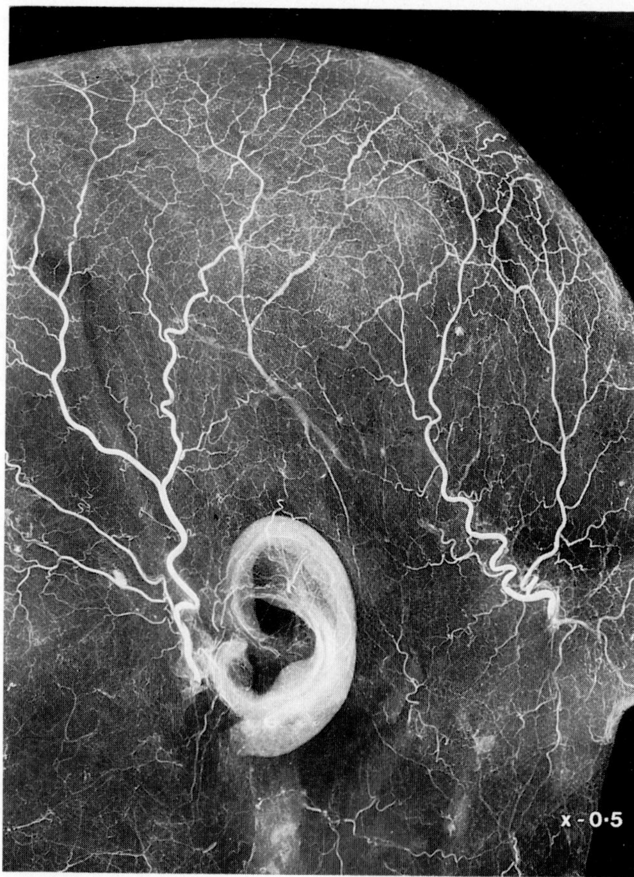

Fig. 7.253 Radiograph of parietal scalp showing the superficial temporal artery and the occipital artery. The posterior auricular artery is either absent or has failed to fill with contrast medium (probably the former). Some contrast has carried through the vascular bed and has produced slight opacification of the posterior auricular vein. Anastomoses between branches of the superficial temporal and the occipital arteries are visible on the original radiograph but have been lost in the reproduction at half size.

Some flaps run counter to the main vessels yet survive with length-to-breadth ratios of 3:1, thereby demonstrating the exceptional vascularity of the scalp and the efficiency of the anastomoses. For example the flap proposed by Nataf in 1976[5] for the treatment of frontal alopecia runs perpendicular to the main axis of the superficial temporal vessels. This flap, designed with its anterior edge in a step-shape so as to permit insertion under a thin layer of frontal epidermis through which the hair from the flap then grows, has become increasingly popular and is known as the inserted flap. It is not described here because it is not based on axial vessels yet it is sufficiently successful to have replaced the Juri and Elliot flaps for some surgeons.

In the bald individual an island flap of scalp skin may be raised on the posterior branch of the superficial temporal artery and used for reconstruction on the face.

Temporo-parietal fascial flaps are not considered here.

Anatomy

The vascular anatomy of the scalp has several particular features. The arteries are confined to the connective tissue layer between the skin and the galea (aponeurosis) where they form a rich network of vessels with numerous anastomoses both between the vessels of one side and between the vessels of opposite sides (Figs 7.253 & 7.254). Arterial branches do not cross the layer of loose areolar tissue beneath the galea, and the pericranium is supplied by vessels from the bone. The venous network also lies above the galea but receives tributaries across the sub-galeal space from diploic veins – a minor route of drainage of the marrow space in the calvarium – and emissary veins which connect with the intracranial venous sinuses. The latter communications are important in so far as they form a potential route for spread of infection from the scalp into the cranial cavity. The extensive anastomoses mean that dynamic and potential territories may greatly exceed anatomical ones. This fact is well demonstrated by the temporo-parieto-occipital flaps.

The anatomy and surface markings of the occipital and superficial temporal arteries are described on pages 136–138.

Flaps

Temporo-parieto-occipital flaps
These flaps are based on the posteriorly directed ramifications of the parietal branch of the superficial temporal artery (Fig. 7.255). Depending on the degree of baldness for which the surgery is required, unilateral or bilateral flaps can be transposed to the frontal region. Preliminary delays are probably advisable although some reports indicate that it is possible to get away without these. If flaps from both sides are required then the operations are separated by an interval of at least one month.

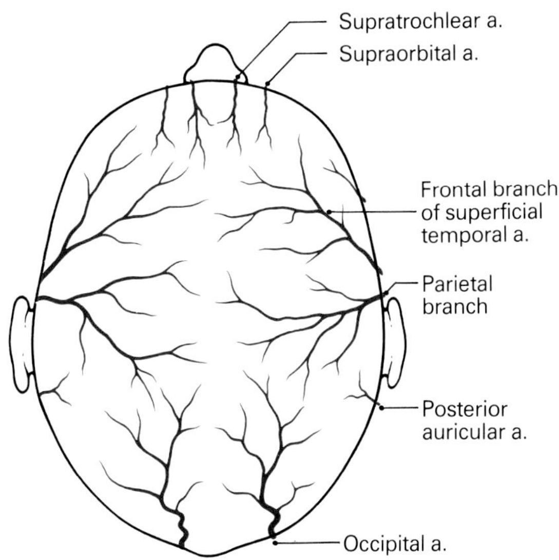

Fig. 7.254 Schematic representation of vessels feeding the scalp.

If done without a delay then it is essential to centre the flap over a significant branch of the superficial temporal artery and this can be achieved by pre-operatively marking out the course of such vessels with a Doppler probe. The flap measures 4 cm in width and elevation is relatively straightforward. The recipient area is prepared by excising a bald area of the same dimensions as the flap and the donor area is closed directly after wide undermining. Modifications of this procedure include extending the flap over to the opposite retro-auricular area in order to create a flap that is sufficiently long enough to be able to turn the end round and inset it into the frontal region. This will then reproduce the normal, i.e. forwardly-inclined, direction of hair growth since with the standard Juri flap the hair growth will be directed backwards from the new anterior hair line. A further modification for the treatment of occipital baldness involves creating an occipito-parieto-temporal flap on an occipital pedicle.

Lateral scalp flap
The 'lateral scalp flap' was developed by Elliot for anterior hairline reconstruction in an endeavour to simplify the method of Juri's flaps and also to reduce their potential for developing complications. The lateral scalp flap is a short flap which aims to reconstruct only one-half of the anterior hairline. The other half can then be completed by a second flap from the opposite side although this should not be transferred until after two months from the first procedure. The average anterior hairline measures between 26 and 30 cm in length and each flap will therefore have to be between 13 and 15 cm long. The base of the flap is 3.0 cm wide and is centred over the main stem of the superficial temporal artery.

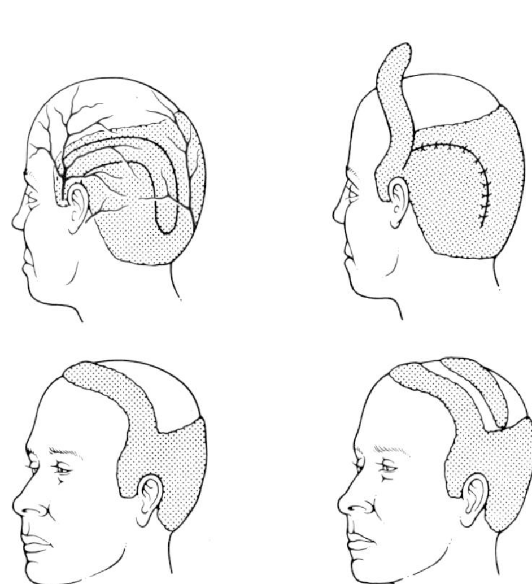

Fig. 7.255 Temporo-parieto-occipital flaps (Juri).

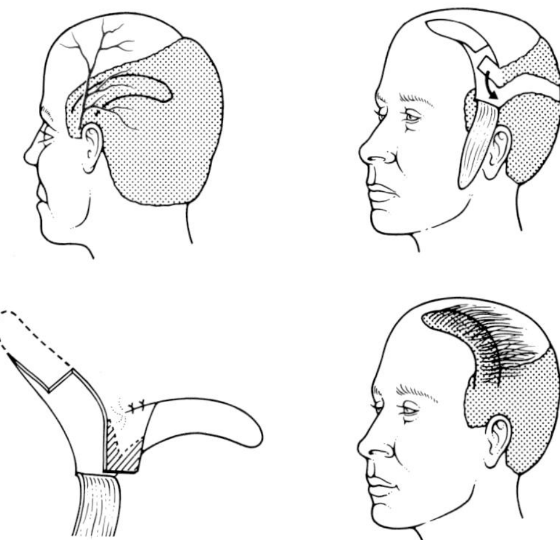

Fig. 7.256 Lateral scalp flaps (Elliot).

The anterior margin of the flap starts at the existing temporal hairline so that when the flap is transposed into the frontal region natural continuity of the new hairline will be obtained. From this point the flap curves posterosuperiorly, becomes horizontal below any balding area, and narrows to 2.5 cm in width. Elliot[2] states that branches of the superficial temporal artery do not require to be identified if the length-to-breadth ratio of the flap is kept to less than 5:1. Figure 7.256 shows how a small flap may be created in the recipient area for rotation into the donor defect in order to reduce tension in the closure at this point.

Island scalp flaps
An island of scalp skin may be carried on the posterior branch of the superficial temporal artery which is accompanied by a reliable venous dranage system. Brent & Byrd[7] have described the technique of dissecting the vessels within the scalp and a useful length of pedicle can be dissected out down to the level of the tragus if the anterior branch of the STA is divided. The bald scalp is much more flexible than hairy scalp thereby allowing the flap to be moulded into various shapes. For example, such an island flap has been used to reconstruct the oral commissure and adjacent parts of the lips with the pedicle passing in a tunnel beneath the cheek skin.

Orticochea triple scalp flaps
This technique is intended for the reconstruction of moderate sized defects located over the occipital or frontal regions. As originally described, the method required the remaining scalp to be elevated as four separate flaps but in a later modification[3] three flaps were found to be superior since their wider pedicles ensured a better blood supply. The flaps depend on the superficial temporal, posterior auricular and occipital arteries for their support in the following manner:

With a *frontal defect* (Fig. 7.257) two flaps are marked out parallel to the superior edge of the defect with widths about half that of the defect, up to a maximum of 6 cm. The ends of these flaps are cut obliquely so that they overlap and the vascular support of both comes from the superficial temporal vessels. The third flap consists of nearly the whole of the remaining scalp based on a postero-lateral pedicle containing the occipital and posterior auricular vessels on one side. If the defect is to one side then the third flap is based on the opposite side; if the defect lies symmetrically about the midline then the third flap may be based on either side.

The flaps are elevated in the avascular plane beneath the aponeurosis which is then incised with multiple incisions about 1 cm apart in the coronal plane avoiding injury to arteries and veins. The first two flaps are now juxtaposed to cover the defect. The third flap covers the defect resulting from having moved the first two. The result is a closure of the defect with equal distribution of tension in the skin flaps over the whole of the vault of the skull.

With an *occipital defect* the first two flaps are based on a combination of branches of the occipital and the posterior auricular arteries. The third flap is based on the superficial temporal vessels of the opposite side.

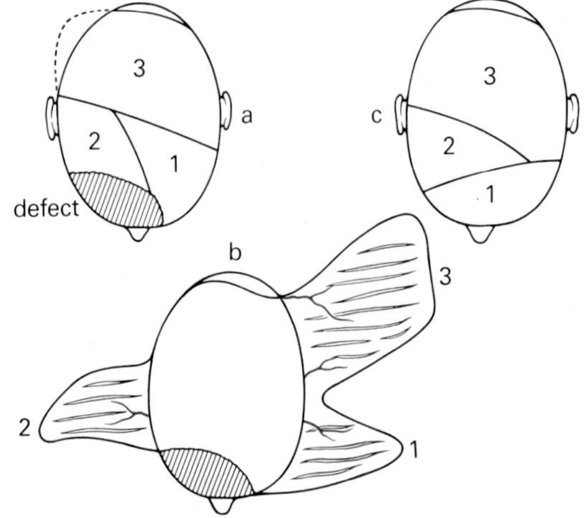

Fig. 7.257 Triple scalp flaps (Orticochea).

References

1. Juri J, Juri C 1982 Temporo-parieto-occipital flap for the treatment of baldness. Clinics in Plastic Surgery 9: 255–261 (This paper lists 11 other publications by the same authors on this subject)
2. Elliot R A 1982 The lateral scalp flap for anterior hairline reconstruction. Clinics in Plastic Surgery 9: 241–253
3. Orticochea M 1971 New three-flap scalp reconstruction technique. British Journal of Plastic Surgery 24: 184–188
4. Harii K, Ohmori K, Ohmori S 1974 Hair transplantation with free scalp flaps. Plastic and Reconstructive Surgery 53: 410–413
5. Nataf J, Elbaz J S, Pollet J 1976 Etude critique des transplantations de cuir chevelu et propositions d'une optique. Annales de Chirurgie Plastique 21: 199–206
6. Corso P F 1961 Variations of the arterial, venous and capillary circulation of the soft tissues of the head. Plastic and Reconstructive Surgery 27: 160–184
7. Brent B, Byrd H S 1983 Secondary ear reconstruction with cartilage grafts covered by axial, random and free flaps of temporoparietal fascia. Plastic and Reconstructive Surgery 72: 141–151

SUPERFICIAL TEMPORAL ARTERY
POSTERIOR AURICULAR ARTERY

Preauricular island flap
Postauricular pedicled flaps
ipsilateral pedicle
contralateral pedicle

The ability of the blood flowing in the superficial temporal and posterior auricular arteries to reverse its direction of flow when the main stems of these vessels are occluded, is a consequence of the excellent anastomoses that the branches of these vessels make across the midline with the contralateral arteries and with the ipsilateral supraorbital and supratrochlear arteries. This reversal of flow can supply blood to flaps situated over the proximal preauricular part of the superficial temporal artery or in the hairless postauricular skin.

Preauricular island flap

This flap was developed by Bostwick et al[1] in response to the problem of a full-thickness forehead skin defect overlying irradiated bare frontal bone.

Anatomy
The flap utilises spare preauricular skin and is really only suited to use in the female where preauricular hair is sparse, although Bostwick et al suggest that some hair-bearing skin in the male may be used for simultaneous eyebrow reconstruction (however hair growth would be in the wrong direction). The blood supply to the flap is from small branches directly off the superficial temporal artery, variably augmented by the zygomatico-orbital or transverse facial arteries depending on their exact sites of origin from the superficial temporal artery (p. 138). The superficial temporal artery is ligated and divided at the level of the tragus and blood flows into it by its numerous anastomoses on the forehead and scalp (Fig. 7.258).

Surgery
The flap is planned in reverse with the desired amount of skin marked out first, with the posterior edge of the territory lying in the preauricular crease. Elevation of the flap commences inferiorly in a plane just superficial to the parotid fascia. The superficial temporal artery and vein are ligated and divided about 5 mm below the zygomatic arch. A vertical extension upwards from the incision around the flap enables the vascular pedicle to be exposed and dissected superiorly. The pedicle is mobilised by dividing only those branches which seriously tether the flap and prevent its transposition. The presence of a tortuous superficial temporal artery may be useful at this point in enabling an extra centimetre of pedicle length to be gained. Once mobilised sufficiently, a subcutaneous tunnel is created to the forehead defect and the flap brought through and inset.

The donor defect is closed in the manner of a rhytidectomy after undermining the cheek skin subcutaneously and advancing it posteriorly.

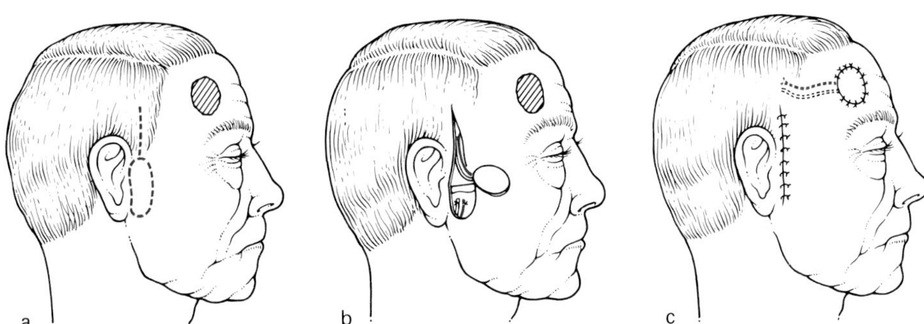

Fig. 7.258 Preauricular island flap (Bostwick): **a.** outline of flap; **b.** superficial temporal artery and vein are divided at the lower border of the zygomatic arch; **c.** the pedicle passes through a subcutaneous tunnel to enable the flap to reach the defect.

Orticochea retro-auricular temporal artery flap

This is an elaborate and lengthy procedure of four stages in which fronto-auricular pedicles are created and the main stem of the superficial temporal artery is transplanted from its position in front of the ear to a position behind the ear[2–4] (Fig. 7.259).

Surgery

The pedicle is prepared and delayed in two stages by parallel incisions which are taken down behind the ear. Here the full thickness of the concha is included by incising the preauricular skin and the cartilage along the anterior, superior and posterior borders of the concha, i.e. an inferior pedicle is left intact which supports both the preauricular and the postauricular skin. The anterior (as viewed with the auricle folded forwards) auricular incision on the back of the ear travels parallel to the helix and about 1 cm from the rim of the ear. The posterior/ cranial incision is carried along the hairline to the lower margin of the mastoid process. At the same stage a vertical preauricular incision is made 1.5 cm in front of the ear and the superficial temporal vessels are dissected free, but the fatty areolar tissue around them is preserved. The superficial temporal vessels are ligated at the level of the lower border of the tragus and the upper ends are then tunnelled through the substance of the flap and sutured to its undersurface. Anastomoses form between the small vessels in the fatty areolar tissue around the temporal vessels and the vessels in the flap thereby increasing the blood supply to the concha.

In the second stage the lower end of the fronto-auricular flap (containing preauricular and retro-auricular skin, conchal cartilage and temporal bone if required), is delayed under local anaesthesia by dividing the skin between the two vertical incisions and raising the lower cutaneous end of the flap.

In the third stage the remaining skin bridges and the inferior attachment of the concha are divided and the flap transferred. In the fourth stage the pedicles are returned to the scalp.

Postauricular flap based on contralateral STA

By utilising the major part of the scalp a larger flap may be taken from the postauricular and mastoid skin (with or without cartilage) with only one delay procedure (Fig. 7.260). The broad base of the flap is necessary for adequate venous drainage.[5]

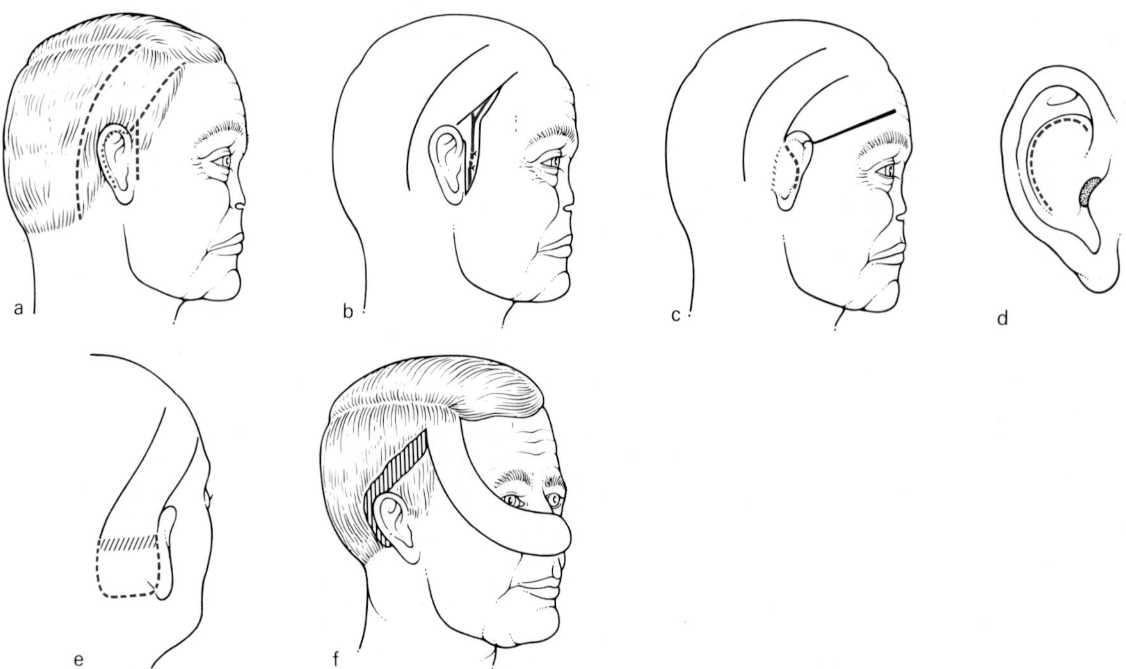

Fig. 7.259 Retroauricular flap (Orticochea). **a–d.** First stage with division of superficial temporal artery and relocation of the superior part beneath the postauricular skin. **e.** Second stage. The inferior end of the flap is completed and undermined except for a strip which remains temporarily attached to skull. **f.** Third stage. Flap brought to defect. Fourth stage (not shown) involves return of the pedicle.

Surgery
The flap is delayed ten days prior to definitive surgery by undermining the upper neck and postauricular skin with division and ligation of the ipsilateral postauricular, occipital and posterior branches of the superficial temporal vessels (Fig. 7.260a). The undermining is carried out in the plane of loose tissue beneath the galea. When raised ten days later by the incisions shown in Figure 7.260b–d the length of the flap is sufficient to allow it to reach any cervicofacial defect, the exposed pericranium being temporarily covered with a split skin graft. A grafted area remains in the postauricular region after return of the scalp pedicle but is relatively inconspicuous.

The PARAS flap

A similar flap to that of Galvao has been described by Dias[7] and termed the post- and retro-auricular scalping flap (the PARAS flap). This differs principally in that the flap is raised without a prior delay and does not extend as far into the neck, the tip of the flap not going beyond the lower margin of the concha of the ear.

References

1. Bostwick J, Briedis J, Jurkiewicz M J 1976 The reverse flow temporal artery island flap. Clinics in Plastic Surgery 3: 441–445
2. Orticochea M 1971 A new method for total reconstruction of the nose: the ears as donor areas. British Journal of Plastic Surgery 24: 225–232
3. Orticochea M 1977 Méthode pour la reconstruction totale du nez. Annales de Chirurgie Plastique 22: 181–188
4. Orticochea M 1980 Refined technique for reconstructing the whole nose with the conchas of the ears. British Journal of Plastic Surgery 33: 68–73
5. Galvao M S L 1981 A postauricular flap based on the contralateral superficial temporal vessels. Plastic and Reconstructive Surgery 68: 891–897
6. Wilson J S P, Galvao M S L, Brough M 1980 The application of hair-bearing flaps in head and neck surgery. Head and Neck Surgery 2: 386–409
7. Dias A D, Chhajlani P 1987 The post- and retro-auricular scalping flap (the PARAS flap). British Journal of Plastic Surgery 40: 360–366

Note:
The term 'postauricular' is used to refer to the mastoid region and 'retro-auricular' to the posterior surface of the ear.

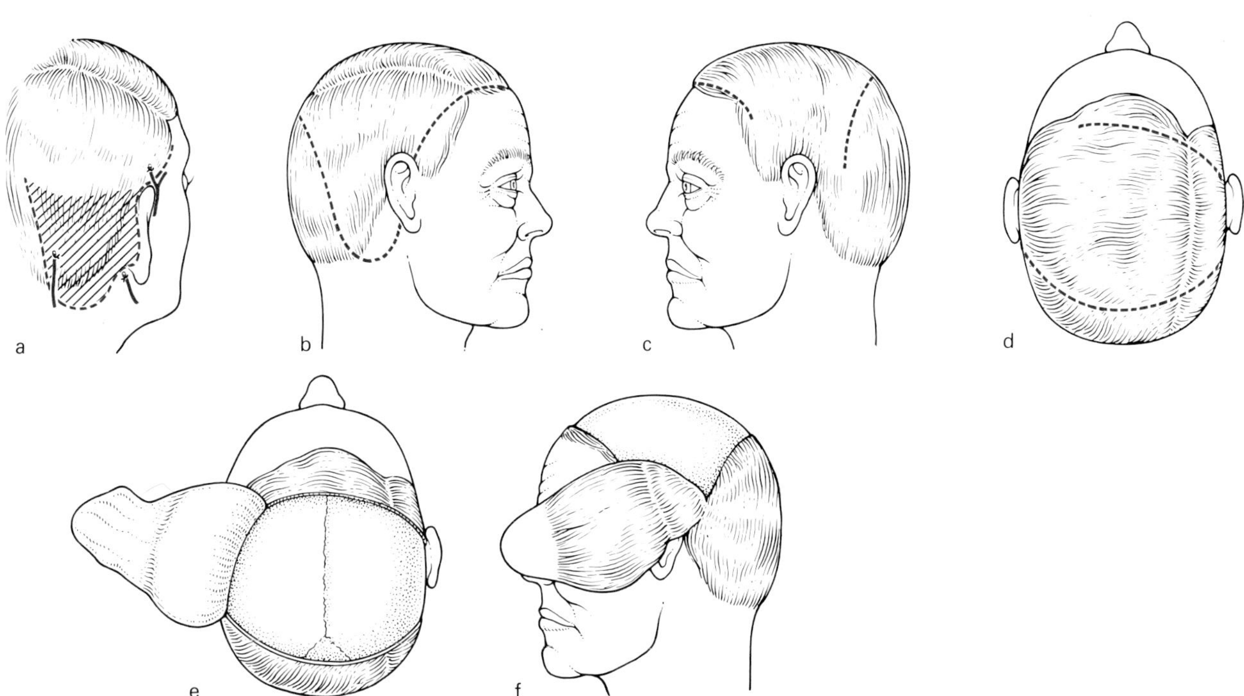

Fig. 7.260 Postauricular flap based on opposite superficial temporal artery (Galvao). **a.** Preliminary delay of postauricular skin and a variable amount of upper neck skin. Superficial temporal, postauricular and occipital arteries are divided and ligated, **b–d.** the incisions for elevating the flap. **e-f.** flap mobilised and brought forward.

SUPERFICIAL TEMPORAL ARTERY

Retro-auricular flaps

Various flaps designed to move retro-auricular skin on a pedicle containing branches of the superficial temporal artery have been described. The three illustrated here span the range from those requiring a delay, through one-stage procedures dependent on a large scalp pedicle, to one-stage procedures using a subcutaneous vascularised fascial pedicle.

Delayed pedicles

Haas & Meyer[1] have modified a method of Maggiore[2] in creating a composite ear flap on a parietal pedicle for partial nasal reconstruction. Figure 7.261 shows how the pedicle extends from the midline frontal scalp to the retro-auricular area. The delay is effected by creating a 7-cm-wide bipedicle flap which is left for three weeks before the retro-auricular skin and underlying conchal cartilage are incised together in the shape best suited to the recipient defect. The compound graft is then transferred on the end of the scalp pedicle to the nasal defect. After another three weeks or so, the pedicle is divided and returned to the parietal region. The donor site may be closed by a local inferiorly-based advancement flap.

Scalp pedicles for immediate transfer

The technique of transferring skin, and sometimes cartilage, from behind the ear was modified by Washio[3,4] who enlarged the base of the pedicle and thereby removed the necessity for delaying a comparatively narrow pedicle to do the same job. The ingenious feature of this flap is the way in which an oblique incision above the ear allows the flap to be folded on itself in such a way as to bring the skin from behind the ear into the anterior area of the face with the raw side facing posteromedially. Figure 7.262a–f show how this is accomplished with a double twist of the flap so that a kind of tubing takes place (Fig. 7.262e) and yet there is no tension on the pedicle.

Subcutaneous pedicles

Guyuron[5] has developed a one-stage retro-auricular island flap for reconstruction of the contracted eye socket which after radiotherapy tends not to accept skin and mucosal grafts very readily.

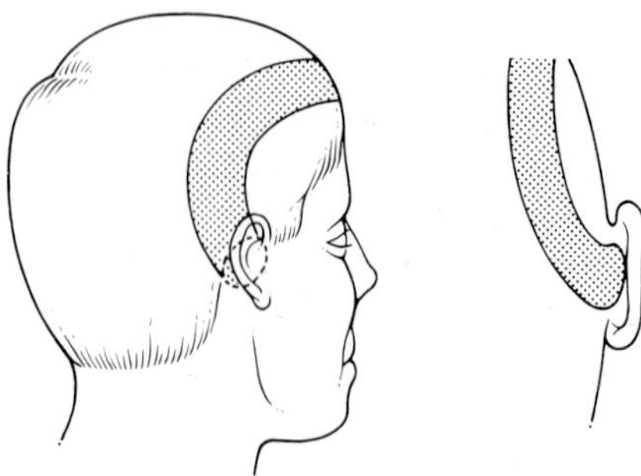

Fig. 7.261 'Frontomastoid' flap (Maggiore). Schematic representation of a method of transferring postauricular skin on a scalp pedicle. This method required a delay.

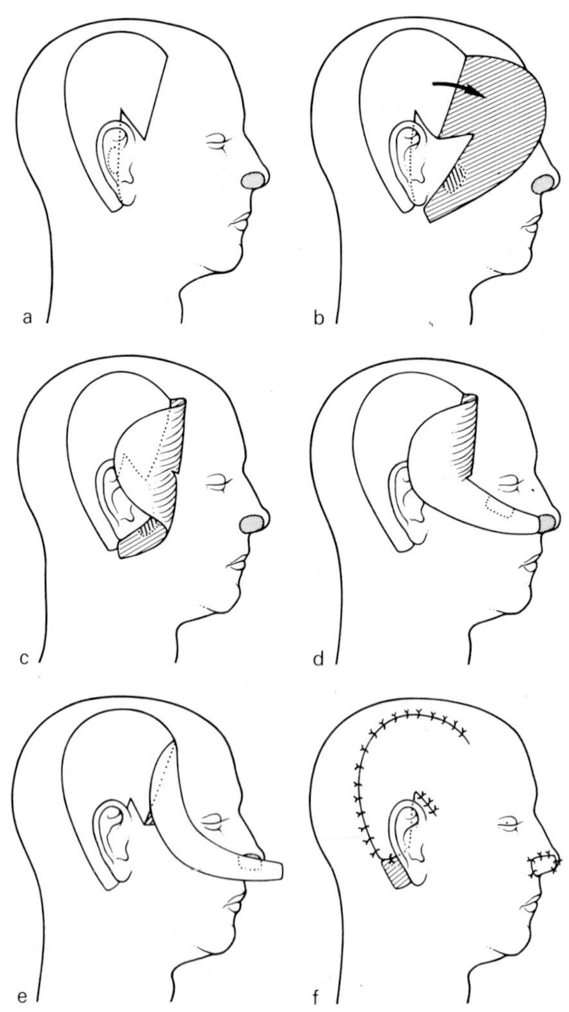

Fig. 7.262 Washio retroauricular flap. Method of carrying postauricular skin and auricular cartilage to the nose by a large pedicle.

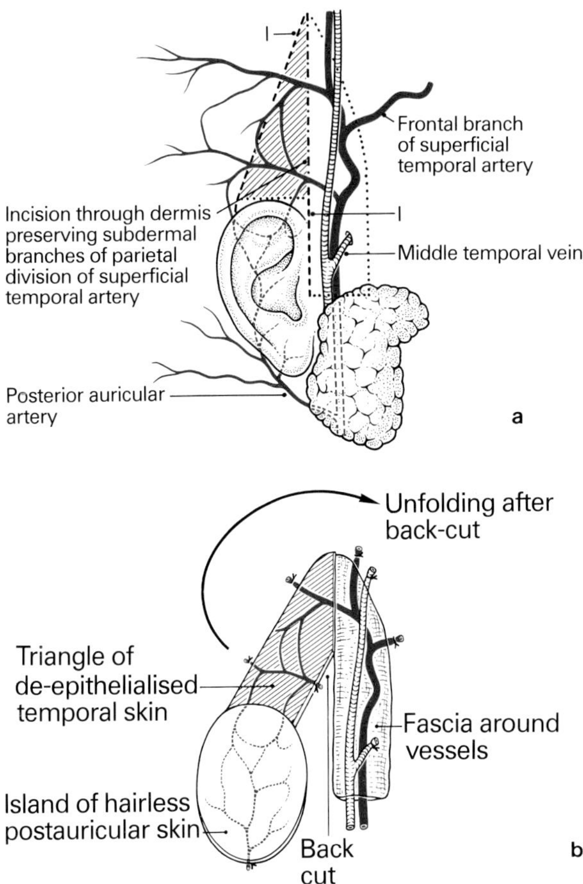

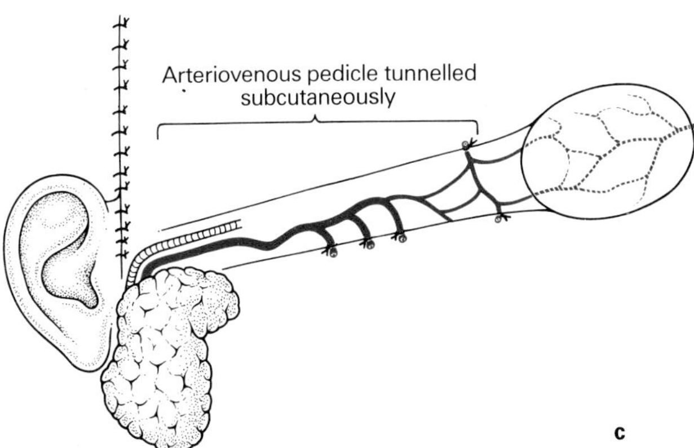

Fig. 7.263 Postauricular fasciocutaneous island flap. **a.** Vascular anatomy and flap planning. **'I'** indicates incisions through the full thickness of the skin. **b.** Schematic representation of skin island on its pedicle to show the limited back-cut which permits unfolding. **c.** Donor site closure. The pedicle may be passed subcutaneously so that the skin island reaches the orbit. (Superficial temporal vein not shown over its full length for clarity.)

Anatomy

The blood supply to the skin on the posterior/cranial surface of the auricle, and the adjacent hairless skin over the mastoid process, comes from the posterior auricular artery. It is less well known that the superficial temporal artery (STA) supplies the uppermost part of the cranial surface of the auricle by a small branch which descends from its posterior terminal division. Because the point at which the superficial temporal artery divides into its two terminal branches is variable (usually 3–4 cm, but occasionally up to 7 cm, above the zygomatic arch), the exact origin of this retro-auricular branch is also variable. In Figure 7.263 there is a high division of the STA and the retro-auricular branch has been shown arising from the main stem of the STA via a branch running back over the ear. A similar branch of the posterior STA lies above this and all the vessels in this area anastomose freely. The superficial temporal vein initially lies anterior to the posterior division of the STA, but as it descends in front of the ear it crosses over the artery to lie posterior to the STA. There is also a good venous plexus in the region above and behind the ear.

The anatomical vascular basis of these flaps depends on two sets of anastomoses. Firstly those between separate branches of the STA above the ear; here not only the dermal branches are important but also the ones on the temporalis fascia. Secondly it depends on those between STA branches and the posterior auricular artery on the cranial surface of the auricle and the postauricular skin.

Surgery

The fasciocutaneous island flap. The flap has three distinct portions which require to be marked out. The first and second encompass the vascular pedicle, the third is the skin island. The first, or fascial, part lies in front of the ear and is made up of the superficial temporal artery and its accompanying vein. The second is a cutaneous and fascial triangle above the ear. This contains the posterior terminal division of the STA and its branches, including the one running onto the cranial surface of the auricle. The base of the triangle is drawn level with the superior attachment of the ear and lies over the postauricular skin. The apex of this triangle lies approximately 5 cm above the base and contains the posterior terminal division of the STA or one of that vessel's posterior branches. This triangle is de-epithelialised. The third portion comprises the non-hair-bearing postauricular skin and the skin from the cranial surface of the auricle.

References

1. Haas E, Meyer R 1968 Konstruktive und rekonstruktive Chirurgie. In: Gohrbandt E, Gabka J, Berndorfer A (eds) Handbuch der Plastichen Chirurgie. W de Gruyter, Berlin
2. Maggiore D L 1960 La ricostruzione del naso con il lembo frontomastoideo. Congress of the International College of Surgeons, Rome
3. Washio H 1969 Retroauricular temporal flap. Plastic and Reconstructive Surgery 43: 162–166
4. Washio H 1972 Further experiences with the retroauricular temporal flap. Plastic and Reconstructive Surgery 50: 160–162
5. Guyuron B 1985 Retroauricular island flap for eye socket reconstruction. Plastic and Reconstructive Surgery 76: 527–530
6. Ohtsuka H 1988 Eye socket and eyelid reconstruction using the combined island frontal flap and retroauricular island flap: a preliminary report. Annals of Plastic Surgery 20: 244–248

SUPERIOR ULNAR COLLATERAL ARTERY

Medial arm flap

The thin, non-hair-bearing skin from the inner aspect of the upper arm forms an ideal donor site for a fasciocutaneous flap based on the fasciocutaneous perforators emerging along the medial intermuscular septum. Flaps from this area may be pedicled or free flaps. The possibility of creating a neurosensory free flap arises because the upper part of the donor area is innervated by the intercostobrachial nerve and the lower part by the medial cutaneous nerve of the arm. An example of such a free flap was first reported by Daniel et al[1] and further examples were subsequently reported by many others.[2–7] Briedenbach et al have reported successful clinical transfer of flaps up to 20 cm × 14 cm in size.

Anatomy

The skin on the medial aspect of the upper arm is supplied by a series of five or six fasciocutaneous perforators which arise from the brachial artery, from the branch it gives to biceps, from the superior ulnar collateral artery, and – when present – from the middle ulnar collateral artery. These perforators emerge along the medial intermuscular septum and fan out over biceps and triceps at the level of the deep fascia. Their internal diameters range from 0.5 to 1.0 mm.

The superior ulnar collateral artery is a considerable vessel with a diameter of 2–3 mm which arises from the brachial artery at about the midpoint of the upper arm

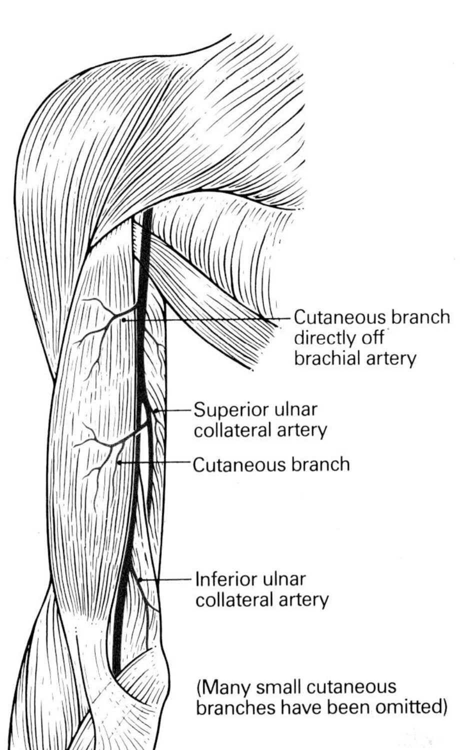

Fig. 7.264 Vascular anatomy. A fasciocutaneous perforator is shown arising from the superior ulnar collateral artery and passing anteriorly over biceps, but it could equally have passed posteriorly.

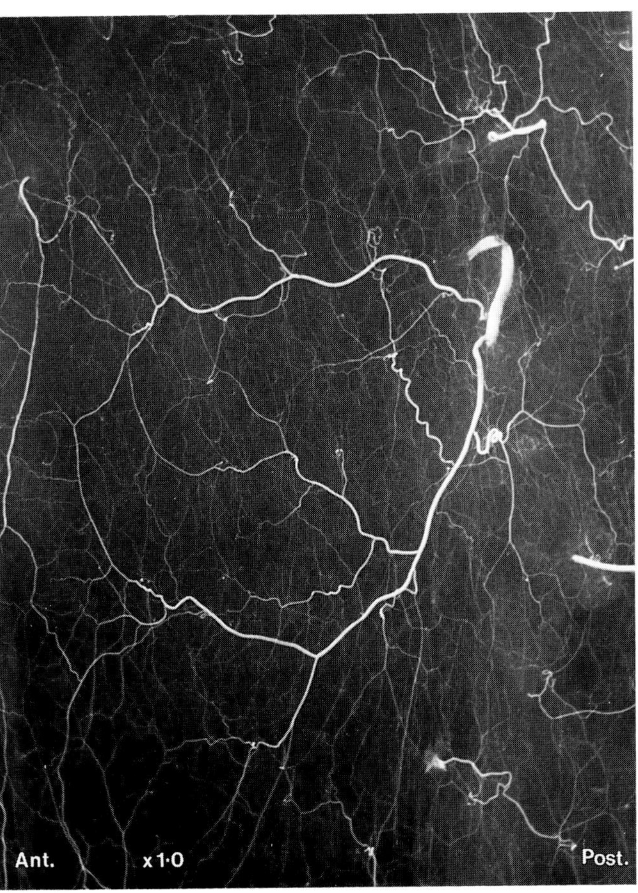

Fig. 7.265 Radiograph of skin showing two cutaneous branches arising from the superior ulnar collateral artery. A 2 cm segment of the artery has been removed.

or slightly lower, pierces the medial intermuscular septum and runs down its posterior aspect to supply the medial head of triceps. (Variations in the origin of this vessel are described on p. 181). It gives off one, sometimes two, fasciocutaneous perforators which supply an area on the medial aspect of the upper arm approximately 7 cm × 13 cm in size (Fig. 7.265). This perforator, with its accompanying venae comitantes, forms the vascular basis of the medial arm free flap and has been consistently described as such. In ~ 20% of cases, however, this vessel is small and then the major supplying vessel to the medial side of the upper arm which replaces it is a branch from the artery to biceps – indeed the sizes of these two perforators appear to be inversely proportional to each other.

The intercostobrachial nerve is the lateral cutaneous branch of the second intercostal nerve although it may often be joined by a branch from the third nerve. Unlike the other lateral intercostal cutaneous branches, the intercostobrachial nerve does not divide into anterior and posterior branches but crosses the axilla to the medial side of the arm where, becoming superficial, it supplies the skin to a point half-way down the arm and in some cases even as far as the elbow.

The medial cutaneous nerve of the forearm and the basilic vein are not raised with the flap, but the medial cutaneous nerve of the arm is included.

Surgery

Free flaps. It is not possible to predict which perforator will be the largest nor in which direction the branches of the fasciocutaneous perforators will fan out, whether anteriorly or posteriorly. Therefore the precise situation of the free flap is largely determined as the dissection proceeds and the anatomy is revealed. A section of the SUCA must be removed where the cutaneous branch takes origin thereby providing a larger diameter of vessel for the anastomosis. If there is more than one branch the appropriate length of SUCA will have to be removed. In raising the flap it will be found

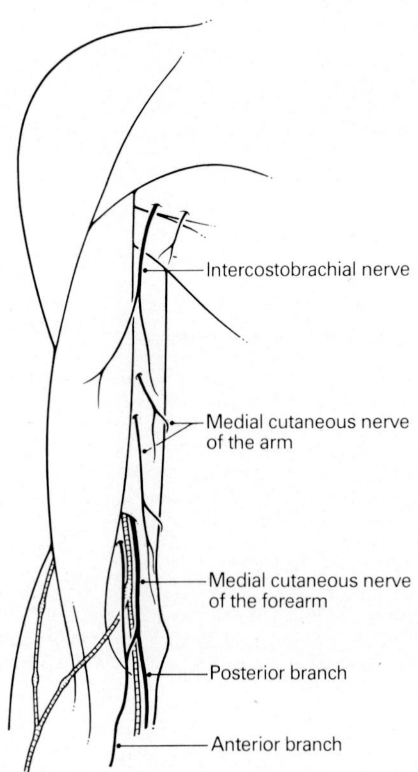

Fig. 7.266 Cutaneous nerves and veins in the area of the flap. The basilic vein may pierce the deep fascia at a higher level and may interfere with the development of the pedicle. Venous drainage of the flap is through the venae comitantes of the superior ulnar collateral artery.

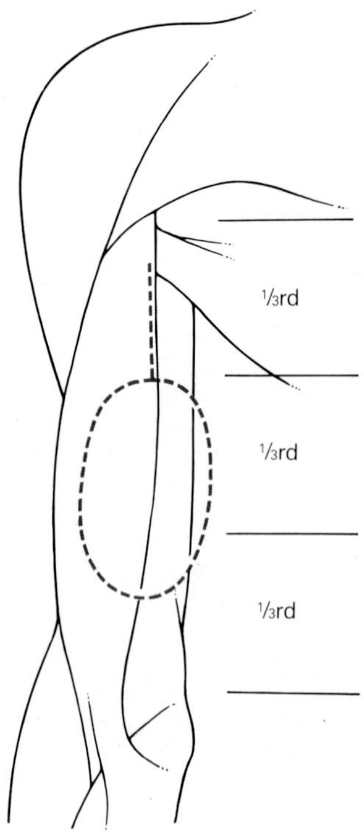

Fig. 7.267 Flap planning. The site of the initial incision in the upper third of the arm is shown. The vascular anatomy is exposed and the flap, which is initially planned to be centred on the medial intermuscular septum, is then developed in such a way as to exploit the local vascular anatomy and may be repositioned more anteriorly or posteriorly. The distal limit is 5 cm above the medial epicondyle.

that the cutaneous branches of the SUCA generally pass posterior to the ulnar nerve but when the vessels are replaced by a direct cutaneous branch from the brachial artery, this may pass either anterior or posterior to the nerve. In the latter situation the vessels are probably too small for anastomosis.

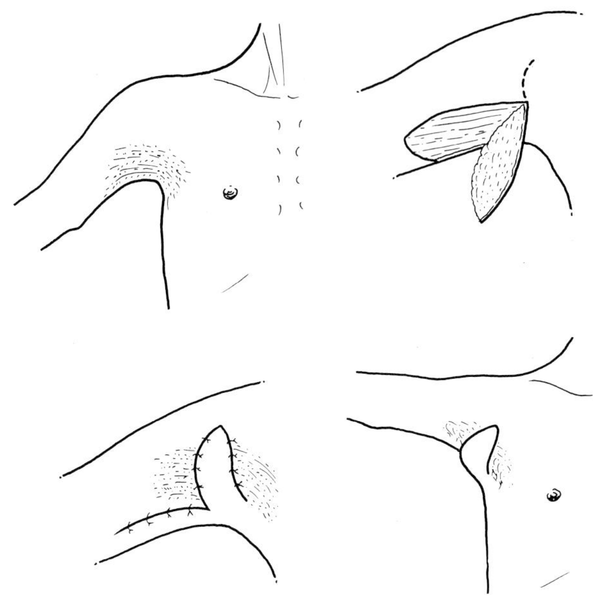

Fig. 7.268 Inner arm flap for release of anterior axillary scar contracture (Budo).

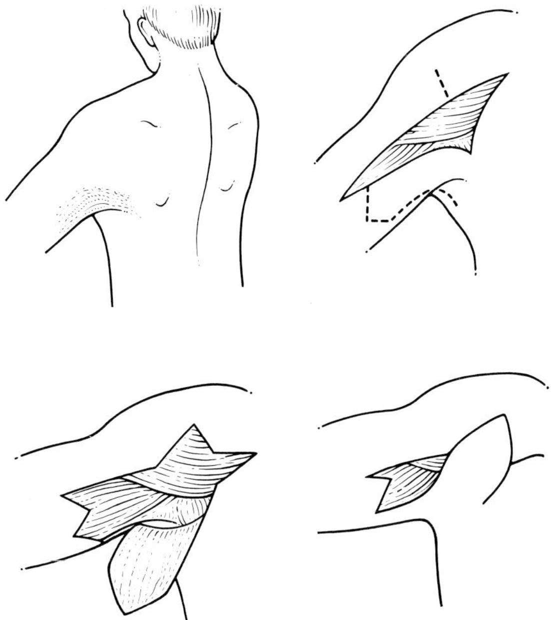

Fig. 7.269 Inner arm flap for release of posterior axillary scar contracture (Beasley).

Conventional pedicled flaps. The area of the inner arm was used in the past as a convenient site for a 'cross-arm' flap for hand reconstruction. The area is also a natural choice for the creation of a flap for transposition into the axilla for release of post-burn scar contractures because the inside of the arm usually escapes being involved in the burn injury through being opposed to the chest wall. Budo et al[8] have reported on the use of such an inner arm flap consisting of skin, subcutaneous fat and deep fascia, for release of post-burn scar contractures of the anterior wall of the axilla. The flap is essentially similar to that which Beasley[9] described for release of a posterior axillary contracture. Neither of these papers documented the anatomy but it is clear that the anastomoses between successive perforators facilitate the flow of blood along the long axis of the flap. An artery accompanies the intercostobrachial nerve (it has no official anatomical name) and helps feed the base of the flap. Although this artery is not intentionally exposed during elevation of the flap, it has been observed by transillumination of the flap at the time of operation. Clinical experience has shown that a flap elevated at this site, with a proximal base in the floor of the axilla, may be safely designed with a length-to-breadth ratio of up to 2.5:1. In Figure 7.269 a method of fish-tailing the end of the flap is shown which helps achieve greater release of the contracture. The donor defect is split skin grafted, or closed primarily if the flap is not too large.

References

1. Daniel R K, Terzis J, Schwarz G 1975 Neurovascular free flaps. A preliminary report. Plastic and Reconstructive Surgery 56: 13–60
2. Dolmans S, Guimberteau J C, Baudet J 1979 The upper arm flap. Journal of Microsurgery 1:162
3. Kaplan E N, Pearl R M 1980 An arterial medial arm flap, vascular anatomy and clinical applications. Annals of Plastic Surgery 4: 205–215
4. Newsom H T 1981 Medial arm flap: Case Report. Plastic and Reconstructive Surgery 67: 63–66
5. Song R, Song Y, Yu Y, Song Y 1982 The upper arm free flap. Clinics in Plastic Surgery 9: 27–35
6. Gao X-S, Mao Z-R, Yang Z-N, Wang B-S 1985 Medial upper arm skin flap: Vascular anatomy and clinical applications. Annals of Plastic Surgery 15: 348–351
7. Briedenbach W C, Adamson W, Terzis J K 1987 Medial arm flap. Annals of Plastic Surgery 18: 156–163
8. Budo J, Finucan T, Clarke J 1984 The inner arm fasciocutaneous flap. Plastic and Reconstructive Surgery 73: 629–632
9. Beasley R W 1977 Burns of axilla and elbow. In: Converse J H (ed) Reconstructive plastic surgery, 2nd edn. W S Saunders, Philadelphia, vol 6: 3391

7 SUPRACLAVICULAR ARTERY

Axial pattern flap

This flap was described by Lamberty[1] in 1979 after noting that certain old anatomical atlases, notably Hochstetter's Edition of Toldt's Atlas (1921),[2] showed a vessel which emerged between sternomastoid and trapezius in the lower part of the posterior triangle, and passed over the acromion and shoulder. Dissection of 15 preserved and 22 fresh cadavers confirmed the presence of this vessel and it was named the supraclavicular artery in the absence of any official designation in *Nomina Anatomica*. It has similarities to the original Mütter flap[3] from this region, and has also been found useful for skin replacement following release of post-burn scar contractures of the anterior neck.

Anatomy

Since the Anatomical Society of Great Britain reported on the thyrocervical trunk in 1891[4] there have been several studies[5,6,7] of the vessels in this area. The situation is greatly obscured by the changes in nomenclature that have taken place over the years but the authors advocate the system described on page 132. On this basis the supraclavicular artery is a perforator which arises from either the suprascapular artery or the superficial cervical artery or the ramus superficialis of the transverse cervical artery. (The latter two are essentially the same vessel in terms of terminal distribution). The vessel is given off beneath or lateral to the posterior belly of omohoid and may also supply the supraclavicular fat pad. (See the Transverse cervical artery based neurovascular free flap, p. 487)

The vessel averages 1.0–1.5 mm in diameter and reaches the deep fascia just behind the medial or middle third of the clavicle (Fig. 7.272). It passes directly laterally towards the acromioclavicular joint where it divides, the branches passing over the superior part of the deltoid. Here it anastomoses with cutaneous branches of the posterior circumflex humeral artery, especially the posterior deltoid perforator (arteria deltoidea subcutanea posterior). Throughout most of its course the vessel lies at the level of the deep fascia.

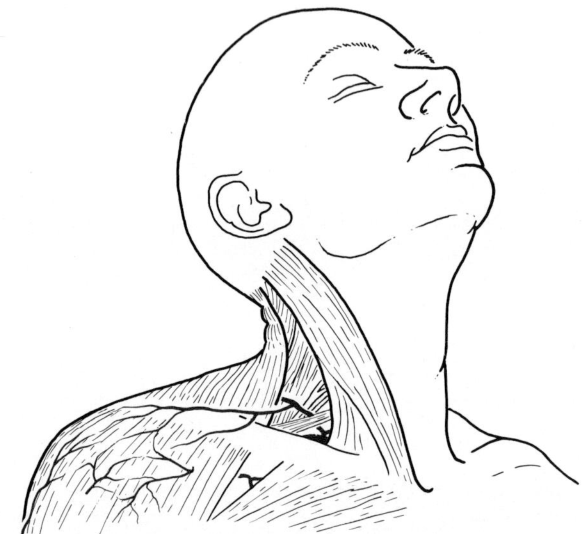

Fig. 7.270 Vascular anatomy. The supraclavicular artery is shown passing over the shoulder and anastomosing with perforators from the posterior circumflex humeral artery and with perforators from the deltoid branch of the thoraco-acromial axis.

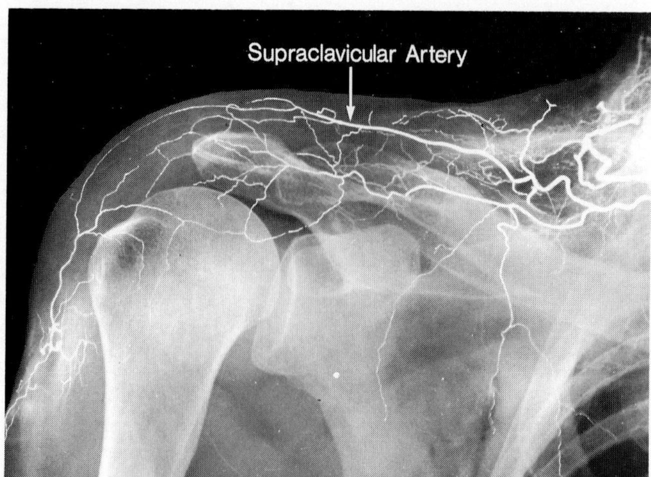

Fig. 7.271 Cadaver injection study of the supraclavicular artery. Note retrograde filling of branches of the posterior circumflex humeral artery via anastomoses over the point of the shoulder. (Slightly retouched illustration.)

Flap planning

An area of skin 6 cm × 16 cm can be safely elevated on this vessel. The extent to which this territory can be extended down the upper arm is uncertain and depends on the variable nature of the anastomoses with the perforators from the posterior circumflex humeral artery. In the cervico-humeral flap, which also contains musculocutaneous perforators from trapezius at its base, the territory extends down to the midpoint of the upper arm.[8] The territory has not been investigated by in vivo fluorescein injection techniques for two reasons: firstly, in raising the flap, the thyrocervical trunk is not visualised and the cutaneous vessel is too small for injection; secondly, the deep cervical artery may anastomose with the anterior spinal artery and it seems that there may be a very small risk of fluorescein damage to the cord although this has not been reported.

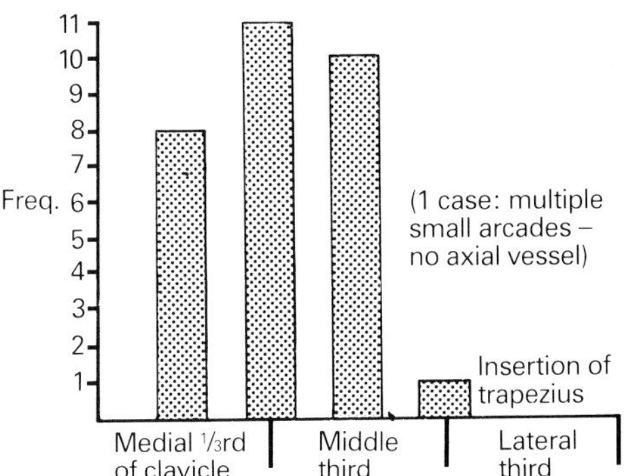

Fig. 7.272 Surface marking of the point of origin of the supraclavicular artery in 31 cadaver dissections (Lamberty, 1979).

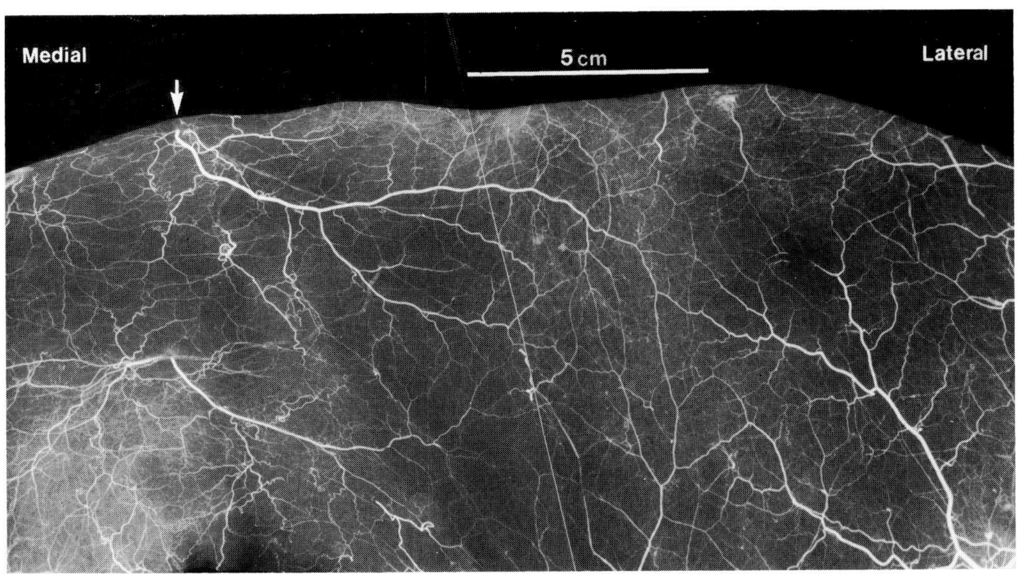

Fig. 7.273 Radiograph of skin specimen showing part of a supraclavicular artery (arrow). The skin incision which resulted in the upper margin of this specimen passed along the clavicle and divided the vessel so that only the portion lying below the clavicle is seen but this shows its anastomoses with a posterior deltoid subcutaneous artery.

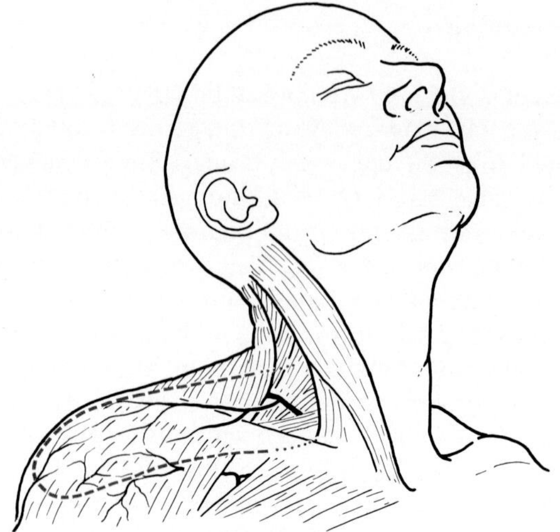

Fig. 7.274 Flap planning. Inferior incision (broken line) initially ends below clavicle but may be extended later (dotted line). Superior incision initially ends at mid-clavicular line but may also be extended medially at a later stage when the position of the artery has been established.

Surgery

The medially based flap is raised so as to include fat, platysma and deep fascia. The base lies along part of a line drawn from the sternoclavicular joint to the middle of the anterior border of the trapezius muscle. The anterior border of the flap lies anterior to the clavicle and does not cross it. It passes onto the deltoid muscle and the lateral aspect of the upper arm. The posterior incision initially does not extend medial to the mid-clavicular line although after visualising the vessel and avoiding the accessory nerve it may be extended or a back-cut made to facilitate rotation of the flap into the anterior neck. Note that branches of the thoraco-acromial axis are divided by the anterior incision. The donor site may be closed directly after extensive undermining.

References

1. Lamberty B G H 1979 The supraclavicular axial patterned flap. British Journal of Plastic Surgery 32: 207–212
2. Toldt 1921 Anatomischer Atlas. Urban & Schwarzenberg, Berlin
3. Mütter T D 1843 Cases of deformity from burns relieved by plastic surgery. Merrihew & Thomson, Philadelphia
4. Committee of Collective Investigation of the Anatomical Society of Great Britain and Ireland 1891 Second Annual Report. Journal of Anatomy and Physiology 26
5. Bean R B 1905 A composite study of the subclavian artery in man. American Journal of Anatomy 4: 303–328
6. Huelke D F 1958 A study of the transverse cervical and dorsal scapular arteries. The Anatomical Record 132: 233–243
7. Daseler E H, Anson B J 1959 Surgical anatomy of the subclavian artery, and its branches. Surgery, Gynaecology and Obstetrics 108: 149–174
8. Lamberty B G H, Cormack G C 1983 Misconceptions regarding the cervico-humeral flap. British Journal of Plastic Surgery 36: 60–63

SUPRATROCHLEAR (AND SUPRAORBITAL) ARTERIES

Forehead flaps

Since the earliest Indian midline forehead rhinoplasty flaps, a plethora of flap designs have evolved based on the supratrochlear, supraorbital and superficial temporal arteries. A selection of those depending mainly for their support on the supratrochlear artery are described here. Some, because of the complexity of their shape, require a preliminary delay procedure. (For forehead flaps based on the superficial temporal artery see p. 443.)

Anatomy

The supraorbital artery is present in 85% of cases, and leaves the orbit through the supraorbital notch or foramen in the company of veins and the supraorbital nerve. This notch/foramen lies an average 29 mm from the midline (range 23–38 mm). In Hayreth's series of cases[1] the artery was described as abnormally large in size in 20%, medium sized in 70% and very small in 10%. It is usually smaller than the supratrochlear artery, and only as strong or stronger in less than 10% of cases. Many of its branches lie beneath frontalis.

The supratrochlear or frontal artery is usually the largest of the terminal divisions of the ophthalmic artery (the medial palpebral and external nasal being the other two). Note that it emerges by piercing the orbital septum above the medial palpebral ligament and does not accompany the supratrochlear nerve which lies lateral to it. The nerve passes through the frontal foramen/notch which lies on average 20 mm from the midline (range 13–25 mm). The supratrochlear artery emerges between the origin of the superior fibres of orbicularis oculi and the depressor supercilii, and is the more significant of the two vessels in supplying central forehead skin.

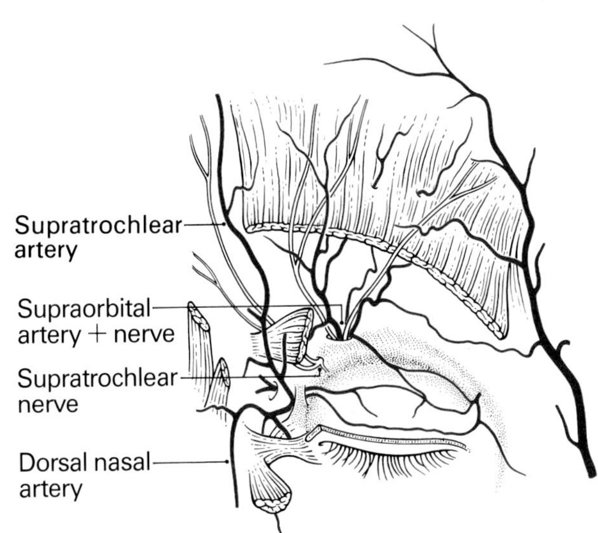

Fig. 7.275 Points of emergence of supratrochlear and supraorbital arteries from the orbit are shown. Orbicularis oculi and part of frontalis have been removed. Veins also omitted for clarity.

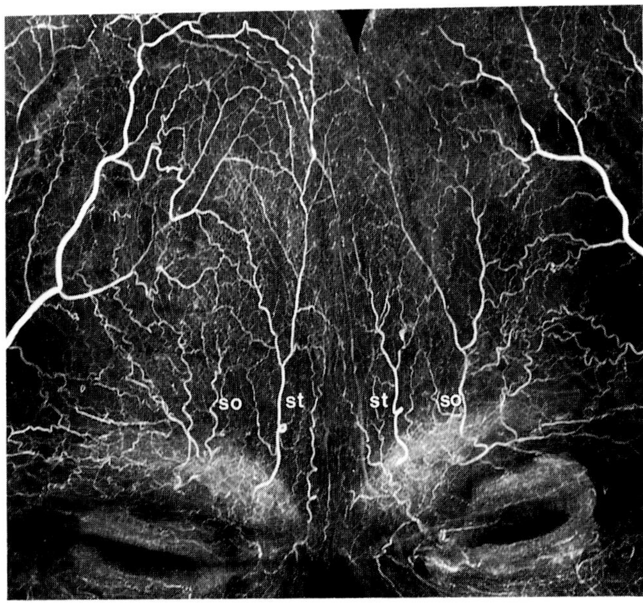

Fig. 7.276 Radiograph of forehead skin showing supratrochlear artery (**st**) and branches of supraorbital artery (**so**).

Flaps

Gillies 'up and down' forehead flap (Fig. 7.277). These flaps have now been superseded but were undoubtedly dependent on the supratrochlear and supraorbital vessels of one side.[2]

Midline flaps (Fig. 7.278). The midline forehead flap is extremely reliable and can be based on a remarkably narrow pedicle that can be turned safely through 180°. The flap is 2–2.5 cm wide and is based on two supratrochlear and dorsal nasal arteries at the root of the nose, extending vertically up to the hairline. The flap is elevated in the subgaleal plane (there is a midline gap between the two parts of the frontalis muscle and therefore postoperative expressive functions of the forehead are not interfered with). The maximum width of defect which can be closed on the forehead without resorting to a graft is 3.5 cm and this limits the maximum width of the flap. After ten days the pedicle may be divided and the proximal part returned to its bed in order to replace the eyebrows in their correct position.

A variation on the midline flap involves creating a de-epithelialised subcutaneous pedicle for it and tunnelling the flap to the defect beneath an intervening skin bridge (Fig. 7.279).

Glabellar flap (Fig. 7.280). This flap, also known as the Mitre flap because of the shape of the midline extension, is useful for reconstruction of defects on the side of the nose adjacent to the medial canthus. The design of the flap allows direct closure of the donor defect.

Extended midline forehead flap (Fig. 7.281).[3] This flap is narrow at the root of the nose and widens as it passes up to the hairline. It is usually situated in the midline but may be orientated slightly obliquely to gain more length on a short forehead. It is extended downwards along the medial border of the eyebrow on one side, cutting across the supratrochlear artery of that side. On the other side the extended incision is carried through skin alone and then careful dissection is carried out in the subdermal plane guarding the supratrochlear artery. The width of the flap at the upper end can be 4 cm or more and to enable direct closure of this large defect incisions are extended laterally within the hairline from each side of the upper end of the flap. The incisions may extend downwards in front of the ear as far as the tragus. The lateral flaps can then be elevated in the subgaleal plane as far as the level of the eyebrows, rotated and advanced to meet together in the midline. The loose skin in front of the ear facilitates advancement and this is also aided by multiple vertical incisions through the galea perpendicular to the line of stretching. In the final insetting of the flap only sufficient of the pedicle is returned between the eyebrows as is necessary to recreate a normal gap between the medial ends of the eyebrows. This triangle of skin results in an inverted V-shaped scar extending down from the vertical midline scar.

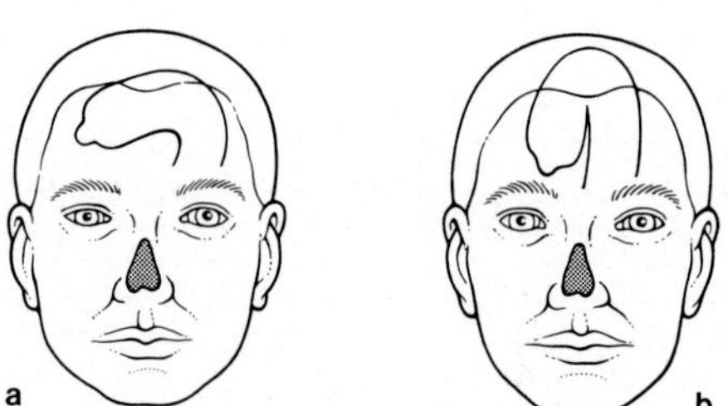

Fig. 7.277 a. Gillies 'up and down', **b.** Gillies 'more up, more down'

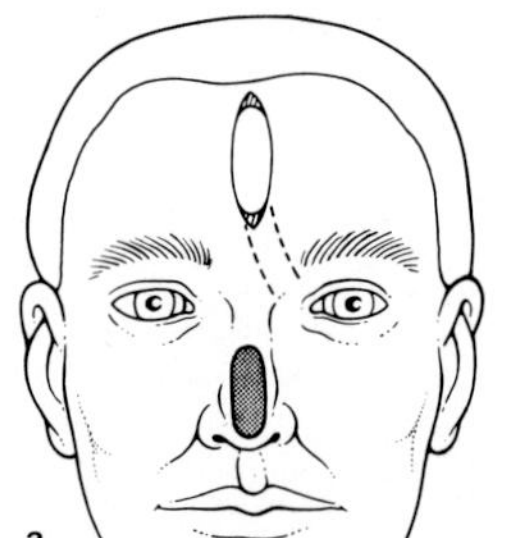

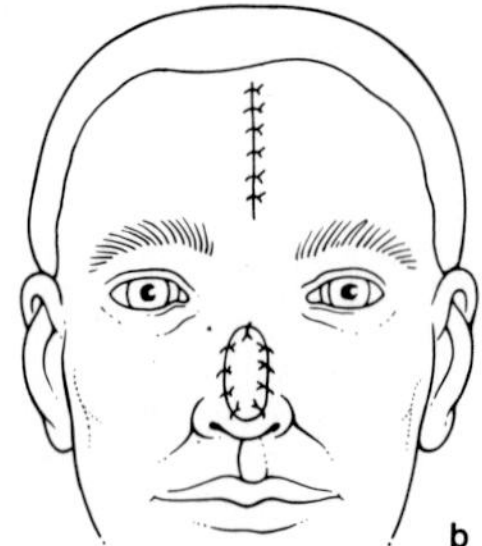

Fig. 7.279 Subcutaneously pedicled version of the midline flap.

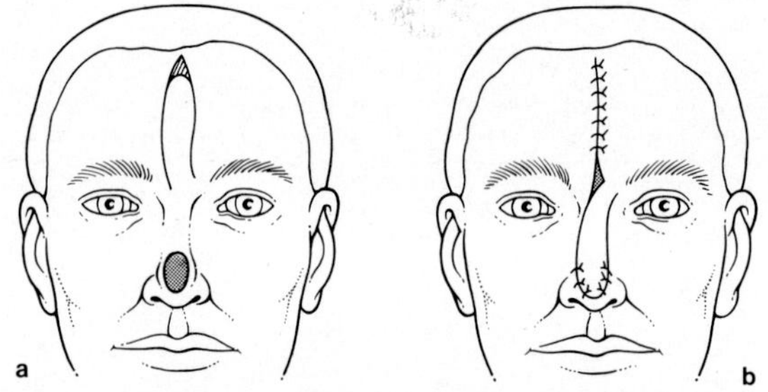

Fig. 7.278 Midline forehead flap: **a.** maximum width permitting direct closure is about 3 cm; **b.** after first stage and before return of pedicle.

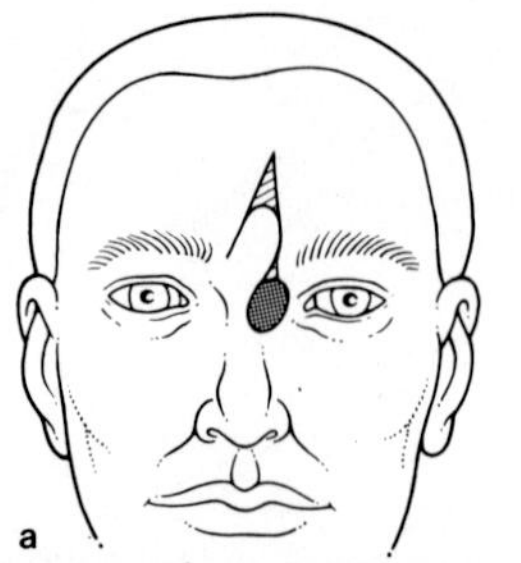

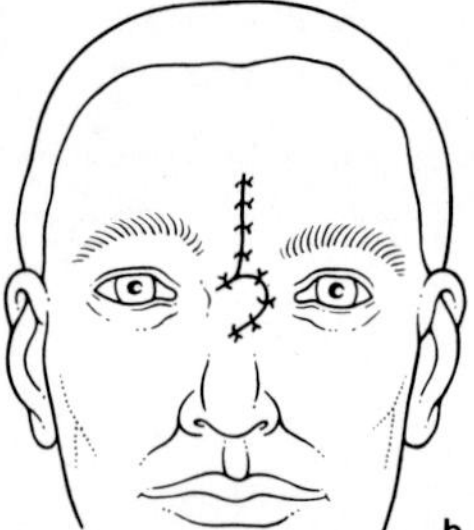

Fig. 7.280 Mitre of glabellar flap: **a.** defect on side of nose adjacent to medial canthus; **b.** one-stage repair.

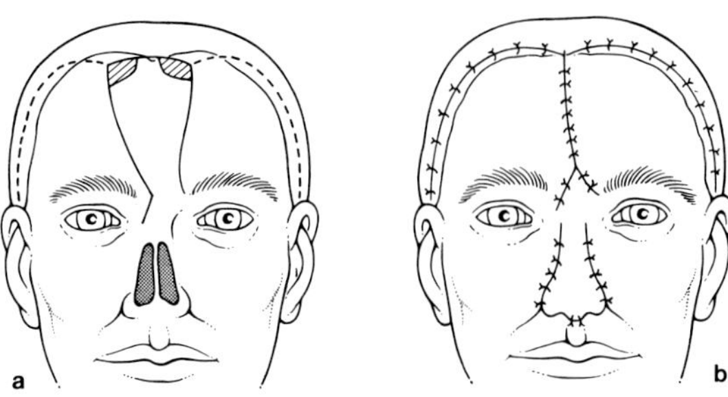

Fig. 7.281 Extended midline flap: **a.** note incisions in the hairline to permit donor site closure (local flaps for nasal lining are not shown); **b.** after third stage when pedicle has been returned to glabellar region.

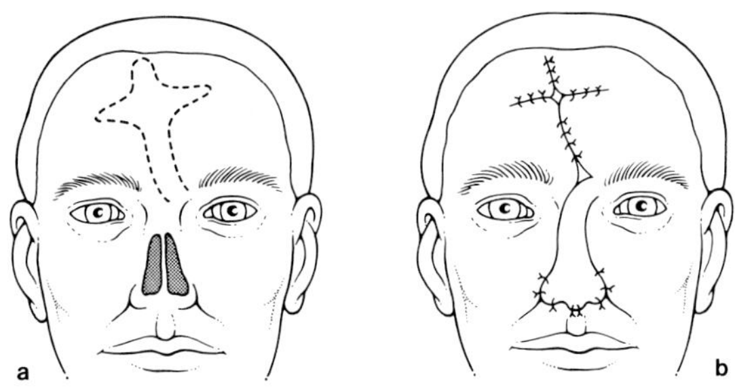

Fig. 7.282 'Seagull' flap (Millard). **a.** Primary delay required. Local flaps must be turned in for lining, **b.** after second stage and before division of pedicle.

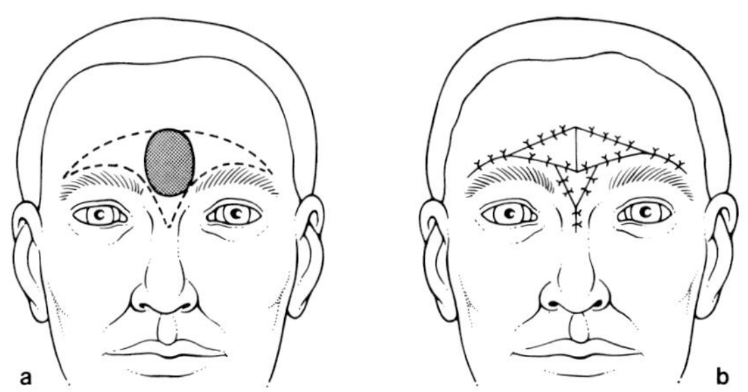

Fig. 7.283 Subcutaneously pedicled V–Y advancement flaps. **a.** Midline defect. Inferior pedicles to flaps, **b.** direct one-stage closure.

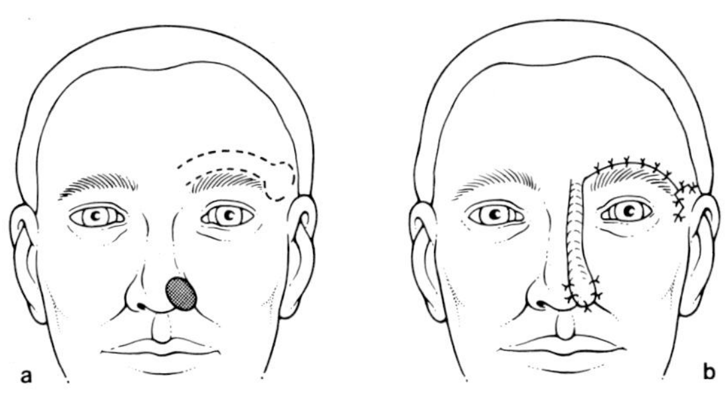

Fig. 7.284 Frontotemporal flap: **a.** first stage – delay of temporal and supraciliary parts; **b.** second stage – flap transferred. Direct donor site closure. Pedicle to be excised later.

The seagull flap (Fig. 7.282). For total nasal reconstruction (excluding lining) Millard has devised a seagull-shaped flap based on the supratrochlear vessels of one side.[4] This provides a regional unit of tissue for the bridge, tip, alae and columella, but is a three-stage procedure requiring a preliminary delay of three weeks.

The stem of the flap is about 2.5 cm wide and lies vertically with its base over the medial end of one eyebrow, while the wings are spread out along the natural horizontal furrows of the forehead. The wings are tapered but are shaped wide and long enough to construct the alae and curl into the nostril floor as alar bases. The more rounded superior end of the flap is destined for the tip and columella.

Subcutaneously pedicled V–Y advancement flaps (Fig. 7.283). A somewhat unusual solution to the problem of a midline defect but it illustrates the use of skin islands with an inferior subcutaneous pedicle containing the supratrochlear vessels.[5]

The frontotemporal flap (Fig. 7.284). This flap was introduced by Schmid in 1952 and subsequently modified by Meyer & Kesselring.[6] It has applications in subtotal rhinoplasty but has the disadvantage of requiring a preliminary delay. The flap consists of a horizontal pedicle situated above one eyebrow and a temporal portion which can be tailored by the addition of ear cartilage and split skin grafts to replace missing structures on the nose. In the first stage the temporal component of the flap is prepared and the pedicle is cut in a bevelled fashion with angled incisions so that the skin layer is narrow (about 5 mm) while the subcutaneous width of the flap is twice as large (approximately 10 mm). This carrier flap is then covered on its raw surfaces with a split skin graft and the supraciliary defect closed by direct approximation after undermining the frontal skin. Two to three weeks later the prefabricated tip and carrier flap are transposed to the recipient site. The pedicle is divided two weeks later.

References

1. Hayreh S S 1962 The ophthalmic artery. III Branches. British Journal of Ophthalmology. 46: 212–247
2. Gillies H D, Millard D R Jr 1957 Principles and art of plastic surgery. Little Brown, Boston
3. Sawhney C P 1979 Use of a larger midline forehead flap for rhinoplasty with new design for closure of donor site. Plastic and Reconstructive Surgery 63: 395–397
4. Millard D R Jr 1974 Reconstructive rhinoplasty for the lower half of the nose. Plastic and Reconstructive Surgery 53: 133–139
5. Zook E G, Van Beek A L, Russel R C, Moore J B 1979 V–Y advancement flap for facial defects. Plastic and Reconstructive Surgery 65: 786–797
6. Meyer R, Kesselring U K 1981 Reconstructive surgery of the nose. Clinics in Plastic Surgery 8: 435–469

7

SURAL ARTERIES

Gastrocnemius musculocutaneous flaps

Prior to the development of the musculocutaneous flap concept there had been extensive experience with the gastrocnemius muscle as a locally transposed muscle for coverage of the tibia in the treatment of traumatic injuries and residual ulcers from chronic osteomyelitis.[1,2] The realisation that the muscle could carry skin[3] led to the use of musculocutaneous flaps based either on the medial head[4] or the lateral head of the muscle. In addition to the standard version in which the skin island overlies the muscle, more useful extended versions have evolved. However, because of the donor site deformity and the inability to close it directly these flaps are reserved only for serious salvage problems, and even then a free flap – when the facilities are available – is a better choice. For this reason, as microsurgical expertise has become more widely available, the use of this flap has declined.

Although it is generally accepted that each head has only one pedicle entering at its superior end and that therefore inferiorly-based flaps are precluded, three cases have been reported in which inferiorly-based flaps have been successfully used based on the vascular communications between the lower ends of the two parts of the muscle.

Before they enter the muscle the sural arteries may give off superficial branches which run through the deep fascia overlying the muscles. These superficial sural arteries are the basis for fasciocutaneous flaps described on page 440.

Anatomy

In terms of flap potential, gastrocnemius is considered as being made up of two anatomically distinct muscles. Each head arises by a strong tendon from the upper part of its respective femoral condyle and the adjacent capsule of the knee joint. Each tendon expands in an aponeurotic fan on the surface of the muscle and the muscle fibres arise from this to form the muscle bellies. Both tendons are separated from the knee by bursae and that under the medial head usually communicates with the knee joint cavity. The larger medial head descends further than the lateral and the fibres of both insert into the superficial surface of a broad aponeurosis which faces soleus – this aponeurosis narrows to join the tendon of soleus in the Achilles tendon.

Each head is supplied by a sural artery (approximately 3 mm in diameter) which arises from the popliteal artery at, or slightly above, the level of the joint line and after a course of 2–5 cm enters the deep surface of the muscle along an elongated interfascicular hilum at the level of the tibial condyles. In over 90% of cases the nerves also enter with the arteries, with the nerves generally lying more posteriorly. Each artery is accompanied by two venae comitantes of which one tends to be larger than the other and measures up to 4 mm D. The artery to the medial head runs directly to the muscle, that to the lateral head passes anterior to the popliteal vein and the tibial nerve, and may give off branches to plantaris and soleus as well as a small vessel accompanying the lateral sural nerve. Occasionally the two sural arteries arise by a common trunk or the lateral sural artery arises by a common trunk with the inferior lateral or middle genicular artery.

Within the muscles each sural artery divides into two branches which run longitudinally between the muscle fibre bundles and often subdivide further. Accessory sural arteries may be given off by the popliteal below the main sural arteries and one of these is seen contributing to the lateral head in the radiograph on the opposite page.

The presence of anastomotic vessels between the arteries of the two heads or cross-supply of one artery to the opposite side is denied in anatomical texts but is illustrated in Figure 7.286 where an example can be seen of a lateral sural artery crossing over into the distal part of the larger medial head to supply it. This is the anatomical vascular basis for the inferiorly pedicled muscle flap described by Bashir.[6] Its reliability in a large number of cases has not been demonstrated.

Most of the branches of the sural arteries give off musculocutaneous perforators to the overlying skin and some end by piercing the surface of the muscle to reach overlying skin. The vessels do not continue on into the Achilles tendon and there is no blood supply from the tendon to overlying skin.

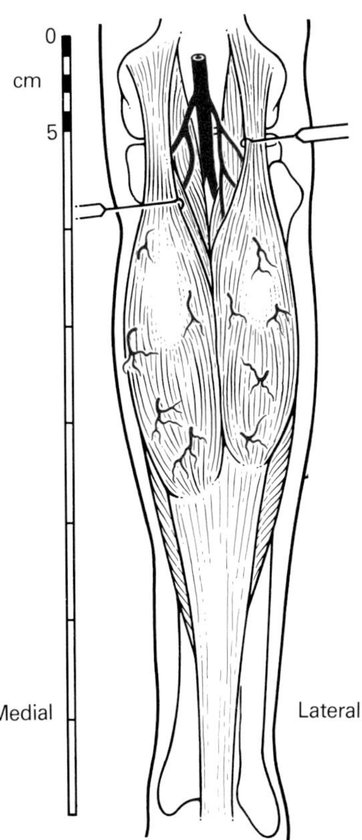

Fig. 7.285 Vascular anatomy. Sural arteries are shown arising from the popliteal artery and entering the deep surfaces of the two heads of gastrocnemius. Musculocutaneous perforators emerge from the muscle to supply overlying skin.

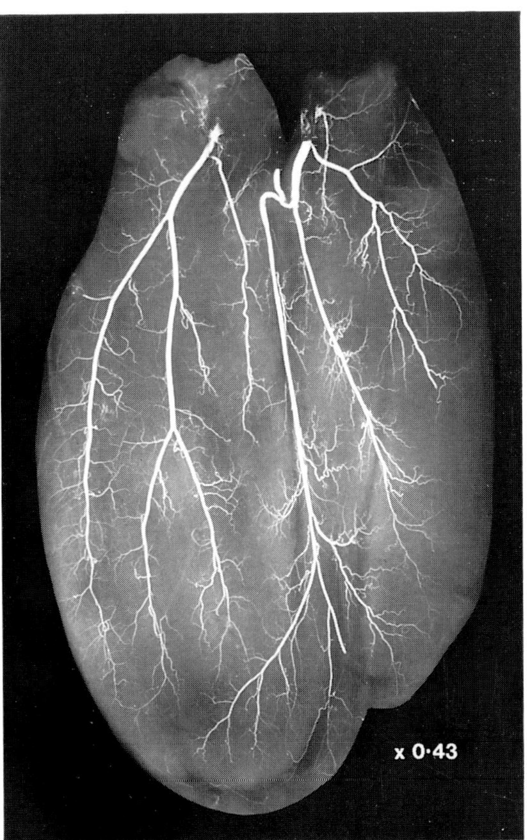

Fig. 7.286 Radiograph of injected gastrocnemius muscle. Note the abrupt terminations of some of the vessels. At these points the vessels exit from the surface of the muscle as musculocutaneous perforators; they were transected when the overlying skin was removed.

7

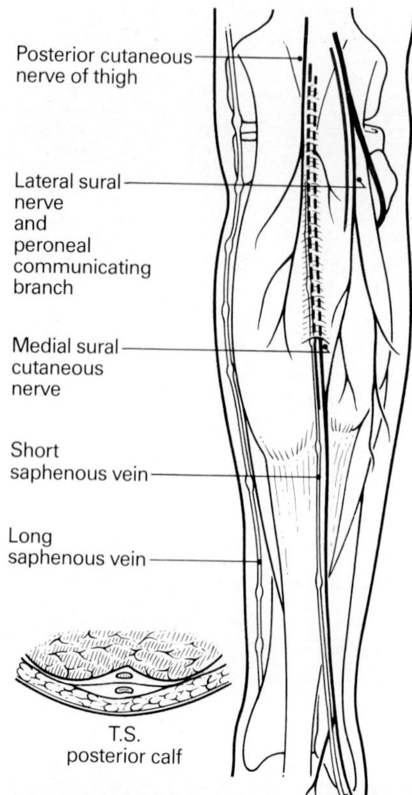

Fig. 7.287 Cutaneous nerves, veins and arteries in the area of the flaps are shown. (See also superficial sural arteries on p. 440.) Small diagram shows how the short saphenous vein may lie between the two layers of the deep fascia separate from the medial sural cutaneous nerve.

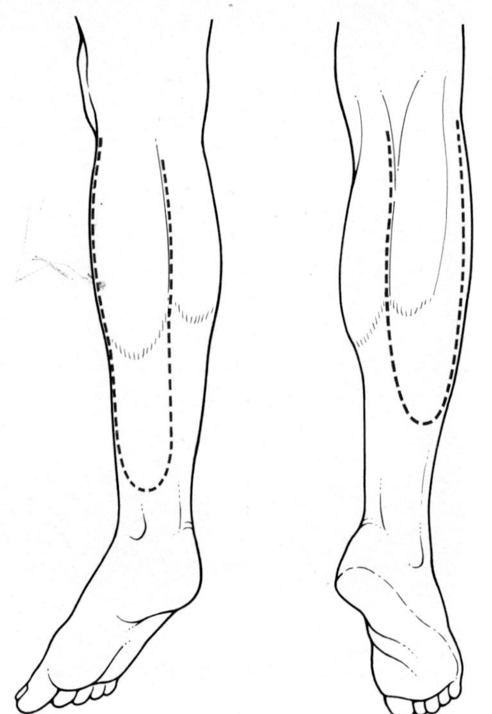

Fig. 7.288 Flap planning. On the left the medial gastrocnemius musculocutaneous flap which may be extended further distally than the lateral flap which is shown on the right.

Surgery

Medial flap. The posterior margin is formed by the midline of the calf and the anterior margin lies along the medial edge of the tibia. By incorporating the deep fascia, the length of the flap may be extended beyond the lower end of the muscle to within 5 cm of the medial malleolus.

Lateral flap. The posterior margin also lies in the midline, while the anterior margin overlies the fibula. The flap may be extended to within 8 cm of the lateral malleolus.

The skin incision starts in the posterior midline just below the popliteal skin crease. A guide to the plane between the medial and lateral heads of gastrocnemius is the short saphenous vein. It lies deep to fat most often on the surface of deep fascia but sometimes beneath it. The sural nerve always lies subfascially in the midline and a longitudinal incision of the fascia will lead to it and the midline between the muscle bellies. By starting superiorly the muscles can then be separated by blunt dissection which is carried down to the underlying soleus. Further finger dissection in this avascular plane separates the chosen head of gastrocnemius from soleus. The sides of the flap are next incised and then the distal part is elevated from distal to proximal beneath the deep fascia but leaving paratenon over the tendo calcaneus. When elevation of the distal part reaches the stage where the lower fibres of gastrocnemius are revealed then the insertion of the muscle is divided and the elevation continues at the previously defined plane on the surface of soleus.

The short saphenous vein should be preserved throughout but the long saphenous vein will be encroached on by the medial flap and will require to be ligated.

References

1. Ger R 1971 The technique of muscle transposition and the operative treatment of traumatic and ulcerative lesions of the leg. Journal of Trauma 2: 502–510
2. Pers M, Medgyesi S 1973 Pedicle muscle flaps and their application in the surgery of repair. British Journal of Plastic Surgery 26: 313–321
3. McCraw J B, Dibbell D G, Carraway J H 1977 Clinical definition of independent myocutaneous vascular territories. Plastic and Reconstructive Surgery 60: 341–352
4. Feldman J J, Cohen B E, May J W Jr 1978 Medial gastrocnemius myo-cutaneous flap. Plastic and Reconstructive Surgery 61: 531–539
5. McCraw J B, Fishman J H, Sharzer L A 1978 The versatile gastrocnemius myocutaneous flap. Plastic and Reconstructive Surgery 62: 15–23
6. Bashir A H 1983 Inferiorly based gastrocnemius muscle flap in the treatment of war wounds of the middle and lower third of the leg. British Journal of Plastic Surgery 36: 307–309

THORACO-ACROMIAL AXIS – deltoid branch

Pectoralis major clavicular head free flap
Free flap on direct cutaneous branch of deltoid artery

The anatomy of the thoraco-acromial axis has been described by Reid & Taylor[1] with particular reference to the pectoral branch and its communications with the vessels of the rib cage, but also with regard to the deltoid branch. The anatomy of the deltoid branch and the possibility of raising an osteo-myo-cutaneous free flap on this vessel has been demonstrated in three clinical cases by Reid et al.[2] The flap has a rich blood supply and the advantages of hairless skin and a good donor site, but suffers from a short pedicle and a relatively small size although it could be made larger at the expense of direct closure of the donor site.

Anatomy

The pectoralis major muscle may be considered as having four heads of origin, namely clavicular, manubrial, sternal and costal. The clavicular head is functionally distinct, sharing with the anterior fibres of deltoid a role in flexion of the shoulder. The difference in function between the clavicular and sternal parts of pectoralis major is emphasised by the differential nerve supply consisting of a branch from the lateral cord of the brachial plexus to the clavicular head and branches mainly from the medial cord to the rest of the muscle. It is therefore to be expected that the clavicular head will also have an independent blood supply.

The thoraco-acromial axis is classically described as dividing into four main branches – the clavicular, deltoid, pectoral and acromial arteries. In the majority of cases the arrangement is one of a major bifurcation into deltoid and pectoral branches with the acromial artery arising from the deltoid branch. The clavicular branch has a variable origin from the main trunk or any of its branches and most frequently (60%) arises at the point of bifurcation of the main artery. In addition, a cutaneous branch about 1.0 mm in diameter is given off by one of the branches in ~50% of cases and pierces the fascia over the infraclavicular fossa to reach the overlying skin (Fig. 7.290). The distribution of the pectoral branch is fully described on page 166. The deltoid branch at its origin measures approximately 2.5 mm in external diameter (range 1.5–3.5 mm). It runs laterally to supply the anterior fibres of deltoid. In its course it gives off several branches which supply the lateral part of the clavicular head of pectoralis major while the most medial part of the clavicular head is supplied by its own vessel usually from the clavicular branch. The length of the deltoid branch measured from the axillary artery to the clavicular head is around 5–7 cm. There are only a few perforators through the lateral part of the clavicular head of pectoralis major to the overlying skin since this area may also be supplied by the direct cutaneous branch emerging from the infraclavicular fossa. However, the terminal branches of the deltoid artery run along the fascial septa between the muscle fibre bundles of the anterior part of deltoid and emerge as two to four small perforators to supply the overlying skin. A single particularly large perforator emerges in the middle of the deltopectoral groove,

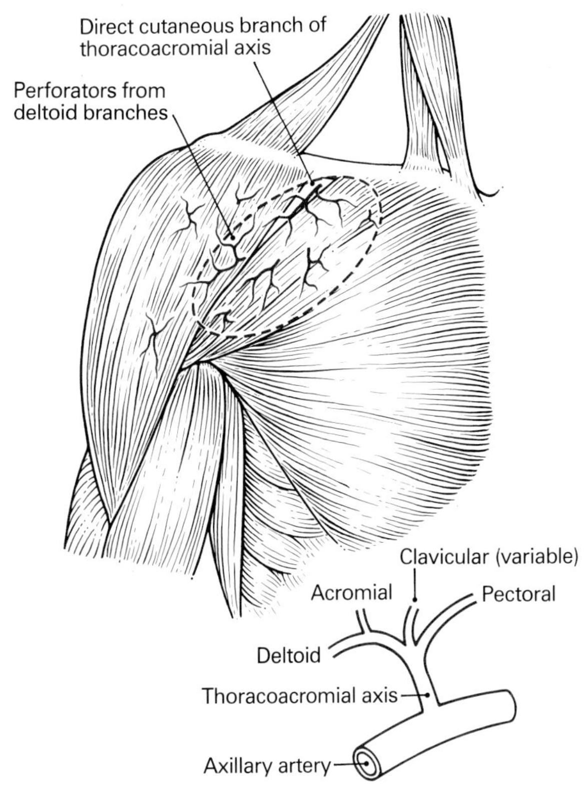

Fig. 7.289 Vascular antomy. Musculocutaneous perforators from the deltoid branch of the thoraco-acromial axis are shown in the main illustration. Inset shows the most common pattern of branching of the thoraco-acromial axis.

pierces the deep fascia and spreads out in the manner of a musculocutaneous perforator at the subcutaneous level. It divides into branches which ascend towards the clavicle, descend towards the deltoid insertion and others which fan out over the clavicular fibres of deltoid. Manchot named this vessel the Arteria subcutanea deltoidea anterior. It is not present with the same regularity as the posterior deltoid perforator and when underdeveloped it is replaced by musculocutaneous perforators from the deltoid artery either emerging from the deltopectoral groove or through the deltoid muscle. The intramuscular branches of the deltoid artery also anastomose with periosteal vessels covering the clavicle.

The venous pattern is less constant than the arterial pattern in that it tends to be more plexiform but it matches the corresponding arteries. The vein accompanying the deltoid artery has an external diameter of about 4 mm (range 1–6 mm). A significant point is that the cephalic vein which lies in the deltopectoral groove and runs through the territory of the deltoid artery, has virtually no significant tributaries from the pectoralis major or deltoid muscles in this part of its course although all the veins become confluent immediately prior to their entry into the axillary vein.

Flap elevation

The outlines of a possible flap are shown in Figure 7.289 within the territory of the deltoid branch. The incision of the margin of the flap commences superolaterally and the flap is elevated up to the deltopectoral groove where any cutaneous arteries emerging from between deltoid and pectoralis major to enter the flap are preserved. The cephalic vein is left in the groove and the dissection is deepened to reveal the deltoid artery branch passing from pectoralis major into deltoid—this artery is divided distally. The distal and medial margins of the flap overlying the pectoralis major are now incised and the clavicular head transected at the distal limit of the skin island. Any part of the skin flap lying on the sternal part of pectoralis major is dissected off the muscle up to the medial margin of the clavicular head where the muscle fibres of the clavicular head are split from the remainder of the muscle. This permits upward elevation of the compound flap, division of the upper branch of the lateral pectoral nerve which supplies the clavicular head, and exposure of the thoraco-acromial axis where the pedicle is dissected out. Separation of the clavicular head from the clavicle may be carried out before or after dissection and division of

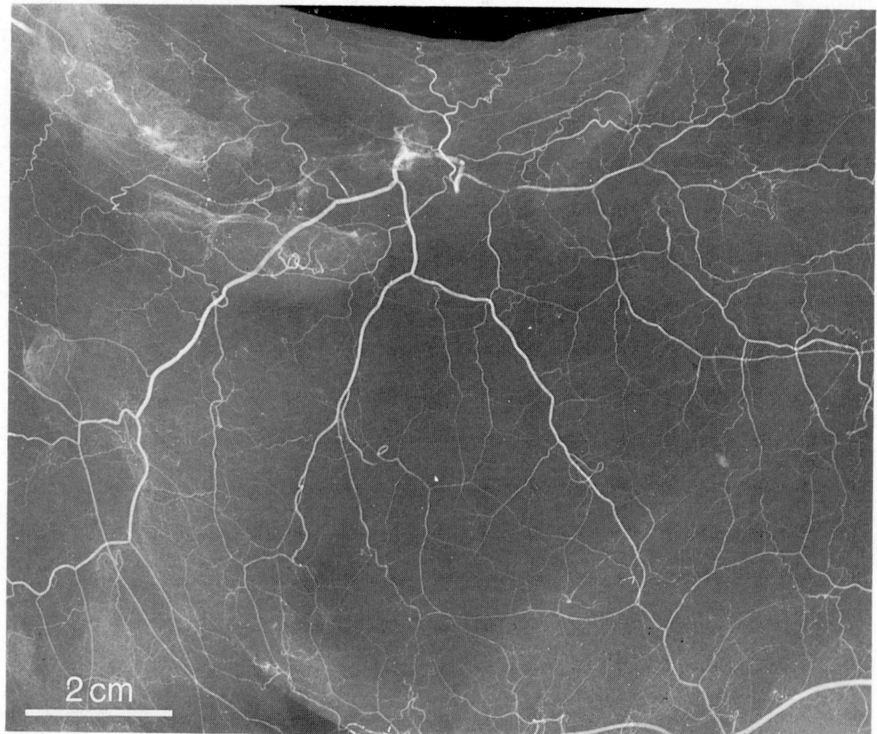

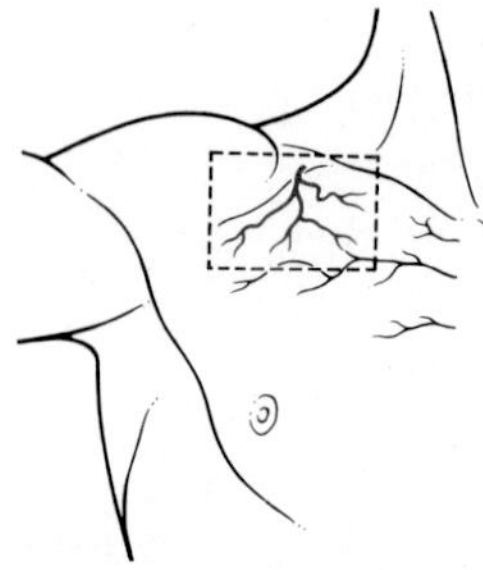

Fig. 7.290 Radiograph of skin showing direct cutaneous branch over infraclavicular fossa. Line drawing shows the area from which the specimen was taken.

the pedicle. The anterior fibres of deltoid lying lateral to the thoraco-acromial axis, and attached to the clavicle, may also be removed with the flap if a larger area of skin is required but this creates a more problematic donor defect. The attachment of the muscle to the clavicle may be preserved and an approximately 7 cm long strut of split clavicle may be removed as a compound flap.

Free flap on cutaneous perforator from deltoid artery. A purely cutaneous flap based on only the anterior subcutaneous branch of the deltoid artery has also been described.[3] (In this report the terminology of the vessels was different as the artery of the flap was termed the acromial branch but this in fact lies in the upper part of the deltoid as can be seen in Fig. 7.291). The artery of the flap pierces the anterior edge of the deltoid muscle and fans out over the muscle as shown in Figure 7.289 and in the radiograph (Fig. 6.43) in which the vessel is labelled as number 7. The vessels are small and the pedicle short. Nine flaps were transferred without loss and only the largest measuring 9 cm × 8 cm suffered superficial blistering.

References

1. Reid C D, Taylor G I 1984 The vascular territory of the acromiothoracic axis. British Journal of Plastic Surgery 37: 194–212
2. Reid C D, Taylor G I, Waterhouse N 1986 The clavicular head of pectoralis major musculocutaneous free flap. British Journal of Plastic Surgery 39: 57–65
3. Zhou L-Y, Cao Y-L 1989 Clincial application of the free flap based on the cutaneous branch of the acromiothoracic artery. Annals of Plastic Surgery 23: 11–16
4. Milroy B C, Korula P 1988 Vascularised innervated transfer of the clavicular head of the pectoralis major muscle in established facial paralysis. Annals of Plastic Surgery 20: 75–81
5. Knudsen F W, Andersen M, Krag C 1989 The arterial supply of the clavicle. Surgical and Radiologic Anatomy 11: 211–214

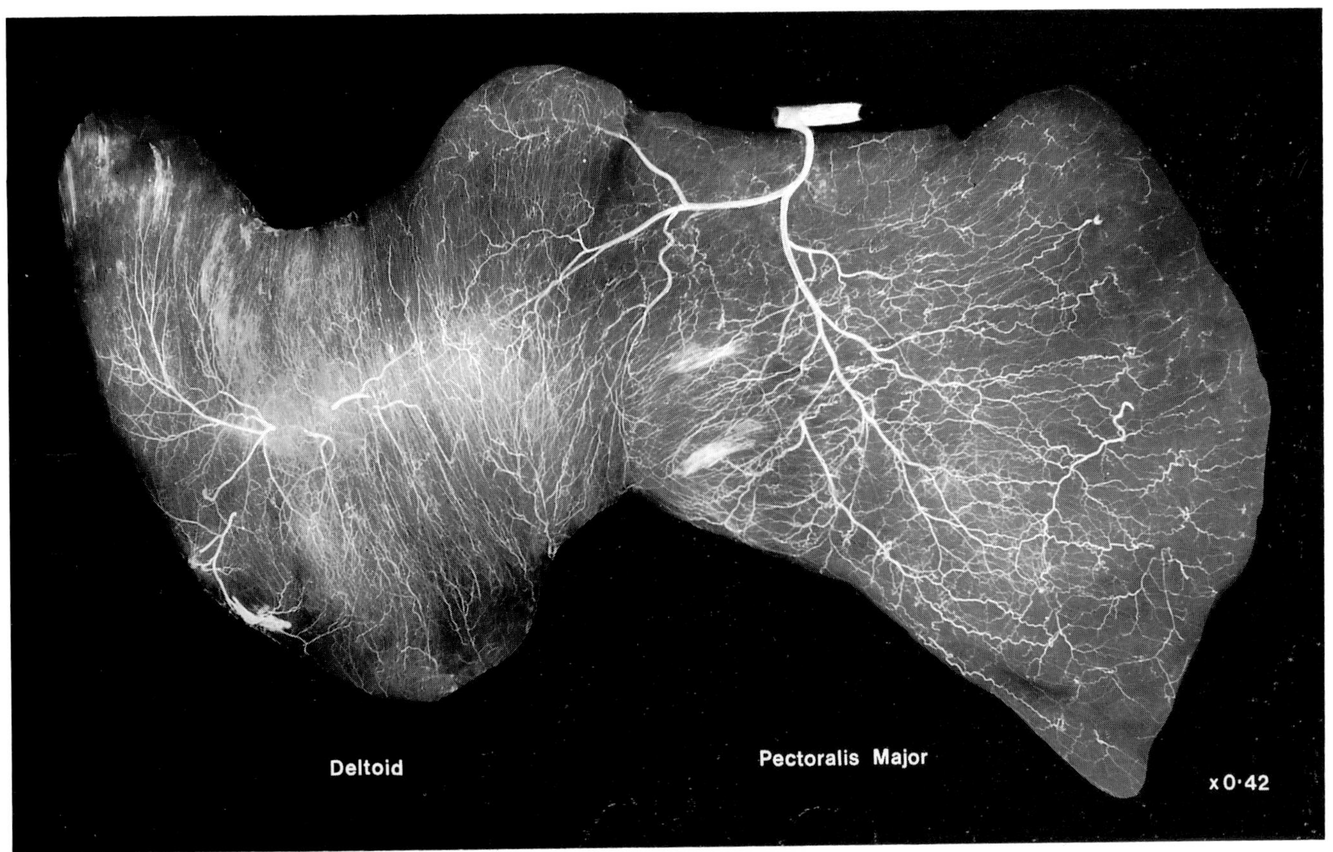

Fig. 7.291 Radiograph of deltoid and pectoralis major in continuity showing the deltoid branch of the thoraco-acromial axis passing laterally to supply the clavicular head of deltoid and, via perforators, the overlying skin (not shown).

7

THORACO-ACROMIAL AXIS – pectoral branch

Pectoralis major musculocutaneous flap

A laterally based deltopectoral skin flap which included part of the underlying pectoralis major was described by Hueston & McConchie in 1968[1] but it was Ariyan[2] who popularised the pectoralis musculocutaneous flap pedicled on the branches of the thoraco-acromial axis. He reduced the amount of muscle around the vascular pedicle and converted the skin component to an island flap or 'paddle' located over the inferomedial part of the muscle.

Anatomy

The thoraco-acromial axis arises from the second part of the axillary artery, pierces the clavipectoral fascia medial to the tendon of pectoralis minor and classically divides into four branches – acromial, clavicular, deltoid and pectoral. The commonest pattern of division is indicated in Figure 7.292. The deltoid branch is the largest (~ 2.5 mm D) and gives off the acromial branch to the tip of the shoulder. The pectoral branch (~ 2.0 mm D) gives off the clavicular branch although this vessel may arise from the trunk itself or from any other branch. The approximate cutaneous territories of these four vessels are indicated in Figure 7.293.

The pectoral branch descends on the posterior surface of pectoralis major within the epimysial sheath of the muscle and supplies it by branches which pass between the fibre bundles. Some of these vessels pierce the surface of the muscle to reach the overlying skin, while the terminal branches of the pectoral artery pass round the infero-lateral border of pectoralis major to reach the skin. Within the muscle many of the arterial branches pass medially along the fascial septa between the fibre bundles and anastomose with the segmental anterior

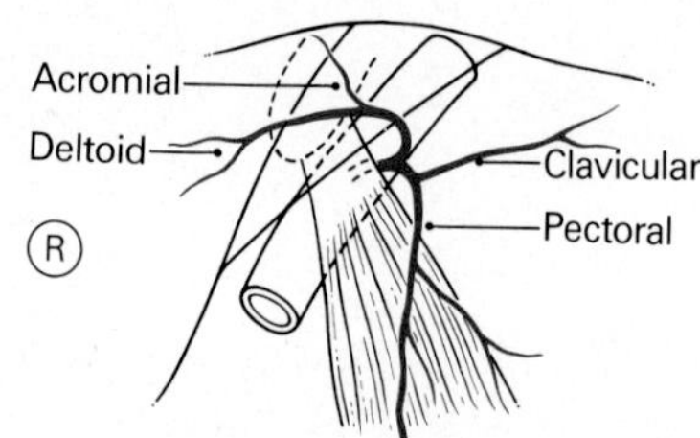

Fig. 7.292 Commonest branching pattern of the thoraco-acromial axis.

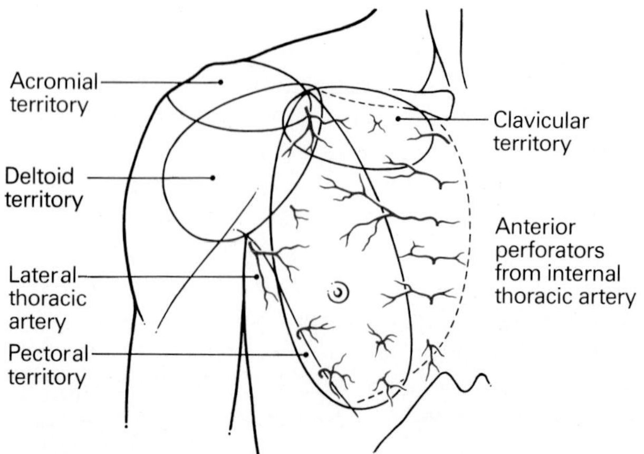

Fig. 7.293 Schematic representation of the blood supply to the skin on the anterior chest wall.

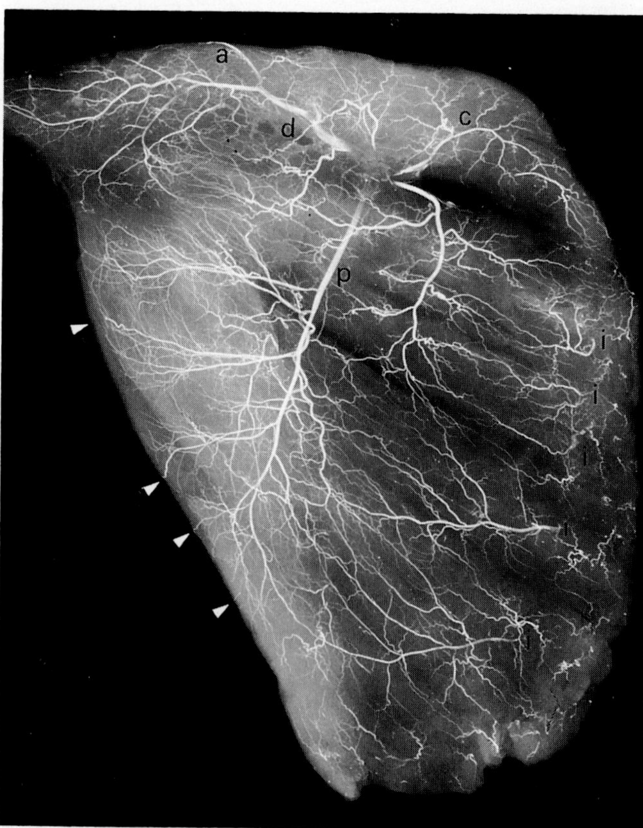

Fig. 7.294 Radiograph of right pectoralis major muscle. Arrows indicate points at which the terminal branches of the pectoral division end abruptly as they pass round the lateral edge of the muscle. Here the vessels were divided as they passed up to the overlying skin.

perforators from the internal thoracic artery which penetrate the medial part of pectoralis to reach the overlying skin as direct cutaneous vessels. Further anastomoses may exist with a branch of the lateral thoracic artery which runs along beneath the lateral edge of the muscle.

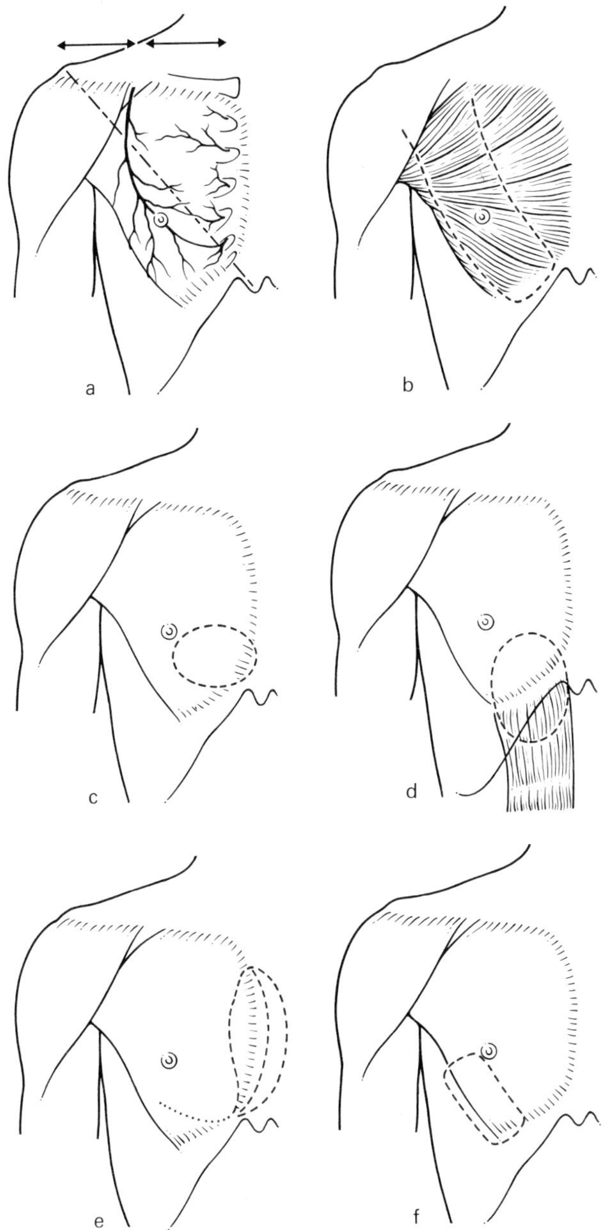

Fig. 7.295 Variations on the pectoralis musculocutaneous flap: **a.** approximate method of surface marking the vascular pedicle; **b.** original laterally-based pectoral compound flap; **c.** inferomedial skin paddle; **d.** extended pectoralis paddle (incorporates anterior rectus sheath); **e.** parasternal paddle with variable extension over sternum; **f.** laterally situated paddle supplied by terminal branches passing round the edge of the muscle (see arrows in Fig. 7.294).

In the method for surface marking the vascular axis described by Ariyan, the vascular pedicle follows a vertical line drawn downwards from a point half-way along the clavicle until it meets a line between shoulder tip and xiphoid along which it then runs in a medial direction (Fig. 7.295a). More commonly the vessels pursue a course that lies lateral to both these lines and approaches the free lateral border of the muscle before curving medially as demonstrated by the specimen in Figure 7.294.

In addition, in about 25% of cases the pectoral branch of the thoraco-acromial axis gives off a significant cutaneous artery which pierces the deep fascia in the infraclavicular fossa and runs in the subcutaneous fat in an inferior direction.

Flap planning

The laterally pedicled compound skin and muscle flap (Fig. 7.295b) has been superseded by various versions of the island flap:

1. The original model designed by Ariyan placed the skin island in an inferomedial position where it was supplied by perforators from the muscle and by the lower internal thoracic artery perforators with which the pectoral branch anastomoses[1] (Fig. 7.295c).
2. Others have extended the skin island to include the uppermost part of the anterior rectus sheath and overlying skin which are supported, albeit somewhat precariously, by distal anastomoses at the level of the sheath[5] (Fig. 7.295d).
3. In order to reduce the thickness of the inferomedial island and to reduce the distorting effect on the breast of the donor site scar in this position, a further modification has been to site the skin island in a parasternal position.[6] Here it is entirely dependent on the anterior perforating branches of the internal thoracic artery and the anastomoses which these vessels make within pectoralis major with the pectoral branch of the thoraco-acromial axis. The skin island may overlie the sternum and even extend across the midline (Fig. 7.295e). The principal advantage is that the thickness of muscle and subcutaneous tissue beneath the skin island is much reduced but the pedicle is larger because the whole sternocostal part of the muscle must be included.
4. The most recent modification results from a more thorough understanding of the vascular anatomy, and sites the skin island over the lower lateral edge of the muscle so that it is supplied directly by the terminal branches of the pectoral artery which pass round the border of the muscle (Fig. 7.295f).
5. The parasternal paddle may include the outer table of the sternum.[7]

6. The standard island may be modified to include a segment of the fourth or fifth rib since pectoralis major has been shown to have an attachment to these ribs and costal cartilages in the mid-clavicular line.[3] The supply from pectoralis to the sixth rib is poor and unreliable.

Surgery

The muscle may be exposed in one of three ways. Firstly, by dissecting out the muscle pedicle subcutaneously by a relatively blind approach leaving an intact skin bridge between the island and the neck incision. This may involve unnecessary risk to the vessels.[5] Secondly, by an open approach through a skin incision between the island and the base of the pedicle which allows direct visualisation of the full length of the muscle pedicle. Thirdly, and more desirably, the territory of the deltopectoral flap may be preserved by elevating this first to gain exposure of the pedicle. This provides excellent visualisation but has the disadvantage of restricting the deltopectoral flap to the length raised at the time of surgery. Carrying out a prior bipedicle delay of the deltopectoral flap has been recommended as a means of solving this problem.

Exposing the muscle will also have involved incising the outline of the skin island. There are then three options for dealing with the pedicle: (1) The vascular pedicle can be dissected free of the muscle by dividing the overlying muscle fibres and thereby gaining direct access to the pedicle. (2) The clavicular head can be preserved intact and the pedicle freed from the undersurface of the muscle by working from the infraclavicular fossa above and from an incision through the muscle below. This allows the upper part of the pectoralis major to be preserved intact although its nerve supply is likely to have been destroyed in dissecting the pedicle. (3) The third option is to make two incisions in the muscle all the way up to the clavicle and remove a strip of muscle in continuity with and overlying the pedicle. This confers no advantage other than removing the need to carefully divide offshoots of the pectoral branch going to the upper part of the muscle and has the disadvantages of totally destroying the pectoralis and of adding to the bulk of the pedicle when it is turned up over the clavicle.

When maximum length of pedicle is required the skin island will be positioned in a low parasternal position. A broad muscle pedicle with the same vertical width as the skin paddle should then be dissected horizontally towards the free lateral border of pectoralis. The incision for the lower edge of this horizontal pedicle is carried through to the lateral edge of the muscle. The upper edge is only taken half-way across the muscle and then the free lateral edge of the muscle is raised from the chest wall. This plane is developed until the pectoral branch comes into view on the posterior surface of the muscle. It can then be seen where the upper edge of the horizontal muscle pedicle incision should turn to a vertical line immediately medial to the pectoral pedicle. The muscle pedicle can then be developed towards the clavicle and as the elevation proceeds superiorly the vessel pedicle will reach a substantial size on the back of the muscle and at this point the pedicle can be reduced to the vessels and surrounding fatty connective tissue only. This approach with a low parasternal paddle actually creates an L-shaped pedicle which, when straightened out, creates extra length. If pedicle length is not crucial then the skin island is preferentially positioned nearer the lateral edge of the muscle. The disadvantage of this position is that it may include the nipple. The lateral edge of the skin island is incised and dissection proceeds by locating the lateral edge of the muscle and raising it off the chest. The remainder of the muscle round the edge of the skin island is incised and the pedicle developed in any of the aforementioned ways.

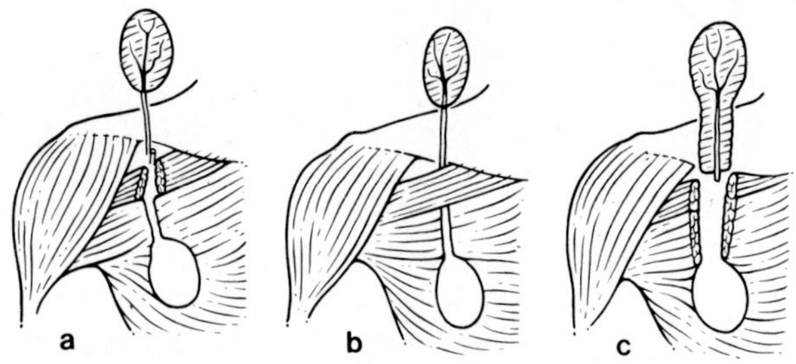

Fig. 7.296 Methods of passing the pedicle upwards over the clavicle: **a.** by dividing the clavicular head; **b.** by tunnelling beneath it; **c.** by incorporating part of the clavicular head in the pedicle.

References

1. Hueston J T, McConchie H A 1968 A compound pectoral flap. Australian and New Zealand Journal of Surgery 38: 61–63
2. Ariyan S 1979 The pectoralis major myocutaneous flap. Plastic and Reconstructive Surgery 63: 73–81
3. Reid C D, Taylor G I 1984 The vascular territory of the acromiothoracic axis. British Journal of Plastic Surgery 37: 194–212
4. Freeman J L, Walker E P, Wilson J S P, Shaw H J 1981 The vascular anatomy of the pectoralis major myocutaneous flap. British Journal of Plastic Surgery 34: 3–10
5. Magee W P, Gilbert D A, McInnis W D 1980 Extended muscle and musculocutaneous flaps. Clinics in Plastic Surgery 7: 57–70
6. Sharzer L A, Kalisman M, Silver C E, Strauch B 1981 The parasternal paddle; a modification of the pectoralis major myocutaneous flap. Plastic and Reconstructive Surgery 67: 753–762
7. Green M F, Gibson J R, Bryson J R, Thomson E 1981 A one-stage correction of mandibular defects using a split sternum pectoralis major osteo-musculocutaneous transfer. British Journal of Plastic Surgery 34: 11–16
8. Baek S M, Lawson W, Biller H F 1982 An analysis of 133 pectoralis major myocutaneous flaps. Plastic and Reconstructive Surgery 69: 460–467

Latissimus dorsi musculocutaneous flap

Tansini was the first to use a superiorly based flap of skin and latissimus dorsi muscle in 1895.[1] The method was used sporadically until the late 1970s when McCraw and others developed the true latissimus musculocutaneous flap in which an island of skin is carried on the muscle. A further development was its use as a free musculocutaneous flap or osteo-myo-cutaneous tissue transfer when combined with a segment of the ninth or tenth rib.[2] Recently a more thorough understanding of the neurovascular anatomy of the muscle has enabled various refinements to be developed, including splitting of the muscle with preservation of motor function.[3]

Anatomy

Latissimus dorsi is a Type V muscle with a single dominant vascular pedicle from the thoracodorsal artery at its insertion, and multiple secondary segmental pedicles originating from some of the lumbar and lower six intercostal arteries, at its origin. The thoracodorsal artery enters the muscle together with the thoracodorsal nerve at a point approximately 8.5 cm distal to the origin of the subscapular artery (range 6.0–11.5 cm) and 2.5 cm from the lateral border of the muscle (range 1.0–4.0 cm). The diameter of the subscapular artery is 3–4 mm and of the thoracodorsal 2–3 mm at its origin. Within the muscle, nerves and arteries follow a similar pattern of branching. In 94% of cases the thoracodorsal artery bifurcates into a medial and a slightly larger lateral branch.[3] The lateral branch characteristically parallels the lateral border of the muscle running approximately 2.5 cm from its edge as seen in Figure 7.298. The upper or medial branch separates from it at an angle of about 45° and parallels the upper muscle border.[4] Within the muscle both branches divide into lesser branches which run medially and anastomose with perforators from the intercostal and lumbar arteries. A very significant feature of these anastomoses is their large diameter. In the remaining 6% of cases the neurovascular tree splits into three or four major branches. Both branching patterns supply the muscle with long, parallel neurovascular branches which run in the fascia between bundles of muscle fibres and thereby enable the muscle to be split into independent vascularised innervated units.

The skin over the upper part of latissimus dorsi is supplied from these arteries by large musculocutaneous perforators which lie about 3–5 cm apart. Over the middle third of the muscle the supply is by smaller perforators and also through the lateral dorsal cutaneous branches of the intercostal and lumbar vessels; these enter the muscle approximately 8 cm from the midline (just lateral to the edge of the thoracolumbar fascia) and anastomose within the muscle with the ramifications of the thoracodorsal artery. Adjacent to the midline the supply is from segmental medial dorsal cutaneous branches and over the lower third of the muscle, just above the iliac crest, the supply is entirely from segmental perforators which do not connect so well with the thoracodorsal pedicle. This means that a skin island isolated over the lower one-third may not be

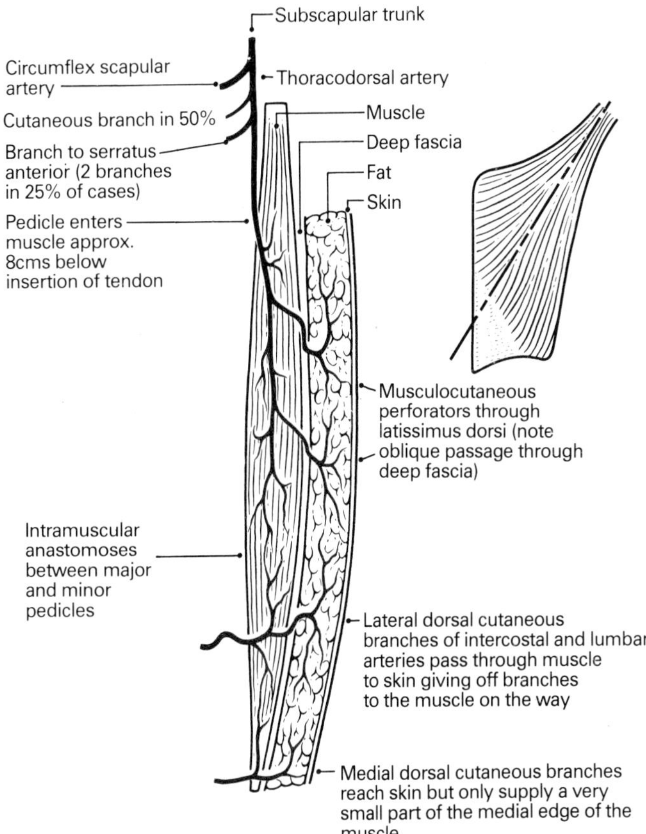

Fig. 7.297 Vascular anatomy. Schematic section through muscle and overlying skin along the section indicated top right.

consistently viable, though a portion of skin from the distal third area may be safely carried as an extension of a more superiorly based island.

Near the humeral insertion of the muscle a number of significant vessels connect with the thoracodorsal artery and these vessels play an important part in the development of a collateral circulation following division of the thoracodorsal artery during radical mastectomy.[6] The thoracodorsal artery gives off one to three branches of about 1 mm diameter to serratus anterior which penetrate the muscle in its midportion along the course of the long thoracic nerve. Reversal of flow may take place in these vessels and also in vessels from teres major in the paratenon around the insertion and perhaps in other direct vessels entering from axillary and intercostal vessels.

The venous drainage of the muscle parallels the arterial supply but the presence of venous valves has important implications for flap design. The lower and medial parts of the muscle preferentially drain through the intercostal and lumbar venous systems and not via the thoracodorsal system. Valves within the veins ensure this direction of flow. Whereas in the arteries reversal of flow can easily take place and blood can reach the extreme parts of the muscle, on the venous side there are problems in draining the inferior end of the muscle into the thoracodorsal system (see Fig. 7.299). The result is that the muscle-only flap suffers venous compromise in its lower part and any areas that appear suspect after reperfusing a free flap should be excised as experience has shown that these areas, which initially have an arterial inflow but which ooze dark deoxygenated blood, do not survive. By contrast, the musculocutaneous flap fares better in its distal part, perhaps because venous blood from the muscle can find an additional pathway of return through the subcutaneous venous network.

Compound osteo-musculocutaneous flap

It is possible to harvest the flap in conjunction with a portion of the lateral edge of the scapula which is vascularised by branches of the circumflex scapular artery (Fig. 7.305). Alternatively a segment of the 9th rib may be taken at the site of attachment of one of the slips of origin of the latissimus muscle. As can be seen from Figure 7.298 the vascular connections between the thoracodorsal branches and the vessels in these muscle slips at their sites of origin are not great.

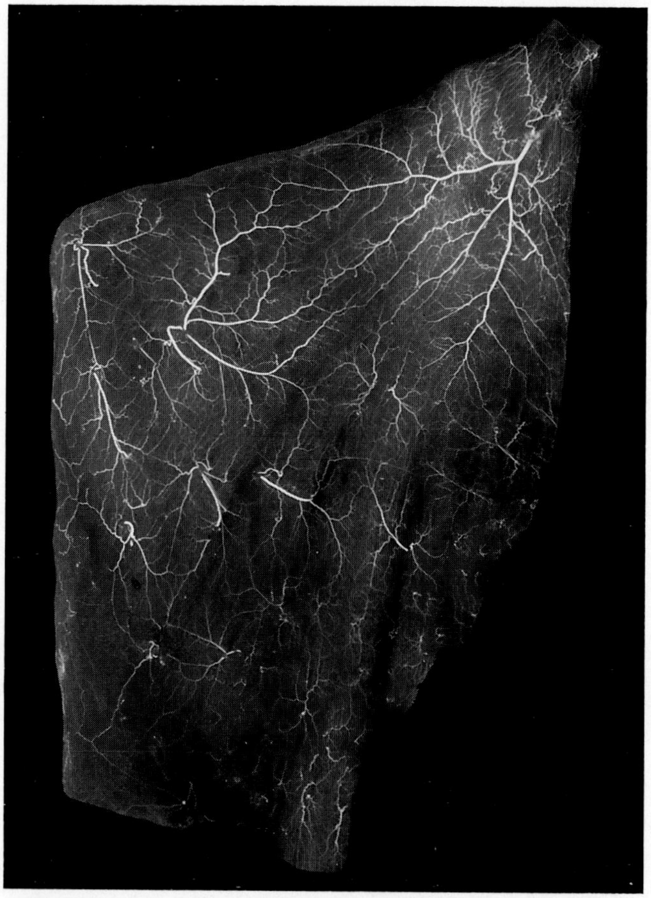

Fig. 7.298 Arterial anatomy. Radiograph of latissimus dorsi muscle after injection of the arterial tree.

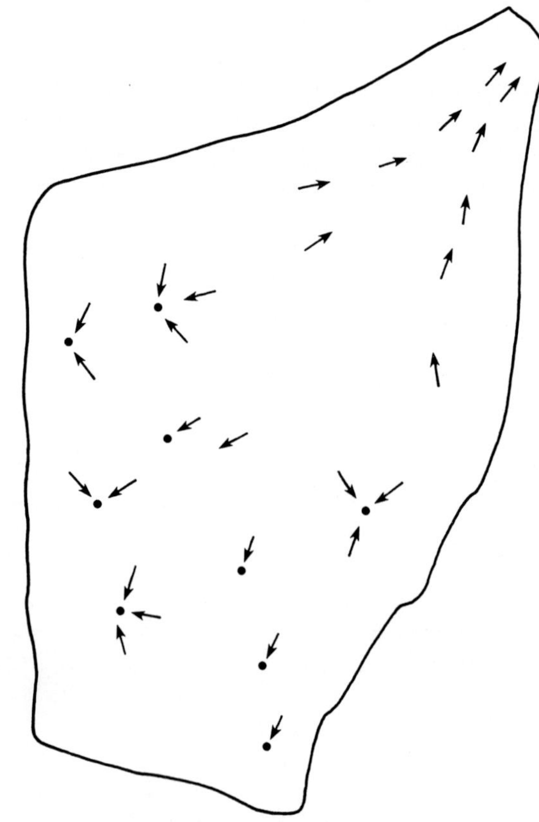

Fig. 7.299 Venous anatomy. The directions of the valves are indicated. The inferior part of the muscle can only drain into the thoracodorsal system by flowing counter to the direction of the venous valves.

Planning

Early designs of the flap orientated the elliptical skin island longitudinally along the anterolateral border of the muscle and this is still the best situation for a flap destined for head and neck or upper arm reconstruction. The flap may overlap the lateral edge of the muscle by 3 cm (Fig. 7.300). A more appropriate design for breast reconstruction is with the skin island orientated transversely below the upper border of the muscle, thereby leaving a transverse scar which can be more easily concealed (Fig. 7.301). If a reconstruction of an infraclavicular area necessitates the use of the whole latissimus muscle then the skin island will need to be placed superomedially on the back since the muscle cannot be rotated independently of the skin island and the muscle will need to lie initially lateral and inferior to the flap (Fig. 7.302) so that when moved round to the anterior chest the muscle will lie in the infraclavicular area above the skin island. Maximum dimensions of the skin island which permit direct closure are about 12 cm × 35 cm.

Most breast reconstructions using the latissimus flap replace the breast volume with a prosthesis, but it is possible to increase the bulk of the flap by including the

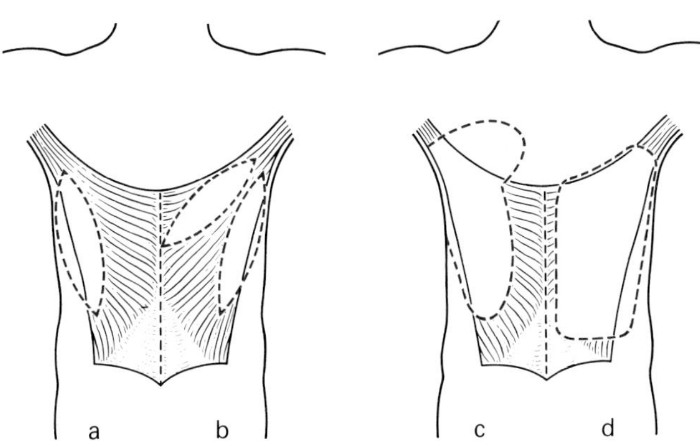

Fig. 7.300 Various possible flap designs. **a.** Vertical flap slightly overlapping the anterior edge of the muscle. **b.** Split latissimus flap with two skin islands separate from each other. This exploits the major bifurcation of the intramuscular part of the thoracodorsal artery. **c.** A large regional flap created by combining the scapular flap based on the horizontal branch of the circumflex scapular artery with the latissimus flap. Teres major would need to be divided in order to preserve the continuity of the vascular pedicles of the two flaps with each other and with the subscapular trunk. **d.** A large flap with dimensions of up to 35 cm × 20 cm based on the entire muscle.

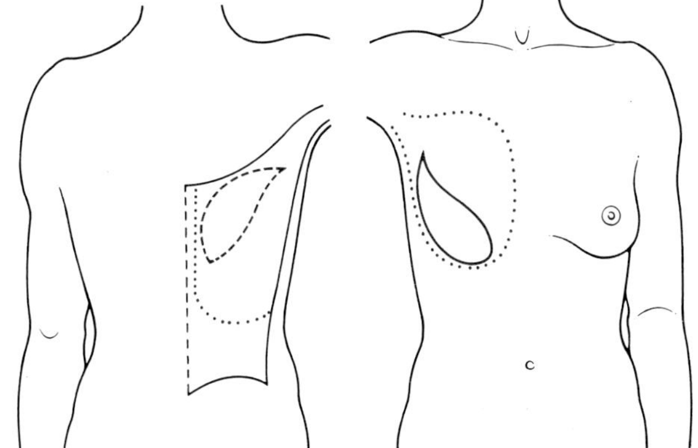

Fig. 7.302 Design of flap in a medial and superior position on the posterior chest wall in combination with maximum utilisation of the muscle when reconstructing the pectoral fullness after a radical mastectomy (after Wolf & Biggs, 1982). The flap is inset obliquely irrespective of the orientation of the mastectomy scar so as to produce vertical and transverse relaxation and act as a sling supporting the fullness of the breast.

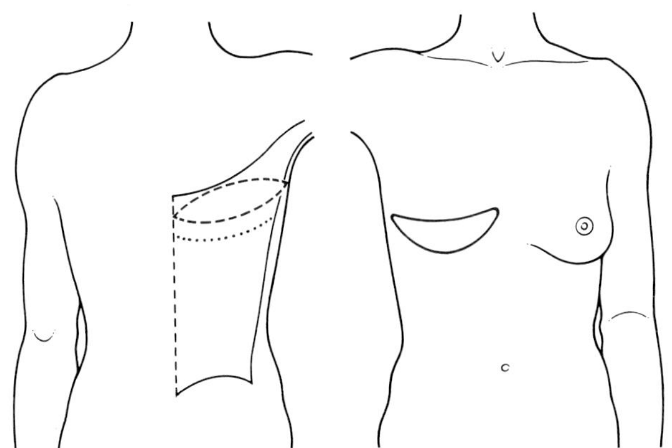

Fig. 7.301 Horizontal ellipse of skin combined with the upper part of the muscle for breast reconstruction. Donor site closes as a single line that is of a convenient orientation for camouflage by a brassiere.

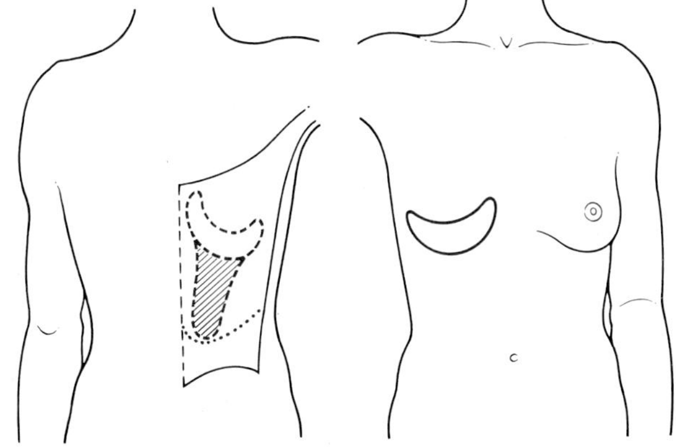

Fig. 7.303 Sickle-shaped flap. Additional fullness may be obtained in the reconstructed breast by taking a dart of skin and subcutaneous fat from a position inferior to the skin island. When de-epithelialised this may be buried beneath the skin flaps on the anterior chest to provide added bulk.

whole of the muscle and a large volume of subcutaneous tissue from the region above the iliac crest where it tends to be thick. A sickle-shaped skin island, positioned lower than usual on the back, is taken with a large dart of skin and subcutaneous tissue which extends down from the island over latissimus dorsi to the iliac crest. This is de-epithelialised and is turned beneath the skin and muscle flap to provide adequate bulk in the reconstructed breast (Fig. 7.303).

Surgery

The patient will generally be positioned on the side with the arm of the donor side abducted 90° and suspended in this position by the forearm resting supported in a horizontal position on a floor-standing Mayo table or some appropriate table-mounted support. The skin island is incised down to the muscle fascia widening the base of attachment to the muscle. The skin around the flap is dissected off the muscle and the edges of the muscle defined. The muscle is then dissected off the chest wall commencing at the free lateral edge. During this process large perforators from the intercostal and lumbar vessels are divided. Medial and inferior incisions through the muscle are made with the positions of these incisions dictated by how much muscle is required in the flap. Attention can then be turned to the pedicle. Initially this is best dissected by leaving the muscle insertion intact and turning the flap upwards so as to expose the pedicle on the undersurface of the muscle. This avoids undue traction on the pedicle. An alternative approach is to leave the flap in place on the chest (securing it with a few sutures if it has already been fully mobilised) and to carefully divide the thin flat tendon of insertion of the muscle so as to expose the pedicle. Either way, the pedicle is dissected free with isolation and division of the branches of the thoracodorsal artery that pass to serratus anterior and teres major. The thoracodorsal nerve is divided and the sole remaining attachments are then the thoracodorsal artery and vein. Depending on the size and position of the skin island, an additional incison over the anterior edge of the muscle extending up to the axilla will be required for this exposure of the pedicle.

If the intention is to split the muscle and retain half of it on the chest with an intact nerve supply, then the dissection is obviously more complicated. The vascular basis for splitting the flap is the known bifurcation of the thoracodorsal artery within the muscle which enables either the superior horizontal part of the muscle or the anterior vertical part to be harvested on the thoracodorsal pedicle. In this situation the part of the muscle left on the chest is detached from the thoracodorsal pedicle and receives its blood supply from the intercostal perforators. If this part of the muscle is left in continuity with the tendon of insertion and its innervation is preserved, then some function should be retained in it. The bifurcation of the thoracodorsal artery is on average 8.7 cm from the point where the subscapular artery arises from the axillary artery.

When raising the flap with bone from the scapula there are variations in the anatomy to be considered. The general scheme is shown in Figure 7.305a with the angular branch supplying the lower pole and the circumflex scapular artery the middle and upper thirds of the lateral border. The angular branch arises directly from the thoracodorsal artery just proximal to the origin of the branch to serratus anterior (Fig. 7.305b), or it arises from the branch of the thoracodorsal to serratus (Fig. 7.10). The angular artery is 4 to 5 cm long and lies over the serratus anterior muscle in the interval between teres major and the latissimus dorsi.[9] It divides into small branches 1 to 2 cm lateral to the edge of the scapula approximately 2 or 3 cm above the lower pole and vascularises the bone through musculoperiosteal vessels. The circumflex scapular artery generally gives off a nutrient vessel to the lateral border of the scapula which enters the costal side of the scapular border in its upper two- to three-tenths. If this vessel is not present, a supply from periosteal branches substitutes for it.[10] Using this anatomy the latissimus muscle can be combined with a strut of vascularised bone.[10] In elevating the flap the

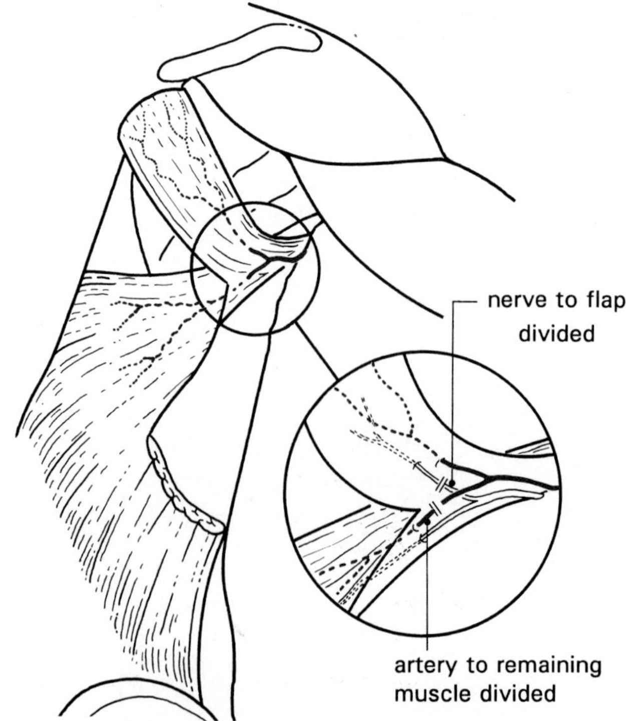

Fig. 7.304 Splitting the flap. Key points are indicated in this diagram showing the upper part of the muscle retained on the chest wall.

7

plane between teres major and latissimus dorsi is opened to expose the angular branch. Above the teres major the circumflex scapular artery is identified. The teres major must then be divided and retracted laterally to expose the lateral border of the scapula and establish the vascular anatomy. Mobilisation of the scapular border requires the detachment of serratus at the lower pole, and parts of subscapularis on the undersurface, and infraspinatus on the superficial surface. The donor defect is repaired by suturing the serratus anterior and teres major back to the infraspinatus and subscapularis muscles, which then enclose the remaining scapula.

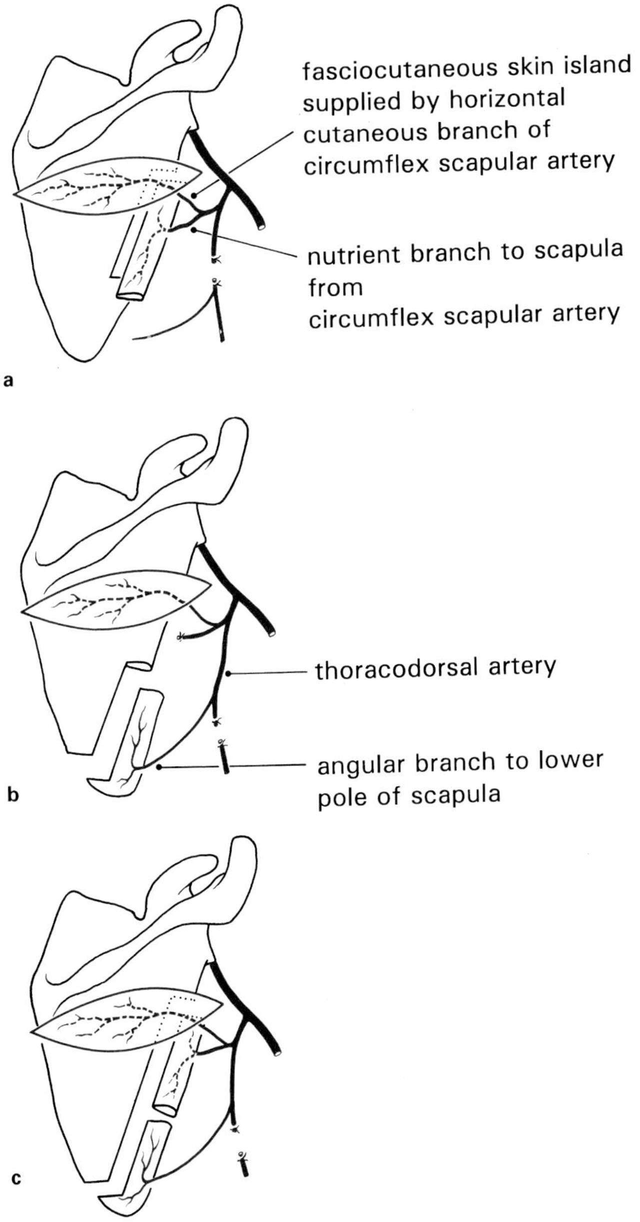

Fig. 7.305 Vascular basis of the compound flap incorporating lateral border of scapula. These diagrams show the bone segment which is supplied by the angular branch of the thoracodorsal artery raised in combination with a scapular flap but the bone could equally well be combined with a latissimus flap.

References

1. Tansini I 1896 Nuovo processo per l'amputazione della mammella per cancre. La Reforma Medica 12:3. Reprinted in Langenbeck's Archiv für Klinische Chirurgie 1896
2. Schmidt D R, Robson M C 1982 One stage composite reconstruction using the latissimus myo-osteo-cutaneous free flap. American Journal of Surgery 144: 470–472
3. Tobin G R, Schusterman M, Peterson G H, Nichols G, Bland K I 1981 The intramuscular neurovascular anatomy of the latissimus dorsi muscle: the basis for splitting the flap. Plastic and Reconstructive Surgery 67: 637–641
4. Bartlett S P, May J W, Yaremchuk M J 1981 The latissimus dorsi muscle: a fresh cadaver study of the primary neurovascular pedicle. Plastic and Reconstructive Surgery 67: 631–636
5. Marshall D R, Anstee E J, Stapleton M J 1984 Soft tissue reconstruction of the breast using an extended composite latissimus dorsi myocutaneous flap. British Journal of Plastic Surgery 37: 361–368
6. Fisher J, Bostwick J, Powell R W 1983 Latissimus dorsi blood supply after thoracodorsal vessel division: the serratus collateral. Plastic and Reconstructive Surgery 72: 502–509
7. Wolf L E, Biggs T M 1982 Aesthetic refinements in the use of the latissimus dorsi flap in breast reconstruction. Plastic and Reconstructive Surgery 69: 788–793
8. Maxwell G P, Stueber K, Hoopes J E 1978 A free latissimus dorsi myocutaneous flap. Plastic and Reconstructive Surgery 62: 462–466
9. Coleman J J and Sultan M R 1991 The bipedicled osteocutaneous scapular flap. Plastic and Reconstructive Surgery 87: 682–691
10. Sekiguchi J, Kobayashi S, Ohmori K 1993 Use of the osteocutaneous free scapular flap on lower extremities. Plastic and Reconstructive Surgery 91: 103–112
11. Elliot L F, Raffel B, Wade J 1989 Segmental latissimus dorsi free flap: clinical applications. Annals of Plastic Surgery 23: 231–238
12. Maruyama Y, Urita Y, Ohnishi K 1985 Rib latissimus dorsi free flap in reconstruction of a mandibular defect. British Journal of Plastic Surgery 38: 234–237

7 THORACODORSAL ARTERY – cutaneous branch

Thoracodorsal axillary flap
Subaxillary pedicled flap

The thoracodorsal artery gives off a cutaneous branch which may be used as the basis for a flap from the lateral chest wall. (Note that cutaneous vessels in this area are very variable and flaps in this region may also be based on the lateral thoracic artery or on the superficial thoracic artery – these are described on p. 371.) The name thoracodorsal axillary flap is derived from both the vessel of supply and the topographical site, but flaps based on this vessel sometimes go under another name in the literature. The feasibility of raising a flap on this artery was first investigated anatomically by de Coninck et al[1] and Taylor & Daniel.[2] Clinical transfer as free flaps has been described by Baudet et al[3] and Irigaray et al.[4] The latter case was carried out in a child where the authors found the flap convenient for microvascular transfer on account of the large size of the thoracodorsal artery (compared to the vessels in a groin flap which they considered to be the alternative). The anatomy has been described by Cabanié et al.[5] Chandra et al have standardised the design of a pedicled flap based on this vessel and have termed it the subaxillary pedicled flap.[7] A wider and longer version of this pedicled flap, based on the cutaneous branch of the thoracodorsal together with any of the other vessels present on the lateral chest wall is described under the lateral thoracic artery on page 373.

Anatomy

The subscapular artery generally arises from the third part of the axillary artery and passes down behind the axillary vein sometimes giving off the posterior circumflex humeral artery. At a level between 0.5 and 5 cm (mode 3 cm) below its point of origin, it divides into the circumflex scapular artery and the thoracodorsal artery. The thoracodorsal artery gives off a cutaneous branch in about 75% of cases, before it continues on to penetrate and supply latissimus dorsi (Fig. 7.306). The cutaneous branch arises between 0.5 and 2 cm beyond the bifurcation of the subscapular artery. Therefore the maximum possible length of vascular pedicle made up of the subscapular and thoracodorsal vessels, varies between 1 and 7 cm. A further component to the vascular pedicle is provided by the cutaneous branch itself, which is either of a long type or a short type, making the total length of the surgically anastomosable vascular trunk between 3 and 10 cm long with a mean of 6 cm.

In eight cadaver dissections Chandra et al found that the artery tended to pierce the deep fascia at the level of the fourth intercostal space in the posterior axillary line; thereafter becoming progressively more superficial as it ran downwards approximately 1 cm anterior and parallel to the free border of latissimus dorsi.

The venous drainage of the flap is by a small cutaneous vein which drains into the vena comitans (sometimes two venae comitantes) of the thoracodorsal artery. These drain latissimus dorsi and also receive tributaries from the serratus anterior, thereby reaching a diameter of up to 3.5 mm. The thoracodorsal veins join

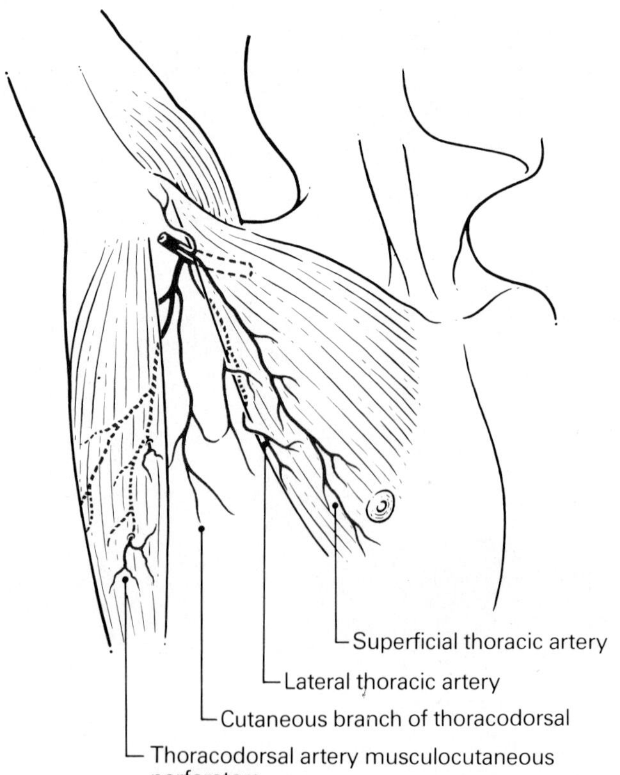

Fig. 7.306 Vascular anatomy. A schematic representation of the blood supply to the axilla and lateral chest wall in which all the possible vessels which may supply skin in this area are shown.

with circumflex scapular veins to form the subscapular venous trunk of about 3–6 mm in diameter. A further means of drainage of the flap is via the lateral thoracic vein. This is larger than the cutaneous vein described above but tends to drain straight into the axillary vein and is therefore smaller in diameter for microanastomosis than the subscapular venous trunk. The nerve supply of the flap is from lateral cutaneous branches of the third and fourth intercostal nerves. The motor nerve to latissimus dorsi (thoracodorsal nerve) lies anterior to the thoracodorsal artery.

Planning

Pedicled flap

In planning the pedicled flap, e.g. for a two-stage reconstruction of a defect on the opposite hand, Chandra uses the horizontal continuation of a line drawn through the nipples (with the arm by the side) to surface mark the base of the flap. The long axis of the flap then has its centre line 1 cm anterior and parallel to the edge of the latissimus dorsi. The largest flap described by Chandra was 7 cm × 20 cm and all donor sites were capable of direct closure.

Free flap

Due to variability in the site of origin of the cutaneous branch which may even be absent, it is best to dissect the axilla first and establish the anatomy. If the cutaneous branch is too small or totally absent, then the muscle branch together with a piece of the edge of latissimus dorsi will be needed to support the flap and the outline of the flap will be in the more posterior of the positions shown in Figure 7.309. With a strong cutaneous branch the flap may be positioned more anteriorly.

For the cutaneous branch flap, the territory is bounded by the edge of pectoralis major anteriorly, by a line 2 cm medial to the edge of latissimus dorsi posteriorly, and by the 8th intercostal space inferiorly.

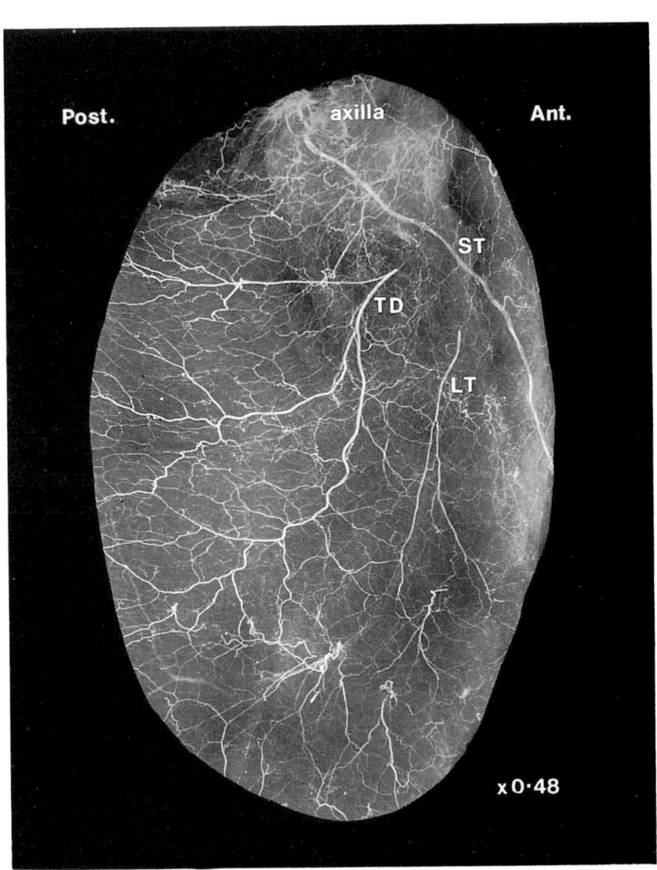

Fig. 7.307 Radiograph showing several cutaneous vessels supplying skin over the lateral thorax. Precise nomenclature of these vessels is uncertain but they have been labelled: **ST.** superficial thoracic, **TD.** cutaneous branch of thoracodorsal, **LT.** branch of lateral thoracic.

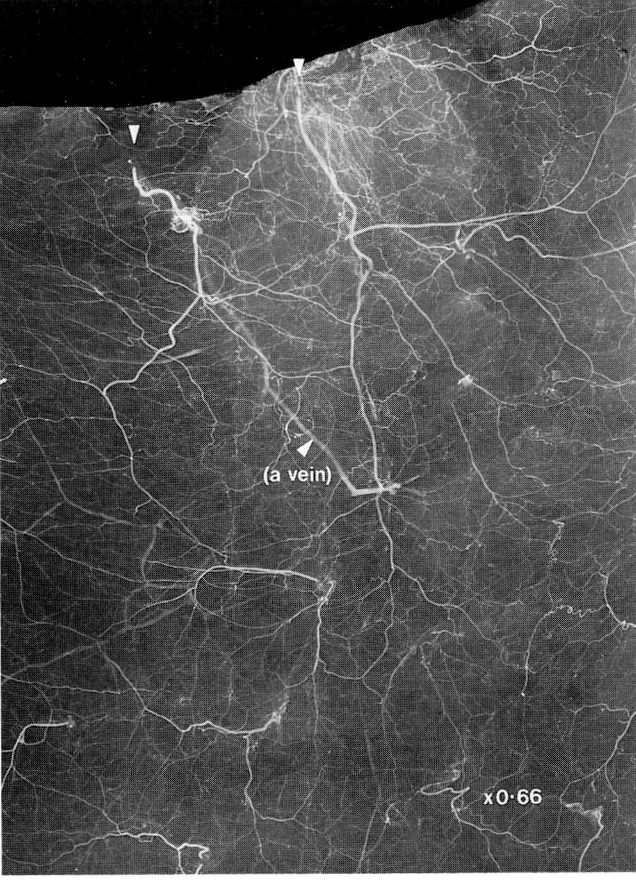

Fig. 7.308 Radiograph of skin showing two cutaneous vessels supplying lateral thoracic skin. Precise nomenclature of these vessels is uncertain.

Surgery

Free flap

The patient is placed supine with the donor side elevated 45° and the arm abducted 130°. A mid-axillary incision is made to expose the axillary vein which is traced proximally to reveal the subscapular vein. The subscapular artery is identified posteromedial to this and traced distally to establish the position and course of the thoracodorsal artery and its cutaneous branch. Small cutaneous nerves are divided but the long thoracic nerve is preserved. The incision for the anterior border of the flap follows a line sloping obliquely distally and slightly anteriorly from the axilla downwards along the lateral border of pectoralis major. The incision curves round the distal end of the flap and passes up over the edge of latissimus dorsi. The fascia over the muscle is included with the flap. For a left-sided flap Cabanie et al recommend an anticlockwise dissection from the axilla whereas Yang et al a clockwise one. A skin graft may be needed for the donor site.

References

1. De Coninck A, Boeckx W, Vanderlinden E, Claessen G 1975 Autotransplants avec microsutures vasculaires. Anatomie des zones donneuses. Annales de Chirurgie Plastique 20: 163–170
2. Taylor G I, Daniel R K 1975 The anatomy of several free flap donor sites. Plastic and Reconstructive Surgery 56: 243–253
3. Baudet J, Guimberteau J C, Nascimento E 1976 Successful clinical transfer of two free thoracodorsal axillary flaps. Plastic and Reconstructive Surgery 58: 680–688
4. Irigaray A, Roncagliolo A, Fossati G 1979 Transfer of a free lateral thoracic flap in a child: Case Report. Plastic and Reconstructive Surgery 64: 259–263
5. Cabanié H, Garbé J-F, Guimberteau J-C 1980 Anatomical basis of the thoracodorsal axillary flap with respect to its transfer by means of microvascular surgery. Anatomia Clinica 2: 65–73
6. Yang Z N, Shih H-R, Chao L, Shih T-S 1983 Free transplantation of sub-axillary lateral thoracodorsal flap in burn surgery. Burns 10: 164–169
7. Chandra R, Kumar P, Abdi S H M 1988 The subaxillary pedicled flap. British Journal of Plastic Surgery 41: 169–173

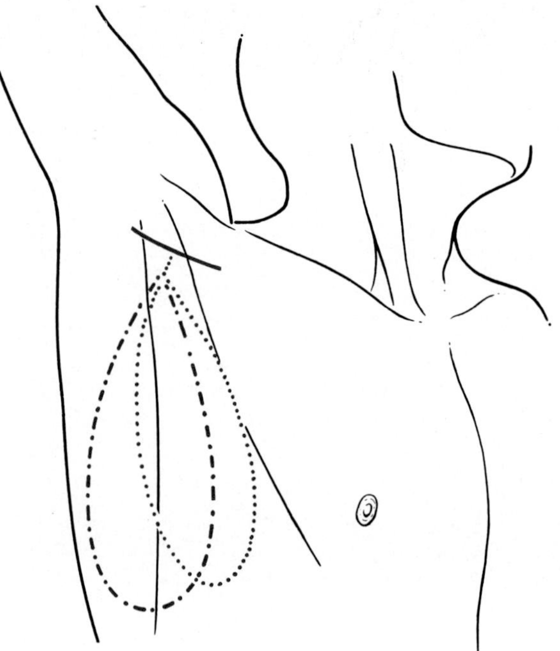

Fig. 7.309 Flap planning. The more posteriorly situated flap is based on musculocutaneous perforators and cutaneous branches of the thoracodorsal artery. This flap includes a portion of the latissimus dorsi muscle. The more anteriorly situated flap is based solely on the cutaneous branch of the thoracodorsal artery.

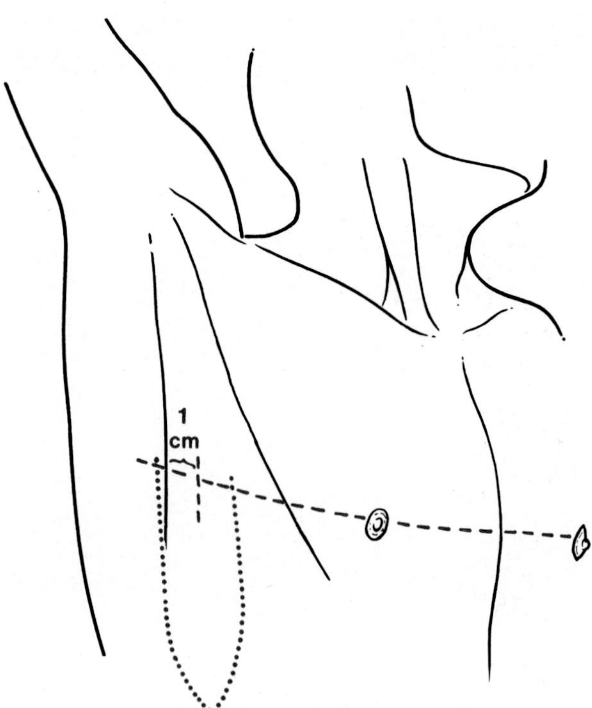

Fig. 7.310 Flap planning. The pedicled flap has its base at the level of the fourth rib (marked by a line through the nipples with the arm by the side) and its centre line 1 cm anterior to the free edge of latissimus dorsi.

TRANSVERSE CERVICAL ARTERY

Cervico-humeral flap

An undelayed pedicled flap based in the lateral neck and extending over deltoid onto the upper arm was designed by Wilson in 1969.[1] The blood supply of the flap was investigated by Mathes & Vasconez[2] who published their findings and some examples of its clinical applications in reconstruction of the head and neck. The vascular support of this flap was originally thought to be the musculocutaneous perforators through the lateral part of trapezius but the flap also contains a significant fasciocutaneous element.[3]

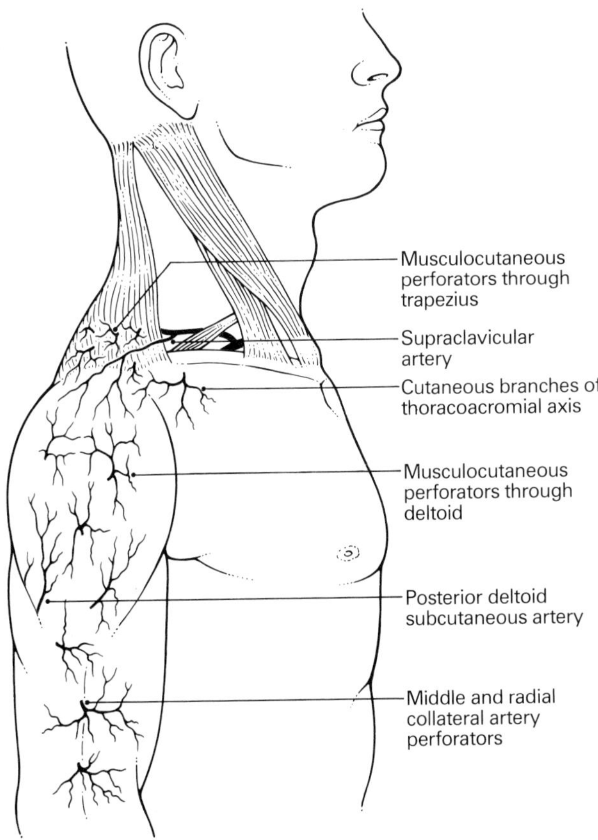

Fig. 7.311 Vascular anatomy. Vessels at the top of the shoulder feed into a potential longitudinal plexus formed by anastomoses between multiple separate perforators.

Anatomy

Although basically an extended lateral trapezius musculocutaneous flap there are several other vascular factors contributing to the reliability of this flap and failure to appreciate all these details of anatomy may be the underlying explanation for the widely different failure rates which have been reported for this flap.[1,2,4] The dominant vascular pedicle of the trapezius muscle is the transverse cervical artery. Its superficial branch supplies the middle and lateral parts of the muscle while its deep branch supplies the lower part of the muscle. Perforators through the lateral part of the muscle feed the base of the flap. In addition, the superficial branch of the transverse cervical artery commonly gives off a branch which runs laterally over the acromioclavicular joint at the level of the deep fascia. This vessel was demonstrated by Mathes & Vasconez as an 'ascending branch of the artery cephalad to the clavicular insertion of the trapezius muscle', and has been named the supraclavicular artery by Lamberty.[5] Perforators from the acromial and deltoid branches of the thoraco-acromial axis may also contribute to the base of the flap. The skin over deltoid is supplied by musculocutaneous perforators from the deltoid branch of the thoraco-acromial axis anteriorly, and laterally and posteriorly by perforators from the posterior circumflex humeral artery. These are divided in elevating the flap. The perforators anastomose with each other and with the supraclavicular artery thereby forming a longitudinal vessel plexus which will be incorporated in the flap if the dissection is carried out at the subfascial level. If the flap is extended down the anterolateral aspect of the upper arm beyond the deltoid insertion, perforators from the radial and middle collateral arteries will be divided. It is inadvisable to spiral the flap round the front of the arm in order to use skin on the medial aspect because this is a separate territory supplied mainly by the superior ulnar collateral artery, and flaps raised in this manner are very liable to undergo necrosis.[6]

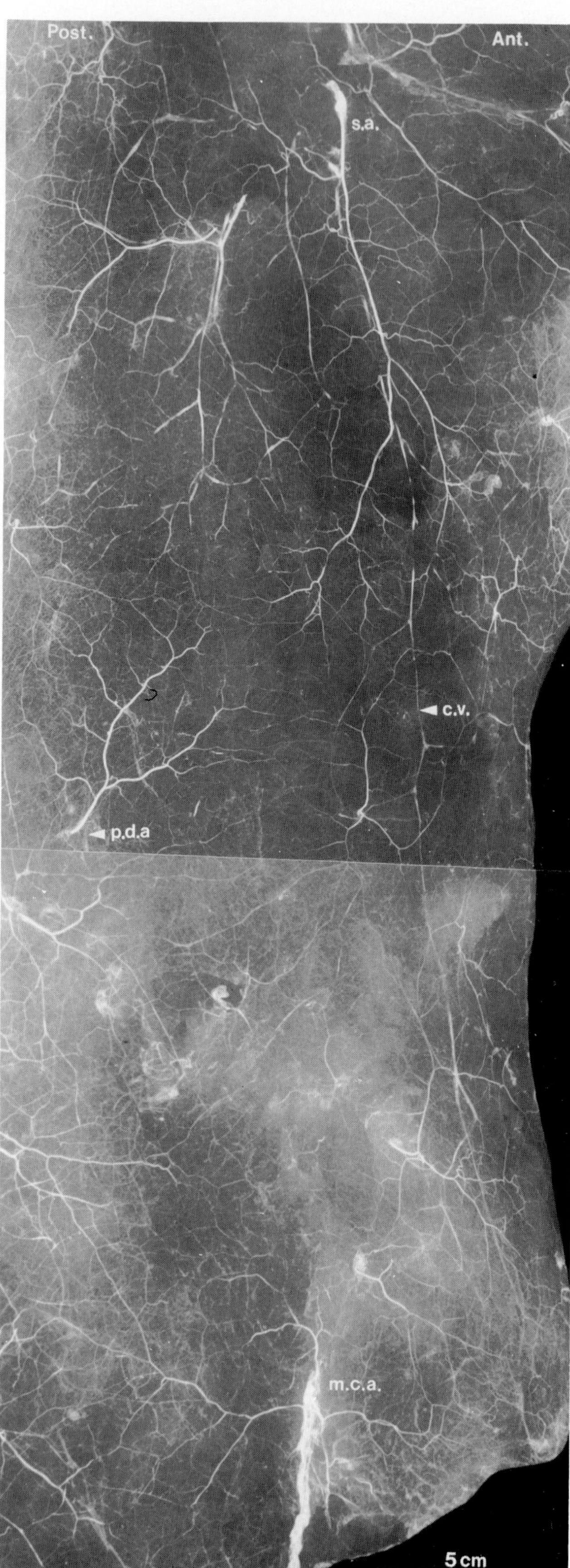

Fig. 7.312 Radiograph of skin over shoulder and lateral aspect of upper arm. The cutaneous branch of the thoraco-acromial axis is small and the main vessels running over the top of the shoulder are branches of the supraclavicular artery (**sa**), one of which follows the course of the cephalic vein (**cv**). (The full diameter of the vein is not revealed since only a small amount of contrast has penetrated through into the venous side of the circulation and has settled out in the bottom of the vein.) Longitudinal anastomoses are not well shown in this specimen, which illustrates the fact that long flaps are unreliable. (**pda.** posterior deltoid subcutaneous artery, **mca.** middle collateral artery)

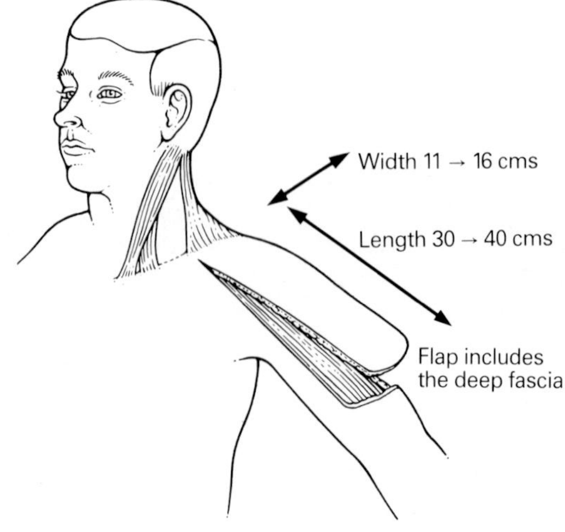

Fig. 7.313 Flap planning. (After Mathes & Vasconez, 1978.)

Surgery

Undelayed flaps can be raised with length-to-breadth proportions of 2:1 or 3:1. The base of the flap is centred over the acromioclavicular joint and is between 11 and 16 cm wide. The flap extends down the lateral aspect of the arm for a distance of 35–40 cm and is elevated in the subfascial plane. It has an arc of rotation which takes in the floor of the mouth, the neck and the anterior chest. Wilson successfully used this flap undelayed in 90% of his cases. Mathes & Vasconez had partial necrosis in one case out of six – possibly through problems in tubing it – while Blevins & Luce[4] had 40% distal necrosis despite prior delays. This difference may be accounted for by different treatment of the supraclavicular artery. Mathes & Vasconez, having identified it, took measures to preserve it, as shown by their diagram and cases in which the anterior incision clearly does not cross the clavicle. By contrast, Blevins & Luce endeavoured to gain additional length by carrying out proximal muscle mobilisation by an anterior skin incision extending up into the neck together with elevation of the trapezius muscle at its clavicular insertion; a manoeuvre which is likely to divide the supraclavicular artery with the consequence that instead of the cervico-humeral flap being a combined musculocutaneous and fasciocutaneous flap it then becomes purely musculocutaneous with a random extension. We feel that preservation of the supraclavicular artery is a crucial point in ensuring maximum reliability and safety of the flap.[3]

However, irrespective of the way in which this flap is raised, it should be appreciated that limitations remain regarding the use of this flap in head and neck reconstructive surgery, especially for malignant disease.

References

1. Wilson C A 1978 The cervico-humeral flap – letter to the Editor. Plastic and Reconstructive Surgery 62: 288
2. Mathes S J, Vasconez L O 1978 The cervico-humeral flap. Plastic and Reconstructive Surgery 61: 7–12
3. Lamberty B G H, Cormack G C 1983 Misconceptions regarding the cervico-humeral flap. British Journal of Plastic Surgery 36: 60–63
4. Blevins P K, Luce E A 1980 Limitations of the cervicohumeral flap in head and neck reconstruction. Plastic and Reconstructive Surgery 66: 220–225
5. Lamberty B G H 1979 The supraclavicular axial patterned flap. British Journal of Plastic Surgery 32: 207–212
6. Vasconez L O 1978 The cervico-humeral flap – letter to the Editor. Plastic and Reconstructive Surgery 62: 288

7 TRANSVERSE CERVICAL ARTERY

Lateral trapezius musculocutaneous flap
Cervicodorsal skin flap
Cervicoscapular skin flap

The use of the lateral part of trapezius as the vascular support and pedicle for an undelayed island of lateral neck and shoulder skin was described by Demergasso.[1] This part of the muscle is supplied by the transverse cervical artery and the muscle, through its attachment to the spine of the scapula, acromion and clavicle, provides a blood supply to these bones which enables parts of them to be incorporated in the flap. Such an osteo-myocutaneous pedicled flap may be used for mandibular reconstruction.[1,3,4,5,6]

Flaps of dorsal skin based on a single large perforator through the middle of the muscle, possibly incorporating a small block of muscle around the perforator but essentially leaving the trapezius undisturbed, have been described by Nakajima & Fujino, and by Hayakusoku et al. These are termed the cervicodorsal and cervicoscapular flaps.[7,8]

Anatomy

The skin situated over the lateral part of trapezius receives its blood supply by multiple musculocutaneous perforators from the underlying muscle. These perforators arise from the superficial branch of the transverse cervical artery which is the supplying vessel of the lateral part of trapezius. This artery arises from the thyrocervical trunk and passes laterally deep to omohyoid and enters the deep surface of trapezius approximately two fingers' breadths medial to the medial edge of the acromion. The descending branch (dorsal scapular artery) of the transverse cervical artery frequently passes between the trunks or divisions of the brachial plexus. The transverse cervical vein travels in the same fascial plane as the artery but may drain into the subclavian vein 2 or 3 cm lateral to the thyrocervical

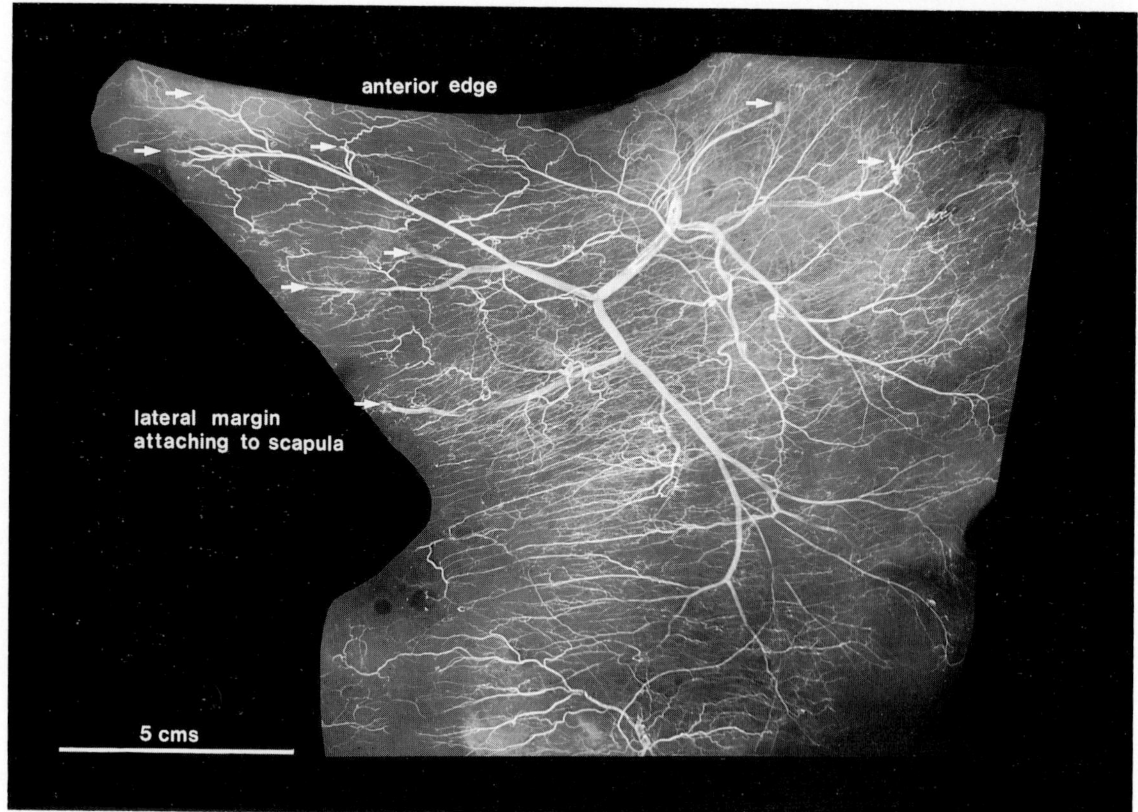

Fig. 7.314 Radiograph of the middle section of trapezius supplied by the superficial branch of the transverse cervical artery. The occipital part supplied by the occipital artery, and the lower part supplied from the dorsal scapular artery are not included. Arrows indicate the points at which branches appear to end abruptly – these are the points at which the vessels pierce the surface of the muscle to supply the overlying skin.

trunk or even into the lowest segment of the external jugular vein. The eleventh cranial nerve passes beneath the anterior edge of the muscle at a more superior level than the vascular pedicle, corresponding to a point one-third of the way up the anterior edge of the muscle. It is possible to preserve the accessory nerve supply to the major part of the muscle unless a very large segment of trapezius is required in which case the nerve will have to be transected. The cutaneous innervation of the skin overlying the acromioclavicular joint comes from the most lateral of the supraclavicular nerves and by identifying and preserving these fibres useful sensory function may potentially be obtained in the flap.

Surgery

Lateral trapezius musculocutaneous flap

The anatomical landmarks are outlined pre-operatively. The skin island is centred over the acromioclavicular joint and an incision for exposure of the neck appropriate to the type of resection being performed, is linked to the incision around the flap. This provides the exposure of the contents of the posterior triangle and the transverse cervical artery is first identified in the supraclavicular area and followed into the trapezius. The anterior part of the skin island is now elevated off deltoid up to the acromioclavicular joint. Beyond this point the skin is elevated with the trapezius muscle by detaching the insertion of trapezius from the lateral third of the clavicle and from the acromion. As the posterior part of the skin island is elevated, trapezius is detached from the upper border of the spine of the scapula. Sutures anchor the skin island to the underlying muscle and the muscle pedicle is then mobilised to the required degree by splitting the fibres upwards towards the occiput and partially or completely transecting the muscle pedicle depending on the adequacy of the vascular pedicle, the degree of mobility required and the nature of the surgical defect. If the mandible is to be reconstructed then the entire acromion and spine of scapula may be removed in continuity with the muscle by dividing the spine with an osteotome and disarticulating the acromioclavicular joint.

Cervicodorsal and cervicoscapular flaps

The cervicodorsal flap takes the form of a long skin ellipse situated adjacent to the midline and overlying the trapezius muscle with its upper end at the level of the vertebra prominens. Flaps of up to 30 cm × 7 cm have survived. The flap includes the fascia over the muscle and is raised so as to preserve a vascular pedicle at its upper end. This pedicle is formed by a perforator from the

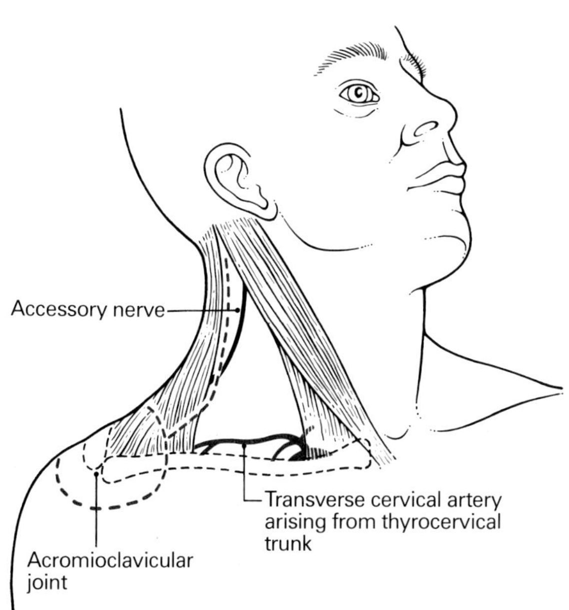

Fig. 7.315 Flap planning. Initial incision passes along the anterior edge of trapezius and leads down to the flap which is centred over the acromioclavicular joint and adjacent part of the trapezius.

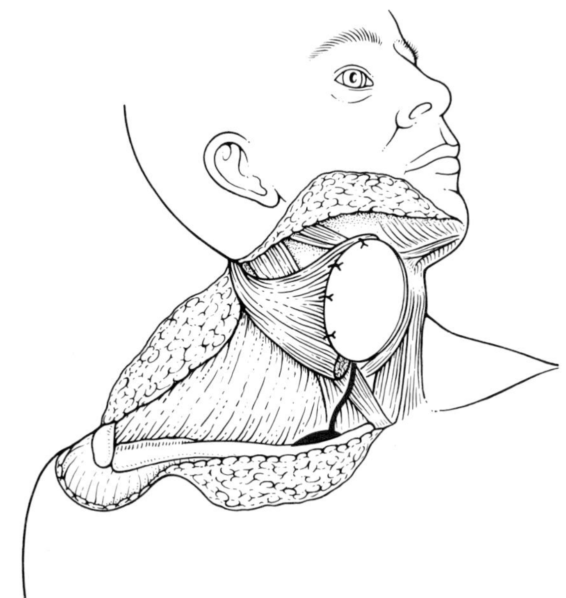

Fig. 7.316 Skin island carried on the lateral part of trapezius. (The structures in the floor of the posterior triangle have not been indicated.)

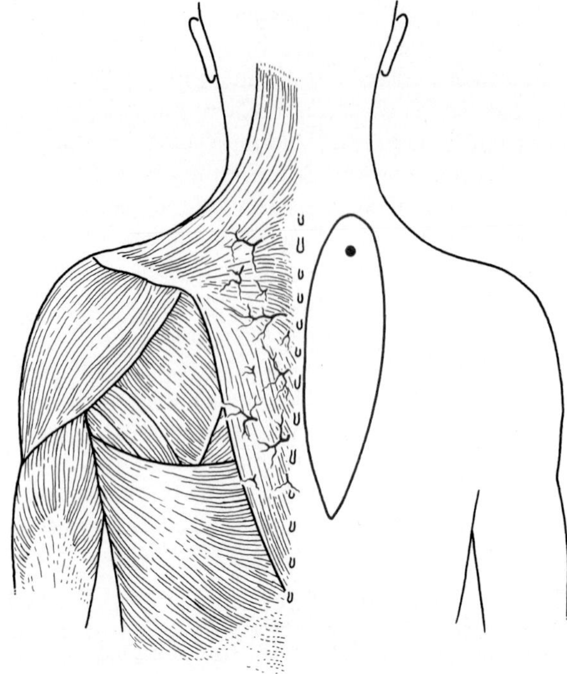

Fig. 7.317 Vascular anatomy and planning of cervicodorsal flap.

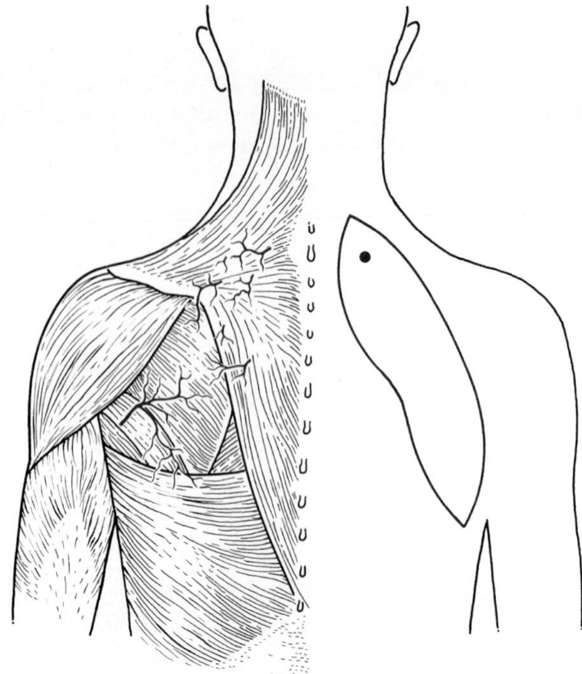

Fig. 7.318 Vascular anatomy and planning of cervicoscapular flap.

superficial branch of the transverse cervical artery and its accompanying venae comitantes. It is not possible to be precise about the location of the pedicle which has to be developed by careful dissection at the proximal end of the flap. It may not be possible to skeletonise the pedicle and protection of the vessels is recommended by retaining a broad fascial pedicle to the flap even if the skin component is islanded. On occasion it may be necessary to cut out around the pedicle a muscle block from trapezius to protect the vessels and give adequate mobility to the base of the pedicled flap.

The cervicoscapular flap has an oblique orientation and has been reported as surviving to a larger size (32 cm × 12 cm) as it makes use of the fasciocutaneous territory of the circumflex scapular artery branches. The pedicle is the same. Hyakusoku et al reported the use of these flaps principally for extensive burn cases where other flap options were limited.

References

1. Demergasso F, Piazza M V 1979 Trapezius myocutaneous flap in reconstructive surgery for head and neck cancer: an original technique. American Journal of Surgery 138: 533–536
2. Panje W 1980 Myocutaneous trapezius flap. Head and Neck Surgery 2: 206–212
3. Panje W, Cutting C 1980 Trapezius osteomyocutaneous island flap for reconstruction of the anterior floor of mouth and mandible. Head and Neck Surgery 3: 66–71
4. Gantz B J, Panje W R 1981 Trapezius myocutaneous island flap. The Laryngoscope 91: 1196–1199
5. Guillamondegui O M, Larson D L 1981 The lateral trapezius musculocutaneous flap: its use in head and neck reconstruction. Plastic and Reconstructive Surgery 67: 143–150
6. Bem C, O'Hare P M 1986 Case Report: reconstruction of the mandible using the scapular spine pedicled upon trapezius muscle; description of the posterior approach to the transverse cervical vessels. British Journal of Plastic Surgery 39: 473–477
7. Nakajima H, Fujino T, Adachi S 1986 A new concept of vascular supply to the skin and classification of skin flaps according to their vascularisation. Annals of Plastic Surgery 16: 1–17
8. Hyakusoku H, Yoshida H, Okubo M, Hirai T, Fumiiri M 1990 Superficial cervical artery skin flaps. Plastic and Reconstructive Surgery 86: 33–38

TRANSVERSE CERVICAL ARTERY

Neurovascular posterior triangle cutaneous free flap

The skin over the base of the posterior triangle of the neck is innervated by the supraclavicular nerves and receives its blood supply by branches of the transverse cervical artery. An ellipse of skin, including platysma and part of the underlying supraclavicular fat pad, may be taken from this area and used as a free flap. Free flaps of this design, with dimensions of up to 8 cm × 15 cm, were first described by McCabe[1] and by Morris et al,[2] while pedicled flaps based on branches of the transverse cervical artery have been described by Lamberty.[3,4]

Anatomy

The transverse cervical artery arises from the thyrocervical trunk, passes laterally deep to sternomastoid, crosses the phrenic nerve on scalenus anterior and crosses the trunks of the brachial plexus to reach levator scapulae where it divides into superficial and deep parts. The presence of branches to platysma and to skin from either the transverse cervical artery or its superficial branch, or less commonly from the suprascapular artery, is well established and these vessels form the basis of several flaps. The flap described here is based on a small branch 1–1.5 mm in diameter which is often given off deep to omohyoid and reaches the superficial structures by passing round the superior border of the lower belly of the muscle. The vessel rapidly divides into many small branches which enter the supraclavicular fat pad and the platysma and skin over the base of the posterior triangle of the neck (Fig. 7.319). The vessel may end in this way or may

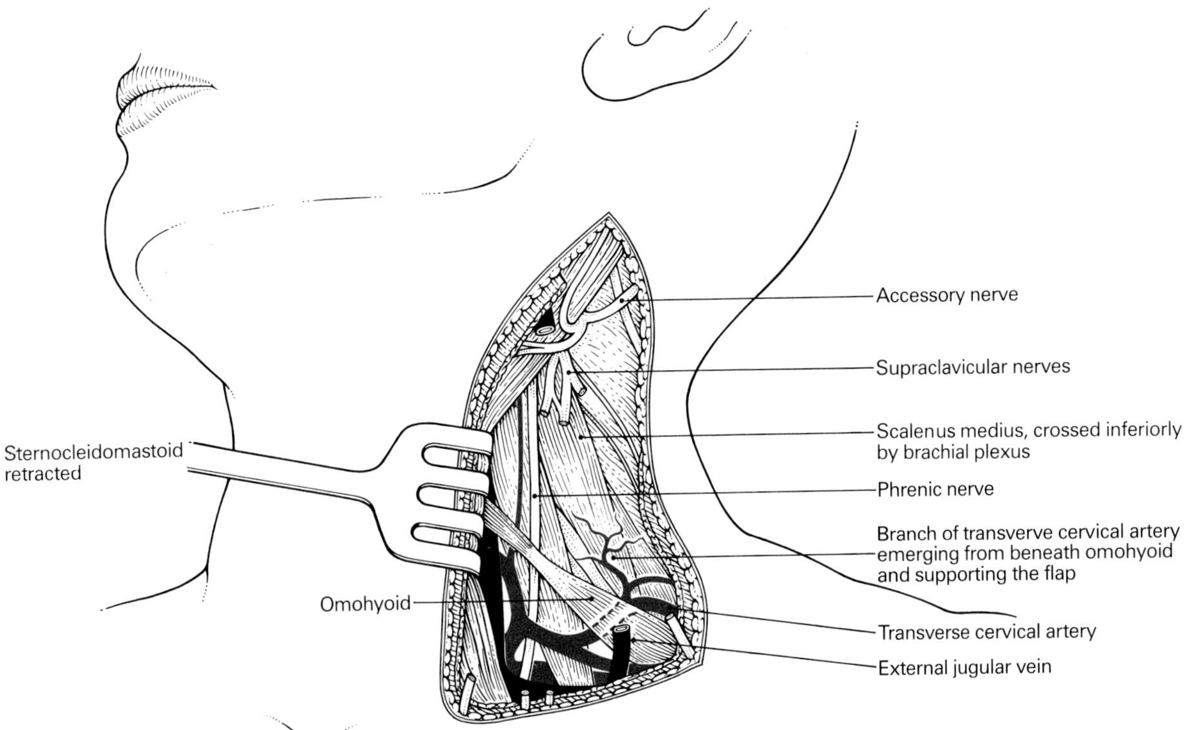

Fig. 7.319 Anatomy underlying the posterior triangle free flap. The outline of the area displayed does not coincide with the margins of the flap.

continue in an axial manner at the level of the deep fascia over the acromion (see Supraclavicular artery axial pattern flap, p. 458). A segment of the transverse cervical artery which includes the portion giving off these branches is removed and provides a relatively large vessel for microvascular anastomosis with a reasonable length of pedicle.

The venous anatomy is less reliable. Venae comitantes of the transverse cervical artery are very variable and when used as the sole venous drainage of a free flap tend to be inadequate. A better means of drainage is provided by the external jugular vein which passes vertically through the flap lying in the tissue plane just deep to platysma (Fig. 7.320). The external jugular vein may be absent.

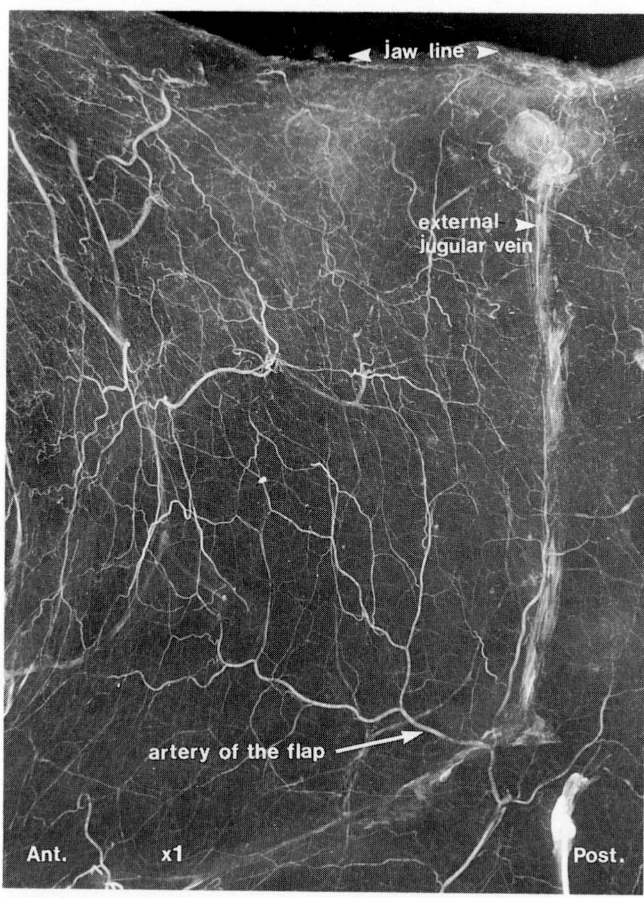

Fig. 7.320 Radiograph of skin from area over base of posterior triangle.

The skin over the lower part of the posterior triangle is supplied by the supraclavicular nerves (C3, C4). Their common trunk emerges from below the posterior border of sternomastoid and divides, deep to platysma, into divergent medial, intermediate and lateral branches. These descend, interweaving in the superficial part of the supraclavicular fat pad with branches of the arteries and veins, and pierce the deep fascia above the clavicle. The medial supraclavicular nerves cross sternomastoid and the external jugular vein; the intermediate supraclavicular nerves cross the clavicle to supply the skin over pectoralis major and deltoid; the lateral nerves reach and supply the skin on the upper part of the shoulder over trapezius and the acromion. It is therefore the intermediate/middle supraclavicular nerve whose branches innervate the flap. Two-point discrimination of the intact skin in this area has been found to lie between 17 and 24 mm.[2]

Significant anatomical variations occur among the muscles of this region and 'extra' muscles of varying degrees of development may be found in the roof of the posterior triangle in about 15% of cases[5,6] (Fig. 7.321). These muscles insert into the middle of the clavicle and either arise from the superior nuchal line of the occipital bone just lateral to trapezius (occipito-cleidalis), or they arise from the transverse processes of the upper cervical vertebrae just in front of the origins of levator scapulae (levator claviculi or cleidocervicalis). Fascial thickenings may occur in association with the muscles or form tendinous bands across the posterior triangle to which stray parts of trapezius or sternomastoid insert[5] (Fig. 7.321c). The variability of these muscles is such that no guidance can be given as to where they are likely to lie in relation to the flap, and any problem relating to one of these muscles can be dealt with only when it arises. It is worth noting that these muscles, when they exist, are generally bilateral.[6]

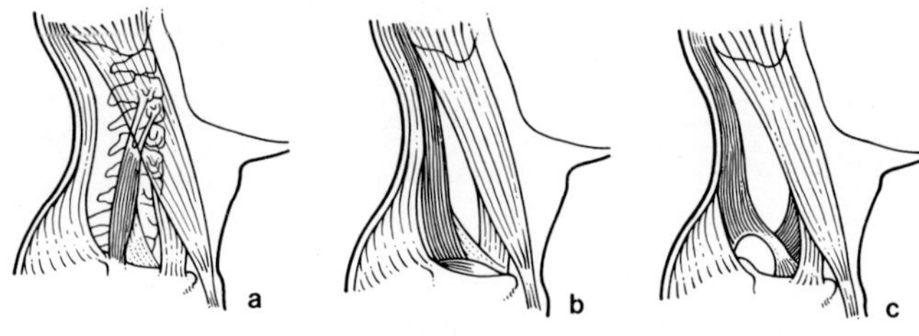

Fig. 7.321 Unusual muscle arrangements occasionally encountered in the floor of the posterior triangle: **a.** cleidocervicalis and fascial thickening; **b.** occipito-cleidalis, supraclavicularis and fascial thickening; **c.** trapezius and sternomastoid joined by a tendinous arch. (After Eisler, 1912.)

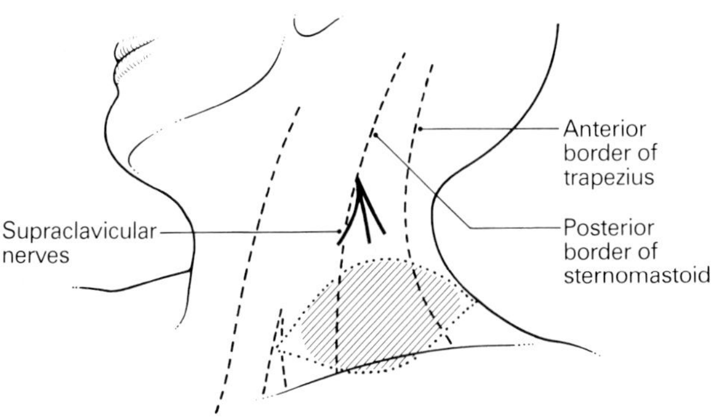

Fig. 7.322 Flap planning.

References

1. McCabe J S April 1980 Presentation at the Senior Residents' Conference, USA (Winner of the Reconstructive Category).
2. Morris R L, Dillman D, McCabe J S, Holdredge T, Carson L, Given K S 1983 The transverse cervical neurovascular free flap. Annals of Plastic Surgery 10: 90–98
3. Lamberty B G H 1979 The supraclavicular axial patterned flap. British Journal of Plastic Surgery 32: 207–212
4. Lamberty B G H 1982 The cutaneous arterial supply of cervical skin in relation to axial skin flaps. Anatomia Clinica 3: 317–324
5. Eisler P (ed) 1912 Die Muskeln des Stammes. Bardeleben's Handbuch der Anatomie Des Menschen. Gustav Fischer, Jena
6. Wood J 1870 On a group of varieties of the muscles of the human neck, shoulder and chest. Philosophical Transactions 160: 83–116

Planning

The area of the flap is confined within a transverse ellipse situated just above the clavicle between the posterior margin of sternomastoid and the anterior edge of trapezius (Fig. 7.322). The ends of the ellipse overlap the borders of these muscles which should be surface marked. The external jugular vein may be surface marked pre-operatively by the patient performing the Valsalva manoeuvre, and the supraclavicular nerves may sometimes be brought into prominence by active extension and lateral flexion of the neck. They emerge from behind sternomastoid at its midpoint whereas the accessory nerve emerges at the junction of the upper one-third with the lower two-thirds of the muscle.

Surgery

Morris' method involves making the inferior incision first and deepening it through platysma in order to expose the external jugular vein. The supraclavicular fat pad is swept superiorly, and the posterior belly of omohyoid is retracted anteriorly in order to expose the transverse cervical artery. The artery is traced proximally to its origin and distally to trapezius where the posterior part of the flap is incised and the transverse cervical artery ligated. The flap can then be elevated from posterior to anterior with the superior border being incised and the external jugular vein identified, ligated and divided. The supraclavicular nerves are identified and divided as necessary depending on which one(s) supplies the flap and whether or not a neurovascular flap is required. Care is taken not to damage the phrenic nerve. The anterior part of the flap now remains to be dissected free from sternomastoid and omohyoid, so that only the transverse cervical vessels and the external jugular vein remain linking the flap with the neck. These are ligated, microclips applied and the vessels divided.

7

ULNAR ARTERY

Ulnar forearm free flap
Becker flap – ulnodorsal perforator islanded flap

An ulnar artery forearm fasciocutaneous flap has been developed along the same lines as the Chinese radial forearm flap. It mirrors the versatility of the radial flap in permitting a skin island to be raised either as a free flap (with or without bone) or as a distally pedicled island flap with reversed flow in the artery. The flap may include muscle (flexor carpi ulnaris) or tendon (palmaris longus)[1] in much the same way as the radial flap may include muscle (flexor pollicis longus) or tendon (palmaris longus and split brachioradialis tendon).[2] The single most significant advantage of the ulnar artery flap over the radial forearm flap is that the skin on the medial side of the forearm is relatively much less hairy than on the radial side. This gives the flap particular virtues in intra-oral reconstruction.

Becker[8] has described a flap from the ulnar border of the distal forearm which is islanded on a single ulnar artery dorsal perforator at its distal end. This allows it to be turned through 180° to reconstruct defects on the dorsum of the hand without disruption of the ulnar artery. This is often known as the Becker flap and is a Type B fasciocutaneous flap. Becker termed his flap the ulnar flap but this fails to differentiate it from the ulnar flap removed in continuity with the ulnar artery (a Type C fasciocutaneous flap).

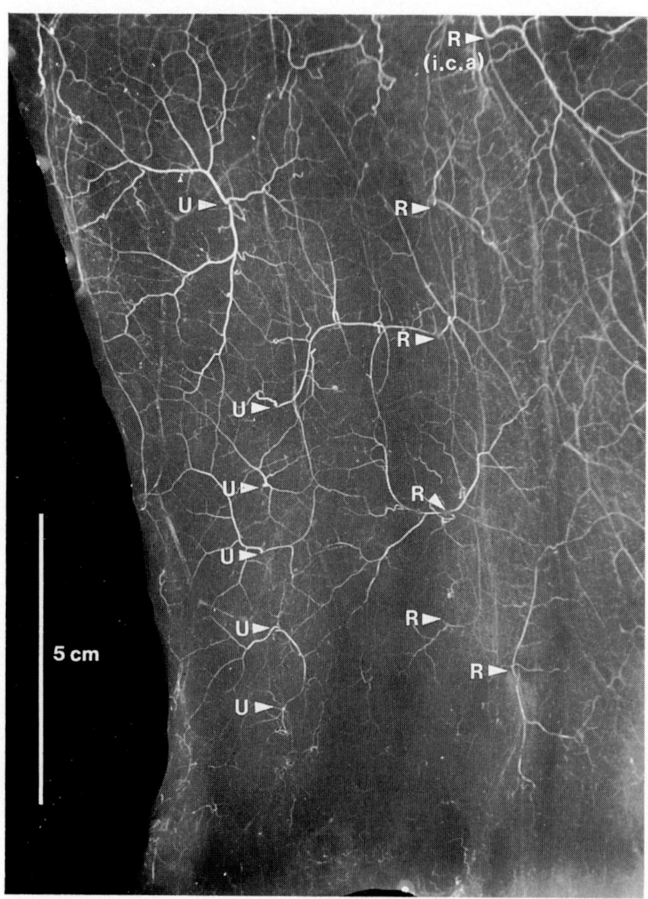

Fig. 7.323 Radiograph of a section of anterior forearm skin. The left edge of the specimen was created by an incision overlying the subcutaneous border of the ulna. **R.** denotes perforators from the radial artery, **U.** denotes perforators from the ulnar artery.

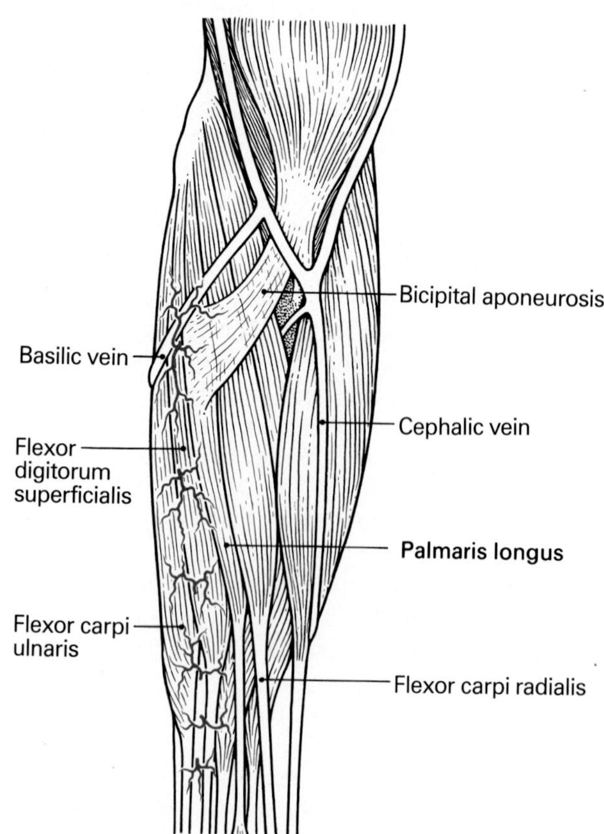

Fig. 7.324 Vascular anatomy. Fasciocutaneous perforators from the ulnar artery are shown.

Anatomy

Ulnar artery flap (Type C fasciocutaneous)
In the distal three-quarters of the forearm the ulnar artery gives rise to a series of fasciocutaneous perforators which pass up to the surface between flexor carpi ulnaris and flexor digitorum superficialis. These perforators fan out predominantly on the superficial surface of the deep fascia and anastomose laterally with similar fasciocutaneous perforators from the radial artery, and on the medial side with one or two small musculocutaneous perforators through flexor carpi ulnaris but mainly with branches of the posterior interosseous artery on the dorsum of the forearm. Of the perforators given off by the ulnar artery the most proximal one tends to be the largest (Figs. 7.323 & 7.324) and arises from the ulnar artery approximately 3–4 cm beyond the point where it gives origin to the common interosseous artery.

The basilic vein provides the main venous drainage of the area of the flap, although the median forearm vein may be well developed in the anterior midline and may be incorporated in the lateral part of the flap. Venae comitantes of the ulnar artery may be removed with the flap and, as with the radial forearm flap, these may permit venous drainage by reversed flow in distally pedicled island flaps. Generally, however, the superficial veins will be used in free flaps and therefore the venae comitantes have been omitted in Figure 7.325.

The potential for a sensate reconstruction is inherent in the flap since the medial cutaneous nerve of the forearm runs adjacent to the basilic vein. Lovie et al[1] have also clearly described the possibility of including flexor carpi ulnaris and a segment of the ulna in this flap (Fig. 7.326). The flexor carpi ulnaris may be carried with its motor nerve which may be split off the ulnar nerve.

Ulnodorsal perforator flap (Type B fasciocutaneous)
Between 2 and 5 cm proximal to the pisiform the ulnar artery gives off a dorsal branch which accompanies the dorsal branch of the ulnar nerve deep to flexor carpi ulnaris (diameter 0.8 to 1.3 mm). This arterial branch gives off branches proximally to the muscle and distally to the pisiform bone (Fig. 7.327) and then reaches the deep fascia where it gives off distal and proximal branches. This vessel does not appear in Figure 7.323 due to the line of division of the skin specimen. The proximally-directed branches may run in close proximity to the posterior branch of the medial cutaneous nerve of the forearm and some of these vessel branches appear to be running just inside the edge of the proximal half of the specimen in Figure 7.323. The distal branch runs onto the back of the hand and anastomoses with the dorsal carpal arch.

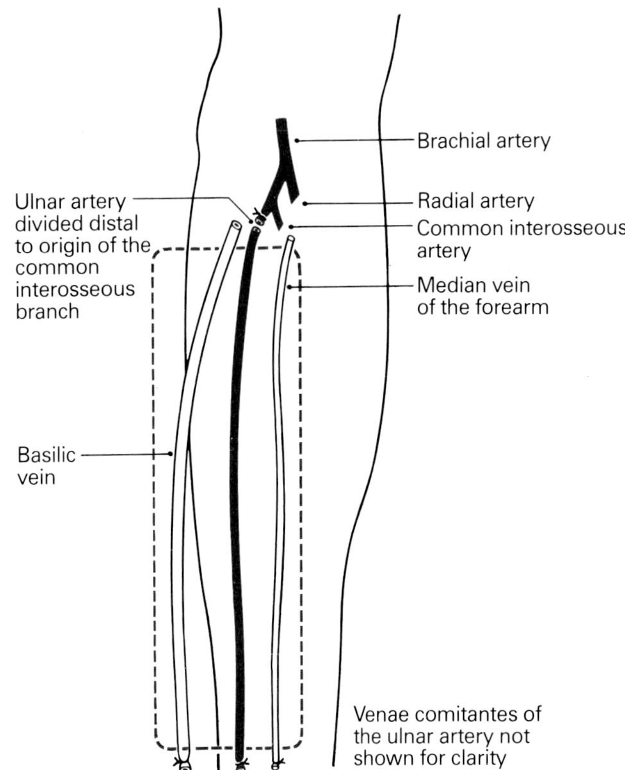

Fig. 7.325 Flap planning. The outline of a possible flap is indicated by the interrupted line.

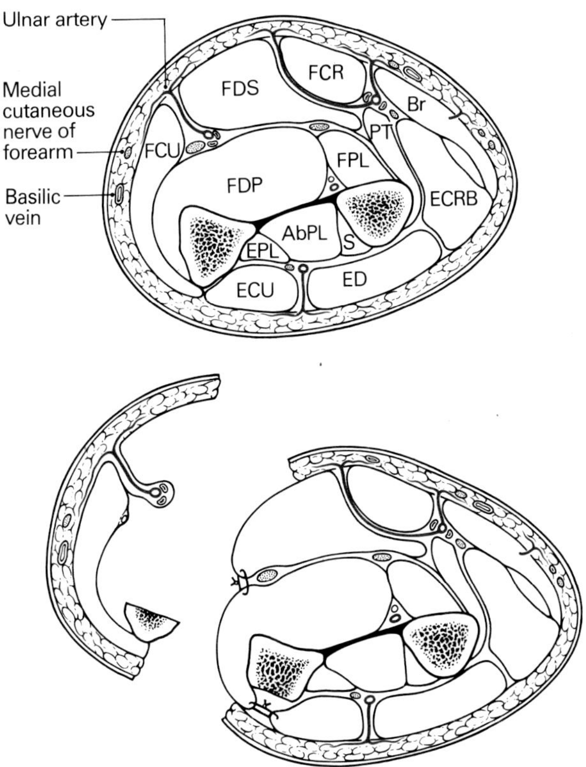

Fig. 7.326 Myo-osteo-fasciocutaneous tissue transfer.

7

Flap planning and surgery

Ulnar artery flap (Type C)

The ulnar artery fasciocutaneous perforators, through their anastomoses with the radial and posterior interosseous arteries, are able to support the skin of the anterior and medial aspects of the forearm down to the wrist. The proximal margin of this potential territory is uncertain but does not extend as far proximally as that of the radial artery which, through its inferior cubital and radial recurrent branches, supplies the skin over and lateral to the antecubital fossa and may support a flap extending onto the upper arm. The ulnar forearm flap is restricted to the forearm skin, and the ulnar artery may be removed only from a point distal to the origin of its common interosseous branch since the posterior compartment is entirely dependent on this vessel.

Elevation is straightforward and, as with the radial flap, proceeds deep to the deep fascia. Over the proximal part of the forearm flexor muscles, an artery approximately 1.5 mm in diameter will usually be encountered running medially from the antecubital fossa over the muscles deep to the fascia and then sinking into them. This vessel does not contribute to the blood supply of the skin and should be left behind intact on the muscle when the deep fascia is elevated off it.

Vein replacement of the ulnar artery does not appear to be necessary in the presence of a good radial pulse.

The ulnar nerve will be left exposed if the flexor carpi ulnaris is removed with the overlying skin. It may be covered by suturing flexor digitorum superficialis and flexor digitorum profundus together (Fig. 7.326).

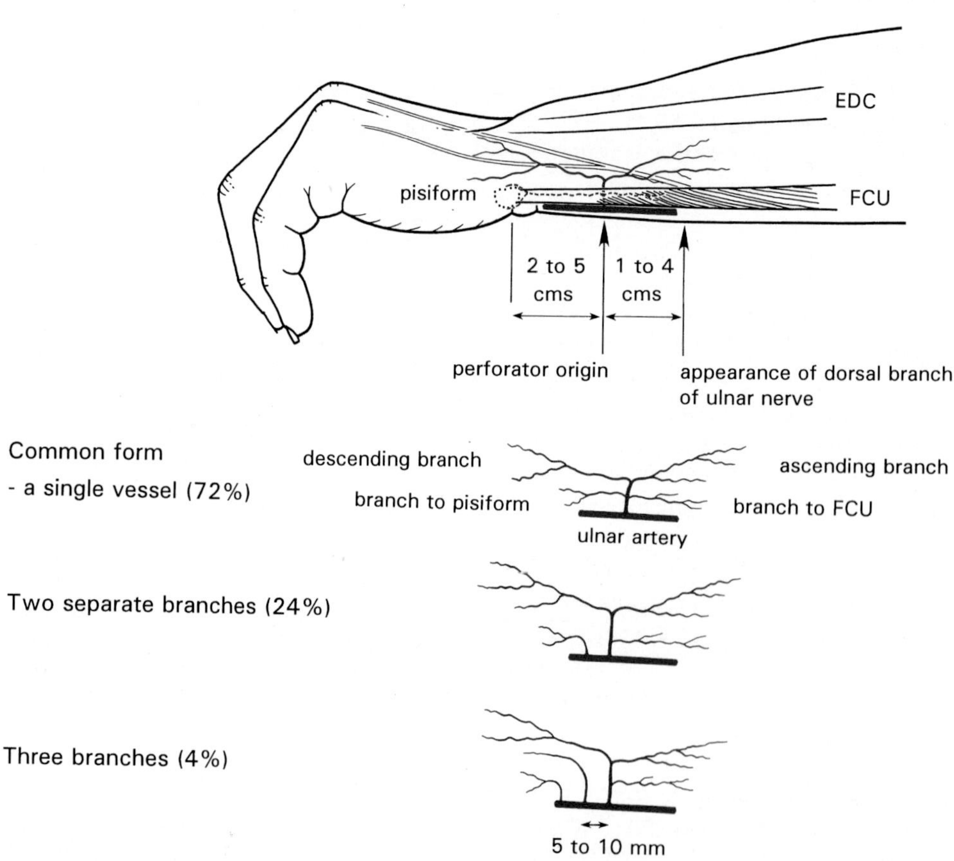

Fig. 7.327 Vascular anatomy of the Becker flap and variations in the ulno-dorsal perforator. Percentage figures are those from Becker based on 100 dissections (no perforator present in one case).

Ulnodorsal perforator flap (Type B)
The total territory that can be supported by this vessel measures 10 to 20 cm in length and 5 to 9 cm in width with the boundaries being the tendon of palmaris longus anteriorly and the tendons of extensor digitorum communis posteriorly. The flap is elevated from proximal to distal including the deep fascia. As the pedicle is approached care is taken to preserve the dorsal branch of the ulnar nerve and this also applies if a distal incision has to be made 1 cm from the pisiform to convert the flap from a pedicled to an islanded version. An islanded flap is able to reach further distally than one with a skin pedicle.

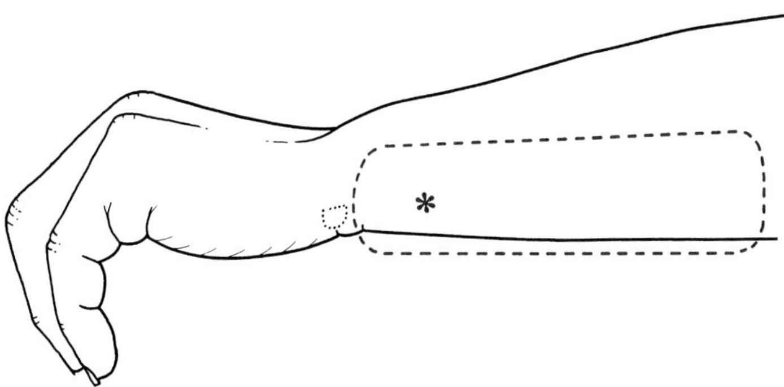

Fig. 7.328 Flap planning of the ulno-dorsal perforator based flap.

References

1. Lovie M J, Duncan G M, Glasson D W 1984 The ulnar artery forearm free flap. British Journal of Plastic Surgery 37: 486–492
2. Reid C D, Moss A L H 1983 One stage repair with vascularised tendon grafts in a dorsal hand injury using the 'Chinese' forearm flap. British Journal of Plastic Surgery 36: 473–479
3. Glasson D W, Lovie M J, Duncan G M 1986 The ulnar forearm flap in penile reconstruction. Australian and New Zealand Journal of Surgery 56: 477–479
4. Glasson D W, Lovie M J 1988 The ulnar island flap in hand and forearm reconstruction. British Journal of Plastic Surgery 41: 349–353
5. Koshima I, Iino T, Fukuda H, Soeda S 1987 The free ulnar forearm flap. Annals of Plastic Surgery 18: 24–29
6. Li Z, Liu K, Cao Y 1989 The reverse flow ulnar artery island flap: 42 clinical cases. British Journal of Plastic Surgery 42: 256–259
7. Guimberteau J C, Goin J L, Panconi B, Schuhmacher B 1988 The reverse ulnar artery forearm island flap in hand surgery: 54 cases. Plastic and Reconstructive Surgery 81: 925–932
8. Becker C, Gilbert A 1988 Le lambeau cubital. Annales de Chirurgie de la Main 7: 136–142
9. Oppikofer C, Büchler U, Schmid E 1992 The surgical anatomy of the dorsal carpal branch of the ulnar artery: basis for a neurovascular dorso-ulnar pedicled flap. Surgical and Radiologic Anatomy 14: 97–101

7

ULNAR RECURRENT ARTERIES

Reverse medial arm flap

This island fasciocutaneous flap was designed by Maruyama et al principally for the release of antecubital scar contractures. Although distally based flaps from the medial side of the arm with a skin and deep fascia pedicle had previously been used for these cases, they had the disadvantage of creating an unsightly dog-ear on transposition. The great advantage of the ulnar recurrent flap based on specific vascular anatomy is that the base of the flap may be reduced to vascular pedicle only and the skin island may then be brought into the recipient defect via a subcutaneous tunnel thereby eliminating all dog-ears.

Anatomy

Shortly after its origin the ulnar artery gives off either an ulnar recurrent artery which divides into anterior and posterior branches or it gives off separate anterior and posterior ulnar recurrent arteries. The anterior passes in front of the medial epicondyle to anastomose with the inferior ulnar collateral artery, and the posterior recurrent passes behind the epicondyle to anastomose with branches of the superior ulnar collateral artery. Arteries are accompanied by veins.

The posterior recurrent artery is the larger of the two and passes between the two heads of flexor carpi ulnaris to lie alongside the ulnar nerve between brachialis and triceps. Here it lies posterior to the ulnar nerve. In its course it gives off branches which pass along the medial intermuscular septum to reach the deep fascia and supply the skin. Dye injections in cadavers stain a territory measuring 15 cm × 7 cm.

Flap planning

The limits of the flap are defined by the midanterior and midposterior lines. Proximally the flap may reach to the axilla. However, if direct closure of the donor site is to be achieved then the flap will have to be much narrower than this.

Surgery

The sides of the flap are incised down to deep fascia and elevated up to the septum. The medial cutaneous nerves of the arm and forearm should be preserved if possible. The intermuscular septum between biceps and triceps is then dissected and the ulnar nerve and the posterior recurrent vessels exposed. At the distal end of the flap (proximally on the arm) the septum and the vessels are divided. This part of the flap can then be lifted up and the the deep surface of the septum containing the vessels dissected free down towards the elbow. The flap is transposed or tunnelled through to the recipient defect. The donor site can generally be closed directly.

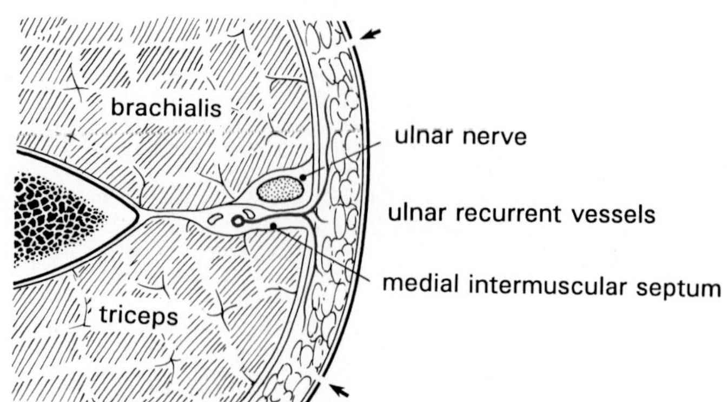

Fig. 7.329 Vascular anatomy. Schematic transverse section through the lower part of the medial intermuscular septum showing posterior ulnar recurrent vessels and their relationship to the ulnar nerve.

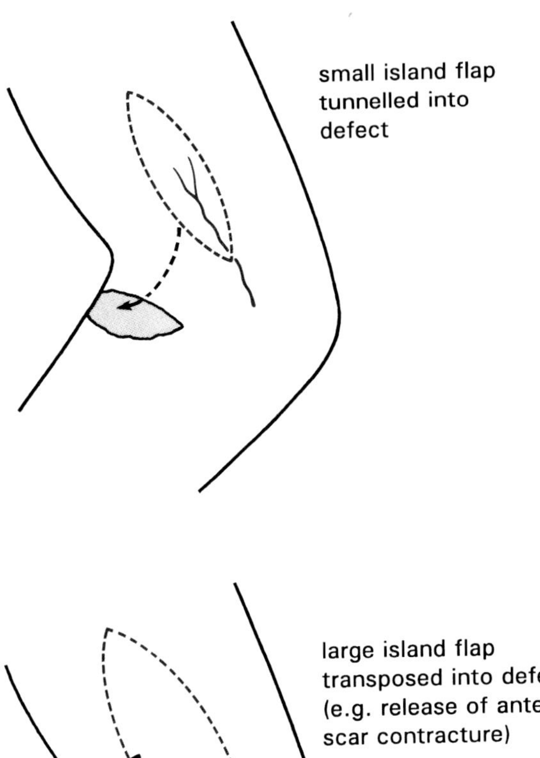

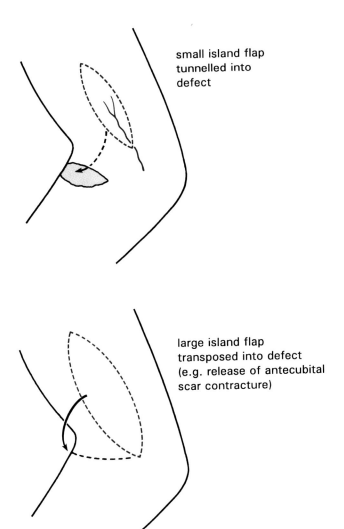

Fig. 7.330 Flap planning. Two typical flap outlines are shown.

Reference

1. Maruyama Y, Onishi K, Iwahira Y 1987 The ulnar recurrent faciocutaneous island flap: reverse medial arm flap. Plastic and Reconstructive Surgery 79: 381–387

Composite flaps incorporating bone

8

8

During the decade 1980–1990 significant progress was made in understanding the principles of the blood supply to bone and in applying this knowledge to the design of composite tissue transfers in which skin ± muscle was combined with bone segments. Such composite free tissue transfer has now become commonplace for reconstructing complex defects in which there are both bone and soft tissue losses. Transfer purely of vascularised bone without an accompanying skin flap has also found numerous indications: bone loss in the upper or lower limb due to trauma; reconstruction of massive bone defects after resection of localised malignant tumours or osteo-myelitis; congenital pseudoarthrosis; congenital failure of development of one or other of the forearm bones are examples. It is remarkable what a variety of sites on the skeleton have been exploited for these purposes. It is therefore appropriate to consider this topic in its own chapter although many of these composite flaps have been mentioned briefly in Chapter 7.

There is now a large literature on the subject of the blood supply to bone, largely because of its relevance to fracture healing, and as might be expected much of this is in orthopaedic rather than plastic surgery publications. The principal points of interest in the context of reconstructive plastic surgery are presented here. For a fuller discussion the references in the orthopaedic research literature should be consulted.

BLOOD SUPPLY TO LONG BONES AND TO PERIOSTEUM

General principles

Bone has long been regarded as being supplied by two systems of blood vessels, indeed the presence of a *circulus vasculosus articuli* around the epiphyseal plate was described by William Hunter in 1743. These two systems are:

1. Nutrient vessels entering nutrient foramina which are located in the midshaft and metaphyseal regions of long bones, and – in immature bones prior to closure of the growth plate – in a ring around the epiphysis. In the limbs these vessels are branches of the principal compartmental arteries.

2. A network of much smaller arteries lying on the periosteum in regions of heavy fascial attachment, these being largely the sites of origin or insertion of muscle fibres, or attachment of intermuscular fascial septa.

This is an essentially anatomical view of bone vascular supply with the emphasis being on the locations of vessels. This is an appropriate viewpoint to take for someone wishing to raise a composite flap but an alternative approach which is favoured by some authors, classifies vessels in functional terms as being *afferent vascular system, efferent vascular system, intermediate vascular system of compact bone*, and *the extraosseous blood supply of healing bone* (Rhinelander, 1972). These terms are self-explanatory except, perhaps, for the last which refers to the new and transitory blood supply derived from surrounding soft tissues that supplements the normal supply in a bone undergoing repair. Note that the term ‘vascular system’ is used rather than ‘vessels’ because a true capillary bed does not exist in the bone. The ‘vessels’ within compact bone, which are intermediate between afferent and efferent systems, are not true capillaries of variable size and are better referred to as ‘cortical sinusoids’ (Brookes, 1971). However, like capillaries, they are part of the functional vascular lattice where ion exchange occurs between the blood and the surrounding tissues. In the medullary cavity, medullary sinusoids replace the usual capillaries and the haemopoietic elements receive an arterial supply from the same ascending and descending branches of the nutrient artery as supply the diaphyseal cortex, but their venous drainage is distinct and different in that the medullary sinusoids drain to central veins which retrace the path of the nutrient arteries or sometimes pierce the cortex elsewhere as emissary veins.

By regarding the anatomical and functional classifications as complimentary rather than alternatives to each other, we are forced to think about the direction of blood flow between the two anatomical systems.

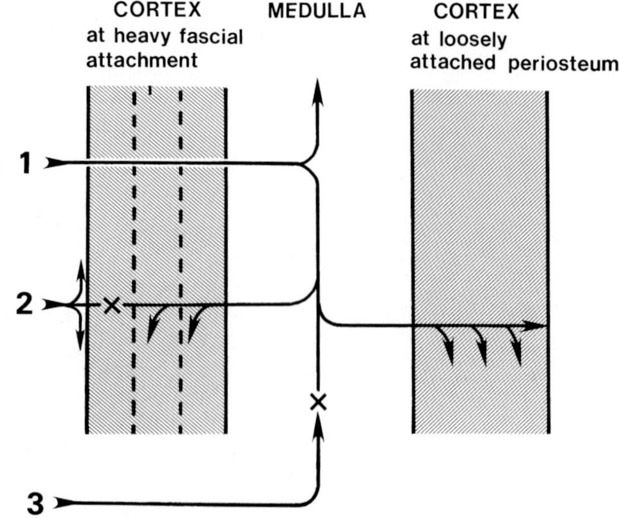

Fig. 8.1 Blood flow through cortical bone (modified after Gothman 1960 and Rhinelander 1974). **1, 2** and **3** are different parts of the afferent vascular system: **1** = principal nutrient artery; **2** = periosteal arterioles; **3** = metaphyseal arteries. **X** marks sites of anastomoses.

Classically the flow of blood through the cortex connecting the two anatomical systems (nutrient vessel and periosteal plexus) was thought to be centripetal but more recent evidence suggests a centrifugal pattern of flow. On the surface of the bone the cortical vessels form connections with capillaries and venules of the periosteal plexus. In areas of loose soft tissue attachment to the periosteum the flow is probably centrifugal through the full thickness of the cortex whereas at sites where the fascial attachment is strong, probably the outer third of the cortex is supplied from the periosteal vessels (Rhinelander, 1974). This is represented diagrammatically in Figure 8.1. Since the flow is centrifugal, the majority of the foramina penetrating the surface of the bone are occupied by thin-walled veins rather than arteries. At certain points on bones, such as near the ends of long bones, the proportion of foramina occupied by arteries will be higher, and it is these metaphyseal and epiphyseal arteries that are able to maintain perfusion of the medullary cavity when the contribution from the diaphyseal nutrient artery has been obliterated either naturally or surgically.

In the skeletally immature the blood supply of the bone is more complex because of the presence of the epiphyseal plate. Several arteries enter an epiphysis and their terminal capillary loops supply the epiphyseal surface of the growth plate. Ramifications of the diaphyseal nutrient artery provide the metaphyseal supply and are evenly distributed over the central part of the growth plate. The cartilagenous epiphyseal plate acts as a barrier and cross-anastomosis between the epiphyseal and metaphyseal circulations is the exception rather than the rule. Such transphyseal vessels may be found in the large epiphyses (Crock, 1967), near their periphery, and become less frequent as the secondary ossification centre enlarges (Ogden, 1979). The outer fringe of the epiphyseal plate is supplied from perichondrial vessels which, by their connections with the periosteal vessels, are a further possible route of communication between the epiphyseal and metaphyseal circulations.

In a manner analogous to that in which the skin may be regarded as being supplied by three different systems, so the periosteal plexus of arteries appears to be fed by three routes (Simpson, 1985). These may be designated as direct periosteal, musculoperiosteal and fascioperiosteal (Fig. 8.2). Direct periosteal vessels arise from nutrient

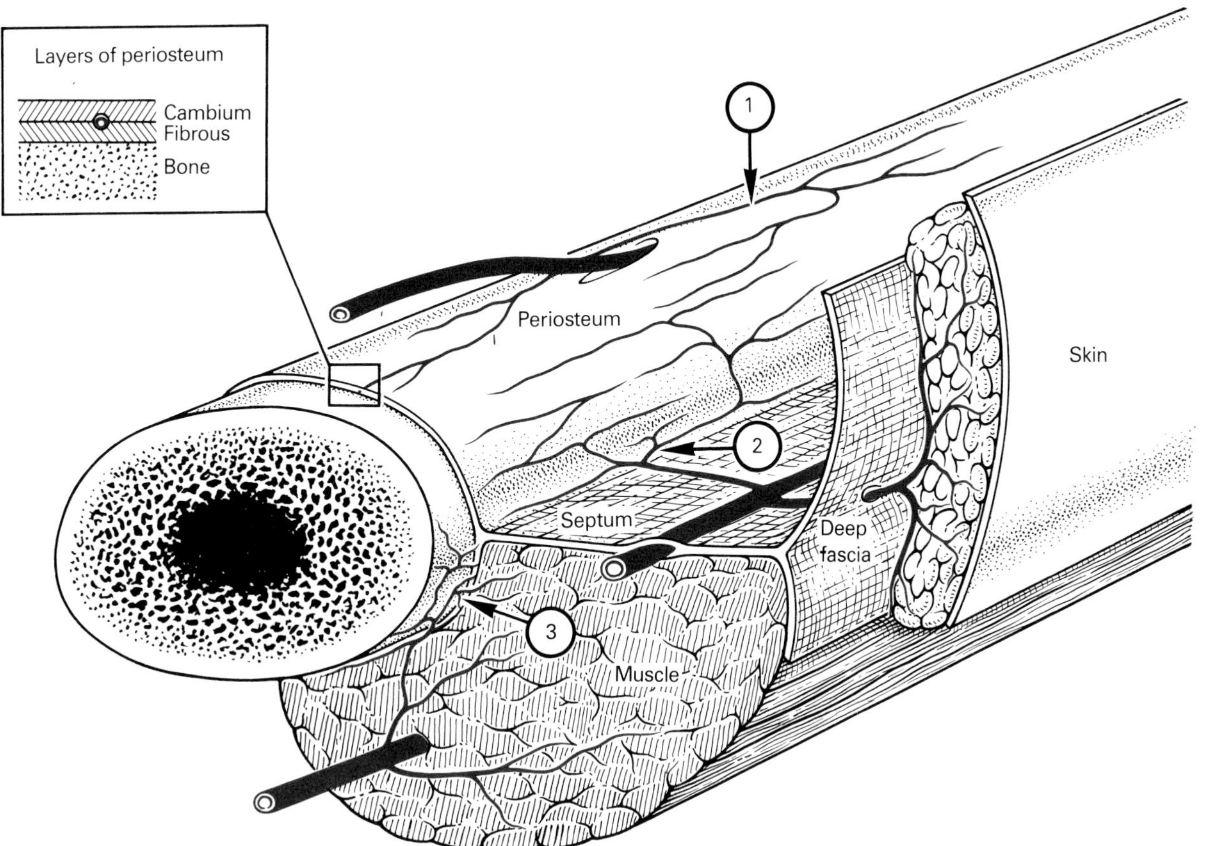

Fig. 8.2 Schematic illustration of the principles of blood supply to periosteum. **1.** Direct periosteal branches of a nutrient artery which is penetrating the cortex. **2.** Fascioperiosteal branches passing along an intercompartmental septum to reach the periosteum from a compartmental artery. **3.** Musculoperiosteal branches arising from the blood vessels of a muscle at the point of its attachment to the bone.

arteries entering foramina and come directly from segmental (trunk) or compartmental (limb) arteries without passing through muscles first; musculoperiosteal vessels arise from arteries within muscles that attach directly to bone without intervening tendon; fascioperiosteal arteries pass along intermuscular fascial septa that are attached to bone, generally arising from the same compartmental vessels as supply fasciocutaneous perforators to overlying skin.

Details of specific long bones

The anatomical literature contains a number of investigations into the *direction* of the nutrient canals on long bones, but only a few regarding the *number* and the *positions* of the foramina on the diaphysis; arterial and venous foramina in the metaphyseal regions are multiple and are ignored in the literature (Lütken, 1950; Mysorekar, 1967; Forriol Campos et al, 1987; Sendemir & Çimen, 1991). In this section the nutrient foramina of the diaphysis of the principal long bones of the upper and lower extremities will be considered.

Direction of the canal is determined by the growth of the bone and the pull of the periosteum. The simple rule is that as it goes in the canal is directed obliquely away from the principal growing end of the bone, i.e. in the upper limb towards the elbow, and in the lower limb away from the knee.

Numbers of nutrient foramina are summarised in Table 8.1. There may be more than one foramen on the diaphysis with the exception of the radius which seems always to have only one. Some bones, such as the femur and the clavicle, commonly have two. Absence of a nutrient foramen is also a well-recognised occurrence, particularly in the shorter 'long bones' such as the metatarsals and metacarpals (Patake & Mysorekar, 1977).

Table 8.1 Number of nutrient foramina in long bones: for the metacarpals and metatarsals the figures vary slightly for each bone

Bone	None	One foramen	Two foramina	Three foramina
humerus		75%	25%	
radius		100%		
ulna		91%	9%	
femur		30%	60%	10%
tibia		93%	7%	
fibula	6%	86%	8%	
clavicle	the 'foramen' is probably for venous drainage			
metatarsals	6–8%	>90%	1–7%	
metacarpals	2–9%	>90%	1–6%	

Position of a nutrient foramen is best expressed with reference to the overall length of a long bone and this is known as the foraminal index which is expressed as a percentage:

$$FI = \frac{\text{distance from proximal end of bone to foramen}}{\text{total length of bone}} \times 100$$

Figure 8.3 shows the mean foraminal indices of the six major long bones together with the range of values observed. Table 8.2 indicates the constancy with which a foramen is found on a particular aspect of a bone.

Table 8.2 Anatomical situation of the nutrient foramina

Bone	Site of foramen on bone	% of diaphyseal foramina on that bone
humerus	anteromedial	81%
	posterior	16%
	anterolateral	3%
radius	anterior	100%
ulna	anterior	100%
femur	linea aspera	44%
	medial lip	48%
	lateral lip	8%
tibia	posterior	100%
fibula	posterior	68%
	medial	32%

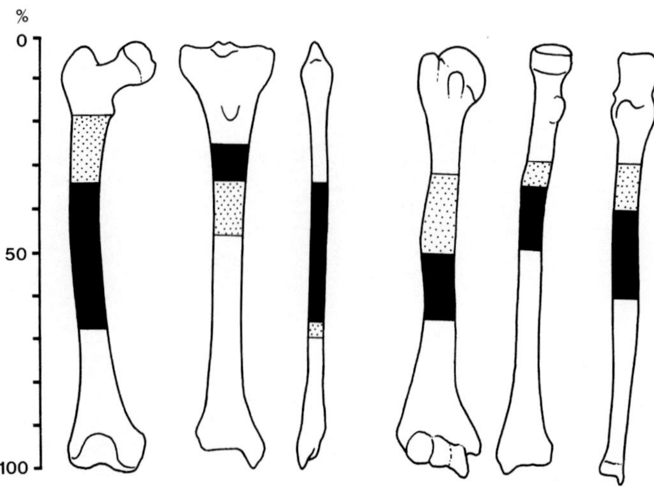

Fig. 8.3 Location of nutrient foramina in long bones. Dark areas represent the usual positions, stippled areas the less frequent positions.

Shaft of fibula
Because of its relative dispensability, the fibula has been the long bone most used for free vascularised bone transfer based on a nutrient artery pedicle. As a result there are more studies in the recent literature on this bone than any other. Using three hundred fibulas, McKee et al (1984) found the nutrient foramen was absent in 6% and in the middle third in 96% of the remaining cases. Restrepo et al (1980) found the foramen absent in 4%. Bonnel et al (1981) also sited the vascular foramen in the middle third of the bone. Forriol Campos et al (1987) in 33 fibulas sited the foramen in the middle third, equally distributed between the posterior and medial surfaces. It is often visible on plain radiographs and this may take the guesswork out of locating it in clinical situations.

The head of fibula
Because of the wish in certain circumstances (e.g. radial club hand) to transfer a growth plate as well as a length of bone, the head of the fibula has also received much attention. Classical anatomical texts clearly identify the arterial supply to the head of the mature fibula as derived from six arteries arising from the popliteal and the anterior tibial arteries (Table 8.3.). Of these vessels the principal two are a branch of the inferior lateral genicular artery coming down onto the epiphysis from above, and a recurrent branch from the anterior tibial (recurrens fibularis anterior) coming on to the anteromedial aspect from below as shown in Figure 8.4 (Bonnel et al, 1981; Chen & Zhang, 1987). In the adult these vessels have an average diameter of around 1.1 mm and in young children they are even smaller, and hence not anastomosable unless a short segment of the anterior tibial artery is also removed (with the gap either filled by direct anastomosis or by vein graft).

Table 8.3 Arterial supply to the head of the fibula. The inferior lateral genicular artery usually arises from the popliteal artery, and the rest from the anterior tibial artery although other origins sometimes apply. See also Figure 8.4 where the same numbering is applied. Terminology in the literature is inconstant and is not translated consistently from the Latin

Artery	Diameter at origin (mm)	Range (mm)
1. inferior lateral genicular	1.7	1.2–2.3
2. anterior tibial recurrent branch	1.1	0.7–1.5
3. posterior fibular recurrent*	1.3	0.5–2.1
4. anterior tibial recurrent		
5. posterior tibial recurrent		
6. medial fibular recurrent		

*also known as Weber's artery of the head of the fibula.

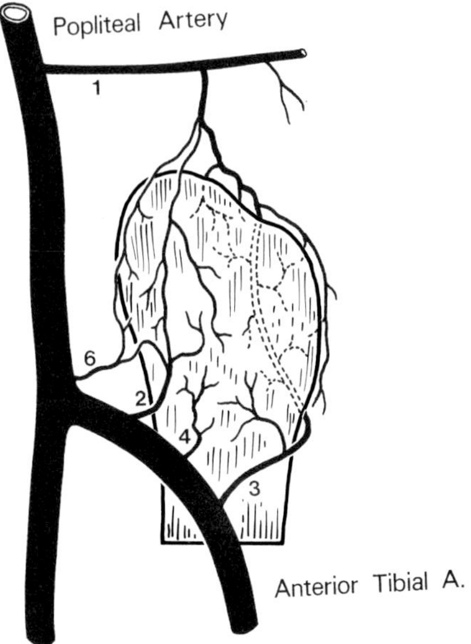

Fig. 8.4 Blood supply to the head of the fibula. See Table 8.3 for code.

Metacarpals and metatarsals
Metatacarpals and metatarsals can be considered as miniature long bones but they are peculiar in generally having an epiphysis at only one end, typically at the base of the first metacarpal or metatarsal, and in the heads in the remainder. However, additional epiphyses have been described for the head of the first metacarpal, base of the second metacarpal, and, rarely, for the bases of the other metacarpals. In the foot there may be an epiphysis for the head of the first metatarsal, while the epiphyses normally appearing in the heads of the others may be replaced by epiphyses in their bases. These considerations may be relevant to transfer of vascularised metatarsophalangeal joints to the hand. The nutrient foramina have been little studied other than by Patake & Mysorekar (1977) who confirmed the textbook description of foramina located in the middle third. In metacarpals they are on the medial side of the first (from the princeps pollicis) and second (from 2nd palmar metacarpal artery) and on the lateral sides of the remaining ones. In the foot the pattern is the reverse of this since the limb rotates during development. The relevance of the foramina to flaps is questionable as vascularised bone transfer is mainly dependent on periosteal vessels (see p. 506.)

Clavicle
The clavicle is atypical of a long bone in that it is formed by membranous ossification and has almost nothing in the way of a medullary cavity in its middle portion (Knudsen et al, 1989). Vascularised transfer is achieved by taking the bone in continuity with the clavicular head of pectoralis major (Reid et al, 1986).

VASCULARISED BONE TRANSFER

Vascularised bone transfer has been demonstrated to be superior to conventional bone grafting in several respects, namely time to union at the juncture sites, earlier hypertrophy, and higher mechanical strength (Weiland et al, 1984). On the negative side it must be said that if a free vascularised bone graft undergoes anastomotic failure then the bone does not behave as a conventional bone graft but often becomes resorbed or infected. Infection is particularly likely if the bone is surrounded by a cuff of (dead) muscle which prevents revascularisation from the bed and acts as a further nidus for infection. Vascularised bone grafts that remain vascularised appear to be fairly resistant to infection, perhaps because prophylactically administered antibiotics are better able to penetrate the vascularised bone.

Reconstructive techniques have moved on a long way from the traditional idea that vascularised bone grafts have to be attached to portions of muscle. The majority of microvascular bone grafts still rely on musculoperiosteal vessels or on nutrient arteries of the diaphysis but transfer of bone on direct periosteal vessels or on fascioperiosteal systems is increasingly used. As a result it is possible to carry out basically four types of vascularised bone transfer:

1. diaphyseal – based on the nutrient artery of the shaft
2. epiphyseal – based on a variety of vessel arrangements including metaphyseal and epiphyseal perforators
3. apophyseal – there are only a few possible sites for this and they are based on specific vessels
4. cortical plate – based on periosteal vessels.

Some of these may also be combined with a skin flap (see Table 8.6).

Diaphyseal transfer

The principle underlying transfer of bone on the nutrient artery pedicle accompanied by draining veins is clear. However, what is not clear is whether all of these osteocytes survive in a successfully revascularised bone graft since circulation may not be preserved in all portions of the cortex. Similar concepts apply to the transfer of rib segments fed through the nutrient branch of the posterior intercostal artery although ribs are not generally regarded as 'long bones'. The main bone from which it is possible to harvest a diaphyseal segment is the fibula and this has been utilised as a free vascularised graft for all the purposes mentioned in the introduction. Generally it is the bone of first choice when the defect to be filled is over 10 cm in length. However, it has also been used in a variety of other situations as diverse as replacing vertebral bodies, bridging gaps in the pelvis (Yajima et al, 1992), and augmenting the blood supply in the neck of the femur in young patients with osteonecrosis of the femoral head (Malizos et al, 1992).

When used as a single strut it is generally carried on the nutrient artery of the diaphysis (Taylor et al, 1975; Gilbert 1979). The diaphyseal supply is also used if the graft is to be used as a local transfer without anastomosis, as in reconstruction of pseudoarthrosis of the tibia. Here the middle of the fibular shaft may be transferred distally on a 'reverse-flow' peroneal pedicle and inset into the tibial defect (Townsend, 1990).

If the fibula is to be osteotomised the periosteal circulation must be preserved by dissecting out the bone in continuity with branches of the peroneal artery and with a cuff of muscle around the bone. Osteotomy may then be carried out once, for example, to produce a more substantial double strut for filling a femoral shaft defect, or several times to contour a mandibular reconstruction (Fig. 8.5).

When removing the fibula the distal 5 cm should be left intact, and in a child the ankle mortice is best stabilised to reduce the potential for development of a valgus deformity. This may be done by cross-screwing through the proximal end of the fibular remnant into the tibial cortex. Free fibular transfer was first carried out in 1975 but the majority of cases of diaphyseal transfer have only been carried out since 1982 and and the long-term effects on the ankle are unclear. In the last few years reports have been slowly appearing in the literature suggesting that as the years go by problems may appear in some cases. These problems include instability, muscle weakness, and pain in the ankle (see Gore et al, 1987; Ganel & Yaffe, 1990; de Boer et al, 1990; Anderson & Green, 1991) and there have been cases of deformity of the ankle and talus

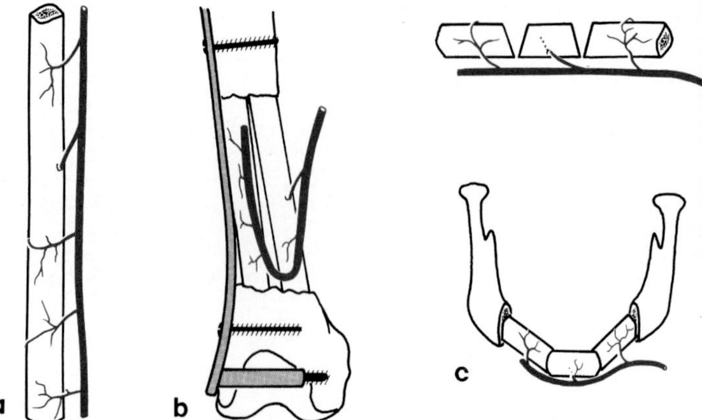

Fig. 8.5 Fibular shaft: **a.** on nutrient artery pedicle for single strut; **b.** single osteotomy; **c.** multiple osteotomies. (Venae comitantes not shown.)

in infants (Vilkki, 1991). Removing part of the shaft may allow the fibular head to move superiorly and the lateral knee ligament to become slightly slack. In one study moderate symptomatic lateral knee laxity occurred in half the cases (Murray & Schlafly, 1986).

Epiphyseal transfer

Transplantation of epiphyses without vascular anastomoses has been carried out since the turn of the century (Helferich, 1899) with mixed results (see Table 8.4). The best results have followed transplantation with only a thin plate of attached metaphysis which allows for rapid incorporation. During this early avascular period, which probably lasts for up to 10 days, the growth plate relies for its nutrition on diffusion of tissue fluids and therefore for this form of grafting to be successful the mass of tissue must be small. The haphazard nature of revascularisation, particularly if the graft is beyond a critical volume, is one of the factors which may account for the variable and unpredictable results of transplantation. When microsurgical techniques became available it became inevitable that vascularised epiphyseal transplantation would be developed in order to try to make epiphyseal grafting a more reliable process in terms of survival of the open growth plate and future growth.

Table 8.4 Results of free non-vascularised epiphyseal transfer. Even in those cases where growth reportedly continued, the segment rarely grew normally and at maturity was usually smaller than the equivalent contralateral epiphysis. An 'open plate' on a radiograph is not necessarily indicative of function

Date	Author	Subject	Outcome (growth)
1929	Straub	human	some growth
1931	Haas	human	failure
1945	Wenger	human	success
1954	Barr	human	success
1954	Graham	human	plate open at 2 years
1955	Ring	rabbits	5 of 18 normal growth
1955	Riordan	human	no growth
1956	Peacock	human	normal at 2 years
1963	Erdelyi	humans	success (whole joints)
1964	Spira et al	human	no growth
1965	Freeman	77 human toes	success in 42%
1965	Harris et al	rabbit	< 80% of normal growth
1966	Wilson	humans (11)	3 had some growth
1966	Eades & Peacock	human	normal growth
1967	Spira & Farin	human	failed
1972	Hoffman et al	dogs (tubed flap)	some growth
1974	Calderwood	rabbits	some growth
1977	Whitesides	human	normal growth
1978	Rank	humans	1 failed, 1 grew
1982	Goldberg, Watson	human	90% patency and growth

Transfer of vascularised epiphyses was first carried out in dogs and reported in 1979. These and other experimental results (see Table 8.5) indicated nearly normal growth of epiphyses post-transplantation. Subsequently transfer of vascularised epiphyses in the clinical situation concentrated on the head of the fibula and on phalanges in the form of whole-toe-to-hand transfers in children.

Table 8.5 Results of experimental vascularised epiphyseal transfer. This table does not differentiate between heterotopic transplants and orthotopic revascularisations. Code for blood supply to epiphysis is: **d** = nutrient artery pedicle; **m** = metaphyseal supply, **e** = epiphyseal artery supply, **j** = whole joint transfer

Date	Author	Subject	Blood supply	Outcome (growth)
1979	Donski et al	dogs	d	63% of normal
1979	Hurwitz	dogs	j	near normal
1980	Donski, O'Brien	dogs	m	69% of normal
1982	Zaleske et al	rabbits	j	near normal
1983	Brown et al	dogs	dme	82% of normal
1984	Nettleblad et al	dogs	me	normal growth
1986	Teot et al	dogs	de	50% of normal

The head of the fibula may in theory be transferred either (1) on an epiphyseal supply, or (2) on a metaphyseal supply, or (3) on a diaphyseal/metaphyseal supply with a soft tissue cuff providing connections to the perichondrial vessels of the epiphysis.

1. An epiphyseal supply requires identifiable vessels and these have been described above.

2. A metaphyseal supply from the peroneal artery should support the epiphysis if there are functional anastomoses. Donski et al (1979) found that experimental epiphyseal transplantation based on a medullary blood supply produced 63% of normal growth and they felt that this supported the trans-epiphyseal anastomosis theory, as little growth would be have been expected if this did not exist. Ideally, however, the integrity of both metaphyseal and epiphyseal circulations should be preserved, especially as the current concept is that the epiphyseal arteries supply the germinal layer of the physis and the metaphyseal arteries support ossification (Tomita et al, 1986).

3. In theory the preservation of a cuff of soft tissue around metaphysis and epiphysis should provide an effective route for cross-communication between the metaphyseal and epiphyseal circulations. In practice, the peroneal artery is available for anastomosis and its branches to the shaft and metaphysis appear able to supply the epiphysis via the intercommunicating branches along musculo-periosteal and perichondrial vessels and vessels of the soft tissue cuff. The first clinical transfers designed on these principles, reported transplantation of the superior epiphysis and superior half of the diaphysis in a 7-year-old boy to stabilise a radial club hand (Weiland & Daniel, 1979). The graft was vascularised only by the peroneal artery. The clinical and radiologic results were excellent, epiphyseal cartilage remained

visible and ulnar deflection was stabilised. Three years later the epiphyseal plate was still open. Gori et al (1981) used the same technique with successful outcome. Pho et al (1988) have similarly reported three cases and highlighted many of the intrinsic and extrinsic factors which may influence the growth of the epiphysis in its new location and which are in many instances not yet fully understood.

Obviously there are difficulties associated with removing the head of the fibula. The tendon of insertion of biceps femoris and the fibular collateral ligament of the knee must be divided prior to disarticulation of the superior tibio-fibular joint and must then be inserted by a staple onto the tibia. The leg frequently remains mildly symptomatic with residual weakness and knee laxity (Anderson & Green, 1991).

Phalanges

Epiphyseal growth occurs in replanted digits in children (Van Beek et al, 1979) and in toe-to-hand transfers (Gilbert, 1982). Vascularised epiphyses or joints that are isolated so that they are not part of a digit may also be transferred. Mathes et al (1980) reported successful microvascular transplantation of a second metatarso-phalangeal joint with associated epiphyses in a 4-year-old child. $2\frac{1}{2}$ years later there were open epiphyseal plates and growth had been near normal. Ischida & Tsai (1991) reported 19 joint transfers in children with the principal indication being injury of the MCP or IP joint of the thumb with associated epiphyseal injury.

Apophyseal transfer

An apophysis is a growth centre which does not participate in forming a joint the way an epiphysis does. Vascularised apophyses may be harvested from the iliac crest and the lateral border and inferior pole of the scapula. Teot et al (1982) first developed the iliac crest transfer but found it to be deforming and went on to develop the scapular apophyseal transfer based on branches of the subscapular axis (Teot et al, 1981, 1992). The chondro-osseous tissue can be combined with a scapular skin flap or a latissimus dorsi muscle or musculocutaneous flap. The advantages of the scapula over the fibula are less potential morbidity at the donor site, the possibility of combination with a muscle or skin flap, and the increased plasticity of the apophysis which is thought to have greater potential for remodelling. The donor scapula remains small but the subglenoid growth centre hypertrophies and partially compensates for the absence of the lower growth plate, while the reinserted muscles seem to contribute to new scapular bone formation by the effect of pulling on the periosteum.

Cortical bone transfer

Pieces of cortical bone must generally be transferred through their periosteal supply since the medullary supply will have been disrupted. As usual there are exceptions and as an example one might consider the transfer of a strut of cortex from the lateral border of the scapula on a perforating nutrient artery from the circumflex scapular artery. The majority of pieces of cortex will however be carried on direct periosteal, musculoperiosteal or fascioperiosteal afferent systems.

Direct periosteal branches are available at certain sites, e.g. metacarpal, medial condylar plate of femur (Martin et al, 1991), and lateral aspect of distal half of radius (Cormack et al, 1986). The femur is one of the most interesting sites since it may – given favourable vascular anatomy – be possible to carry out transfer to a more distal location on the tibia without an anastomosis (Hertel & Masquelet, 1989). This is shown in Figure 8.6.

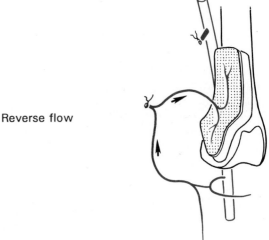

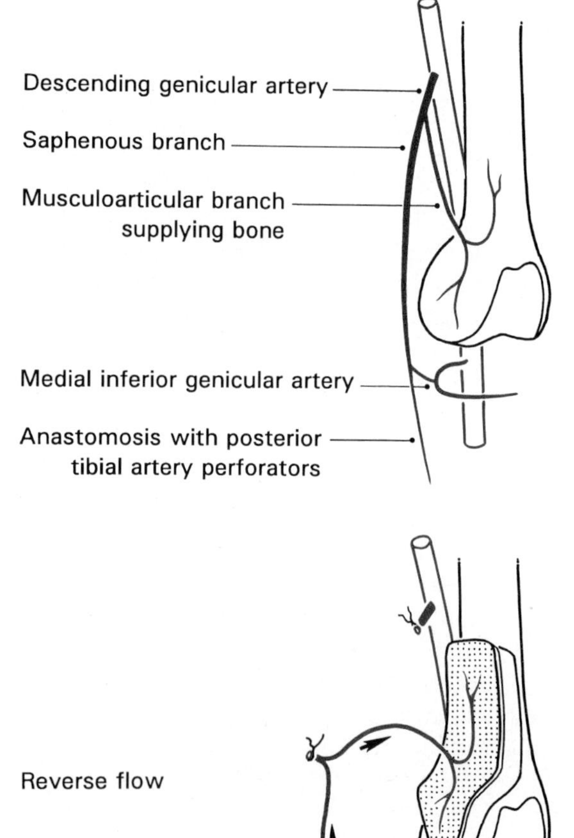

Fig. 8.6 Medial femoral cortex pedicled transfer.

Musculoperiosteal vessels are small, lack robustness and their connections with the vessels of the muscle may be further narrowed by tension on the muscle. Indeed many such grafts probably derive as much benefit from lying within their bed of vascularised muscle, as they do through putative connections between the vascular systems of the muscle and the periosteum. Many pieces of the skeleton may be transferred by this means and examples would be sternum, rib or clavicle on parts of pectoralis major and rib on latissimus dorsi.

Fascioperiosteal vessels are fed by arteries travelling along relatively inextensible intermuscular fascial septa and provide a fairly robust means of carrying a segment of that bone. The combination of a skin flap with a segment of bone supplied by fascioperiosteal perforators from the same compartmental artery (Fig. 8.7) provides an elegant antomical example of how knowledge of the periosteal and skin supplies can be used in the design of a clinically successful composite osteo-fasciocutaneous flap, e.g. on the lateral side of the upper arm based on the middle collateral artery (= posterior radial collateral A.).

The various sites on the skeleton that have been used for vascularised bone transfer are summarised in Figure 8.8 and Table 8.6.

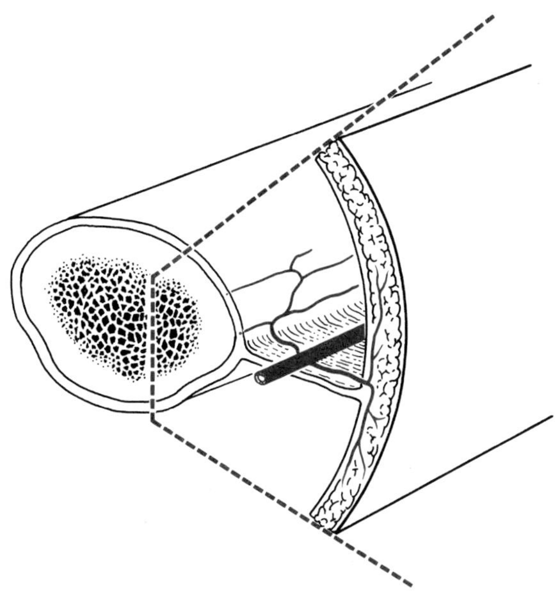

Fig. 8.7 Fascioperiosteal vessels to bone and associated fasciocutaneous Type C flap.

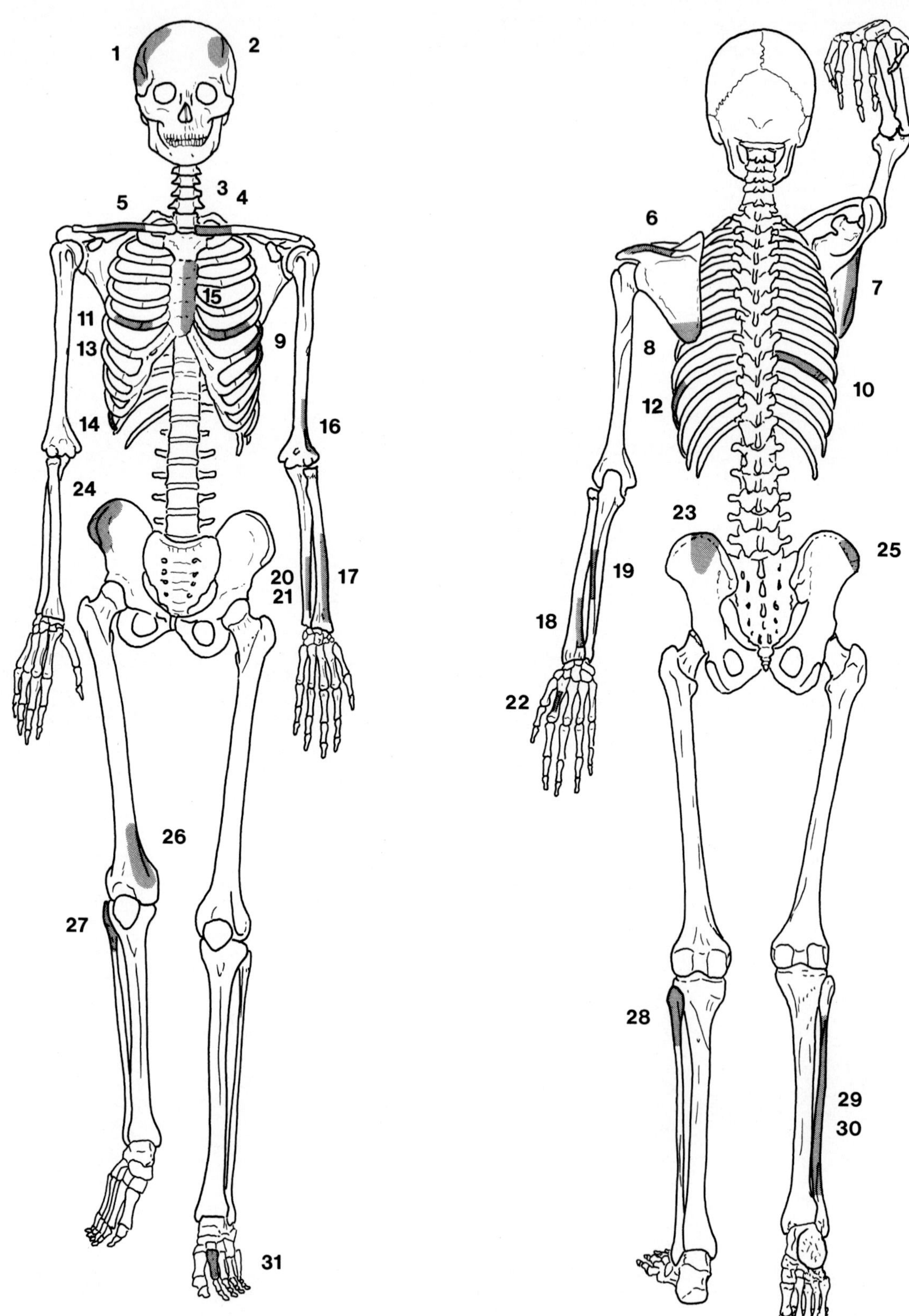

Fig. 8.8 Areas of the skeleton that have been used for vascularised bone harvest. Numbers correlate with Table 8.6.

Table 8.6 Possible sites for harvesting of either bone-only or skin + bone composite flaps. The numbers in the left-hand column correspond with the numbers on Figure 8.8. Code to vascular supply: mp = musculoperiosteal; dp = direct periosteal; na = nutrient artery of diaphysis or endosteal supply (e.g. rib); fp = fascioperiosteal. In column headed skin island, nd = not described but theoretically possible

	Bone		Arterial supply	System	Skin island	Described by
1	frontal bone		sup. temporal A., post. b.	fp	yes	McCarthy & Zide 1984
2	frontal bone	*	deep temporal A.	mp	no	Watson-Jones 1933
3	medial clavicle	*	sternomas. & occip. A.	mp (SCM)**	no	Siemssen et al 1978
4	medial clavicle	*	tubed delayed skin	dp	tube	Snyder et al 1970
5	middle clavicle		acromio-thoracic axis	mp (Pec Mj)	yes	Reid et al 1986
6	spine of scapula		sup. b. trans. cervical A.	mp (Trap)	yes	Panje & Cutting 1980
7	lateral border scapula		nutrient b. circ. scap. A.	na	yes	Sekiguchi et al 1993
8	inferior pole scapula		angular b. of thoracod.	dp	yes	Coleman & Sultan 1991
9	6th & 7th ribs, laterally		serratus anterior b's	mp (SA)	yes	Richards et al 1985
10	rib, posteriorly		posterior intercostal A.	na	yes	Buncke et al 1977
11	5th rib anteriorly	*	pectoral b. thor.-ac. axis	mp (Pec Mj)	yes	Jones & Sommerlad 1983
12	10th rib laterally		thoracodorsal A.	mp (Lat D)	yes	Schmidt & Robson 1982
13	5th rib anteriorly		anterior intercostal A.	mp (Intercost)	yes	Ariyan & Finseth 1978
14	10th rib anteriorly		deep inf. epigastric A.	mp (Intercost)	yes	Taylor et al 1983
15	sternum outer table	*	pectoral b. thor.-ac. axis	mp (Pec Mj)	yes	Green et al 1981
16	humerus lat. ridge		middle collateral A.	fp	yes	Katsaros et al 1991
17	radius, distal lateral		radial A.	dp	yes	Soutar et al 1983
18	radius anteromedial	*	anterior interosseous A.	dp	no	Pagliei et al 1991
19	ulna – posterior	*	post. interosseous A.	mp (EPL)	yes	Costa et al 1988
20	ulna – anterior		ulnar artery	mp (FCU)	yes	Lovie et al 1984
21	ulna – anteromedial	*	anterior interosseous A.	dp	no	Pagliei et al 1991
22	second metacarpal	*	1st dorsal metacarpal A.	dp	nd	Bertelli et al 1992
23	ilium lateral	***	sup. gluteal A., deep b.	mp (G Medius)	nd	Huang et al 1985
24	ilium anterolateral		deep circumflex iliac A.	mp (Iliacus)	yes	Taylor et al 1979
25	ilium anterior		asc. b. of lat. circ. fem. A.	mp (TFL)	yes	Baker 1980
26	femur, medial condyle		desc. genicular A.	dp	yes	Hertel & Masquelet 1989
27	fibular epiphysis		anterior tibial A.	dp	no	Chen & Zhang 1987
28	fibular epiphysis		peroneal A.	mp na pc a	no	Pho et al 1988
29	fibular shaft		peroneal A.	na	no	Taylor et al 1975
30	fibular shaft		peroneal A.	mp fp	yes	Schusterman et al 1992
31	second metatarsal		dorsalis pedis A.	na fp	yes	MacLeod & Robinson1982

Notes

* These sites are not generally regarded as free flap donor sites but are more applicable to pedicled local or loco-regional transfer.

** The vascular connection from the muscular attachment of sternocleidomastoid to the clavicle described by Siemssen who used the muscle as a pedicle to a clavicular bone graft, has not been demonstrated by injection studies. The medial one-fifth of the clavicle is usually vascularised by branches from the internal thoracic artery.

*** In addition to these recognised iliac bone vascularised grafts the Chinese have described a variety of other vascular pedicles such as the iliac branches of iliolumbar vessels, or the third and fourth lumbar vessels. See also Zhao 1986, Yelizarov et al 1993, in the Western literature. All the references in the Chinese literature are quoted by Zhong & Kong (1991). See also Zhao 1986, Yelizarov et al 1993, in the Western literature.

Zhenman & Zhiguang (1986) have described small pieces of bone pedicled solely on periosteum and used as local transfers – these are probably only partially vascularised (if at all).

Free toe transfers and second metatarsophalangeal joint transfers have not been included in this list.

8

VASCULARISED PERIOSTEAL TRANSFER

The osteogenic potential of periosteum has been recognised since Ollier in 1867 concluded that transplanted periosteum and bone could, under certain circumstances, become osteogenic. This classical study was later re-evaluated and developed clinically by Scandinavian surgeons (Skoog, 1965; Ritsilä et al, 1972).

Successful free vascularised periosteal transfer has been demonstrated clinically and experimentally (see Table 8.7) although contradictory views exist concerning osteogenic capability. In the experimental situation pure periosteal flaps show no or very little bone formation in some studies (Puckett et al, 1979) while in other studies tibial periosteal grafts and especially composite musculo-periosteal grafts do show cortical bone formation(Takato et al, 1986; Van den Wildenberg et al, 1984). The explanation for these variable findings is probably related to two main factors: (1) the position of the donor site, and (2) the mechanical stresses present at the recipient site, but other factors such as age are obviously also important in so far as they relate to osteogenic capacity.

1. The donor site of the vascularised periosteal graft has been demonstrated to be important in experimental animal studies. Tibial periosteum has greater osteogenic capacity than mandibular periosteum, calvarial periosteum (Uddströmer, 1978), and rib periosteum (Van den Wildenberg et al, 1984).

2. The degree of bone formation by periosteal grafts is better when the recipient area is subjected to mechanical stresses. Revascularised rib periosteum transplanted to a tibial site in dogs can bridge a 5 cm defect (Finley et al, 1978) whereas the same periosteum applied to ulna and cranial defects is worthless (Acland, 1978). Although non-vascularised, it is probably still relevant that calvarial periosteum transferred to the tibia forms five times as much bone as calvarial periosteum in situ and tibial periosteum in situ forms twice as much bone as when grafted to a calvarial defect (Uddströmer & Ritsilä, 1978).

3. It is generally recognised that the periosteum of adults has less osteogenic capacity than that of children. Regeneration of a terminal phalanx from periosteum only has been described in a child (Vidal & Dickson, 1993).

Table 8.7 Experimental free vascularised periosteal transfer

Year	Author	Site of periosteum	Subject
1978	Finley et al	from rib to tibia	dogs
1978	Acland	from rib to cranium	dogs
1979	Puckett et al	from rib to fibula	dogs
1984	Wildenberg et al	rib and tibia	goats
1986	Takato	from tibia to face or tibia	rabbits

It can therefore be seen that the therapeutic effectiveness of periosteal grafting is likely to be heavily influenced by making the right choice of graft for the right location.

Clinical transfer of vascularised periosteal grafts may take two forms: (i) free vascularised transfer, and (ii) local pedicled transfer. So far there have been only a handful of cases reported in the literature.

Clinical free vascularised periosteal transfer

Satoh et al (1983) have successfully treated a comminuted fracture of the tibia using a vascularised musculo-periosteal free flap from the inner aspect of the ilium supported by the deep circumflex iliac artery. Bone union was demonstrably accelerated and the patient was permitted full weight bearing within 6 months of the operation.

Penteado et al (1990) have investigated a variety of sites for free periosteal flaps. In anatomical studies they have shown that the distal posterior third of the humerus, and the distal third of the femur are other good potential sites.

Clinical local pedicled periosteal transfer

Local pedicled transfer of vascularised periosteal flaps has been demonstrated anatomically by Crock in the lower limb and applied clinically to a tibial fracture (Crock & Morrison, 1992). Crock has shown that a periosteal flap may be raised on the lateral surface of the middle third of the tibial shaft where the periosteum receives a blood supply from several branches of the anterior tibial artery. A ‘flap’ of periosteum attached to the anterior tibial vascular bundle may be transferred either distally to the foot (retrograde flow in vessels) or proximally to the knee (orthograde flow).

Hertel & Masquelet (1989) have demonstrated the anatomy of transferring medial femoral condyle periosteal and osteo-periosteal flaps into a more distal situation in the leg such as a tibial defect, based on the anatomy of the descending genicular artery as described above in the section on condylar bone.

Other potential sites for local pedicled periosteal transfer are the radius and the ulna based on the anterior interosseous artery supply (Pagliei et al, 1991).

References

Acland R D 1978 Caution about clinical use of vascularised periosteal grafts. Plastic and Reconstructive Surgery 62: 290

Anderson A F, Green N E 1991 Residual function deficit after partial fibulectomy for bone graft. Clinical Orthopaedics and Related Research 267: 137–140

Ariyan S, Finseth F J 1978 The anterior chest approach for obtaining free osteocutaneous rib grafts. Plastic and Reconstructive Surgery 62: 676–685

Baker S R 1980 Reconstruction of mandibular defects with the revascularized free tensor fascia lata osteomyocutaneous flap. Archives of Otolaryngology 107: 414–418

Barr J S 1954 Autogenous epiphyseal transplant. Abstract of a case report in Proceedings of The American Academy of Orthopaedic Surgeons. Journal of Bone and Joint Surgery 36A: 688

Bertelli J A, Pagliei A, Lassau J-P 1992 Role of the first dorsal metacarpal artery in the construction of pedicled bone grafts. Surgical and Radiologic Anatomy 14: 275–277

de Boer H H, Wood M B, Hermans J 1990 Reconstruction of large skeletal defects by vascularised fibula transfer. International Orthopaedics 14: 121–128

Bonnel F, Lesire M, Gomis R, Allieu Y, Rabischong P 1981 Arterial vascularisation of the fibula: microsurgical transplant techniques. Anatomia Clinica 3: 13–22

Brookes M 1971 The blood supply of bone. Butterworths, London

Brown K, Marie P, Lyszakowski T, Daniel R, Cruess R 1983 Epiphyseal growth after free fibular transfer with and without microvascular anastomosis. Journal of Bone and Joint Surgery 65B: 493–501

Brunelli F, Brunelli G, Nanfito F 1991 An anatomical study of the vascularisation of the first dorsal interosseous space in the hand, and a description of a bony pedicle graft arising from the second metacarpal bone. Surgical and Radiologic Anatomy 13: 73–75

Buncke H J, Furnas D W, Gordon L, Achauer B M 1977 Free osteocutaneous flap from a rib to the tibia. Plastic and Reconstructive Surgery 59: 799–805

Calderwood J W 1974 The effect of hyperbaric oxygen on the transplantation of epiphysial growth cartilage in the rabbit. Journal of Bone and Joint Surgery 56B: 753–759

Chen Z W, Zhang G J 1987 Epiphyseal transplantation. In: Pho R W H (ed) Microsurgical techniques in orthopaedics. Butterworths, London

Coleman J J, Sultan M R 1991 The bipedicled osteocutaneous scapular flap. Plastic and Reconstructive Surgery 87: 682–691

Cormack G C, Duncan M-J, Lamberty B G H 1986 The blood supply of the bone component of the compound osteocutaneous radial artery forearm flap: an anatomical study. British Journal of Plastic Surgery 39: 173–175

Costa H, Smith R, McGrouther D A 1988 Thumb reconstruction by the posterior interosseous osteocutaneous flap. British Journal of Plastic Surgery 41: 228–233

Crock H V 1967 The blood supply of the lower limb bones in man. Churchill Livingstone, Edinburgh

Crock J G, Morrison W A 1992 Case Report: A vascularised periosteal flap: an anatomical study. British Journal of Plastic Surgery 45: 474–478

Donski P K, Carwell G R, Sharzer L A 1979 Growth in revascularised bone grafts in young puppies. Plastic and Reconstructive Surgery 64: 239–243

Donski P K, O'Brien B M 1980 Free microvascular epiphyseal transplantation: an experimental study in dogs. British Journal of Plastic Surgery 33: 169–178

Eades J W, Peacock E E 1966 Autogenous transplantation of an interphalangeal joint and proximal phalangeal epiphysis. Case Report and ten year follow up. Journal of Bone and Joint Surgery 48A: 775–778

Erdelyi R 1963 Reconstruction of ankylosed finger joints by means of transplantation of joints from the foot. Plastic and Reconstructive Surgery 31: 140–150

Finley J M, Alland R D, Wood M B 1978 Revascularised periosteal grafts. A new method to produce functional new bone without bone grafting. Plastic and Reconstructive Surgery 61: 1–6

Forriol Campos F, Gomez Pellico L, Gianonatti Alias M, Fernandez-Valencia R 1987 A study of the nutrient foramina of human long bones. Surgical and Radiologic Anatomy 9: 251–255

Freeman B S 1965 The results of epiphyseal transplant by flap and by free graft: a brief survey. Plastic and Reconstructive Surgery 36: 227–230

Ganel A, Yaffe B 1990 Ankle instability of the donor site following removal of the vascularized fibula bone graft. Annals of Plastic Surgery 24: 7–9

Gilbert A 1979 Surgical technique – vascularised transfer of the fibular shaft. International Journal of Microsurgery 1–2: 100–102

Gilbert A 1982 Toe transfers for congenital hand defects. Journal of Hand Surgery 7: 118–124

Goldberg N H, Watson H K 1982 Composite toe (phalanx and epiphysis) transfers in the reconstruction of the aphalangic hand. Journal of Hand Surgery 7: 454–459

Gore D R, Gardner G M, Sepic S B, Mollinger L A, Murray M P 1987 Function following partial fibulectomy. Clinical Orthopaedics and Related Research 220: 206–210

Gori Y, Tatsumi Y, Nakamuray S, Fukai A 1981 An experience of vascularised fibular head transplantation in a child with radial club hand (in Japanese). Seikeigeka 32: 1645

Gothman L 1960 The normal arterial pattern of the rabbit's tibia. An angiographic study. Acta Chirurgica Scandinavica 120: 211

Graham W C 1954 Transplantation of joints to replace diseased or damaged articulations in the hand. American Journal of Surgery 88: 136–141

Green M F, Gibson J R, Bryson J R, Thomson E R E 1981 A one-stage correction of mandibular defect using a split sternum pectoralis major osteomusculocutaneous transfer. British Journal of Plastic Surgery 34: 11–16

Haas S L 1931 Further observation on transplantation of the epiphyseal cartilage plate. Surgery, Gynaecology and Obstetrics 52: 958–963

Harris W R, Martin R, Tile M 1965 Transplantation of epiphyseal plates. Journal of Bone and Joint Surgery 47A: 897–914

Helferich H 1899 Versuche uber die transplantation des intermediarknorpels wachsender rohrenknochen. Deutsche Zeitschrifte der Chirurgie 51: 564–573

Hertel R, Masquelet A C 1989 The reverse flow medial knee osteoperiosteal flap for skeletal reconstruction of the leg. Surgical and Radiologic Anatomy 11: 257–262

Hoffman S, Siffert R S, Simon B E 1972 Experimental and clinical experiences in epiphyseal transplantation. Plastic and Reconstructive Surgery 50: 58–65

Huang G K, Liu Z Z, Shen Y L, Hu R Q, Miao H, Yin Z Y 1980 Microvascular free transfer of iliac bone based on the deep circumflex iliac vessels. Journal of Microsurgery 2: 113

Huang G K, Hu R Q, Miao H, Yin Z Y, Lan T D, Pan G P 1985 Microvascular free transfer of iliac bone based on the deep superior branches of the superior gluteal vessels. Plastic and Reconstructive Surgery 75: 68–74

Hurwitz P J 1979 Experimental transplantation of small joints by microvascular anastomoses. Plastic and Reconstructive Surgery 64: 221–231

Ishida O, Tsai T-M 1991 Free vascularised whole joint transfer in children. Microsurgery 12: 196–206

Jones N F, Sommerlad B C 1983 Reconstruction of the zygoma, temporo-mandibular joint and mandible using a compound pectoralis major osteo-muscular flap. British Journal of Plastic Surgery 36: 491–497

Katsaros J, Tan E, Zoltie N, Barton M, Venugopalsrinivasan, Venkataramakrishnan 1991 Further experience with the lateral arm free flap. Plastic and Reconstructive Surgery 87: 902–910

Knudsen F W, Andersen M, Krag C 1989 The arterial supply of the clavicle. Surgical and Radiologic Anatomy 11: 211–214

Lovie M J, Duncan G M, Glasson G W 1984 The ulnar artery forearm free flap. British Journal of Plastic Surgery 37: 486–492

Lütken P 1950 Investigation into the position of the nutrient foramina and the direction of the vessel canals in the shafts of the humerus and femur in man. Acta Anatomica 9: 57–68

McCarthy J G, Zide B M 1984 The spectrum of calvarial bone grafting: introduction of the vascularised calvarial bone flap. Plastic and Reconstructive Surgery 74: 10–18

McKee N H, Haw P, Vettese T 1984 Anatomic study of the nutrient foramen in the shaft of the fibula. Clinical Orthopaedics and Related Research 184: 141–144

MacLeod A M, Robinson D W 1982 Reconstruction of defects involving the mandible and floor of mouth by free osteo-cutaneous flaps derived from the foot. British Journal of Plastic Surgery 35: 239–246

Malizos K N, Beris A E, Xenakis T A, Korobilias A B, Soucacos P N 1992 Free vascularized fibular graft: a versatile graft for reconstruction of large skeletal defects and revascularisation of necrotic bone. Microsurgery 13: 182–187

Martin D, Bitonti-Grillo C, De Biscop J, Schott H, Mondie J M, Baudet J, Peri G 1991 Mandibular reconstruction using a free vascularised osteocutaneous flap from the internal condyle of the femur. British Journal of Plastic Surgery 44: 397–402

Mathes S J, Buchannan R, Weeks P M 1980 Microvascular joint transplantation with epiphyseal growth. Journal of Hand Surgery 5: 586–589

Murray J A, Schlafly B 1986 Giant-cell tumours in the distal end of the radius: Treatment by resection and fibular interposition arthrodesis. Journal of Bone and Joint Surgery 68A: 687–694

Mysorekar V R 1967 Diaphysial nutrient foramina in human long bones. Journal of Anatomy 101: 813–822

Nettelblad H, Randolph H A, Weiland A J 1984 Free microvascular epiphyseal plate transplantation. Journal of Bone and Joint Surgery 66A: 1421–1430

Nettelblad H, Randolph H A, Weiland A J 1986 Heterotopic microvascular growth plate transplantation of the proximal fibula: an experimental canine model. Plastic and Reconstructive Surgery 77: 814–820

Ogden J A 1979 The development and growth of the musculoskeletal system. In: Albright J A, Brand R A (eds) The scientific basis of orthopaedics. Appleton-Century-Crofts, New York, p 41–103

Ollier L 1867 Traité expérimental et clinique de la régénération des os et la production artificielle du tissu osseux. Masson, Paris, Part I, p 79, Part II, p 461

Panje W, Cutting C 1980 Trapezius osteomyocutaneous island flap for reconstruction of the anterior floor of the mouth and the mandible. Head and Neck Surgery 3: 66–71

Pagliei A, Brunelli F, Gilbert A 1991 Anterior interosseous artery: anatomic basis of pedicled bone grafts. Surgical and Radiologic Anatomy 13: 152–154

Patake S M, Mysorekar V R 1977 Diaphysial nutrient foramina in human metacarpals and metatarsals. Journal of Anatomy 124: 299–304

Peacock E E 1956 Reconstructive surgery of hands with injured central metacarpophalangeal joints. Journal of Bone and Joint Surgery 38A: 291–302

Penteado C V, Masquelet A C, Romana M C, Chevrel J P 1990 Periosteal flaps: anatomical bases of sites of elevation. Surgical and Radiologic Anatomy 12: 3–7

Pho R W H, Patterson M H, Kour A K, Kumar V P 1988 Free vascularised epiphyseal transplantation in upper extremity reconstruction. The Journal of Hand Surgery 13B: 440–447

Pierer G, Steffen J, Hoflehner H 1992 The vascular blood supply of the second metacarpal bone: anatomic basis for a new vascularised bone graft in hand surgery. An anatomical study in cadavers. Surgical and Radiologic Anatomy 14: 103–112

Puckett C L, Hurvitz J S, Metzler M H, Silver D 1979 Bone formation by revascularised periosteal and bone grafts, compared with traditional bone grafts. Plastic and Reconstructive Surgery 64: 361–365

Rank B K 1978 Long term results of epiphyseal transplants in congenital deformities of the hand. Plastic and Reconstructive Surgery 61: 321–329

Reid C D, Taylor G I, Waterhouse N 1986 The clavicular head of pectoralis major musculocutaneous free flap. British Journal of Plastic Surgery 39: 57–65

Restrepo F, Katz D, Gilbert A 1980 Arterial vascularisation of the proximal epiphysis and the diaphysis of the fibula. International Journal of Microsurgery 2: 49–54

Rhinelander F W 1968 The normal microcirculation of diaphyseal cortex and its response to fracture. Journal of Bone and Joint Surgery 50A: 784–800

Rhinelander F W 1972 Circulation in bone. In: Bourne G H (ed) The biochemistry and physiology of bone, 2nd edn. Academic Press, New York and London, vol 2: 1–77

Rhinelander F W 1974 Tibial blood supply in relation to fracture healing. Clinical Orthopaedics and Related Research 105: 34–81

Richards M A, Poole M D, Godfrey A M 1985 The serratus anterior/rib composite flap in mandibular reconstruction. British Journal of Plastic Surgery 38: 466–477

Ring P A 1955 Excision and reimplantation of the epiphyseal cartilage of rabbit. Journal of Anatomy 89: 231–237

Ring P A 1955 Transplantation of epiphyseal cartilage: an experimental study. Journal of Bone and Joint Surgery 37B: 642–657

Riordan D C 1955 Congenital absence of the radius. Journal of Bone and Joint Surgery 37A: 1129–1140

Ritsilä V, Alhopuro S, Rintala A 1972 The use of free periosteum for bone formation in congenital clefts of the maxilla. Scandinavian Journal of Plastic and Reconstructive Surgery 6: 57–60

Satoh T, Tsuchiya M, Harii K 1983 A revascularised iliac musculoperiosteal free flap transfer: a case report. British Journal of Plastic Surgery 36: 109–112

Schmidt D R, Robson M C 1982 One-stage composite reconstruction using the latissimus myo-osteocutaneous free flap. The American Journal of Surgery 144: 470–472

Schusterman M A, Reece G P, Miller M J, Harris S 1992 The osteocutaneous free fibula flap: is the skin paddle reliable. Plastic and Reconstructive Surgery 90: 787–793

Sekiguchi J, Kobayashi S, Ohmori K 1993 Use of the osteocutaneous free scapular flap on the lower extremities. Plastic and Reconstructive Surgery 91: 103–112

Sendemir E, Çimen A 1991 Nutrient foramina in the shafts of lower limb bones: situation and number. Surgical and Radiologic Anatomy 13: 105–108

Serafin D, Villarreal-Rios A, Georgiade N G 1977 A rib-containing free flap to reconstruct mandibular defects. British Journal of Plastic Surgery 30: 263–266

Siemssen S O, Kirkby B, O'Connor T P F 1978 Immediate reconstruction of a resected segment of the lower jaw, using a compound flap of clavicle and sternomastoid muscle. Plastic and Reconstructive Surgery 61: 724–735

Simpson A H R W 1985 The blood supply of the periosteum. Journal of Anatomy 140: 697–704

Skoog T 1965 The use of periosteal flaps in the repair of the primary palate. Cleft Palate Journal 2: 332

Snyder C C, Bateman J M, Davis C W, Warden G D 1970 Mandibulofacial restoration with live osteocutaneous flaps. Plastic and Reconstructive Surgery 45: 14–19

Soutar D S, Scheker L R, Tanner N S B, McGregor I A 1983 The radial artery forearm flap: a versatile method for intraoral reconstruction. British Journal of Plastic Surgery 36: 1–8

Spira E, Farin I 1967 The vascular supply to the epiphyseal plate under normal and pathological conditions. Acta Orthopaedica Scandinavica 38: 1–22

Spira E, Farin I, Hashomer T 1964 Epiphyseal transplantation: a case report. Journal of Bone and Joint Surgery 46A: 1278–1282

Straub G F 1929 Anatomical survival, growth and physiological function of an epiphyseal bone transplant. Surgery, Gynaecology and Obstetrics 48: 687–690

Takato T, Hari K, Nakatsuka T, Ueda K, Dotake T 1986 Vascularised periosteal grafts: an experimental study using two different forms of tibial periosteum in rabbits. Plastic and Reconstructive Surgery 78: 489–497

Taylor G I, Townsend P, Corlett R 1979 Superiority of the deep circumflex iliac vessels as the supply for free groin flaps: experimental work. Plastic and Reconstructive Surgery 64: 595–604

Taylor G I, Townsend P, Corlett R 1979 Superiority of the deep circumflex iliac vessels as the supply for free groin flaps. clinical work. Plastic and Reconstructive Surgery 64: 745–759

Taylor G I, Miller G D H, Ham F J 1975 The free vascularised bone graft. Plastic and Reconstructive Surgery 55: 533–544

Taylor G I, Corlett R, Boyd J B 1983 The extended deep inferior epigastric flap: a clinical technique. Plastic and Reconstructive Surgery 72: 751–764

Teot L, Bosse J P, Mouffarrege R, Papillon J, Beauregard G 1981 The scapular crest pedicled bone graft. International Journal of Microsurgery 3: 257–262

Teot L, Bosse J P, Gilbert A, Tremblay G-R 1982 Pedicle iliac crest epiphysis transplantation. Clinical Orthopaedics and Related Research 180: 206–218

Teot L, Charissou J-L, Pous J-G, Arnal F 1986 Pedicled scapular apophysis transplantation. Growing grafts studied in dogs. Acta Orthopaedica Scandinavica 57: 163–167

Teot L, Souyris F, Bosse J P 1992 Pedicle scapular apophysis transplantation in congenital limb malformations. Annals of Plastic Surgery 29: 332–340

Tomita Y, Tsai T M, Steyers C, Ogden L, Jupiter J, Kutz J E 1986 The role of the epiphyseal and metaphyseal circulations on longitudinal growth in the dog: An experimental study. Journal of Hand Surgery 11A: 375–382

Townsend P L G 1990 Vascularised fibula graft using reverse peroneal flow in the treatment of congenital pseudoarthrosis of the tibia. British Journal of Plastic Surgery 43: 261–265

Uddströmer L 1978 The osteogenic capacity of tubular and membranous bone periosteum. Scandinavian Journal of Plastic and Reconstructive Surgery 12: 195–205

Uddströmer L, Ritsilä V 1978 Osteogenic capacity of periosteal grafts. Scandinavian Journal of Plastic and Reconstructive Surgery 12: 207–214

Urken M L 1991 Composite free flaps in oromandibular reconstruction: review of the literature. Archives of Otolaryngology, Head and Neck Surgery 117: 724–732

Van Beek A L, Wavak P W, Zook E G 1979 Microvascular surgery in young children. Plastic and Reconstructive Surgery 63: 457–461

Van den Wildenberg F A J M, Goris R J A, Tutein Noltheniu-Puylaert M C B J E 1984 Free revascularised periosteum transplantation: an experimental study. British Journal of Plastic Surgery 37: 226–235

Vidal P, Dickson M G 1993 Regeneration of the distal phalanx – case report. The Journal of Hand Surgery 18B: 230–233

Vilkki S K 1991 Microvascular epiphyseal transplantation and distraction lengthening in the treatment of radial club hand. Presented at the 10th Symposium of the International Society of Reconstructive Microsurgery, Munich, 1991

Watson-Jones R 1933 The repair of the skull defects by a new pedicle bone-graft operation. British Medical Journal 1: 780–781

Wenger H L 1945 Transplantation of epiphyseal cartilage. Archives of Surgery 50: 148–151

Weiland A, Daniel R 1979 Micro-vascular anastomoses for bone grafts in treatment of massive defects in bone. Journal of Bone and Joint Surgery 61: 98–104

Weiland A J, Phillips T W, Randolph M A 1984 Bone grafts: a radiologic, histologic and biomechanical model comparing autografts, allografts, and free vascularized bone grafts. Plastic and Reconstructive Surgery 74: 368–379

Whitesides E S 1977 Normal growth in a transplanted epiphysis: a case report with thirteen-year follow up. Journal of Bone and Joint Surgery 59A: 546–548

Wilson J N 1966 Epiphyseal transplantation: a clinical study. Journal of Bone and Joint Surgery 48A: 245–256

Wray J C, Mathes S J M, Young V L, Weeks P M 1981 Free vascularised whole-joint transplants with ununited epiphyses. Plastic and Reconstructive Surgery 67: 519–525

Yajima H, Tamai S, Mizumoto S, Sugimura M, Horiuchi K 1992 Vascularized fibular graft for reconstruction after resection of aggressive benign and malignant bone tumours. Microsurgery 13: 227–233

Yelizarov V G, Minachenko V K, Gerasimov O R, Pshenisnov K P 1993 Vascularized bone flaps for thoracolumbar spinal fusion. Annals of Plastic Surgery 31: 532–538

Zaleske D J, Ehrlich M G, Piliero C, May J W, Mankin H J 1982 Growth-plate behavior in whole joint replantation in the rabbit. Journal of Bone and Joint Surgery 64A: 249–258

Zhao J 1986 Free iliac skin flap transplantation by anastomosing the fourth lumbar blood vessel. Plastic and Reconstructive Surgery 77: 836–842

Zhenman S, Zhiguang X 1986 Experimental study and clinical use of the fasciosteal flap. Plastic and Reconstructive Surgery 78: 201–208

Zhong S Z, Kong J M 1991 Microsurgical anatomy in China. Surgical and Radiologic Anatomy 11: 115–122

Alternative flap nomenclature and classification

9

Introduction

Over the last 100 years numerous different approaches have been suggested for classifying the anatomy of cutaneous vessels with many authors focusing on the concept of direct or primary perforators and indirect or secondary perforators (Table 9.1). There are historical grounds for describing the vessels to the integument as direct and indirect if only as a tribute to the pioneering work of Spalteholz in this field in 1893. Taylor (1987) has been an advocate of this scheme of classification in the modern era. At first glance this looks beguilingly simple, with the indirect vessels being the 'terminal spent branches of arteries whose main purpose is to supply the muscles and other deep tissues', while the direct vessels are branches to the integument straight off the source arteries. But then the indirect branches are also ultimately arising from the source arteries, and the scheme tells us little about the inter-relationship of these vessels with other tissues and to clarify this further four unnamed subdivisions of the direct vessels have been described, which are really quite difficult to distinguish from each other.

It is probably impossible to devise a nomenclature that is universally acceptable. Even if a single system were widely adopted there would still be flaps that defied classification and there would be arguments about which category they belonged to. Unfortunately there is no *effective* official authority overseeing matters of nomenclature in general in plastic surgery. Even simple anatomical terms which one would imagine as coming within the sphere of influence of the *Nomina Anatomica*, are in disarray. An example is the fascia lying beneath the extension of the galea in the temporoparietal region – this has been given 13 names in five separate languages and a new one has recently been proposed bringing the grand total to 14 (Tolhurst et al, 1991). Even when there are recognised anatomical terms in *Nomina Anatomica* they may be disregarded; for example the middle collateral artery is regularly termed the posterior radial collateral in the American literature (actually a better name for it). In recognition of the fact that the definitive classification has not yet been devised we are presenting in this chapter some of the alternative schemes that have been put forward.

To some pragmatists the concept of classification may at first glance seem an esoteric matter, best reserved for academics, but for many surgeons classification is a useful tool in everyday practice. One needs to have various mental systems so that a full range of alternative solutions for a given problem can be readily brought to mind. Thorough familiarity with a classification allows an almost subconscious scan and decision to be made as well as being useful as a teaching aid which permits one to explain options and choices in a logical way.

Tripartite system

We did not find the simple division into direct and indirect to be sufficiently informative and in writing this book chose to use a system of classification that was simple, that used similar terms for the anatomical system of perforators as for the clinical varieties of flaps (Table 9.2) and also conveyed by those terms some information. The advantage of this approach is that it also reflects the three stages in the historical evolution of the flap concept as outlined in Chapter 1. It also avoids the confusion engendered by numerous flap types designated by numerals I to X (or whatever).

Table 9.1 Some of the terms used over the last 100 years in connection with the vessels supplying the integument

Spalteholz	1893	Directe Aeste grosser Arterienstämme; Endverzweigungen der Aeste der Muskeln
McGregor & Morgan	1973	Random and axial pattern vessels
Daniel & Williams	1973	Segmental, perforating and direct cutaneous vessels
Wilson & Behan	1973	Prop arteries and angiotomes
Cormack & Lamberty	1986	Direct cutaneous, musculocutaneous, fasciocutaneous
Taylor & Palmer	1987	Direct and indirect vessels; angiosomes; choke vessels
Tolhurst	1987	Atomic system of flaps (tripartite system of vessels)
Saijo	1988	Vessel Types A to E
Nakajima	1986	10 vessel types and subtypes
Satoh	1990	Septocutaneous versus fasciocutaneous vessels
Kunert	1991	Reticular, segmental and axial vessels

In addition to the flaps falling within the tripartite scheme there are various random-pattern flaps which may be created without due regard for local patterns of blood supply and assume a reliance on subcutaneous and subdermal plexi. These flaps include some skin flaps, de-epithelialised turn-over flaps (Thatte, 1981, 1982), and some random subcutaneous tissue and adipofascial flaps.

The angiosome approach (Taylor & Palmer, 1987) with its emphasis on anatomical territories linked through reduced calibre 'choke' vessels and through true anastomoses, fits well with the tripartite classification because both are founded on vascular anatomy. Because of the differences outlined in Chapter 1 between anatomical territories and potential territories, neither of these schemes is able to define the maximum territories that may be transferred on a given vessel but they do define the minimum-sized volume of tissue that can be safely raised. In fact it is reasonably safe to say that no scheme of classification at the present time is able to define the maximum limits to which flaps may be reliably raised.

A further potential criticism of these schemes is that with their emphasis on anatomy they fail to address some of the practicalities involved in the actual physical elevation of the flap. Part of this issue is tackled on pages 126–128 with respect to flaps based on the fasciocutaneous system of perforators, out of which arises the suggestion that the term 'septocutaneous' should be used, not to describe anatomy, but to define those flaps whose elevation involves physically dissecting out the fascial septum containing the perforators.

This aspect of correlating the way in which flaps are mobilised with the structure of the vessel pattern in the tissues, has been attempted by Kunert.

The Kunert system

Kunert presented a theoretical model, rather than an anatomical description, which was based on analysis of vascular morphology on the one hand and the way in which flaps were raised on the other. This scheme is internally quite consistent and shows a simple functional correlation between the two variables, but the manner in which it is presented means that it is really a concept rather than a practical and useful scheme.

According to Kunert there are three elementary vascular patterns located in the subcutaneous tissue, the deep fascia (including septa) and the muscles. These are (Fig. 9.1):

1. large vessels running horizontally
2. vertical ascending vessel branches
3. horizontal two- or three-dimensional vessel networks.

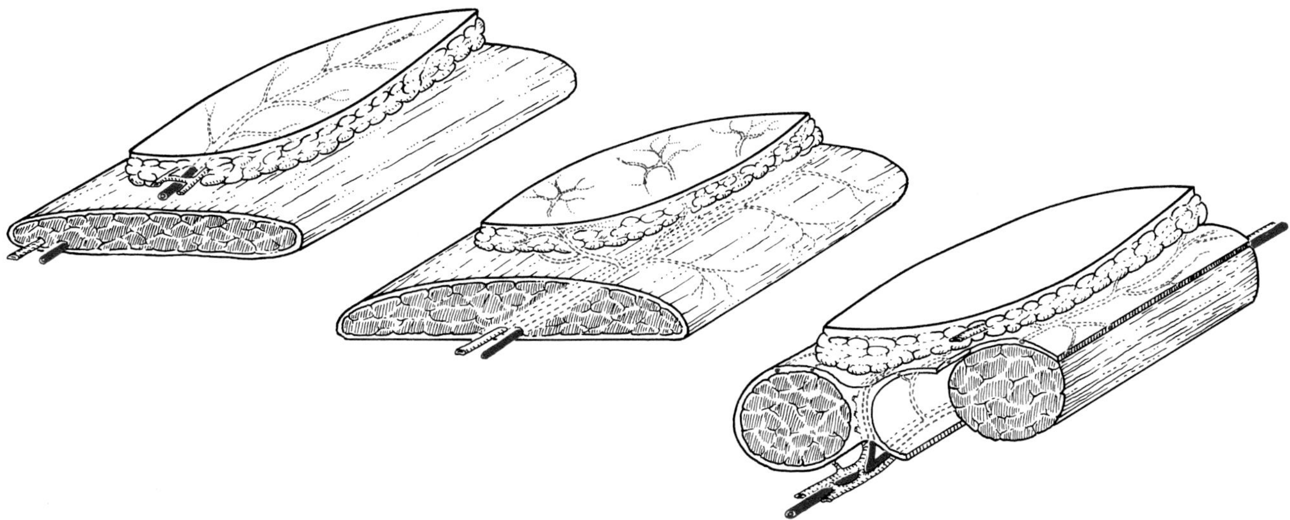

Fig. 9.1 Schematic form of the Tripartite classification

Table 9.2 The basic tripartite classification of skin flaps based on defined vasculature

Anatomical system	Clinical type of flap	Defined
direct cutaneous arteries	axial pattern flaps	up to 1970
musculocutaneous perforators	musculocutaneous flaps	1970–1980
fasciocutaneous perforators	fasciocutaneous flaps	1980–1990

These are termed axial, segmental and reticular. (Segmental in this context has nothing to do with the way in which this term is applied, in the sense of somite-related, in other classifications.)

This recognises the basic concept that big blood vessels in the body run parallel to the surface, then branch out into smaller ones that run vertically to the surface and again branch out into a vascular plexus that lies parallel to the body surface. However, much the same descriptive arrangement could be applied to the fascial plexus, the branches ascending from this to the skin, and the subdermal plexus.

The 'elementary' flap types are then based on the axial, reticular and segmental parts in a pure form. The second level of flap complexity combines elementary flap types in one of two ways, either in a 'sequential' or in a 'parallel' mode. In both arrangements the key to flap viability is maintaining continuity between the elementary patterns. Finally, the level beneath the surface at which these vascular elements lie is recorded as subcutaneous, fascial or muscular. By this means the blood supply of any flap can be indicated and various examples are given by Kunert in his paper.

This scheme looks workable on paper but is difficult to use in speech and unfortunately is unlikely to be helpful to the surgeon in his clinical practice.

Other classifications

The simple approach of the Tripartite classification is easy for the newcomer to the subject to assimilate, but once one has progressed to a more sophisticated level of understanding it is easy to see that there are many ways in which this simple approach can be improved.

Because flap surgery is so complex, with a multitude of choices from which only a small number are applicable for any given problem, it follows that a classification made solely on the basis of blood supply will be inadequate in many circumstances. As well as the Circulation of the flap, attention may have to be paid to its tissue Constituents, its Construction in terms of pedunculated or circumscribed, its Conformation or geometry, its Contiguity or otherwise to the defect, and the effect of any Conditioning in the form of delay or expansion. These may be termed the six Cs of flap design (see Table 9.3). Exactly the same concepts underpin Tolhurst's atomic system of flap classification.

Table 9.3 The six Cs of flap design

Circulation
Constituents
Construction
Conformation
Contiguity
Conditioning

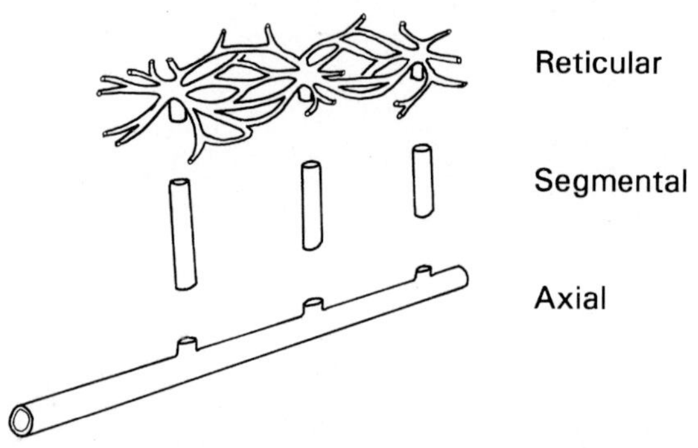

Fig. 9.2 Breakdown of the vascular supply to skin into elementary vascular patterns.

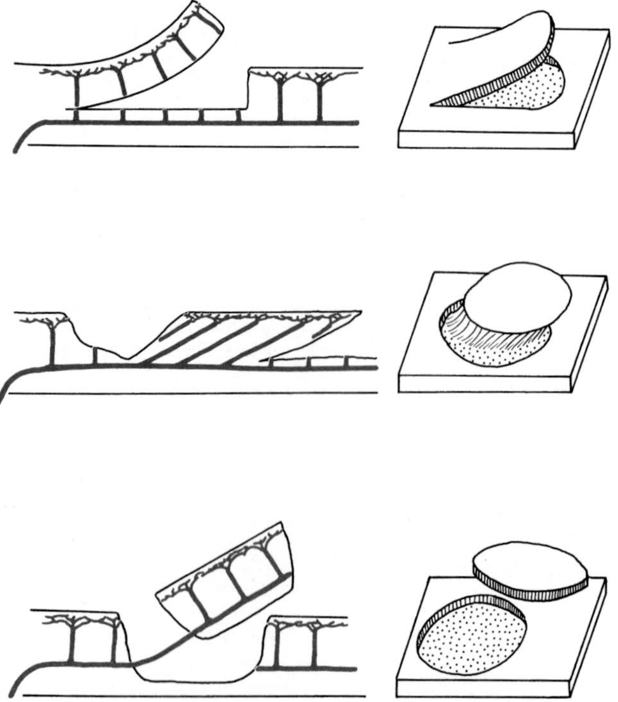

Fig. 9.3 The three basic flap types. (Top) The reticular flap, partially circumcised, totally mobilised. (Middle) The segmental flap, totally circumcised, partially mobilised. (Bottom) The axial flap, totally circumcised, totally mobilised.

Atomic system

As originally proposed by Tolhurst (1987) this consisted of two main parts, a nucleus, comprising the tissue components of the flaps, and an outer shell system, in which the secondary characteristics are listed. This is really less of a formula for description and more of a list of headings with the atomic format avoiding the need to list them in a specific rank or order. This is reproduced in Figure 9.4. Tolhurst's original scheme is perhaps best modified by placing the anatomical vascular system supporting the flap at the heart of the classification since without an adequate blood supply the other considerations are likely to become meaningless.

To be practical, some further heirarchy needs to be imposed on this system and an example of how this might be done is given in Figure 9.5. Application of this scheme to the group of flaps known as anterior tibial fasciocutaneous flaps was given in Figure 7.3 to show how this can be helpful in practice.

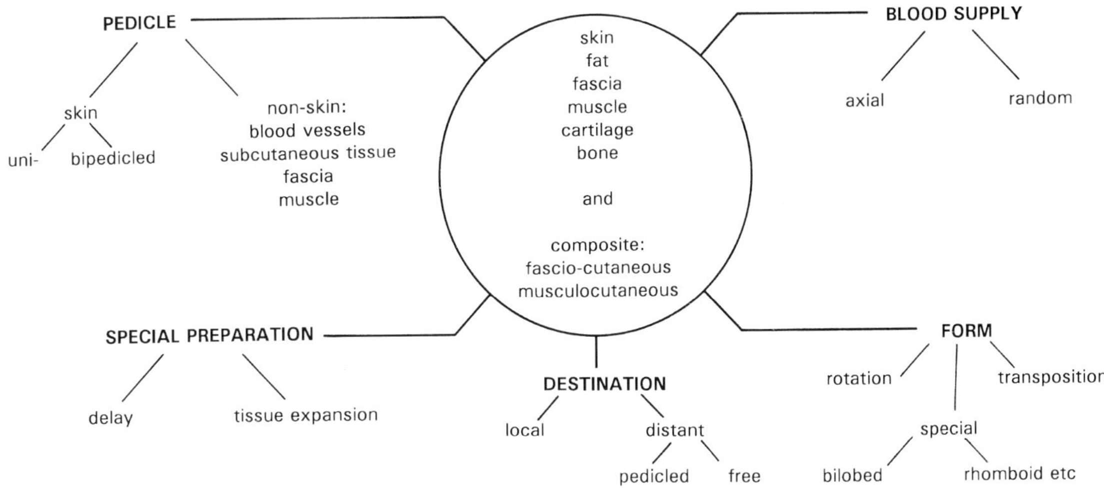

Fig. 9.4 The atomic system.

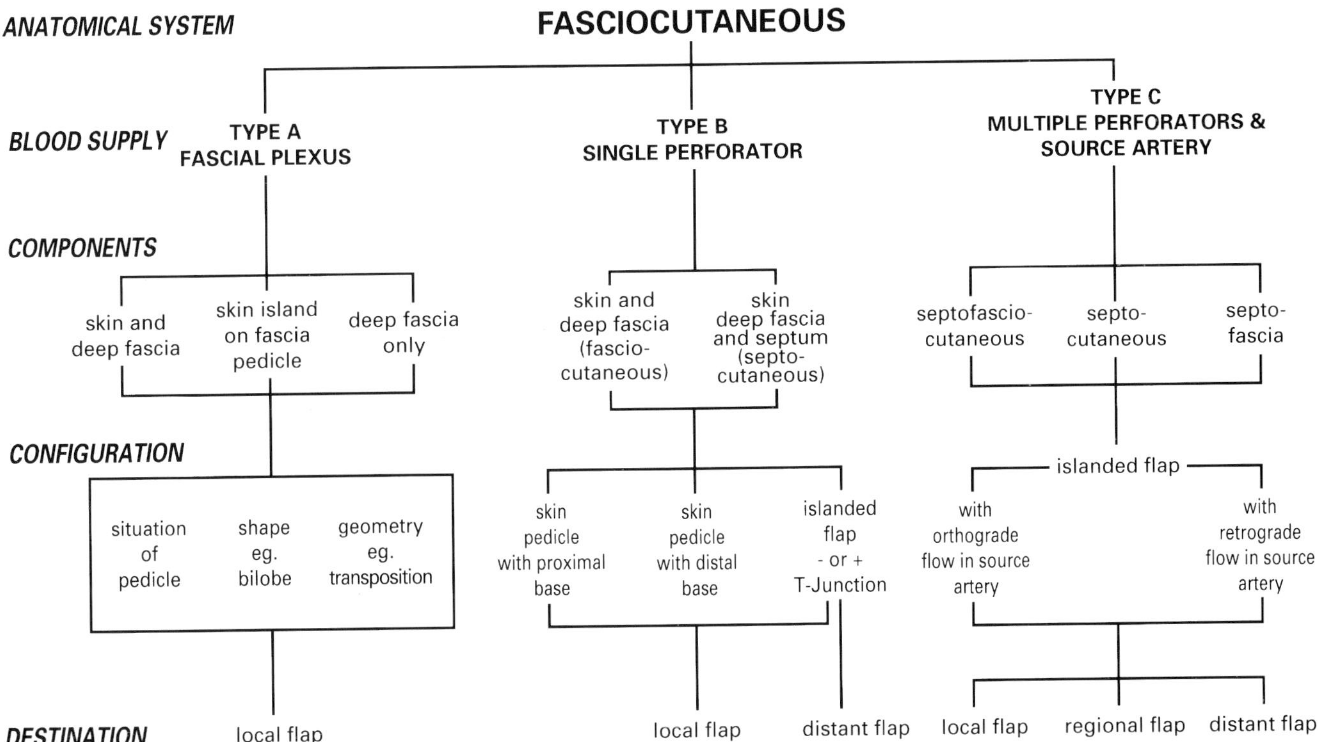

Fig. 9.5 A method of applying a heirarchy to the main features of the atomic system.

Nakajima classification

This classification by Nakajima, Fujino & Adachi was published in 1986. Leaving aside random-pattern and adipofascial flaps this scheme recognises three main types of flap which are termed fasciocutaneous, septocutaneous and musculocutaneous on the basis of their *tissue constituents.* The key to understanding this terminology is contained in the fact that the authors label the entire subcutaneous network of vessels throughout the body as 'the fasciocutaneous plexus' and therefore fasciocutaneous flaps are ones which include the skin and the subcutaneous network – the pattern of blood supply does not contribute to this definition of fasciocutaneous. Septocutaneous flaps are ones which include the skin, the 'fasciocutaneous'/subcutaneous network, *and* an intermuscular/intercompartmental fascial septum. Musculocutaneous flaps are ones which include skin, fasciocutaneous network and muscle.

All of these flaps are supplied by one or more of six basic vessel types which are designated Types A to F and this is indicated in Table 9.4. Fasciocutaneous flaps are supplied by each of the six types resulting in six fasciocutaneous flaps designated Types I to VI. With the inclusion of the septocutaneous and musculocutaneous flaps this makes a total of eight flap types.

Since correct identification of the vessel type is essential for correctly allocating a flap to the right Type I to VI it is worth describing these in more detail:

A Fed by what are classically regarded as the direct cutaneous arteries such as the superficial circumflex iliac artery.

B Intermuscular septocutaneous. The authors attribute a number of vessels to this type which to us do not appear homogeneous. The cutaneous branch of the superior ulnar collateral artery might be in this category.

C Cutaneous branch of a muscular artery given off before it enters the muscle, e.g. cutaneous branch of the thoracodorsal artery.

D Perforating cutaneous branch of a muscular artery. These would appear to be the larger musculocutaneous perforators which possess axiality.

E Small perforators passing up along intermuscular fascial septa, e.g. the radial artery perforators. Sometimes these are septomuscular, i.e. perforating a muscle at its margin where it may be adherent to the fascial septum.

F These are the classical musculocutaneous perforators.

In summary Types A and B supply large axial territories. Types C and D axially supply skin over a muscle and in some instances beyond the edge of it. And Types E and F individually have small territories of supply but may combine to supply large ones.

There are many good points to this scheme, particularly the emphasis on axiality in what are elsewhere known as musculocutaneous vessels but the main problem is that it can be difficult to allocate a vessel to one of the six types with certainty. Types B and E are hard to separate and D and F can also be problematic. For example, the authors ascribed B status to the radial collateral artery, the superior ulnar collateral artery, the posterior circumflex humeral artery, and the inferior cubital artery which do not immediately appear to be similar vessels.

Table 9.4 Classification after Nakajima et al 1986. Key to tissue types: **D** = skin and subdermal plexus; **F** = subcutaneous tissue with 'fasciocutaneous' network; **S** = intermuscular fascial septum; **M** = muscle

Flaps	Tissue	Vessel type	Pattern	Clinical form
Fasciocutaneous	D,F			
Type I		Type A	axial	free, island
Type II		Type B	axial	free, island
Type III		Type C	axial	free, island
Type IV		Type D	axial	free, island
Type V		Type E	random	pedicled
Type VI		Type F	random	pedicled
Septocutaneous	D,F,S	Type E	axial	free, island
		Type B		
Musculocutaneous	D,F,M	Type F	axial	free, island
		Type D		

Saijo classification

Saijo, in his classification published in Japanese in 1988, adopted the conventional tripartite approach to vascular anatomy but built on this to emphasise some useful points. He followed Nakajima et al in identifying three different types of musculocutaneous perforator, namely intramuscular, intermuscular and musculocutaneous as shown in Figure 9.6. From this it can be seen that the intermuscular perforator is identified as being something different from the septocutaneous perforator which passes along an intermuscular septum. This enables three different types of 'musculocutaneous' flap to be identified and these are designated as Flap Types B, C, and E, with only Type E necessarily always including muscle (see Fig. 9.7). This classification therefore allows for the possibility of a flap of skin supported by musculocutaneous perforators but which does not include muscle – an entity that creates a problem for other classifications. This problem has been referred to previously; for example, the muscle component of the extended deep inferior epigastric flap may be reduced to virtually nothing by careful dissection of the vascular pedicle free from the muscle yet the flap remains in its principles of vascularisation a musculocutaneous flap. Such a flap falls into the category of a Type B Flap as described by Saijo.

This classification also highlights the fact that the concept of axiality can be applied to more than just direct cutaneous vessels running in the subcutaneous fat. Figure 9.7 is adapted from Saijo's paper and this illustrates that whilst direct cutaneous arteries tend to produce axial pattern flaps with the greatest length-to-breadth ratios, the axial musculocutaneous perforators, the axial anastomoses of successive fasciocutaneous perforators, and the longitudinal pattern of perforators along the length of a muscle all confer axiality on Type B, D and E flaps.

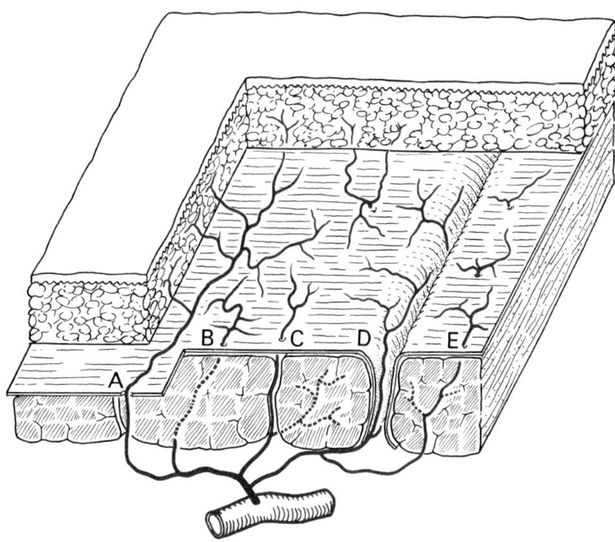

Fig. 9.6 Saijo's approach to vessels supplying skin: **A.** direct cutaneous branch; **B.** intramuscular branch; **C.** intermuscular branch; **D.** septocutaneous branch; **E.** musculocutaneous perforator.

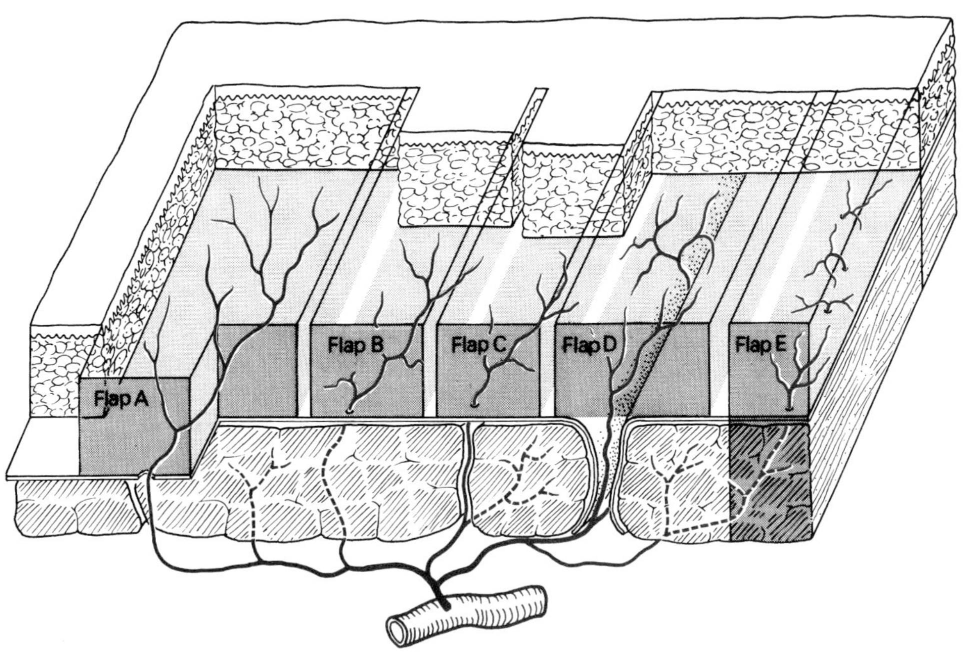

Fig. 9.7 Axiality of the various flaps based on the five types of vessel.

Compound flaps

The term 'compound', when applied to flaps, implies that the flap contains more than one tissue type, and that these different tissues are linked in their dependence on a single common blood supply. Composite is applied in much the same way although it is perhaps more used specifically in the context of bone-containing flaps.

In the majority of compound flaps the maintenance of the vascular link between the different tissues means that a degree of physical contact must be maintained between them that limits the degree to which the different tissue components can be individually manoeuvred into position when carrying out a reconstruction. The need to have different tissue types in a flap reconstruction and yet to have full independence of positioning can only be achieved by either (1) using two completely independently vascularised flaps; (2) having two different flaps on separate branches of a single major vascular axis; (3) by having two separate flaps linked together by microsurgery on a single vascular axis. In addition there is the entity of two flaps of different tissues which are physically joined but which have entirely separate blood supplies. Clearly there is a need for some sort of terminology to distinguish these different types of compound flap.

Table 9.5 lists the main four compound flap types and these are illustrated in Figure 9.8.

Simple compound flap. This refers to a flap where the different tissue types are interdependent and physically linked by their blood supply. The different tissues may be physically close such as the latissimus dorsi muscle and its overlying skin island, or they may be slightly separated yet linked to the common vascular pedicle as, for example, in the lateral arm skin flap taken with a piece of the lateral supracondylar ridge of the humerus. Simple compound flaps are the commonest variety of compound flap.

Chimeric flaps. This term was introduced by Hallock (1991) to describe two or more different tissues carried on separate branches of a single more major vascular axis. For example the subscapular axis can supply a scapular flap through the circumflex scapular artery at the same time as a latissimus dorsi muscle through the thoracodorsal artery. A segment of the lateral border or lower pole of the scapula could also be simultaneously carried on this vessel group as could part of the serratus anterior muscle with a section of rib. Other examples are given in Table 9.5. The term 'chimeric' is derived from Greek mythology in which the Chimera was a goat with a lion's head and a serpent's tail – the concept of mixing of different tissues being the basis on which this

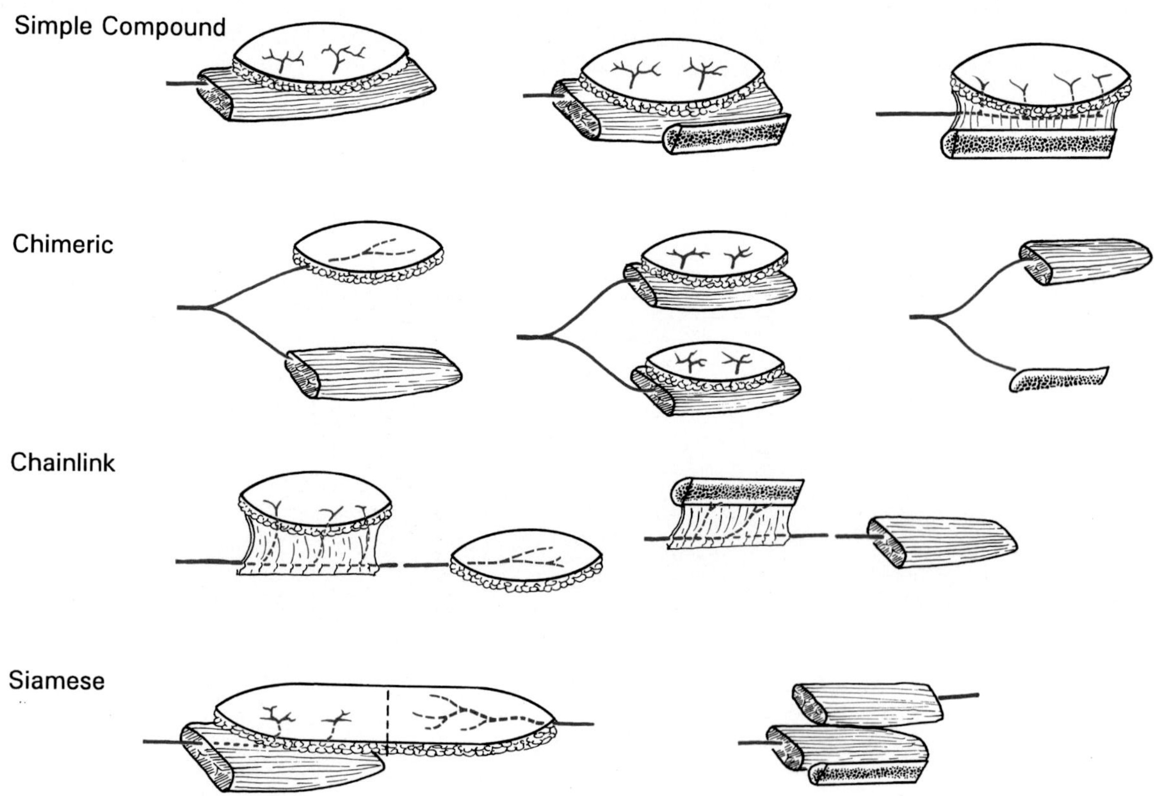

Fig. 9.8 Various types of compound flap.

term was introduced to plastic surgery. In modern usage a chimera is also a wild impossible scheme or an unreal conception, but hopefully this does not apply to flap classifications.

Chainlink or bridge flaps. This describes two separate flaps linked together by microsurgery on a single vascular axis, probably with a through-flow arrangement on one of the vascular pedicles. We proposed the term 'Siamese flaps' for this arrangement in 1984 but in retrospect this is not a good label and the chainlink concept applied to these flaps as described by Chen et al in 1989 is probably more appropriate. The obvious arrangement is where a Type C fasciocutaneous flap such as the radial forearm flap is used with one end of the radial artery connected in the recipient site and a further free flap (of the same or a different type) is then anastomosed to the other end of the radial artery. Two radial artery forearm flaps were used in such a manner and formed into a long tube for oesophageal reconstruction by Chen et al.

Siamese flaps. This term is probably best reserved for flaps which are physically linked at some point but which have separate blood supplies. For example the combined latissimus dorsi/groin island free flap described by Harii et al (1981) falls into this category. Blood supply to both components must be re-established independently.

These different compound flap types are illustrated diagramatically in Figure 9.8

Conclusion

For trainee surgeons the principal message to be read from this is that there is no substitute for acquiring the necessary anatomical knowledge, both by reading and by cadaver dissections, and then making up your own mind. Equally it is clear that there is now so much known about the blood supply of skin that the truly random flap can only be considered to be the last refuge of the anatomically destitute surgeon.

Table 9.5 Compound flap types with a few examples; this is not intended to be a comprehensive list of all possibilities

Simple compound	
skin and muscle	latissimus dorsi and overlying skin island
skin, muscle and bone	latissimus dorsi musculocutaneous flap and rib
muscle and bone	tensor fasciae latae and attached iliac crest
skin and bone	lateral arm flap and supracondylar ridge of humerus
Chimeric	
skin and muscle	anterolateral thigh flap and tensor fasciae latae or rectus femoris
skin + muscle, and bone	latissimus dorsi musculocutaneous flap and lateral border of scapula
muscle and bone	part of vastus lateralis and anterior iliac crest
skin and bone	scapular flap and lower pole of scapula
skin + muscle, and muscle	latissimus dorsi musculocutaneous flap and serratus anterior
Chainlink	
skin and skin	Type B or C fasciocutaneous flap and any skin or fasciocutaneous flap
skin + bone, and muscle	radial forearm flap with radius and any appropriate muscle flap
bone and muscle	fibula on peroneal artery and any muscle flap
Siamese	
skin + muscle, and skin	latissimus dorsi musculocutaneous flap and groin flap
muscle + bone, and muscle	tensor fasciae latae and gluteus medius

References

Chen H C, Tang Y B, Noordhoff M S 1989 Reconstruction of the entire oesophagus with 'chain flaps' in a patient with severe corrosive injury. Plastic and Reconstructive Surgery 84: 980–984

Cormack G C, Lamberty B G H 1984 A classification of fasciocutaneous flaps according to their patterns of vascularisation. British Journal of Plastic Surgery 37: 80–87

Hallock G G 1991 Simultaneous local transposition of anterior thigh and fascia flaps: an introduction to the chimera flap principle. Annals of Plastic Surgery 27: 126–131

Harii K, Iwaya T, Kawaguchi N 1981 Combination myocutaneous flap and microvascular free flap. Plastic and Reconstructive Surgery 68: 700–710

Kunert P 1991 Structure and construction: the system of skin flaps. Annals of Plastic Surgery 27: 509–518

Tolhurst D E 1987 A comprehensive classification of flaps. The Atomic System. Plastic and Reconstructive Surgery 80: 608–609

Saijo M 1988 Skin flap surgery – the basis of pedicled skin flap transfer. In: New encyclopedia of surgical science 29A. (In Japanese), Nakajama Co, 141–159

Nakajima H, Fujino T, Adachi S 1986 A new concept of vascular supply to the skin and classification of skin flaps according to their vascularization. Annals of Plastic Surgery 16: 1–17

Taylor G I, Palmer J H 1987 The vascular territories (angiosomes) of the body; experimental study and clinical applications. British Journal of Plastic Surgery 40: 113–141

Taylor G I, Caddy C M, Watterson P A, Crock J G 1990 The venous territories (venosomes) of the human body: experimental study and clinical implications. Plastic and Reconstructive Surgery 86: 185–213

Thatte R L 1981 Random-pattern de-epithelialised 'turn-over' flaps to replace skin loss in the upper third of the leg. British Journal of Plastic Surgery 34: 312–314

Thatte R L. 1982 One-stage random-pattern de-epithelialised 'turn-over' flaps in the leg. British Journal of Plastic Surgery 35: 287–292

Tolhurst D, Carstens M H, Greco R J, Hurwitz D J 1991 The surgical anatomy of the scalp. Plastic and Reconstructive Surgery 87: 603–612

Appendices

Appendix I
Terminology

Appendix II
Technical data

APPENDIX I
Terminology

Note: This is *not* intended for plastic surgeons. It is included in the hope that some anatomists and others interested in the blood supply of skin may consult this book; in which eventuality a word of explanation about some of the probably unfamiliar technical surgical terms used in the text may be appropriate.

Pedicled flap

This is an area of skin, usually rectangular in shape, which is detached from its surroundings on three sides and separated from the underlying structures. The fourth side of the rectangle forms the bridge through which blood enters and leaves the flap and is known as its base.

Random pattern flap

For many years this was considered to be a pedicled skin flap which did not incorporate an axial cutaneous vessel entering the flap through its base, and was therefore limited in its dimensions to length-to-breadth proportions of 2:1 at the very most. The blood vessels supplying, and contained within, the flap were considered to be randomly orientated although in point of fact some predominating axiality was probably present at the site where the flap was raised. However, a flap orientated and raised without due regard for the local patterns of blood supply (or in ignorance of them) may still be considered a random flap.

Island flap

This is an area of skin which is isolated from all its attachments except for the single artery supplying it and the veins draining it. These may be dissected out to provide a long pedicle so that the skin island may either be transposed locally or may be detached for reattachment elsewhere by microvascular anastomosis. In some instances the sensory innervation of the skin island is preserved together with the supplying artery and veins thereby constituting a *neurovascular island flap.*

Axial pattern flap

This is a flap of skin and subcutaneous tissue raised so as to include a direct cutaneous vessel and its accompanying venae comitantes within it in such a way that the vessels run along the long axis of the flap. Such a flap might be expected to survive with length-to-breadth proportions several times greater than those of a random pattern flap, e.g. 3:1 or more, up to 5:1 commonly. Some doubt remains as to what a flap should be called which is dependent for its survival not on a single axial vessel but on an anastomosis of vessels at the level of the deep fascia which is such that the plexus of vessels has a marked axial pattern aligned parallel to the long axis of the flap. Clearly this is also an axial pattern type of flap but should be further qualified to indicate the fascial component by calling it an *axial fasciocutaneous flap*. In our classification of flaps we have called this a Type A fasciocutaneous flap.

Microvascular graft

This is a piece of tissue which may consist of, for example, skin only, or skin and muscle, or skin, muscle and bone, which is supplied by an identifiable artery and drained by identifiable veins, and which is removed from one site (the donor site) and transferred to another site on the same individual (the recipient site). This has, somewhat inaccurately, come to be known as a *free flap*.

Tube pedicle

This is a bipedicled flap, the edges of which have been sewn together, thereby converting the flap into a tube with no exposed raw area. The tube remains attached by its ends to the donor site for three weeks during which time an axial flow becomes established within it.

This is a technique that was mainly used before the details of the blood supply to skin were worked out and the skin strip was therefore basically a random pattern flap situated somewhere on the trunk. Occasionally conscious efforts were made to orientate the flap along lines of venous drainage. After an interval of approximately three weeks, one end could be detached and transferred into the recipient site. Sometimes the tube pedicle was used to carry a square of skin which was fashioned at one end by means of carefully staged delay procedures spaced out over a long time period. As can be readily imagined this method of reconstruction was lengthy and expensive in terms of hospitalisation. In a review of 196 tube pedicles raised in the ten-year period 1960–1970, 5.8 months was the average time taken to complete the reconstruction and on average five operations were necessary. Even then 6% of tube pedicles were never used, 14% failed to achieve their planned objective and 80% were successful.

Wrist carrier

Tube pedicles may be transferred from the trunk to a distant location on the head, neck, or limbs by using a wrist carrier. One end of the matured tube pedicle is attached to the wrist where a 'trapdoor' is elevated to provide a raw area from which the tube pedicle may derive a blood supply. After three or four weeks, when the tube has picked up a blood supply from the wrist, it is detached from its attachment to the trunk and may then be readily transferred to any other part of the body, there to be anchored, for a final period of three weeks before it is severed from the wrist. After a final period of a further three weeks the tubed portion of the flap may be spread and finally set into the recipient defect.

II

APPENDIX II
Technical data

Injection procedure

Radio-opaque medium
Barium sulphate suspension as Micropaque Liquid 100% w/v of Barium Sulphate
Volume for whole cadaver injections
1200–1800 ml
Pressure
7–9 lb per sq inch
Injection site
Carotid artery
Apparatus
Lear embalming pump or other source of compressed air used with a 2-litre reservoir.

Radiography

Equipment
General Radiological Electronic Mark II c. 1945
Film
Kodak Industrex CX 30 cm × 40 cm (ready packaged) a medium-speed, fine-grain, high-contrast, direct-exposure film (i.e. film used without cassette or intensifying screens)
Exposures
At 42 inches FFD

skin – 250 mA	0.2 sec	44–46 kV
fascia – 250 mA	0.16 sec	40 kV
muscle – 250 mA	0.2 sec	48–52 kV

(All ratings nominal due to antiquated nature of the equipment)
Development
Hand processed in Kodak LX 24 for 4 minutes
Fixation
May and Baker Amfix for 10 minutes

Photography

Prints from radiographs
Radiographs masked with opaquing fluid (Winsor and Newton). Radiographs copied onto Ilford Pan F 50 ASA film using standard Kodak twin-tube radiograph viewing box. Film development in ID 11 for 4 minutes 30 seconds, and fixed in Amfix for 3 minutes
Standard exposure
2 seconds with appropriate aperture between f3.5 and f22
Camera
Canon AE1 with FD 50 mm f/3.5 macro lens
Prints
On Kodabrome II RC Grades F1 to F3 developed for 60 sec in Ilford Ilfospeed developer

Indexes

Subject index

Author index

Only the first-named author of multi-author papers is listed.